Pelvic Floor Disorders

G.A. Santoro • A.P. Wieczorek • C.I. Bartram
Editors

Pelvic Floor Disorders

Imaging and Multidisciplinary Approach to Management

Forewords by
Jim Fleshman
András Palkó
Peter K. Sand

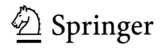 Springer

Giulio Aniello Santoro
Head, Pelvic Floor Unit and Colorectal Service
1ˢᵗ Department of General Surgery
Regional Hospital
Treviso, Italy

Andrzej Paweł Wieczorek,
Department of Pediatric Radiology
Children's Teaching Hospital
Skubiszewski Medical University of Lublin
Lublin, Poland

Clive I. Bartram
Diagnostic Imaging
Princess Grace Hospital
London, UK

ISBN 978-88-470-1541-8   e-ISBN 978-88-470-1542-5

DOI 10.1007/978-88-470-1542-5

Springer Dordrecht Heidelberg London Milan New York

Library of Congress Control Number: 2010926927

Cover design: Simona Colombo, Milan, Italy
Typesetting: Ikona S.r.l., Milano
Printing and binding: Printer Trento S.r.l., Trento
Printed in Italy

Springer-Verlag Italia S.r.l., Via Decembrio 28, 20137 Milan
Springer is a part of Springer Science+Business Media (www.springer.com)

The glory of medicine is that it is constantly moving forward,
that there is always more to learn.

William J. Mayo (1861-1939)

*To the most important people in my life – my wife Anna and my children
Giuseppe, Paolo, and Marco for their love and support*

To my mother and my father, to whom I will be eternally grateful

To the memory of my friend Bjorn Fortling

G.A. Santoro

To my family

C.I. Bartram

To my family

A.P. Wieczorek

Foreword

Drs. Santoro, Wieczorek, and Bartram have honored me by asking me to write the foreword for this comprehensive text about pelvic floor disorders. The editors have raised the bar for the rest of us with this new publication. In the past, rectal and anal issues with pelvic disorders have been evaluated separately, away from urologic and gynecologic issues. Other books have addressed these issues in more isolated format. In this comprehensive text, the anterior and posterior pelvis are evaluated and managed as a unit, with obvious improvement in our approach to both areas.

Pelvic Floor Disorders provides us with the theory behind disorders, the normal and abnormal functional issues, as well as testing and imaging methodology. Not since the classic *Coloproctology and the Pelvic Floor* by Henry and Swash, has there been a textbook that dealt so thoroughly with the specifics of pelvic floor diseases or disorders. The book contains everything that any starting colon and rectal surgeon will need to develop a practice in pelvic floor disorders, as well as being a reference book for those of us who have been experts in the pelvic floor for many years.

The book is extremely thorough, with comprehensive coverage of all approaches, new technology, and practical guides to performance of specific procedures. The step-by-step description of operations, with excellent intraoperative photographs, make this almost an atlas of techniques. The outstanding quality of reproduced images from ultrasonography and magnetic resonance imaging allows us to compare the imaging modalities to the illustration models, which use different colors to make anatomic relationships easy to comprehend.

The book is well referenced, with an extensive up-to-date bibliography for each chapter. The editors have gathered a spectacular collection of expert international authors. The table of contents is clear and well organized, and the chapters are of manageable length with the latest of techniques and references. This will be a must-have and must-read text for all of us who deal with pelvic floor abnormalities. I want to congratulate the editors on a job well done and look forward to this as a beginning of a longstanding educational effort on their behalf as we see edition after edition in the future.

Prof. Dr. Jim Fleshman MD
Professor of Surgery, Chief of Colon and Rectal Surgery
Washington University in St Louis, MO, USA
Past-President of American Society of Colon and Rectal Surgeons

Foreword

The pelvic floor is a rather complex system, comprising active and passive components, bestowing mechanical support but at the same time preserving continence and managing coordinated relaxation during bladder and bowel voiding. Its malfunction may manifest in the form of pain, constipation, incontinence, and prolapse.

As a result of increasing awareness of clinical conditions resulting from dysfunction and anatomical disorders of the pelvic floor, with respect to the rather high, although frequently hidden, prevalence of these changes that compromise the quality of life of many patients, together with the rapidly developing and increasingly widely available technical-technological solutions, pelvic floor imaging has become an extensively required segment of imaging diagnostics. However, some of the techniques are available at relatively few centers only, and members of the community of radiologists, including even specialists of abdominal and urogenital imaging, are far less aware of the therapeutic and diagnostic implications of these conditions than their significance deserves.

A group of renowned experts, as editors and authors, with the assistance of many professionals from different fields of medicine, have thus chosen the optimal time and format to present most diagnostic and therapeutic aspects of pelvic floor disorders. The decision to discuss the subject in such a comprehensive structure, compiling not only the traditional radiological but also the clinical approach, has been highly fruitful; as a result, the content of the volume covers not only the imaging but also the clinical management of this condition and, beyond this, it presents the topic in a "multicompartmental", integrated fashion. The conventional "setting the ground" chapters (anatomy, ultrasonographic and magnetic resonance anatomy of the pelvic floor) are followed by those describing not only the multimodality imaging (with special emphasis on multiplanar visualization), but also the multidisciplinary management of pathologic conditions affecting one or more of the pelvic compartments (damage caused by childbirth, urinary incontinence and voiding dysfunctions, fecal incontinence, pelvic organ prolapse, pelvic pain, fistulae and the diagnostics and management of complications of surgery).

The target group of this volume therefore includes interested radiologists, but the book reaches beyond this expert group and encourages clinicians to better understand not only the reports but also the images resulting from ultrasonographic and/or magnetic resonance imaging of the pelvic structures, which is necessary to fully understand the diagnostic capacity (and of course the limitations) of these modalities. While these examinations may today be considered as "exotic" by many radiologists and clinicians, proper training, standardized imaging and evaluation technique, and well-established diagnostic and therapeutic protocols will shift their performance from the art of a few talented experts to the routine of many abdominal and urogenital imaging specialists.

The need for detailed anatomical and functional imaging of the pelvic floor structures is likely to increase, on the one hand because of the growing patient and physician consciousness, on the other hand because of the improvement in available therapeutic solutions. Since this book fills a void in the current literature, giving those interested in the topic the opportunity to have an up-to-date source of knowledge, it may be offered for thorough reading not only to radiologists and other experts deeply immersed in this special segment of their profession, but also to all those interested in new developments of their discipline.

Prof. Dr. András Palkó PhD
Head and Chairman of the Department of Radiology,
University of Szeged, Hungary
Vice-president of the European Society of Radiology

Foreword

This new book *Pelvic Floor Disorders,* is an exciting, novel contribution by Drs. Giulio Aniello Santoro, Andrzej Paweł Wieczorek, and Clive Bartram that should greatly add to our understanding of diagnosing and treating women with pelvic floor dysfunction. This is a unique contribution that has brought together experts from around the world from multiple disciplines (urogynecology, urology, colorectal surgery, radiology, physical therapy, gynecology, and oncology), to give their opinions on how to diagnose urinary and fecal incontinence, fistulae, pelvic pain, and prolapse. This multidisciplinary approach and commentary from subspecialists in different fields offers the reader a different perspective than textbooks that just present the opinion of one specialty. This is further enhanced by the integration of imaging chapters covering all aspects of pelvic floor dysfunction.

This multidisciplinary approach, with authors recruited from all around the world, is particularly attractive to me. As a member of the International Urogynecological Association for the last 25 years, and the current president of this organization, I have learned the importance of soliciting opinions and knowledge from specialists throughout the world. The tendency of editors to publish work that just represents singular provincial views from one nation or continent often cheats readers of knowledge and different perspectives from different parts of the world. While subspecialists often share many common approaches to the diagnosis and treatment of pelvic floor dysfunction around the world, the subtle differences to the approach to these problems can improve the care of women being treated for pelvic floor dysfunction around the globe. However, without books like *Pelvic Floor Disorders* or participation in international organizations, like the International Urogynecological Association, many clinicians would never be exposed to the diversity of opinions and approaches to all of these disorders. These three editors from different countries and backgrounds are to be complimented for their foresight in preparing an excellent book and soliciting contributions from experts from around the world with diverse perspectives. It is an excellent book that sets a new standard for diversity.

Prof. Dr. Peter K. Sand, MD, FACOG
Professor of Obstetrics & Gynecology
Director, Evanston Continence Center
Director, Fellowship in Female Pelvic Medicine, NorthShore University HealthSystem
University of Chicago, Pritzker School of Medicine, Chicago, IL, USA
President of the International Urogynecological Society

Preface

Major developments in medicine over last few years have resulted in more reliable and accessible diagnostics and treatment of pelvic floor disorders. A unique aspect of the pelvic floor is the number of specialties involved (urology, gynecology, gastroenterology, colorectal surgery, radiology, rehabilitation medicine) and how often patients have problems that transgress the boundaries of any single specialty. Given the complex multicompartmental physiopathology of pelvic floor disorders, we felt that the approach in this volume should not be limited to the assessment of one compartment but should involve the three compartments (anterior, central, and posterior) in an integrated fashion. The subtitle of this book "Imaging and Multidisciplinary Approach to Management" encompasses this concept of cutting across boundaries to expand our knowledge base with regard to both imaging and the clinical management of incontinence, prolapse, pelvic pain, and fistula. We have endeavored, with the help of an international group of contributors, to provide an up-to-date and authoritative account of the imaging and clinical issues involved in the expert management of pelvic floor disorders.

Our starting point (Section I) is the anatomy of the pelvic floor, and this section addresses not only what it is in anatomical terms, but also how it works throughout life, with chapters on its musculo-elastic and neurophysiological control, and the changes associated with ageing and the menopause.

Imaging, particularly ultrasonography and magnetic resonography, knows no bounds and will take the specialist into regions of the pelvis that may be unfamiliar territory. Many clinicians undertake their own ultrasonography, and the whole of Section II is devoted to the various techniques (conventional two-dimensional, and three/four-dimensional endovaginal, endoanal, and transperineal ultrasonography) that may be employed to image the pelvic floor, in the hope that more clinicians will be encouraged to expand their repertoire of these more specialized examinations. Standardization of these techniques, fundamental for reliability and repeatability, the development of new software options, and increasing availability of training, will take pelvic floor ultrasonography from a niche application and lead to more general acceptance of this modality as a standard diagnostic option in pelvic floor disorders. Considerable space has been dedicated to drawings illustrating anatomy and techniques and to two-dimensional and three-dimensional echographic images, in order to help the reader to learn how to see and interpret ultrasound images, and provide more experienced examiners with an opportunity to review and reassess their techniques.

Childbirth represents the single most important cause of damage to the female pelvic floor, and in recognition of this, Section III is devoted to the mechanisms involved and preventative measures. The next three sections (Sections IV, V, and VI) focus on urinary incontinence and voiding dysfunction, fecal incontinence, and pelvic organ prolapse, considered as a global entity. Surgical principles of reconstructive surgery are aimed at either restoring anatomy with a presumed restoration of function, or creating compensatory anatomical mechanisms. Thus far, decision making in relation to operative treatment has been based mainly on clinical assessment. The purpose of these sections is to describe how pelvic floor imaging, providing an extensive understanding of the pathomorphologic changes leading to these disorders, influences the selection of different forms of treatment. An important feature throughout is that every section, or group of chapters, is accompanied by an invited commentary. We hope that these expert overviews may highlight and balance the individual contributions, to add to the reader's depth of understanding.

Two issues that often cause undue concern in management and tend to be overlooked in the literature are pelvic pain and what to do when it all goes wrong surgically. These are dealt with in detail in Sections VII and Section IX, to complete what the editors trust is an interesting and very practical work to further our knowledge and care of these disorders.

We wish to express our deep appreciation to Springer-Verlag for supporting the idea of publishing a book in such an innovative form. Special thanks are due to Dr. Alessandra Born, a representative of the publisher, for her constant assistance throughout the development of the project, organizing every stage of the editorial work. Special acknowledgements must be given to the authors, who are among the foremost experts with outstanding qualifications in this complex field, and who have contributed to the many diverse chapters and provided critical commentaries of the individual sections of this volume. Without their experience and cooperation, this book would not have been possible. Further, thanks must go to our hospitals, whose advanced technological support made it possible to accomplish this new project, to the medical illustrators Mrs. Nadia Simeoni, Lisa Belhange, and Primal Pictures, who have created the numerous artistic drawings, and to Mr. Steffen Jorgensen, Mr. Gert Karlsson, and Mrs. Anne Mitchell of B-K Medical, for gathering much of the data and photographic material showing the technological equipment as well as for their contribution to organizing meetings of the editors' team.

We are confident that this textbook will be met with great interest from all clinicians involved in the care of patients suffering from pelvic floor disorders.

London, May 2010   *Giulio Aniello Santoro*
                                                                                     Andrzej Paweł Wieczorek
                                                                                              Clive I. Bartram

Contents

Section IV   Urinary Incontinence and Voiding Dysfunction

Section VI   Pelvic Organ Prolapse

Investigation

Section IX   Failure or Recurrence after Surgical Treatment: What to Do When it All Goes Wrong

Contributors

Paul Abrams, **MD** Bristol Urological Institute, Southmead Hospital, Bristol, UK

A. Muti Abulafi, **MD** Department of Colorectal Surgery, Mayday University Hospital, Croydon, Surrey, UK

Pier Francesco Almerigi, **MD** Unit of General Surgery, Department of General Surgery and Organ Transplantation, S. Orsola-Malpighi Hospital, University of Bologna, Bologna, Italy

Donato F. Altomare, **MD** Colorectal Unit, Department of Emergency and Organ Transplantation, University of Bari, Bari, Italy

Luca Amadio MD Department of Oncological and Surgical Science, 2nd Surgical Clinic, University of Padova, Padova, Italy

Clive I. Bartram, **MD** Diagnostic Imaging, Princess Grace Hospital, London, UK

Gabriele Bazzocchi, **MD** Unit of Visceral Disorders and Autonomic Dysfunction, Montecatone Rehabilitation Institute, University of Bologna, Imola, Italy

Francesco Beniamin, **MD** Division of Urology, Regional Hospital, Treviso, Italy

Roberto Bergamaschi, **MD** Division of Colon and Rectal Surgery, State University of New York, Stony Brook, NY, USA

Francesco Bianco, **MD** Division of Colon and Rectal Surgery, Department of Oncologic Surgery, National Cancer Institute "G. Pascale", Napoli, Italy

Kari Bø, **PhD** Department of Sports Medicine, Norwegian School of Sport Sciences, Oslo, Norway

Michał Bogusiewicz, **MD** 2nd Department of Gynecology, Medical University of Lublin, Lublin, Poland

Ingeborg Hoff Brækken, **PhD** Department of Sports Medicine, Norwegian School of Sport Sciences, Oslo, Norway

Luisa Caggiano, **MD** Division of General Surgery, Military Policlinic "Celio", Roma, Italy

Luca Cancian, **MD** Department of Radiology, Regional Hospital, Treviso, Italy

Marcello Caria, **MD** Urogynecology Unit, Department of Obstetrics and Gynecology, University of Brescia, Brescia, Italy

Maria Angela Cerruto, **MD** Urology Clinic, Department of Biomedical and Surgical Sciences, University of Verona, Verona, Italy

Mauro Cervigni, **MD** Division of Urogynecology, San Carlo-IDI Hospital, Roma, Italy

Michał Chlebiej, **MSc** Department of Parallel and Distributed Computing, Faculty of Mathematics and Computer Science, Nicolaus Copernicus University, Torun, Poland

Valentina Ciaroni, **MD** Unit of General Surgery, Department of General Surgery and Organ Transplantation, S. Orsola-Malpighi Hospital, University of Bologna, Bologna, Italy

Filip Claerhout, **MD** Pelvic Floor Unit, UZ Gasthuisberg, Leuven, Belgium

Silvia Cornaglia, **MD** Department of General Surgery, U. Parini Hospital, Aosta, Italy

Filippa Cuccia, **MD** Colorectal Unit, Department of Emergency and Organ Transplantation, University of Bari, Bari, Italy

Pierpaolo Curti, **MD** Urology Clinic, Department of Surgery, A.O.U.I., Policlinic Hospital, Verona, Italy

G. Willy Davila, **MD** Department of Gynecology, Urogynecology and Reconstructive Pelvic Surgery, Cleveland Clinic Florida, Weston, FL, USA

Gian Gaetano Delaini, **MD** Department of Surgery and Gastroenterology, University of Verona, Verona, Italy

John O.L. DeLancey, **MD** Department of Obstetrics and Gynecology, University of Michigan Medical School, Pelvic Floor Research Group, Ann Arbor, MI, USA

Conor P. Delaney, **MD** Division of Colorectal Surgery, Case Medical Center, Cleveland, OH, USA

Jan Deprest, **MD** Pelvic Floor Unit, UZ Gasthuisberg, Leuven, Belgium

Dirk De Ridder, **MD** Pelvic Floor Unit, UZ Gasthuisberg, Leuven, Belgium

Paolo Di Benedetto, **MD** Department of Rehabilitation Medicine, Institute of Physical Medicine and Rehabilitation, University of Udine, Udine, Italy

Hans Peter Dietz, **MD** Department of Obstetrics, Gynecology and Neonatology, Sydney Medical School-Nepean, University of Sydney, Sydney, Australia

Giuseppe Di Falco, **MD** 1st Department of Surgery, Regional Hospital, Treviso, Italy

Giuseppe Dodi, **MD** Department of Oncological and Surgical Science, 2nd Surgical Clinic, University of Padova, Padova, Italy

Peter L. Dwyer, **MD** Department of Urogynaecology, Mercy Hospital for Women, Merlbourne, VIC, Australia

Tim W. Eglington, **MD** Division of Colorectal Surgery, Department of Academic Surgery, University of Otago, Christchurch, New Zealand

Anton Emmanuel, **MD** GI Physiology Unit, University College Hospital, London, UK

Dee E. Fenner, **MD** Department of Obstetrics and Gynecology, University of Michigan Medical School, Pelvic Floor Research Group, Ann Arbor, MI, USA

Julia R. Fielding, **MD** Department of Radiology, University of North Carolina at Chapel Hill, Chapel Hill, NC, USA

Frank A. Frizelle, **MD** Division of Colorectal Surgery, Department of Academic Surgery, University of Otago, Christchurch, New Zealand

Gamal M. Ghoniem, **MD** Department of Urology, Cleveland Clinic Florida, Weston, FL, USA

Giuseppe Gizzi, **MD** Department of Medicine and Gastroenterology, S. Orsola-Malpighi Hospital, University of Bologna, Bologna, Italy

Philippe Grange, **MD** Laparoscopic Urology, Department of Urology, Kings College Hospital, London, UK

W. Thomas Gregory, **MD** Female Pelvic Medicine and Reconstructive Surgery, Departments of Obstetrics and Gynecology and Urology, Oregon Health and Science University, Portland, OR, USA

Sara Grosso, **MD** Urogynecology Unit, Department of Obstetrics and Gynecology, University of Brescia, Brescia, Italy

Steve Halligan, **MB** Department of Gastrointestinal Radiology, University College, London, UK

Yvonne Hsu, **MD** Department of Obstetrics and Gynecology, University of Utah, Salt Lake City, UT, USA

Aldo Infantino, **MD** Department of Surgery, "Santa Maria dei Battuti" Hospital, San Vito al Tagliamento, Italy

Patrizia Inselvini, **MD** Urogynecology Unit, Department of Obstetrics and Gynecology, University of Brescia, Brescia, Italy

Wiesław Jakubowski, **MD** Department of Diagnostics Imaging, General Brodnowski Hospital, Medical University of Warsaw, Warsaw, Poland

Marek Jantos, **PhD** Behavioural Medicine Institute of Australia, Adelaide, Australia

Joshua R. Karas, **MD** Division of Colon and Rectal Surgery, State University of New York, Stony Brook, NY, USA

Gevorg Kasyan, **MD** Department of Urology, Moscow State Medical Stomatological University (MSMSU), Moscow, Russia

Kimberly Kenton, **MD** Female Pelvic Medicine & Reconstructive Surgery, Departments of Obstetrics and Gynecology and Urology, Loyola University Stritch School of Medicine, Chicago, IL, USA

Dennis H. Kim, **MD** Department of Urology, Cleveland Clinic Florida, Weston, FL, USA

Małgorzata Kołodziejczak, **MD** Department of Surgery with Subdepartment of Proctology, Hospital at Solec, Warsaw, Poland

Ewa Kuligowska, **MD** Department of Radiology, Boston Medical Center, Boston University School of Medicine, Boston, MA, USA

Filippo La Torre, **MD** Department of Surgical Sciences, University "La Sapienza", Roma, Italy

Andrea Lauretta, **MD** Department of Surgery, "Santa Maria dei Battuti" Hospital, San Vito al Tagliamento, Pordenone, Italy

Joseph K.-S. Lee, **MD** Department of Urogynaecology, Mercy Hospital for Women, Victoria, Australia

Luigi Maccatrozzo, **MD** Division of Urology, Regional Hospital, Treviso, Italy

Andrea Maier, **MD** Department of Radiology, Medical University of Wien, Wien, Austria

Albert Mako, **MD** Division of Urogynecology, San Carlo-IDI Hospital, Roma, Italy

Mauro Menarini, **MD** Unit of Visceral Disorders and Autonomic Dysfunction, Montecatone Rehabilitation Institute, University of Bologna, Imola, Italy

Gianfranco Minini, **MD** Urogynecology Unit, Department of Obstetrics and Gynecology, University of Brescia, Brescia, Italy

Giovanni Morana, **MD** Department of Radiology, Regional Hospital, Treviso, Italy

Elizabeth R. Mueller, **MD** Female Pelvic Medicine & Reconstructive Surgery, Departments of Obstetrics and Gynecology and Urology, Loyola University Stritch School of Medicine, Chicago, IL, USA

Sthela M. Murad-Regadas, **MD** Department of Surgery, School of Medicine, Federal University of Ceará, Fortaleza, Ceará, Brazil

Loredana Nasta Italian Interstitial Cystitis Association, Roma, Italy

Franca Natale, **MD** Division of Urogynecology, San Carlo-IDI Hospital, Roma, Italy

Thang Nguyen, **MD** Division of Colorectal Surgery, Department of Academic Surgery, University of Otago, Christchurch, New Zealand

Edoardo Ostardo, **MD** Division of Urology, "Santa Maria degli Angeli" Hospital, Pordenone, Italy

Claudio Pastore, **MD** 1st Department of Surgery, Regional Hospital, Treviso, Italy

Luciano Pellegrini, **MD** Gastroenterology and Endoscopy Service, "MF Toniolo" Hospital, Bologna, Italy

Francesco Pesce, **MD** Neuro-Urology Unit, CPO Hospital, Roma, Italy

Peter Papa Petros, **MD** Formerly Department of Gynecology, Royal Perth Hospital, Perth, Australia, School of Engineering, University of Western Australia, Crawley, Australia

Johann Pfeifer, **MD** Department of General Surgery, Medical University of Graz, Graz, Austria

Vittorio L. Piloni, **MD** Diagnostic Imaging Centre, "Villa Silvia" Clinic, Senigallia, Italy

Rodrigo A. Pinto, **MD** Division of Colon and Rectal Surgery, Cleveland Clinic Florida, Weston, FL, USA

Filippo Pucciani, **MD** Department of Medical and Surgical Critical Care, University of Firenze, Firenze, Italy

Dmitry Pushkar, **MD** Department of Urology, Moscow State Medical Stomatological University (MSMSU), Moscow, Russia

Davide Quaresmini, **MD** Urogynecology Unit, Department of Obstetrics and Gynecology, University of Brescia, Brescia, Italy

Amrith Raj Rao, MS Laparoscopic Urology, Department of Urology, Kings College Hospital, London, UK

Carlo Ratto, **MD** Department of Surgical Sciences, Catholic University, Roma, Italy

Tomasz Rechberger, **MD** 2nd Department of Gynecology, Medical University of Lublin, Lublin, Poland

Caecilia S. Reiner, **MD** Institute of Diagnostic and Interventional Radiology, University Hospital, Zurich, Switzerland

Marcella Rinaldi, **MD** Colorectal Unit, Department of Emergency and Organ Transplantation, University of Bari, Bari, Italy

Paul Riss, **MD** Department of Obstetrics and Gynecology, Landesklinikum Thermenregion Moedling, Moedling, Austria

Joan Robert-Yap, **MD** Proctology Unit, University Hospital, Geneva, Switzerland

Bruno Roche, **MD** Proctology Unit, University Hospital, Geneva, Switzerland

Rebecca G. Rogers, **MD** Department of Obstetrics and Gynecology, University of New Mexico, Albuquerque, NM, USA

Giovanni Romano, **MD**, Division of Colon and Rectal Surgery, Department of Oncologic Surgery, National Cancer Institute "G. Pascale", Napoli, Italy

Maurizio Roveroni, **MD** Department of General Surgery, U. Parini Hospital, Aosta, Italy

Andrea Rusconi, **MD** Department of General Surgery, "San Pio X" Hospital, Milano, Italy

Beatrice Salvioli, **MD** Department of Clinical Medicine, S. Orsola-Malpighi Hospital, University of Bologna, Bologna, Italy, Humanitas Institute, Rozzano (MI), Italy

Giulio Aniello Santoro, **MD** Pelvic Floor Unit and Colorectal Service, 1st Department of General Surgery, Regional Hospital, Treviso, Italy

Jakob Scholbach, Dipl Math Mathematisches Institut, Albert-Ludwigs-Universität, Freiburg, Germany

S. Abbas Shobeiri, **MD** Section of Female Pelvic Medicine and Reconstructive Surgery, Department of Obstetrics and Gynecology, The University of Oklahoma Health Sciences Center, Oklahoma City, OK, USA

Aleksandra Stankiewicz, **MD** Department of Pediatric Radiology, Children's Teaching Hospital, Medical University of Lublin, Lublin, Poland

Erica Stocco, **MD** Department of Oncological and Surgical Science, 2nd Surgical Clinic, University of Padova, Padova, Italy

Jaap Stoker, **MD** Department of Radiology, Academic Medical Center, University of Amsterdam, Amsterdam, The Netherlands

Iwona Sudoł-Szopińska, **MD** Department of Proctology, Hospital at Salte, Warsaw; Department of Diagnostic Imaging, Medical University of Warsaw, Warsaw, Poland

Abdul H. Sultan, **MD** Department of Obstetrics and Gynaecology, Mayday University Hospital, Croydon, Surrey, UK

Natalia Sumerova, **MD** Department of Urology, Moscow State Medical Stomatological University (MSMSU), Moscow, Russia

Sondra L. Summers, **MD** Department of Obstetrics and Gynecology, Loyola University Medical Center, Chicago, IL, USA

Michael Swash, **MD** Department of Neurology and Neuroscience, The Royal London Hospital, Barts and The London School of Medicine and Dentistry, Queen Mary University of London, London, UK

Stuart Taylor, **MD** Department of Clinical Radiology, University College, London, UK

Ranee Thakar, **MD** Department of Obstetrics and Gynaecology, Mayday University Hospital, Croydon, Surrey, UK

Mario Trompetto, **MD** Colorectal Eporediensis Centre, "Santa Rita" Clinic, Vercelli, Policlinic of Monza, Italy

Giuseppe Tuccitto, **MD** Division of Urology, Regional Hospital, Treviso, Italy

Frank Van der Aa, **MD** Pelvic Floor Unit, UZ Gasthuisberg, Leuven, Belgium

Joan Veldman, **MD** Pelvic Floor Unit, UZ Gasthuisberg, Leuven, Belgium

Jasper Verguts, **MD** Pelvic Floor Unit, UZ Gasthuisberg, Leuven, Belgium

Dominik Weishaupt, **MD** Institute of Radiology, Triemli Hospital Zurich, Zurich, Switzerland

Erika Werbrouck, **MD** Pelvic Floor Unit, UZ Gasthuisberg, Leuven, Belgium

Steven D. Wexner, **MD** Division of Colon and Rectal Surgery, Cleveland Clinic Florida, Weston, FL, USA

Andrzej Paweł Wieczorek, **MD** Department of Pediatric Radiology, Children's Teaching Hospital, Medical University of Lublin, Lublin, Poland

Magdalena Maria Woźniak, **MD** Department of Pediatric Radiology, Children's Teaching Hospital, Medical University of Lublin, Lublin, Poland

Silvia Zanelli, **MD** Urogynecology Unit, Department of Obstetrics and Gynecology, University of Brescia, Brescia, Italy

Andrew P. Zbar, **MD** Division of Colon and Rectal Surgery, Universities of New England and New Castle, New South Wales, Australia

Guillaume Zufferey, **MD** Proctology Unit, University Hospital, Geneva, Switzerland

Section I
Pelvic Floor Anatomy

State of the Art Pelvic Floor Anatomy

1

John O.L. DeLancey and S. Abbas Shobeiri

Abstract We frequently associate pelvic floor injury with parity, ageing, hysterectomy, and chronic straining. Exactly what structures are injured remains the focus of intense research. Therefore, basic understanding of pelvic floor anatomy is essential to effective communication between pelvic floor specialists. The goal of the current chapter is to lay a firm anatomic foundation for interpreting different imaging modalities by emphasizing pelvic floor innervations, morphology of the levator ani muscle by origin-insertion pairs, and fascial and muscular support of the anterior and posterior compartments.

Keywords Anatomy • Incontinence • Innervation • Levator ani • Pelvic floor

1.1 Introduction

Pelvic floor disorders, including pelvic organ prolapse and urinary incontinence, are debilitating conditions that result in surgery in 1 out of 9 women [1]. In the US the National Center for Health Statistics estimates 400,000 operations are performed for pelvic floor dysfunction each year, with 300,000 occurring in the in-patient setting [2, 3]. This is six to eight times more operations than for radical prostatectomies performed each year. Although there is wide recognition of urinary incontinence, pelvic organ prolapse is responsible for twice as many operations, yet its causes are largely unknown. Prolapse arises because of injuries and deterioration of the muscles, nerves, and connective tissue that support and control normal pelvic function. This chapter addresses the *functional* anatomy of the pelvic floor in women and specifically focuses on how the

pelvic organs are supported by the surrounding muscles and fasciae. It also considers the pathophysiology of pelvic organ prolapse as it relates to changes in these structures.

1.1.1 Support of the Pelvic Organs: Conceptual Overview

The pelvic organs rely on (1) their connective tissue attachments to the pelvic walls, and (2) support from the levator ani muscles that are under neuronal control from the peripheral and central nervous systems. In this chapter, the term "pelvic floor" is used broadly to include all the structures supporting the pelvic cavity, rather than the restricted use of this term to refer to the levator ani group of muscles.

The pelvic floor consists of several components lying between the peritoneum and the vulvar skin. From above downward, these are the peritoneum, pelvic viscera and endopelvic fascia, levator ani muscles, perineal membrane, and superficial genital muscles. The

J.O.L. DeLancey
Department of Obstetrics and Gynecology, University of Michigan Medical School, Ann Arbor, MI, USA

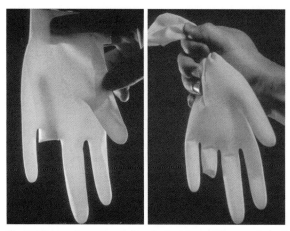

Fig. 1.1 Bonney's analogy of vaginal prolapse. The eversion of an intussuscepted surgical glove finger by increasing pressure within the glove is analogous to prolapse of the vagina

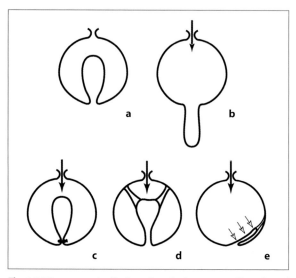

Fig. 1.2 Diagrammatic display of vaginal support. **a** Invaginated area in a surrounding compartment; **b** the prolapse opens when the pressure (*arrow*) is increased; **c** closing the bottom of the vagina prevents prolapse by constriction; **d** ligament suspension; **e** flap valve closure where suspending fibers hold the vagina in a position against the wall allowing increases in pressure to pin it in place

support for all these structures comes from connections to the bony pelvis and its attached muscles. The pelvic organs are often thought of as being supported by the pelvic floor, but are actually a part of it. The pelvic viscera play an important role in forming the pelvic floor through their connections with structures such as the cardinal and uterosacral ligaments.

In 1934, Bonney pointed out that the vagina is in the same relationship to the abdominal cavity as the inturned finger of a surgical glove is to the rest of the glove (Fig. 1.1) [4]. If the pressure in the glove is increased, it forces the finger to protrude downwards in the same way that increases in abdominal pressure force the vagina to prolapse. Fig. 1.2a,b provides a schematic illustration of this prolapse phenomenon. In Fig. 1.2c, the lower end of the vagina is held closed by the pelvic floor muscles, preventing prolapse by constricting the base of the invaginated finger closed. Fig. 1.2d shows suspension of the vagina to the pelvic walls. Fig. 1.2e demonstrates that spatial relationships are important in the "flap valve" closure, where the suspending fibers hold the vagina in a position against the supporting walls of the pelvis; increases in pressure force the vagina against the wall, thereby pinning it in place. Vaginal support is a combination of constriction, suspension, and structural geometry.

The female pelvis can naturally be divided into anterior, posterior, and lateral compartments (Fig. 1.3). The genital tract (vagina and uterus) divides the anterior and posterior compartments through lateral connections to the pelvic sidewall and suspension at its apex. The levator ani muscles form the bottom of the pelvis. The

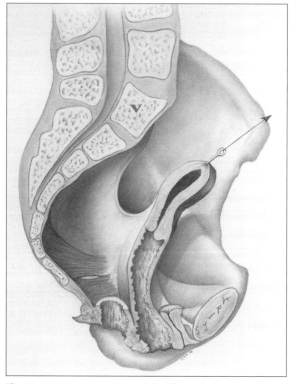

Fig. 1.3 Compartments of the pelvis. The vagina, connected laterally to the pelvic walls, divides the pelvis into an anterior and posterior compartment. *V*, fifth lumbar vertebra

organs are attached to the levator ani muscles when they pass through the urogenital hiatus, and are supported by these connections.

1.2 Functional Anatomy and Prolapse

1.2.1 Overview

The pelvic organ support system is multifaceted and includes the endopelvic fascia, the perineal membrane, and the levator ani muscles that are controlled by the central and peripheral nervous system. The supports of the uterus and vagina are different in different regions (Fig. 1.4) [5]. The cervix (when present) and the upper one-third of the vagina (level I) have relatively long suspensory fibers that are *vertically* oriented in the standing position, while the mid-portion of the vagina (level II) has a more direct attachment *laterally* to the pelvic wall (Fig. 1.5). In the most caudal region (level III), the vagina is attached directly to the structures that surround it. In this level, the levator ani muscles and the perineal membrane have important supportive functions.

In the upper part of the genital tract, a connective tissue complex attaches all the pelvic viscera to the pelvic sidewall. This endopelvic fascia forms a continuous sheet-like mesentery, extending from the uterine artery at its cephalic margin to the point at which the vagina fuses with the levator ani muscles below. The fascial region that attaches to the uterus is called the parametrium, and that which attaches to the vagina the

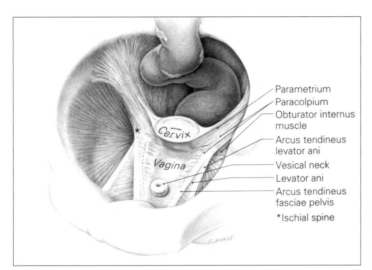

Fig. 1.4 Attachments of the cervix and vagina to the pelvic walls demonstrating different regions of support with the uterus in situ. Note that the uterine corpus and the bladder have been removed

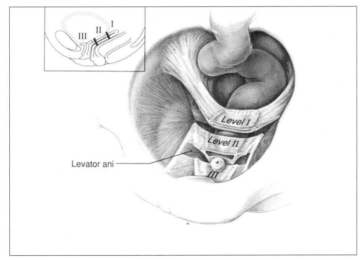

Fig. 1.5 Levels of vaginal support after hysterectomy. Level I (suspension) and level II (attachment). In level I the paracolpium suspends the vagina from the lateral pelvic walls. Fibers of level I extend both vertically and also posteriorly towards the sacrum.
In level II the vagina is attached to the arcus tendineus fasciae pelvis and the superior fascia of the levator ani

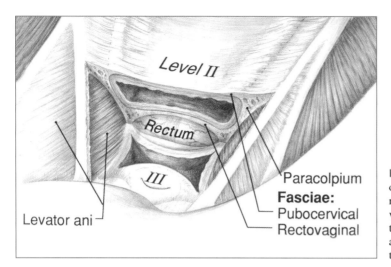

Fig. 1.6 Close up of the lower margin of level II after a wedge of vagina has been removed (inset). Note how the anterior vaginal wall, through its connections to the arcus tendineus fascia pelvis, forms a supportive layer clinically referred to as the pubocervical fascia

paracolpium. Level I is composed of both parametrium and paracolpium. The uterosacral and cardinal ligaments together form the parametrium and support the uterus and upper one-third of the vagina. The paracolpium portion of level I consists of a relatively long sheet of tissue that suspends the superior aspect of the vagina by attaching it to the pelvic wall. This is true whether or not the cervix is present. The uterosacral ligaments are important components of this support. At level II, the paracolpium changes configuration and forms more direct lateral attachments of the mid-portion of the vagina to the pelvic walls (Fig. 1.6). These lateral attachments have functional significance, i.e. they stretch the vagina transversely between the bladder and the rectum. In the distal vagina (level III), the vaginal wall is directly attached to surrounding structures without any intervening paracolpium. Anteriorly, the vagina fuses with the urethra, posteriorly with the perineal body, and laterally with the levator ani muscles.

Damage to level I support can result in uterine or vaginal prolapse of the apical segment. Damage to the level II and III portions of vaginal support results in anterior and posterior vaginal wall prolapse. The varying combinations of these defects are responsible for the diversity of clinically encountered problems and will be discussed in the following sections.

1.2.2 Apical Segment

In level I, the cardinal and uterosacral ligaments attach the cervix and the upper one-third of the vagina to the pelvic walls [6, 7]. Neither are true ligaments in the

sense of a skeletal ligament that is composed of dense regular connective tissue similar to knee ligaments. They are "visceral ligaments" that are similar to bowel mesentery. They are made of blood vessels, nerves, smooth muscle, and adipose tissue intermingled with irregular connective tissue. They have a supportive function in limiting the excursion of the pelvic organs, much as the mesentery of the small bowel limits the movement of the intestine. When these structures are placed on tension, they form condensations that surgeons refer to as ligaments.

The uterosacral ligaments are bands of tissue running under the rectovaginal peritoneum, composed of smooth muscle, loose and dense connective tissue, blood vessels, nerves, and lymphatics [6]. They originate from the posterolateral aspect of the cervix at the level of the internal cervical os and from the lateral vaginal fornix [6]. While macroscopic investigation observed insertion of the ligament to the levator ani, coccygeus, and the presacral fascia [8], magnetic resonance imaging (MRI) examination showed the uterosacral ligaments overlie the sacrospinous ligament and coccygeus in 82% of cases and over the sacrum in only 7% of cases [9]. The difference between the appearance of these structures in MRI and on dissection may be related to the tension placed on the structures during dissection and will require further research to clarify.

The cardinal ligament is a mass of retroperitoneal areolar connective tissue in which blood vessels predominate; it also contains nerves and lymphatic channels [7]. It has a configuration similar to that of "chicken wire" or fishing net in its natural state, but when placed under tension assumes the appearance

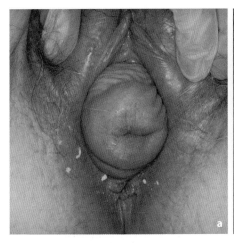 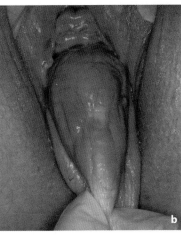

Fig. 1.7 Uterine prolapse showing the cervix protruding from the vaginal opening (**a**) and vaginal prolapse where the puckered scar indicates where the cervix used to be (**b**). Note the upper vaginal prolapse

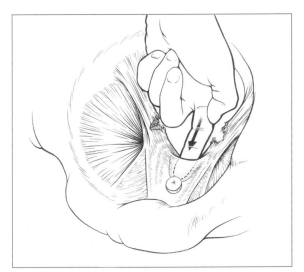

Fig. 1.8 Damage to the suspensory ligaments can lead to eversion of the vaginal apex when subjected to downward forces

ward descent of the vaginal apex after hysterectomy is resisted by the paracolpium. Damage to the upper suspensory fibers of the paracolpium (cardinal and uterosacral ligaments) allows uterine or apical segment prolapse (Fig. 1.8).

Although descriptions of uterine support often imply that the uterus is suspended by the cardinal/uterosacral complex much like a light suspended by a wire from the ceiling, this is not the case. The suspensory ligaments hold the uterus in position over the levator muscles, which in turn reduce the tension on the ligaments and protect them from excessive tension. This will be discussed later in the section on interactions between muscle and ligaments.

1.2.3 Anterior Compartment

Anterior compartment support depends on the connections of the vagina and periurethral tissues to the muscles and fascia of the pelvic wall via the arcus tendineus fascia pelvis (Fig. 1.9). On both sides of the pelvis, the arcus tendineus fascia pelvis is a band of connective tissue attached at one end to the lower one-sixth of the pubic bone, one centimeter lateral to the midline, and at the other end to the ischium, just above the spine.

The anterior wall fascial attachments to the arcus tendineus fascia pelvis have been called the paravaginal fascial attachments by Richardson and colleagues [10]. Lateral detachment of the paravaginal fascial connections from the pelvic wall is associated with stress incontinence and anterior prolapse (Fig. 1.10). Further details of the structural mechanics of anterior wall

of a strong cable as the fibers align along the lines of tension [7]. It originates from the pelvic sidewall and inserts on the uterus, cervix, and upper one-third of the vagina. Both the uterosacral and cardinal tissues are critical components of level I support and provide support for the vaginal apex following hysterectomy (Fig. 1.5). The cardinal ligaments are oriented in a relatively vertical axis (in the standing posture), while the uterosacral ligaments are more dorsal in their orientation.

The nature of uterine support (Fig. 1.7) can be understood when the cervix is pulled downward with a tenaculum during dilation and curettage. After a certain amount of descent, the level I supports become tight and arrest further cervical descent. Similarly, down-

support will be provided later. In addition, the upper portions of the anterior vaginal wall are affected by the suspensory actions of level I. If the cardinal and uterosacral ligaments fail, the upper vaginal wall prolapses downward while the lower vagina (levels II and III) remains supported.

Anterior vaginal wall prolapse can occur either because of lateral detachment of the anterior vaginal wall at the pelvic sidewall, referred to as a displacement "cystocele", or as a central failure of the vaginal wall

itself that results in distension "cystocele" (Fig. 1.11). Although various grading schemes have been described for anterior vaginal prolapse, they are often focused on the degree of prolapse rather than the anatomic perturbation that results in this descent; therefore, it is important to describe anterior prolapse with regard to the location of the fascial failure (lateral detachment versus central failure). At present, although a number of investigators have described techniques to distinguish central from lateral detachment, validation of these techniques remains elusive.

Defects of the midline fascia resulting in cystocele are easy to understand, but understanding how lateral

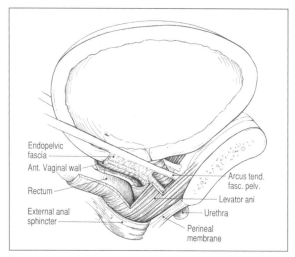

Fig. 1.9 Lateral view of the pelvic floor structures related to urethral support seen from the side in the standing position, cut just lateral to the midline. Note that windows have been cut in the levator ani muscles, vagina, and endopelvic fascia so that the urethra and anterior vaginal walls can be seen

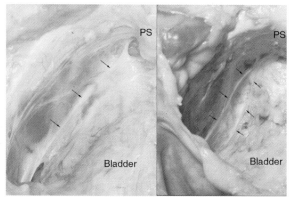

Fig. 1.10 Left panel shows the attachment of the arcus tendineus pelvis to the pubic bone (arrow). Right panel demonstrates a paravaginal defect where the cervical fascia has separated from the arcus tendineus (arrow points to the sides of the split). PS, pubic symphysis

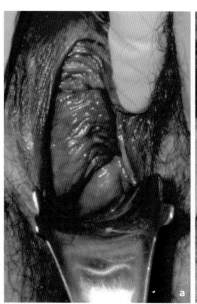
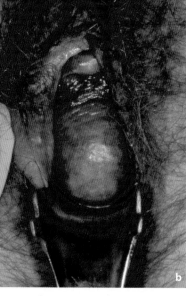

Fig. 1.11 a Displacement "cystocele" where the intact anterior vaginal wall has prolapsed downward due to paravaginal defect. Note that the right side of the patient's vagina and cervix has descended more than the left because of a larger defect on this side. b Distension "cystocele" where the anterior vaginal wall fascia has failed and the bladder is distending the mucosa

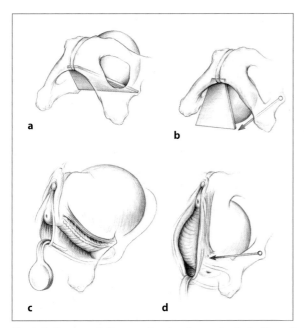

Fig. 1.12 Conceptual diagram showing the mechanical effect of detachment of the arcus tendinous fascia pelvis from the ischial spine. **a** The trapezoidal plane of the pubocervical fascia. The attachments to the pubis and the ischial spines are intact. **b** The connection to the spine has been lost, allowing the fascial plane to swing downward. **c** Normal anterior vaginal wall as seen with a weighted speculum in place. **d** The effect of dorsal detachment of the arcus from the ischial spine

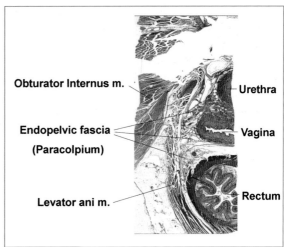

Fig. 1.13 Histologic cross-section of pelvis at the level of mid-urethra, from the collection of Dr Thomas E. Oelrich

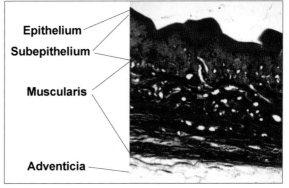

Fig. 1.14 Higher magnification of a section of vaginal wall. Note the lack of a fascial layer. The endopelvic fascia is not seen at this magnification

detachment results in cystocele is not as obvious. The fact that lateral detachment was associated with cystourethrocele was first established by Richardson et al (Fig. 1.10) [10]. A study of 71 women with anterior compartment prolapse has shown that paravaginal defect usually results from a detachment of the arcus tendineus fascia pelvis from the ischial spine, and rarely from the pubic bone [11]. A visual analogy is that of a swinging trapezoid (Fig. 1.12). The mechanical effect of this detachment allows the trapezoid to rotate downward. When this happens, the anterior vaginal wall protrudes through the introitus. Upward support of the trapezoid is also provided by the cardinal and uterosacral ligaments in level I. For this reason, resuspension of the vaginal apex at the time of surgery in addition to paravaginal or anterior colporrhaphy helps to return the anterior wall to a more normal position.

Anatomically, the endopelvic fascia refers to the areolar connective tissue surrounding the vagina. It continues down the length of the vagina as loose areolar tissue surrounding the pelvic viscera (Fig. 1.13). The term "fascia" is often used by surgeons to refer to the strong tissue that they sew together during anterior repairs. This has led to confusion and misunderstanding of the anatomy. Repeat histologic examination shows that the vagina is made up of three layers – epithelium, muscularis, and adventitia (Fig. 1.14) [12–14]. The adventitial layer is loose areolar connective tissue made up of collagen and elastin. These layers form the vaginal tube. The tissue that a surgeon plicates during repairs is not what an anatomist would refer to as endopelvic fascia but rather is the vaginal muscularis and the adventitial layer of the vaginal tube. Also, many basic science studies that we will address later in the pathophysiology section use biopsies from the vaginal tube and not from the endopelvic fascia that connects the vaginal wall to the pelvic sidewalls.

1.2.4 Perineal Membrane (Urogenital Diaphragm)

Spanning the anterior part of the pelvic outlet, below the levator ani muscles, there is a dense triangular membrane called the perineal membrane. The term "perineal membrane" replaces the old term "urogenital diaphragm", reflecting the fact that this layer is not a single muscle layer with a double layer of fascia ("diaphragm"), but rather a set of connective tissues that surround the urethra [15]. The orientation consists of a single connective tissue membrane, with muscle lying immediately above. The perineal membrane lies at the level of the hymen and attaches the urethra, vagina, and perineal body to the ischiopubic rami (Fig. 1.15). The compressor urethrae and urethrovaginal sphincter muscles are associated with the cranial surface of the perineal membrane.

1.2.5 Posterior Compartment and Perineal Membrane

The posterior vagina is supported by connections between the vagina, the bony pelvis, and the levator ani muscles [16]. The lower one-third of the vagina is fused with the perineal body (level III) (Fig. 1.16a), which connects the perineal membranes on either side. The mid-posterior vagina (level II) is connected to the inside of the levator ani muscles by sheets of endopelvic fascia (Fig. 1.17). These connections prevent vaginal descent during increases in abdominal pressure. The most medial aspects of these paired sheets are the rectal pillars. In its upper one-third, the posterior vagina is connected laterally by the paracolpium of level I. Separate systems for anterior and posterior vaginal support do not exist at level I.

The fibers of the perineal membrane connect through the perineal body, thereby providing a layer that resists downward descent of the rectum. If this attachment becomes broken, then the resistance to downward descent is lost (Fig. 1.16b). This situation is somewhat like an incisional hernia seen after disruption of a vertical incision where the bowel protrudes through a defect between the rectus abdominus muscles when

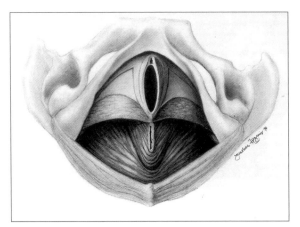

Fig. 1.15 Position of the perineal membrane and its associated components of the striated urogenital sphincter, the compressor urethra, and the urethrovaginal sphincter

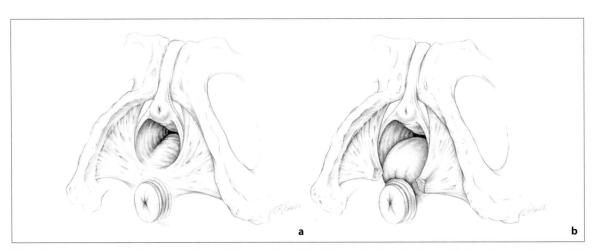

a   b

Fig. 1.16 a The perineal membrane spans the arch between the ischiopubic rami with each side attached to the other through their connection in the perineal body. **b** Note that separation of the fibers in this area leaves the rectum unsupported and results in a low posterior prolapse

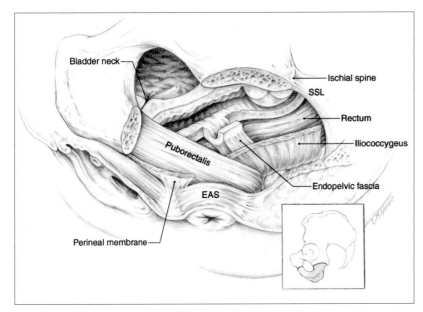

Fig. 1.17 Lateral view of the pelvis showing the relationships of the puborectalis, iliococcygeus, and pelvic floor structures after removal of the ischium below the spine and sacrospinous ligament (*SSL*) (*EAS*, external anal sphincter). The bladder and vagina have been cut in the midline yet the rectum is left intact. Note how the endopelvic fascial "pillars" hold the vaginal wall dorsally preventing its downward protrusion

due to a defect in the rectus sheath. In the same way, protrusion of the rectum between the levator ani muscles can be seen when a disruption of the perineal body and connections of the perineal membrane occurs (Fig. 1.18). Re-attachment of the separated structures during perineorrhaphy corrects this defect and is a mainstay of reconstructive surgery. Because the levator ani muscles are intimately connected with the cranial surface of the perineal membranes, this reattachment also restores the muscles to a more normal position under the pelvic organs in a location where they can provide support.

Three muscular structures that maintain fecal continence consist of the internal anal sphincter (IAS), the external anal sphincter (EAS), and the puborectalis muscle. The anal canal is 2–4 cm long. The spatial relationships between the internal and external anal sphincters are such that the internal anal sphincter is always extended above the external anal sphincter for a distance of greater than 1 cm. The internal sphincter lies consistently between the external sphincter and the anal mucosa, usually overlapping by 17.0 mm (standard deviation (SD) 6.9 mm). In the majority of cases, the external anal sphincter begins inferiorly to the internal anal sphincter by a few millimeters (Fig. 1.19) [17].

The IAS extends 1 cm below the dentate line. The striated muscle fibers from the levator ani become fibroelastic as they extend caudally to merge with the conjoined longitudinal layer (CLL) that is inserted

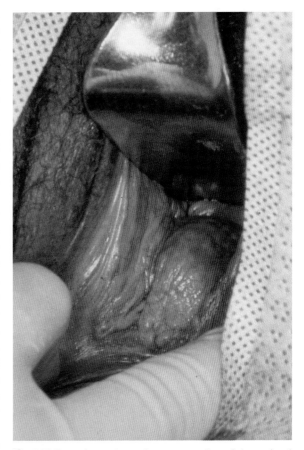

Fig. 1.18 Posterior prolapse due to separation of the perineal body. Note the end of the hymenal ring that lies laterally on the side of the vagina, no longer united with its companion on the other side

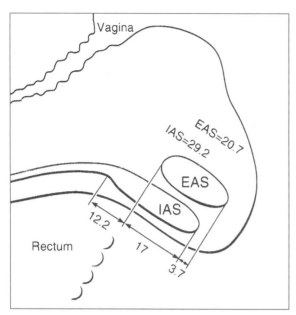

Fig. 1.19 Dimensions and spatial relationships between the internal anal sphincter (*IAS*) and the external anal sphincter (*EAS*) in the midline of the perineal body, expressed in millimeters

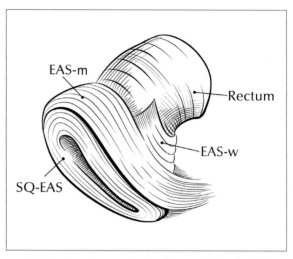

Fig. 1.20 Drawing of external anal sphincter (*EAS*) subdivisions. Anterior portion of model is to the left, posterior to the right. Notice decussation of fibers toward the coccyx posteriorly. The main body of the external anal sphincter also has a concentric portion posteriorly that is not shown in this view. *EAS-m*, main body of *EAS*; *EAS-w*, winged portion of *EAS*; *SQ-EAS*, subcutaneous *EAS*

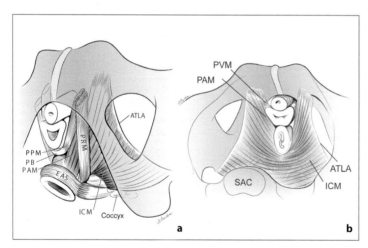

Fig. 1.21 a Schematic view of the levator ani muscles from below after the vulvar structures and perineal membrane have been removed showing the arcus tendineus levator ani (*ATLA*); external anal sphincter (*EAS*); puboanal muscle (*PAM*); perineal body (*PB*) uniting the two ends of the puboperineal muscle (*PPM*); iliococcygeal muscle (*ICM*); and puborectalis muscle (*PRM*). Note that the urethra and vagina have been transected just above the hymenal ring. **b** The levator ani muscle seen from above looking over the sacral promontory (*SAC*) showing the pubovaginalis muscle (*PVM*). The urethra, vagina, and rectum have been transected just above the pelvic floor. (The internal obturator muscles have been removed to clarify the levator muscle origins)

between the external and internal anal sphincters [18]. The external anal sphincter includes a subcutaneous portion (SQ-EAS), a visibly separate deeper portion (EAS-m), and a lateral portion that has lateral winged projections (EAS-w). The SQ-EAS is the distinct part of the EAS. A clear separation does not exist between concentric portions of the EAS-m and the winged EAS-w. The EAS-w fibers have different fiber directions than the other portions, forming an open "U-shaped" configuration. These fibers are contiguous with the EAS but visibly separate from the puborectalis muscle, whose fibers they parallel (Fig. 1.20) [19].

1.2.6 Lateral Compartment and Levator Ani Muscles

Below and surrounding the pelvic organs are the levator ani muscles (Fig. 1.21) [20]. When these muscles and their covering fascia are considered together, the combined structures are referred to as the pelvic diaphragm (not to be confused with the urogenital diaphragm, i.e. perineal membrane – discussed in the previous section).

There are three major components of the levator ani muscle. The iliococcygeal portion forms a thin, relatively flat, horizontal shelf that spans the potential

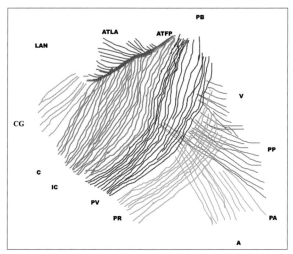

Fig. 1.22 The levator ani muscle is color coded: from left to right, light brown = coccygeus muscle (*CG*), brown = iliococcygeus muscle (*IC*), magenta = arcus tendineus levator ani/arcus tendineus fascia pelvis (*ATLA/ATFP*), red = pubovisceralis muscle (*PV*), green = puborectalis muscle (*PR*), pink = puboperinealis muscle (PP), orange = puboanalis muscle (*PA*). The labels are placed to orient the viewer to the relative position of the other structures in the pelvis. *A*, anus; *C*, coccyx; *LAN*, levator ani nerve; *PB*, pubic bone; *V*, vagina. Reproduced from [18], with permission

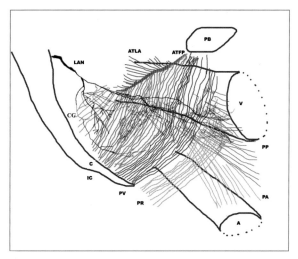

Fig. 1.23 The levator ani nerve (LAN) in relation to the levator ani muscle complex and pelvic structures. For abbreviations, see Fig. 1.22. Reproduced from [18], with permission

gap from one pelvic sidewall to the other. The pubovisceral (also known as the pubococcygeus) muscle attaches the pelvic organs to the pubic bone, while the puborectalis muscle forms a sling behind the rectum. The origins and insertions of these muscles as well as their characteristic anatomical relations are shown in Table 1.1 and Fig. 1.21 [21]. The lesser-known subdivisions of the levator are the pubovaginal, puboanal, and puboperineal muscles (Fig. 1.22) [18].

The opening between the levator ani muscles through which the urethra, vagina, and rectum pass is the levator hiatus. The portion of the levator hiatus ventral to the perineal body is referred to as the uro-

genital hiatus, and it is through this that prolapse of the vagina, uterus, urethra, and bladder occurs. The urogenital hiatus is bounded anteriorly by the pubic bones, laterally by the levator ani muscles, and posteriorly by the perineal body and external anal sphincter. The baseline tonic activity of the levator ani muscle keeps the hiatus closed by compressing the urethra, vagina, and rectum against the pubic bone, pulling the pelvic floor and organs in a cephalic direction [22]. This continuous muscle action, similar to the external anal sphincter, closes the lumen of the vagina much as the anal sphincter closes the anus. This constant action eliminates any opening within the pelvic floor through which prolapse could occur and forms a relatively horizontal shelf on which the pelvic organs are supported [23]. Damage to the levators resulting from nerve or connective tissue damage will leave the urogenital hiatus open and results in prolapse.

Table 1.1 International standardized terminology (Nomina Terminologica) divisions of the levator ani muscle

Nomina Terminologica	Origin/insertion
Pubovisceral muscle ("pubococcygeus")	
Puboperinealis muscle (PPM)	Pubis/perineal body
Pubovaginalis muscle (PVM)	Pubis/vaginal wall at the level of the midurethra
Puboanalis muscle (PAM)	Pubis/intersphincteric groove between internal and external anal sphincter
	to end in the anal skin
Puborectalis muscle (PRM)	Pubis/forms sling behind the rectum
Iliococcygeus muscle (ICM)	Tendinous arch of the levator ani/the two sides fuse in the iliococcygeal raphe

1.2.7 Endopelvic Fascia and Levator Ani Interactions

The interaction between the levator ani muscles and the endopelvic fascia is one of the most important biomechanical features of pelvic organ support. As long as the muscles maintain their constant tone closing the pelvic floor, the ligaments of the endopelvic fascia have very little tension on them even with increases in abdominal pressure. If the muscles become damaged so that the pelvic floor sags downward, the organs are pushed through the urogenital hiatus. Once they have fallen below the level of the hymenal ring, they are unsupported by the levator ani muscles and the ligaments must carry the entire load. Although the endopelvic fascia can sustain these loads for short periods of time, if the pelvic muscles do not close the urogenital hiatus, the connective tissue eventually fails, resulting in prolapse. The support of the vagina has been likened to a ship in its berth, floating on the water and attached by ropes on either side to a dock [24]. The ship is analogous to the vagina, the ropes to the ligaments, and the water to the supportive layer formed by the pelvic muscles. The ropes function to hold the ship (pelvic organs) in the center of its berth as it rests on the water (pelvic muscles). If, however, the water level were to fall far enough that the ropes would be required to hold the ship without the supporting water, the ropes would all break.

Once the pelvic musculature becomes damaged and no longer holds the organs in place, the ligaments are subjected to excessive forces. These forces may be enough to cause ligament failure over the course of time. A young woman sustaining an injury to her pelvic floor muscles when she is young must depend to a greater extent on the strength of her ligaments to prevent pelvic organ prolapse over the subsequent years of her life. An individual with injured muscles may have strong connective tissue that compensates and therefore never develops prolapse, while another woman who has the same degree of muscular damage but was born with weaker connective tissue may experience prolapse as she ages.

In addition, the interaction between the pelvic floor muscles and endopelvic fascia is responsible for maintaining the "flap valve" configuration in the pelvic floor that lessens ligament tension because of the supportive nature of the levator plate (Fig. 1.2e). The flap valve requires the dorsal traction of the uterosacral ligaments, and to some extent the cardinal ligaments, to hold the cervix back in the hollow of the sacrum. It also requires the ventral pull of the pubovisceral portions of the levator ani muscle to swing the levator plate more horizontally to close the urogenital hiatus. It is therefore this interaction between the directions of these two forces that is so critical in maintaining the normal structural relationships that lessen the tension on ligaments and muscles.

1.2.8 Nerves

There are two main nerves that supply the pelvic floor relative to pelvic organ prolapse. One is the pudendal nerve that supplies the urethral and anal sphincters and perineal muscles, and the other is the nerve to the levator ani that innervates the major musculature that supports the pelvic floor. These are distinct nerves with differing origins, courses, and insertions. The nerve to the levator originates from S3 to S5 foramina, runs inside of the pelvis on the cranial surface of the levator ani muscle, and provides the innervation to all the subdivisions of the muscle (Fig. 1.23). The pudendal nerve originates from S2 to S4 foramina and runs through Alcock's canal which is caudal to the levator ani muscles. The pudendal nerve has three branches: the clitoral, perineal, and inferior hemorrhoidal, which innervate the clitoris, the perineal musculature, and inner perineal skin, and the external anal sphincter respectively [25]. Motor nerves to the internal anal sphincter are derived from (1) L5 to presacral plexus sympathetic fibers, (2) S2–4 parasympathetic fibers of the pelvic splanchnic nerve. The levator ani muscle often has a dual somatic innervation, with the levator ani nerve as its constant and main neuronal supply [18, 26]. Blockade of the pudendal nerve decreases resting and squeeze pressures in the vagina and rectum, increases the length of the urogenital hiatus, and decreases electromyogram (EMG) activity of the puborectalis muscle [27].

References

1. Olsen AL, Smith VJ, Bergstrom JO et al. Epidemiology of surgically managed pelvic organ prolapse and urinary incontinence. Obstet Gynecol 1997;89:501.
2. Boyles SH, Weber AM, Meyn L. Procedures for pelvic organ prolapse in the United States, 1979–1997. Am J Obstet Gynecol 2003;188:108.

3. Boyles SH, Weber AM, Meyn L. Procedures for urinary incontinence in the United States, 1979–1997. Am J Obstet Gynecol 2003;189:70.
4. Bonney V. The principles that should underlie all operations for prolapse. Obstet Gynaecol Br Emp 1934;41:669.
5. DeLancey JO. Anatomic aspects of vaginal eversion after hysterectomy. Am J Obstet Gynecol 1992;166:1717–1724.
6. Campbell RM. The anatomy and histology of the sacrouterine ligaments. Am J Obstet Gynecol 1950;59:1.
7. Range RL, Woodburne RT. The gross and microscopic anatomy of the transverse cervical ligaments. Am J Obstet Gynecol 1964;90:460.
8. Blaisdell FE. The anatomy of the sacro-uterine ligaments. Anat Record 1917;12:1–42.
9. Umek WH, Morgan DM, Ashton-Miller JA, DeLancey JO. Quantitative analysis of uterosacral ligament origin and insertion points by magnetic resonance imaging. Obstet Gynecol 2004;103:447.
10. Richardson AC, Edmonds PB, Williams NL. Treatment of stress urinary incontinence due to paravaginal fascial defect. Obstet Gynecol 1981;57:357.
11. DeLancey JO. Fascial and muscular abnormalities in women with urethral hypermobility and anterior vaginal wall prolapse. Am J Obstet Gynecol 2002;187:93.
12. Ricci JV, Thom CH. The myth of a surgically useful fascia in vaginal plastic reconstructions. Q Rev Surg Obstet Gynecol 1954;11:253.
13. Gitsch E, Palmrich AH. Operative Anatomie. De Gruyter, Berlin, 1977.
14. Weber AM, Walters MD. Anterior vaginal prolapse: review of anatomy and techniques of surgical repair. Obstet Gynecol 1990;89:311.
15. Oelrich TM. The striated urogenital sphincter muscle in the female. Anat Rec 1983;205:223–232.
16. DeLancey JO. Structural support of the urethra as it relates to stress urinary incontinence: the hammock hypothesis [comment]. Am J Obstet Gynecol 1994;170:1713.
17. DeLancey JO, Toglia MR, Perucchini D. Internal and external anal sphincter anatomy as it relates to midline obstetric lacerations. Obstet Gynecol 1997;90:924.
18. Shobeiri SA, Chesson RR, Gasser RF. The internal innervation and morphology of the human female levator ani muscle. Am J Obstet Gynecol 2008;199:686.e1–6.
19. Hsu Y, Fenner DE, Weadock WJ, DeLancey JO. Magnetic resonance imaging and 3-dimensional analysis of external anal sphincter anatomy. Obstet Gynecol 2005;106:1259.
20. Lawson JO. Pelvic anatomy. I. Pelvic floor muscles. Ann R Coll Surg Engl 1974;54:244.
21. Kearney R, Sawhney R, DeLancey JO. Levator ani muscle anatomy evaluated by origin-insertion pairs. Obstet Gynecol 2004;104:168–173.
22. Taverner D. An electromyographic study of the normal function of the external anal sphincter and pelvic diaphragm. Dis Colon Rectum 1959;2:153.
23. Nichols DH, Milley PS, Randall CL. Significance of restoration of normal vaginal depth and axis. Obstet Gynecol 1970;36:251.
24. Paramore RH. The uterus as a floating organ. In: Paramore RH. The statistics of the female pelvic viscera, vol 1. HK Lewis and Co, London, 1918, pp 12–15.
25. Barber MD, Bremer RE, Thor KB et al. Innervation of the female levator ani muscles. Am J Obstet Gynecol 2002;187:64.
26. Wallner C, van Wissen J, Maas CP et al. The contribution of the levator ani nerve and the pudendal nerve to the innervation of the levator ani muscles; a study in human fetuses. Eur Urol 2008;54:1136.
27. Noelani M, Guaderrama NM, Liu J et al. Evidence for the innervation of pelvic floor muscles by the pudendal nerve. Obstet Gynecol 2005;106:774.

The Integral Theory: A Musculo-elastic Theory of Pelvic Floor Function and Dysfunction

2

Peter Papa Petros and Michael Swash

Abstract The Integral Theory (1993) stated: "Stress, urge, and abnormal emptying are mainly caused by connective tissue laxity in the suspensory ligaments of vagina, a result of altered connective tissue". More recently, the theory has been amended to include pelvic pain, fecal incontinence, and defecation difficulties. According to the theory, therefore, accurate diagnosis and reconstruction of the suspensory ligaments will cure such symptoms. Essential to understanding the theory are the following concepts: the organs are suspended by ligaments; the organs are opened or closed by neurologically coordinated muscle forces contracting against these ligaments; lax ligaments may invalidate the muscle forces causing organ prolapse, and dysfunctions in closure (incontinence) or opening (evacuation symptoms); a symptom-based diagnostic algorithm helps to locate ligament laxity; these are confirmed by a three-zone structured examination system; and organ prolapse and abnormal symptoms are both addressed by using tapes to reinforce damaged suspensory ligaments.

Keywords Integral Theory • Ligaments • Nocturia • Pelvic pain • Pictorial algorithm • Prolapse • Stress incontinence • TFS • Urge incontinence

2.1 Introduction

The Integral Theory (1993) stated: "Stress, urge, and abnormal emptying are mainly caused by connective tissue laxity in the suspensory ligaments of vagina, a result of altered connective tissue" [1]. More recently, the theory has been amended to include pelvic pain, fecal incontinence, and defecation difficulties [2–4]. According to the theory, therefore, accurate diagnosis and reconstruction of the suspensory ligaments will cure such symptoms.

P. Papa Petros
Formerly Department of Gynecology, Royal Perth Hospital, School of Engineering, University of Western Australia, Crawley, Australia

2.1.1 Origins and Development of the Integral Theory

The Integral Theory evolved from the investigation of a series of discordant findings following the prototype midurethral sling operations performed at Royal Perth Hospital in 1986–9 [5]. Patients were cured with x-ray evidence of no bladder base elevation, an obvious contradiction of the "Pressure Equalization Theory". Abdominal ultrasound studies in Uppsala in 1990 demonstrated distal urethral closure from behind by muscle forces [5]. This was described as the "hammock closure mechanism". It was also hypothesized that there was a second more powerful proximal closure mechanism, the "bladder neck closure mechanism". This was demonstrated in 1993 [1] with electromyography

(EMG) and with dynamic x-ray studies following injection of radio-opaque dye into the bladder, vagina, rectum, and levator plate. These studies indicated that proximal urethral closure was activated by a musculoelastic mechanism, not intra-abdominal pressure. OAB ("overactive bladder") in the non-neurological patient was defined as a premature activation of the micturition reflex [6]. Urodynamic studies demonstrated an identical sequence of events to that seen in a normal micturition reflex – first, sensory urgency, then a fall in urethral pressure, then detrusor contraction, then urine loss [6].

The second (1993) publication of the Integral Theory [1] presented radiological and urodynamic studies and brought a higher level of proof. The "posterior fornix syndrome" was described, a symptom complex resulting from laxity in the uterosacral ligaments, "posterior zone" (see below, 2.3). Reconstruction of the posterior ligaments improved symptoms of urge, nocturia, abnormal emptying, and pelvic pain [1].

The years 1994 to 2009 have seen a consolidation and international acceptance of many parts of the Integral Theory, in particular, the treatment of stress incontinence with a midurethral sling, and apical prolapse and posterior zone symptoms (see 2.3) with a posterior

sling. The theory framework has expanded to include fecal incontinence [3], abnormal bladder emptying, and some types of pelvic pain. Validation of these symptoms by more objective data, and by other investigators is slowly emerging. One major criticism of the theory, failure to locate anatomical evidence of "bladder base stretch receptors", has been recently answered by the description of transient receptor potential channels, "TRPs", in the bladder epithelium [7]. These function as stretch, volume, and pain receptors [7]. The theory is now more accurately described as the "integral system". It has four components – function, dysfunction, diagnosis, and management.

2.2 Function

2.2.1 The Organs

The bladder, uterus, and rectum (Fig. 2.1) are receptacles, connected to the outside by an emptying tube, the urethra, vagina, and anus.

2.2.2 The Ligaments

There are four suspensory ligaments (Fig. 2.1). They suspend the organs from above, and act as anchoring points for muscle forces. The perineal body (PB) is not a suspensory ligament, but it also supports the organs and acts as an anchoring point for muscle contractions.

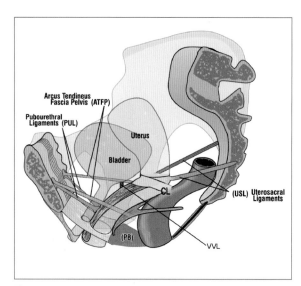

Fig. 2.1 The organs and suspensory ligaments. The organs are separated by organ spaces, allowing them to move freely. They are closely attached to each other 2–3 cm at their distal ends. The four suspensory ligaments are pubourethral (PUL), arcus tendineus fascia pelvis (ATFP), cardinal (CL), and uterosacral (USL). The vesico-vaginal ligament (VVL) is the attachment between the bladder base and proximal vagina. The perineal body (PB), though not a ligament, functions as an important anchoring point for muscle forces

2.2.3 The Muscles

The muscles support the organs from below, and contract against the suspensory ligaments to stretch the organs for both opening and closure (Fig. 2.2) [8, 9]. So if a ligament is lax, the muscles will not function optimally, and the organs may have dysfunction in opening (evacuation), closure (continence), or both.

2.2.4 The Nerves

The nerves have two main functions, as a sensor of organ fullness or muscle tension, and as a 'motor' to coordinate and accelerate the complex series of events involved in organ retention or emptying (Fig. 2.3).

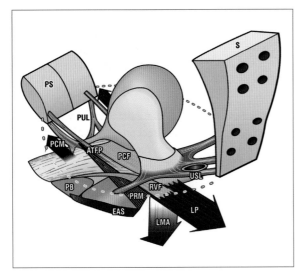

Fig. 2.2 The muscle forces. Forward force (*arrow*): the *PCM* (anterior part of pubococcygeus muscle) contracts against the pubourethral ligament (*PUL*). Backward force (*arrow*): the levator plate (*LP*) contracts against the *PUL*, uterosacral ligament (*USL*), and perineal body (*PB*). Downward force (*arrow*): the longitudinal muscle of the anus (*LMA*) contracts against the *USL* external anal sphincter (*EAS*). The puborectalis is a separate muscle which surrounds the rectum, and can pull all the organs upwards during voluntary contraction ("squeezing"). *ATFP*, arcus tendineus fascia pelvis; *PRM*, puborectalis muscle; *PS*, pubic symphysis; *RVF*, rectovaginal fascia; *S*, sacrum

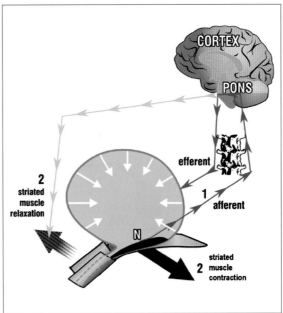

Fig. 2.3 Function of nerves – as an afferent sensor of bladder fullness. "1", from the stretch receptors (*N*), or as an efferent coordinator for muscle action during emptying or retention, "2". Continence: forward and backward muscles contract. Micturition: forward muscles relax and backward muscles contract

2.2.5 Role of Urethral Resistance Incontinence Control

External muscle forces (levator plate/longitudinal muscle of the anus (LP/LMA), Fig. 2.4) stretch and narrow the evacuation tube (urethra, Fig. 2.4) against a firm pubourethral ligament (PUL), then close it by angulating it downwards against the PUL. Narrowing a tube increases the resistance to flow inversely by the fourth power of the radius (Poisseuille's Law) [10]. A lax PUL prevents closure by the muscle forces, exponentially reducing resistance to flow of urine within the urethral tube – incontinence.

2.2.6 Role of Urethral Resistance in Organ Evacuation

Relaxation of the forward vector force (Fig. 2.5) allows the two backward vectors, LP/LMA, to contract against the uterosacral ligaments (USL), to open out the posterior urethral wall (Fig. 2.5). External opening of the

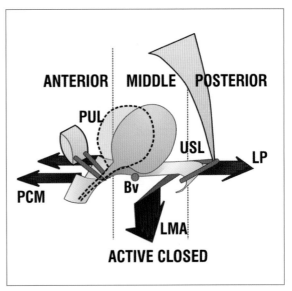

Fig. 2.4 Urethral tube closure. The *PCM* (anterior portion of pubococcygeus muscle) contracts against the pubourethral ligament (*PUL*) to narrow the distal urethra. *LP/LMA* (levator plate/longitudinal muscle of the anus) vectors stretch the vagina backwards to narrow the proximal urethra, then rotate it around the *PUL* to "kink" and close the proximal urethra. *Broken lines* = resting phase; *Bv*, fibromuscular attachment of the bladder base to the vagina

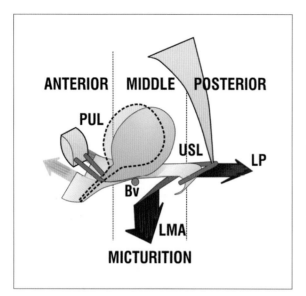

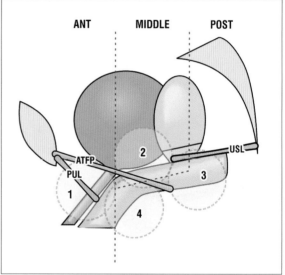

Fig. 2.5 Urethral tube opening (micturition): schematic representation of opening forces, *PCM* (anterior portion of pubococcygeus muscle) relaxes. This allows *LP/LMA* (levator plate/longitudinal muscle of the anus) vectors to stretch the vagina backwards/downwards against the uterosacral ligaments (*USL*), opening out the proximal urethra to "funnel" it, vastly reducing the resistance to flow, and therefore, expulsion pressure. *Broken lines* = resting phase; *Bv*, fibromuscular attachment of the bladder base to the vagina

Fig. 2.6 Connective tissue damage at childbirth (*circles*). Schematic representation of damaged structures ligaments and fascia. *1: PUL* = pubourethral ligament (stress incontinence); *2, ATFP* = arcus tendineus fascia pelvis and pubocervical fascia (cystocoele); *3, USL* = uterosacral ligament (uterine prolapse); *4,* perineal body/rectovaginal fascia (rectocele). Surgery in one area may, in time, cause dislocation and prolapse in another subclinically damaged area

tube decreases the resistance to flow inversely by the fourth power of the radius [10].

It follows that a lax USL will exponentially affect resistance and, therefore, emptying.

2.2.7 Anorectal Function and Dysfunction

Similar muscles and ligaments activate anorectal closure and evacuation. The reader is referred to reference [3].

2.3 Dysfunction: Causation of Lax Connective Tissue

Fig. 2.6 schematically represents the fetal head descending through the birth canal, distending the supporting ligaments and fascia laterally in three zones of the vagina. Though the collagen depolymerizes to 5% of its original strength 24 hours before labour [11], tolerances for damage are low. The anterior–posterior (A–P) diameter of the pelvis is 12–13 cm. A flexed head measures 9.4 cm, and a deflexed head 11.2 cm.

Tissues may overstretch, and incompletely restitute, leaving the ligaments in a lax distended state. Lateral separation of ligaments may allow the organs to prolapse through the gap. As the ligaments are the effective insertion point of the three muscle forces, deficiencies in closure (continence), i.e. evacuation, may occur. The ligaments and associated fascial structures also provide support for stretch receptors (Fig. 2.7), and provide structural support for nerves within the uterosacral ligaments. The symptomatic expressions of these dysfunctions are detailed in Fig. 2.8, which also acts as a guide to diagnosis.

2.4 Diagnosis

2.4.1 Diagnosis of Damaged Ligaments (by Symptoms)

The association of symptoms with the prolapses in the three zones of the vagina in Fig. 2.8 is not absolute. Some patients may have prolapse with no symptoms, and others major symptoms with minimal prolapse. The explanation of this apparent paradox lies in the

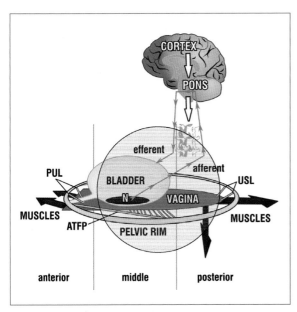

Fig. 2.7 Schematic representation of a fetal head pressing into the pelvic brim, against the vagina and its suspensory ligaments, uterosacral (*USL*), pubourethral (*PUL*), and arcus tendineus fascia pelvis (*ATFP*). There may be no major separation of ligaments. Even minor damage may cause urgency, as this symptom is neurologically determined; a lax vaginal membrane may not be able to support sensitive stretch receptors "*N*", so that these activate the micturition reflex prematurely. The patient senses this as urgency and frequency, and, at night, nocturia

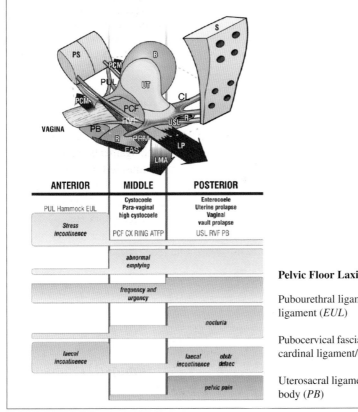

Pelvic Floor Laxities which can be repaired

Pubourethral ligament (*PUL*); hammock; external urethral ligament (*EUL*)

Pubocervical fascia (*PCF*); arcus tendineus fascia pelvis (*ATFP*); cardinal ligament/cervical ring (*CL*)

Uterosacral ligament (*USL*); rectovaginal fascia (*RVF*); perineal body (*PB*)

Fig. 2.8 The pictorial diagnostic algorithm schematically indicates the sites of connective tissue defects (laxities of ligaments or fascias), which can be repaired by surgery, and the association of each zone with symptoms of pelvic floor dysfunction. The area of the symptom rectangle indicates the estimated frequency of symptom causation in each zone. Anterior zone: external meatus to bladder neck; middle zone: bladder neck to anterior cervical ring; posterior zone: posterior vaginal wall from the cervix to the perineal body. *B*, bladder; *EAS*, external anal sphincter; *LMA*, longitudinal muscle of the anus; *LP*, levator plate; *PCM*, pubococcygeus muscle; *PS*, pubic symphysis; *R*, rectum; *S*, sacrum; *UT*, uterus

widely variable sensitivity of the nerve endings for urgency and pelvic pain.

2.4.2 Diagnosis of Damaged Ligaments (by Vaginal Examination)

Not all symptoms are zone specific. For example, urgency may occur with damage in all three zones, fecal incontinence in the anterior or posterior zones, and abnormal bladder emptying in the middle or posterior zones. In such cases, associated symptoms are used to assist the diagnosis of site of damage. Vaginal examination confirms the site of damage. The only way to diagnose pubourethral damage is to digitally support the midurethra during coughing ("simulated operation"). Control of stress incontinence (SI) indicates that the pubourethral ligament (PUL) is weak, and that the SI is amenable to cure with a midurethral sling.

2.4.2.1 "Simulated Operations"

Digital support of the PUL may also alleviate urge symptoms, and this explains the cure of mixed incontinence. Alleviation of urgency following support of the bladder base (middle zone) or posterior fornix (posterior zone) indicates that laxity in these structures may be causing the urgency, and that repair of these structures may cure such symptoms.

Often the definitive examination (Fig. 2.9) needs to be made in the operating room, as it can be difficult to make a precise diagnosis of each zone in an outpatient setting.

2.5 Management: Surgery

The principles of surgical repair are simple: avoid excision of vaginal tissue and hysterectomy where possible, and repair the ligaments using polypropylene tapes inserted in the precise position of the damaged ligaments (Fig. 2.10).

2.6 Conclusions

Lax ligaments may invalidate the muscle forces that support the organs, their opening and closure mechanisms, and their nerves and stretch receptors. Prolapse, symptoms, and abnormal urodynamic findings are mainly secondary manifestations of connective tissue

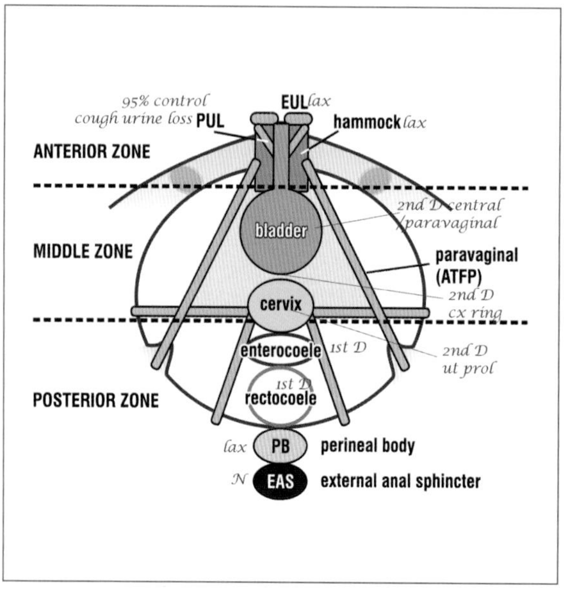

Fig. 2.9 Structured examination record. Actual patient. The state of the three structures in each zone as detailed in Fig. 2.8 is examined and recorded. *ATFP*, arcus tendineus fascia pelvis; *EAS*, external anal sphincter; *EUL*, external urethral ligament; *PB*, perineal body

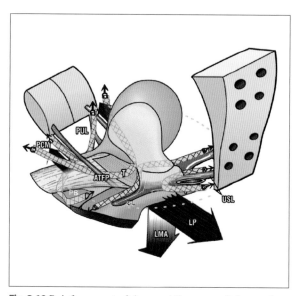

Fig. 2.10 Reinforcement of damaged ligaments. Polypropylene tapes *T* may be used to reinforce the three main suspensory ligaments – pubourethral (*PUL*), uterosacral (*USL*), cardinal (*CL*) and arcus tendineus fascia pelvis (*ATFP*), and also the perineal body (*PB*). *LMA*, longitudinal muscle of the anus; *LP*, levator plate; *PCM*, pubococcygeus muscle

defects in the suspensory ligaments. The challenge is how to accurately diagnose and repair the damaged structures in a manner that does not distort the anatomy to cause new dysfunctions.

References

1. Petros PE, Ulmsten U. An Integral Theory and its method, for the diagnosis and management of female urinary incontinence, Scand J Urol Nephrol 1993;2(suppl 153):1–93.
2. Petros PE. Severe chronic pelvic pain in women may be caused by ligamentous laxity in the posterior fornix of the vagina. Aust NZ J Obstet Gynaecol 1996;36:351–354.
3. Petros PE, Swash M. The Musculoelastic Theory of anorectal function and dysfunction. Pelviperineology 2008; 27:89–93. www.pelviperineology.org/ano_rectal_function/musculo_elastic_theory_of_anorectal_function_dysfunction.html (accessed 17 September 2009).
4. Abendstein B, Brugger BA, Furtschegger A et al. Role of the uterosacral ligaments in the causation of rectal intussusception, abnormal bowel emptying, and fecal incontinence – a prospective study. Pelviperineology 2008; 27:118–121.
5. Petros PE, Ulmsten U. An Integral Theory of female urinary incontinence. Acta Obstet Gynecol Scand Suppl 1990; 153:1–79.
6. Petros PE, Ulmsten U. Bladder instability in women: a premature activation of the micturition reflex. Neurourol Urodyn 1993;12:235–239.
7. Everaerts W, Gevaert T, Nilius B, De Ridder D. On the origin of bladder sensing: Tr(i)ps in urology. Nerourol Urodyn 2008;27:264–273.
8. Petros PE, Ulmsten U. Role of the pelvic floor in bladder neck opening and closure: I muscle forces. Int Urogynecol J Pelvic Floor Dysfunct 1997;8:74–80.
9. Petros PE, Ulmsten U. Role of the pelvic floor in bladder neck opening and closure: II vagina. Int Urogynecol J Pelvic Floor Dysfunct 1997;8:69–73.
10. Bush MB, Petros PEP, Barrett-Lennard BR. On the flow through the human urethra. Biomech 1997;30:967–969.
11. Rechberger T, Uldbjerg N, Oxlund H. Connective tissue changes in the cervix during normal pregnancy and pregnancy complicated by a cervical incompetence. Obstet Gynecol 1988;71:563–567.

Pathophysiology of the Pelvic Floor: Basic Physiology, Effects of Ageing, and Menopausal Changes

3

Dee E. Fenner and Yvonne Hsu

Abstract The etiologic risk factors and associations contributing to pelvic floor disorders include vaginal parity, ageing, hormonal status, pelvic surgery, collagen diseases, and depression. Many of these relationships, including hormonal status, are poorly understood. In addition, not all pelvic floor disorders are explained by the same risk factors or mechanisms. For example, vaginal parity appears to be the greatest risk factor for developing pelvic organ prolapse, while urinary incontinence has many other risks factors with equal or greater influence, including obesity and ageing. The basic mechanisms of disease and structural failure, both gross and microscopic, which lead to pelvic floor disorders need further investigation. A better understanding of the muscular, collagen, and neuronal components of the pelvic organs and their supports would provide targeted areas for prevention and treatment.

Keywords Ageing • Collagen • Hormones • Pelvic floor muscles • Vaginal parity

3.1 Introduction

Pelvic floor dysfunctions (PFD) are common, affecting approximately one-third of adult women, with significant impact on their quality of life, emotional well-being, and ability to actively participate in society. Etiologic risk factors and associations contributing to PFD include vaginal parity, ageing, hormonal status, pelvic surgery, collagen diseases, and depression. Many of these relationships, including hormonal status, are poorly understood, and have conflicting reports in the current literature.

The structural components that include the pelvic floor musculature, connective tissue condensations, and fibromuscular walls of the pelvic viscous work together to provide pelvic organ support. The current scientific literature regarding possible causes of structural failure that lead to pelvic organ prolapse and the inciting factors, including birth, ageing and hormonal changes, is complex in nature and often lacking in completeness.

In order to organize this topic, we have broken the sections into components that are thought to be important in pelvic support and function: connective tissue supports and the vaginal wall, levator ani muscles, and nerves. At the end of each component section, we discuss the challenges and questions that confront future research. In addition to the three major components, we will discuss the pathophysiology of vaginal delivery on the development of prolapse because of its special importance in the natural history of prolapse, and the relationships of hormonal changes and

D.E. Fenner
Department of Obstetrics and Gynecology, University of Michigan Medical School, Ann Arbor, MI, USA

ageing on the pathophysiology of pelvic floor dysfunction, specifically urinary incontinence and pelvic organ prolapse.

3.2 Connective Tissue Supports and the Vaginal Wall

The adventitial layer of the vagina, referred to as the endopelvic fascia, is composed of collagen and elastin that separates the muscular wall of the vagina and the paravaginal tissues. Investigators have studied the biology of pelvic connective tissue whose structural support comes from its composition, which includes collagen and elastin arranged in different fiber orientations and embedded in a dynamic ground substance. Much of the distensibility of collagen and connective tissues comes from rearrangement of the fibers. A collagen fiber by itself is relatively inelastic, only able to stretch 4% longitudinally compared to an elastin fiber which can stretch up to 70% [1]. Therefore, if the fibers were arranged longitudinally, they would not be able to stretch much before rupture. Instead, collagen and elastin fibers are arranged in different directions, so that, when placed under strain, they can stretch much more before being subject to rupture. An analogy can be made in comparing a cotton ball to a cotton dress shirt. When you pull on a cotton ball, there is a great deal of stretch that occurs until all the individual fibers become aligned in the same direction. After fiber alignment occurs, there is little stretch prior to rupture, as the mechanical properties of the individual fibers come into play. In a cotton dress shirt, the individual fibers are already in alignment and little stretch can occur prior to rupture.

Several studies have explored whether differences in the vaginal tissues of women with prolapse and normal support explain the pathophysiology of prolapse. Researchers have focused on collagen, elastin, smooth muscle, and hormone receptors as the major factors in vaginal support.

3.2.1 Collagen

Collagen provides much of the tensile strength for the endopelvic fascia and vaginal epithelium. Over the years, collagen studies have yielded varying, and at times conflicting, results. In early histochemical studies

using fibroblasts cultures, women with prolapse had just as high, if not higher, rates of collagen synthesis compared to women without prolapse [2]. In contrast, Jackson et al found women with prolapse had a 25% reduction in total collagen compared to controls [3]. Types I and III are the most common collagen fibers in vaginal tissues. Type I fibers are the most abundant while type III contributes more of the elastic properties of the tissue [4]. Liapis et al found a modest reduction in collagen type III in women with prolapse and a more significant decrease in women with stress incontinence, suggesting an altered ratio could lead to pelvic floor dysfunction [4]. However, other researchers have found no difference in the collagen ratios [3].

Recently, attention has turned towards collagen metabolism and turnover as markers of prolapse. There does seem to be consistent evidence that collagen metabolism is significantly altered in the pelvic tissues of women with prolapse. Collagen fibers are stabilized by intermolecular covalent cross-link. The formation of cross-links and glycation lead to maturation and inhibit turnover. Degradation depends on the activity of proteinases secreted from connective tissue cells [3]. While women with prolapse have collagen with more cross-links and other signs of maturation, they also have increased synthesis of new collagen, which is degraded in preference to older material because it has fewer cross-links [3].

Chen et al found increased expression of matrix metalloproteinase mRNA was responsible for collagen breakdown and decreased expression of inhibitors of metalloproteinases in women with stress incontinence and prolapse [5].

3.2.2 Elastin

Elastin provides much of the elastic properties of the pelvic connective tissue [1]. Compared to collagen, fewer studies have examined the role of elastin in the development of prolapse. Jackson et al did not find a difference in elastin content between premenopausal women with prolapse and controls [3]. Chen et al examined elastolytic activity in women with both stress incontinence and prolapse compared with controls. They found little difference in elastolytic activity but a decrease in alpha-1 antitrypsin, an inhibitor of elastin turnover, in women with prolapse, suggesting that there may be higher elastin turnover in prolapse [6].

3.2.3 Smooth Muscle

Smooth muscle is another important aspect of the endopelvic fascia, since it is a major component of the vaginal wall. Smooth muscle analysis of the anterior vaginal wall sections from the urethrovesical junction of fresh cadavers shows quantifiable variations in thickness and density. Morphometric analysis of the anterior and posterior vaginal walls showed a decreased fraction of smooth muscle in the muscularis of women with pelvic organ prolapse compared to controls [7–9]. Other markers suggest that women with prolapse have less smooth muscle contractility and force maintenance [10].

3.2.4 Challenges

There has been a significant body of basic scientific research regarding the components of the vaginal wall (vaginal tube). However, relatively little has been done to investigate the connections of the vagina to the pelvic walls, e.g. the endopelvic fascia. Most of the studies reviewed used either partial or full-thickness vaginal biopsies. It is difficult to make any assumptions about the endopelvic fascia as it is not included in samples of the vaginal wall (Fig. 3.1). Therefore, as there is no objective research that identifies whether it is the connection between the vagina and the pelvic sidewall that fails, or whether it is the vaginal wall itself that is involved in prolapse, these questions remain scientifically unresolved. Also, while some of the differences found in women with prolapse suggest that biochemical changes in the connective tissue may play an important role in prolapse, these studies are unable to explain the sequence of prolapse progression. In other words, we are left to wonder whether alterations in connective tissue lead to prolapse or are a response to the mechanical effects of prolapse.

3.3 Levator Ani Muscles

Magnetic resonance imaging (MRI) has been established as a technique for examinations of the levator ani muscle [11, 12]. Using MRI, visible levator ani defects are beginning to be linked to the development of prolapse. Up to 20% of primiparous women have a visible defect in the levator ani muscle, probably as a result of birth injury [13]. Also, computer-generated birth models using MRI have found that the medial pubovisceral muscle is at greatest risk for stretch-induced injury [14]. A few investigations have found that the levator ani muscles of women with prolapse have different morphologic characteristics compared to controls [15–17]. The changes in morphoglogy are beginning to be quantified. Investigators have found that women with prolapse have smaller overall levator volumes [15, 16], larger levator symphysis gap, and wider levator hiatus [17]. Aside from these MRI findings, histologic evidence of muscle damage has been found as well [18] and is associated with operative failure [19].

3.3.1 Challenges

Quantification of levator ani differences or defects in prolapse have so far been limited to measurements of volume or thickness [15, 16, 20]. The maximal force that a muscle generates depends on the cross-sectional area of the muscle perpendicular to its fiber direction [21]. This is challenging, due to the complex shape of the levator ani muscles, with different sections having differing fiber directions. Continued advances in imaging will hopefully make it possible for us to relate levator ani appearance to function.

3.4 Nerves

A unifying neurogenic hypothesis has been well established as a contributor to pelvic floor dysfunction.

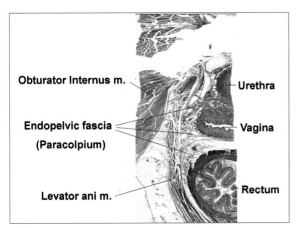

Fig. 3.1 Histologic cross-section of pelvis at the level of mid-urethra, from the collection of Dr Thomas E. Oelrich. Reproduced with permission from J.O.L. DeLancey

Although there is a significant body of literature regarding neurogenic causes of fecal incontinence and urinary incontinence, there is comparatively little exploring the relation between nerve damage and prolapse. Prospective study of perineal descent on defecography and pudendal nerve terminal motor latency failed to show any relationship between pudendal nerve damage and increased degree of perineal descent [22]. Two studies where prolapse patients were included did not show any difference in the pudendal nerve terminal motor latencies in patients with prolapse [23, 24]. However, electromyographic (EMG) studies of women with pelvic floor dysfunction, including prolapse and incontinence, found changes consistent with motor unit loss or failure of central activation [25]. More EMG and nerve studies will need to be done to establish a link between neurogenic injury and pelvic organ prolapse.

3.5 Vaginal Birth

Although it is clear that incontinence and prolapse increase with age [26], there is no time during a woman's life when these structures are more vulnerable than during childbirth. Vaginal delivery confers a four- to eleven-fold higher risk of prolapse that increases with parity [27]. Increased descent of vaginal wall points after vaginal delivery has been found using a combined method of clinical examination and functional cine-MRI [28]. There are two studies that suggest that pregnancy alone may be a risk factor for worsening

prolapse; however, both of these studies used definitions of prolapse that many would consider clinically normal [29, 30]. Several studies using MRI or transperineal ultrasound have looked at levator ani muscle damage or pelvic organ prolapse [31, 32]. A recent study by DeLancey et al has linked the presence of levator ani muscle damage, a known injury associated with vaginal delivery, to pelvic organ prolapse (Fig. 3.2). Major levator defects of the pubovisceral muscle were found in 55% of women with pelvic organ prolapse compared to 16% of women with normal support [31].

3.6 Hormones, Menopause, and Ageing

It has long been assumed that pelvic floor dysfunction is related to changes in menopause and is influenced by hormones. Untangling loss of hormonal action from age-related changes is extremely difficult. Epidemiologic studies have found pelvic organ prolapse (POP) to be consistently related to increasing age, vaginal parity, operative vaginal delivery, and chronic straining. Clinically, the use of perioperative vaginal estrogen therapy has been a mainstay of care for many gynecologic surgeons. Despite this traditional use, there is a lack of data supporting or refuting better or faster healing or improved surgical outcome with the use.

Several studies have looked at the presence or absence of hormone receptors in tissues that are involved in pelvic organ support [33, 34]. Other studies have examined the effects of estrogen on biologic markers

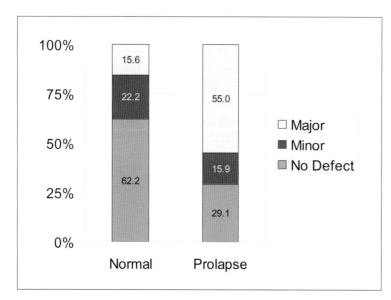

Fig. 3.2 Major levator defects are three times more common in women with pelvic organ prolapse compared to controls. Reproduced from [31], with permission

such as collagen [35–37]. Estrogen receptors are present throughout the body and yet there are important differential effects. For example, the endometrium is highly sensitive to fluctuations in estrogen, while the skin is much less responsive. Any supposition that hormones play a major role in pelvic organ prolapse must be based upon human studies that actually prove differences in prolapse occurring in those with and without hormonal supplementation or administration of hormonal antagonists.

3.6.1 Tissue Factors and Mechanisms of Action

Several studies have evaluated vaginal tissues and supportive tissues, including the uterosacral ligaments and lateral vaginal attachments to the arcus tendineus fascia pelvis in pre- and postmenopausal women with and without prolapse. Differences in collagen content, collagen metabolism, tissue deformation, and elasticity have been compared using various in vitro methods. Goh evaluated vaginal wall samples from pre- and postmenopausal women with prolapse for biomechanical properties [1]. He found little to no differences regarding elongation or long-term tissue deformation between groups. There was, however, a significant loss of elasticity and increased stiffness in the tissue from postmenopausal women. Comparisons to prior studies suggested these changes were related to ageing and were not necessarily hormone mediated [1]. Jones et al examined uterosacral ligament resilience (UsR) for menopause-associated connective tissue changes [38]. Using a tensinometer, they measured tissue resilience (load × tissue extension) in uterosacral ligaments from pre- and postmenopausal women with and without POP. UsR was significantly reduced in women with POP. There was a significant decrease in UsR with vaginal delivery (P = 0.003), menopause (P = 0.009), and older age (P = 0.005). The uterosacral ligaments were significantly thinner and contained fewer estrogen and progesterone receptors after menopause, but this did not affect UsR [38].

Moalli et al compared biopsies of arcus tendineus fascia pelvis from women with POP from three groups, (1) premenopausal, (2) postmenopausal, and (3) postmenopausal on hormone replacement therapy (HRT). They found a decrease in the ratio of collagen type I/collagen types III + IV in postmenopausal women not on

HRT compared to premenopausal women, due to a 75% decrease in type I collagen (P = 0.046). The decrease in type I collagen and change in collagen ratios was not seen in the postmenopausal women on HRT. The amount of elastin and smooth muscle did not differ between groups. Type 1 collagen is the stronger collagen type and primarily determines tensile strength. These changes in collagen type may provide a plausible link between menopause, estrogen and POP [37].

3.6.2 Hormone Use and Prevention of POP

Several large cohort studies and randomized controlled trials (RCTs) evaluating contraceptive hormone use and HRT have examined the impact of estrogen replacement therapy on the development of POP. Mant et al, in the annual survey of a cohort in the Oxford Family Planning Association study, found no difference in the risk of POP eight years after stopping oral contraceptive pills, comparing cases and controls [27]. In a case control study comparing women undergoing surgery for POP with women seen during a similar time in the same office for routing gynecologic care, cases were more likely than controls to have a higher body mass index (BMI, 28.6 ± 6.3 vs. 26.4 ± 6.1 kg/m², P = 0.1), to have undergone forceps delivery (64% vs. 44%, P ≤ 0.001), and to have had previous gynecologic surgery (34% vs. 16%, P = 0.003). After menopause, use of HRT for five or more years was protective (P = 0.001) [39]. In the Women's Health Initiative (WHI), past use of hormones at study enrollment was associated with a slight decrease in risk in uterine prolapse, odds ratio (OR) 0.84 (95% confidence interval (CI) 0.74–0.96) and cystocele, OR 0.92 (95% CI 0.86–0.99) [40]. Follow-up studies evaluating longitudinal changes in POP with and without HRT from the WHI should provide some further insights.

Overall, there is a paucity of literature evaluating the link between menopause and prolapse that has been able to separate hormone status from ageing. Biomechanical evidence supports a link between collagen type and hormone status. In contrast to tissue studies from women with urinary incontinence, collagen studies from women with POP may indicate estrogen is protective. Clinical trials and cohort studies provide some evidence that hormone use may be protective. No data exist supporting the improvement or treatment of POP with systemic or vaginal estrogen therapy. In exploring the literature for other hormonal influences, there are several blinded randomized placebo controlled studies of two selective estrogen receptor modulators (SERMs); idoxifene and levormeloxifene were felt to be associated with an increased incidence of pelvic organ prolapse in postmenopausal women participating in clinical trials of osteoporosis [41]. In contrast, neither tamoxifen nor toremifene, two clinically available SERMs, have been associated with pelvic floor relaxation [42, 43]. More recently, there has been evidence that raloxifene reduced the likelihood of or need for prolapse surgery by 50% [44]. Paradoxically, Vardy et al suggested an increase in prolapse in women receiving raloxifene and tamoxifen, but the status of support in the population was not given and most changes were small (1 cm) with only one individual having a change in prolapse stage [45]. This might be due to minor differences in vaginal pliability and may not reflect structural changes such as connective tissue rupture and muscle damage that are associated with actual prolapse.

3.6.3 Urinary Incontinence

The role of menopause and HRT use in the treatment of urinary incontinence is by far the most widely studied relationship between hormone status and pelvic floor dysfunction. Loss of estrogen and the subsequent urogenital atrophy associated with menopause has long been considered as a factor contributing to the increased prevalence of urinary incontinence in ageing women. The interaction between estrogen and progesterone, types of hormones given, and wide range of tissue levels achieved depending on route of delivery, contribute to our lack of understanding of how HRT impacts urinary incontinence.

3.6.3.1 Tissue Factors and Mechanisms of Action

The presence of alpha and beta estrogen receptors (ER-α and ER-β) throughout the urogenital tract suggests that estrogen has a role in the continence mechanism, and many observational studies have supported positive physiologic effects of exogenous estrogens [46]. Estrogen has been shown to increase urethral blood flow [47] and urethral closure pressures [48, 49]. Cellular maturation index values increase in the urethra and vagina with systemic and topical estrogen therapy, and have been shown to correlate with the resolution of urogenital atrophy symptoms [50, 51].

Estrogen receptors have been identified in the epithelial cells of the bladder, bladder base or trigone, urethra, and vaginal mucosa, as well as the central and peripheral nervous system. The concentration of the two types of receptors, the ER-α and ER-β, varies depending on hormone status. The ER-α predominates over the ER-β after menopause and the alpha receptor density varies with estrogen use, where the ER-β does not [39, 52]. How these changes in receptor number and type impact urinary incontinence is not known.

A possible mechanism to explain a relationship between hormone levels and urinary incontinence is estrogen's impact on collagen metabolism. Exogenous estrogen affects the remodeling of collagen in the urogenital tissues, changing both the quantity and quality of collagen in postmenopausal women [46]. Contrary to popular thought, several studies have found that exogenous estrogen causes a reduction in the total collagen concentration, a decrease in the cross-linking of collagen, and an increase in the levels of collagen turnover markers in the periurethral tissues of both continent and incontinent women [53, 54]. In addition, expression of transforming growth factors and elastin microfibril components in periurethral connective tissue has been shown to vary with hormone changes during the menstrual cycle and to differ between continent and incontinent women [36].

3.7 Conclusions

Understanding the functional anatomy of prolapse lays the necessary groundwork for understanding the mechanisms in pelvic organ prolapse and other pelvic floor disorders. When the components of pelvic support and how they relate to each other have been identified, we will be able to understand how disruptions result in failure and the resulting symptoms. Compared to stress incontinence, prolapse has received relatively little scientific attention. While basic scientific research on vaginal connective tissue and levator ani muscles has started, little has been done on other vital structures such as the endopelvic fascia. In addition, investigations into the biomechanical processes of prolapse are lacking. In summary, HRT clinically does not improve urinary incontinence and may in fact promote symptoms and increase the severity of incontinence. In contrast, HRT may protect from developing POP. Much work is needed at the molecular, cellular, and clinical levels to understand the mechanisms and associations between HRT, ageing, and the impact of vaginal birth on pelvic floor dysfunction.

References

1   Goh JT. Biomechanical and biochemical assessments for pelvic organ prolapse. Curr Opin Obstet Gynecol 2003; 15:391–394.

2. Makinen J, Kahari VM, Soderstrom KO et al. Collagen synthesis in the vaginal connective tissue of patients with and without uterine prolapse. Eur J Obstet Gynecol Reprod Biol 1987;24:319–325.

3. Jackson SR, Avery NC, Tarlton JF et al. Changes in metabolism of collagen in genitourinary prolapse. Lancet 1996;347:1658–1661.

4. Liapis A, Bakas P, Pafiti A et al. Changes of collagen type III in female patients with genuine stress incontinence and pelvic floor prolapse. Eur J Obstet Gynecol Reprod Biol 2001;97:76–79.

5. Chen BH, Wen Y, Li H, Polan ML. Collagen metabolism and turnover in women with stress urinary incontinence and pelvic prolapse. Int Urogynecol J Pelvic Floor Dysfunct 2002;13:80–87.

6. Chen B, Wen Y, Polan ML. Elastolytic activity in women with stress urinary incontinence and pelvic organ prolapse. Neurourol Urodyn 2004;23:119–126.

7. Morgan DM, Iyengar J, DeLancey JO. A technique to evaluate the thickness and density of nonvascular smooth muscle in the suburethral fibromuscular layer. Am J Obstet Gynecol 2003;188:1183–1185.

8. Boreham MK, Wai CY, Miller RT et al. Morphometric analysis of smooth muscle in the anterior vaginal wall of women with pelvic organ prolapse. Am J Obstet Gynecol 2002;187:56–63.

9. Boreham MK, Wai CY, Miller RT et al. Morphometric properties of the posterior vaginal wall in women with pelvic organ prolapse. Am J Obstet Gynecol 2002;187:1501–1508; discussion 1508–1509.

10. Boreham MK, Miller RT, Schaffer JI, Word RA. Smooth muscle myosin heavy chain and caldesmon expression in the anterior vaginal wall of women with and without pelvic organ prolapse. Am J Obstet Gynecol 2001; 185:944–952.

11. Tunn R, DeLancey JO, Quint EE. Visibility of pelvic organ support system structures in magnetic resonance images without an endovaginal coil. Am J Obstet Gynecol 2001; 184:1156–1163.

12. Singh K, Reid WM, Berger LA. Magnetic resonance imaging of normal levator ani anatomy and function. Obstet Gynecol 2002;99:433–438.

13. DeLancey JO, Kearney R, Chou Q et al. The appearance of levator ani muscle abnormalities in magnetic resonance images after vaginal delivery. Obstet Gynecol 2003;101:46–53.

14. Lien KC, Mooney B, DeLancey JO, Ashton-Miller JA. Levator ani muscle stretch induced by simulated vaginal birth. Obstet Gynecol 2004;103:31–40.

15. Hoyte L, Schierlitz L, Zou K et al. Two- and 3-dimensional MRI comparison of levator ani structure, volume, and integrity in women with stress incontinence and prolapse. Am J Obstet Gynecol 2001;185:11–19.

16. Hoyte L, Fielding JR, Versi E et al. Variations in levator ani volume and geometry in women: the application of MR based 3D reconstruction in evaluating pelvic floor dysfunction. Arch Esp Urol 2001;54:532–539.

17. Singh K, Jakab M, Reid WM et al. Three-dimensional magnetic resonance imaging assessment of levator ani morphologic features in different grades of prolapse. Am J Obstet Gynecol 2003;188:910–915.

18. Koelbl H, Saz V, Doerfler D et al. Transurethral injection of silicone microimplants for intrinsic urethral sphincter deficiency. Obstet Gynecol 1998;92:332–336.

19. Hanzal E, Berger E, Koelbl H. Levator ani muscle morphology and recurrent genuine stress incontinence. Obstet Gynecol 1993;81:426.

20. Hoyte L, Jakab M, Warfield SK et al. Levator ani thickness variations in symptomatic and asymptomatic women using magnetic resonance-based 3-dimensional color mapping. Am J Obstet Gynecol 2004;191:856–861.

21. Ikai M, Fukunaga T. Calculation of muscle strength per unit cross-sectional area of human muscle by means of ultrasonic measurement. Int Z Angew Physiol 1968;26:26–32.

22. Jorge JM, Wexner SD, Ehrenpreis ED et al. Does perineal descent correlate with pudendal neuropathy? Dis Colon Rectum 1993;36:475–483.

23. Beevors MA, Lubowski DZ, King DW, Carlton MA. Pudendal nerve function in women with symptomatic utero-vaginal prolapse. Int J Colorectal Dis 1991;6:24–28.

24. Bakas P, Liapis A, Karandreas A, Creatsas G. Pudendal nerve terminal motor latency in women with genuine stress incontinence and prolapse. Gynecol Obstet Invest 2001; 51:187–190.

25. Weidner AC, Barber MD, Visco AG et al. Pelvic muscle electromyography of levator ani and external anal sphincter in nulliparous women and women with pelvic floor dysfunction. Am J Obstet Gynecol 2000;183:1390–1399; discussion 1399–1401.

26. Olsen AL, Smith VJ, Bergstrom JO et al. Epidemiology of surgically managed pelvic organ prolapse and urinary incontinence. Obstet Gynecol 1997;89:501–506.

27. Mant J, Painter R, Vessey M. Epidemiology of genital prolapse: observations from the Oxford Family Planning Association Study. Br J Obstet Gynaecol 1997;104:579–585.

28. Dannecker C, Lienemann A, Fischer T, Anthuber C. Influence of spontaneous and instrumental vaginal delivery on objective measures of pelvic organ support: assessment with the pelvic organ prolapse quantification (POPQ) technique and functional cine magnetic resonance imaging. Eur J Obstet Gynecol Reprod Biol 2004;115:32–38.

29. Sze EH, Sherard GB 3rd, Dolezal JM. Pregnancy, labor, delivery, and pelvic organ prolapse. Obstet Gynecol 2002; 100:981–986.

30. O'Boyle AL, Woodman PJ, O'Boyle JD et al. Pelvic organ support in nulliparous pregnant and nonpregnant women: a case control study. Am J Obstet Gynecol 2002;187:99–102.

31. Delancey JOL, Morgan DM, Fenner DE et al. Comparison of levator ani muscle defects and function in women with

and without prolapse. Obstet Gynecol 2007;109:296–302.

32. Dietz HP, Lanzarone V. Levator trauma after vaginal delivery. Obstet Gynecol 2005;106:707–712.

33. Fu X, Rezapour M, Wu X et al. Expression of estrogen receptor-alpha and -beta in anterior vaginal walls of genuine stress incontinent women. Int Urogynecol J Pelvic Floor Dysfunct 2003;14:276–281.

34. Ewies AA, Thompson J, Al-Azzawi F. Changes in gonadal steroid receptors in the cardinal ligaments of prolapsed uteri: immunohistomorphometric data. Hum Reprod 2004; 19:1622–1628.

35. Jackson S, James M, Abrams P. The effect of oestradiol on vaginal collagen metabolism in postmenopausal women with genuine stress incontinence. BJOG 2002;109:339–344.

36. Chen B, Wen Y, Wang H, Polan ML. Differences in estrogen modulation of tissue inhibitor of matrix metalloproteinase-1 and matrix metalloproteinase-1 expression in cultured fibroblasts from continent and incontinent women. Am J Obstet Gynecol 2003;189:59–65.

37. Moalli PA, Talarico LC, Sung VW et al. Impact of menopause on collagen subtypes in the arcus tendineous fasciae pelvis. Am J Obstet Gynecol 2004;190:620–627.

38. Jones NHJR, Healy JC, King LJ et al. Pelvic connective tissue resilience decreases with vaginal delivery, menopause and uterine prolapse. Br J Surg 2003;90:466–472.

39. Moalli PA, Ivy SJ, Meyn LA, Zyczynski HM. Risk factors associated with pelvic floor disorders in women undergoing surgical repair. Obstet Gynecol 2003;101:869–874.

40. Hendrix SL, Clark A, Nygaard EI et al. Pelvic organ prolapse in the WHI; gravity and gravidity. Am J Obstet Gynecol 2002;186:1160–1166.

41. Silfen SL, Ciaccia AV, Bryant HU. Selective estrogen receptor modulators: Tissue specificity and differential uterine effects. Climacteric 1999;2:268–283.

42. Fisher B, Costantino JP, Wickerham DL et al. Tamoxifen for prevention of breast cancer: Report of the National Surgical Adjuvant Breast and Bowel Project P-1 Study. J Natl Cancer Inst 1998;90:1371–1388.

43. Maenpaa JU, Ala-Fossi SL. Toremifene in postmenopausal breast cancer. Efficacy, safety and cost. Drugs Aging 1997;11:261–270.

44. Goldstein SR, Neven P, Zhou L et al. Raloxifene effect on frequency of surgery for pelvic floor relaxation. Obstet Gynecol 2001;98:91–96.

45. Vardy MD, Lindsay R, Scotti RJ et al. Short-term urogenital effects of raloxifene, tamoxifen, and estrogen. Am J Obstet Gynecol 2003;189:81–88.

46. Waetjen LE, Dwyer PL. Estrogen therapy and urinary incontinence: what is evidence and what do we tell our patients? Int Urogynecol J 2006;17:541–545.

47. Jarmy-Di Bella ZI, Girao MJ, Sartori MF et al. Doppler of the urethra in continent and incontinence, pre- and postmenopausal women. Int Urogynecol J 2000;11:148–154.

48. Sacco F, Rigon G, Carbone A, Sacchini D. Transvaginal estrogen therapy in urinary stress incontinence. Merva Ginecol 1990;42:539–544.

49. Elia G, Bergman A. Estrogen effects on the urethra: beneficial effects in women with genuine stress incontinence. Obstet Gynecol Surv 1993;48:509–517.

50. Bergman A, Karram M, Bhatia N. Changes in urethral cytology following estrogen administration. Gynecol Obstet Invest 1990;29:211–213.

51. Bhatia N, Bergman A, Karram M. Effects of estrogen on urethral function in women with urinary incontinence. Am J Obstet Gynecol 1989;160:176–181.

52. Gebhardt J, Richard D, Barrett T. Expression of estrogen receptor isoforms alpha and beta messenger RNA in vaginal tissue of premenopausal and postmenopausal women. Am J Obstet Gynecol 2001;185:1325–1330.

53. Keane DP, Sims TJ, Abrams P, Bailey AJ. Analysis of collagen status in premenopausal nulliparous women with genuine stress incontinence. Br J Obstet Gynecol 1997; 104:994–998.

54. Falconer C, Ekman-Ordeberg G, Blomgren B. Paraurethral connective tissue in stress incontinent women after menopause. Acta Obstet Gynecol Scand 1998;77:95–100.

Michael Swash

Abstract The background to the development of current ideas of pelvic floor function is reviewed. The importance of understanding motor control mechanisms of pelvic floor responsiveness in health and disease is an underlying theme of the response to all forms of treatment in pelvic floor disorders. This is an adaptive response based on the capacity of the system to respond when there is significant functional damage.

Keywords Incontinence • Ligamentous stretch • Motor control • Neurogenic • Pelvic floor • Sphincter tear

4.1 Introduction

The concept that the pelvic floor should be considered as a holistic functional entity, rather than three separate anterior, middle, and posterior perineal systems or structures, arose during studies of fecal continence begun at St Mark's Hospital, then located at its original site on the City Road, London, not far from the London Hospital (now the Royal London Hospital) and St Bartholomew's Hospital. I had become involved, or perhaps was recruited is a better term, in the general problem of the pathophysiology of so-called "idiopathic fecal incontinence" [1] by my late colleague at the London Hospital, Sir Alan Parks (Fig. 4.1). Sir Alan was then a senior colorectal surgeon at the London and St Mark's Hospitals, who had developed ideas that led to his introduction of the postanal repair operation for the management of fecal incontinence [2]. At that time, this postanal procedure seemed superior to other sur-

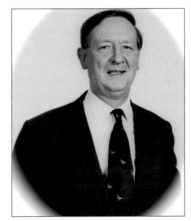

Fig. 4.1 Sir Alan Parks 1920–1982

gical operations in restoring fecal continence in women with idiopathic fecal incontinence. The term "idiopathic fecal incontinence" was used at that time to distinguish the idiopathic form of fecal incontinence, largely a disorder of women, implying fecal incontinence developing without evident cause, from other recognizable causes, including particularly neurological disease, and sphincter tears or other forms of direct sphincter damage, such as local anal infection or inflammation, direct trauma, anal fissures, and cancer [1, 3].

M. Swash
Department of Neurology and Neuroscience, The Royal London Hospital, Barts and The London School of Medicine and Dentistry, Queen Mary University of London, UK

At this time, ultrasound imaging and magnetic resonance (MR) scanning had not been developed, and the preferred investigation after clinical examination was anorectal manometry [4], which itself was relatively underdeveloped and unstandardized. Thus, detection of muscle weakness, muscle damage, and muscle dysfunction was difficult, but it was clear from the work of many earlier surgeons and investigators [5] that something was wrong with these muscles in incontinence, and perhaps in some patients with organ prolapse. We therefore introduced quantitative neurophysiological procedures, derived from my ongoing association with Dr Erik Stålberg in Uppsala, Sweden [6], together with quantitative enzyme histochemical studies of muscle biopsies [7], which had become standard techniques in my clinical and research practice in the investigation of neuromuscular diseases at the London Hospital. Both these techniques were then relatively new and not generally used in clinical practice. Regular teatime conversations with Sir Alan in the staff room at the London Hospital resulted in an agreement that I would study any biopsy material he might obtain during his operative repair procedures at St Mark's, from muscles presumed to be involved in anal continence, including some material from non-incontinent subjects. So began a long period of pelvic floor research with the assistance and intellectual stimulus of a series of talented and energetic research fellows from the UK and other European countries, and from Australia and New Zealand, Japan, and the USA, which continued long after Sir Alan's untimely death in 1982.

4.2 The Pelvic Floor

Muscle biopsies obtained during postanal repair and other procedures [8] were usually derived from the external anal sphincter, the puborectalis muscle, and sometimes the lowermost component of the levator ani muscle; the anatomical separation of the puborectalis from the lowermost fibers of the levator ani was itself often dubious [9, 10]. Smooth muscle from the internal anal sphincter was sometimes included in external anal sphincter biopsies, especially when little remaining external anal sphincter tissue could be identified. At that time, the most attractive concept for understanding normal fecal continence was the "flap-valve theory", by which it was thought that the puborectalis acted as a lever, tensing and making more

acute the normal angulation between the rectum and anal canal so that the weight of the abdominal contents closed the lumen of the anorectum at the angulation, resulting in a passive mechanism for continence [1]. The length of the anal canal was critical for this mechanism. Sensory input from receptors in the upper anal canal [11] was conceived of as signaling the ingress of fecal matter or gas into the upper anal canal (the sampling reflex), thus triggering relaxation of the puborectalis and external sphincter, leading, by a voluntary nervous control system, to defecation or release of flatus [12]. The internal sphincter was suggested as a sensitive regulator of the ingress of material into the upper anal canal rather than a primary sphincter necessary for continence. Actually, defecation itself was not well understood. It seemed to imply shortening of the anorectum and straightening of the anorectal angle from relaxation of the puborectalis, and often involved or was triggered by "mass movements" (gut contraction) of the rectum and descending colon; thus, defecation required a combination of coordinated smooth and voluntary muscle activity. The role of associated pelvic floor muscles, such as the pubococcygeus and levator ani, was considered to be important but was not readily demonstrable by the techniques for investigation then available.

The role of the anterior pelvic floor musculature, and the importance of the suspensory ligaments of the urethra, bladder, vagina, and uterus, was scarcely acknowledged in this formulation, although these were recognized as an essential component of normal function, especially in micturition. Indeed, the importance of pelvic floor descent [13] on simulated straining at stool, as a sign of weakness of the pelvic floor musculature in women with either "idiopathic" fecal incontinence or stress urinary incontinence, was an essential part of the formulation of the "weak muscles" concept for fecal incontinence.

But the role of ligamentous stretch and weakness was not fully appreciated at that time, although it was well recognized by clinicians.

4.3 Functional Abnormalities in Idiopathic Fecal Incontinence

The starting point for our studies in the anorectal lab at St Marks was the monograph of Kerremans, published in 1969 [4]. Kerremans, working in Leuven, had developed clinical methods for evaluating anorectal function, including radiological images of the anorectal angle, and anorectal pressure studies. In addition he had used histological methods, in a small number of patients, to investigate the pelvic floor muscles. In these early studies, however, Kerremans was unable to derive a satisfactory understanding of normal function or of a distinctive pattern of dysfunction leading to fecal incontinence. We set out to systematically investigate this problem.

4.3.1 Clinical Issues

Idiopathic fecal incontinence is principally a disorder afflicting women. It is related to the experience of a difficult childbirth [14], but usually develops some years later, or a few years after the menopause [1, 15]. Clinical examination discloses weakness and laxity of the pelvic floor, with abnormal descent of the perineum during defecation straining [13]; sometimes there is associated anorectal or genital prolapse [1, 8]. Digital anal examination reveals weakness of anal sphincter tone and contraction force.

There is usually no reduction in anal and perianal sensory acuity to ordinary clinical examination, although slight sensory abnormality in the distribution of the perineal nerve innervation has been observed with semi-quantitative examination techniques [16]. Although there are many recognized causes of anorectal incontinence [1], including neurological disorders, these are by definition excluded from this syndrome [17]. Finally, we recognized that anorectal incontinence is a progressive disorder [14], with increasing disability developing over a period of several years.

It is important to recognize that terms such as stress urinary incontinence, urge incontinence, and idiopathic fecal incontinence are no more than clinical descriptions of functional abnormality and do not in themselves imply any causative mechanisms, although, especially in the context of urinary incontinence of women, a theory of causation has come to be associated with the functional disorder, largely based on the interpretation of cystometrography.

The rigidity implied by this functional classification, which is generally accepted in urogynecological practice, does not necessarily aid understanding of causation, although, undeniably, it has proved useful in clinical practice in determining management options from the medical and surgical methods hitherto available.

4.3.2 Anorectal Pressure Measurements

The first step in our studies was to establish normative values for anorectal pressures, using a balloon manometric technique, in normal subjects, and then in women with incontinence, anorectal prolapse, and other functional anorectal disorders [18]. These measurements showed marked variability even in apparently normal women [19] – that is, women with no declared symptoms of anorectal or urinary voiding dysfunction, referred to us for study as volunteers. Nonetheless, as others had shown before us, we found that both the resting anal pressure and the squeeze anal pressure were reduced in patients with anorectal incontinence. In many patients there was almost no discernible rise in anal pressure during a maximal voluntary squeeze, or during a cough [18, 20, 21]. Clearly, there was weakness of the pelvic floor muscles, together with laxity of the pelvic floor's suspensory ligaments.

4.3.3 Muscle Biopsies

These biopsies, studied with a series of standardized enzyme histochemical methods, revealed features of chronic partial denervation [8], with fiber type grouping and fiber atrophy. In addition, there was muscle fiber loss, and in some biopsies fibrous scarring was observed [8]. Abnormalities were particularly marked in external anal sphincter and puborectalis biopsies [8, 9], and less evident in the lowermost part of the levator ani muscle. The internal anal sphincter showed loss of smooth muscle fibers and disruption and fibrosis of the muscle architecture.

Elastic tissue within the internal anal sphincter was strikingly stretched and disrupted. In addition, there was direct histological evidence of damage to nerve fibers within small nerve bundles innervating the external anal sphincter and puborectalis muscles. Thus, the inferior rectal nerves innervating the external anal sphincter and the direct S2–3 nerves innervating the puborectalis were both damaged [9]. These features seemed to suggest chronic partial denervation, with fibrosis, of the affected muscles.

4.3.4 Electromyographic Evidence

Electromyography (EMG) studies using quantitative single-fiber EMG [22, 23] revealed an increased fiber density, and concentric needle EMG [24, 25] showed abnormalities typical of chronic partial denervation in the external anal sphincter and puborectalis muscles, features consistent with the abnormalities seen in the histological studies of these muscles. In subsequent studies of patients with a range of functional abnormalities in the pelvic floor, an incremental degree of EMG abnormality was documented [26], which could be loosely correlated with the functional disorder.

4.3.5 Pudendal Nerve Terminal Motor Latency Measurements

An intra-anal electrode array, mounted on the examiner's finger glove, was used to directly measure the conduction time (terminal motor latency) in the distal segment of the pudendal innervation of the external anal sphincter muscle, testing each side of this circular muscle separately [27, 28]. Although in the initial recordings there was variation in the resultant latencies, with practice, the technique was shown to be reliable and reproducible, providing direct evidence of slowed conduction in the distal segment of this nerve, often asymmetrically. It was recognized that no direct correlation between EMG abnormality and terminal motor latency was to be expected, since EMG measures reinnervation, a compensatory process that follows damage to a muscle's innervation through its motor nerve, and terminal motor conduction time is largely a measure of conduction velocity in large myelinated axons in the segment of a motor nerve under test. There is thus no direct relation between the two measures [26], although both can be considered as techniques that provide evidence of damage to a muscle's innervation. In addition, it was evident that this technique would be difficult to reproduce, even with the development of a standardized finger glove-mounted electrode array, since there was neither direct visualization of the point of stimulation of the nerve nor visualization of the recording electrodes' proximity to the muscle under test. The course of the pudendal nerve within the pelvis was likely to be anatomically variable [27].

Nevertheless, it proved possible to show that the test–retest reliability of the terminal motor latency in this nerve was satisfactory in practiced hands [29]. In women with anorectal incontinence, the pudendal nerve terminal motor latency was not only increased, but it further and temporarily increased following a maximal strain as if defecating [30], and the degree of abnormality at rest correlated with the extent of perineal descent occurring during this voluntary defecatory strain [31]. This observation was consistent with the hypothesis that in this form of idiopathic fecal incontinence there was stretch injury to this nerve. Thus, a number of research approaches suggested that stretch injury to the nerve supply of the pelvic floor muscles was likely to be an important factor leading to denervation of these muscles, with resultant weakness of the pelvic floor, and so to the development of "stress" fecal incontinence – to use a functional term borrowed from urogynecology.

The value of this method of measuring pudendal nerve function, which was derived from Giles Brindley's use of a similar technique to excite parasympathetic nerve fibers in the lumbosacral plexus in order to obtain sperm in paraplegic men, has more recently been disputed [32]. Certainly, the technique is likely to be unreliable without assiduous attention to the stimulation and recording sites, and it is theoretically not likely to directly reflect nerve function in the same way that quantitative EMG will reflect muscle function. It should be remembered that the electrophysiological evidence of damage to the motor nerves and chronic partial denervation of the pelvic floor muscles is also shown by the histological data.

4.4 Stress Urinary Incontinence

Similar neurophysiological observations have been made regarding EMG evidence of chronic partial denervation of the external urinary sphincter muscle, using concentric needle EMG in women with stress urinary incontinence [33], and in the external anal sphincter and external urinary sphincter, using single-fibre EMG [34]. Genital prolapse was also associated with EMG abnormality [34]. The terminal motor latency in the perineal branch of the pudendal nerve, innervating the external urinary sphincter muscle, was found to be selectively increased in women with stress urinary incontinence, in that the inferior rectal branch of this nerve was normal when urinary incontinence was not associated with fecal incontinence [35]. A relationship between idiopathic fecal incontinence and stress urinary incontinence is well recognized [8], although these functional disorders can, and often do, occur separately.

In women with idiopathic anorectal incontinence, we found that there was often a slight increase in the perineal terminal motor latency, but not to the extent noted in women with frank stress urinary incontinence [28]. However, the characteristic laxity of the pelvic floor, together with a propensity to develop genital and organ prolapse, and increased perineal descent during straining, implied lax ligamentous support of the pelvic floor itself, over and above the presence of neurogenic weakness of the pelvic floor muscles, a concept that has subsequently been described in detail by Petros et al [36–38].

4.5 Childbirth and the Pelvic Floor

A quantitative study of the effect of vaginal delivery, with and without prolonged labor, the use of forceps extraction, and cesarean section, and the role of multigravid experience, was required to unravel these risk factors, all of which appeared to be important in the histories of many of the women with fecal incontinence. The study revealed acute post-partum damage to the innervation of the external anal sphincter that was evident within a few days of childbirth, and gradually resolved, at least partially, over a period of several months [39]. This was not always present, but correlated with difficult deliveries, especially those requiring forceps assistance, and it was much more marked in multipara. Women delivering by elective cesarean section did not develop this EMG abnormality. There was a correlation between the abnormality found in the external anal sphincter muscle and increase in the pudendal nerve terminal motor latency [39]. These observations suggested that damage, presumably stretch induced, occurred to the pudendal innervation during the process of vaginal delivery, perhaps as the fetal head passed through the birth canal.

This prospective investigation also revealed that damage to the pelvic floor innervation was most likely to occur in women in whom a sphincter tear had occurred during delivery, although not in women in whom episiotomy had been carried out [40]. The coincidence of sphincter tear, itself a well-recognized cause of fecal incontinence, with EMG evidence of sphincter dener-

vation, termed a "double lesion" [41], was particularly significant in leading to intractable fecal incontinence, whether because the occurrence of a sphincter tear was an index of a particularly difficult delivery, or because the combination of damage to the pelvic floor and sphincter innervation and direct damage to the sphincter muscle itself was a double lesion much more likely to lead to incontinence than either injury alone. Clearly, the latter notion was the more likely explanation, particularly since surgical experience indicated that overlapping repair of sphincter tears was recognized as an effective management strategy for fecal incontinence associated with sphincter tear, even if, in some cases, only in the short or medium term, but that the results of sphincter repair were less good when there was evidence of coincident nerve damage [42].

Subsequent studies have provided more detailed information. With the advent of diagnostic ultrasound imaging of the anal sphincter, direct injury (anal sphincter tears) to the internal and external anal sphincter muscles and to the puborectalis muscles was revealed much more accurately than by clinical examination and anorectal manometry. Anal sphincter injury during childbirth was revealed as more common than had previously been surmised [43–45]. Ultrasound studies of the anal sphincter in older women with idiopathic fecal incontinence often reveal quite marked fibrosis in these muscles, as was reported in our original histological studies. This fibrosis must be acquired over time, from the combined effect of sphincter damage during parturition, pelvic floor laxity from ligamentous damage, and denervation of the pelvic floor muscles, together with age-related effects [46]. Pollack et al [14] found that 44% of women with anal sphincter tears had some anal incontinence 9 months after delivery, a number that rose to 53% 5 years after delivery. That this was not the only factor was shown by an incidence of anal incontinence in 25% of women without anal sphincter tears 9 months after delivery, rising to 32% at 5 years. "Idiopathic" dysfunction of the pelvic floor is therefore caused by multiple factors.

4.6 Other Factors Leading to "Idiopathic" Fecal Incontinence

The introduction of high-resolution MR imaging (MRI) has led to new concepts of pelvic floor function in health and disease. The role of ligamentous support in maintaining the appropriate vectors for muscle action has been shown to be crucial for pelvic floor function [36, 37]. Indeed, this support is particularly important in enabling effective muscle action when the muscles themselves are weakened by damage to their innervation, and by scarring from direct injury. These concepts have led to the musculo-elastic concept of normal pelvic floor function [36, 37] and to the introduction of new relatively non-invasive surgical approaches to pelvic floor weakness and laxity. Many of these procedures, for example the tape suspension procedure for correction of urinary or fecal incontinence, are relatively non-invasive day-case procedures, and promise in time to revolutionize management. These aspects of pelvic floor disorders are described in later chapters of this book. It is important to recognize, nonetheless, that even a muscle of normal strength will be acting at a disadvantage when contracting against lax ligaments and deformed tendinous insertions, since it will not be able to transmit a normal force in its direction of action, and will not enable normal muscle tone at rest to be developed.

In a study of 47 women with urinary incontinence [38], biopsies of the pubococcygeus muscle made at the time of a tape insertion procedure revealed extensive fibrosis of this muscle, with little remaining muscle tissue in 21 of 38 women with stress urinary incontinence. Of the remainder, 15 showed muscle damage with neurogenic change and fibrosis. The tape-suspension procedure relieved the laxity of the pelvic floor and enabled the weakened muscles to function more effectively, thus relieving incontinence. Standardized assessment and measurement, including cystometry, will be required preoperatively and postoperatively to delineate the precise interventions required to effect the best result in such patients.

The internal anal sphincter itself has an important function in sampling anorectal contents [12], but is not essential as a muscular sphincter in achieving continence [46], although its muscle fibers show abnormalities in fecal incontinence [47].

4.7 Central Control Mechanisms of the Pelvic Floor

How do the brain and the central nervous system modulate pelvic floor and sphincter activity? This has been studied using functional MRI of the brain, and by MR and ultrasound studies of the pelvic floor itself in nor-

mal subjects [48], but there is little understanding of the neuro-coordinative adaptations that must occur when there is pelvic floor weakness, an abnormality that differs slightly from patient to patient.

4.7.1 Physiological Principles of Motor Control

There are certain principles in the physiology of central motor control that apply to all motor systems [49]. In the case of the pelvic floor, these include an effective muscular system that is relatively undamaged and capable of acting in synergy across the pelvic floor anteriorly, posteriorly, and laterally, with central support in the region of the perineal body. Focal weakness in any plane would be expected to impose distorted vectors and therefore to lead to pelvic floor dysfunction, but little is known about this concept at present. An example in gait studies is the foot drop that occurs with common peroneal neruropathy, which leads to loss of plantigrade foot function and secondarily to disabling genu recurvatum and disorganization and destabilization of the knee joint, with increasing and preventable loss of the ability to walk easily.

Muscles cannot function in a coordinated fashion without sensory input to the nervous system. This is supplied by muscle spindles, which are stretch receptors found in all striated muscles, including pelvic floor muscles, and which signal the extent of stretch of a muscle (static stretch) and the rate of stretch of the muscle (dynamic stretch). In addition, the tension developed in a muscle during contraction is signalled by Golgi tendon organs, thus indicating the force applied to the muscle during contraction or during eccentric stretch; that is, stretch applied to a contracting muscle under load.

Pacinian corpuscles signal pressure in the muscle, but also respond to external forces, for example deformatory forces and, specifically, to vibration. Muscles also contain free nerve endings that signal pain and changes in pH, the latter reflecting lactic acidosis. Sensory input, especially with regard to static and dynamic stretch and to tension, is integrated with the neural drive delivered through the motor nerve innervating the muscle to regulate the speed and force of the contraction necessary for the task. This integration requires central modulation of the output from specific motor neurons in the spinal cord in the S2–4 segments, mainly from Onuf's nucleus. Sensory input from receptors as described above can induce an immediate response from these motor neurons, but this can only occur after a short delay due to conduction time delays to and from the spinal cord, and to processing time at synapses in the spinal cord. Therefore, voluntary movement is directed from higher centers, and the sensory response is fed back into the nervous system, where the progress of the intended movement is followed and integrated with the subsequent sequence of motor commands to the muscles.

This is part of the process termed "efference copy" that allows the nervous system to monitor motor output and to modulate its progress in relation to the intended goal. Integrated motor actions require central processing at brainstem and cerebral levels, especially in the basal ganglia and motor cortex.

The pelvic floor sphincters are represented on the cortical motor map at the vertex, close to the interhemispheric fissure.

It has been suggested that the brainstem neural system works as a tonic "neural switch" between storage and voiding [50]. In the urinary system, voiding requires integration between contractile activity in the bladder detrusor muscle, an involuntary smooth muscle innervated by parasympathetic nerve fibers, and relaxation of the smooth muscle of the internal urinary sphincter, and also of the striated muscle components of the urinary sphincter. These two components of the urinary sphincter are innervated by autonomic and somatic efferent nerve fibers respectively. Integration of these functional systems can be conceived as occurring at brainstem level in response to cortically derived decision programs. A similar mechanism accounts for the switch between fecal continence and defecation (fecal voiding).

One example of this integrated activity in the pelvic floor is pelvic floor contraction occurring in response to a cough. The pressure wave of the cough is transmitted to the pelvic floor via the abdominal contents, and results in stimulation of muscle spindles. This muscle spindle signal reflexly evokes a contraction of the pelvic floor musculature. This response is reflex; it does not consist of a programmed or integrated contraction occurring at the same time as the cough itself but occurs a little later [51]. Little is known about the range of integration of pelvic floor functional activity occurring in relation to defecation, micturition, or other pelvic floor functions [52, 53]. Although it is clear that these voluntary and semi-reflex activities require graded and coordinated muscle contraction and relaxation, the range of such activities in normal subjects and the compensatory patterns of activity of these same muscles in the presence of weakness, fibrosis, and ligamentous laxity are largely unknown. Hopefully, with real-time ultrasonography it will be possible to address these issues, and this understanding will itself inform future treatment options.

4.7.2 The Brain and Spinal Cord

Clearly, continence and evacuation, whether of feces or urine, are under the control of the will, and therefore of the brain. Ultimately, the frontal lobes determine storage of urine and feces, and the voluntary decision to allow evacuation to occur. The necessity to initiate evacuation, however, is almost always triggered by sensory input from the bladder or lower colon and rectum, indicating a need to switch from storage to evacuation. The concept of a "neural switch" between these two functions has proved useful in understanding these processes. The neural switch concept was first developed in studies of the control of micturition [50], when it was recognized that there was a brainstem (pontine) center that determined whether the urinary sphincter opened in concert with detrusor muscle activity, leading to bladder emptying. Although at first a reflex mechanism, this micturition switch comes under voluntary control from higher centers with brain maturation in late infancy, and a similar process leads to control of defecation.

The initial studies in the cat nervous system were later complemented by case descriptions of patients with brainstem and cortical lesions, often of vascular cause, and then by functional MRI (fMRI) and positron emission tomography (PET) studies showing activation of centers in the brainstem during micturition in normal men and women [48, 54, 55].

The pathogenesis of detrusor-sphincter dyssynergia, and of inability to micturate occurring in young women, the latter associated with abnormal repetitive EMG activity in the external urinary sphincter muscle [56], however, are not yet clearly understood. It remains unclear whether these are acquired disorders or in some way reflect abnormalities in hard-wiring of the neural circuits involved in micturition. A somewhat similar abnormality in coordination of colonic activity and of external anal sphincter and puborectalis contraction has been reported in anismus and in patients with Parkinson's disease [57]. Furthermore, the role of the smooth muscle of the internal urinary (or anal) sphincter in this coordinated mechanism of normal evacuation remains largely undetermined; whether these smooth muscle components of the sphincters have a role other than in facilitating sensory input from the rectum or urethra is especially controversial.

Although the brainstem and spinal neural control mechanisms for the pelvic floor and its sphincters may be considered relatively simple, it is a system that is able to respond in a graded fashion to the functional demands placed upon it. This plasticity of response depends on the integration of sensory input and of motor responses from the evacuatory musculature, and this is modulated at both a spinal and a brainstem level. The overall sensitivity of the response is controlled by descending input derived from the basal ganglia and frontal cerebral cortex. This modulation enables a healthy person to resist, for a time, the call to stool or to urination. When the pelvic floor is dysfunctional, whether because of stretch injury to its ligamentous framework, causing pelvic floor laxity and inefficient muscular action, or because of denervation-induced weakness to the pelvic floor musculature, especially to the external sphincters and inferior support musculature, or as a result of direct injury to these muscles (and their ligamentous support and insertions) during childbirth – and there is usually a combination of these factors rather any single one of them – the central nervous system is capable of redirecting output controlling muscular action in maintaining continence, so long as there are sufficient muscular forces available to allow this. Thus, the CNS can adapt the action of the weakened muscular system to maintain function, even when the damage to the effector system is quite severe. Similar adaptations take place in limb muscle systems in people with peripheral neuropathies, spasticity muscular dystrophy, or poliomyelitis – conditions in which the central nervous system is intact and capable of modulating its output to compensate for weakness.

4.8 Feedback Modulation Therapy

Biofeedback has been enthusiastically propounded as a treatment for fecal incontinence [58]. The technique utilizes one or more of several methods of biofeedback, in most instances involving feedback of EMG signals derived from surface EMG recordings of pelvic floor muscle activity in order to "teach" the subject how better to activate and control these muscles. In mild dysfunctional states, it can be quite effective. It utilizes the ability of the central nervous system to learn modified responses to sensory input from a damaged effector system, in this case the pelvic floor.

4.9 Conclusions

The pelvic floor and its related organs is a complex, but unitary structure that normally functions almost unnoticed. Derangements are difficult to tolerate however, and effective management is therefore very important. This requires a full understanding of the factors leading to symptoms, and effective, relatively non-invasive procedures to alleviate the functional abnormalities. While much has been learned in recent years, a full understanding of the effects of weakness in specific muscular systems, and of the effects of loss of elastic resistance in pelvic floor ligaments, is not yet accomplished. In addition, the compensatory capacity of the central nervous system to modulate pelvic floor function in the context of pelvic floor pathology is also not yet well understood. Only a full knowledge of this capacity will enable appropriate and testable procedures to be developed. Much progress has been made, but there is much more to be learned.

References

1. Parks AG. Anorectal incontinence. Proc R Soc Med 1975; 68:681–690.
2. Browning GGP, Parks AG. Post-anal repair for neuropathic incontinence; correlation of clinical results and anal canal pressures. Br J Surg 1983;70:101–104.
3. Womack N, Morrison J, Williams NS. Prospective study of the effects of post-anal repair in neurogenic faecal incontinence. Br J Surg 1985;75:48–52.
4. Kerremans R. Morphological and physiological aspects of anal continence and defaecation. Editions Arscia, Brussels, 1969.
5. Denny-Brown D, Robertson EG. An investigation in to the nervous control of defaecation. Brain 1935;38:256–310.
6. Stalberg E, Trontelj J. Single fibre electromyography. Mirvalle Press, Old Woking, 1979.
7. Swash M, Schwartz MS. Neuromuscular disorders; a practical approach to diagnosis and management. Springer-Verlag, London, 1981.

8. Parks AG, Swash M, Urich H. Sphincter denervation in ano-rectal incontinence and rectal prolapse. Gut 1977;18:656–665.
9. Beersiek F, Parks AG, Swash M. Pathogenesis of anorectal incontinence: histometric study of the anal sphincter musculature. J Neurol Sci 1979;42:111–127.
10. Swash M. Histopathology of the pelvic floor. In: Henry MM, Swash M (eds) Coloproctology and the pelvic floor. Butterworths, London, 1985, pp129–150.
11. Duthie HL, Bennett RL. The relation of sensation in the anal canal to the functional anal sphincter: a possible factor in anal incontinence. Gut 1963;4:179–182.
12. Miller R, Bartolo D, Cerveto F, Mortensen NJ. Anorectal sampling: comparison of normal and incontinent subjects. Br J Surg 1988;75:44–47.
13. Henry MM, Parks AG, Swash M. Electrophysiological and histological studies of the pelvic floor in the descending perineum syndrome. Br J Surg 1982;69:470–472.
14. Pollack J, Nordenstam J, Brismar S et al. Anal incontinence after vaginal delivery: a five-year prospective study. Obstet Gynecol 2004;1297–1402.
15. Bartolo DC, Paterson HM. Anal incontinence. Best Pract Res Clin Gastroenterol 2009;23:505–515.
16. Rogers J, Henry MM, Misiewicz JJ. Combined sensory and motor deficit in primary neuropathic faecal incontinence. Gut 1988;29:5–9.
17. Henry MM, Swash M. Pathogenesis and clinical features. In: Henry MM, Swash M (eds) Coloproctology and the pelvic floor. Butterworths, London, 1985, pp 222–228.
18. Neill ME, Parks AG, Swash M. Physiological studies of the anal sphincter musculature in faecal incontinence and rectal prolapse. Br J Surg 1981;68:531–536.
19. Kumar D, Hallan RI, Womack N et al. Measurement of ano-rectal function. In: Kumar D, Waldron J, Williams NS (eds) Clinical measurement in coloproctology. Springer-Verlag, London, 1991, pp 37–42.
20. Read NW, Haynes WG, Bartolo DCC et al. Use of anorectal manometry during rectal infusion of saline to investigate sphincter function in incontinent patients. Gastroenterology 1979;85:105–113.
21. Read NW, Bannister JJ. Anorectal manometry: techniques in health and anorectal disease. In: Henry MM, Swash M (eds) Coloproctology and the pelvic floor. Butterworths, London, 1985, pp 65–87.
22. Neill ME, Swash M. Increased motor unit fibre density in the external anal sphincter muscle in anorectal incontinence: a single fibre EMG study. J Neurol Neurosurg Psychiatry 1980;43:343–347.
23. Snooks SJ, Barnes RPH, Swash M. Damage to the voluntary anal and urinary sphincter musculature in incontinence. J Neurol Neurosurg Psychiatry 1984;47:1269–1273.
24. Bartolo DCC, Jarratt JA, Read NW. The use of conventional electromyography to assess external sphincter neuropathy in man. J Neurol Neurosurg Psychiatry 1983;46:1115–1118.
25. Bartolo DCC, Jarratt JA, Read NW et al. The role of partial denervation of the puborectalis in idiopathic faecal incontinence. Br J Surg 1983;70:664–667.
26. Kiff ES, Swash M. Slowed conduction in the pudendal nerves in idiopathic (neurogenic) faecal incontinence. Br J Surg 1984;71:614–616.
27. Wunderlich M, Swash M. The overlapping innervation of

the two sides of the external sphincter by the pudendal nerve. J Neurol Sci 1983;59:91–109.
28. Swash M, Snooks SJ, Henry MM. A unifying concept of pelvic floor disorders and incontinence. J Roy Soc Med 1985;78:906–911.
29. Rogers J, Laurberg S, Henry MM et al. Anorectal physiology validated. Br J Surg 1969;76:607–609.
30. Lubowski DZ, Swash M, Nicholls RJ, Henry MM. Increase in pudendal nerve terminal motor latency with defaecation straining. Br J Surg 1988;75:1095–1097.
31. Jones PN, Lubowski DZ, Swash M, Henry MM. Relation between perineal descent and pudendal nerve damage in idiopathic faecal incontinence. Int J Colorectal Dis 1987; 2:93–95.
32. Roberts MM. Neurophysiology in neurourology. Muscle Nerve 2008;38:815–836.
33. Fowler CJ, Kirby RS, Harrison MJ et al. Individual motor unit analysis in the diagnosis of disorders of urethral sphincter innervation. J Neurol Neurosurg Psychiatry 1984;47: 637–641.
34. Smith ARB, Hosker GL, Warrell DW. The role of partial denervation of the pelvic floor in the aetiology of genito-urinary prolapse and stress incontinence of urine: a neuro-physiological study. Br J Obstet Gynaecol 1989;96: 244–248.
35. Snooks SJ, Badenoch D, Tiptaft R, Swash M. Perineal nerve damage in genuine stress urinary incontinence: an electro-physiological study. Br J Urol 1985;57:422–426.
36. Petros PE, Woodman PJ. The integral theory of continence. Int Urogynecol J Pelvic Floor Dysfunct 2008;19:35–40.
37. Petros P, Swash M. The musculo-elastic theory of anorectal function and dysfunction. Pelviperineology 2008;27:89–93.
38. Petros P, Kakulas B, Swash M. Stress urinary incontinence results from muscle weakness and ligamentous laxity in the pelvic floor. Pelviperineology 2008;27:107–109.
39. Snooks SJ, Swash M, Setchell M Henry MM. Injury to in-nervation of pelvic floor sphincter musculature in childbirth. Lancet 1984;2:546–550.
40. Snooks SJ, Swash M, Henry MM, Setchell M. Risk factors in childbirth causing damage to the pelvic floor innervation: a precursor of stress incontinence. Int J Colorect Dis 1986;1:20–24.
41. Snooks SJ, Henry MM, Swash M. Faecal incontinence due to external anal sphincter division in childbirth is associated with damage to the innervation of the pelvic floor muscu-lature: a double pathology. Br J Obstet Gynaecol 1985; 92:824–828.
42. Laurberg S, Swash M, Henry MM. Delayed external sphincter repair for obstetric tear: pudendal nerve damage im-plies a poor result from sphincter repair. Br J Surg 1988;75:786–788.
43. Sultan AH, Kamm MA, Hudson CN et al. Anal sphincter disruption during vaginal delivery. N Engl J Med 1993; 329:1905–1911.
44. Nordenstam J, Altman D, Brismar S, Zetterstrom J. Natural progression of anal incontinence after childbirth. Int Uro-gynecol J Pelvic Floor Dysfunct 2009;20:1029–1035.
45. Snooks SJ, Swash M, Mathers SE, Henry MM. Effect of vaginal delivery on the pelvic floor: a five year follow-up. Br J Surg 1990;77:1358–1360.

46. Petros P, Anderson J. Role of internal anal sphincter damage in the causation of idiopathic faecal incontinence – a prospective study. Aust N Z J Obstet Gynaecol 2005;45:77–78.

47. Swash M, Gray A, Lubowski DZ, Nicholls J. Ultrastructural changes in internal sphincter in neurogenic faecal incontinence. Gut 1988;29:1692–1698.

48. Holstege G, Sie JAML. The central control of the pelvic floor. In: Pemberton JH, Swash M, Henry MM (eds) The pelvic floor: its function and disorders. WB Saunders, London, 2001, pp 94–101.

49. Porter R, Lemon RL. Corticospinal function and voluntary movement. Monographs of the Physiological Society 45. Clarendon Press, Oxford, 1995.

50. Fowler CJ, Griffiths D, de Groat WC. The neural control of micturition. Nat Rev Neurosci 2008;9:453–466.

51. Chan CL, Ponsford S, Swash M. The anal reflex elicited by cough and sniff: validation of a clinical sign. J Neurol Neurosurg Psychiatry 2004;75:1449–1451.

52. Uher E-M, Swash M. Human sacral reflexes; physiology and clinical application. Dis Colon Rectum 1998;41:1165–1177.

53. Vodusek DB. Sacral reflexes. In: Pemberton JH, Swash M, Henry MM (eds) The pelvic floor: its function and disorders. WB Saunders, London, 2001, pp 237–247.

54. Blok BFM, Willemsen AT, Holstege G. A PET study on brain control of micturition in humans. Brain 1997;120:111–131.

55. Blok BFM, Sturms LM, Holstege G. Brain activation during micturition in women. Brain 1998;121:2033–2042.

56. Fowler CJ, Kirby RS. Electromyography of urethral sphincter in women with urinary retention. Lancet 1986;1:1455–1477.

57. Mathers SE, Kempster PA, Swash M, Lees AJ. Constipation and paradoxical puborectalis contractions in anismus and Parkinson's disease: a dystonic phenomenon? J. Neurol Neurosurg Psychiatry 1988;51:1503–1507.

58. Enck P, Musial F. Biofeedback in pelvic floor disorders. In: Pemberton JH, Swash M, Henry MM (eds) The pelvic floor: its function and disorders. WB Saunders, London, 2001, pp 393–402.

Clinical Neurophysiology of the Pelvic Floor 5

W. Thomas Gregory and Kimberly Kenton

Abstract Electrodiagnostic testing of the pelvic floor is becoming increasingly common in clinical pelvic medicine and pelvic floor research. Clinically, it can be used with history, physical examination, and urodynamic testing to aid in the diagnosis of certain pelvic floor disorders and to determine if a central or peripheral neurologic problems exists. Electrodiagnostic testing is also emerging in studies investigating the etiology of pelvic floor disorders. A basic understanding of the principles and techniques used in electrodiagnostic medicine is essential for reconstructive pelvic surgeons. However, most pelvic surgeons will never have the skills or expertise to perform pelvic floor neurophysiologic testing. Multidisciplinary teams including urogynecologic, urologic, and colorectal surgeons, physiatrists, neurologists, and physical therapists are imperative if we are going to improve our understanding of pelvic floor disorders and improve treatment outcomes.

Keywords Electromyography • EMG • Nerve conduction studies • Pudendal nerve terminal motor latency

5.1 Introduction

As discussed in previous chapters, pelvic organ support and function rely on the complex interplay of connective tissues, nerves, and muscles. Imaging modalities described in this textbook help define normal and abnormal anatomic relationships in asymptomatic women and those with pelvic floor disorders. Many imaging modalities can also provide information on the function and integrity of the neuromuscular system. However, neurophysiologic studies remain the gold standard for neuromuscular evaluation and are often required to complete the evaluation of the sacral and central nervous systems.

Electrodiagnostic testing of the pelvic floor is becoming increasingly common in clinical pelvic medicine and pelvic floor research. Clinically, it can be used with history, physical examination, and urodynamic testing to aid in the diagnosis of certain pelvic floor disorders and to determine if a central or peripheral neurologic problem exists. Electrodiagnostic testing is also emerging in studies investigating the etiology of pelvic floor disorders. A basic understanding of the principles and techniques used in electrodiagnostic medicine are essential for reconstructive pelvic surgeons. However, most pelvic surgeons will never have the skills or expertise to perform pelvic floor neurophysiologic testing. Multidisciplinary teams including urogynecologic, urologic, and colorectal surgeons, physiatrists, neurologists,

W.T. Gregory
Female Pelvic Medicine and Reconstructive Surgery,
Departments of Obstetrics and Gynecology and Urology,
Oregon Health and Science University, Portland, OR, USA

and physical therapists are imperative if we are going to improve our understanding of pelvic floor disorders and improve treatment outcomes.

5.2 Neuroanatomy

The somatic nerve supply to the pelvic floor muscles is provided by the pudendal nerve and by direct sacral branches. The lower motor neuronal cell bodies for these nerves are found in Onuf's nucleus in the anterior horn of the 2nd to 4th sacral spinal cord segments, which terminate as the conus medullaris. The descending rami for these nerves travel together prior to exiting the sacral foramina as the cauda equina. The pudendal nerve exits the pelvis via the greater sciatic foramen, passes around the sacrospinous ligament, and re-enters the pelvis via the lesser sciatic foramen. In the pelvis, the pudendal nerve passes along the pelvic sidewall in Alcock's canal before branching into its three terminal branches:

1. inferior hemorrhoidal nerve (mixed sensory and motor nerve) – provides efferent fibers to the external anal sphincter muscle and afferent fibers to the perianal skin
2. perineal nerve (mixed sensory and motor nerve) – provides efferent fibers to the striated urethral sphincter muscle and afferent fibers to the perineum
3. dorsal nerve to the clitoris (sensory nerve) – provides afferent innervation to the clitoris and erectile tissue.

Direct somatic branches from S3 and S4 serve the levator ani. Autonomic afferent and efferent nerves travel in the pelvic plexus anterior to the pelvic muscles to reach the various viscera.

Neurologic diseases or direct injury to the central or peripheral nervous system can alter pelvic organ function.

Clinicians and researchers utilize certain neurophysiologic tests to explore and better understand the neurologic basis of certain symptoms or identify the etiology of pelvic floor dysfunction. When neural or neuromuscular etiologies are the suspected causes of illness or disease in other regions of the body, clinicians focus the neuromuscular evaluation around the following questions: (1) what is the problem? (2) is it acute or chronic? and (3) can the injury or disease be localized? Electrodiagnostic studies are a valuable tool, but must be an extension of the clinical examination, and an adjunct to other diagnostic studies.

5.3 Role of Neurophysiologic Studies

Neurophysiologic testing in the pelvis is different than testing performed elsewhere in the body. This is due to the unique difficult-to-access to anatomical characteristics of the pelvis, as well as the special features of the pelvic floor and sphincter muscles. However, the utility of electrodiagnostic testing in the pelvis may be better understood by discussing more commonly recognized types of neuromuscular disorders. For example, consider the evaluation of a patient with hand numbness and/or weakness.

The first portion of the diagnostic evaluation is to determine which portions of the nerve and muscle are intact. Symptoms of hand numbness and weakness may result from a lesion in the neuron, the axon, the neuromuscular junction, or the muscle fibers, so the evaluation must assess whether each is functioning correctly. Additionally, determining the precise location of the injury is important. For instance, the diagnostic evaluation of hand numbness and weakness must assess the following: (1) are the symptoms secondary to a median nerve entrapment in the carpal tunnel? (2) are the symptoms from an ulnar nerve lesion? (3) are sensory and motor fibers affected? and (4) is the muscle function affected?

Three common tests are frequently utilized in the evaluation of neuromuscular disorders:

- nerve conduction studies, which evaluate the velocity of propagation of an action potential along different nerve segments
- repetitive nerve stimulation, which tests the consistency of transmission across the neuromuscular junction (not typically utilized for pelvic floor studies)
- electromyography, which evaluates the intramuscular response to inherent neuronal signals.

These tests are complementary to one another; no one test provides all the diagnostic information. In addition, multiple testing sites are required not only to localize the injury, but also to describe the extent of affected anatomy.

5.4 Types of Neurophysiologic Studies

5.4.1 Nerve Conduction Studies

A nerve conduction study is the introduction of an action potential in the peripheral nervous system and the subsequent recording of the neural impulse at some location distant to the site of stimulation. Nerve conduction studies measure the velocity of action potential propagation and the magnitude of the response, thereby allowing one to make clinical judgments about the health of a particular nerve. Depending on the type of nerve stimulated and where the recording electrodes are placed, one can measure three different types of response. Pure sensory nerve action potentials, compound nerve action potentials from mixed sensory and motor nerves, and pure motor nerve evaluations by measuring compound muscle action potentials (CMAPs).

CMAPs have been traditionally used to evaluate neuropathies in women with pelvic floor disorders. Nerve conduction studies allow one to identify precise neural injuries or more generalized neuropathic injuries along portions of the peripheral nervous system. As with all electrodiagnostic tests, it is important to have a thorough understanding of peripheral neuromuscular anatomy prior to performing nerve conduction studies.

5.4.1.1 Stimulating

When performing nerve conduction studies, a stimulus is given at a predefined site using a surface or monopolar needle electrode. Most pelvic floor electromyographers use surface electrodes to stimulate, reserving needle electrodes for nerves that are hard to stimulate with surface electrodes because of excess fat or edema. The magnitude of stimulus used in routine nerve conduction studies is referred to as the supramaximal stimulus.

The supramaximal stimulus is approximately 20–30% above the stimulus that does not produce any further increase in CMAP response because all the nerve fibers to the muscle are being depolarized. The larger, myelinated axons are depolarized first, and then at supramaximal stimulation, the smaller, myelinated axons are depolarized. The pulse width is the duration over which the stimulus is delivered and typically ranges from 0.05 to 1 ms.

5.4.1.2 Recording

After stimulating the nerve, it is necessary to record the response. Surface or monopolar needle electrodes can be used. When recording a muscle response, three electrodes are necessary – an active, a reference, and a ground electrode. The active electrode should be placed directly over the muscle being studied, and the reference electrode should be placed some distance from the muscle. The responses recorded from the active and reference electrodes undergo differential amplification, resulting in the CMAP displayed on the electrodiagnostic instrument. The ground electrode should ideally be placed between the active and reference electrodes.

This is frequently not possible in pelvic floor nerve conduction studies and the ground electrode can be placed on the inner thigh. To decrease impedance from the skin and improve the recorded response, the skin under the electrodes should be gently abraded with fine sandpaper prior to placing the electrodes with a small amount of electrode gel.

5.4.1.3 Compound Muscle Action Potential

A CMAP is the biphasic waveform obtained from stimulating a nerve proximal to a muscle and recording the potential directly over the muscle. A CMAP, or M response, is a summation of all the muscle fibers that are depolarized by a single stimulated nerve. Several parameters recorded from the CMAP are useful in electrodiagnostic testing (Fig. 5.1): Onset latency is the time from nerve stimulation to the initial upward deflection of the CMAP. It reflects neural activation at the cathode, propagation of the action potential along the nerve, and transmission at the neuromuscular junction. Therefore, an abnormality at any of these sites can result in prolonged latency. Latency measures only the large, heavily myelinated, fastest-conducting axons in a nerve. If a nerve has lost many axons but a few myelinated axons remain intact, the onset latency will be normal. When the latency is prolonged, one can assume significant loss of neuromuscular function. However, if only a few axons conduct the nerve impulse at a normal velocity, the latency can be normal despite significant neural injury. Therefore, latency is not a sensitive measure of nerve injury. Amplitude is measured from the baseline to the maximum point of the waveform. Amplitude reflects the total number of

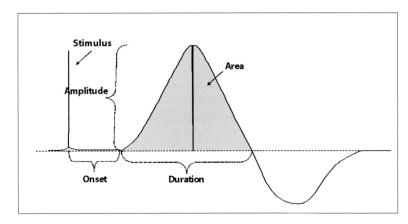

Fig. 5.1 Compound muscle action potential (CMAP); parameters measured from the CMAP are depicted

axons and muscle fibers being tested and provides an estimate of the amount of functioning tissue. For the pelvic floor, it is less reliable than latency because the distance between the electrode and muscle can significantly attenuate the signal. Area is the space under the portion of the waveform above the baseline and provides the most direct estimate of functioning tissue. Compound muscle action potential duration is typically measured from the onset latency to where it crosses the baseline. Duration and shape of the waveform measure the temporal dispersion of all the individual fibers. Nerve conduction velocity is the rate at which an action potential propagates along the stimulated nerve. It is calculated by dividing the length of nerve over which the action potential travels by the time required to travel the distance. However, in motor nerve conduction studies the latencies between two different sites of stimulation are subtracted from one another to account for the delay at the neuromuscular junction. Nerve conduction velocities are difficult to obtain on the pudendal nerve due to the nerve's anatomic course and the inability to stimulate at two well-defined sites.

If the anticipated CMAP response is not obtained, the electromyographer should not assume it is absent before troubleshooting and trying to elicit a response. Make sure stimulation is supramaximal. Also, check to ensure proper placement of both the active and reference electrodes. Verify continuity of the electrode leads and that the preamplifier is turned on. If the expected response is small, most electrodiagnostic instruments have programs to distinguish the waveform from baseline noise. Nerve conduction velocities are affected by the diameter of the nerve (large nerves conduct more quickly), temperature (cooler temperatures increase latency and amplitude), and age (age

greater than 60 years decreases nerve conduction velocity and amplitude). Therefore, delayed nerve conduction velocities in these instances may not be abnormal.

5.4.1.4 Pudendal Nerve Terminal Motor Latency

Pudendal nerve conduction studies are the most commonly reported electrodiagnostic tests carried out on the pelvic floor. First described by Kiff and Swash in 1984 to study patients with fecal incontinence [1], they have been used to investigate the role of pudendal neuropathy in stress urinary incontinence and pelvic organ prolapse [2–8]. Pudendal nerve terminal motor latency (PNTML) is a study in which sensory and motor fibers from the pudendal nerve are stimulated, and the CMAP response recorded at one of the muscles served by the pudendal nerve (external anal sphincter, striated urethral sphincter, or bulbocavernosus muscle).

PNTML is performed by using a specially designed electrode called the St Mark's electrode, which consists of two stimulating electrodes and two recording electrodes (Fig. 5.2). The St Mark's electrode is attached to a gloved index finger, so the stimulating electrodes are located at the tip of the index finger and the recording electrodes at the base. The pudendal nerve is then stimulated at the level of the ischial spine. If stimulation is applied transrectally, the recording electrodes are located at the external anal sphincter. In women, it is preferable to stimulate the pudendal nerve using a transvaginal approach with surface electrodes placed over the external anal sphincter at the 3 and 9 o'clock positions, with the patient in dorsal lithotomy. Normative data using this technique in 42 continent women have been established [9]. Older age, more vaginal deliveries, and a wide genital hiatus were associated with longer pudendal and perineal nerve terminal motor latencies.

Unlike nerve conduction studies in limbs, only two parameters are typically reported in pudendal nerve conduction studies: amplitude and onset latency (Fig. 5.1). CMAP amplitude reflects the total number of axons and muscle fibers being tested and provides an estimate of the amount of functioning tissue. It is less reliable than latency because the distance between the electrode and muscle influences it; therefore, it has not been utilized to follow loss of motor axons or muscle fibers in the pelvis.

Latency is the time from the delivery of the current over the axons to create an action potential and the onset of the action potential in the muscle of interest. The PNTML measures the large, heavily myelinated, fastest-conducting axons in a nerve, and therefore may not provide information about loss of the slower-con-

ducting units in the system. The CMAP latencies recorded with this technique have good reproducibility; however, CMAP amplitudes vary with the size of the examiner's index finger.

The clinical usefulness of pudendal and perineal nerve terminal motor latencies is hotly debated. They should not be used in isolation from other electrodiagnostic tests when evaluating pelvic floor injuries. Generally, electromyography (EMG) follows nerve conduction studies since EMG is more sensitive for detecting neuropathic injury.

5.4.1.5 Perineal Nerve Conduction Studies

The amplitude and latency of fibers to the urethral sphincter can be measured at the same time that pudendal nerve conduction studies are being done. Ring electrodes (Fig. 5.3) consisting of two pieces of plat-

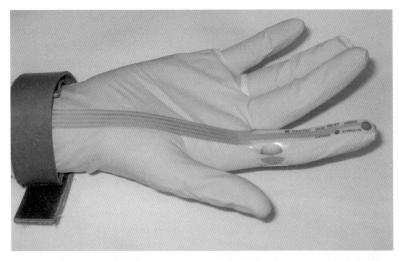

Fig. 5.2 St Mark's electrode. The stimulating cathode and anode are at the tip of the finger, while the recording electrode pair (when used transrectally) is wrapped around the base of the finger

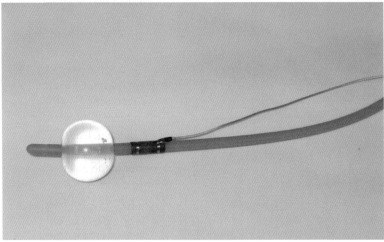

Fig. 5.3 Ring electrode. The paired electrode arrangement over a Foley catheter allows it to be used as either a stimulating or recording electrode

inum wire wound onto a small cylinder are available, which slip onto the end of a Foley catheter. When the electrode is placed 1 cm distal to the Foley balloon and the balloon is secured at the level of the urethrovesical junction, the electrode can record neuromuscular activity from the striated urethral sphincter. Stimulating the pudendal nerve at the ischial spine and recording from the urethral sphincter and external anal sphincter simultaneously, allows one to record a CMAP from the pudendal (inferior hemorrhoidal) and perineal branches.

Fig. 5.4 shows typical waveforms from pudendal and perineal nerve conduction studies from a vaginally parous woman with stress incontinence.

5.4.1.6 Sacral Reflexes

The commonly performed clinical reflex tests of the sacral nervous system are the "bulbocavernosus reflex" and the "anal reflex". Stated another way, the reflex is the contraction of a perineal muscle in response to a previous stimulation. A reflex that is present suggests intact afferent and efferent innervation. The electrophysiologic congeners are the sacral reflexes, and are commonly named based on the site of stimulation and recording. In females they are: clitoral–anal, urethral–anal, and bladder–anal reflexes. Depending on the site of stimulation for the reflex, the afferent pathway can be somatic or visceral, but the efferent pathway is somatic (namely the pudendal nerve).

For the clitoral–anal reflex, the stimulus is applied directly to the dorsal nerve of the clitoris utilizing a bipolar anode/cathode stimulator. To facilitate the appropriate early, oligosynaptic response, a dual, square-wave stimulus (3–5 ms apart) is delivered. The intensity of the stimulus is typically 3–4 times the sensory threshold (i.e. the lowest current that produced sensation). The response to the stimulus is recorded at the external anal sphincter using either surface or needle electrodes. Ideally, this test is done separately for the right and left sides, to explore any evidence of asymmetry.

The urethral stimulation in the urethral–anal reflex is delivered via a specially made bipolar montage affixed on a ring that is slipped around a Foley catheter. To perform the bladder–anal reflex, the catheter is inserted more deeply, to allow the electrodes to come into direct contact with the bladder mucosa.

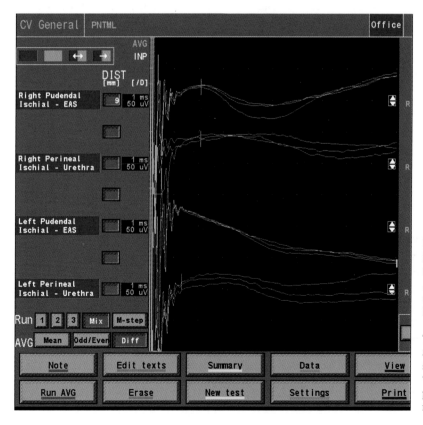

Fig. 5.4 PNTML and PeNTML. Stimulus is applied with the St Mark's electrode. A two-channel system allows for simultaneous recording of CMAP latency at the anal (PNTML) and urethral (PeNTML) sphincter. Typical small-amplitude responses are seen. Occasionally, due to the short latency, there is no return to "baseline" after the shock artifact prior to the onset of the CMP, making measurement difficult

5.4.2 Electromyography

The term electromyography (EMG) refers to the study of the patterns of electrical activity moving along the muscle fibers. EMG studies the inherent electrical activity that originates from a nerve, and therefore is generally thought to be a test of nerve function. However, in its complete utility, EMG is used to discriminate between normal, denervated, and reinnervated, as well as myopathic (local or systemic) muscle. In addition, it can demonstrate subclinical disease, and define the evolution, stage, and prognosis of a disease.

5.4.2.1 Kinesiologic EMG

The pelvic floor muscles are tonically contracting to maintain continence and support. Evaluation of voluntary increases and decreases in pelvic floor muscle contractions during certain activities yields helpful information. Kinesiologic EMG assesses the presence or absence of muscle activity during certain maneuvers.

Surface electrodes are placed on the skin over the muscle being evaluated and can be used to evaluate patterns of muscle activity. Surface electrodes record a summation of electrical activity from the muscle, but cannot distinguish individual motor unit action potentials (MUAPs), and therefore, cannot be used to diagnose or quantify neuropathy or myopathy. They are easier to use and less painful than needle electrodes, but provide less reliable information due to signal distortion by intervening skin, subcutaneous tissue, and volume conduction from other muscles.

Surface electrodes are commonly used during urodynamic studies to assess striated urethral sphincter activity. Electrodes are placed on either side of the perineal body or anal sphincter, and neuromuscular activity is recorded during the cystometry and voiding portions of the study. An increase in activity is normally seen during filling, with an absence of activity during voiding or episodes of detrusor overactivity. This set-up records neuromuscular activity of multiple pelvic floor muscles, not just the striated urethral sphincter, making it difficult to differentiate which muscle is contributing to the signal. A recent study comparing perineal surface to urethral needle electrodes during urodynamics demonstrated that needle tracings were consistently more interpretable than surface recordings [10]. Needle tracings demonstrated urethral relaxation with voiding 79% of the time, while surface recordings only demonstrated urethral relaxations 28% of the time.

Urethral EMG performed during urodynamic voiding studies can be used to diagnose detrusor sphincter dyssynergia, a potential cause of urinary retention. Similarly, EMG activity assessed for disorders such as obstructed defecation can demonstrate non-relaxing puborectalis or anal sphincters during defecation.

5.4.2.2 Needle EMG

Electromyographers consider needle EMG the gold standard for studying peripheral striated neuromuscular disease. Needle electrodes are inserted directly into the muscle, allowing an accurate portrayal of the electrical signals to diagnose neuropathy or myopathy. A variety of needle electrodes are available – monopolar, single fiber, and concentric – each with unique recording properties.

Unlike kinesiologic EMG, needle EMG can uncover electrical patterns that help delineate the location of a neuromuscular lesion, its chronicity, and expected recovery.

Understanding the motor unit is essential to interpreting needle EMG. A motor unit is a neuron, its axon, and all the muscle fibers it serves. In the case of most pelvic floor sphincter muscles, the neuronal cell bodies lie in a special location of the anterior horn of the spinal cord known as Onuf's nucleus. Near and within the muscle, the axon branches and innervates muscle fibers scattered throughout the muscle. Under normal circumstances, given muscle fibers from different motor units are intermingled, creating a mosaic pattern.

Most commonly, a concentric needle electrode (CNE) is used. At the beveled tip of the needle is a fine platinum wire (active electrode) surrounded by a steel cannula (reference electrode). The "uptake area" of the small active electrode is equivalent to about 20 muscle fibers. Therefore, the local arrangement of motor unit mosaicism, as well as the level of muscle contraction, will dictate how many motor units can be observed.

To fully appreciate the utility of needle EMG, a brief review of a few of the EMG concepts germane to pelvic floor disorders is warranted. More information can be gleaned from the needle EMG examination than is presented here, but the details are beyond the scope of this text. Although the sampling area of the needle electrode is small, the bioelectric signal detected still represents a summation of detected action potentials from multiple muscle fibers in its vicinity. An action potential is a sequence of depolarizations and repolarizations along the length of a membrane capable of supporting an energy-dependent voltage potential. The analyzed output from the electrode is a complex waveform with time on the x axis and voltage on the y axis. An action potential in a muscle originates at the neuromuscular junction. If an action potential begins at a distance from rather than adjacent to the needle, the "arriving" voltage potential will be relatively positive (when compared to the reference electrode). As the action potential continues toward the needle electrode, the polarity will at some point switch to negative and then again to positive (Fig. 5.5).

At the appropriate level of muscle contractility and activity, a single motor unit's waveform can be sampled. In a normal muscle, the majority of action potential waveforms take on the triphasic morphology just alluded to. When increased force is required, more (and larger) motor units contribute to the increase in muscle contractility. Electrically, these waveforms coalesce, overlap, and interfere with one another. No single MUAP waveform is visible, and a so-called "interference pattern" is created.

The MUAP waveform created can provide information about the multiple neuronal axons and muscle fibers transmitting the signal. Following partial nerve injury (for example), myelin sheaths and axons themselves may become dysfunctional. Neighboring axons might provide reinnervation to muscle fibers that lost their connection following the injury. During the time of nerve regrowth, myelin recreation, and re-establish-

ment of neuromuscular junctions, the coordinated summation of the bioelectric signal for that motor unit can become altered. Two main things occur. First, temporal dispersion of the action potential detected by the needle electrode prolongs and increases the complexity of the waveform. Secondly, the scattered mosaicism of the motor unit distribution changes. More muscle fibers in a given location may belong to the same motor unit, leading to a higher-amplitude signal. The interference pattern created for higher muscle forces is similarly affected. Typically fewer motor units (each with larger-amplitude signal) contribute to the pattern, subjectively referred to as "reduced". This can be quantified using advanced algorithms on modern EMG instruments.

With complete denervation (but prior to complete atrophy of the muscle fiber should no reinnervation occur), the muscle attempts to create its own pacemaker, leading to characteristic (but small) waveforms known as fibrillation potentials or positive sharp waves that eventually disappear if successful reinnervation occurs.

5.4.2.3 The Anal Sphincter

The largest and most accessible muscle of the sacral myotome is the external anal sphincter. Anatomists describe it in multiple discrete layers: subcutaneous, superficial, and deep. The two deeper layers are the substantive portions of the sphincter complex, and work in concert to create closure and apposition. The subcutaneous layer inserts directly onto the dermal junction and is partly responsible for creating the radial grooves in the skin beyond the mucocutaneous junction. This superficial layer can be easily sampled by

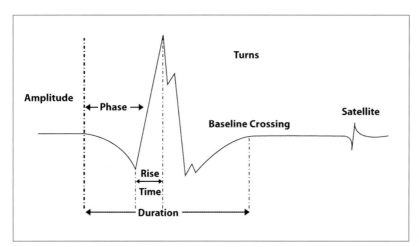

Fig. 5.5 Motor Unit Action Potential (MUAP) waveform. The main parameters of a MUAP are depicted

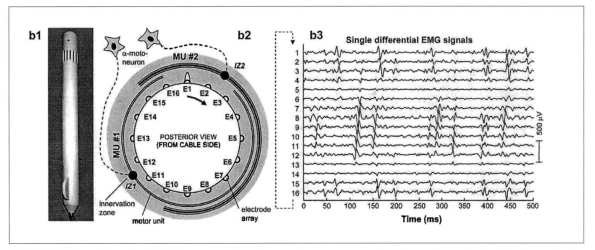

Fig. 5.6 Multi-electrode surface EMG. An array such as this prototype can, among other things, demonstrate the location and extent of innervation zones and overlapping innervation. In this simple system, 16 equally spaced electrodes around the plastic cylinder are referenced to their closest neighbor to create 16 channels. Channel 1 = E1–E2, Channel 2 = E2–E3, etc. In this set-up, motor unit 1 (MU#1) would have an action potential start in channel 11, then "evolve" bilaterally toward channel 16 (clockwise) and channel 1 (counterclockwise). A separately identifiable motor unit would initiate in channel 2, and likewise evolve clockwise and counterclockwise. With today's fast processors, multiple arrays can be utilized simultaneously. Reprinted with permission of S Karger AG (Basel) and Prof Merletti, LISIN, Politecnico di Torino, from [12]

the EMG electrode for a radius of about 1 cm outside the mucocutaneous junction, at a depth of 3 mm. There do not appear to be any electrophysiologic differences between the subcutaneous layers and the deeper layers; therefore some neurophysiologists choose to analyze this layer alone in their quest to determine the presence and extent of sacral injuries (e.g. cauda equina or conus medullaris lesions) that affect all of the sacrally innervated muscles. The deeper portions of the anal sphincter can be analyzed by advancing the needle at a 30 degree angle to the anal axis starting just at the mucocutaneous junction.

Quantitative EMG algorithms have made the analysis of MUAP waveforms and interference patterns previously introduced much less time-consuming, thereby reducing patient discomfort. During MUAP analysis, a representative sample of MUAPs should be obtained from the left and right side of the muscle separately. Standardized methods for doing this have been published [11]. High- and low-frequency filter settings can drastically alter these quantitative parameters. Commonly used settings for concentric needle EMG of the anal sphincter are 5 Hz and 10 kHz, meaning the instrument filters all frequencies below 5 Hz and above 10 kHz. Sweep and gain settings are typically 50–500 µV per division and 10 ms per division.

Recently, multiple small surface electrodes have been circumferentially mounted on an appropriately sized cylinder. Each electrode serves as both an "active" electrode and a "reference" electrode to its neighbor. In this fashion, discriminating electrical and spatial resolution of single MUAPS has been accomplished for the anal sphincter (Fig. 5.6). Initial reports using this technology have revealed that, unlike most striated muscles of the appendicular skeleton that have a discrete "neuromuscular junction zone", the innervations zones for the anal sphincter are spread rather diffusely throughout the circumference of the sphincter complex in women [12, 13]. Further studies using this less invasive technique are ongoing.

5.4.2.4 The Striated Urethral Sphincter

The urethra is composed of striated and smooth muscles, which are innervated by somatic and autonomic nerves, respectively. The striated urethral sphincter is composed of three separate muscles that function together as a single unit to maintain continence. The sphincter urethrae is a striated band of muscle that surrounds the proximal two-thirds of the urethra, while the compressor urethrae and urethrovaginal sphincter arch over the distal one-third of the urethra [14, 15]. A concentric needle electrode can be inserted into the striated urethral sphincter muscle at 12 o'clock (5 mm above the external urethral meatus), then at 3 o'clock, and 9 o'clock. The electrode is advanced approximately 1.5 cm at each insertion site. Alternatively, a transvaginal approach is used in an effort to decrease the discomfort of needle insertion. A speculum is used to maneuver the posterior vaginal wall away, so that the needle can be introduced just off midline, approximately 2 cm proximal to the external meatus. Standard filter settings (10 Hz to 10 kHz) and an amplifier gain of 50 μV per division are used.

5.4.2.5 The Levator Ani

The levator ani complex is probably innervated by direct sacral branches rather than by branches from the pudendal nerve [16]. Access to the most distal and medial muscles of the levator ani complex can be achieved in two ways. The muscle is palpated transvaginally and the needle can be directed through the vaginal mucosa posterolaterally, until EMG activity is detected. Using a longer needle (75 mm at times), the muscle can alternatively be accessed following anal sphincter EMG. This is done by directing the needle in the posterior portion of the anal sphincter (6 o'clock position) beyond to the anal sphincter. Initially, as the needle is advanced beyond the anal sphincter, one encounters an area of electrical silence in the medial limits of the ischiorectal fossa, then EMG activity resumes when the needle reaches the levator ani.

5.5 Clinical Applications

Electrodiagnostic testing has both clinical and research applications in pelvic floor disorders.

5.5.1 Fecal Incontinence

Most of this text is dedicated to the imaging techniques used for pelvic floor disorders. Anal ultrasound is important in demonstrating anal sphincter integrity and disruption as it applies to fecal incontinence. Prior to the more widespread use of anal ultrasound, investigators would utilize EMG to "map" the location of functioning anal sphincter muscle. Neurophysiologic tests have been used to determine the neurologic component of incontinence in both intact and disrupted sphincters.

Using a technique called single-fiber EMG, patients with anal incontinence had evidence of denervation and reinnervation when compared with patients without incontinence [17].

Pudendal and perineal nerve conduction studies have established a link between pudendal neuropathy and stress urinary incontinence and fecal incontinence [4, 7, 8, 18, 19]. Pudendal nerve terminal motor latencies are most frequently reported in case series of women undergoing anal sphincteroplasty. Authors have attempted to predict surgical outcomes based on normal versus abnormal pudendal nerve function, with varying results [20–22].

One hundred subjects underwent anterior overlapping anal sphincteroplasty after pudendal nerve testing. Sixty-two per cent of subjects with normal nerve terminal motor latencies had "successful" outcomes versus only 17% of subjects with unilateral or bilateral pudendal nerve terminal motor latencies [20]. Other authors have reported good postoperative success in patient with prolonged pudendal nerve terminal motor latencies [22].

Quantitative anal sphincter EMG also reveals significant difference in sphincter innervations after vaginal delivery. Motor unit action potentials from 23 parous (12-week postpartum) women had significantly higher amplitudes, longer durations, and increased phases than nulliparous women, lending further evidence that vaginal childbirth results in pudendal neuropathy [23].

5.5.2 Urinary Incontinence

Similar to the anal sphincter, ultrasound has been used to study the integrity of the striated urethral sphincter. Transvaginal ultrasound was used to measure the striated urethral sphincter in 19 continent and 55 stress-incontinent Japanese women. A significant decrease in sphincter thickness was noted in the stress-incontinent women [24]. Similarly, intraurethral ultrasound showed a decreased thickness in women with urodynamic stress incontinence compared to continent women [25].

Concentric needle EMG has been used in pelvic floor muscles to confirm the association between pelvic nerve injury, and vaginal delivery, stress incontinence, and fecal incontinence. Needle EMG of the levator ani and external anal sphincter muscles has shown EMG evidence of denervation with reinnervation in women with stress urinary incontinence. Two studies have used quantitative CNE of the urethral sphincter in women undergoing incontinence surgery [26]. Women with severe urinary incontinence or intrinsic sphincter deficiency have urethral EMG evidence of more severe neuromuscular injury [27]. Fischer et al demonstrated more advanced neuropathic changes in women with persistent stress urinary incontinence [27]. Kenton et al studied 89 women undergoing Burch urethropexy with CNE and found significant differences in EMG parameters of women with successful incontinence surgery, suggesting that these women had better innervations of their urethral sphincters. Specific EMG criteria were established, which could predict surgical success 100% of the time [26].

5.5.3 Pelvic Organs Prolapse

Much has been posited about the important role that the pelvic floor muscles play in maintaining support and function of the pelvic organs. Women with enlarged levator hiatus or severe alterations in the muscular integrity/attachments are seen to have more advanced uterovaginal prolapse, or stress incontinence. However, due to the challenge of access to these important striated muscles, there are little data that can be cited.

There are a few reports that document the presence of abnormal EMG patterns and activity following childbirth, but little to no data that focus on the levator ani complex (pubovisceralis, pubococcygeus, iliococcygeus) in women with and without measurable or symptomatic uterovaginal prolapse.

As such, many important questions remain. If neurophysiologic evidence of neuropathic changes exists in the urethral or anal sphincter muscles, can we assume the same of the levator ani muscles? Does injury occur symmetrically? Is injury similar in the more medial and distal portion of the muscle group, when compared to the more lateral muscles?

5.5.4 Post-operative Assessment

Clinical evidence suggests that certain types of reconstructive surgery may affect pelvic floor innervation. Zivkovic et al measured perineal nerve terminal motor latencies before and after vaginal reconstructive surgery and found significantly prolonged terminal motor latencies in women who underwent vaginal needle suspension procedures [28]. Similarly, Benson et al found significantly prolonged pudendal and perineal nerve terminal motor latencies in 27 women undergoing vaginal repair, while the terminal motor latencies of 21 women undergoing abdominal repair were not different [29]. They then compared postoperative perineal terminal motor latencies of the women with "optimal" and "suboptimal" repairs. Pudendal neuropathy was significantly more common in the women with "suboptimal" repairs. In a well-conducted randomized controlled trial of abdominal versus vaginal reconstructive surgery, Benson et al found superior anatomic results in the abdominal group [30]. Another randomized controlled trial also demonstrated anatomic superiority of the abdominal approach [31]. These data suggest that vaginal reconstructive surgery results in denervation of the pelvic floor musculature, which may affect the anatomic success of the surgery. There are also increasing data showing that preoperative pelvic floor denervation may impact surgical outcomes, particularly for continence procedures. Two recent studies demonstrated a relationship between urethral sphincter neuropathy and outcome of continence surgery.

5.5.5 Childbirth

To anyone who has witnessed vaginal childbirth, it will come as no surprise that there is neurophysiologic evidence of mechanical and stretch injury. The pudendal nerve is tethered by the ischial spine, with potential traction or direct laceration-type injury at that location. However, distal nerve branches may be stretched or compressed with resultant ischemia that also leads to nerve dysfunction.

Several different types of studies have demonstrated this. In over 40% of women, following vaginal delivery, prolongation of PNTML (with eventual recovery in most) and increased fiber density of the anal sphincter was seen immediately. Abnormal PNTML was also seen in women who had a cesarean delivery after 8 cm of dilation [32]. Increased MUAP parameters in the anal sphincter and levator ani were seen immediately after birth, but similar differences did not seem to persist for women studied many years after their deliveries [33].

5.5.6 *Neurologic Conditions*

There are many neurologic conditions that can affect pelvic floor function. Lesions of the brain can affect the coordination of signaling required for urinary voiding and storage, leading to hyperreflexia of the detrusor, sphincter dyssynergia, and uncoordinated sphincter relaxations. Kinesiologic EMG during urodynamics or anal manometry may be useful.

To the practicing neurologist, a clinical dilemma of trying to differentiate Parkinson's disease from multiple system atrophy can arise. Like multiple sclerosis, both diseases can have bladder or bowel symptoms present. One way to differentiate the two conditions is by using EMG. The neurons in Onuf's nucleus are affected by multiple system atrophy, but not in Parkinson's disease. Therefore, as neurons degenerate, features typical of acute and chronic denervation can develop in the anal sphincter.

Multiple complex relationships and reflexes exist between the higher central nervous system and the pelvic floor. This is especially relevant with respect to bladder function and dysfunction. For lesions cephalad to the conus medullaris, an "upper motor neuron" lesion exists.

This interrupts the signal processing and alters the coordination of sphincter relaxation that needs to be associated with detrusor contraction. Kinesiologic EMG studies performed during urodynamics may be abnormal, whereas the remainder of the studies highlighted in this textbook would be normal.

Anything that affects the pelvic plexus can potentially disrupt the urethral and bladder anal reflexes. This can be seen in peripheral neuropathies with significant autonomic components and after radical pelvic surgery or radiation. The clitoral anal reflex should be preserved because the course of this branch is not involved. Pudendal neuropathy typically results in prolonged or absent clitoral anal reflex with preservation of the urethral and bladder anal reflexes. The afferent limb of the pathway through the pelvic plexus is less affected and is a temporally longer portion of the pathway. Lesions in the conus medullaris and cauda equina frequently produce abnormalities in all sacral reflexes.

Suppression of the urethral anal reflex by actively trying to void is a measure of upper motor neuron function. If a patient is unable to suppress the response during voiding, she may have a lesion in the suprasacral spinal cord.

5.6 Conclusions

Much of our current understanding of the etiology of pelvic floor disorders has come from both nerve conduction studies and EMG of the pelvic floor muscles in women with stress incontinence, fecal incontinence, or pelvic organ prolapse. We understand that surgery can affect pelvic innervations, and electrodiagnosis has also confirmed the relationship between vaginal childbirth and pudendal neuropathy. The degree of denervation and pelvic floor injury can be measured, and therefore studied.

Such measurements have some correlation with clinical outcomes, but further research refining techniques and establishing normative electrodiagnostic parameters for the urethral sphincter, anal sphincter, and levator ani are imperative.

Pelvic floor electrodiagnostic studies may aid in the clinical diagnosis of some pelvic floor disorders and help to predict outcomes of incontinence surgery. However, confirmatory studies are necessary. Clinicians who wish to add electrodiagnosis to their clinical evaluation of patients with pelvic floor disorders should have proper training in nerve conduction studies and EMG, or work in a multidisciplinary setting with a neurologist or physiatrist trained in electrodiagnosis.

References

1. Kiff ES, Swash M. Slowed conduction in the pudendal nerves in idiopathic (neurogenic) faecal incontinence. Br J Surg 1984;71:614–616.
2. Snooks SJ, Swash M, Mathers SE, Henry MM. Effect of vaginal delivery on the pelvic floor: A 5-year follow-up. Br J Surg 1990;77:1358–1360.
3. Snooks SJ, Swash M, Henry MM, Setchell M. Risk factors in childbirth causing damage to the pelvic floor innervation. Int J Colorectal Dis 1986;1:20–24.
4. Snooks SJ, Badenoch DF, Tiptaft RC, Swash M. Perineal nerve damage in genuine stress urinary incontinence. An electrophysiological study. Br J Urol 1985;57:422–426.
5. Snooks SJ, Henry MM, Swash M. Faecal incontinence due to external anal sphincter division in childbirth is associated with damage to the innervation of the pelvic floor musculature: A double pathology. Br J Obstet Gynaecol 1985; 92:824–828.
6. Snooks SJ. Risk factors in childbirth causing damage to the pelvic floor innervation. Br J Surg 1985;72(suppl):S15–17.
7. Snooks SJ, Barnes PR, Swash M. Damage to the innervation of the voluntary anal and periurethral sphincter musculature in incontinence: an electrophysiological study. J Neurol Neurosurg Psychiatry 1984;47:1269–1273.

8. Snooks SJ, Swash M. Abnormalities of the innervation of the urethral striated sphincter musculature in incontinence. Br J Urol 1984;56:401–405.

9. Olsen AL, Ross M, Stansfield RB, Kreiter C. Pelvic floor nerve conduction studies: Establishing clinically relevant normative data. Am J Obstet Gynecol 2003;189:1114–1119.

10. Mahajan ST, Fitzgerald MP, Kenton K et al. Concentric needle electrodes are superior to perineal surface-patch electrodes for electromyographic documentation of urethral sphincter relaxation during voiding. BJU Int 2006;97:117–120.

11. Podnar S, Vodusek DB. Standardization of anal sphincter electromyography: Utility of motor unit potential parameters. Muscle Nerve 2001;24:946–951.

12. Enck P, Franz H, Azpiroz F et al. Innervation zones of the external anal sphincter in healthy male and female subjects. Preliminary results. Digestion 2004;69:123–130.

13. Merletti R, Bottin A, Cescon C et al. Multichannel surface EMG for the non-invasive assessment of the anal sphincter muscle. Digestion 2004;69:112–122.

14. Oelrich TM. The striated urogenital sphincter muscle in the female. Anat Rec 1983;205:223–232.

15. Junemann KP, Schmidt RA, Melchior H, Tanagho EA. Neuroanatomy and clinical significance of the external urethral sphincter. Urol Int 1987;42:132–136.

16. Barber MD, Bremer RE, Thor KB et al. Innervation of the female levator ani muscles. Am J Obstet Gynecol 2002;187:64–71.

17. Snooks SJ, Barnes PR, Swash M. Damage to the innervation of the voluntary anal and periurethral sphincter musculature in incontinence: an electrophysiological study. J Neurol Neurosurg Psychiatry 1984;47:1269–1273.

18. Snooks SJ, Swash M, Henry MM. Abnormalities in central and peripheral nerve conduction in patients with anorectal incontinence. J R Soc Med 1985;78:294–300.

19. Snooks SJ, Barnes PR, Swash M, Henry MM. Damage to the innervation of the pelvic floor musculature in chronic constipation. Gastroenterology 1985;89:977–981.

20. Gilliland R, Altomare DF, Moreira H Jr et al. Pudendal neuropathy is predictive of failure following anterior overlapping sphincteroplasty. Dis Colon Rectum 1998;41:1516–1522.

21. Sangwan YP, Coller JA, Barrett RC et al. Unilateral pudendal neuropathy. Impact on outcome of anal sphincter repair. Dis Colon Rectum 1996;39:686–689.

22. Chen AS, Luchtefeld MA, Senagore AJ et al. Pudendal nerve latency. Does it predict outcome of anal sphincter repair? Dis Colon Rectum 1998;41:1005–1009.

23. Gregory WT, Lou JS, Stuyvesant A, Clark AL. Quantitative electromyography of the anal sphincter after uncomplicated vaginal delivery. Obstet Gynecol 2004;104:327–335.

24. Kondo Y, Homma Y, Takahashi S et al. Transvaginal ultrasound of urethral sphincter at the mid urethra in continent and incontinent women. J Urol 2001;165:149–152.

25. Heit M. Intraurethral sonography and the test–retest reliability of urethral sphincter measurements in women. J Clin Ultrasound 2002;30:349–355.

26. Kenton K, FitzGerald MP, Shott S, Brubaker L. Role of urethral electromyography in predicting outcome of burch retropubic urethropexy. Am J Obstet Gynecol 2001; 185:51–55.

27. Fischer JR, Hale DS, McClellan E, Benson JT. The use of urethral electrodiagnosis to select the method of surgery in women with instrinsic sphincter deficiency. Int Urogynecol J 2001;12(suppl 1):51.

28. Zivkovic F, Tamussino K, Ralph G et al. Long-term effects of vaginal dissection on the innervation of the striated urethral sphincter. Obstet Gynecol 1996;87:257–260.

29. Benson JT, McClellan E. The effect of vaginal dissection on the pudendal nerve. Obstet Gynecol 1993;82:387–389.

30. Benson JT, Lucente V, McClellan E. Vaginal versus abdominal reconstructive surgery for the treatment of pelvic support defects: A prospective randomized study with long-term outcome evaluation. Am J Obstet Gynecol 1996; 175:1418–1421; discussion 1421–1422.

31. Maher CF, Qatawneh AM, Dwyer PL et al. Abdominal sacral colpopexy or vaginal sacrospinous colpopexy for vaginal vault prolapse: A prospective randomized study. Am J Obstet Gynecol 2004;190:20–26.

32. Fynes M, Donnelly VS, O'Connell PR, O'Herlihy C. Cesarean delivery and anal sphincter injury. Obstet Gynecol 1998;92:496–500.

33. Podnar S, Lukanovic A, Vodusek DB. Anal sphincter electromyography after vaginal delivery: Neuropathic insufficiency or normal wear and tear? Neurourol Urodyn 2000;19:249–257.

Section II
Pelvic Floor Imaging

Pelvic Floor Imaging: Introduction

Giovanni Morana and Luca Cancian

The pelvic floor is a sophisticated anatomical and functional unit, with a complex interaction of multiple structures. Its main functions are to ensure stable pelvic continence and control of defecation and urination.

Disruption of this balance due to functional problems has major personal impact for the patient, who suffers psychological distress in addition to the physical difficulties; it has a major social impact as a result of the high incidence of such problems in the population, with greater frequency among multiparous women.

Until recently, anatomical knowledge of this region was derived only from the study of anatomical dissection, which made joint assessment of morphological and functional aspects very difficult. Thorough knowledge of the anatomy of the pelvic floor is crucial for the identification and understanding of disorders. Historically, the pelvic floor is divided into three compartments: anterior, medial, and posterior, to which is added a fourth segment, the peritoneal cavity and the fascia [1]. Technological advances in diagnostic imaging have led to a more precise understanding of the anatomy and function. The advent of endorectal ultrasonography (ERUS), developed further with three-dimensional (3D) visualization, and magnetic resonance imaging (MRI) with both endorectal and phased array coils, and with the ability to perform dynamic imaging of defecography by magnetic resonance angiography. In applying the advances from this revolution in anatomical imaging, traditional defecography should not be forgotten – an investigation that was born in the 1960s, which still continues to provide important anatomical and functional information for an appropriate surgical evaluation.

Ultrasonography is taking an increasingly central role in defining the diagnosis of pelvic floor disorders. The approach using a rotating endorectal probe, a method that was developed in England in the 1990s, allows accurate recognition of the anatomic structures of the complex sphincter, with clear definition of the distinct layers of the rectal wall, the mucosa, submucosa, and internal sphincter, which are continuous with the circular muscle layer of the rectum, and the external sphincter muscle, which is continuous with the puborectalis [2]. Externally, these structures are still identified by the puborectalis muscle, the anococcygeal ligament, the ischiopubic fat space, and the anus, vagina, and urethra. Technological development has led to the possibility of ultrasound scans with 3D reconstruction, with consequent improvements in diagnostic accuracy – the sensitivity and specificity of anal endosonography for the diagnosis of anal sphincter defect is over 90% [3].

Ultrasound examination of the pelvic floor also includes the possibility of an intravaginal or perineal approach. The latter involves the use of a 5–7 MHz convex-type translabial probe with support along the sagittal axis, with the patient supine, and allows visualization of the bladder neck and the mobility of the urethra. During the examination, the patient performs a Valsalva maneuver and contraction of the pelvic muscles to facilitate examination of the effect of altered position of the anatomical structures [4]. A transvaginal approach with use of high-resolution and 3D reconstruction provides adequate visualization of the area that surrounds the urethral sphincter, and details of anatomy that are not visible with other approaches [5].

Used in a complementary way, these two methods give excellent information on anatomical and functional disorders of the genitourinary tract such as incontinence and prolapse.

L. Cancian
Department of Radiology, Regional Hospital, Treviso, Italy

G.A. Santoro, A.P. Wieczorek, C.I. Bartram (eds.) *Pelvic Floor Disorders*
© Springer-Verlag Italia 2010

MRI is a technique that has become valuable in the management of pelvic floor problems. Magnetic resonance studies have significantly changed knowledge of the anatomy of the pelvic floor [6]. Use of an endorectal coil appears to have high accuracy in visualization of the sphincter complex, and particularly in identification of atrophy of the external anal sphincter. In clinical practice, MRI uses mainly the coil "phased array" surface which does not disturb the patient and allows good study of the sphincter complex, with only a slight loss of accuracy in the assessment of the internal sphincter when compared to endorectal MR and ultrasound techniques, and the added advantage of a larger field of view. Thus, when the examination is conducted in different planes, it allows an assessment of all the pelvic floor structures with a large field of view that includes the levator ani muscles and allows visualization of all the pelvic support structures [6].

A defecography-functional MRI examination allows dynamic study of the pelvic floor structures. This examination can be performed with an open scanner, with the patient in a sitting position, or using standard equipment with the patient supine. Standard scanners (closed-magnet system) give valuable information for the diagnosis of significant changes as they have a better signal-to-noise ratio as a result of using a strong magnetic-field (1.5 T vs. 0.5 T in open units) [7]. The procedure has evolved since 1991 as a result of a study by Yang and Krutt, which described the movement of the bladder, vagina, and rectum in relation to the pubococcygeus muscle and between the symphysis pubis and the sacrum. Over time, a technique has evolved with the ability to perform ultrafast sequences that can be repeated 15–25 times in the same position to capture the various stages of defecation (relaxation and contraction of pelvic muscles). The protocol includes the anatomical sequences of the structures visualized, and the latter phases – both static and dynamic – in order to generate anatomical and functional assessment of all three compartments involved in the pathology of the pelvic floor. Some studies have compared the traditional defecography, urethrocystography, and colpocistorecto-graphy with MRI, demonstrating that the techniques overlap in concurrent dynamic assessment [8]. However, MRI allows more accurate assessment of the condition of muscle and ligaments, not only from the anatomical point of view but also revealing changes that are secondary, for example, to muscle denervation.

In the future, complex evaluation of pelvic floor anatomy and function is priority and seems to be already achieved by MRI sequences as a result of increased speed and volume acquisition, which may soon allow assessment of the entire pelvic volume during the phases of contraction and relaxation. On the other hand, ultrasonography with 3D reconstruction with a transrectal and vaginal approach allows excellent evaluation of the pelvic structures, with high spatial resolution. These complex techniques facilitate understanding of the complex disorders of the pelvic floor and related treatment decisions, as there is a need for a multidisciplinary approach to diagnosis and therapy.

The radiologist that deals with diagnosis of pelvic floor disorders should have a knowledge of all the modalities that could be used for pelvic floor imaging, should know how to conduct and interpret each of the examinations, and should be a dedicated specialist who introduces a single common language for the various medical specialties involved in the process of diagnosing pelvic floor disorders.

References

1. Weber AM, Abrams, Brubaker L et al. The standardization of terminology for researchers in female pelvic floor disorders. Int Urogynecol J 2001;12:178–186.
2. Nielsen MB, Pedersen JF, Hauge C et al. Endosonography of the anal sphincter: findings in healthy volunteers. AJR Am J Roentgenol 1991;157:1199–1202.
3. Dobben AC, Terra MP, Slors JF et al. External anal sphincter defects in patients with fecal incontinence: comparison of endoanal MR imaging and endoanal US. Radiology 2007;242:463–471.
4. Tunn R, Petri E. Introital and transvaginal ultrasound as the main tool in the assessment of urogenital and pelvic floor dysfunction: an imaging panel and practical approach. Ultrasound Obstet Gynecol 2003;22:205–213.
5. Santoro GA, Wieczorek AP, Stankiewicz A et al. High-resolution three-dimensional endovaginal ultrasonography in the assessment of pelvic floor anatomy: a preliminary study. Int Urogynecol J Pelvic Floor Dysfunct 2009;20:1213–1222.
6. Stoker J, Halligan S, Bartram CI et al. Pelvic floor imaging. Radiology 2001;218:621–641.
7. Bertschinger KM, Hetzer FH, Roos JE et al. Dynamic MR imaging of the pelvic floor performed with patient sitting in an open-magnet unit versus with patient supine in a closed-magnet unit. Radiology 2002;223:501–508.
8. Constantinou CE. Dynamics of female pelvic floor function using urodynamics, ultrasound and Magnetic Resonance Imaging (MRI). Eur J Obstet Gynecol Reprod Biol 2009;144(suppl 1):S159–165.

Endovaginal Ultrasonography: Methodology and Normal Pelvic Floor Anatomy

6

Giulio Aniello Santoro, Andrzej Paweł Wieczorek, S. Abbas Shobeiri and Aleksandra Stankiewicz

Abstract High-resolution three-dimensional endovaginal ultrasonography (EVUS) provides a detailed evaluation of the pelvic floor muscles and the levator ani complex, the lower urinary tract, and the anorectal region in planes that cannot be determined by conventional two-dimensional EVUS. Multiplanar reconstruction and rendering techniques allow the investigator to correctly recognize and measure specific anatomic elements of the pelvic floor and to understand their true spatial relationships (anterior, lateral, and posterior compartments). This modality is relatively easy to perform and is time efficient, correlates well with other imaging modalities, and delivers relevant information in patients with pelvic floor disorders.

Keywords Anal sphincters • Endovaginal ultrasonography • Levator ani • Levator hiatus • Pelvic floor • Perineal muscles • Pubovisceral muscle • Three-dimensional ultrasonography • Urethral complex • Urogenital hiatus

6.1 Introduction

Endovaginal ultrasonography (EVUS) has become a valuable tool in the diagnostic workup of patients with pelvic floor disorders, and it provides sufficient information for clinical decision making in many cases [1, 2]. However, with the conventional two-dimensional (2D) ultrasound (US), there are many elements of the image that cannot be correctly recognized as components of a three-dimensional (3D) structure, or at least not perceived in their true spatial relationships, and a good deal of relevant information may remain hidden.

As the transition towards total digital image acquisition continues, 3D ultrasound, constructed from a synthesis of a high number of parallel transaxial 2D images, has been developed [3]. After a 3D dataset has been acquired, it is immediately possible to select coronal anterior–posterior or posterior–anterior as well as sagittal right–left views, together with any oblique image plane. Three-dimensional US, particularly developed for obstetric applications during the last 15 years, has been shown to be a useful adjunct to conventional 2D-US for evaluation of the lower urinary tract, the levator ani complex, pelvic organ prolapse (POP), and anal sphincter imaging [4–7].

In this chapter we will review the methodology of 3D-EVUS (equipment, patient preparation, and patient position, technique of examination, manner of performing measurements) and evaluate the anatomy of the female pelvic floor (anterior, lateral, and posterior compartments) with this technique, providing a standardization both with regard to which levels of the pelvic floor and on which scan planes key anatomic structures can be described and measured.

G.A. Santoro
Pelvic Floor Unit and Colorectal Service, 1st Department of General Surgery, Regional Hospital, Treviso, Italy

G.A. Santoro, A.P. Wieczorek, C.I. Bartram (eds.) *Pelvic Floor Disorders*
© Springer-Verlag Italia 2010

6.2 Technical Aspects of 3D Endovaginal Ultrasound

We currently use the UltraView B-K Medical scanner (B-K Medical A/S, Mileparken 34, DK-2730 Herlev, Denmark) (Fig. 6.1). In order to obtain meaningful ultrasonic images, the operator must have an overall understanding of the technique and know how to use the controls available on the ultrasound device correctly. It is important to be aware that inadequate regulation of the equipment produces poor images and can lead to false-positive or false-negative diagnosis. Many types of ultrasound transducers have been developed for endovaginal assessment of the pelvic floor. The types of endoluminal probes include mechanical radial probes with a full 360° field, electronic biplanar probes with linear and transverse curved arrays, and endfire probes. The rotational transducer (type 2050, B-K Medical, Herlev, Denmark) has a shaft length of 270 mm, with a double crystal rotating at its tip. This probe has a frequency range from 6 to 16 MHz, with a focal length of 2–5 cm and a 90° scanning plane; it is rotated at 4–6 cycles/s, to give a radial scan of the surrounding structures (Figs. 6.2, 6.3).

The 2050 transducer has a built-in 3D automatic motorized system (the proximal–distal actuation mechanism and the electronic mover are fully enclosed

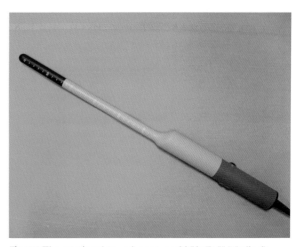

Fig. 6.2 The rotational transducer type 2050 (B-K Medical)

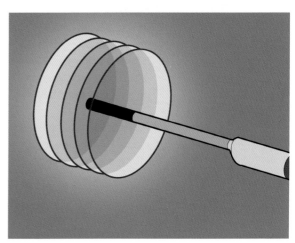

Fig. 6.3 The 2050 transducer is a mechanical radial probe with a full 360° field. It is rotated at 4–6 cycles per second and has a 90° scanning plane

within the housing of the probe) that allows acquisition of 300 transaxial images over a distance of 60 mm in 60 s, at the touch of a button, without requiring any movement relative to the investigated tissue (Fig. 6.4). The data from a series of closely spaced 2D images are combined to create a 3D volume displayed as a cube (Fig. 6.5) [3]. With the conventional 2D-US, the screen resolution is measured in number of pixels (display matrix: 700 × 700 pixel elements), with each pixel having a value between 0 and 255 (256 levels of grey). The result seen on the ultrasound monitor is a 2D image (X and Y plane only) with no depth information. Adding the third dimension means that the pixel is transformed in a small 3D picture element called a voxel, which will also have an assigned value

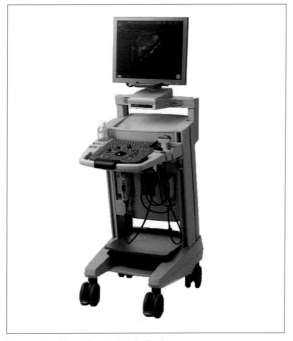

Fig. 6.1 The UltraView B-K Medical scanner

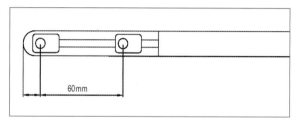

Fig. 6.4 The 2050 transducer has a built-in 3D automatic motorized system. The proximal–distal actuation mechanism and the electronic mover are fully enclosed within the housing of the probe; therefore, the 3D acquisition does not require any movement relative to the investigated tissue

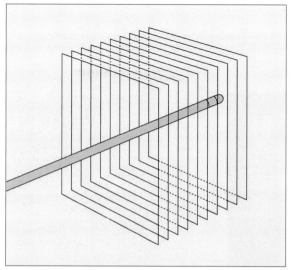

Fig. 6.5 A 3D volume, displayed as a cube, is created from a series of closely spaced 2D images (300 transaxial images over a distance of 60 mm)

between 0 and 255. Ideally, a voxel should be a cubic structure; however, the dimension in the Z plane is often slightly larger than that in the X and Y planes. The depth of the voxel is critical to the resolution of the 3D image, and this depth is directly related to the spacing between two adjacent images [3]. As already stated, the voxel should ideally form an exact cube, however sampling in the Z plane generally has slightly lower resolution than in the 700 × 700 matrix, due to acquisition speed. High-resolution 3D-US acquires four to five transaxial images sampled per millimeter of acquisition length in the Z plane. This means that an acquisition based upon sampling of transaxial images over a distance of 60 mm in the human body will result in a data volume block consisting of between 240 and 300 transaxial images. High-resolution data volumes will consist of typical voxel sizes around

0.15 × 0.15 × 0.2 mm. Because of this resolution in the longitudinal plane, which is close to the axial and transverse resolution of the 2D image, this technique ensures the true dimensions of the 3D data cube are also present in the reconstructed Z plane and provides accurate distance, area, angle, and volume measurements [8].

The ability to visualize information in the 3D image depends critically on the rendering technique [7]. Three basic types of technique are used.

1. *Surface render mode (SRM):* an operator or algorithm identifies the boundaries of the structures to create a wire-frame representation. It is the most commonly known version of render mode and is extensively used by some medical centers in producing perhaps the very first images of an unborn baby's facial contours. Surface rendering techniques only give good results when a surface is available to render, such as is possible for the pubovisceral muscle assessed by 3D transperineal US (see Chapter 7) [9]. This technique, however, fails when a strong surface cannot be found such as in the subtly layered structures within the pelvic floor. SRM is, by its requirements, mainly a superficial postprocessed topographical presentation of an often rapidly acquired 4D dataset, with a lesser degree of information inside the depth of the 3D volume of data compared to high-resolution 3D data volumes.

2. *Multiplanar reconstruction (MPR):* three perpendicular planes (axial, coronal, and longitudinal) are displayed simultaneously (Figs. 6.6, 6.7) and can be moved and rotated to allow the operator to infinitely vary the different section parameters and visualize the lesion at different angles (Fig. 6.8).

3. *Volume render mode (VRM):* this is a special feature that can be applied to high-resolution 3D-US [7]. Under normal circumstances, an US image has no depth information because the lateral resolution of the image must be kept as high as possible. The image may be compared to looking at a photographic image on a piece of paper. Three-dimensional US does not change this fact. All three of the surfaces visible on the screen when viewing a 3D volume also have no depth information. This can be compared to looking at a cardboard box from the outside. The contents of the box remain unknown. Volume rendering changes the depth information

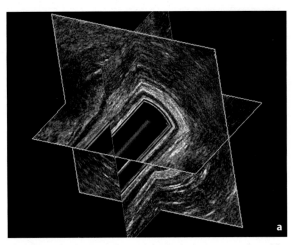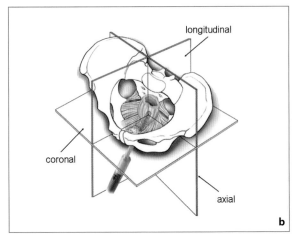

Fig. 6.6 Three-dimensional endovaginal ultrasonography with multiplanar reconstruction. **a** The axial, coronal, and longitudinal planes are simultaneously displayed in the same ultrasonographic image. **b** Schematic illustration. Image obtained using the 2050 probe (B-K Medical). Reproduced from [3]

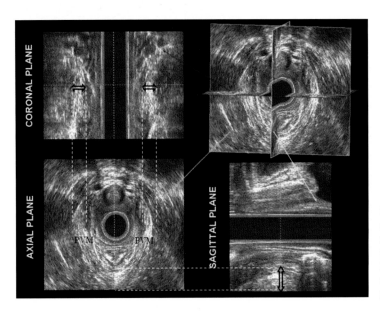

Fig. 6.7 Three-dimensional endovaginal ultrasonography with multiplanar reconstruction. The pubovisceral muscle (PVM) thickness can be measured at the 3 o'clock and 9 o'clock positions on the coronal plane, and at the 6 o'clock position on the sagittal plane (*arrows*)

of a 3D data volume so information inside the cube is reconstructed to some extent (Fig. 6.9). This technique uses a ray tracing model as its basic operation. A beam is projected from each point on the viewing screen (the display) back into and through the volume data. As the beam passes through the volume data, it reaches the different elements (voxels) in the dataset. Depending on the various render mode settings, the data from each voxel may be discarded, may be used to modify the existing value of the beam, or may be stored for reference to the next voxel and used in a filtering calculation. All of these calculations result in the current color or intensity

of the beam being modified in some way. In normal VRM, the following four different postprocessing display parameters can be used [7]:

a. *opacity*: sets the relative transparency of the volume. The higher the value, the further into the volume the ray can travel before being terminated. Because of accumulated brightness as the ray traverses the volume, the net effect is to make the volume appear brighter as this control value is increased

b. *luminance*: sets the inverse of the self-luminance value for the pixels, and should be used in conjunction with the opacity control for displaying

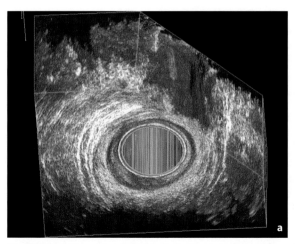
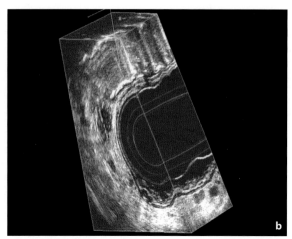

Fig. 6.8 Three-dimensional endovaginal ultrasonography with multiplanar reconstruction: oblique sections (**a**, **b**). Images obtained using the 2050 probe (B-K Medical)

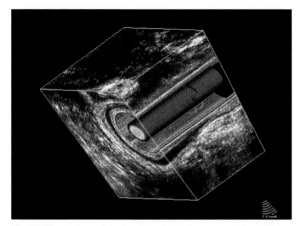

Fig. 6.9 Three-dimensional endovaginal ultrasonography with volume rendering modality. This technique changes the depth information of a 3D data volume, so information inside the cube is reconstructed to some extent

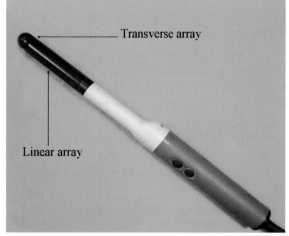

Fig. 6.10 The electronic linear transducer type 8848 (B-K Medical). This probe has a linear and a curved transverse array

certain voxel values for optimal visualization. The final image impression should be adjusted to the reader's requirements by setting the normal brightness and contrast controls

c. *thickness*: sets an upper limit to the penetration of the rays into the volume. This value is used in conjunction with the opacity parameter to determine when the ray traversal is terminated. Increasing the thickness setting allows deeper penetration, and the result is often a slightly smoother presentation together with a significant increase in the visual depth impression of a lesion

d. *filter*: sets the lower threshold value for pixel intensities. Pixel values less than the filter value are not included in determining the intensity of

the final ray value. In normal VRM, the rendering mode stops each ray when the value found reaches a specified value of opacity. This is affected by the setting of some of the controls (opacity, thickness, and to some extent luminance).

Endovaginal US can also be performed with an electronic linear transducer 21 mm in diameter (type 8848, B-K Medical), frequency range 5–12 MHz, focal range 3–60 mm. The 8848 is a biplane transducer with linear and curved transverse arrays (Fig. 6.10). The linear array of this transducer has a long contact surface (65 × 5.5 mm) and a 90° imaging orientation to the longitudinal axis. A computer-controlled acquisition of 350 parallel longitudinal 2D images in 25 s is obtained by connecting

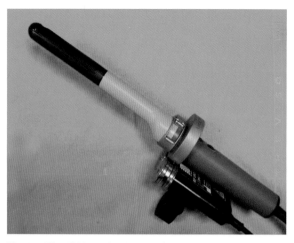

Fig. 6.11 The 180° rotational mover for 3D motorized acquisition is connected to the transducer type 8848 (B-K Medical) by using a magnetic disk

the probe to a 180° rotation mover (UAO513 B-K Medical) (Fig. 6.11). For assessment of the anterior compartment, rotation is performed from the right side (9 o'clock position) to the left side (3 o'clock position) of the patient, and for assessment of the posterior compartment from the 3 o'clock to the 9 o'clock position (Fig. 6.12).

The 8848 transducer also provides evaluation of the vascular pattern of the urethra by the use of color Doppler, and allows a dynamic assessment to be performed by asking the patient to squeeze, or to make a Valsalva maneuver.

6.3 3D Ultrasonographic Anatomy of the Pelvic Floor

No patient preparation is required. We recommend the patient has a comfortable volume of urine in the bladder. No rectal or vaginal contrast is used. The patient is placed in dorsal lithotomy and the probe is inserted into the vagina in a neutral position to avoid excessive pressure on surrounding structures that might distort the anatomy.

Assessment is initially performed with the 2050 transducer to provide a topographical overview of the pelvic floor anatomy (Fig. 6.13). The 3D-data automatic acquisition starts slightly above the bladder neck to end below the external meatus of the urethra. We define four standard levels of assessment in the axial plane (Fig. 6.14) [8].

- *Level I*: at the highest level the bladder base can be visualized on the screen at the 12 o'clock position and the inferior one-third of the rectum at the 6 o'clock position.
- *Level II*: corresponds to the bladder neck, the intramural region of the urethra, and the anorectal junction.
- *Level III*: corresponds to the midurethra and to the upper one-third of the anal canal. To facilitate assessment of the position of these structures and for evaluation of the symmetry between the urethra and

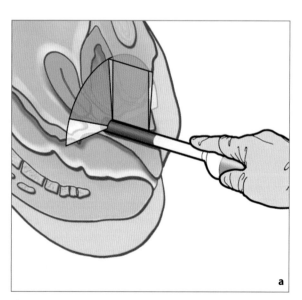
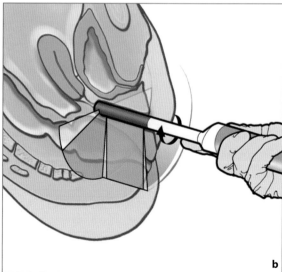

Fig. 6.12 Schematic illustrations of the technique of endovaginal ultrasonography performed by 8848 probe (B-K Medical) for the assessment of the anterior (**a**) and posterior compartment (**b**)

anal canal, a geometric reference point, termed "gothic arch", is defined at the 12 o'clock position, specifically at the point where the inferior branches of the pubic bone join at the symphysis pubis (SP). At this level, the muscles of the lateral compartment can be accurately evaluated. The pubovisceralis muscle (PVM) is completely visualized as a multilayer highly echoic sling, lying posteriorly to the anal canal and attaching to the pubic bone (Fig. 6.15) [9, 10]. The fiber directions of the PVM are oblique to the axial scan plane, such that the entire muscle loop is not visible in any one slice. For this reason, we use a plane parallel to the PVM, tilting the reconstructed axial plane from the most protruding surface of the SP, anteriorly, to the lowest border of the PVM surrounding the anus posteriorly (Fig. 6.16). The thickness of the PVM can be measured in the coronal plane at the 3 o'clock (left branch) and 9

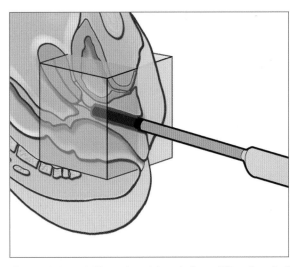

Fig.6.13 Schematic illustration of the technique of 3D endovaginal ultrasonography performed by 2050 probe (B-K Medical) for assessment of the pelvic floor

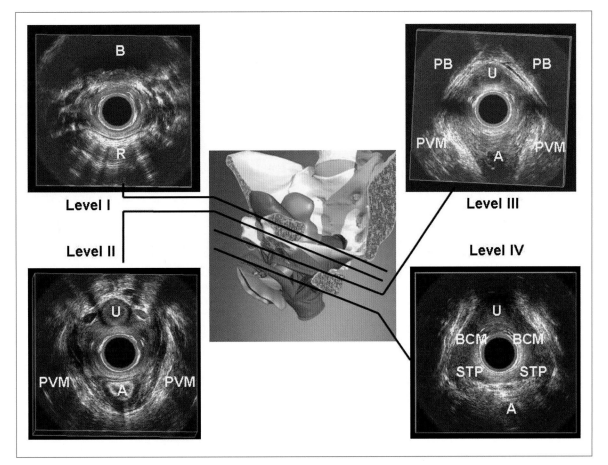

Fig.6.14 Four standard levels of assessment of the female pelvic floor with endovaginal ultrasound (2050 transducer, B-K Medical). Right side of the image is left side of the patient. *A*, anal canal; *B*, bladder; *BCM*, bulbocavernosus muscle; *PB*, pubic bone; *PVM*, pubovisceral muscle; *R*, rectum; *STP*, superficial transverse perinei muscle; *U*, urethra

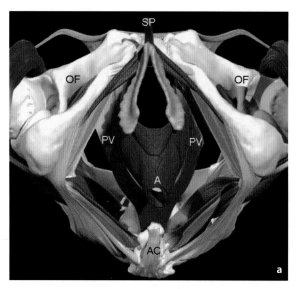

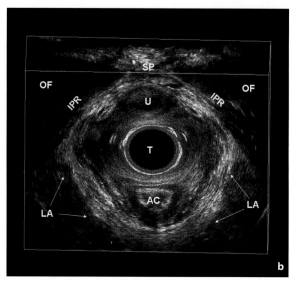

Fig. 6.15 Female pelvic floor: Level III. **a** Schematic illustration (© Primal Pictures Ltd., with permission). **b** Ultrasonographic images obtained by 2050 probe (B-K Medical). Reference point of symmetry between the urethra and anal canal is the symphysis pubis. *A*, anal canal; *AC*, anococcygeal ligament; *IPR*, inferior pubic rami; *LA*, levator ani; *OF*, obturator foramen; *PV*, pubovisceral muscle; *SP*, symphysis pubis; *T*, transducer; *U*, urethra

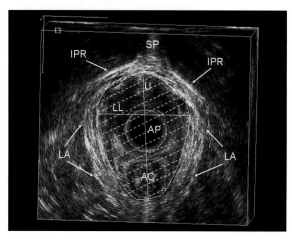

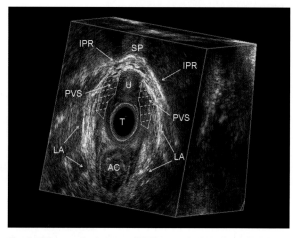

Fig. 6.16 The levator hiatus (*LH*) indices are measured at level III. In this 28-year-old female the anteroposterior diameter (*AP*) was 42.6 mm, the transverse diameter (*LL*) was 32.2 mm and LH area was 12.8 cm^2. Scan obtained by 2050 transducer. *AC*, anal canal; *IPR*, inferior pubic rami; *LA*, levator ani; *SP*, symphysis pubis; *U*, urethra

Fig. 6.17 Paravaginal spaces (*PVS*) measured on the right (*1*) and left (*2*) sides (1.69 cm^2 and 1.55 cm^2, respectively). Scan obtained by 2050 transducer (*T*) (B-K Medical). *AC*, anal canal; *IPR*, inferior pubic rami; *LA*, levator ani; *SP*, symphysis pubis; *U*, urethra

o'clock position (right branch), and in the sagittal plane at the 6 o'clock position (Fig. 6.7). In the same tilted axial plane, levator hiatus (LH) measurements are determined. The distance between the inferior margin of the SP and the inner margin of the PVM is defined as the anteroposterior (AP) diameter of the LH. The transverse diameter of the LH is measured between the inner margins of the lateral branches of the PVM at the level of their attachment

to the pubic bone. The levator hiatus area can also be calculated (Fig. 6.16). In the same scan, we determine the area of the paravaginal spaces, located between the lateral border of the vaginal wall and the medial border of the PVM (Fig. 6.17).

In a study on 20 nulliparous females we found that increasing LH area was correlated with an increase in LH anteroposterior diameter ($\rho = 0.7$; $P = 0.0007$) and LH laterolateral (LL) diameter

Table 6.1 Biometric indices of the relevant pelvic floor structures assessed by 3D-EVUS with 360° rotating transducer [8]

Parameter	Plane of examination	Mean	SD
Levator hiatus			
AP diameter (cm)	Tilted axial plane	4.85	0.46
LL diameter (cm)	Tilted axial plane	3.29	0.18
Area (cm²)	Tilted axial plane	12.0	1.70
Paravaginal space (cm²)			
Left side	Tilted axial plane	1.05	0.10
Right side	Tilted axial plane	1.05	0.10
Pubovisceral muscle thickness (mm)			
3 o'clock	Coronal plane	6.0	0.5
9 o'clock	Coronal plane	6.0	0.6
6 o'clock	Sagittal plane	5.5	0.7
Urogenital hiatus			
AP diameter (cm)	Tilted axial plane	3.0	0.45
Ischiocavernosus muscle length (cm)			
Left side	Tilted axial plane	3.32	0.22
Right side	Tilted axial plane	3.32	0.27
Superficial transverse perinei muscle length (cm)			
Left side	Tilted axial plane	2.5	0.20
Right side	Tilted axial plane	2.6	0.18
Bulbocavernosus muscles thickness (mm)			
Left side	Tilted axial plane	3.15	0.40
Right side	Tilted axial plane	3.11	0.28

AP, anteroposterior; *LL*, laterolateral; *SD*, standard deviation

($\rho = 0.58$; $P = 0.008$). Statistically significant correlations were also found between LH area and age ($\rho = 0.5$; $P = 0.03$) and between the area of the paravaginal spaces and age ($\rho = 0.7$; $P = 0.00038$) (Table 6.1) [8].

- *Level IV:* at the outer level, the superficial perineal muscles, the perineal body, the distal urethra, and the middle and inferior one-third of the anal canal can be evaluated. To visualize these structures in their entirety, the reconstructed axial plane is tilted from the most protruding surface of the SP anteriorly, to the ischiopubic rami laterally so that the different insertion points of the perineal muscles can be seen (Fig. 6.18). The ischiocavernosus muscles are visualized as two hypoechoic bands extending from the SP to the ischiopubic rami. The superficial transverse perinei muscles (STP) are visualized as two hypoechoic bands lying transversely between the ischial tuberosity and the perineal body. The bulbocavernosus muscles appear as an oval hypoechoic structure surrounding the vaginal wall and extending from the SP to the perineal body.

In the same scan, we can determine the anteroposterior diameter of the urogenital hiatus (UGH), corresponding to the SP–perineal body distance [11]. We have also found that the UGH AP diameter significantly correlated with LH area ($\rho = 0.58$; $P = 0.008$) (Table 6.1) [8].

6.3.1 Assessment of the Anterior Compartment

Using the sagittal plane of the 3D volume acquired by 2050 transducer, we can obtain a longitudinal view of the anterior compartment and can assess the bladder neck and the urethra (Fig. 6.19). Additional information is provided by using the 8848 transducer (Fig. 6.10) [8]. Assessment of the anterior compartment in the midsagittal section includes measurements of the length (from the bladder neck to the external urethral orifice) and thickness of the urethra, bladder–symphysis distance (from the bladder neck to the lowest margin of the SP), rhabdosphincter (RS) length and thickness,

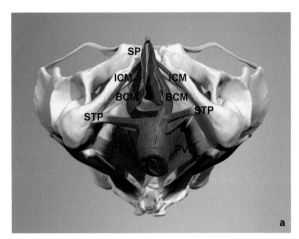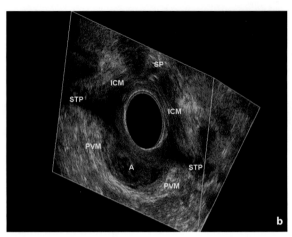

Fig. 6.18 Superficial structures of the lower pelvis: Level IV. **a** Schematic illustration (© Primal Pictures Ltd., with permission). **b** Ultrasonographic image obtained by 2050 transducer (B-K Medical). *A*, anal canal; *BCM*, bulbocavernosus muscles; *ICM*, ischiocavernosus muscles; *PVM*, pubovisceral muscle; *SP*, symphysis pubis; *STP*, superficial transverse perinei muscle

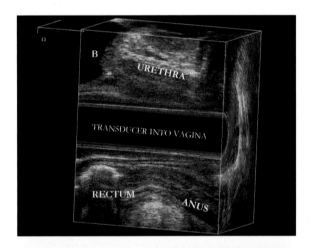

Fig. 6.19 Three-dimensional reconstruction of the longitudinal plane allows assessment of the anterior and posterior compartments. *B*, bladder. Image obtained by 2050 transducer (B-K Medical)

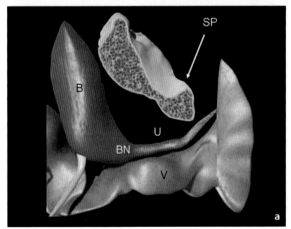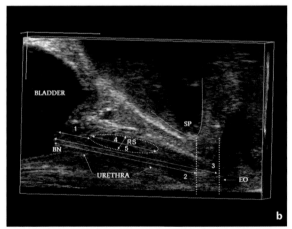

Fig. 6.20 Longitudinal view of the anterior compartment. **a** Schematic illustration (© Primal Pictures Ltd., with permission). **b** Ultrasonographic image obtained by 8848 transducer (B-K Medical) using the linear array. Measurements include: bladder neck-rhabdosphincter distance (*1*), bladder-symphysis distance (*2*), urethral length (*3*), rhabdosphincter length (*4*) and thickness (*5*). *B*, bladder; *BN*, bladder neck; *EO*, external urethral orifice; *RS*, rhabdosphincter; *SP*, symphysis pubis; *U*, urethra; *V*, vagina

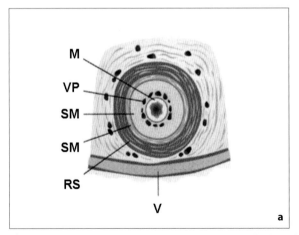
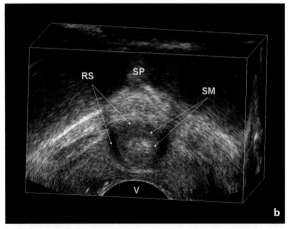

Fig. 6.21 a Schematic representation of the midurethra in the axial plane. b Ultrasonographic image obtained by 8848 transducer (B-K Medical) using the axial array. Rhabdosphincter (*RS*) appears as a slightly echoic structure overlapping a more echoic smooth urethral muscle (*SM*). *M*, mucosa; *SP*, symphysis pubis; *V*, vagina; *VP*, vascular plexus

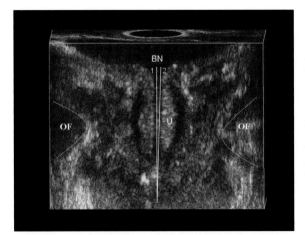

Fig. 6.22 Coronal view of the urethra (*U*). In this plane, the omega angle, formed by the vertical line passing through the bladder neck (*BN*) (*1*) and the long axis of the urethra (*2*), can be measured. Image obtained by 8848 transducer. *OF*, obturator foramen

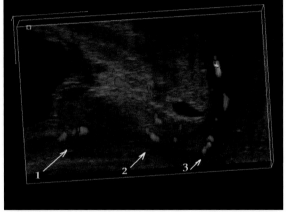

Fig. 6.23 Vessels supporting the urethral complex form three levels (1.intramural part of the urethra, 2.midurethra, 3.distal part of the urethra) in the longitudinal plane. Scan obtained by 8848 transducer (B-K Medical) using the linear array

and the distance between the bladder neck and the RS (Fig. 6.20). The striated urethral sphincter (RS) starts in the upper part of the urethra approximately 9.1 mm (range: ± 0.94 mm) from the urinary bladder neck. In transverse section it has a typical omega shape, surrounding the ventral and lateral sides of the midurethra and creating a raphe connected to the anterior vaginal wall. Its echogenicity is slightly lower than that of smooth urethral muscle (Fig. 6.21).

In our study on 20 nulliparous females, significant correlations were found among the following parameters: urethral width with urethral length ($\rho = 0.65$; $P = 0.002$) and urethral thickness ($\rho = 0.5$; $P = 0.02$); urethral volume with urethral thickness ($\rho = 0.7$; $P =$

0.002), urethral width ($\rho = 0.87$; $P = 0.0001$), urethral length ($\rho = 0.75$; $P = 0.00005$) and RS volume ($\rho = 0.5$; $P = 0.03$) [8]. The position of the urethra is determined in the reconstructed coronal plane by measuring the angle that we term "omega angle", between the vertical line passing through the bladder neck and the long axis of the urethra (Fig. 6.22).

The urethra is surrounded by connective tissue containing numerous vessels. In the reconstructed longitudinal plane these vessels appear to form three levels (Fig. 6.23). The first level, situated cranially, is seen below the urinary bladder neck. The second level is situated in the middle region of the urethra penetrating from the ventral side to reach the RS. The vessels pen-

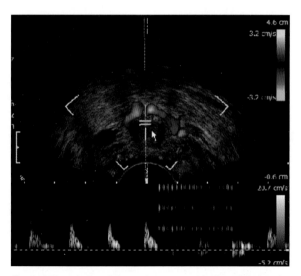

Fig. 6.24 Vascularity of the urethra assessed in the axial plane by color Doppler. Scan obtained by 8848 transducer (B-K Medical)

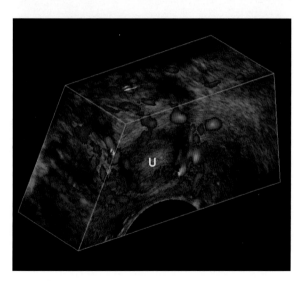

Fig. 6.25 Three-dimensional color Doppler imaging. Spatial distribution of the urethral vessels. Image obtained by 8848 transducer (B-K Medical). *U*, urethra

etrating here, on transverse section, have a typical "V" shape (Fig. 6.24). The third and lowest level is situated below the lower margin of the SP, in the area of the external ostium.

Using 3D color Doppler imaging, we can observe the global vascularization of the urethra (Fig. 6.25). It is possible to visualize the spatial distribution of blood flow, to demonstrate vessel continuity and vessel branching in different planes, and to evaluate the pattern of vascularization (density of vessels, branching, caliber changes and tortuosity).

6.3.2 Assessment of the Lateral Compartment

The area posterior to the pubic bone is dense with bands of intertwined levator ani muscles which defy conventional description of the levator ani being made up of the puborectalis, pubococcygeus, and iliococcygeus muscles. The anatomy of distal subdivisions of the levator ani muscle was further described in a recent study [12]. Using a nomenclature based on the attachment points of different subdivisions of the levator ani muscles, the muscles posterior to the pubic bone are identified as the pubovaginalis, puboanalis, and puboperinealis as the subdivisions of the PVM [13]. Margulies et al demonstrated excellent reliability and reproducibility in visualizing major portions of the levator ani in nulliparous volunteers with magnetic resonance imaging (MRI) [14]. However, because the puboanalis, pubovaginalis, and puboperinealis are small, they have proved to be difficult to visualize in the rigid axial, coronal, and sagittal views of MRI.

Shobeiri et al [15] identified the subdivisions of the distal levator ani as seen on 3D-EVUS in cadaveric dissections. Endovaginal scanning was performed as described earlier in this chapter. Echogenic structures suspicious for being STP, pubovaginalis, puboperinealis, puboanalis, puborectalis, and iliococcygeus muscles were tagged with biopsy needles (MPM Medical, Elmwood Park, NJ) and marked with 1 mL indigo carmine dye for localization. Additionally, any other unknown structures and possible defects were tagged in the same manner (Fig. 6.26). After each pelvis was scanned with US, the findings were recorded digitally, and each pelvis

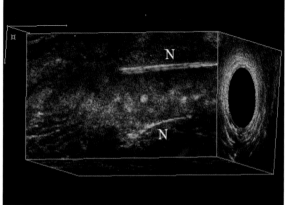

Fig. 6.26 Ultrasound needle (*N*) localization of muscles. Sagittal view of two needles inserted into the iliococcygeus muscle. Image obtained by 2050 transducer (B-K Medical)

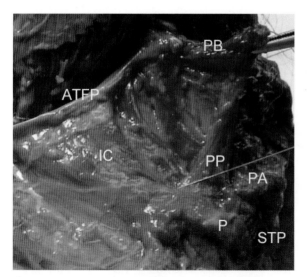

Fig. 6.27 Gross cadaveric dissection. A needle is seen inserted into the puboperinealis muscle (*PP*). The other structures are identified: *ATFP*, arcus tendineus fascia pelvis; *IC*, iliococcygeus muscle; *PA*, puboanalis muscle; *PB*, pubic bone or pubic bone insertion; *P*, perineum; *STP*, superficial transverse perinei muscle

dissected to locate each of the numbered needles in all the cadaveric specimens (Fig. 6.27) [15].

In the US imaging and the correlative dissections of the fresh-frozen pelvis, the STP was the first muscle visualized (Fig. 6.28). Immediately cephalad to it was the puboperinealis insertion into the perineal body. In the dissections, the puboanalis was located deep and lateral to the puboperinealis and had a wide base inserting itself into the anorectal fibers. Puboanalis fibers intermixed with lateral supportive fibers of the rectum to form the posterior arcus, which in turn fused with laterally located fibers of the iliococcygeus [16]. The pubovaginalis was a short band 3 cm cephalad to the ischiopubic rami, causing an indentation in the anterior vaginal epithelium. The puborectalis insertion was lateral, wrapping itself around the rectum 3 cm cephalad to the anus. By US, the puboperinealis had mixed echogenicity and was located immediately cephalad to superficial transverse perinei. The puboanalis was identified as a triangular hypoechoic area lateral to puboperinealis. The pubovaginalis was identified as dense muscular bands at the level of the midurethra in cadavers, and as hypoechoic areas causing heart-shaped angulation of the anterior vaginal mucosa. All these structures and the iliococcygeus were accurately identified by needle identification during 3D-EVUS, and authenticated by gross dissection (Fig. 6.28) [15].

Shobeiri et al [15] also performed the 3D scans in

50 nulliparous volunteers to develop a scoring system for visualization of the pelvic floor muscles. The characteristic features of each of the five separate levator subdivisions were determined on a three-level system. Level 1 contained the muscles that insert into the perineal body, namely the STP, puboperinealis, and puboanalis muscles. Superficial transverse perinei served as the reference point. Level 2 contained the attachment of the pubovaginalis, puboperinealis, puboanalis, puborectalis, and iliococcygeus to the pubic bone. Level 3 contained subdivisions visible cephalad to the inferior pubic ramus, namely the iliococcygeus which winged out towards the ischial spine. The visualization of the pubococcygeus was debatable, and since this structure was not reliably visualized during pelvic floor dissection, it was not included. Using this system (muscle subdivisions "visible" or "not visible" at three levels), they calculated the inter-rater reliability. There was 98% (95% CI: 0.92–1), 96% (95% CI: 0.95–0.99), and 92% (95% CI: 0.88–0.95) agreement for level 1, 2, and 3 muscles respectively. κ values for agreement were calculated for individual muscles as follows: STP and puborectalis, κ = 1 (excellent agreement); puboperinealis, pubovaginalis, and puboanalis: κ = 0.645 (good agreement); iliococcygeus, κ = 0.9 (excellent agreement) [15].

6.3.3 Assessment of the Posterior Compartment

The posterior compartment is evaluated by using the axial, sagittal, and coronal planes of the 3D volume acquired by 2050 (Fig. 6.19) or 8848 transducers (Fig. 6.12) [8]. Assessment includes measurements of the internal (IAS) and external anal sphincters (EAS). In the axial plane the IAS appears as a concentric hypoechoic ring surrounding a more echogenic central mucosa, and the EAS appears as a concentric band of mixed echogenicity surrounding the IAS (Fig. 6.29). The thickness of the internal and external sphincters is taken in the coronal plane at the 3 o'clock and 9 o'clock positions. An echogenic disruption is defined as a gap. The location of any defect is described using a clock-face notation. The longitudinal plane allows examination of the perineal body, appearing as a triangular-shaped, slightly hyperechoic structure anterior to the anal sphincter, and of the rectovaginal septum (RVS), visualized as a three-layer-structure (hyperechoic,

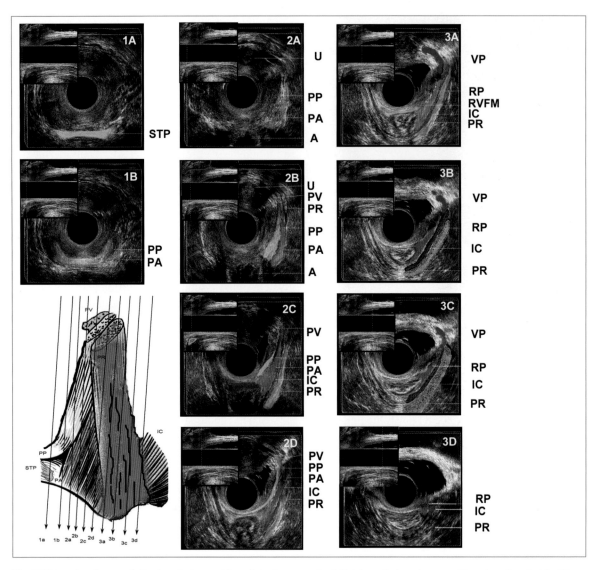

Fig. 6.28 Drawing (bottom left): the relative position of the levator ani subdivisions during ultrasound imaging: Levels 1A–3D are identified in the individual panels. Midline structures are identified in lateral views with corresponding colors in the picture insert at the upper left corner of the ultrasound images at each level. The dotted green vertical line in the insert corresponds to the relative position in the vagina where the image is obtained. Level 1A: at 0 cm, the first muscle seen is the superficial transverse perinei muscle (*STP*; green) with mixed echogenicity. Level 1B: immediately cephalad to the superficial transverse perinei is the puboperinealis muscle (*PP*; yellow) that can be traced to pubic bone with manipulation of the 3D cube. It comes in at a 45° angle as a mixed echoic band to join the perineal body. Lateral to it, the puboanalis muscle (*PA*, pink) is seen as a hypoechoic triangle. Level 2A: this level marks the attachment of the muscles to the pubic arch. The external urethral meatus is visible (dark red). The puboperinealis and puboanalis insertions are highlighted (*A*, anus; *U*, urethra). Level 2B: the pubovaginalis (*PV*, blue) and puborectalis muscles (*PR*, mustard) insertions come into view. The urethra (*U*) and the bladder are outlined (red) in the lateral view. Level 2C: the heart-shaped vaginal sulcus (outlined in red) marks the pubovaginalis insertion. Iliococcygeus (*IC*) fibers (red) come into view. The perineal body is outlined in the lateral view. Level 2D: the puboanalis (*PA*) is starting to thin out. The puborectalis (*PR*) is seen in the lateral view. Level 3A: the puboperinealis (*PP*) and puboanalis (*PA*) become obscure. Anatomically, the puboanalis becomes a thick fibromuscularis layer forming a tendineus sheet, the rectal pillar (*RP*). The perivesical venous plexus (*VP*) is prominent (purple). The rectovaginal fibromuscularis (*RVFM*, green) is shown in sagittal view as a continuous mixed echogenic structure approaching the perineal body and laterally attaching to the RP. Level 3B: the rectal pillar (orange) is easily seen. The iliococcygeus (*IC*) becomes prominent and widens. Level 3C: the iliococcygeus (*IC*) widens further and inserts into the arcus tendineus fascia pelvis. Level 3D: the puborectalis (*PR*) fades out of view. The puborectalis (mustard) and iliococcygeus (red) are outlined in the lateral view showing their entire course

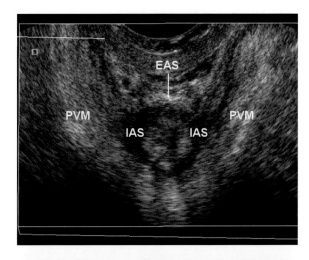

Fig. 6.29 Axial view of the anal complex obtained by 8848 transducer (B-K Medical) using the transverse array. The external anal sphincter (*EAS*) appears as a hyperechoic ring surrounding the hypoechoic ring of the internal anal sphincter (*IAS*); *PVM*, pubovisceral muscle

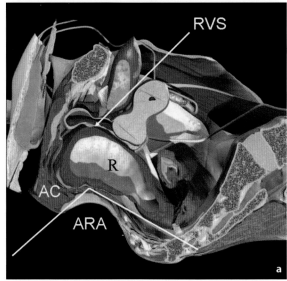
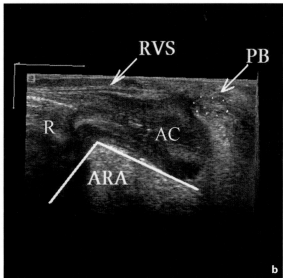

Fig. 6.30 Longitudinal view of the posterior compartment. **a** Schematic illustration (© Primal Pictures Ltd., with permission). **b** Ultrasonographic image obtained by 8848 transducer (B-K Medical) using the linear array. *AC*, anal canal; *ARA*, anorectal angle; *PB*, perineal body; *R*, rectum; *RVS*, rectovaginal septum

hypoechoic, and hyperechoic layers) between the external margin of the vagina and the external part of the rectal wall (Fig. 6.30). An RVS defect is defined as a discontinuity in this echographic pattern. In the midsagittal plane, the anorectal angle (ARA), formed by the longitudinal axis of the anal canal and the posterior rectal wall, can also be measured.

6.4 Discussion

The pelvic floor is a 3D mechanical apparatus with a complex job description [17]. When we display a nor-

mal 2D-US cross-sectional view, there are many elements of the image that will not be correctly recognized as components of a 3D structure, or at least not perceived in their true spatial relationships. With ultrasound imaging we are usually looking at a 3D structure that contains a solid volume of echoes and which therefore does not readily translate onto a 2D projection. In routine clinical scanning, the operator forms a mental representation of the 3D anatomic or pathological structure, while viewing a large series of 2D slices interactively. In this case the operator is using manual sense information about the physical location of the individual slices in building up 3D subjective impressions.

3D- and indeed 4D-US has been promoted by different ultrasound companies for several years. The acquisition of a 3D data volume and the underlying techniques are, however, different from application to application. The pelvic floor requires extremely high-resolution 3D volumes of data for adequate and precise diagnostic evaluation. An advantage of working with high-resolution 3D-US is that the 3D image does not remain fixed, rather, it can be freely rotated, rendered, tilted, and sliced to allow the operator to infinitely vary the different section parameters and visualize the different structures at different angles to obtain the most information from the data. After data are acquired, it is possible to select coronal anterior–posterior or posterior–anterior as well as sagittal right–left views, together with any oblique image plane. The multiview function allows the reader to see up to six different and specialized views at once with multiplanar reconstruction. Three-dimensional US allows us to assess directly the different planes in which the significant anatomic structures of the pelvic floor (pelvic bones, pelvic organs, pelvic floor muscles, fascia, and ligaments) are located.

Two structures extensively evaluated by 3D-EVUS imaging are the LH and PVM [8]. Assessment of these structures is important because significant correlations have been reported between levator ani defects and increased LH size and pelvic organ descent [18] (see Chapter 37). Tilting the axial plane in the acquired 3D data volume provides a maximal transverse section of the PVM, not otherwise obtainable with conventional 2D-EVUS, thus avoiding the artifacts due to its oblique shape. Our measurements of PVM thickness (6.0 mm on both sides) were comparable with those reported by Tunn et al [19] with MRI (6.3 mm on both sides). As the lateral attachments of the PVM to the pubic bone are also clearly visualized, 3D-EVUS can be utilized to document major levator ani trauma, in a similar way to 3D translabial ultrasound (TLUS) [20] and MRI [13, 18]. This technique also allows a detailed evaluation of the levator ani subdivisions [15] which are not visualized by TLUS [20]. Although it may be argued that these subdivisions of the levator ani muscle are not important, knowing exactly which muscles are damaged may not be inconsequential in clinical practice. Many of the functions of the pelvic floor governing micturition, defecation, and intercourse are only recently understood by describing the subdivisions of the levator ani muscle. Attachments are important

because the muscles exert their action by contraction. For example, a patient with defecatory dysfunction due to a detached puboperinealis will not benefit from a posterior repair. Also, reattachment of the puboperinealis does not address defecatory dysfunction due to loss of anorectal angle from a damaged puborectalis.

Biometric indices of the LH determined in the axial tilted plane in our preliminary study on 20 nulliparous females (AP diameter 4.84 cm, LL diameter 3.28 cm, hiatal area 12 cm^2) [8] were comparable to the results published by Dietz et al [9] in 49 nulliparous females with 3D-TLUS (AP diameter 4.52 cm, LL diameter 3.75 cm, hiatal area 11.25 cm^2), and Tunn et al [19] in 20 nulliparous females with MRI (AP diameter 4.1 cm, LL diameter 3.3 cm, hiatal area 12.8 cm^2). In the same tilted axial plane, the paravaginal spaces and urethral symmetry can be assessed [8]. This has clinical relevance, as a lateral paravaginal defect can be suspected when a wider paravaginal space or an asymmetry of the urethra is observed . It has been hypothesized that paravaginal defects, due to separation of the endopelvic fascia from the arcus tendineus fascia pelvis, are the underlying anatomical abnormalities in anterior vaginal wall descent [21, 22] (see Chapter 37).

Understanding the anatomy of the pelvic diaphragm is important for urogynecologists and proctologists. Damage to the perineal muscles and/or perineal body, frequently occurring during vaginal childbirth, is associated with pelvic organ prolapse [14]. As reported by Orno et al [23], these muscles cannot be visualized in their entirety by using 2D-EVUS because they originate from the walls of the pelvis and converge at the perineal body from different angles. Three-dimensional EVUS could overcome this limitation. Tilting the reconstructed axial plane from the SP, anteriorly, to the ischiopubic rami laterally, we are able to evaluate the different insertion points and to determine the dimensions of the superficial perineal muscles. In contrast with these findings, 3D-TLUS cannot properly assess the perineal structures due to the shape of the transducer, its position on the introital area, and a limited field of view of the acquired volume [22]. In the same scan, the AP diameter of the UGH can also be measured. Our study confirmed that this diameter had a positive correlation with LH area [8].

In the diagnostics of the anterior compartment, it is very important to assess the morphology and location of the urethra and to evaluate its supportive structures [19]. High-resolution 3D-EVUS gives the opportunity to assess the urethral position in three different planes and allows the anatomy and morphology of the bladder neck and urethral complex to be quantified [8] (see Chapter 15). Biometric indices of the urethral complex determined in our study [8] were comparable to the results reported by Umek et al [6] with 3D transrectal US, with regard to both urethral thickness (11 mm on vaginal vs. 11.5 mm on rectal scans) and width (14 mm on vaginal vs. 15 mm on rectal scans) and to RS thickness (3.0 mm on vaginal vs. 2.7 mm on rectal scans) and volume (0.46 cm^3 on vaginal vs. 0.5 cm^3 on rectal scans). Additionally, the mean bladder neck–RS distance determined in our study (9.1 mm) was consistent with the measurement reported by using MRI (10 mm) [24].

The current gold standard for assessment of the posterior compartment is considered to be endoanal US (EAUS) [3, 7]. Endovaginal US offers an alternative imaging modality of the anal sphincter complex and has proven to be as accurate as EAUS [2]. Our preliminary results using this method [8] confirmed that the thickness of the anal sphincter was comparable to the measurements reported in the literature by using EAUS, TLUS, or MRI [25–27]. However, regardless of the absolute dimensions of the anal sphincters, the most relevant utility of EVUS applies in the detection of localized EAS defects when EAUS cannot depict any sphincter damage, in order to confirm or exclude EAUS findings in patients with idiopathic fecal incontinence, passive fecal incontinence, or obstructive defecation disorders. The most important advantage of EVUS compared to EAUS is the access to the longitudinal plane that allows assessment of the ARA, rectovaginal septum, and perineal body [8].

High-resolution 3D-EVUS provides a detailed assessment of the pelvic floor for both identifying and measuring specific anatomic structures and for understanding their complex spatial arrangements. It is relatively easy to perform, time efficient, correlates well with other imaging modalities, and delivers additional information on urethral complex and superficial perineal structures at the same time.

References

1. Tunn R, Petri E. Introital and transvaginal ultrasound as the main tool in the assessment of urogenital and pelvic floor dysfunction: an imaging panel and practical approach. Ultrasound Obstet Gynecol 2003;22:205–213.

2. Sultan AH, Loder PB, Bartram CI et al. Vaginal endosonography. New approach to image the undisturbed anal sphincter. Dis Colon Rectum 1994;37:1296–1299.

3. Santoro GA, Fortling B. New technical developments in endoanal and endorectal ultrasonography. In: Santoro GA, Di Falco G (eds) Benign anorectal diseases. Diagnosis with endoanal and endorectal ultrasonography and new treatment options. Springer-Verlag Italy, Milan, 2006, pp 13–26.

4. Dietz HP, Steensma AB. Posterior compartment prolapse on two-dimensional and three-dimensional pelvic floor ultrasound: the distinction between true rectocele, perineal hypermobility and enterocele. Ultrasound Obstet Gynecol 2005;26:73–77.

5. Mitterberger M, Pinggera GM, Mueller T et al. Dynamic transurethral sonography and 3-dimensional reconstruction of the rhabdosphincter and urethra: initial experience in continent and incontinent women. J Ultrasound Med 2006; 25:315–320.

6. Umek WH, Lami T, Stutterecker D et al. The urethra during pelvic floor contraction: observations on three-dimensional ultrasound. Obstet Gynecol 2002;100:796–800.

7. Santoro GA, Fortling B. The advantages of volume rendering in three-dimensional endosonography of the anorectum. Dis Colon Rectum 2007;50:359–368.

8. Santoro GA, Wieczorek AP, Stankiewicz A et al. High-resolution three-dimensional endovaginal ultrasonography in the assessment of pelvic floor anatomy: a preliminary study. Int Urogynecol J 2009;20:1213–1222.

9. Dietz HP, Shek C, Clarke B. Biometry of the pubovisceral muscle and levator hiatus by three-dimensional pelvic floor ultrasound. Ultrasound Obstet Gynecol 2005; 25:580–585.

10. Ashton-Miller JA, DeLancey JO. Functional anatomy of the female pelvic floor. Ann N Y Acad Sci 2007;1101:266–296.

11. DeLancey JOL, Hurd WW. Size of the urogenital hiatus in the levator ani muscles in normal women and women with pelvic organ prolapse. Obstet Gynecol 1998;91:364–368.

12. Shobeiri SA, Chesson RR, Gasser RF. The internal innervation and morphology of the human female levator ani muscle. Am J Obstet Gynecol 2008;199:686.e1–6.

13. Kearney R, Sawhney R, DeLancey JO. Levator ani muscle anatomy evaluated by origin-insertion pairs. Obstet Gynecol 2004;104:168–173.

14. Margulies RU, Hsu Y, Kearney R et al. Appearance of the levator ani muscle subdivisions in magnetic resonance images. Obstet Gynecol 2006;107:1064–1069.

15. Shobeiri SA, LeClaire E, Nihira MA, et al. Appearance of the levator ani muscle subdivisions in endovaginal three-dimensional ultrasonography. Obstet Gynecol 2009; 114: 66–72.

16. Lien KC, Mooney B, DeLancey JO et al. Levator ani muscle stretch induced by simulated vaginal birth. Obstet Gynecol 2004;103:31–40.

17. DeLancey JO. The hidden epidemic of pelvic floor dysfunction: achievable goals for improved prevention and treatment. Am J Obstet Gynecol 2005;192:1488–1495.

18. DeLancey JO, Morgan DM, Fenner DE et al. Comparison of levator ani muscle defects and function in women with and without pelvic organ prolapse. Obstet Gynecol 2007; 109:295–302.

19. Tunn R, DeLancey JOL, Howard D et al. Anatomic variations in the levator ani muscle, endopelvic fascia and urethra in nulliparas evaluated by magnetic resonance imaging. Am J Obstet Gynecol 2003;188:116–121.

20. Dietz HP. Quantification of major morphological abnormalities of the levator ani. Ultrasound Obstet Gynecol 2007;29:329–334.

21. DeLancey JO. Fascial and muscular abnormalities in women with urethral hypermobility and anterior vaginal wall prolapse. Am J Obstet Gynecol 2002;187:93–98.

22. Dietz HP, Steensma AB, Hastings R. Three-dimensional ultrasound imaging of the pelvic floor: the effect of parturition on paravaginal support structures. Ultrasound Obstet Gynecol 2003;21:589–595.

23. Orno AK, Marsal K, Herbst A. Ultrasonographic anatomy of perineal structures during pregnancy and immediately following obstetric injury. Ultrasound Obstet Gynecol 2008; 32:527–534.

24. Umek WH, Kearney R, Morgan DM. The axial location of structural regions in the urethra: a magnetic resonance study in nulliparous women. Obstet Gynecol 2003;102:1039–1045.

25. Williams AB, Cheetham MJ, Bartram CI et al. Gender differences in the longitudinal pressure profile of the anal canal related to anatomical structure as demonstrated on three-dimensional anal endosonography. Br J Surg 2000;87:1674–1679.

26. Hall RJ, Rogers RG, Saiz L, Qualls C. Translabial ultrasound assessment of the anal sphincter complex: normal measurements of the internal and external anal sphincters at the proximal, mid and distal levels. Int Urogynecol J 2007;18:881–888.

27. Schaefer A, Enck P, Furst G et al. Anatomy of the anal sphincters. Comparison of anal endosonography to magnetic resonance imaging. Dis Colon Rectum 1994;37:777–781.

Translabial Ultrasonography: Methodology and Normal Pelvic Floor Anatomy

7

Hans Peter Dietz

Abstract Translabial or transperineal ultrasound is fast becoming the standard imaging method for the assessment of women with symptoms of lower urinary tract dysfunction and pelvic organ prolapse. Three/four-dimensional (3D/4D) imaging has greatly added to the utility of the method, and suitable equipment is becoming widely available. This chapter describes the technical requirements and equipment as well as the basic and advanced methodology of 2D-, 3D-, and 4D-ultrasound in the investigation of pelvic floor and lower urinary tract disorders.

Keywords 3D • Female pelvic organ prolapse • Incontinence • Lower urinary tract • Pelvic floor • Ultrasound

7.1 Introduction

More than 20 years have passed since the introduction of ultrasound imaging into the clinical evaluation of pelvic floor disorders, and this technique is still not regarded as standard by many clinicians working in this field. If this appears odd, then one should consider the fate of transvaginal ultrasound – first described in the late 1960s, and finally generally accepted in the 1990s. Physicians have been slow in realizing that clinical assessment alone is a very inadequate tool for assessing pelvic floor function and anatomy, but then this resistance to new technology is not exactly unusual in clinical medicine. In the age of evidence-based medicine, the standards of proof are becoming higher all the time, and it is notoriously difficult to prove that a given diagnostic intervention substantially improves patient care. I am not aware of any such proof for any of the currently used diagnostic interventions in pelvic floor medicine, and the same is true for imaging, regardless of the route and technology.

However, we are tasked to provide optimal care to patients seeking our help, and it is hard to see how this could be achieved, in the year 2009, without utilizing imaging. Our examination skills are poor, focusing on surface anatomy rather than true structural abnormalities, and recurrence after pelvic reconstructive surgery is common [1], proving that there is ample room for improvement. I have no doubt that, in theory, clinical assessment skills could be improved to such a degree as to make imaging unnecessary in many cases. However, this clearly is not the case at present, and it is unlikely to happen unless we allow imaging techniques to demonstrate what (and where) the actual problems are. To give just one example: the missing link between vaginal childbirth and prolapse – major levator trauma in the form of avulsion of the anteromedial aspects of the puborectalis muscle off the pelvic sidewall [2, 3] – is palpable, but palpation

H.P. Dietz
Department of Obstetrics, Gynecology and Neonatology,
Sydney Medical School-Nepean, University of Sydney,
Australia

- Recurrent urinary tract infections
- Symptoms of the overactive bladder: urgency, frequency, nocturia and/or urge urinary incontinence
- Stress urinary incontinence
- Insensible urine loss
- Bladder-related pain
- Persistent dysuria
- Symptoms of voiding dysfunction: hesitancy, straining to void, stop–start voiding, slow stream
- Symptoms of prolapse, i.e. the sensation of a lump or a dragging sensation
- Symptoms of obstructed defecation: straining at stool, chronic constipation, vaginal or perineal digitation, and the sensation of incomplete bowel emptying
- Fecal incontinence
- Pelvic or vaginal pain after anti-incontinence or prolapse surgery
- Vaginal discharge or bleeding after anti-incontinence or prolapse surgery

of levator trauma requires considerable skill and teaching [4–6], preferably with imaging confirmation. My personal experience with dozens of trainees would suggest a learning curve of about 100 cases and months of training. Certainly, diagnosis by imaging is more reproducible than diagnosis by palpation [6], and much easier to teach, and suspected levator trauma and abnormal distensibility ("ballooning") are by no means the only reason to perform pelvic floor imaging (see Box 7.1).

This chapter will summarize the basic methodology

of translabial or transperineal/introital ultrasound. This was, with the exception of abortive attempts to use transabdominal ultrasound [7], the first imaging technique described in the investigation of lower urinary tract disorders and prolapse [8, 9], and the basic methodology has remained the same since 1986.

7.2 Methodology and Instrumentation

7.2.1 Two-dimensional Imaging

A basic two-dimensional (2D) translabial pelvic floor ultrasound (US) examination can be performed with a system manufactured in the mid- to late 1980s, that is, with a simple B mode-capable 2D-US system with cine loop function, a 3.5–6 MHz curved array transducer, and a videoprinter. The field of view or aperture angle should be at least 70 degrees, and higher angles will allow simultaneous imaging of both the symphysis pubis and all three compartments, even on maximal Valsalva. A midsagittal view is obtained by placing a transducer (usually a curved array with frequencies between 3.5 and 8 MHz) on the perineum (Fig. 7.1), after covering the transducer with a glove, condom, or thin plastic wrap. Sterilization, as for intracavitary transducers, is generally considered unnecessary. We use alcoholic wipes to clean the transducer between patients, taking care to remove any gel before disinfection, but regulations may vary between jurisdictions.

Powdered gloves can impair imaging quality due to reverberations, and should be avoided. It is worth-

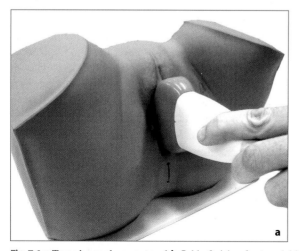
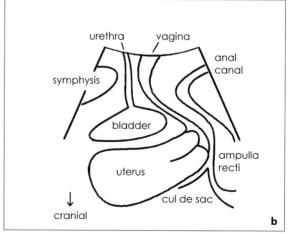

Fig. 7.1 a Transducer placement and **b** field of vision for translabial/perineal ultrasound, midsagittal plane. Reproduced from [10], with permission

while testing several types of probe covers for their effect on image quality and ease of application, and if there are ongoing problems then a thin plastic wrap such as is used in the kitchen may serve the purpose. It is essential to remove all air bubbles from between the transducer and probe cover since even a small air pocket can produce substantial reverberation artifact. Imaging is performed in dorsal lithotomy, with the hips flexed and slightly abducted, or in the standing position. The latter is particularly useful in patients who are unable to relax the levator on performing a Valsalva maneuver. Requiring the patient to place the heels close to the buttocks and then move the hips towards the buttocks will result in an improved pelvic tilt. Bladder filling should be specified; usually prior voiding is preferable since a full bladder will impede organ descent and increase the likelihood of leakage, making the patient reluctant to perform a proper Valsalva maneuver. The presence of a full rectum can impair diagnostic accuracy and sometimes necessitates a repeat assessment after bowel emptying. Parting of the labia can improve image quality, which is generally best in pregnancy and poorest in menopausal women with marked atrophy, most likely due to varying hydration of tissues. Vaginal scar tissue can also impair visibility, but obesity virtually never seems to be a problem. Vaginal meshes create an acoustic shadow and may interfere with imaging of more cranial regions as well as imaging of the pelvic sidewall.

The transducer can usually be placed firmly on the perineum and the symphysis pubis without causing discomfort, unless there is marked atrophy. Due to the location of the transducer one is unlikely to compress the clitoral area. The resulting image includes the symphysis anteriorly, the urethra and bladder neck, the vagina, cervix, rectum, and anal canal (Fig. 7.1). Posterior to the anorectal junction a hyperechogenic area indicates the central portion of the levator plate, i.e. the puborectalis muscle. The cul de sac may also be seen, filled with a small amount of fluid, echogenic fat, or peristalsing small bowel. Parasagittal or transverse views may yield additional information, e.g. enabling assessment of the puborectalis muscle and its insertion on the inferior pubic ramus, and for imaging of implants.

While there has been disagreement regarding image orientation in the midsagittal plane, the author prefers an orientation as on conventional transvaginal US (cranioventral aspects to the left, dorsocaudal to the right). The latter also seems more convenient when using 3D/4D systems, and is the orientation used in the first two publications on the subject [8, 9].

7.2.2 Three-dimensional Imaging

The introduction of 3D-US has had a major impact on pelvic floor imaging. One could argue that 3D enhances our diagnostic capabilities to a greater degree than in any other area of obstetrics and gynecology. This is mainly due to the fact that 4D-US gives access to the axial plane to a degree and with an ease that far surpasses what is possible using intracavitary transducers. While 3D transvaginal or transrectal probes are still used in research and clinical practice, a short review of the current literature will serve to demonstrate the obvious limitations of such an approach in clinical diagnostic use, except for niche applications such as the investigation of urethral diverticulae. The most substantial disadvantage is the fact that intracavitary transducers interfere with the normal movement of pelvic organs on Valsalva maneuver and pelvic floor muscle contraction.

A single volume obtained at rest with an acquisition angle of 70 degrees or higher will include the entire levator hiatus with the symphysis pubis, urethra, paravaginal tissues, the vagina, anorectum, and lower aspects of the levator ani muscle from the pelvic sidewall to the posterior aspect of the anorectal junction.

Basic requirements for 3D pelvic floor US include a system that allows acquisition, reconstruction, and analysis of volume datasets including the capability to measure distances and areas in this volume. This implies motorized acquisition or freehand acquisition with an external position sensor, although the latter is now regarded as obsolete. Currently, the commonest 3D probes are those that combine an electronic curved array of 3–8 MHz with mechanical sector technology, allowing fast motorized sweeps through a field of vision. Any 3D system that allows imaging using an abdominal obstetric probe for visualizing the fetus will be suitable, provided the acquisition angle and field of view are sufficient to include the entire levator hiatus (i.e. at least 70 degrees). Optimally, one should be able to obtain volumes at an acquisition angle of 80–85 degrees.

Volume datasets (especially if saved as cine loops of volumes, i.e. as '4D'), should be stored on a separate server with a storage capacity in the terabyte range, since they can be rather large and will soon fill up the hard disk drive of the US system. Tomographic or multislice imaging capability is highly useful, since it will allow assessment of the entire puborectalis muscle at a glance.

7.2.3 Display Modes

Fig. 7.2 demonstrates the two basic display modes commonly used on modern 3D-US systems. The multiplanar or orthogonal display mode shows cross- sectional planes through the volume in question. For pelvic floor imaging, this most conveniently means the midsagittal (Fig. 7.2a), coronal (Fig. 7.2b) and axial (Fig. 7.2c) planes. Imaging planes on 3D-US can be varied in a completely arbitrary fashion in order to enhance the visibility of a given anatomical structure, either at the time of acquisition or offline at a later time. The levator ani at rest, for example, often requires an axial plane that is slightly tilted in a ventrocaudal to dorsocranial direction. This is obtained by rotating the A-plane by about 20 degrees in an anticlockwise direction.

The three orthogonal images (Fig. 7.2a–c) are complemented by a 'rendered image', i.e. a semitransparent representation of all voxels in an arbitrarily definable 'region of interest' or 'ROI' (Fig. 7.2d). In essence, the rendered image is obtained by assigning varying brightness to voxels encountered at varying depths at varying thresholds. The results can be quite striking, emphasizing surfaces, soft tissue, bone, or even fluid-filled spaces, depending on the chosen rendering settings. The inferior aspects of the levator ani muscle are highly echogenic, since the fibre direction is almost perpendicular to the incident beam, and as a result rendering techniques are highly suitable to enhance the visibility of the puborectalis muscle and of the levator hiatus. Fig. 7.2d shows a standard rendered image of the levator hiatus, with the rendering direction set from caudally to cranially, which is the most appropriate for imaging the hiatus and the inferior aspects of the levator ani muscle.

7.2.4 Four-dimensional Imaging

4D imaging implies the real-time acquisition of volume US data, which can then be represented in orthogonal planes or rendered volumes. Many systems (not only the top of the range 'flagship' systems) are now capable of storing cine loops of volumes, which is of major importance in pelvic floor imaging as it allows enhanced documentation of functional anatomy. Even on 2D single-plane imaging, a static assessment at rest gives little information compared with the evaluation of maneuvers such as a levator contraction and Valsalva.

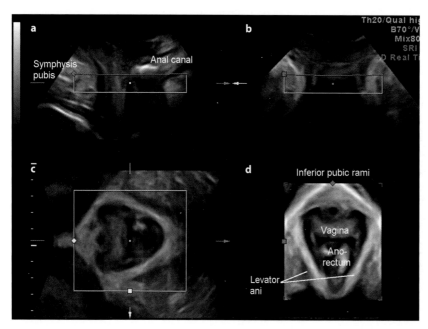

Fig. 7.2 Standard representation of 3D pelvic floor ultrasound. The usual acquisition/evaluation screen on Voluson type systems shows the three orthogonal planes: sagittal (**a**), coronal (**b**), and axial (**c**), as well as a rendered volume (**d**) which is a semi-transparent representation of all grayscale data in the rendered volume (i.e. the box visible in **a-c**). Reproduced from [11], with permission

Their observation will allow assessment of levator function and delineate levator or fascial trauma more clearly. Incidentally, pattern recognition is much easier on observing moving structures, since our eyes and visual cortex are substantially better at evaluating them compared to stills – a sign of our ancestors' priorities for survival in the jungle or savannah.

The ability to perform a real-time 3D (or 4D) assessment of pelvic floor structures makes the technology clearly superior to magnetic resonance imaging (MRI). Prolapse assessment by MRI requires ultrafast acquisition [12], which is of limited availability and will not allow optimal resolutions – and which is possible only in predetermined slices, not volumes. Some 'open' systems allow imaging of the sitting or erect patient, but accessibility is very limited. The physical characteristics of MRI systems make it difficult for the operator to ensure efficient maneuvers, as over 50% of all women will not perform a proper pelvic floor contraction when asked [13], and a Valsalva maneuver is commonly confounded by concomitant levator activation [14]. Without real-time imaging, these confounders are impossible to control for. Therefore, ultrasound has major potential advantages when it comes to describing prolapse, especially when associated with fascial or muscular defects, and in terms of defining functional anatomy. Offline analysis packages allow distance, area, and volume measurements in any user-defined plane (oblique or orthogonal), which is much superior to what is possible with conventional 2D DICOM viewer software on a standard set of single-plane MRI images.

7.3 Functional Assessment

7.3.1 Valsalva Maneuver

The Valsalva maneuver, i.e. a forced expiration against a closed glottis and contracted diaphragm and abdominal wall, is routinely used to effect downwards displacement of the pelvic organs, to reveal symptoms and signs of female pelvic organ prolapse, and to demonstrate distensibility of the levator hiatus. A Valsalva maneuver can also be used to mimic defecation in an effort to demonstrate anatomical causes of obstructed defecation. The maneuver results in dorsocaudal diaplacement of the urethra and bladder neck that can be quantified using a system of coordinates based on the inferoposterior symphyseal margin [15] (Fig. 7.3) or on the central axis of the symphysis pubis [16]. There also is downwards movement of the uterine cervix and the rectal ampulla towards the vaginal introitus or beyond. In the axial plane the hiatus is distended, and the lateral and posterior aspects of the levator plate are displaced caudally, resulting in a varying degree of perineal descent. All this can be observed on pelvic floor US, but it is important to let the transducer move with the tissues, avoiding undue pressure on the perineum which would prevent full development of a prolapse.

Attempts have been made to standardize Valsalva pressure, since this factor is considered by some to be the main confounder for measures of pelvic organ descent [17]. However, any direct intra-abdominal measurement of pressure would require invasive instrumen-

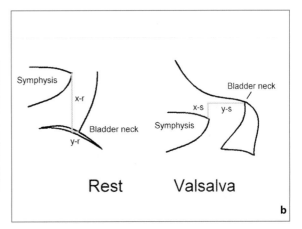

Fig. 7.3 Perineal ultrasound image (**a**) and line drawing (**b**), illustrating some of the measured parameters (distances between bladder neck and symphysis pubis at rest (*x-r, y-r*) and on Valsalva maneuver (*x-s* and *y-s*) required to obtain bladder neck descent (BND). BND = (*x-r*) – (*y-r*); i.e. 28.1 mm – 10.0 mm = 38.1 mm

tation. Some authors have used a spirometer to standardize intra-abdominal pressures, but this allows only rather low Valsalva pressures up to 30–40 cmH$_2$O and probably causes levator co-activation, since forced expiration necessarily requires contraction of the diaphragm. At any rate, most women can achieve Valsalva pressures of 100 cmH$_2$O, and it seems that even pressures of about 60 cmH$_2$O are sufficient to produce near-maximal descent [18], provided they are sustained for at least 5-6 seconds [own unpublished data]. This is supported by the generally good repeatability reported for measures obtained on Valsalva (see Chapter 38).

It is likely that another confounder, generally ignored until recently, is of far greater importance. In young nulliparous women, but also in older women with good pelvic floor function, a Valsalva maneuver is frequently confounded by levator activation [14],

which is visible as a reduction in the anteroposterior diameter of the levator hiatus on Valsalva (Fig. 7.4). This has to be avoided in order to obtain an accurate measure of pelvic organ descent. Any imaging assessment of organ descent requires real-time observation of the effect of a Valsalva maneuver, in order to correct suboptimal efforts, especially if leakage from the bladder or bowel is likely. At times, involuntary levator co-activation can prevent adequate assessment in the supine position, particularly in women with a strong, intact levator shelf. Sometimes it is necessary to repeat imaging in the standing position, which seems to increase the likelihood of an adequate bearing-down effort.

The effect of a Valsalva maneuver is also evident in the axial plane as increasing distension of the levator hiatus. In order to measure this effect it is necessary to identify the "plane of minimal hiatal dimensions" [19]

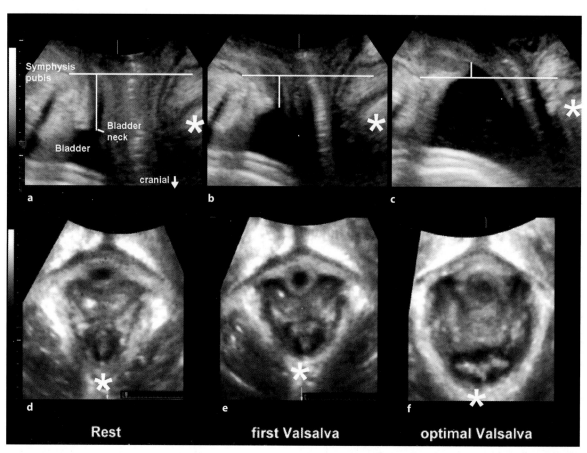

Fig. 7.4 Evidence of levator co-activation as seen in the midsagittal plane (top three images) and the axial plane (bottom three images). The left images of each group (**a** and **d**) show the situation at rest, the central ones (**b** and **c**) show findings on a suboptimal Valsalva maneuver with levator co-activation, evident in a narrowed hiatus visible in **e**. The right image (**c** and **f**) of each group demonstrates the effect of an adequate Valsalva maneuver without levator co-activation, as evidenced by an enlarged hiatus. The * marks the posterior aspect of the puborectalis loop in all images. Reproduced from [14], with permission

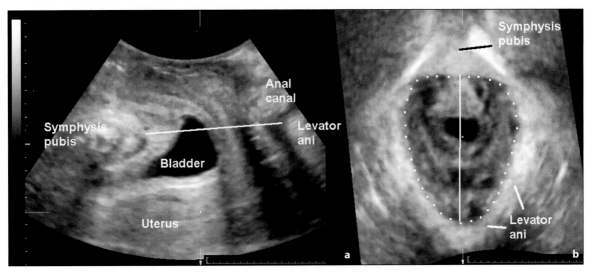

Fig. 7.5 Determination of the plane of minimal hiatal dimensions: the minimal distance between the posterior symphyseal margin and the levator ani immediately posterior to the anorectal angle (**a**, midsagittal plane) serves to identify the correct axial plane (**b**)

(Fig. 7.5). Measurements of diameters and areas in this plane seem to be highly repeatable [19–21] and correlate well with similar measures obtained on MRI [20]. Due to the non-Euclidean or "warped" nature of this plane [22], especially in women with marked prolapse, it may be more valid and repeatable to obtain measurements of the plane of minimal hiatal dimensions in rendered volumes [23], although this is not currently possible on all 3D/4D-capable US systems. A hiatal area of over 25 cm^2 has been defined as "ballooning" or abnormal hiatal distensibilty [24] on the basis of receiver operating characteristic (ROC) curves in women complaining of symptoms of prolapse [24]. Interestingly, this cut-off seems close to the mean plus two standard deviations in young nulliparous Caucasian women [19], confirming its validity.

7.3.2 Pelvic Floor Muscle Contraction

Ultrasound is a highly useful tool in the assessment of the pelvic floor musculature, both in purely anatomical terms (see later) and for function. A levator contraction will reduce the size of the levator hiatus in the sagittal plane and elevate the anorectum, changing the angle between the levator plate and symphysis pubis. As an indirect effect, other pelvic organs such as the uterus, bladder, and urethra are displaced cranially (Fig. 7.6), and there is compression of the urethra, vagina, and anorectal junction [25], an effect that probably explains

the role of the levator ani in urinary and fecal continence as well as for sexual function.

Even transabdominal B mode imaging can demonstrate elevation of the bladder base on pelvic floor muscle contraction (PFMC), but quantification is difficult and repeatability lower than for translabial US [26]. The latter has been employed for the quantification of pelvic floor muscle function, both in women with stress incontinence and continent controls [27] as well as before and after childbirth [28, 29]. A cranioventral shift of pelvic organs imaged in a sagittal midline orientation is taken as evidence of a levator contraction. The resulting displacement of the internal urethral meatus is measured relative to the inferoposterior symphyseal margin (Fig. 7.6). Care has to be taken to avoid concomitant activation of the abdominal muscles, especially of the rectus abdominis or the diaphragm, as this would tend to cause caudal displacement of the bladder neck.

Another means of quantifying levator activity is to measure reduction of the levator hiatus in the midsagittal plane, or to determine the changing angle of the hiatal plane relative to the symphyseal axis. The method can also be utilized for teaching pelvic floor muscle exercises by providing visual biofeedback [30] and has helped validate the concept of 'the knack', i.e. of a reflex levator contraction immediately prior to increases in intra-abdominal pressure such as those resulting from coughing [31]. Correlations between cranioventral shift of the bladder neck on the one hand

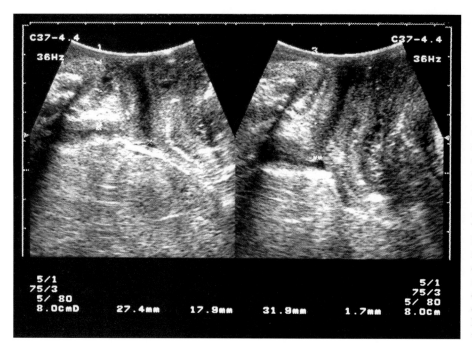

Fig. 7.6 Quantification of levator contraction: cranioventral displacement of the bladder neck is measured relative to the inferoposterior symphyseal margin. The measurements indicate 4.5 (31.9 – 27.4) mm of cranial displacement and 16.2 (17.9 – 1.7) mm of ventral displacement of the bladder neck. Reproduced from [32], with permission

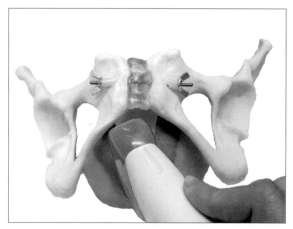

Fig. 7.7 Probe placement for assessment of the inferior aspects of the levator ani by 2D translabial ultrasound

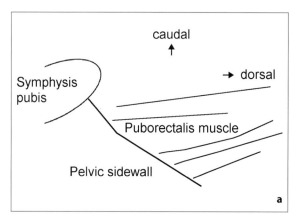

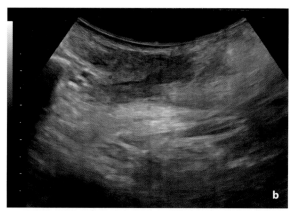

Fig. 7.8 Normal puborectalis muscle as imaged on 2D translabial ultrasound. **a** A schematic drawing. **b** The image demonstrates normal findings on ultrasound

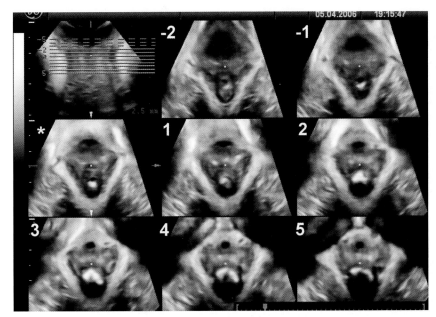

Fig. 7.9 Multislice or tomographic ultrasound imaging of the puborectalis muscle in a nulliparous asymptomatic patient, obtained on maximal pelvic floor muscle contraction. The reference slice (marked by a *) is obtained in the plane of minimal hiatal dimensions (see Fig. 7.6), with the interslice interval set at 2.5 mm. Two slices (−2 and −1) are placed at 2.5 and 5 mm below the plane of minimal hiatal dimensions, and five more at 2.5, 5, 7.5, 10, and 12.5 mm above the reference plane. In this way the entire insertion of the puborectalis muscle can be visualized in a highly repeatable fashion

and palpation/perineometry on the other hand have been shown to be good [33].

The inferior aspects of the levator muscle can be imaged directly by 2D-US, using an oblique parasagittal approach (Figs. 7.7, 7.8). With this method, the integrity of the muscle can be ascertained with very basic systems, and in a few seconds. A contraction of the puborectalis muscle can be observed directly and confirm the presence and function of this muscle. However, repeatability as regards the detection of trauma is lower than for 3D-US [34], probably because there is no clear point of reference. If the transducer is placed too medially in a patient with a normal, intact muscle, one may obtain appearances typical of an avulsion, and if the approach is too lateral one may mistake the bulbocavernosus or the perineal membrane for the puborectalis muscle.

The identification of levator trauma was first described using rendered volumes, with the rendering direction set from caudally to cranially, and this method seems fairly repeatable [35, 36]. However, the use of rendered volumes can result in artifactual appearances of bilateral trauma if the ROI is placed too caudally. The most reproducible method for identifying abnormalities of the puborectalis muscle at present seems to be tomographic or multislice imaging [37] (Fig. 7.9). This is usually obtained on maximal pelvic floor muscle contraction, in order to optimize visibility of the muscle, which is of course thicker on contraction, and to better define the insertion of the muscle on the inferior pubic

ramus [38]. As for the assessment of hiatal distensibility, the plane of minimal hiatal dimensions is determined in the axial plane, and a set of eight axial plane slices is generated from 5 mm below to 12.5 mm above this plane. An interslice interval of 2.5 mm has been proposed which allows bracketing of the main area of interest representing the insertion of the puborectalis muscle on the inferior pubic ramus [37]. The extent of defects can be described as a "TUI (tomographic ultrasound) score", with the highest score being $2 \times 8 = 16$. However, it is evident that abnormalities found above or below the insertion of the puborectalis are of lesser importance [39], which reduces the usefulness of any linear scoring system. In addition, there are multiple patterns of partial trauma: both thinning of muscle as well as complete absence or retraction of full-thickness muscle may occur at any particular level. The distance between the centre of the urethra and the most medial aspect of the insertion of the puborectalis, the "levator–urethra gap" or LUG, seems useful in distinguishing an abnormal muscle insertion in difficult cases [40]. LUG measurements of over 2.5 cm in the plane of minimal hiatal dimensions and in the slices immediately above this plane are strongly associated with an abnormal insertion [40]. This is in agreement with data obtained on magnetic resonance [41], showing there is a significant association between a similar measurement, the "levator–symphysis gap", and pelvic organ prolapse.

Incomplete trauma, whether incomplete in the craniocaudal dimension, or in the sense of globally or partially reduced muscle thickness, necessarily limits the repeatability of any assessment for levator trauma, and palpation is often helpful to clarify findings in patients with less than complete trauma, allowing mapping of more complex patterns of muscle damage [6].

Chapter 38 will discuss the main clinical and research uses of translabial/transperineal US, including 3D/4D imaging.

References

1. DeLancey J. The hidden epidemic of pelvic floor dysfunction: achievable goals for improved prevention and treatment. Am J Obstet Gynecol 2005;192:1488–1495.
2. Dietz H, Lanzarone V. Levator trauma after vaginal delivery. Obstet Gynecol 2005;106:707–712.
3. Kearney R, Miller J, Ashton-Miller J, DeLancey J. Obstetric factors associated with levator ani muscle injury after vaginal birth. Obstet Gynecol 2006;107:144–149.
4. Dietz HP, Hyland G, Hay-Smith J. The assessment of levator trauma: a comparison between palpation and 4D pelvic floor ultrasound. Neurourol Urodyn 2006;25:424–427.
5. Kearney R, Miller JM, Delancey JO. Interrater reliability and physical examination of the pubovisceral portion of the levator ani muscle, validity comparisons using MR imaging. Neurourol Urodyn 2006;25:50–54.
6. Dietz HP, Shek KL. Validity and reproducibility of the digital detection of levator trauma. Int Urogynecol J 2008;19:1097–1101.
7. White RD, McQuown D, McCarthy TA, Ostergard DR. Real-time ultrasonography in the evaluation of urinary stress incontinence. Am J Obstet Gynecol 1980;138:235–237.
8. Grischke EM, Dietz HP, Jeanty P, Schmidt W. [A new study method: the perineal scan in obstetrics and gynecology.] Ultraschall Med 1986;7:154–161.
9. Kohorn EI, Scioscia AL, Jeanty P, Hobbins JC. Ultrasound cystourethrography by perineal scanning for the assessment of female stress urinary incontinence. Obstet Gynecol 1986;68:269–272.
10. Dietz HP. Pelvic floor ultrasound: a review. Am J Obstet Gynecol 2009; in press.
11. Dietz HP. Pelvic floor ultrasound. ASUM Ultrasound Bulletin 2007;10:17–23.
12. Yang A, Mostwin JL, Rosenshein NB, Zerhouni EA. Pelvic floor descent in women: dynamic evaluation with fast MR imaging and cinematic display. Radiology 1991;179:25–33.
13. Bo K, Larson S, Oseid S et al. Knowledge about and ability to do correct pelvic floor muscle exercises in women with urinary stress incontinence. Neurourol Urodyn 1988;7:261–262.
14. Oerno A, Dietz H. Levator co-activation is a significant confounder of pelvic organ descent on Valsalva maneuver. Ultrasound Obstet Gynecol 2007;30:346–350.
15. Dietz HP, Wilson PD. Anatomical assessment of the bladder outlet and proximal urethra using ultrasound and videocystourethrography. Int Urogynecol J 1998;9:365–369.
16. Schaer GN. Ultrasonography of the lower urinary tract. Curr Opin Obstet Gynecol 1997;9:313–316.
17. King JK, Freeman RM. Is antenatal bladder neck mobility a risk factor for postpartum stress incontinence? Br J Obstet Gynaecol 1998;105:1300–1307.
18. Martan A, Masata J, Halaska M et al. The effect of increasing of intraabdominal pressure on the position of the bladder neck in ultrasound imaging. Proceedings of the 31st Annual Meeting, International Continence Society, 18–21 September 2001, Seoul, Korea.
19. Dietz H, Shek K, Clarke B. Biometry of the pubovisceral muscle and levator hiatus by three-dimensional pelvic floor ultrasound. Ultrasound Obstet Gynecol 2005;25:580–585.
20. Yang J, Yang S, Huang W. Biometry of the pubovisceral muscle and levator hiatus in nulliparous Chinese women. Ultrsound Obstet Gynecol 2006;26:710–716.
21. Kruger J, Dietz H, Murphy B. Pelvic floor function in elite nulliparous athletes and controls. Ultrasound Obstet Gynecol 2007;30:81–85.
22. Kruger J, Heap X, Murphy B, Dietz H. Pelvic floor function in nulliparous women using 3-dimensional ultrasound and magnetic resonance imaging. Obstet Gynecol 2008;111:631–638.
23. Wong V, Shek KL, Dietz HP. A simplified method for the determination of levator hiatal dimensions. Int Urogynecol J 2009;20(S2):S145–146.
24. Dietz H, De Leon J, Shek K. Ballooning of the levator hiatus. Ultrasound Obstet Gynecol 2008;31:676–680.
25. Jung S, Pretorius D, Padda B et al. Vaginal high-pressure zone assessed by dynamic 3-dimensional ultrasound images of the pelvic floor. Am J Obstet Gynecol 2007;197:52.e1–7.
26. Thompson JA, O'Sullivan PB, Briffa K et al. Assessment of pelvic floor movement using transabdominal and transperineal ultrasound. Int Urogynecol J 2005;16:285–292.
27. Wijma J, Tinga DJ, Visser GH. Perineal ultrasonography in women with stress incontinence and controls: the role of the pelvic floor muscles. Gynecol Obstet Invest 1991;32:176–179.
28. Peschers UM, Schaer GN, DeLancey JO, Schuessler B. Levator ani function before and after childbirth. Br J Obstet Gynaecol 1997;104:1004–1008.
29. Dietz H. Levator function before and after childbirth. Aust N Z J Obstet Gynaecol 2004;44:19–23.
30. Dietz HP, Wilson PD, Clarke B. The use of perineal ultrasound to quantify levator activity and teach pelvic floor muscle exercises. Int Urogynecol J Pelvic Floor Dysfunct 2001;12:166–168; discussion 168–169.
31. Miller JM, Perucchini D, Carchidi LT et al. Pelvic floor muscle contraction during a cough and decreased vesical neck mobility. Obstet Gynecol 2001;97:255–260.
32. Dietz HP. Ultrasound Imaging of the pelvic floor, part I: two-dimensional aspects. Ultrasound Obstet Gynecol 2004;23:80–92.
33. Dietz HP, Jarvis SK, Vancaillie TG. The assessment of levator muscle strength: a validation of three ultrasound techniques. Int Urogynecol J 2002;13:156–159.
34. Dietz HP, Shek KL. Levator trauma can be diagnosed by 2D translabial ultrasound. Int Urogynecol J 2009;20:807–811.
35. Dietz HP, Steensma AB. The prevalence of major abnorma-

lities of the levator ani in urogynaecological patients. BJOG 2006;113:225–230.

36. Weinstein MM, Pretorius D, Nager CW, Mittal R. Inter-rater reliability of pelvic floor muscle imaging abnormalities with 3D ultrasound. Ultrasound Obstet Gynecol 2007; 30:538.

37. Dietz H. Quantification of major morphological abnormalities of the levator ani. Ultrasound Obstet Gynecol 2007;29:329–334.

38. Dietz H. Ultrasound imaging of the pelvic floor: 3D aspects. Ultrasound Obstet Gynecol 2004;23:615–625.

39. Dietz H, Shek K. Tomographic ultrasound of the pelvic floor: which levels matter most? Neurourol Urodyn 2008; 27:639–640.

40. Dietz H, Abbu A, Shek K. The levator urethral gap measurement: a more objective means of determining levator avulsion? Ultrasound Obstet Gynecol 2008; 31:941–945.

41. Singh K, Jakab M, Reid W et al. Three-dimensional magnetic resonance imaging assessment of levator ani morphologic features in different grades of prolapse. Am J Obstet Gynecol 2003;188:910–915.

Endoanal and Endorectal Ultrasonography: Methodology and Normal Pelvic Floor Anatomy

8

Giulio Aniello Santoro and Giuseppe Di Falco

Abstract High-resolution three-dimensional endoanal ultrasonography (3D-EAUS) clearly demonstrates the anatomy of the anal canal. All relevant structures, including the puborectalis muscle, the internal and external sphincter, the conjoined longitudinal layer, and the transverse perinei muscles, are visualized and any sphincter disruptions or defects can be detected. The asymmetrical shape of the anal canal and the gender differences in the ventral part of the external sphincter are also easily evaluated in the different reconstructed planes of the three-dimensional volume. High-resolution three-dimensional endorectal ultrasound (3D-ERUS) provides an accurate visualization of the five-layer structure of the rectal wall and of the all pelvic organs adjacent to the rectum. The purpose of this chapter is to present the technique of 3D-EAUS and 3D-ERUS and to revise the ultrasonographic anatomy of the anorectal region.

Keywords Endoanal ultrasound • Endorectal ultrasound • External anal sphincter • Internal anal sphincter • Puborectalis muscle • Three-dimensional ultrasound

8.1 Introduction

The anal canal is surrounded by the internal sphincter (IAS), the longitudinal muscle layer (LM), and the external sphincter (EAS) [1–3] (Fig. 8.1). The anatomy of the anorectal region is currently of clinical interest. An intact anal sphincter complex has a decisive role for continence. It is very important for gynecologists to know where birth damage may occur, leading to rupture of the IAS or EAS as well as the puborectalis muscle (PR). Knowledge of the correct anatomy helps to identify defects and to reconstruct them in a meticulous way to achieve as good a functional result as possible. With the help of endoanal (EAUS) and endorectal ultrasonography (ERUS), it has become possible to demonstrate clearly the morphology of the anal sphincter complex and to detect sphincter disruptions or defects. The results of ultrasound studies have also demonstrated the sexual differences in the ventral part of the EAS [4–10].

The purpose of this chapter is to present the techniques of EAUS and ERUS and to revise the ultrasonographic anatomy of the anal sphincter complex in axial, longitudinal, and coronal planes with the use of high-resolution three-dimensional reconstruction.

8.2 Ultrasonographic Technique

Endoanal ultrasound is performed by using the same 12–16 MHz rotational 360° transducer (type 2050, B-K Medical, Herlev, Denmark) described in Chapter 6

G.A. Santoro
Pelvic Floor Unit and Colorectal Service, 1st Department of General Surgery, Regional Hospital, Treviso, Italy

G.A. Santoro, A.P. Wieczorek, C.I. Bartram (eds.) *Pelvic Floor Disorders*
© Springer-Verlag Italia 2010

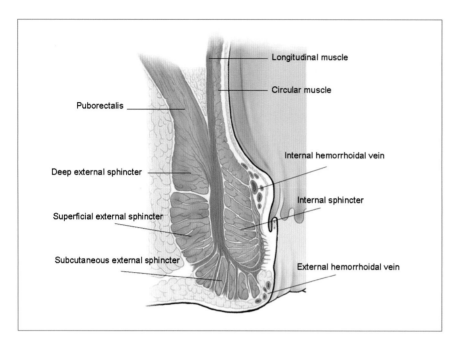

Puborectalis

Deep external sphincter

Superficial external sphincter

Subcutaneous external sphincter

Longitudinal muscle

Circular muscle

Internal hemorrhoidal vein

Internal sphincter

External hemorrhoidal vein

Fig. 8.1 Normal anatomy of the anal canal. The muscularis propria of the rectal wall consists of both circular and longitudinal smooth muscle fibers. The circular layer is continuous with the circular internal anal sphincter muscle. The longitudinal layer extends into the intersphincteric space of the anal canal. The external sphincter extends further down than the internal sphincter

for the endovaginal technique. During examination the patient is placed in dorsal lithotomy or in the left lateral decubitus position. Before the probe is inserted into the anus, a digital rectal examination should be performed. If there is an anal stenosis, the inserted finger can be used to check whether easy passage of the probe will be possible.

A gel-containing condom is placed over the probe, and a thin layer of water-soluble lubricant is placed on the exterior of the condom. Any air interface will cause a major interference pattern. The patient should be instructed before the examination that no pain should be experienced. Under no circumstances should force be used to advance the probe.

By convention, the transducer is positioned to provide the following image: the anterior aspect of the anal canal will be superior (12 o'clock) on the screen, right lateral will be left (9 o'clock), left lateral will be right (3 o'clock), and posterior will be inferior (6 o'clock). Some adjustments may be necessary in the gain of the ultrasound unit to provide optimal imaging. It is always possible to perfectly depict all layers of the anal canal circumferentially. This is very important when assessing the canal at different levels. At the origin of the anal canal, the "U"-shaped sling of the puborectalis is the main landmark and should be used for final adjustment.

Three-dimensional ultrasound (3D-US) is constructed from a synthesis of a high number of parallel

transaxial two-dimensional (2D) images. The 2050 transducer has a built-in 3D automatic motorized system that allows an acquisition of 300 transaxial images over a distance of 60 mm in 60 s, without requiring any movement relative to the investigated tissue (see Chapter 6) [11] (Fig. 8.2). After a 3D dataset has been acquired, it is immediately possible to select coronal anterior–posterior or posterior–anterior as well as sagittal right–left views, together with any oblique image plane. The 3D image can be rotated, tilted, and sliced

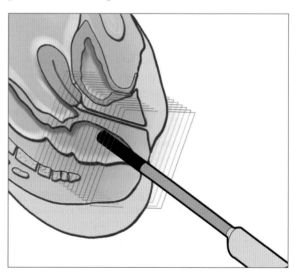

Fig. 8.2 Schematic illustration of the technique of three-dimensional endoanal ultrasonography performed by 2050 transducer (B-K Medical) for the assessment of the anorectal region

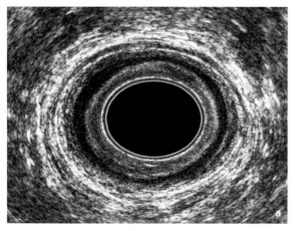
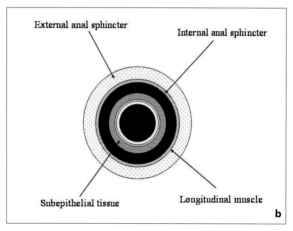

Fig. 8.3 Normal ultrasonographic five-layer structure of the mid-anal canal. **a** Axial image obtained by 2050 transducer (B-K Medical). **b** Schematic representation

to allow the operator to infinitely vary the different section parameters, visualize the assessed region at different angles, and measure accurately distance, area, angle, and volume [11].

8.3 Endosonographic Anatomy of the Anal Canal

On ultrasound, five hypoechoic and hyperechoic layers can be seen in the normal anal canal [12, 13]. The ultrasonographer must have a clear understanding of what each of these five layers represents anatomically (Fig. 8.3).

1. The first hyperechoic layer, from inner to outer, corresponds to the interface of the transducer with the anal mucosal surface.
2. The second layer represents the subepithelial tissues and appears moderately reflective. The mucosa as well the level of dentate line is not visualized. The muscularis submucosae ani can be sonographically identified in the upper part of the anal canal as a low reflective band.
3. The third hypoechoic layer corresponds to the IAS. The sphincter is not completely symmetric, either in thickness or termination. It can be traced superiorly into the circular muscle of the rectum, extending from the anorectal junction to approximately 1 cm below the dentate line. In older age groups, the IAS loses its uniform low echogenicity, which is characteristic of smooth muscle through-

out the gut, to become more echogenic and inhomogeneous in texture [13].
4. The fourth hyperechoic layer represents the LM. It presents a wide variability in thickness and is not always distinctly visible along the entire anal canal. The LM appears moderately echogenic, which is surprising as it is mainly smooth muscle; however, an increased fibrous stroma may account for this. In the intersphincteric space the LM conjoins with striated muscle fibers from the levator ani, particularly the puboanalis, and a large fibroelastic element derived from the endopelvic fascia to form the "conjoined longitudinal layer" (CLL) (Fig. 8.4) [14]. Its fibroelastic component, permeating through the subcutaneous part of the EAS, terminates in the perianal skin. According to the "Integral Theory" proposed by Papa Petros, the CLL creates the downward force for bladder neck closure during effort, and stretches open the outflow tract during micturition [15].
5. The fifth mixed echogenic layer corresponds to the EAS. The EAS is made up of voluntary muscle that encompasses the anal canal. It is described as having three parts [16]: (1) the deep part is integral with the PR. Posteriorly there is some ligamentous attachment. Anteriorly some fibers are circular and some decussate into the deep transverse perinei; (2) the superficial part has a very broad attachment to the underside of the coccyx via the anococcygeal ligament. Anteriorly there is a division into circular fibers and a decussation to the superficial transverse perinei; (3) the subcutaneous part lies below the internal anal sphincter.

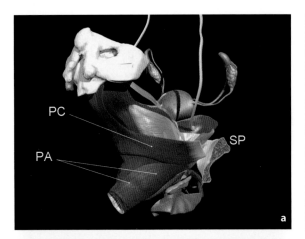

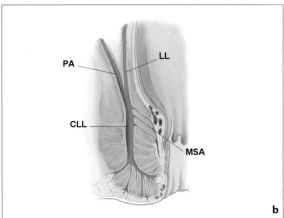

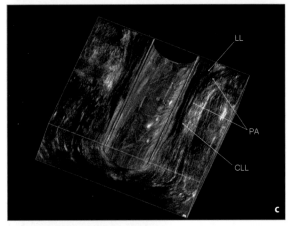

Fig. 8.4 a The puboanalis (*PA*) rises from the medial border of the pubococcygeous muscle (*PC*) (©Primal Pictures Ltd, with permission). **b** Fibers from the longitudinal muscle run through the internal anal sphincter to form the muscularis submucosae ani (*MSA*). **c** Coronal image of the anal canal obtained by 2050 transducer (B-K Medical). SP, symphysis pubis. The PA joins the longitudinal muscle layer (*LL*) of the rectum to form the conjoined longitudinal layer (*CLL*).

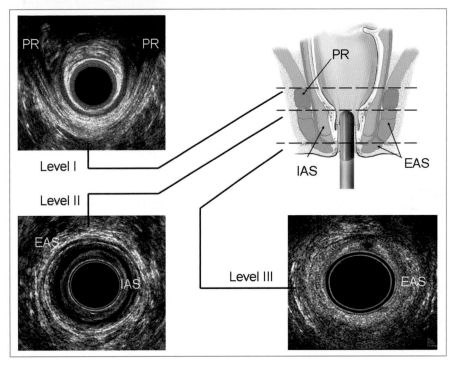

Fig. 8.5 Three levels of assessment of the anal canal in the axial plane. Right side of the image is left side of the patient. *EAS*, external anal sphincter; *IAS*, internal anal sphincter; *PR*, puborectalis.
Scan obtained by 2050 transducer (B-K Medical)

Ultrasound imaging of the anal canal can be divided into three levels of assessment in the axial plane (upper, middle, and lower levels), referring to the following anatomical structures (Figs. 8.5, 8.6) [12, 17–19]:

- upper level: the sling of the PR, the deep part of the EAS and the complete ring of IAS
- middle level: the superficial part of the EAS (complete ring), the CLL, the IAS (complete ring), and the transverse perinei muscles
- lower level: the subcutaneous part of the EAS.

The muscles of the lower and the upper part of the anal canal are different. The first ultrasonographic image recorded is normally the PR muscle and is labeled upper level. The PR slings the anal canal instead of completely surrounding it. At its upper end, the PR is attached to the funnel-shaped levator ani muscle and the levator ani anchors the sphincter complex to the inner side of the pelvis. The deep part of the EAS is similar in echogenicity to the PR and cannot be differentiated from it posteriorly. Anteriorly, the circular fibers of the deep part of the EAS are not recognizable in females, whereas in males thin arcs of muscle from the deeper part of the sphincter may be seen extending anteriorly.

Moving the probe a few millimeters in the distal direction will show an intact anterior EAS forming just below the superficial transverse perinei muscles, imaged at 11 o'clock and 1 o'clock (Fig. 8.7). This image is a mid-anal projection where the IAS, CLL, and superficial EAS all are identified. This image will be labeled middle level. In females, fibers between the transverse perinei fuse with the EAS, so that there is

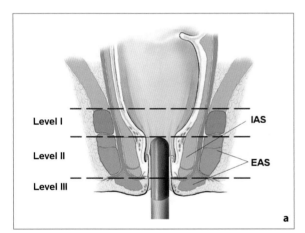
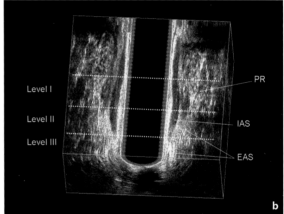

Fig. 8.6 Three levels of assessment of the anal canal. The internal sphincter ends at the level of the junction between the superficial (level II) and subcutaneous (level III) external sphincter. **a** Schematic representation. **b** Coronal image obtained by 2050 transducer (B-K Medical). *EAS*, external anal sphincter; *IAS*, internal anal sphincter; *PR*, puborectalis muscle

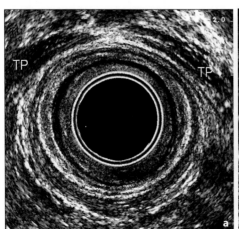
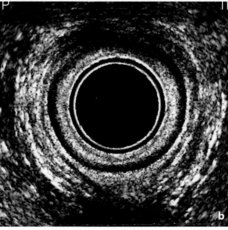

Fig. 8.7 Images of the transverse perinei muscles (*TP*) in the axial plane in male (**a**) and female (**b**). The anoccoccygeal ligament (ACL) is seen as a posterior hypoechoic triangle. Scan obtained by 2050 transducer (B-K Medical)

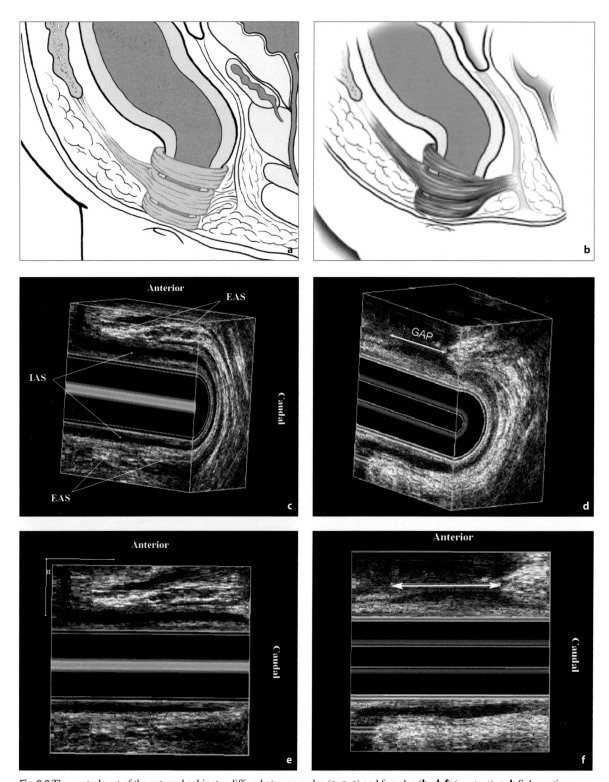

Fig. 8.8 The ventral pert of the external sphincter differs between males (**a**, **c**, **e**) and females (**b**, **d**, **f**) (see text). **a**, **b** Schematic representations; **c–f** Three-dimensional endosonographic reconstructions in the longitudinal plane. The distance between the anterior anorectal junction and the external sphincter is called the gap (*arrows*). *EAS*, external anal sphincter; *IAS*, internal anal sphincter. Scans obtained by 2050 transducer (B-K Medical)

no plane of dissection between these two structures. In males a plane of fat persists between the transverse perinei and the EAS. EAUS is not able to precisely assess the perineal body because of the lack of clear limits. Also the proposed use of a finger introduced into the vagina as a landmark seems to be of poor benefit, altering its normal configuration due to the digital compression on the central perineum [20, 21]. At this level, the anococcygeal raphe is seen as a posterior hypoechoic triangle (Fig. 8.7).

When the probe is pulled further out, the image of the IAS will disappear and only the subepithelium and the subcutaneous segment of the LM + EAS will be seen. This last image will be labeled lower level (Fig. 8.6).

The anterior part of the EAS differs between genders, and anatomic studies have shown that this difference is already present in the fetus. In males, the EAS is symmetrical at all levels; in females, it is shorter anteriorly, and there is no evidence of an anterior ring high in the canal (Fig. 8.8). In examining a female subject, the ultrasonographic differences between the natural gaps (hypoechoic areas with smooth, regular edges) and sphincter ruptures (mixed echogenicity,

due to scarring, with irregular edges) occurring at the upper anterior part of the anal canal must be kept in mind. Three-dimensional longitudinal images are particularly useful to assess these anatomic characteristics of the EAS [22–25] (Figs. 8.8, 8.9).

8.4 Endosonographic Anatomy of the Rectum

The normal rectum is 11–15 cm long and has a maximum diameter of 4 cm. It is continuous with the sigmoid colon superiorly at the level of the third sacral segment and courses inferiorly along the curve of the sacrum to pass through the pelvic diaphragm and become the anal canal. It is surrounded by fibrofatty tissue that contains blood vessels, nerves, lymphatics, and small lymph nodes. The superior one-third is covered anteriorly and laterally by the pelvic peritoneum. The middle one-third is only covered with peritoneum anteriorly, where it curves anteriorly onto the bladder in the male and onto the uterus in the female. The lower one-third of the rectum is below the peritoneal reflection and is related anteriorly to the

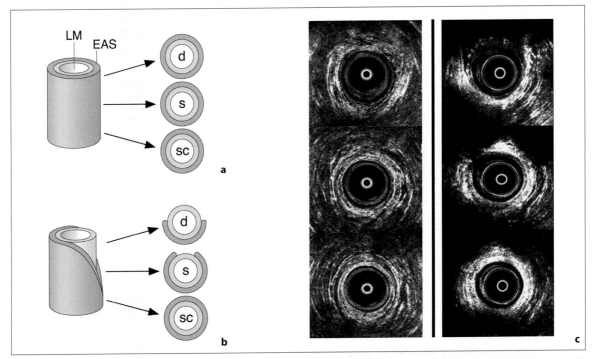

Fig. 8.9 Schematic representations of the external sphincter at three levels of the anal canal in male (**a**) and female (**b**). **c** Ultrasonographic images in the axial plane (*left*, male; *right*, female). *LM*, longitudinal muscle; *EAS*, external anal sphincter; *d*, deep external sphincter; *s*, superficial external sphincter; *sc*, subcutaneous external sphincter. Scans obtained by 2050 transducer (B-K Medical)

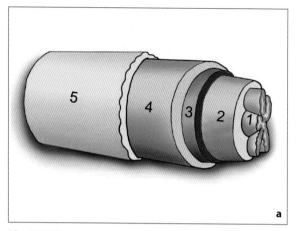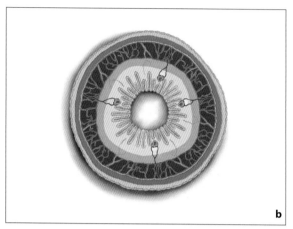

Fig. 8.10 Diagrammatic representation of the five-layer structure of the normal rectal wall. **a, b** *1*, mucosa; *2*, submucosa; *3*, muscularis propria/circular layer; *4*, muscularis propria/longitudinal layer; *5*, serosa/perirectal fat

bladder base, ureters, seminal vesicles, and prostate in the male and to the lower uterus, cervix, and vagina in the female.

The rectal wall consists of five layers surrounded by perirectal fat or serosa (Fig. 8.10). On ultrasound the normal rectal wall is 2–3 mm thick and is composed of a five-layer structure [26]. There is some debate as to what the actual layers represent anatomically. Hildebrandt et al [27] believe that three layers are anatomical, while the other layers represent interfaces between the anatomical layers. Beynon et al [28], however, have produced both experimental and clinical evidence that the five anatomic layers are recognizable. Good visualization depends on maintaining the probe in the center lumen of the rectum and having adequate distension of a water-filled latex balloon covering the transducer to achieve good acoustic contact with the rectal wall. It is important to eliminate all bubbles within the balloon to avoid artifacts that limit the overall utility of the study. The rectum can be of varying diameters and therefore the volume of water in the balloon may have to be adjusted intermittently. The five layers represent (Fig. 8.11):

1. the first hyperechoic layer corresponding to the interface of the balloon with the rectal mucosal surface
2. the second hypoechoic layer to the mucosa and muscularis mucosae
3. the third hyperechoic layer to the submucosa
4. the fourth hypoechoic layer to the muscularis propria (in rare cases seen as two layers: inner circular and outer longitudinal layer)

5. the fifth hyperechoic layer to the serosa or to the interface with the fibrofatty tissue surrounding the rectum (mesorectum). The mesorectum contains blood vessels, nerves, and lymphatics and has an inhomogeneous echo pattern. Very small, round to oval, hypoechoic lymph nodes should be distinguished from blood vessels which also appear as circular hypoechoic structures.

Endorectal ultrasound allows an accurate visualization of all pelvic organs adjacent to the rectum: the bladder, seminal vesicles, and prostate in males (Fig. 8.12), and the uterus, cervix, vagina, and urethra in females. Intestinal loops can also be easily identified as elongated structures (Fig. 8.13).

8.5 Normal Values

The anal canal length is the distance measured between the proximal canal, where the PR is identified, and the lower border of the subcutaneous EAS. It is significantly longer in males than in females, as a result of a longer EAS, whereas there is no difference in PR length. In males the anterior part of the EAS is present along the entire length of the canal (Figs. 8.9 and 8.10). In females the anterior ring of the EAS is shorter. Williams et al [22] reported that the anterior EAS occupied 58% of the male anal canal compared with 38% of the female canal (P < 0.01). In females the PR occupied a significantly larger proportion of the canal than in male (61 vs. 45%; P = 0.02). There was no difference in the length of the IAS between males and

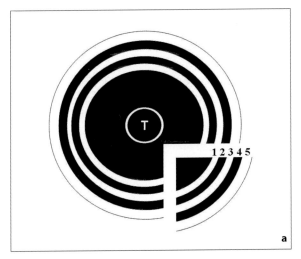

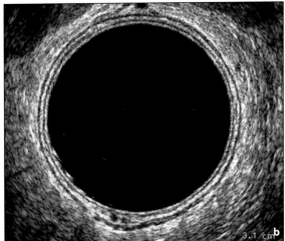

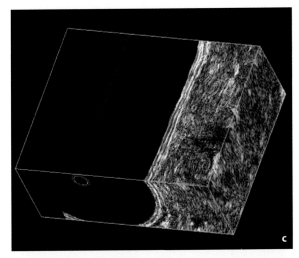

Fig. 8.11 a Schematic ultrasound representation of the rectal wall (*T*, transducer). **b** The five layers in the axial plane correspond to: *1*, acoustic interface with mucosal surface; *2*, mucosa; *3*, submucosa; *4*, muscularis propria; *5*, serosa/perirectal fat interface. **c** Three-dimensional reconstruction of the rectal wall in the coronal plane. Scans obtained by 2050 transducer (B-K Medical)

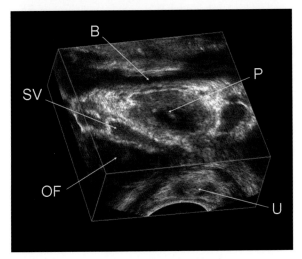

Fig. 8.12 Coronal view of the bladder (*B*), seminal vesicles (*SV*), prostate gland (*P*), urethra (U), and obturator foramen (*OF*). Scans obtained by 2050 transducer (B-K Medical)

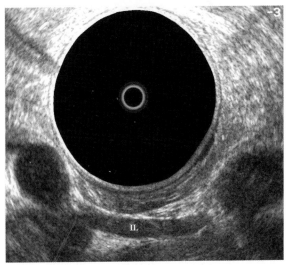

Fig. 8.13 Sonographic view of the intestinal loops (*IL*). Scans obtained by 2050 transducer (B-K Medical)

females (34.4 vs. 33.2 mm), or in the proportion of the anal canal that it occupied (67 vs. 73%; P = 0.12).

Normal values for sphincter dimensions differ between techniques. It is not really relevant to define the true values of sphincter muscle thickness, because the purpose of measuring anal sphincters is to distinguish a normal versus abnormal measurement, regardless of the absolute values. Measurement should be taken at the 3 o'clock and 9 o'clock positions in the midlevel of the anal canal. The IAS thickness varies between 1.8 ± 0.5 mm and increases with age, because of the presence of more fibrous tissue as the absolute amount of muscle decreases, measuring 2.4–2.7 mm in individuals aged less than 55 years and 2.8–3.5 mm in those aged more than 55 years. Any internal anal sphincter > 4 mm thick should be considered abnormal whatever the patient's age; conversely a sphincter of 2 mm is normal in a young patient, but abnormal in an elderly one. The longitudinal muscle is 2.5 ± 0.6 mm in males and 2.9 ± 0.6 mm in females. The average thickness of the EAS is 8.6 ± 1.1 mm in males and 7.7 ± 1.1 mm in females. However, endosonography largely overestimates the size of the EAS due to its failure to recognize and separate the LM. By using the reconstructed 3D coronal plane, the anterior longitudinal extent of the EAS can also be measured (Fig. 8.14).

Many studies have specifically addressed the problems of the reproducibility of EAUS sphincter measurements [10, 29–32]. Enck et al [31] examined a small group of healthy volunteers and concluded that EAUS did not provide reliable measurements of IAS and EAS thicknesses. Gold et al [32] examined 51 patients and found that measurements of the IAS were more reproducible than those of the EAS. These findings are consistent with results from Beets-Tan et al [29], which compared EAUS, endoanal magnetic resonance imaging (MRI) and phased-array MRI for anal sphincter measurement in healthy volunteers. EAUS enabled reliable measurement of only IAS thickness, whereas both MRI modalities enabled reliable measurement of all sphincter components. Measurement errors of the LM and EAS are related to the ultrasonographic features of these muscles, which show low contrast with the surrounding hyperechoic fatty tissue. Both the inner and outer borders of the EAS are more difficult to define, leading to less reliable measurement. In contrast, the IAS is easy to define because it is a hypoechoic structure that is highlighted against hyperechoic fatty tissues. Williams et al [22] reported different results. They found an excellent correlation for the interobserver measurement of the EAS, IAS, and submucosal width on endosonography and poor correlation only for the LM. Frudinger et al [10] also reported that the EAS thickness was difficult to define in only 2% of patients at all three levels examined, and in 3% at the subcutaneous level only. A significant negative correlation with the patients' age was also demonstrated in this study, at all anal canal levels. In particular, the anterior EAS region was found to be significantly thinner in older subjects.

The high inherent soft-tissue contrast makes magnetic resonance a more reliable imaging method to measure anal sphincter components [33–39]. Multiplanar EAUS, however, has enabled detailed longitudinal measurement of the components of the anal canal [7, 11, 40]. Williams et al [22] reported that the anterior EAS was significantly longer in men than women (30.1 mm vs. 16.9 mm; P < 0.001). There was no difference in the length of the PR between men and women, indicating that the gender difference in anal canal length is solely due to the longer male EAS. The IAS did not differ in length between males and females. Regadas et al [23] demonstrated the asymmetrical shape of the anal canal and also confirmed that the anterior EAS was significantly shorter in females. West et al [40] reported similar results, with IAS and EAS volumes found to be larger in males than in females.

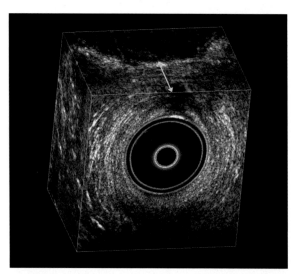

Fig. 8.14 Measurement of the anterior length of the external sphincter in the coronal plane (*arrow*). Scans obtained by 2050 transducer (B-K Medical)

Regardless of the absolute values of the anal sphincter dimensions, the most relevant utility of EAUS application is in the detection of localized sphincter defects, where its benefit has been proven [41–43]. It has been suggested that measuring sphincter thickness is important when EAUS cannot depict any sphincter damage, to exclude diffuse structural sphincter changes associated with idiopathic fecal incontinence, passive fecal incontinence, or obstructive defecation disorders [44–46]. A postulated association between manometric function of the sphincters and their sonographic appearance, however, has remained controversial in the literature. Some authors have found no correlation between muscle thickness and muscle performance – either resting or squeeze pressure. Scanning anal sphincter muscle may allow determination of its integrity, but not its morphometric properties.

References

1. Uz A, Elhan A, Ersoy M, Tekdemir I. Internal anal sphincter: an anatomic study. Clin Anat 2004;17:17–20.
2. Lunniss PJ, Phillips RKS. Anatomy and function of the anal longitudinal muscle. Br J Surg 1992;79:882–884.
3. Fritsch H, Brenner E, Lienemann A, Ludwikowski B. Anal sphincter complex. Reinterpreted morphology and its clinical relevance. Dis Colon Rectum 2002;45:188–194.
4. Bartram CI. Ultrasound. In: Bartram CI, DeLancey JOL (eds) Imaging pelvic floor disorders. Springer-Verlag, Berlin, Heidelberg; 2003, pp 69-79.
5. Williams AB, Bartram CI, Halligan S et al. Endosonographic anatomy of the normal anal canal compared with endocoil magnetic resonance imaging. Dis Colon Rectum 2002; 45:176–183.
6. Konerding MA, Dzemali O, Gaumann A et al. Correlation of endoanal sonography with cross sectional anatomy of the anal sphincter. Gastrointest Endosc 1999;50:804–810.
7. Williams AB, Bartram CI, Halligan S et al. Multiplanar anal endosonography – normal anal canal anatomy. Colorectal Dis 2001;3:169–174.
8. Thakar R, Sultan A. Anal endosonography and its role in assessing the incontinent patient. Best Pract Res Clinic Obstet Gynaecol 2004;18:157–173.
9. Sultan AH, Kamm MA, Talbot IC et al. Anal endosonography for identifying external sphincter defects confirmed histologically. Br J Surg 1994;81:463–465.
10. Frudinger A, Halligan S, Bartram CI et al. Female anal sphincter: age-related differences in asymptomatic volunteers with high-frequency endoanal US. Radiology 2002;224:417–423.
11. Santoro GA, Fortling B. The advantages of volume rendering in three-dimensional endosonography of the anorectum. Dis Colon Rectum 2007;50:359–368.
12. Santoro GA, Di Falco G. Endosonographic anatomy of the normal anal canal. In: Santoro GA, Di Falco G (eds) Benign anorectal diseases. Diagnosis with endoanal and endorectal ultrasonography and new treatment options. Springer-Verlag Italy, Milan; 2006, pp 35–54.
13. Starck M, Bohe M, Fortling B, Valentin L. Endosonography of the anal sphincter in women of different ages and parity. Ultrasound Obstet Gynecol 2005;25:169–176.
14. Shafik A. A new concept of the anatomy of the anal sphincter mechanism and the physiology of defecation III. The longitudinal anal muscle: anatomy and role in sphincter mechanism. Invest Urol 1976;13:271–277.
15. Papa Petros PE. The anatomy and dynamics of pelvic floor function and dysfunction. In: Papa Petros PE. The female pelvic floor. Function, dysfunction and management according to the integral theory, 2 edn. Springer-Verlag, Heidelberg; 2007, pp 14–50.
16. Shafik A. A new concept of the anatomy of the anal sphincter mechanism and the physiology of defecation. The external anal sphincter: a triple-loop system. Invest Urol 1975; 12:412–419.
17. Kumar A, Scholefield JH. Endosonography of the anal canal and rectum. World J Surg 2000;24:208–215.
18. Hussain SM, Stoker J, Schutte HE, Lameris JS. Imaging of the anorectal region. Eur J Radiol 1996;22:116–122.
19. Stoker J, Halligan S, Bartram CI. Pelvic floor imaging. Radiology 2001;218:621–641.
20. Zetterstrom JP, Mellgren A, Madoff RD et al. Perineal body measurement improves evaluation of anterior sphincter lesions during endoanal ultrasonography. Dis Colon Rectum 1998;41:705–713.
21. Oberwalder M, Thaler K, Baig MK et al. Anal ultrasound and endosonographic measurement of perineal body thickness. A new evaluation for fecal incontinence in females. Surg Endosc 2004;18:650–654.
22. Williams AB, Cheetham MJ, Bartram CI et al. Gender differences in the longitudinal pressure profile of the anal canal related to anatomical structure as demonstrated on three-dimensional anal endosonography. Br J Surg 2000;87:1674–1679.
23. Regadas FSP, Murad-Regadas SM, Lima DMR et al. Anal canal anatomy showed by three-dimensional anorectal ultrasonography. Surg Endosc 2007;21:2207–2211.
24. Bollard RC, Gardiner A, Lindow S et al. Normal female anal sphincter: difficulties in interpretation explained. Dis Colon Rectum 2002;45:171–175.
25. Gold DM, Bartram CI, Halligan S et al. Three-dimensional endoanal sonography in assessing anal canal injury. Br J Surg 1999;86:365–370.
26. Santoro GA, Di Falco G. Endosonographic anatomy of the normal rectum. In: Santoro GA, Di Falco G (eds) Benign anorectal diseases. Diagnosis with endoanal and endorectal ultrasonography and new treatment options. Springer-Verlag Italy, Milan; 2006, pp 55–60.
27. Hildebrandt U, Feifel G, Schwarz HP, Scherr O. Endorectal ultrasound: instrumentation and clinical aspects. Int J Colorectal Dis 1986;1:203–207.
28. Beynon J, Foy DM, Temple LN et al. The endosonic appearance of normal colon and rectum. Dis Colon Rectum 1986;29:810–813.
29. Beets-Tan RGH, Morren GL, Betts GL et al. Measurement of anal sphincter muscles: endoanal US, endoanal MR ima-

ging, or phased-array MR imaging? A study with healthy volunteers. Radiology 2001;220:81–89.

30. Nielsen MB, Hauge C, Rasmussen OO et al. Anal sphincter size measured by endosonography in healthy volunteers. Effect of age, sex and parity. Acta Radiol 1992; 33:453–456.

31. Enck P, Heyer T, Gantke B et al. How reproducible are measures of the anal sphincter muscle diameter by endoanal ultrasound? Am J Gastroenterol 1997;92:293–296.

32. Gold DM, Halligan S, Kmiot WA, Bartram CI. Intraobserver and interobserver agreement in anal endosonography. Br J Surg 1999;86:371–375.

33. Williams AB, Bartram CI, Modhwadia D et al. Endocoil magnetic resonance imaging quantification of external sphincter atrophy. Br J Surg 2001;88:853–859.

34. Williams AB, Malouf AJ, Bartram CI et al. Assessment of external anal sphincter morphology in idiopathic fecal incontinence with endocoil magnetic resonance imaging. Dig Dis Sci 2001;46:1466–1471.

35. Hussain SM, Stoker J, Zwamborn AW et al. Endoanal MR imaging of the anal sphincter complex: correlation with cross-sectional anatomy and histology. J Anat 1996; 189:677–682.

36. Rociu E, Stoker J, Eijkemans MJC, Lameris JS. Normal anal sphincter anatomy and age- and sex-related variations at high-spatial-resolution endoanal MR imaging. Radiology 2000;217:395–401.

37. Morren GL, Beets-Tan GH, van Engelshoven MA. Anatomy of the anal canal and perianal structures as defined by phase-array magnetic resonance imaging. Br J Surg 2001; 88:1506–1512.

38. DeSouza NM, Puni R, Zbar A et al. MR imaging of the anal sphincter in multiparous women using an endoanal coil: correlation with in-vitro anatomy and appearances in fecal incontinence. Am J Roentgenol 1996;167:1465–1471.

39. Stoker J, Rociu E, Zwamborn AW et al. Endoluminal MR imaging of the rectum and anus: technique, applications and pitfalls. Radiographics 1999;19:383–398.

40. West RL, Felt-Bersma RJF, Hansen BE et al. Volume measurement of the anal sphincter complex in healthy controls and fecal-incontinent patients with a three-dimensional reconstruction of endoanal ultrasonography images. Dis Colon Rectum 2005;48:540–548.

41. Sentovich SM, Wong WD, Blatchford GJ. Accuracy and reliability of transanal ultrasound for anterior anal sphincter injury. Dis Colon Rectum 1998;41:1000–1014.

42. Sultan AH, Kamm MA, Hudson CN et al. Anal-sphincter disruption during vaginal delivery. N Engl J Med 1993; 329:1905–1911.

43. Burnett SJ, Spence-Jones C, Speakman CT et al. Unsuspected sphincter damage following childbirth revealed by anal endosonography. Br J Radiol 1991;64:225–227.

44. Zetterstrom JP, Mellgren A, Jensen LL et al. Effect of delivery on anal sphincter morphology and function. Dis Colon Rectum 1999;42:1253–1260.

45. Tjandra JJ, Milsom JW, Stolfi VM et al. Endoluminal ultrasound defines anatomy of the anal canal and pelvic floor. Dis Colon Rectum 1992;35:465–470.

46. Nielsen MB, Rasmussen OO, Pedersen JF, Christiansen J. Anal endosonographic findings in patients with obstructed defecation. Acta Radiol 1993;34:35–38.

Technical Innovations in Pelvic Floor Ultrasonography

9

Giulio Aniello Santoro, Aleksandra Stankiewicz,
Jakob Scholbach, Michał Chlebiej and
Andrzej Paweł Wieczorek

Abstract In this chapter the diagnostic potential of evaluating structural and functional interactions of female pelvic floor structures using novel image-processing techniques is presented. Technical innovations include three-dimensional volume render mode, maximum intensity projection, manual segmentation and sculpting, fusion imaging, PixelFlux, framing, color vector mapping, and motion tracking. When introduced into routine clinical practice, these new modalities will improve the management of pelvic floor dysfunctions.

Keywords Framing • Fusion imaging • Maximum intensity projection • Motion tracking • PixelFlux • Render mode • Sculpting • Three-dimensional ultrasonography

9.1 Introduction

Recently, several new ultrasound techniques have been developed that could significantly improve the diagnostic value of ultrasonography (US) in pelvic floor disorders. Three-dimensional (3D) and real-time four-dimensional (4D) imaging have been introduced into routine medical practice [1–4]. These techniques overcome some of the difficulties and limitations associated with conventional two-dimensional (2D) US. Although 2D cross-sectional images may provide valuable information, it is often difficult to interpret the relationship between different pelvic floor structures because the 3D anatomy must be reconstructed mentally. Three-dimensional reconstructions may closely resemble the real 3D anatomy and can therefore significantly improve the assessment of normal and pathologic anatomy. Complex information on the exact location, extent, and relation of relevant pelvic structures can be displayed in a single 3D image. Interactive manipulation of the 3D data on the computer also increases the ability to assess critical details.

In this chapter the new methods of 3D-US, including volume render mode (VRM), maximum intensity projection (MIP), and brush/shaving options with manual segmentation (sculpting) will be described. A variety of other advanced ultrasonographic techniques, including fusion imaging, PixelFlux, framing, and color vector mapping and motion tracking will also be presented. It seems likely that these new diagnostic tools will be increasingly used in the future to provide more detailed information on the morphology and function of examined organs, to facilitate planning and monitoring of operations, and for surgical training.

G.A. Santoro
Pelvic Floor Unit and Colorectal Service, 1st Department
of General Surgery, Regional Hospital, Treviso, Italy

G.A. Santoro, A.P. Wieczorek, C.I. Bartram (eds.) *Pelvic Floor Disorders*
© Springer-Verlag Italia 2010

9.2 Volume Render Mode

Volume render mode is a technique for analysis of the information inside a 3D volume by digitally enhancing individual voxels [1]. It is currently one of the most advanced and computer-intensive rendering algorithms available for computed tomography (CT) scanning [5, 6] and can also be applied to high-resolution 3D-US data volume [1, 6]. The typical ray/beam-tracing algorithm sends a ray/beam from each point (pixel) of the viewing screen through the 3D space rendered. Depending on the various render mode settings, the data from each voxel may be stored as a referral for the next voxel and further used in a filtering calculation, may be discarded, or may modify the existing value of the beam. The final displayed pixel color is computed from the color, transparency, and reflectivity of all the volumes and surfaces encountered by the beam. The weighted summation of these images produces the volume-rendered view [1]. The concept of a classification is based on the Gaussian distribution of intensities around a central peak

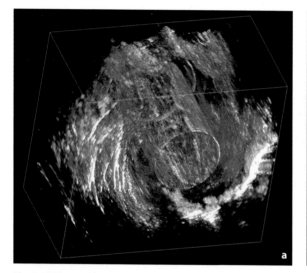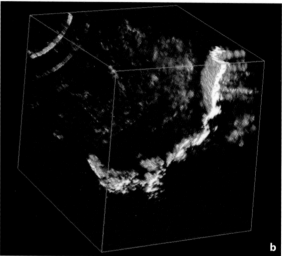

Fig. 9.1 Effects of imaging processing (volume render mode with filtering) on fistula tract views after hydrogen peroxide injection through an external opening (**a**, **b**). Scan obtained by endoanal ultrasound with 2050 transducer (B-K Medical)

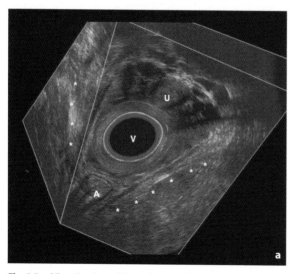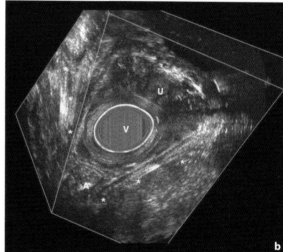

Fig. 9.2 a Visualization of the puborectalis muscle in different oblique planes (*). **b** Post-processing manipulation (volume render mode with high opacity and luminance) improves the visibility of the muscle. *A*, anal canal; *U*, urethra; *V*, transducer into vagina. Scan obtained by endovaginal ultrasound with 2050 transducer (B-K Medical)

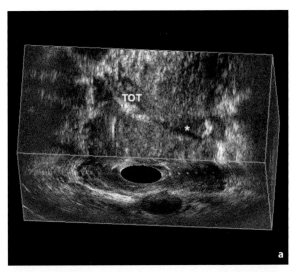 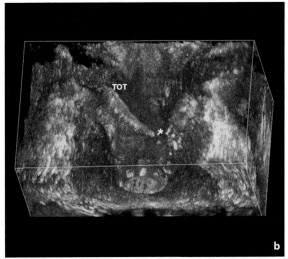

Fig. 9.3 Visualization of the position of a trans-obturator tape (*TOT*) in the coronal plane. In the left side the sling appears dislodged (*). **a** Normal mode, **b** volume render mode. Scan obtained by endovaginal ultrasound with 2050 transducer (B-K Medical)

value, which represents 100% of that tissue (percentage classification). Each voxel may represent one or more tissue types, and the amount of each tissue type as a percentage of the entire voxel ranges from 0% to 100% [1]. As already reported in Chapter 6, four fundamental post-processing functions can be used in VRM: opacity, luminance, thickness and filter. By using these different post-processing display parameters, the volume-rendered image provides better visualization when there are not any large differences in the signal levels of pathologic structures compared with surrounding tissues [1]. Thus, it is successfully applied for more precise assessment of some pathological conditions, such as anal sphincter defects, fistulous tracts in perianal sepsis (Fig. 9.1), and invasiveness of the submucosal layer in early rectal cancer [7]. Moreover, it seems to be a very promising method for detailed evaluation of the integrity of or injuries to the pelvic floor muscles (Fig. 9.2), visualization of the spatial distribution of the vascular networks supplying the urethra, and assessment of the location of tapes or meshes after pelvic floor surgery (Fig. 9.3).

9.3 Maximum Intensity Projection

Maximum intensity projection (MIP) is a 3D visualization modality involving a large amount of computation [3]. It can be defined as the aggregate exposure at each point, which tries to find the brightest or most significant

color or intensity along an ultrasound beam. Once the beam is projected through the entire volume, the value displayed on the screen is the maximum intensity value found (the highest value of gray, or the highest value associated with a color). Conversely, if the value displayed on the screen is the minimum value found, this is termed minimum intensity projection (MinIP).

The application of MIP in a 3D color mode reduces the intensity of the grayscale voxels so that they appear as a light fog over color information, which is in this way highlighted. In a color volume, the colors are mapped to a given value in the volume. Because the pixel color or intensity of the image projected on the display is no longer coded with depth information, the display loses a lot of the 3D appearance. Thus, it seems not to be reliable to use MIP images for location purposes. Moreover, due to the color mapping, a volume with flow information will not display any grayscale information in the MIP mode.

It has been reported in the literature that the application of MIP to 3D color US allows visualization of the distribution of blood vessels in tumors, providing additional information for management. Ohishi et al [8] found that 3D images with MIP mode improved evaluation of the entire vasculature of a tumor compared to cross-sectional 2D-images. Hamazaki et al [9] reported that 3D color Doppler US with MIP mode appeared to be useful for the differential diagnosis of subpleural lesions. Motohide et al [10] considered this technique an efficient and safe modality as an intra-

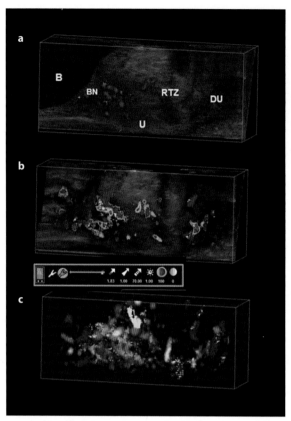

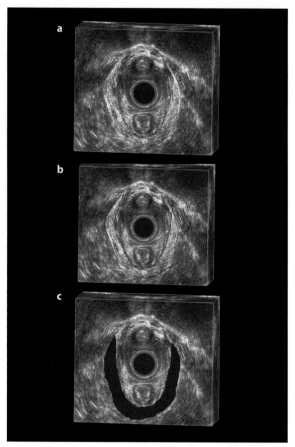

Fig. 9.4 Mid-sagittal view of urethral vasculature with color Doppler mode (**a**), normal render mode (**b**), and maximum intensity projection (**c**). *B*, bladder; *BN*, bladder neck; *DU*, distal urethra; *RTZ*, Retzius plexus; *U*, urethra. Scan obtained by endovaginal ultrasound with 8848 transducer (B-K Medical)

Fig. 9.5 Sculpting of the levator ani muscle. **a** Axial view obtained by endovaginal ultrasound with 2050 transducer. **b** The outlining of the levator ani muscle. **c** The levator ani muscle is removed

operative navigation system for liver surgery. In a preliminary study in nulliparous females, we found that application of MIP reconstruction allowed visualization of the patterns of urethral vessels (spatial distribution and localization of vessels) (Fig. 9.4) [11].

9.4 Brush Options – Segmentation – Sculpting

Sculpting is a post-processing tool that allows the examiner to mark volume voxels, during off-line assessment of 3D-US imaging (version 7.0.0.406 - B-K Medical 3D Viewer), so that they are not displayed in the rendering operations. The marking process uses a standard projection method to map screen locations within a boundary of the volume data. There are two methods available: (1) in the first technique, the voxels are marked in a mirror volume which gives the possibility

of turning the marking on and off or inverting it; (2) in the second technique, the voxels are replaced with some marker value. This method requires reloading of the volume to turn off the sculpting.

Various sculpting tools are possible, giving different degrees of control over what is removed: (1) to draw an outline and then remove everything within that outline to a given depth or through the entire volume; (2) to draw an outline and then remove everything outside the outline; or (3) to use a shaving tool that marks a few voxels at a time around the point of the cursor. The depth of sculpting can be a percentage of the total or a given value in millimeters from the surface of the volume. As pelvic structures vary in shape and lie in different oblique planes, we recommend performing a sculpting on every section of some millimeters' length, or even on every image of 300 transaxial images collected during 3D data acquisition (Figs. 9.5, 9.6). Sculpting was originally developed for enhancing static volumes of the fetus by re-

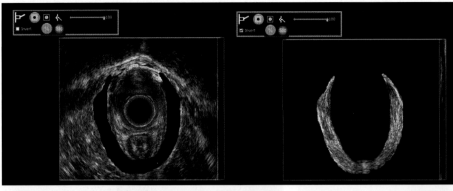

Fig. 9.6 Two methods of sculpting: (1) the levator ani muscle is outlined and is cut off (*left*); and (2) outlining of the levator ani muscle with cut-off of all the structures lying beyond (*right*). Scan obtained by endovaginal ultrasound with 2050 transducer (B-K Medical)

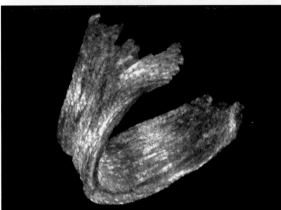

Fig. 9.7 Levator ani muscle reconstruction using the sculpting method. Scan obtained by endovaginal ultrasound with 2050 transducer (B-K Medical)

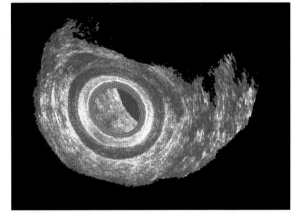

Fig. 9.8 Three-dimensional reconstruction of the middle third of the anal canal using the sculpting method. The two rings of the internal (hypoechoic) and external (hyperechoic) sphincters are clearly visualized. Scan obtained by endoanal ultrasound with 2050 transducer (B-K Medical)

moving the placenta [12]. Its introduction into pelvic imaging might facilitate the assessment of pelvic floor structures (Figs. 9.7, 9.8), allowing comparison of the morphology in different disorders.

9.5 Fusion Imaging

Fusion imaging is based on a simultaneous capturing of scans obtained by two different examinations, e.g. CT/MRI (magnetic resonance imaging), US/MRI, CT-PET (positron emission tomography), MRI-PET, providing the information gathered by both modalities fused. This technique ensures a compensation for the deficiencies of one method and retains the advantages of another one. Fusion imaging is performed by using dedicated software, on a graphic workstation, where the data are transferred using the Digital Imaging and Communications in Medicine (DICOM) system. The volume-rendering mode allows simultaneous projection of the 3D dataset of two different studies to be fused. The datasets are labeled with color to allow the user to identify the separate studies. The color labeling is arbitrary and depends on the user's preference. The registration process requires an individual manipulation and is achieved by superimposing the two datasets with the use of 3D volume projection. It is, however, mostly conducted in the 2D slice views, due to easier visualization of the superimposed datasets, and in the transverse planes, as these provide better scanning resolution. The user works in the standard directions of sagittal, coronal, and transverse, and updates the registration in each of these views. Final image registration is based on anatomical adjustment of the imaging studies.

Fusion imaging is commonly used in the diagnosis of cancer patients. Kim et al [13] showed an additional diagnostic value of fused MR/PET images in comparison with PET/CT in the detection of metastatic lymph

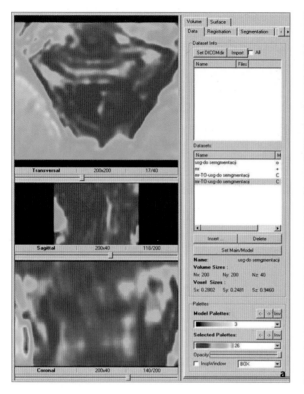

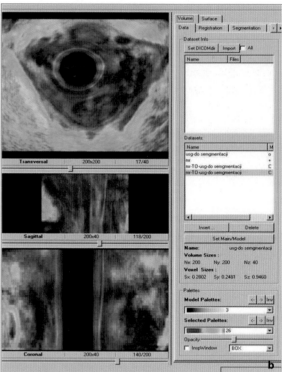

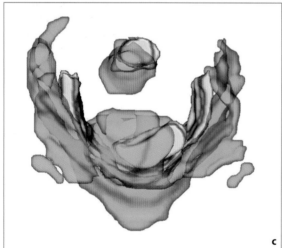

Fig. 9.9 Axial views of the female pelvis. **a** MRI scan.
b Endovaginal ultrasound with 2050 transducer (B-K Medical).
Both images were captured simultaneously to allow fusion
of the information provided by each technique. **c** Fusion
imaging of the three-dimensional reconstruction of the levator
ani muscle (*brown*: US image; *green*: MR image)

nodes in patients with uterine cervical cancer. Another
study reported that the fusion of real-time transrectal
ultrasound (TRUS) and prior MR images of the
prostate facilitated MRI-guided interventions such as
prostate biopsies, cryoablation, brachytherapy, beam
radiation therapy, or direct injection of agents outside
of the MRI suite [14]. Moreover, the image fusion between color-Doppler TRUS and endorectal MRI appeared to improve the accuracy of pathological staging
in patients with prostate cancer [15].

Similarly, CT/MRI fusion imagings were performed for abdominal, cervical, and intracranial regions
assessment [16].

We assessed the application of US/MRI fusion imaging for the visualization of pelvic floor structures
in nulliparous females. Ultrasound examination was
performed by 360° rotational endovaginal transducer
with 3D data acquisition (type 2050, BK Medical),
while MRI was conducted by using 1.0 Tesla MR
scanner (Genesis Signa, GE). For the fusion process,

T_1-weighted axial scans were used. Fusion imaging was performed on a laptop with the use of dedicated software, and once it was completed a 3D reconstruction of the levator ani muscle and the anatomical alignment was conducted (Fig. 9.9). Both methods appeared to be highly concordant in the visualization of this muscle; however, MRI, due to a wider field of view than the ultrasound transducer, provided more information about surrounding structures.

9.6 PixelFlux

PixelFlux is dedicated software that allows an automated calculation of blood perfusion in arbitrary regions of interest (ROIs) of different organs [17, 18]. The basic principle of this software is the requirement that measurements must be reliable. For this reason:

1. Perfusion measurements should not be influenced by the external settings of the US device. Any parameters that impact the perfusion depiction must be kept constant throughout. One of these parameters is pulse repetition frequency (PRF), which is the number of pulses produced per second and is equal to the voltage pulse repetition frequency determined by the ultrasound scanner. Higher PRF permits higher Doppler shifts to be detected and lower PRF allows recording of lower velocities. The calibration of the image, which consists of setting the scale and the maximum Doppler velocity, is automatically provided by the software, particularly when DICOM files are used (Fig. 9.10).
2. Perfusion measurements must not rely on the subjective visual impression of the examiner, as this may lead to serious misinterpretation. To avoid operator dependency, when opening a video or DICOM file the software automatically finds the scale indicating the colors used for perfusion depiction and allows a standardized measurement (Fig. 9.10).
3. Perfusion measurements must yield constant results when comparing the perfusion of the same patient at different times. Measurements should be constant both on a large scale (compatibility between examinations conducted with a delay of some days or weeks, assuming that the patient's physical conditions remain unchanged), and on a small scale (periodic flow pattern of vessels due to cardiac action). In order to assess the perfusion in an authentic way,

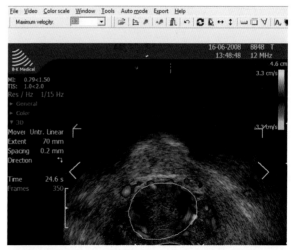

Fig. 9.10 Application of PixelFlux software for perfusion measurements in the female urethra. Data sheet: the setting includes the color scale, the maximum velocity, and the definition of the region of interest. Scan obtained by endovaginal ultrasound with 8848 transducer (B-K Medical)

it is thus crucial either to take into account the perfusion in similar points of the cardiac cycle, e.g. by always comparing the systolic or diastolic perfusion, or to compute the "average perfusion" during a complete heart cycle. As the former approach is both time consuming and error prone, particularly when done by manual definition of the point in question, the latter approach is preferred and is the one predominantly employed in the software.

The key step of the perfusion measurement technique is the definition of the ROI. The ROI can be arbitrarily chosen by the examiner, taking any desired size or shape. In contrast to other methods that assess blood flow, such as spectral Doppler mode, PixelFlux is applicable to both single large vessels and an area of small vessels. In addition to free-hand outlining, a ROI can also be defined as a parallelogram, which has proved useful in measuring renal parenchymal perfusion [18], or can be derived from another free-hand outlined ROI by a dartboard-like scheme, which is adapted to ring-like structures such as the rhabdosphincter muscle or the inner ring of the urethra, including the longitudinal smooth muscle, the circular smooth muscle, and the submucosa layer of the urethra (Fig. 9.11).

After choosing the ROI, the software automatically calculates the perfusion of the region in every frame of the video assessed. The following parameters are computed: (1) the velocity V, which corresponds to

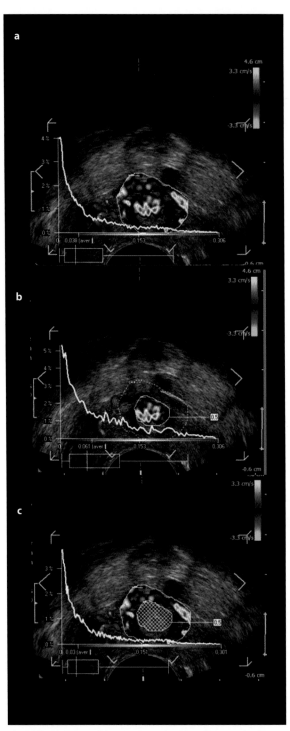

Fig. 9.11 a Region of interest includes the whole urethral complex. Perfusion measurements are calculated, **b** in the inner urethral ring (including the longitudinal smooth muscle, the circular smooth muscle and the submucosa), and **c** in the external urethral ring (corresponding to the rhabdosphincter). Axial scan of the mid-urethra obtained by endovaginal ultrasound with 8848 transducer (B-K Medical)

the color hue of the pixels inside the ROI; (2) the perfused area A, given by the amount of perfused pixels inside the ROI; and (3) the perfusion intensity, I. This parameter is defined as the ratio:

$$I = V \times A / A_{ROI}$$

where A_{ROI} denotes the total area of the ROI. Consequently, the perfusion intensity increases with the perfusion velocity, but decreases if less of the total area of the ROI is globally perfused. These three parameters are computed for each single frame of the video examined. Based on the periodic changes due to the cardiac cycle, the program then automatically calculates the heart period and takes into account only one or multiple full heart cycles. The quantification of complete heart cycles accomplishes the need for a time-independent perfusion measurement as outlined above. Fig. 9.12 shows a heart cycle recognized by the software (the parts of the chart highlighted in red and blue, respectively).

Another key parameter of the PixelFlux software is "perfusion relief". It shows the local distribution of perfusion intensity, like a map depicting the height of mountains (Fig. 9.12). This tool can be used to gain a visual impression of the vasculature, showing areas with different local perfusion (Fig. 9.13). In addition, the spectrum of the measured velocities is also reported, distinguishing areas with higher velocities from those with lower ones. This can help to evaluate whether the perfusion is primarily taking place in larger vessels, where the velocities tend to be higher, rather than in smaller vessels. Using the PixelFlux software for assessment of the blood perfusion in the urethra of nulliparous females, we found that the intramural and distal part of the urethra had poorer vascular intensity than the midurethra. Interestingly, we did not observe any difference between the perfusion intensity in the inner (including the longitudinal smooth muscle, the circular smooth muscle and the submucosa) and outer (corresponding to the rhabdosphincter muscle) rings of the midurethra [19].

The PixelFlux technique enables a quantitative assessment of blood perfusion. The program is completed by an internal database, facilitating the handling of large amounts of patient data, including features for comparison of different patients or examination of the same patient at different times. It appears a very promising method for evaluating the vasculature of pelvic structures

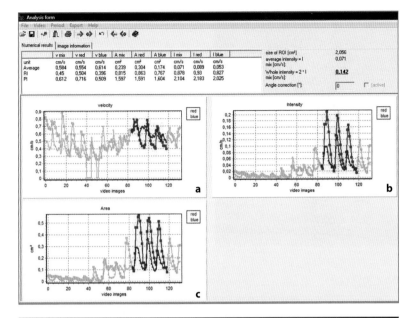

Fig. 9.12 PixelFlux technique. Analysis form shows the heart cycles and the values of velocity (**a**), intensity (**b**), and area (**c**) within the region of interest

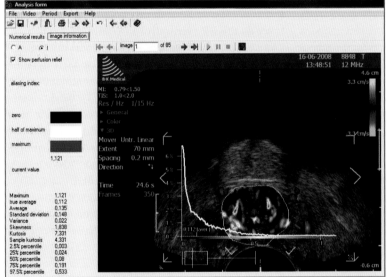

Fig. 9.13 PixelFlux technique. Region of interest includes the mid-urethra. Analysis form showing the local perfusion relief (*red* areas correspond to regions with high perfusion velocity; *white* and *black* areas correspond to regions with moderate or low perfusion velocity). Scan obtained by endovaginal ultrasound with 8848 transducer (B-K Medical)

in females at risk for developing urinary incontinence or organ prolapse. In addition, it could be used to analyze the perfusion intensity in women suffering from any pelvic floor disorder, in order to define whether the severity of their symptoms correlates with perfusion parameters.

9.7 Framing

The motion of pelvic structures can be observed in real-time by using dynamic ultrasound, while asking patients in a supine or standing position to strain or to cough. The data can be registered as video files for off-line examination. Dynamic US, however, provides an abundance of information that cannot be captured by the observer alone, as it occurs too fast.

Framing is a modality that provides a detailed visualization of the motion sequences of specific structures. With use of dedicated software (VIRTUAL-DUB), it is possible to analyze consecutive frames of a video file, by cutting off the frame without decompression. It has potential application in the assessment of functional disorders of the pelvic floor (Fig. 9.14).

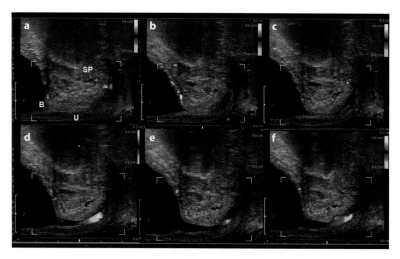

Fig. 9.14 Assessment of urethral complex motion and bladder neck opening in an incontinent female (longitudinal view of the anterior compartment obtained by the endovaginal ultrasound with 8848 transducer). Initially, the rhabdosphincter is flat and the bladder neck is closed (**a**, **b**); then, during Valsalva maneuver, the rhabdosphincter becomes thicker but shorter (**c**, **d**) and the bladder neck opens (**e**, **f**). The data were registered as a video file lasting 33 s. After application of the framing software for evaluation of the timing sequences, the video file was cut into 52 images. *B*, bladder neck; *SP*, symphysis pubis; *U*, urethra

9.8 Motion Tracking and Color Vector Mapping

Our ability to understand pelvic floor dysfunction arises from understanding the complex functional interactions among pelvic organs, muscles, ligaments, and connective tissue. Dynamic US imaging provides a quantitative evaluation of pelvic floor structures. Measurements of bladder neck displacement, urethral inclination, and retrovesical angle at rest and during pushing or straining give important information in patients with urinary incontinence [20]. However, due to small dimensions and different velocities and movements of the pelvic structures, it is not possible to describe their interactions precisely.

Motion tracking is a modality for the assessment of biomechanical properties of tissues and organs [21]. Computer-aided vector-based perineal ultrasound appears to be a feasible and valuable tool for the assessment of bladder neck mobility, allowing the user to distinguish between women with and without stress urinary incontinence [22, 23]. Peng et al [24] reported that motion tracking may be used for the assessment of puborectalis and pubococcygeus contraction, by evaluating the displacement of the anorectal angle (ARA) during perineal US. To map accurately the trajectory of the ARA, every frame was indexed to the same rigid landmark (the symphysis pubis – SP). A template of the SP was initially defined in the first frame of the ultrasonographic video file, then it was compared with the second image with different offset in both the x and y direction. The matching procedure employed some equations

and was repeated until the last image frame. The relative displacement of the ARA to the SP was obtained by subtraction of the SP from the ARA. Results of this study showed that during cough, the ARA moves towards the SP (ventrally) in continent women and away from the SP (dorsally) in urinary-incontinent patients. In addition, the amplitude of ARA maximal caudal displacement was smaller in continent women compared to incontinent patients [24]. Constantinou [25] described the dynamics of female pelvic floor function using urodynamics, ultrasound imaging with motion tracking, and MR, in terms of determining the mechanism of urinary continence. Among these modalities, motion tracking provided quantitative measures (displacement, velocity, acceleration, trajectory, motility, strain) of pelvic floor muscles. On the basis of these parameters, the status of continent and asymptomatic women could be clearly distinguished from those with incontinence.

We developed a novel computer software for quantitative assessment of the motion of pelvic structures. This software was originally applied to 3D echo-cardiographic scans to evaluate the kinetics of the cardiac walls in patients with heart infarction [26, 27]. The process of analysis consisted of several main steps:

- filtering: to improve the US image quality and to remove the noise; the diffusion algorithm was applied, as it dramatically enhances the structure boundaries and reduces the speckle noise
- description of the motion: recovery of transformation, that aligns the reference frame with all the

other frames using intensity-based 3D volume registration; this allows to visualize local deformation of spatial objects

- de-noising procedure using time-averaging technique: the deformation fields are used to generate new datasets elastically aligned with the reference frame T_0; the noise in the datasets is smoothed and the boundaries of the image structures are preserved
- segmentation step using the averaged dataset by iterative deformable boundary approach
- reconstruction of the motion by applying the deformation field operator.

For description of the motion, vector displacement was calculated as a total displacement (relative to the reference frame T_0) and displacement between consequent time frames which can be seen as an instantaneous velocity. To visualize the motion occurring on the surface (twisting), the instantaneous velocity vectors were decomposed into tangential and normal components.

Different techniques can be used to visualize the local variations of the motion as follows:

- Color-based visualization according to length values of displacement vectors. It is the preferred modality when we deal with small moving surfaces.

- Vector-based visualization: for significant motion it is preferred to visualize vector values using the arrows representing the length and spatial orientation of moving matter.
- Line-paths-based visualization: in this method, the small set of surface points is selected and the path of their motion is visualized. Colors of the line segments represent various time frames. This method enables estimation of the viability of the heart using a single image. In addition to the line-paths method, we may also generate the "activity surface". Using this technique, total path length values (in a single cardiac cycle) for every surface point can be visualized. Thus it allows easy detection of moving regions and evaluation of how significant this motion is, as well as estimation of the spatial extent of pathological regions on single static image. Line-paths visualization contains complete information about the motion, whereas activity surfaces show the overall surface activity more clearly [27].

The motion tracking procedure described above can be applied to assessment of the function of pelvic structures. The data are collected using transperineal and endovaginal ultrasound scanning in B mode, during straining and Valsalva maneuver, and registered as video files. The data are then analyzed with the use of

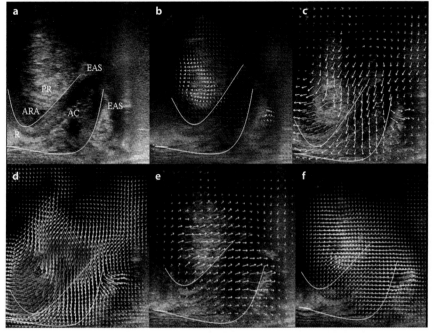

Fig. 9.15 **a** Longitudinal section of the posterior compartment. Color and vector mapping were applied for the assessment of the muscles' motion. *AC*, anal canal; *ARA*, anorectal angle; *EAS*, external anal sphincter; *PR*, puborectalis muscle; *R*, rectum. **b–d** During straining, upward movement of the puborectalis is visualized. This movement closes the anorectal angle, assuring continence. **e, f** During Valsalva maneuver, the puborectalis activity is suppressed, whereas the external sphincter opens. Scans obtained by endovaginal ultrasound with 8848 transducer

color and vector mapping (Fig. 9.15). We believe that this modality could enhance our knowledge of pelvic organ dysfunction, facilitating the diagnosis of injuries or deficiency of pelvic muscles after childbirth that are not detectable by conventional imaging techniques. It can also be useful to evaluate muscle strength after biofeedback treatment.

References

1   Santoro GA, Fortling B. The advantages of volume rendering in three-dimensional endosonography of the anorectum. Dis Colon Rectum 2007;50:359–368.

2. Dietz HP, Steensma AB. Posterior compartment prolapse on two-dimensional and three-dimensional pelvic floor ultrasound: the distinction between true rectocele, perineal hypermobility and enterocele. Ultrasound Obstet Gynecol 2005;26:73–77.

3. Mitterberger M, Pinggera GM, Mueller T et al. Dynamic transurethral sonography and 3-dimensional reconstruction of the rhabdosphincter and urethra: initial experience in continent and incontinent women. J Ultrasound Med 2006; 25:315–320.

4. Santoro GA, Wieczorek AP, Stankiewicz A et al. High-resolution three-dimensional endovaginal ultrasonography in the assessment of pelvic floor anatomy: a preliminary study. Int Urogynecol J 2009;20:1213–1222.

5. Saba L, Pascalis L, Mallagrini G. Multi-detector-row CT of muscles with volume rendering technique. Panminerva Med 2009;51:43–49.

6. Kuo J, Bredthauer JG, Castellucci JB, von Ramm OT. Interactive volume rendering of real-time three-dimensional ultrasound images. IEEE Trans Ultrason Ferroelectr Freq Control 2007;2:54.

7. Santoro GA, Gizzi, G, Pellegrini L et al. The value of high-resolution three-dimensional endorectal ultrasonography in the management of submucosal invasive rectal tumor. Dis Colon Rectum 2009;52:1837–1843

8. Ohishi H, Hirai T, Yamada R et al. Three-dimensional power Doppler sonography of tumor vascularity. J Ultrasound Med 1998;17:619–622

9. Hamazaki N, Kounoike Y, Makinodan K et al. Usefulness of three-dimensional color Doppler sonography for the differential diagnosis of subpleural lesions. Nihon Kokyuki Gakkai Zasshi 2001;39:453–460.

10. Motohide S, Go W, Masahiro O et al. Clinical application of three-dimensional ultrasound imaging as intraoperative navigation for liver surgery. Nippon Geka Gakkai Zasshi 1998;99:203–207.

11. Wieczorek AP, Woźniak MM, Stankiewicz A et al (2009) Quantification of urethral vascularity with high-frequency endovaginal ultrasonography. Preliminary report in nulliparous females (personal communication).

12. Rothenberg F, Fisher SA, Watanabe M. Sculpting the cardiac outflow tract. Birth Defects Res C Embryo Today 2003; 69:38–45.

13. Kim SK, Choi HJ, Park SY et al. Additional value of MR/PET fusion compared with PET/CT in the detection of lymph node metastases in cervical cancer patients. Eur J Cancer 2009;45:2103–2109.

14. Singh AK, Kruecker J, Xu S et al. Initial clinical experience with real-time transrectal ultrasonography-magnetic resonance imaging fusion-guided prostate biopsy. BJU Int 2008;101:841–845.

15. Selli C, Caramella D, Giusti S et al. Value of image fusion in the staging of prostatic carcinoma. Radiol Med 2007; 112:74–81.

16. Mukherji SK, Rosenman JG, Soltys M et al. A new technique for CT/MR fusion for skull base imaging. Skull Base Surg 1996;6:141–146.

17. Scholbach T, Herrero I, Scholbach J. Dynamic color Doppler sonography of intestinal wall in patients with Crohn disease compared with healthy subjects. J Pediatr Gastroenterol Nutr 2004;39:524–528.

18. Scholbach T, Girelli E, Scholbach J. Dynamic tissue perfusion measurement: a novel tool in follow-up of renal transplants. Transplantation 2005;79:1711–1716.

19. Wieczorek AP, Woźniak MM, Stankiewicz A et al. The assessment of normal female urethral vascularity with Color Doppler endovaginal ultrasonography: preliminary report. Pelviperineology 2009;28:59–61.

20. Pregazzi R, Sartore A, Bortoli P et al. Perineal ultrasound evaluation of urethral angle and bladder neck mobility in women with stress urinary incontinence. BJOG 2002; 109:821–827.

21. Rahmanian S, Jones R, Peng Q, Constantinou C. Visualization of biomechanical properties of female pelvic floor function using video motion tracking of ultrasound imaging. Stud Health Technol Inform 2008; 132:390–395.

22. Huang YL, Chen HY. Computer-aided diagnosis of urodynamic stress incontinence with vector-based perineal ultrasound using neural networks. Ultrasound Obstet Gynecol 2007;30:1002–1006.

23. Reddy AP, DeLancey JOL, Zwica LM, Ashton-Miller JM. On-screen vector-based ultrasound assessment of vesical neck movement. Am J Obstet Gynecol 2001;185:65–70.

24. Peng Q, Jones R, Shishido K, Constantinou CE. Ultrasound evaluation of dynamic responses of female pelvic floor muscles. Ultrasound Med Biol 2007;33:342–352.

25. Constantinou C. Dynamics of female pelvic floor function using urodynamics, ultrasound and magnetic resonance imaging. Europ J Obstet Gynecol Reprod Biol 2009;144S:S159–S165.

26. Chlebiej M, Nowiński K, Ścisło P, Bała P. Reconstruction of heart motion from 4D echocardiographic images. In: Kropatsch WG, Kampel M, Hanbury A (eds). Computer analysis of images and patterns. Lecture notes in computer science, volume 4673. Springer-Verlag, Berlin, Heidelberg, 2007, pp 245–252.

27. Chlebiej M, Nowiński K, Ścisło P, Bała P. Heart motion visualization tools for 4D echocardiographic images. J Med Informat Technol 2007;11:177–184.

Invited Commentary

Clive I. Bartram

Our understanding of the sonographic anatomy of the pelvic floor has developed following technical improvements in image quality, and the ability to break free of the restrictions imposed by fixed-plane imaging. Three-dimensional (3D) imaging provides representation of structures in their true anatomical plane, and has allowed direct comparisons to be made with magnetic resonance imaging (MRI). MRI gives hard anatomical detail with striated muscle clearly defined. Using information from a variety of sources such as surgery and cadaveric dissection, but particularly 3D endosonography, to colocate endocoil MRI images, it has been possible to work out the exact anatomical detail of the sphincter. Once the sonographic appearances have been established in this way, greater reliance can be placed on their interpretation. This methodology has been key in developing the sonographic investigation of the pelvic floor.

The quality of a 3D dataset depends on image thickness and separation. Voxel symmetry relates to pixel size and beam width. If non-isometric, the image resolution will vary in different planes. If the gap between images increases, resolution also decreases, as greater interpolation is required that will smooth out fine detail. The current automated transducers represent a considerable advance over previous cumbersome mechanical linear translation devices. It is simple to obtain the dataset and to ensure that the entire length of the canal has been captured. Cine looping through the dataset is exactly the same as continuing the examination, as the dataset stores all the information at maximum resolution. Providing the original dataset is technically adequate, this means that any review will be as informative as re-examining the patient, and far more accurate than looking at a limited selection of images or even a video recording. In routine practice, this is one of the understated advantages of 3D imaging.

The 3D software is also critical, and again this is now highly functional with all the usual volume rendering features one would expect. Unfortunately, ultrasound imposes limitations on dataset analysis. If, for example, the pixel brightness of scarring was within narrow bands distinct from other tissues, it would be simple to seed the dataset for this defined band and then render the overall translucency so that the entire extent of the scarring was revealed. Unfortunately, there is just too much overlap with other structures for this to work. Some enhancement is beneficial, but in practice the main benefits are looking at structures in their correct anatomical plane, measuring length and area, and using some planes to look at specific structures, i.e. the bladder and urethra in the midsagittal plane, and the external sphincter in women in the coronal plane to visualize tears. During review it is often helpful to use two planes, so for the sphincter tears starting in the coronal plane and then moving to the axial plane to have a more complete understanding of the extent of a tear. Fusion imaging automates what was previously a research tool of collocation. Although this is mainly being used in cancer patients, one can foresee the ultrasonography/MRI combination being used in the wider assessment of pelvic floor damage. Perfusion mapping using PixelFlux software may have limited use, but the developments in framing and motion tracking are really very exciting, as these take what has currently to be largely eyeball assessment into the realm of accurate complex measurement that will surely lead to a clearer understanding of normal and abnormal movement, pre and post surgery in the pelvic floor.

C.I. Bartram
Diagnostic Imaging, Princess Grace Hospital, London, UK

Endocavity imaging of the vagina, anus, and rectum is static, as the probe inhibits normal movement. However, this limitation does not apply to external probes and transperineal or translabial imaging has opened a new field of dynamic pelvic floor imaging, aided by dynamic 3D reconstruction. This has been termed "4D" imaging, which really just refers to the dynamic presentation of the 3D data.

The stresses that can be applied to the pelvic floor are the Valsalva and pelvic floor contraction. Dynamic 4D-style imaging during these maneuvers is very informative. Maximal muscle contraction makes the muscle bulkier and further defines the insertion. Changes in the levator hiatus area may also be measured with 3D systems.

The pelvic floor musculature may therefore be analyzed in anatomical and functional terms.

The pelvic floor is a very complex structure. With 3D analysis of endocavity and transperineal sonography we now have relatively simple examination techniques that provide a wealth of information, both static and dynamic, about the pelvic floor.

Magnetic Resonance Imaging: Methodology and Normal Pelvic Floor Anatomy

10

Jaap Stoker

Abstract The female pelvic floor comprises several structures, including anal and urethral sphincters, several anatomical layers, and supportive elements (often constituents of the endopelvic fascia which is an advential layer). The multilayered urethra is supported by several structures such as the endopelvic fascia, compressor urethra, and urethrovaginal sphincter, and has attachment to the pelvic diaphragm. The uterus and vagina are, amongst other, supported by several condensations of the endopelvic fascia (e.g. the uterosacral ligament). The rectum is also supported by endopelvic fascia condensations. The anal sphincter is a multilayered cylindrical structure with an outer striated muscle (external sphincter, puborectal muscle). The perineal body has attachments with multiple structures such as the external sphincter, longitudinal layer, and perineal membrane and therefore has an important role in support. The major constituents of the pelvic diaphragm are the iliococcygeus and pubococcygeus muscles (both part of the levator ani muscle) and the coccygeus muscle.

Keywords Anal sphincter • Magnetic resonance imaging • Pelvic floor • Urethra anatomy

10.1 Introduction

The female pelvic floor region encompasses several structures, including sphincters, several anatomical layers, and supportive elements. Muscular and ligamentous structures are major constituents of these pelvic floor structures and can be visualized by magnetic resonance imaging (MRI). In this chapter the anatomy of the female pelvic floor is described, based on T_2-weighted turbo spin-echo sequences, with images obtained with either an endoluminal coil or an external phased array coil. In this sequence, muscles are relative hypointense (gray), and ligaments and fascia hypointense (black), while fat and smooth muscle are hyperintense (white).

First the urethra, vagina and uterine support, perineal body, and anal sphincter are described, followed by a description of the multilayered pelvic floor itself. The anatomy is presented in a concise manner, describing the prominent pelvic floor structures visualized on MRI. For more details readers are referred to an additional textbook [1].

10.2 The Urethra

The female urethra closes the urinary bladder and is important for maintaining urinary continence. It is

J. Stoker
Department of Radiology, Academic Medical Center,
University of Amsterdam, The Netherlands

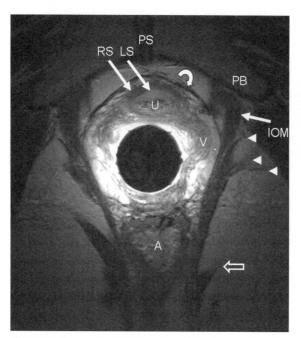

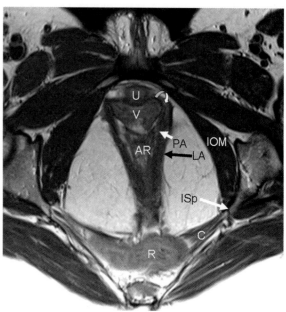

Fig. 10.1 Endovaginal axial oblique T_2-weighted turbo spin-echo. The compressor urethrae (*curved arrow*) is anterior to the urethra and attaches to the levator ani muscle. The urethra has a multi-layered appearance which is central the mucosa/submucosa (*U*), bordered by the relative hyperintense smooth muscle lissosphincter (*LS*) and the relative hypointense striated rhabdosphincter (*RS*). The pubococcygeus muscle part of the levator ani muscle (*arrow*) is attached to the pubic bone (*PB*). Anteriorly the pubococcygeus part of the levator ani muscle courses (*arrowheads*) from the tendineus arc of the levator ani at the internal obturator muscle (*IOM*) (anterior part has origin at pubic bone) and, posteriorly, the iliococcygeus (*open arrow*). A, anorectal junction; *PS*, pubic symphysis; *V*, vaginal wall

Fig. 10.2 External coil axial oblique T_2-weighted turbo spin-echo shows the lateral support of the vagina by the levator ani (*curved arrow*). The puboanalis (*PA*) courses to the longitudinal layer. The triangular-shaped coccygeus muscle (*C*) is visible with its attachment at the ischial spine (*ISp*). AR, anorectal junction; *IOM*, internal obturator muscle; *R*, rectum; *U*, urethra; *V*, vagina

made up two main components: an inner mucosa and an outer muscular coat. The latter comprises an inner smooth muscle layer and an outer striated muscle layer (Fig. 10.1). These layers are easily appreciated on MRI, with their distinct differences in intensity. The smooth muscular layer (lissosphincter) is a cylinder, while the external urethral sphincter (rhabdosphincter) is a ring at the middle of the urethra, but relatively thin posteriorly and deficient superiorly and inferiorly.

10.3 Urethral Support

The precise anatomy of the urethral support as well as the relative contribution of the structures involved are complex and have not yet been fully elucidated. Here the principal structures are discussed.

The urethra is supported by a layer of supportive tissue formed by the endopelvic fascia. The endopelvic fascia – an adventitial layer – (also named pubocervical fascia at this location) is attached at both lateral sides to the tendineus arc of the pelvic fascia. The latter is attached to the levator ani muscle as well as to the pubic bone. This layer of anterior vaginal wall and endopelvic fascia suspended between the tendineus arcs at both sides forms a "hammock" underlying and supporting the urethra [2]. Contraction of the levator ani muscles results in compression of the urethra to the pubic bone, as the tendineus arc of the pelvic fascia, and therefore the vaginal wall, are both elevated. Also the urogenital hiatus is closed.

The urethra is at the level of the pelvic diaphragm, bordered by the most medial part of the pubococcygeus muscle (i.e. the pubovaginal muscle) (Fig. 10.2), which inserts postero-inferiorly into the perineal body.

Anterior to the urethra, a sling-like structure can be identified (Fig. 10.1). This structure courses just anterior to the urethra and has lateral attachments to the levator ani muscle. Although this structure has been identified as the periurethral ligament [3] and the inferior extension of the pubovesical muscle [4], it may also represent the compressor urethrae (see below).

The compressor urethrae and urethrovaginal sphincter are urethral supportive structures with multiple (inter)connections, and have previously been considered part of the deep transverse perineal muscle [5]. The compressor urethrae forms a broad arching muscular sheet close to the urogenital hiatus and adjacent to the rhabdosphincter (Fig. 10.1). It compresses and elongates the urethra. The urethrovaginal sphincter comprises striated muscle fibers encircling the vagina. The urethrovaginal sphincter blends anteriorly with the compressor urethrae and posterior fibers may extend to the perineal body.

10.4 Uterine and Vaginal Support

The uterus and vagina are supported by several structures that, to aid understanding, can be divided into several levels.

The adventitial endopelvic fascia is an important part of the supportive structures for the uterus and vagina. It covers the parametrium (broad ligament), which comprises the most superior layer and gives lateral support. The fascia extends to the paracolpium and has been indicated as level I vaginal support [6]. Support at this level also includes the round ligaments.

The uterosacral and cardinal ligaments are condensations of the endopelvic fascia and form the major constituents of the second level of support [6–8]. The uterosacral ligaments run from the posterolateral aspect of the cervix to the presacral fascia. The cardinal ligament arises from the area of the greater sciatic foramen and courses to the uterine cervix. Both the cardinal and sacrouterine ligaments surround the cervix and envelop the superior part of the vagina. Both ligaments give lateral support. The anteromedial part of the vagina is suspended by the endopelvic fascia (pubocervical fascia), with attachment to the tendineus arc of the pelvic fascia. The vagina also has lateral support from the medial part of the levator ani (level III support) (Fig. 10.2), and from the perineal membrane [6, 8, 9].

10.5 The Perineal Body

The perineal body is situated between the urogenital region and the anal sphincter. Many muscular and fas-

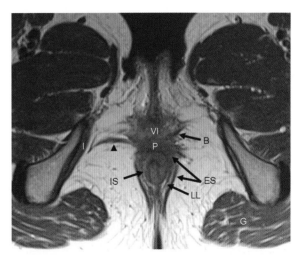

Fig. 10.3 External coil axial oblique T$_2$-weighted turbo spin-echo demonstrates the perineal body (*P*) with attachment of the transverse perineal muscle (*arrowhead*; left transverse perineal muscle visible at contiguous slice), external sphincter (*ES*), and bulbospongiose muscle (*B*). The external sphincter (*arrow*) and internal sphincter (*arrowhead*) show variable degrees of atrophy. *G*, gluteal muscle; *IS*, internal sphincter; *LL*, longitudinal layer in intersphincteric space; *VI*, vaginal introitus

cial structures interconnect: the longitudinal muscle of the anorectum, external anal sphincter, pubococcygeus muscle (pubovaginalis), perineal membrane, superficial transverse perineal muscle, and bulbospongiosus (Fig. 10.3). The perineal body is important for support, as the muscular and fascial constituents of the perineal body have (bony) attachments.

10.6 The Anal Sphincter

The anal sphincter closes the gastrointestinal tract until there is an appropriate time point for evacuation. It is a multilayered cylindrical structure, 5–6 cm in length (average 5 cm) [10] (Figs. 10.4–10.7). The innermost layer is the lining, which changes along the axis of the sphincter (colonic-type epithelium, non-keratinized cuboidal epithelium, keratinized stratified squamous epithelium). The subepithelium seals off the anal canal. Subsequent layers are the cylindrical smooth muscle of the internal sphincter, often separated from the longitudinal layer by a thin fat-containing layer that represents the surgical intersphincteric space. The outermost layer comprises striated muscle, with the external sphincter as the lower half and the sling-like puborectal muscle (part of the pubovisceralis) as the upper half of this layer.

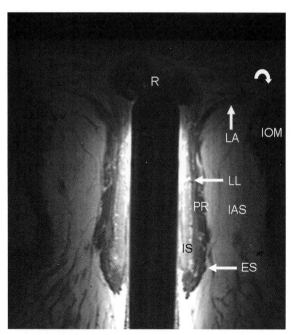

Fig. 10.4 Endoanal coronal oblique T$_2$-weighted turbo spin-echo. The relative hyperintense internal anal sphincter (*IS*) is bordered by the intersphincteric space with the longitudinal layer (*LL*). The outer layer of the anal sphincter is formed by the external sphincter (lower half) and puborectal muscle (*PR*). *LA*, iliococcygeal part of the levator ani which attaches to the internal obturator muscle (*IOM*) fascia at the tendineus arc of the levator ani (*curved arrow*). *ES*, external anal sphincter; *IAS*, ischioanal space; *R*, rectum

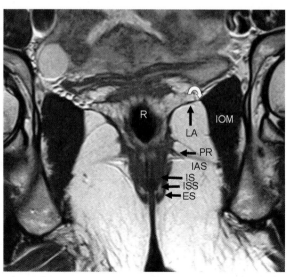

Fig. 10.5 External coil coronal oblique T$_2$-weighted turbo spin-echo. The internal anal sphincter (*IS*) and outer striated muscle layer formed by the external sphincter (*ES*; lower half) and puborectal muscle (*PR*; upper half) are readily appreciated; the intersphincteric space (*ISS*) is in between. *LA*, iliococcygeal part of the levator ani which attaches to the internal obturator muscle (*IOM*) fascia at the tendineus arc of the levator ani (*curved arrow*). *ES*, external anal sphincter; *IAS*, ischioanal space; *R*, rectum

10.6.1 The Internal Anal Sphincter

The internal sphincter is easily recognized on MRI as a circular hyperintense structure. The internal sphincter is approximately 2.9 mm thick on endoluminal MRI [10] (Figs. 10.6, 10.7). The inferior border of the internal sphincter is approximately 1 cm above the inferior edge of the sphincter complex (i.e. inferior edge of the external sphincter) (Fig. 10.6). The internal sphincter is important for the resting tone of the anal sphincter.

10.6.2 The Intersphincteric Space and Longitudinal Layer

The intersphincteric space is the fat-containing space between the internal sphincter and the outer striated muscle layer (i.e. external sphincter, puborectal muscle). The width, and therefore the visibility on MRI, varies considerably. As it contains fat, it is seen as a bright line on T$_2$-weighted MRI (Fig. 10.6).

The longitudinal layer (also named the longitudinal muscle) courses through the intersphincteric space (Figs. 10.4, 10.6). This structure is the continuation of the smooth muscle longitudinal layer of the rectum and has striated muscle contributions from the pubovisceralis (puboanalis) (Figs. 10.2, 10.7) and fibroelastic contributions from the endopelvic fascia [11]. The longitudinal layer is approximately 2.6 mm thick on endoanal MRI.

The longitudinal layer forms a network with extensions to the perineal skin and the ischioanal fossa. These extensions are not visualized on MRI.

10.6.3 The Outer Striated Layer: External Anal Sphincter

The external sphincter is the lower half of the outer striated layer of the anal sphincter [10, 12] (Figs. 10.4, 10.6). The external sphincter extends approximately 1 cm beyond the internal sphincter and forms the lower

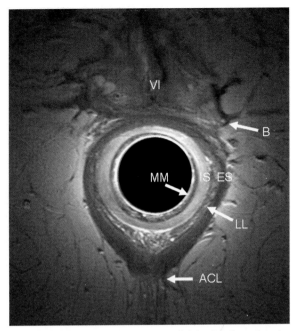

Fig. 10.6 Endoanal axial oblique T$_2$-weighted turbo spin-echo through the lower half of the anal sphincter. Relatively hyperintense mucosa/submucosa with hypointense muscularis submucosae ani (*MM*). The internal anal sphincter (*IS*) is relatively hyperintense and forms a ring. The external sphincter (*ES*) ring is relatively hypointense. The hyperintense fat-containing intersphincteric space is between the internal and external anal sphincter. This space contains the relatively hypointense longitudinal layer (*LL*). *ACL*, anococcygeal ligament; *B*, bulbospongiose muscle; *VI*, vaginal introitus

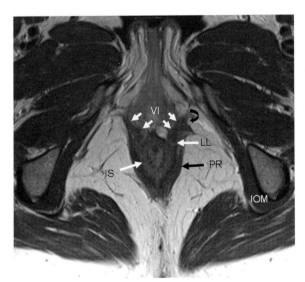

Fig. 10.7 External coil axial oblique T$_2$-weighted turbo spin-echo shows the pubovisceral muscle (*curved arrow*), puborectal muscle (*PR*), and puboanal muscle (*short arrows*). The puboanal muscle courses to the longitudinal layer (*LL*). *IS*, internal sphincter; *IOM*, internal obturator muscle; *VI*, vaginal introitus

edge of the anal sphincter. In females the external sphincter is approximately 2.7 cm high posteriorly and laterally, and approximately 1.4 cm anteriorly [10]. The external sphincter has a thickness of 4.1 mm on endoluminal imaging. Some external sphincter fibers are posteriorly continuous with the anococcygeal ligament, while others extend to the superficial transverse perineal muscle and perineal body anteriorly.

Voluntary closure and reflex closure are the important functions of the external sphincter, while it also adds to the sphincter tone.

10.6.4 The Outer Striated Layer: Puborectal Muscle

The puborectal muscle, which is the principal subdivision of the pubovisceralis part of the levator ani, forms the upper outer striated layer of the anal sphincter (Figs. 10.4, 10.5, 10.7). It is approximately 2.9 cm high and 5.7 mm thick and forms a sling that is open anteriorly [10]. The puborectalis courses anterior oblique, with bilateral attachment to the pubic bone, and borders the urogenital hiatus. The muscle has several functions, most importantly reflex contraction to sudden increase in abdominal pressure.

10.7 Anal Sphincter Support

The anal sphincter is supported anteriorly by the perineal body and related supportive structures, while lateral support is given by the levator ani muscle (pubovisceral muscle) and superficial transverse perineal muscle (Fig. 10.3). Posterior support is given by the anococcygeal ligament and superior support by the continuity with the rectum. The fibroelastic network – which transverses the anal sphincter – is continuous outside the anal sphincter and this gives additional support.

10.8 The Rectum and Rectal Support

The rectum acts as a reservoir at the end of the gastrointestinal tract and is crucial in maintaining continence. Within the mucosa there are distension-sensitive nerve endings, while in the muscular wall, nerve endings are more sensitive to the intensity of distension. The muscularis propria of the rectum comprises two layers: an outer longitudinal layer and an inner circular layer. The latter is continuous with the anal internal sphincter, while the former is continuous as a longitudinal layer of the anal sphincter.

The rectum is supported anteriorly by the anovaginal septum and laterally by the rectal ligaments (or rectal pillars) of the endopelvic fascia. Posterior support is given by the presacral fascia.

10.9 The Pelvic Floor

The pelvic floor comprises four layers, which from external to internal include a superficial muscular layer, perineal membrane, pelvic diaphragm, and endopelvic fascia. The superficial muscular layer is formed by the superficial transverse perineal muscle, bulbospongiosus, and ischiocavernous muscles. For support, the superficial transverse perineal muscle is important and, given the close relation to the perineal membrane, this muscle will be described in the next paragraph. The endopelvic fascia is an adventitial layer covered by parietal peritoneum, enveloping the pelvic organs and supportive structures (e.g. parametrium). This layer is not directly visualized on MRI except for some condensations.

10.9.1 The Perineal Membrane (Urogenital Diaphragm)

The perineal membrane is a fibromuscular layer directly below the pelvic diaphragm. The diaphragm is triangular in shape, spans the anterior pelvic outlet, and is attached to the pubic bones. The perineal membrane is crossed by the urethra and vagina and is attached medially to the lateral vaginal walls.

Formerly it was often referred to as the urogenital diaphragm and described as a trilaminar structure. Two of these three layers (namely the deep transverse perineal muscles and the superior fascia) are currently thought not be present as layers within the perineal membrane. The deep transverse perinei fibers are now thought to be part of the compressor urethrae, and the urethrovaginalis part of the external urethral sphincter muscle which lies above the perineal membrane, or transverse fibers inserting into the vagina (see Urethral Support).

The superficial transverse perinei spans the posterior edge of the perineal membrane (Fig. 10.3). Both insert into the perineal body and external sphincter.

10.9.2 The Pelvic Diaphragm

The pelvic diaphragm is a prominent part of the pelvic floor as visualized on MRI. It constitutes two components of the levator ani muscle (iliococcygeus, pubococcygeus) and the coccygeus muscle. The pelvic diaphragm is a supporting shelf for the pelvic organs (Fig. 10.5). In physiological conditions, the pelvic diaphragm has a dome-shaped form in the coronal plane as a result of the constant muscle tone of the levator ani and coccygeus muscles combined with fascial stability. The pelvic diaphragm is transversed by the urogenital hiatus with the urethra, vagina, and rectum. The urogenital diaphragm is closed by the pelvic diaphragm.

10.10 The Levator Ani Muscle

The levator ani muscle consists of three muscles: the iliococcygeus, pubococcygeus, and pubovisceralis (puborectalis).

The iliococcygeus muscle and pubococcygeus muscle arise from the ischial spine, the tendineus arc of the levator ani muscle, and the pubic bone. The tendineus arc (Figs. 10.4, 10.5) is a linear fascial condensation of the internal obturator muscle, the major constituent of the pelvic sidewall.

The iliococcygeus arises from the posterior half of the tendineus arc (Figs. 10.1, 10.4, 10.5) inserting into the coccyx and the midline anococcygeal raphe. The anococcygeal raphe is formed by the interdigitation of iliococcygeal fibers from both sides [13]. The iliococcygeus forms a sheet-like layer and is often largely aponeurotic.

The pubococcygeus arises from the anterior half of the tendineus arc (Fig. 10.1) and the periosteum of the posterior surface of the pubic bone at the lower border of the pubic symphysis (Fig. 10.1); its fibers are directed posteriorly, inserting into the anococcygeal raphe and coccyx.

The pubovisceralis forms a sling around the urogenital hiatus. This muscle has several constituents. Most important is the puborectalis which is a U-shaped sling around the anorectum (see 10.6) and is attached posteriorly to the anococcygeal ligament. The puboanalis is another part of the pubovisceralis which courses to the anal longitudinal muscle (Figs. 10.2 and 10.7). A further component is the pubovaginal muscle which has attachments to the lateral vaginal walls and courses to the perineal body [14].

10.11 The Coccygeus Muscle

The posterior part of the pelvic diaphragm is formed by the coccygeus.

This muscle arises from the tip of the ischial spine, along the posterior margin of the internal obturator muscle (Fig. 10.2). This triangular shelf-like musculotendinous structure forms the posterior part of the pelvic diaphragm. The sacrospinous ligament is at the posterior edge of the coccygeus muscle and is fused with this muscle.

References

1. Stoker J, Wallner C. Anatomy of the pelvic floor and sphincters. In Stoker J, Taylor SA, DeLancey JOL (eds) Imaging pelvic floor disorders, 2 edn. Springer-Verlag, Berlin Heidelberg, 2008, pp 1–29.
2. DeLancey JOL. Structural support of the urethra as it relates to stress urinary incontinence: the hammock hypothesis. Am J Obstet Gynecol 1994;170:1713–1723.
3. Tan IL, Stoker J, Zwamborn AW et al. Female pelvic floor. Endovaginal MR imaging of normal anatomy. Radiology 1998;206:777–783.
4. Tunn R, DeLancey JOL, Quint EE. Visibility of pelvic organ support system structures in magnetic resonance images without an endovaginal coil. Am J Obstet Gynecol 2001; 184:1156–1163.
5. Oelrich TM. The striated urogenital muscle in the female. Anat Rec 1983;205:223–232.
6. DeLancey JOL. Anatomy and biomechanics of genital prolapse. Clin Obstet Gynecol 1993;36:897–909.
7. DeLancey JOL. Structural aspects of the extrinsic continence mechanism. Obstet Gynecol 1988;72:296–301.
8. DeLancey JOL. Functional anatomy of the female pelvis. In: Kursh ED, McGuire EJ (eds) Female urology, 1 edn. Lippincott, Philadelphia, 1994, pp 3–16.
9. DeLancey JOL, Starr RA. Histology of the connection between the vagina and levator ani muscles. Implications for urinary tract function. J Reprod Med 1990;35:765–771.
10. Rociu E, Stoker J, Eijkemans MJC, Laméris JS. Normal anal sphincter anatomy and age- and sex-related variations at high spatial resolution endoanal MR imaging. Radiology 2000; 217:395–401.
11. Lunniss PJ, Phillips RKS. Anatomy and function of the anal longitudinal muscle. Br J Surg 1992;79:882–884.
12. Hussain SM, Stoker J, Laméris JS. Anal sphincter complex: endoanal MR imaging of normal anatomy. Radiology 1995;197:671–677.
13. Last RJ. Anatomy. Regional and applied, 6 edn. Churchill Livingstone, Edinburgh, 1978.
14. Sampselle CM, DeLancey JO. Anatomy of female continence. J Wound Ostomy Continence Nurs 1998;25:63–74.

Dominik Weishaupt and Caecilia S. Reiner

Abstract Magnetic resonance imaging (MRI) is an excellent tool for understanding the complex anatomy of the pelvic floor and for assessing pelvic floor disorders. Using appropriate imaging protocols, the anatomy of the pelvic floor can be visualized in great detail, without exposing the patient to harmful ionizing radiation. Dynamic MRI allows detection and characterization of functional pelvic floor abnormalities. In this chapter, we review the technical aspects of static and dynamic pelvic floor MRI. We focus on recent technical developments in pelvic floor MRI, which enable a global and integrated approach to the pelvic floor.

Keywords Dynamic magnetic resonance imaging • Magnetic resonance imaging • Magnetic resonance defecography • Magnetic resonance proctography • Pelvic floor • Pelvic floor dysfunction • Pelvic organs

11.1 Introduction

The pelvic floor is a complex anatomic and functional unit. It provides pelvic support, maintains continence, and coordinates relaxation during urination and defecation. Over recent years, magnetic resonance imaging (MRI) has gained increasing acceptance as an imaging modality for evaluation of the pelvic floor. The advantages of MRI are well known and include the lack of radiation, an excellent soft tissue contrast, and multiplanar imaging without superimposition of structures.

MRI of the pelvic floor encompasses static (morphologic) and dynamic MRI. Static MRI means imaging of the anatomical morphology of the pelvic floor with the patient at rest. Dynamic MRI means that the pelvic floor is imaged dynamically, i.e. with the pelvic floor at rest, during squeezing, during straining, and during defecation or urination.

11.2 Static Magnetic Resonance Imaging

Static MRI provides detailed information of the anatomy of the pelvic floor. Current state-of-the art MRI of the pelvic floor includes imaging at a magnetic field strength of 1.5 Tesla (T), with the patient in the supine position and using pelvic or phased-array coils. Using T_2-weighted fast-spin echo (FSE) sequences, the morphology of the pelvic floor can be assessed in great detail [1]. The spatial resolution can be enhanced by using endoluminal (endorectal, endovaginal, endourethral) coils. In combination with T_2-weighted FSE sequences, endoluminal coils provide improved signal-to-noise ratio (SNR) and high-resolution images [2]. However, the drawback of endoluminal coils is

D. Weishaupt
Institute of Radiology, Triemli Hospital Zurich, Switzerland

the limited field of view, since these coils provide sufficient signal for only those structures that are in close proximity to the coil. Therefore, an imaging protocol using an endoluminal coil is always combined with imaging using a phased-array coil. MRI with endoluminal coils has been applied to imaging of the anterior pelvic floor compartment and can be used to delineate the multiple layers of the urethra and its supportive structures. Similarly, endoluminal coils can be used to assess the anal sphincter, particularly subtle changes in the internal sphincter [2]. However, due to the high cost of endoluminal coils, MRI with endoluminal coils has not found broad acceptance for static pelvic floor imaging, and is only used for specific clinical situations, such as high-resolution imaging of the anal sphincter and the supportive structures of the urethra.

Increasingly, 3.0 T MRI systems are being used in clinical practice. The most important advantage of these systems is their increased SNR compared with 1.5 T systems [3]. Because SNR varies linearly with field strength, the SNR at 3.0 T might be expected to be twice of that at 1.5 T. In fact, however, because of technical limitations, the SNR at 3.0 T is usually only 1.7–1.8 times that at 1.5 T [4].

Clinically, the higher SNR obtained at a magnetic field strength of 3.0 T can be used to either increase spatial resolution or decrease acquisition time. For static MRI of the pelvic floor, the potential of 3.0 T to increase spatial resolution is of interest. Admittedly, 3.0 T MRI for static pelvic imaging also has inherent technical limitations, such as standing wave artifact, chemical shift artifact, and susceptibility artifact. In addition, safety issues resulting from the increased energy deposition in the patient's body have to be considered. At this point, it has to be stated that static pelvic imaging at 3.0 T is still in its early stages. At the time of writing this chapter, there is not enough evidence to conclude that, for the pelvic floor, MRI at 3.0 T is superior to MRI at 1.5 T. However, the expected modifications in pulse sequences and hardware components make the future bright for 3.0 T MRI of the pelvic floor.

11.3 Dynamic Magnetic Resonance Imaging

Traditionally, fluoroscopic techniques including dynamic cystoproctography and defecography (also called evacuation proctography) have played an important role in the radiological assessment of patients with functional disorders of the pelvic floor. Whereas cystoproctography requires separate opacification of the bladder, vagina, and rectum, in proctography only the rectum is filled with enema. Although conventional cystoproctography and conventional defecography are still the reference imaging methods for assessing functional pelvic abnormalities, these techniques have some significant limitations. There is considerable irradiation associated with these fluoroscopic techniques, with a mean effective radiation dose of up to 4.9 mSv [5]. Moreover, the conventional techniques are limited from a practical point of view, by their projectional nature and inability to detect soft-tissue structures.

The lack of soft-tissue contrast when using conventional techniques may be a particular disadvantage in those patients who have multicompartment involvement of pelvic floor dysfunction. With the development of fast multislice sequences, MRI has also gained increasing acceptance for dynamic imaging of the pelvic floor. In the following sections, we describe the technique of dynamic pelvic MRI. Because the posterior compartment is traditionally in the focus of interest, dynamic MRI of the pelvic floor is often called MR defecography.

11.4 Patient Positioning

Dynamic pelvic imaging may be performed in an open-configuration MR system in the sitting position, or in a closed-configuration MR system in the supine position. Although the sitting position is the physiological position during defecation, dynamic pelvic MRI is usually performed in the supine position. This is primarily due to the limited availability of open-configuration MR magnets, which would allow examination in the physiological sitting position.

Reports about the influence of body position on defecation are sparse in the literature. A study of patient positioning during MR defecography showed that MR defecography in the supine position and in the seated position are equally effective in identifying most of the clinically relevant abnormalities of the pelvic floor [6]. The absence of influence from gravity when patients are imaged in a supine instead of a sitting position may affect the diagnosis of intussusceptions. In a study by Bertschinger et al [6], all intussusceptions found in upright positions were missed in the supine position. This means that if an intussusception is found in the supine position it should be regarded as clinically relevant, and if it is missing in the supine position, it cannot be reliably regarded as ruled out.

11.5 Patient Preparation

The administration of contrast agent for MRI of the pelvic floor varies in different studies, from use of no contrast agent to filling of the rectum, vagina, urethra, and bladder with contrast agent; placement of markers in the vagina or rectum; or placement of urethral catheters [7–9]. For evaluation of the posterior compartment of the pelvic floor, authorities agree that the rectum should be filled with contrast agent. The rectum is filled with contrast agent not only for better delineation, but mainly in order to study the actual act of defecation. This is of importance, as some disorders of the pelvic floor, such as rectal prolapse or intussusceptions, only appear in their full size during defecation [8].

Immediately before the examination, the rectum is filled with the rectal enema. The volume of enema used is variable and ranges between 120 and 300 mL [10–12]. Some investigators administer contrast agent until the patient feels a sustained desire to defecate. Others use a standardized volume of contrast agent. Although it is not known if the amount of contrast agent administered influences the extent of structural pelvic floor disorders, in our experience, 250–300 mL of enema gives the best results. However, the time needed to evacuate the contrast agent, and thus the assessment of the evacuation ability, depends on the amount of contrast agent. Therefore, it is necessary to standardize the volume administered. The viscosity of the contrast agent should be similar to that of normal rectum content because the manifestations of pelvic floor pathologies vary with different fecal consistency [11, 13, 14]. Authors recommend ultrasound gel (15–18) or mashed potatoes (6, 19, 20). Depending on the sequence used for dynamic MRI, the rectal enema may be doped with a small amount of standard extracellular gadolinium-based MR contrast agent. In general, neither premedication nor oral or rectal preparation for bowel cleansing is necessary before imaging. In our current imaging protocol, we do not perform retrograde filling of the bladder and we do not perform tagging of the vagina. In order to ensure filling of the bladder, we ask the patient not to void the bladder for at least one hour before the examination. With regard to the middle compartment, the soft-tissue contrast is usually high enough to allow identification of all anatomical landmarks. Therefore, we do not perform any tagging of the vagina. Exceptions may be specific queries before surgery is performed, such as reconstruction of the pelvic floor in severe uterus prolapse.

Besides the administration of contrast agent, it is essential to clearly explain to patients the procedure for examination. Because most patients are likely to feel nervous and intimidated, technicians must be trained in placing patients at ease in the MRI unit and giving clear instructions. Patient cooperation is critical for a useful examination. Therefore, patients need to be instructed about imaging at different pelvic positions, including imaging at rest, at squeezing, at straining, and during defecation, before starting the examination.

11.6 Imaging Technique

Dynamic pelvic MRI may be performed in a supine position, using all commercially available closed- or open-configuration MR systems with horizontal access. When dynamic pelvic MR is performed in these MR systems, the patient is placed in a supine position and a pelvic phased-array coil is used for signal transmission and/or reception. After filling the rectum, the examination starts with a localizer sequence. The examination protocol includes non-fat-suppressed static T_2-weighted FSE or fast recovery FSE sequences in the transaxial plane. These sequences are performed to visualize the anatomy of the pelvic floor. Subsequently, dynamic MRI is performed. For dynamic MRI in the different positions (at squeezing, at straining, and during defecation), various MR sequences can be used, with similar results. The basic requirement for the sequence is the necessity for a fast imaging update. Some authors have used T_2-weighted single-shot fast spin echo sequences (SSFSE) in the midsagittal plane, obtained at rest, at squeezing, at straining, and during defecation. Alternatively, balanced steady-state free precession (bSSFP) or a T_1-weighted multiphase gradient recalled echo (GRE) sequence may be used. If the T_1-weighted multiphase GRE sequence is used, the rectal enema is usually tagged with a small amount of an extracellular gadolinium-based contrast agent. Which sequence is used depends on the scanner. For the evacuation phase, it is important to have a sequence that offers the possibility to acquire images over a long time period without the necessity to reload the sequence. This is particularly important in patients with a long prolongation period.

11.7 Image Analysis

Image analysis is performed according to the three-compartment model of the pelvic floor [21]. The three compartments of the pelvic floor are assessed for morphological changes at different pelvic floor positions.

Besides the qualitative assessment, quantitative evaluation of imaging findings is important, because the extent of these findings may influence further management. The use of reference lines for image evaluation is helpful. The most used reference line is the pubococcygeal line (PCL), which is defined on midsagittal images as the line joining the inferior border of the symphysis pubis to the last or second-last coccygeal joint. The length of the base of the bladder (anterior compartment), the cervix, or vaginal vault (middle compartment), and the ano-rectal junction (posterior compartment) is measured at a 90 degree angle to the PCL in the different pelvic floor positions (at rest, squeezing, straining, and evacuation) as shown in Fig. 11.1. The ano-rectal junction (ARJ) is defined as the

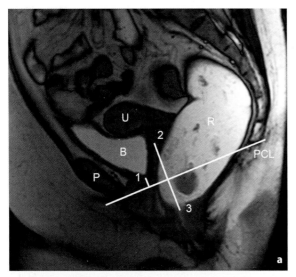

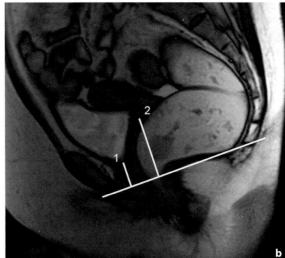

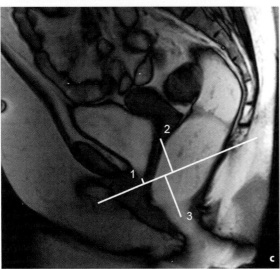

Fig. 11.1 A 54-year old female patient with a moderate descent of the posterior compartment during defecation. On MR images obtained at rest (**a**), at squeezing (**b**), and during evacuation (**c**), the position of the base of the bladder (*1*, anterior compartment), the vaginal vault (*2*, middle compartment), and the ano-rectal junction (*3*, posterior compartment) is measured at a 90° angle to the PCL. *B*, bladder; *P*, symphysis pubis; *PCL*, pubococcygeal line; *R*, rectum; *V*, vaginal vault

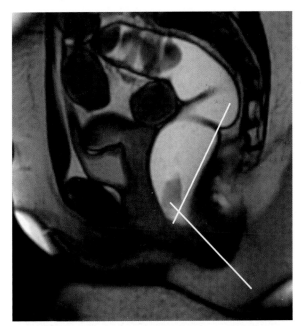

Fig. 11.2 Measurement of the ano-rectal angle (ARA). The ARA is measured as the angle between a line drawn through the posterior border of the distal part of rectum and a line drawn through the central axis of the anal canal

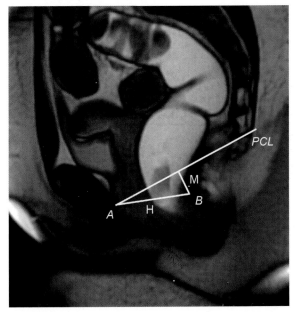

Fig. 11.3 Midsagittal balanced steady-state free precession T$_2$-weighted image obtained at straining shows landmarks used in the HMO system. The landmarks are the inferior aspect of the symphysis pubis (*A*) and the posterior wall of the rectum at the level of the ano-rectal junction (*B*). The H line (*H*) represents the anteroposterior hiatal width and extends from *A* to *B*. The M line (*M*) represents hiatal descent and extends perpendicular from the pubococcygeal line (*PCL*) to the posterior end of the H line

cross-point between a line along the posterior wall of the distal part of the rectum and a line along the central axis of the anal canal. To determine pathologic pelvic floor descent, the measurements are made on the images, which show maximal organ descent, usually during maximal straining or evacuation. In addition, the ano-rectal angle (ARA), which is defined as the angle between the posterior wall of the distal part of the rectum and the central axis of the anal canal, can be measured at rest, squeezing, and straining (Fig. 11.2). It must be noted that the reproducibility of ARA measurements has been debated and questioned in several studies [22, 23], whereas another study found the ARA was a consistent and reliable parameter [24]. Furthermore, the extent of other pathologic conditions such as rectoceles and enteroceles is measured.

Beside the three-compartment-model with the PCL as a reference line, which is mainly used by surgeons and gastroenterologists, the second known system for grading pelvic floor abnormalities is the "HMO system", which is mainly used by urologists and gynecologists [25]. The HMO system distinguishes pelvic organ prolapse and pelvic floor relaxation, which are two separate but often coexistent pathologic entities. In pelvic floor relaxation, the pelvic floor, with its active and passive support structures, becomes weakened, leading to hiatal descent and widening. The degree of pelvic floor relaxation is measured with two reference lines: the H line, which represents hiatal widening and extends from the inferior aspect of the symphysis pubis to the posterior wall of the rectum at the level of the ARJ, and the M line, which represents hiatal descent and extends perpendicular from the PCL to the posterior end of the H line (Fig. 11.3). Lesions of the pelvic musculofascial support result in widening of the hiatus and descent of the levator plate. Thus, the H and M lines tend to elongate with pelvic floor relaxation, representing levator hiatal widening and levator plate descent, respectively. Abnormal pelvic floor relaxation is present, when the H line exceeds 6 cm, and when the M line exceeds 2 cm in length [26].

11.8 Conclusions

Due its inherent physical properties, MRI is a highly suitable imaging modality for imaging the pelvic floor. MRI provides a global integrated approach to the pelvic floor rather than a compartimentalized view. The development of fast MR sequences allows dynamic pelvic MRI to be performed. Dynamic pelvic MRI is an evolving method, which is considered an alternative to conventional techniques. MRI has tremendous potential as a tool for attempts to understand the complex pathophysiology of the large number of disorders of the pelvic floor.

References

1. Stoker J, Halligan S, Bartram CI. Pelvic floor imaging. Radiology 2001;218:621–641.
2. Chou CP, Levenson RB, Elsayes KM et al. Imaging of female urethral diverticulum: an update. Radiographics 2008; 28:1917–1930.
3. Merkle EM, Dale BM, Paulson EK. Abdominal MR imaging at 3T. Magn Reson Imaging Clin N Am 2006;14:17–26.
4. Merkle EM, Dale BM. Abdominal MRI at 3.0 T: the basics revisited. AJR Am J Roentgenol 2006;186:1524–1532.
5. Goei R. Anorectal function in patients with defecation disorders and asymptomatic subjects: evaluation with defecography. Radiology 1990;174:121–123.
6. Bertschinger KM, Hetzer FH, Roos JE et al. Dynamic MR imaging of the pelvic floor performed with patient sitting in an open-magnet unit versus with patient supine in a closed-magnet unit. Radiology 2002;223:501–508.
7. Healy JC, Halligan S, Reznek RH et al. Magnetic resonance imaging of the pelvic floor in patients with obstructed defaecation. Br J Surg 1997;84:1555–1558.
8. Lienemann A, Fischer T. Functional imaging of the pelvic floor. Eur J Radiol 2003;47:117–122.
9. Yang A, Mostwin JL, Rosenshein NB, Zerhouni EA. Pelvic floor descent in women: dynamic evaluation with fast MR imaging and cinematic display. Radiology 1991;179:25–33.
10. Halligan S, Malouf A, Bartram CI et al. Predictive value of impaired evacuation at proctography in diagnosing anismus. AJR Am J Roentgenol 2001;177:633–636.
11. Karlbom U, Nilsson S, Pahlman L, Graf W. Defecographic study of rectal evacuation in constipated patients and control subjects. Radiology 1999;210:103–108.
12. Maglinte DD, Bartram C. Dynamic imaging of posterior compartment pelvic floor dysfunction by evacuation proctography: techniques, indications, results and limitations. Eur J Radiol 2007;61:454–461.
13. Bartram CI, Turnbull GK, Lennard-Jones JE. Evacuation proctography: an investigation of rectal expulsion in 20 subjects without defecatory disturbance. Gastrointest Radiol 1988;13:72–80.
14. Solopova AE, Hetzer FH, Marincek B, Weishaupt D. MR defecography: prospective comparison of two rectal enema compositions. AJR Am J Roentgenol 2008;190:W118–124.
15. Fletcher JG, Busse RF, Riederer SJ et al. Magnetic resonance imaging of anatomic and dynamic defects of the pelvic floor in defecatory disorders. Am J Gastroenterol 2003; 98:399–411.
16. Kelvin FM, Maglinte DD, Hale DS, Benson JT. Female pelvic organ prolapse: a comparison of triphasic dynamic MR imaging and triphasic fluoroscopic cystocolpoproctography. AJR Am J Roentgenol 2000;174:81–88.
17. Lienemann A, Anthuber C, Baron A et al. Dynamic MR colpocystorectography assessing pelvic-floor descent. Eur Radiol 1997;7:1309–1317.
18. Vanbeckevoort D, Van Hoe L, Oyen R et al. Pelvic floor descent in females: comparative study of colpocystodefecography and dynamic fast MR imaging. J Magn Reson Imaging 1999;9:373–377.
19. Dvorkin LS, Hetzer F, Scott SM et al. Open-magnet MR defaecography compared with evacuation proctography in the diagnosis and management of patients with rectal intussusception. Colorectal Dis 2004;6:45–53.
20. Hetzer FH, Andreisek G, Tsagari C et al. MR defecography in patients with fecal incontinence: imaging findings and their effect on surgical management. Radiology 2006; 240:449–457.
21. Roos JE, Weishaupt D, Wildermuth S et al. Experience of 4 years with open MR defecography: pictorial review of anorectal anatomy and disease. Radiographics 2002;22:817–832.
22. Ferrante SL, Perry RE, Schreiman JS et al. The reproducibility of measuring the anorectal angle in defecography. Dis Colon Rectum 1991;34:51–55.
23. Penninckx F, Debruyne C, Lestar B, Kerremans R. Observer variation in the radiological measurement of the anorectal angle. Int J Colorectal Dis 1990;5:94–97.
24. Choi JS, Wexner SD, Nam YS et al. Intraobserver and interobserver measurements of the anorectal angle and perineal descent in defecography. Dis Colon Rectum 2000;43:1121–1126.
25. Comiter CV, Vasavada SP, Barbaric ZL et al. Grading pelvic prolapse and pelvic floor relaxation using dynamic magnetic resonance imaging. Urology 1999;54:454–457.
26. Boyadzhyan L, Raman SS, Raz S. Role of static and dynamic MR imaging in surgical pelvic floor dysfunction. Radiographics 2008;28:949–967.

Invited Commentary

Stuart Taylor and Steve Halligan

Pelvic floor disorders are very common, and although usually not life threatening, they are a considerable cause of patient morbidity, and in some the effects on quality of life can be devastating. The anatomical and functional anatomy of the pelvic floor is highly complex, and imaging techniques are becoming increasingly sophisticated in order to provide the clinician with the necessary structural and functional information to optimize patient management. The Chapters by Professor Stoker, Professor Weishaupt, and Dr Reiner provide an excellent overview of the anatomical and functional information afforded by modern magnetic resonance imaging (MRI) techniques in pelvic floor imaging.

The exquisite anatomical detail provided by the high-resolution T_2-weighted images described by Stoker provides considerable insight into the etiology and functional significance of injury to the muscles and tissues of the pelvic floor beyond the reach of the endoanal ultrasound probe. Such data underline the need to consider the pelvic floor as an integrated functional unit as opposed to the traditional compartmentalized approach; it is now clear that injury often coexists in compartments that are remote to that suggested by the patients' primary symptom complex. Furthermore, specific injury patterns are closely associated with symptoms of prolapse and, importantly, prediction of surgical failure is increasingly possible. Using MRI, DeLancey et al reported 20% of a cohort of 160 women had levator injury after their first vaginal delivery [1], and in a follow-up study Kearney et al reported such injury was associated with forceps use, anal sphincter rupture, and episiotomy but not vacuum delivery [2]. Patients with prolapse are over three times more likely to have a significant levator ani defect than woman with intact pelvic floors [3]. Another important benefit of MRI is its ability to quantify atrophy within pelvic floor muscles, which can predict both surgical treatment failure [4] and pelvic floor function [5].

The advantages of MRI over conventional barium fluoroscopy are well detailed by Professor Weishaupt and Dr Reiner, notably the lack of ionizing radiation, the tri-compartmental overview, and the excellent soft tissue characterization. In our practice, MRI proctography has largely replaced its barium counterpart in the assessment of both rectal evacuatory disorders and pelvic floor prolapse. The literature is reassuring about our ability to assess pelvic floor dynamics in the supine position compared to the more "physiological" erect posture possible with an open MRI magnet system. However, direct comparative studies between MRI and conventional fluoroscopic techniques are relatively lacking and some care must be taken in applying the "rules" of erect barium proctography to supine MRI. For example, is normal evacuatory time the same between both techniques and do our definitions of functional evacuatory disorders remain the same?

A study at our institution compared conventional barium fluoroscopy and supine MRI proctography using rectal ultrasound jelly in over 50 patients undergoing both procedures [6]. The reference standard was a consensus panel of gastroenterologists, surgeons, and radiologists unblinded to all the clinical information and patient follow-up. As would be expected, MRI was superior to fluoroscopy in detecting pelvic organ prolapse, but reassuringly we found no overall difference in the ability of the techniques to diagnose functional disorders or "anismus". However, in certain patients clinically diagnosed with anismus, rectal evacuation was rapid and

S. Taylor
Department of Clinical Radiology, University College, London, UK

complete at MRI, but prolonged and incomplete during upright barium proctography. We must take some care, therefore, in assuming MRI and barium proctography provide identical information in all patients.

In terms of technique, we concur with Professor Weishaupt and Dr Reiner and always undertake rectal filling and formal MRI proctography even if the patients' symptoms are those of prolapse rather than rectal dysfunction. Only by asking the patients to empty the rectum can it be ensured that the straining effort will be sufficient to precipitate organ prolapse, if present. Although some have had some success in imaging prolapse with an unprepared rectum during non-evacuatory straining, in our experience such an approach risks missing significant pathology due to understandable reluctance by the patient to full strain down, fearing "unexpected" incontinence.

We also always prepare the rectum with a clearing enema before the procedure. We have found this is appreciated by patients and MRI staff alike. We use up to 200 mL of ultrasound jelly to fill the rectum and tend to use a fixed volume rather than continuing until the patient expresses a desire to evacuate, although the latter approach arguably may be more physiological. We do not routinely perform contraction and straining views prior to formal evacuation, finding in our practice they add relatively little to the examination. Instead, patients are asked to pass the jelly as rapidly and completely as possible, during which single-shot fast spin echo (SSFSE) images are acquired through the midsagittal plane every second or so. Although there is no standard to define normality, or indeed prolapse, adopted across all imaging modalities used in the assessment of the pelvic floor, like most workers we reference dynamic pelvic floor movement to the pubococcygeal line. It is important for the inexperienced observer not to over-diagnose pelvic floor abnormalities during MRI proctography – a 2 cm rectocele is essentially a normal finding and descent of the bladder base and cervix below the pubococcygeal line on maximum straining can also be normal [7]. The use of vaginal opacification or bladder filling is usually unnecessary.

We undertake static views of the pelvic floor anatomy only in those with clinical concern regarding pelvic floor damage or in those due to undergo pelvic floor or prolapse surgery. In those with only symptoms suggesting a rectal evacuation disorder, we simply undertake the functional dynamic proctographic phase. Patients are therefore in the MR scanner for less than 10 minutes – facilitating a fast and efficient examination.

As described in these two chapters, the technique of MRI pelvic floor imaging is now mature. While higher-strength 3T machines may improve the resolution of our images, in reality it is doubtful if this will impact greatly on our diagnostic abilities. Instead, the focus of research now must be on the clinical and diagnostic impact of the technique as a whole. In whom should we perform MRI? How exactly do findings of pelvic floor disruption on MRI correlate with patient symptoms? How often are they incidental and of little clinical consequence? Do MRI findings influence surgical approach and if so are patient outcomes better? All these questions remain largely unanswered but the onus is on the radiological community to undertake the required clinical studies to begin to address them. Only then will we be better informed how best we can disseminate this powerful imaging technology.

References

1. DeLancey JO, Kearney R, Chou Q et al. The appearance of levator ani muscle abnormalities in magnetic resonance images after vaginal delivery. Obstet Gynecol 2003;101:46–53.
2. Kearney R, Miller JM, Ashton-Miller JA et al. Obstetric factors associated with levator ani muscle injury after vaginal birth. Obstet Gynecol 2006;107:144–149.
3. DeLancey JO, Morgan DM, Fenner DE et al. Comparison of levator ani muscle defects and function in women with and without pelvic organ prolapse. Obstet Gynecol 2007; 109:295–302.
4. Briel JW, Stoker J, Rociu E et al. External anal sphincter atrophy on endoanal magnetic resonance imaging adversely affects continence after sphincteroplasty. Br J Surg 1999; 86:1322–1327.
5. Thiruppathy K, Cohen R, Taylor SA et al. MRI findings of the pelvic floor correlates with function. Gastroenterology 2008;134:A579.
6. Chatoor DR, Emmanuel AV, Elneil S et al. What does MR proctography add in comparison to fluoroscopic proctography in patients with evacuation difficulty? Gut 56;2007:A47.
7. Goh V, Halligan S, Kaplan G et al. Dynamic MR imaging of the pelvic floor in asymptomatic subjects. AJR Am J Roentgenol 2000;174:661–666.

Section III
Pelvic Floor Damage Due to Childbirth

Pelvic Floor Damage Due to Childbirth: Introduction

G. Willy Davila

There is ample scientific evidence that the vaginal childbirth process is associated with neuromuscular and soft tissue injuries to the pelvic floor that are associated with the development of anal and urinary incontinence and pelvic organ prolapse. There is little ongoing debate about these findings, and the focus has been on risk factor assessment and injury-reducing interventions. As would seem natural, the concept of offering all pregnant women an elective cesarean section at term has been the focus of many recent debates and publications. A large clinical trial is probably not needed to document the benefits of prophylactic cesarean section on the pelvic floor – and women are in general very accepting of this proposal, if for no other reason than the practicality of a scheduled cesarean. Indeed, the availability of modern anesthetic techniques, accurate gestational age assessment, and minimization of morbidity associated with cesarean section make an obstetric management protocol of 100% cesarean section rate a feasible and acceptable proposal.

In reality, however, a 100% cesarean section rate is probably not achievable. Not all pregnant women will want to undergo an elective cesarean section, and many women will not have appropriate gestational dating, due to late prenatal care.

Importantly, some women will plan on having more than three children – making the likelihood of placental anomalies, such as placenta accreta, or of uterine rupture during gestation, risks that should be seriously taken into account. Thus, a discussion regarding the effects of vaginal delivery on the pelvic floor, and a review of maneuvers to minimize soft tissue damage and its resultant consequences is always appropriate.

This section of the book will review the current understanding of the mechanisms of pelvic floor trauma during the vaginal delivery process. Understanding these mechanisms can be of great importance in designing injury-reducing interventions – as there are likely simple means of reducing pelvic floor injury, such as early mediolateral episiotomy and avoidance of post-dates gestation.

Much emphasis has recently been placed on protection of the posterior compartment and the anal sphincter during the vaginal delivery process. This focus is of marked importance, as anal incontinence can have a devastating effect on quality of life, and the success rate of anal sphincter repair tends to drop off over time. Thus, efforts to prevent anal sphincter injury, as well as instruction of obstetric practitioners in effective sphincteroplasty techniques are of critical importance; these are the focus of Chapters 13 and 14.

Nothing in medicine is black and white. Avoidance of obstetric pelvic floor damage may seem as simple as avoiding the vaginal delivery process. Unfortunately, in reality there are multiple other non-obstetric factors associated with the development of pelvic floor dysfunction, many of which increase with the ageing process and are thus not fully avoidable. Decisions made regarding obstetric management need to bear in mind the individual patient's risk factors and desires. A well-educated clinician will be best able to provide appropriate advice to his/her patients in making decisions regarding protection of the pelvic floor.

G.W. Davila
Department of Gynecology, Urogynecology and Reconstructive Pelvic Surgery, Cleveland Clinic Florida, Weston, FL, USA

G.A. Santoro, A.P. Wieczorek, C.I. Bartram (eds.) *Pelvic Floor Disorders*
© Springer-Verlag Italia 2010

Mechanisms of Pelvic Floor Trauma During Vaginal Delivery

12

Gianfranco Minini, Silvia Zanelli, Patrizia Inselvini,
Marcello Caria, Sara Grosso and Davide Quaresmini

Abstract Delivery is a crucial event in a woman's life, a landmark in personal fulfillment and biological affirmation. Nevertheless, the physical consequences of vaginal childbirth are important and may vary from mild subclinical conditions to significant severe pathologies either immediately or in the long term. Systematic, exact research has focused on the main risks for pelvic floor damage, providing a theoretical background that can help to eliminate all avoidable damage, aid early detection, define the extent of the effects, and promptly cure these conditions.

Keywords Anal incontinence • Cesarean section • Dyspareunia • Episiotomy • Pelvic floor • Pelvic organ prolapse • Risk factors • Sphincter trauma • Urinary incontinence • Vaginal delivery

12.1 Introduction

Various events during a woman's lifetime affect the muscles of the pelvic floor and other supporting structures of the pelvic organs. Pregnancy, childbirth, menopause, and ageing have a pronounced influence on pelvic anatomy and physiology. The longer-term gynecological sequelae of pelvic floor weakness are pelvic organ prolapse, stress urinary incontinence, and perineal trauma, its subsequent repair, dyspareunia, fecal incontinence, and perineal pain (Box 12.1). In the UK, it is estimated that over 85% of women who have a vaginal birth will sustain some degree of perineal trauma, and among these 60–70% will experience suturing.

Box 12.1 Perineal trauma: 85% of vaginal delivery

Dyspareunia at 3 months	23%
Pain (3–18 months after delivery)	10%
Fecal incontinence	3–10%
Urinary symptoms	24%
Pelvic organ prolapse	32%

12.2 Pelvic Organ Prolapse

Pelvic organ prolapse is a common condition affecting up to 15% of the female population and is responsible for about 20% of women on waiting lists for major gynecological surgery [1]. A woman has an 11.1% lifetime risk of undergoing a single operation for prolapse or incontinence by the age of 80 years. The incidence of women admitted to hospital with prolapse is 2.04 per 1000 persons per year of risk. The main risk factors associated with prolapse are parity and increasing age, while smoking and obesity are secondary factors. Compared to nullipara, the odds ratio was 3.0 for

D. Quaresmini
Urogynecology Unit, Department of Obstetrics and Gynecology, University of Brescia, Italy

G.A. Santoro, A.P. Wieczorek, C.I. Bartram (eds.) *Pelvic Floor Disorders*
© Springer-Verlag Italia 2010

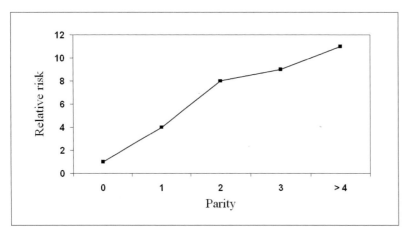

Fig. 12.1 Vaginal parity and relative risk for pelvic organ prolapse surgery

women reporting one vaginal delivery and 4.5 for women with a history of two or more vaginal deliveries [1]. Mant et al analyzed risk factors for prolapse in the 17,032 women enrolled in the Oxford Family Planning Association Study [2]. Cases were identified as women who were given an inpatient diagnosis of prolapse. Parity showed the strongest relation to prolapse. Women who had delivered four or more babies vaginally were found to have 11 times the risk of significant pelvic organ prolapse compared to nulliparous women (Fig. 12.1). Prolapse is more frequent in Caucasian women, due to differences in their connective tissue. The genetic predisposition may be more important than other risk factors such as parity in the development of this pathology.

12.3   Urinary Incontinence

Rates of urinary incontinence incidence range from 20% to 30% in the general population. Risk factors for the development of urinary incontinence are ageing and childbirth. Stress incontinence is more common in parous women compared with nulliparous women. Urinary symptoms are found antenatally in up to 60% of pregnant women. Postnatally, the reported prevalence of urinary incontinence varies from 6% up to 34% [3]. Investigators continue to report both an association with reversible incontinence occurring during pregnancy and the development of chronic incontinence after vaginal delivery [4, 5]. Thorp et al recently reported prospective data showing that the frequency of incontinence episodes peaks during the third trimester, and improves after delivery [6]. A large retrospective study by Foldspang showed increases in

urinary incontinence during pregnancy, immediately after birth, and with age 30 years or greater at the time of the second vaginal delivery [7]. The long-held clinical impression that pregnancy and vaginal childbirth are associated with urinary incontinence in women had been confirmed [8].

12.4   Pelvic Floor Damage

The uterus and vaginal apex are supported by a muscular component, requiring an intact nerve supply, and by a fascial component. Damage to any of these structures can lead to prolapse of the pelvic organs. Three factors are implicated in the etiology of prolapse and stress urinary incontinence: myogenic damage, neuromuscular injury, and damage to the endopelvic fascia.

During pregnancy, pelvi-perineal conditions are unfavorable for contraction and relaxation of the levator ani muscle: this is a consequence not only of the gravidic uterus but also of the direct pressure on the urogenital hiatus, as a reflection of the anteriorization of the endoabdominal pressure vector, in the typically gravidic hyperlordosis. This generates a continuous, abnormal pressure on the weak area of the anterior perineum. Another important moment for pelvic floor damage is the expulsion of the presented part: deflection of the fetal head, as a fulcrum under the pubic symphysis, determines distension of the posterior perineum, forward movement of the central fibrous nucleus, and backwards displacement of the coccyx (Fig. 12.2, Box 12.2). From these dynamics, the precoccygeal region elongates with a great increase of the anovulvar distance. There is histological and magnetic resonance imaging (MRI) evidence that mechanical trauma causes

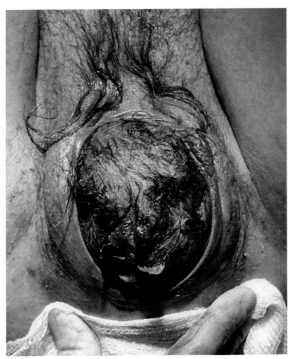

Fig. 12.2 Fetal head at pelvic floor level during vaginal delivery

Box 12.2 Childbirth and pelvic floor: vaginal birth genital trauma

Anterior (periurethral, clitoral, labial)	44%
Anterior and perineal	27%
Perineal	18%

rupture of the pelvic musculature at delivery. Imaging of the pubococcygeal muscle has shown an association between severity of prolapse and loss of muscle size, which correlates with muscle strength. Measurements of the genital hiatus also show a correlation between increasing severity of prolapse and reduction in muscle bulk.

After parturition, histological examination shows direct myogenic damage. The presence and extent of levator trauma is associated with symptoms and signs of pelvic organ prolapse, particularly of the anterior and central compartment. The levator hiatus, which contains the urethra anteriorly, the vagina centrally, and the anorectum posteriorly, varies in young nulliparous women, from an area of 6 cm^2 to 32 cm^2, during Valsalva maneuver. The area of the average fetal head measures 70–90 cm^2, requiring a marked distension and deformation of the levator complex. In parous women with stress incontinence and prolapse, MRI studies have shown a significant decrease in levator muscle volume and an increase in levator hiatus width. There seems to be an association between age at first delivery and levator trauma.

12.5 Damage to the Pelvic Floor Nerve Supply

Damage to the nerve supply of the pelvic floor caused by childbirth may determine progressive denervation of the musculature. Subsequent reinnervation of the pelvic floor leads to an altered function. Pudendal nerve compression is the main mechanism of damage. Nerves pass through the Alcock channel, which is a potential site for compression by the fetal head during childbirth (Box 12.3). Some authors have proposed that the nerve damage is a combination of direct compression injury of the pelvis and traction injury during elongation of the birth canal. Factors associated with greater pelvic floor nerve damage are parity, forceps delivery, prolonged second stage of labor, third-degree perineal tears, and fetal macrosomia. In a 5-year follow-up study, Snooks et al concluded that pudendal nerve damage with partial reinnervation of the external anal sphincter persists, and may become more marked five years after vaginal delivery [9]. Further, this finding was associated with urinary and fecal incontinence. Perineal descent on straining was related to the progression of pelvic floor denervation and reinnervation. Allen et al studied 96 pregnant women prospectively with electromyography (EMG) and pudendal nerve terminal motor latency, and found changes consistent with partial denervation with subsequent reinnervation of pelvic floor muscles [10]. Large fetal size and increase in the length of the second stage correlated with greater damage, whereas forceps use and perineal tears did not. Severe changes of denervation correlated with the onset of stress and fecal incontinence immediately after childbirth. Sultan also studied pudendal nerve terminal motor latency in 122 women before and after childbirth, and reached similar conclusions [11]. Latency

Box 12.3 Neurogenic damage

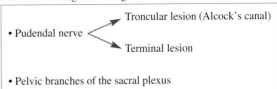

was prolonged after delivery in both nulliparous and multiparous women. It was also prolonged after cesarean section if performed during labor, but not if performed electively. These authors concluded that vaginal delivery, particularly the first one, results in significant pelvic floor tissue stretching and pudendal nerve damage.

12.6   Damage to the Endopelvic Fascia

During parturition, tears in the connective tissue can occur with no clinically apparent signs after delivery. Some women are more susceptible to connective tissue damage due to an inherent weakness in their connective tissue. Prolapse is more common in women with disorders of collagen metabolism. Pregnancy itself has an effect on the connective tissue: the fascia becomes more elastic and weaker. In the past, it has long been assumed that childbirth may result in disruption of the endopelvic fascia, in particular of paraurethral and paravaginal structures. According to data, such defects are considered to be multiple and analogous to striae gravidarum.

12.7   Vascular Damage

Another very important cause of pelvic floor damage is vascular damage: a significant increase in creatine phosphokinase (CPK) has been demonstrated in vaginal versus cesarean delivery, and longer second stages of labor have been shown to be associated with significant increase in CPK.

12.8   Anal Sphincter Injury

Anal sphincter injury is a frequent form of pelvic floor obstetric trauma. Surprising evidence has emerged from modern diagnostic techniques that the incidence of traumas to the posterior perineum (anal sphincter) is higher than the rates suggested by clinical observation. Ultrasound alterations of the anal sphincter after normal vaginal delivery occur in 35% of women presenting with symptoms (incontinence to either gases or feces), and in 13% of pluriparas. Risk factors for anal sphincter damage are the same as the factors for common pelvic floor damage, including median episiotomy that provokes anorectal tears when extended towards the anal region [12, 13]. The main risk factor is considered to

be instrumental vaginal delivery. Fecal incontinence has a clear association to vaginal childbirth. Ryhammer et al studied pelvic floor function in 144 perimenopausal Danish women [14]. They found that increasing parity was associated with: (1) lowered perineal position at rest and during strain; (2) an increased threshold of anal mucosal electrosensitivity; and (3) prolongation of pudendal nerve terminal motor latency bilaterally. The authors concluded that repeated vaginal deliveries have a long-term adverse effect on anorectal physiology in women.

12.9   Chronic Pelvic Pain

Another negative consequence of trauma in vaginal delivery is chronic pelvic pain, which can persist for 6 months after delivery, and is associated with dyspareunia and unsatisfying sexual intercourse in 20% of women.

12.10   Episiotomy

Some special attention must be paid to the role of episiotomy: historically, it has always been considered a positive factor that could protect against wide tears by reducing perineal and anal sphincter lacerations. Evidence now shows that non-selective episiotomy does not protect the perineum: 50% of third-degree lacerations are associated with episiotomy [15]. Thranov reported on Scandinavian women undergoing their first vaginal delivery: 61% of women experienced some incontinence postpartum, with 18% having this symptom for more than 6 months [16]. There was no difference in the incidence of urinary incontinence in women undergoing episiotomy or delivery without episiotomy. Medial episiotomy is associated with a weaker perineum and a higher incidence of anorectal lacerations, which are 50 times more frequent than those caused by mediolateral episiotomy. Thus, mediolateral episiotomy is now considered preferable, if case-selected and carefully performed.

12.11   Cesarean Section

The role of cesarean section has been revised by recent literature [17], showing that it does not protect the pelvic floor, despite past considerations, if performed after the second stage of labor, whereas it affords some level of protection if carried out electively: stress urinary incontinence rates reduce from 10% after a vaginal birth to 3% after elective cesarean delivery. It should also be stressed that pregnancy itself is an important risk factor for pelvic floor dysfunction.

12.12 Conclusions

Many women undergo significant trauma to pelvic floor structures as a consequence of attempts at vaginal delivery. Trauma may affect the pudendal nerve and its branches, the anal sphincter, the levator ani complex, or the pelvic fascial structures. Many risk factors for perineal damage at delivery have been identified, among which the most important are multiparity, forceps application during operative delivery, sacral rotation of the occiput, prolonged second stage of labor, epidural analgesia, third-degree tears, and fetal macrosomia. Some forms of trauma may also occur as a result of rapid labor. Vaginal operative delivery is a risk factor for all forms of pelvic trauma [18]. Regarding prolapse, pregnancy and childbirth are well documented as major risk factors.

The identification of women at high risk for delivery-related pelvic floor trauma should be a priority for everyday good clinical practice. Obstetric perineal damage cannot be avoided, but it certainly can be limited, by means of preventive strategies and therapeutic improvement [12, 19]: that is, identifying perineal risk factors, improving assistance, and timely rehabilitation.

References

1. Drutz HP, Alarab M. Pelvic organ prolapse: demographics and future growth prospects. Int Urogynec J 2006;17(suppl 1):S6–S9.
2. Mant J, Painter R, Vessey M. Epidemiology of genital prolapse: observations from the Oxford Family Planning Association Study. Br J Obstet Gynaecol 1997;104:579–585.
3. Rogers RG. Postpartum genitourinary changes. Urol Clin N Am 2007;34:13–21.
4. Cardozo L, Cutner A. Lower urinary tract symptoms in pregnancy. Br J Urol 1997;80:14–23.
5. Stanton SL, Kerr-Wilson R, Harris GV. The incidence of urological symptoms in normal pregnancy. Br J Obstet Gynecol 1980;87:897–900.
6. Thorp JM Jr, Norton PA, Wall LL et al. Urinary incontinence in pregnancy and the puerperium: a prospective study. Am J Obstet Gynecol 1999; 8:266–273.
7. Foldspang A, Mommsen S, Djurhuus JC. Prevalent urinary incontinence as a correlate of pregnancy, vaginal childbirth and obstetric techniques. Am J Public Health 1999; 89:209–212.
8. Beck RP, Hsu N. Pregnancy, childbirth and the menopause related to the development of stress incontinence. Am J Obstet Gynecol 1965;91:820–823.
9. Snooks SJ, Swash M, Mathers SE et al. Effect of vaginal delivery on the pelvic floor: a five-year follow-up. Br J Surg 1990; 2:1358–1360.
10. Allen RE, Hosker GL, Smith AR, Warrell DW. Pelvic floor damage and childbirth: a neurophysiological study. Br J Obstet Gynecol 1990;97:770–779.
11. Sultan AH, Kamm MA, Hudson CM. Pudendal nerve damage during labour: prospective study before and after childbirth. Br J Obstet Gynecol 1994; 1:22–28.
12. Dandolu F, Chatwani A, Harmanli O et al. Risk factors for obstetrical anal sphincter lacerations. Int Urogynecol J 2007;16:304–307.
13. Sultan AH, Kamm MA, Hudson CM. Anal sphincter disruption during vaginal delivery. N Eng J Med 1993;23:1956–1957.
14. Ryhammer AM, Laurberg S, Hermann AP. Long term effect of vaginal deliveries on anorectal function in normal perimenopausal women. Dis Colon Rectum 1996;39:852–859.
15. Rizk DEE, Abadir MN, Thomas LB et al. Determinants of the length of episiotomy or spontaneous posterior perineal laceration in vaginal birth. Int Urogynecol J 2005; 16:395–400.
16. Thranov I, Kringelbach AM, Melchior E et al. Postpartum symptoms. Episiotomy or tear at vaginal delivery. Acta Obstet Gynecol Scand 1990;99:260–262.
17. Richter HE. Caesarean delivery on maternal request versus planned vaginal delivery: impact on development of pelvic organ prolapse. Semin Perinatol 2006;30:272–275.
18. Toozs-Hobson P, Balmforth JB, Cardozo L et al. The effect of mode of delivery on pelvic floor functional anatomy. Int Urogynecol J 2008;19:407–416.
19. Patel DA, Xu X, Thomason AD et al. Childbirth and pelvic floor dysfunction: assessment of prevention opportunities at delivery. Am J Obstet Gynecol 2006;195:23–28.

Posterior Compartment Disorders and Management of Acute Anal Sphincter Trauma

13

Abdul H. Sultan and Ranee Thakar

Abstract Trauma sustained during childbirth is not always recognized, and damage to tissues and nerves may lead to long-term sequelae that can have a huge impact on the physical, social, and psychological well-being of women. However, even when trauma is recognized and repaired, the outcome may be suboptimal. Focused training in identification and appropriate repair is therefore mandatory. The two most important principles in primary repair of acute anal sphincter injuries are repair of the internal sphincter and restoration of the anal canal length. Subsequent vaginal delivery is not associated with adverse outcome in the majority of women.

Keywords Anal sphincter repair • Cesarean section • Childbirth • Fecal incontinence • Perineal trauma • Rectocele • Third- and fourth-degree tears

13.1 Introduction

The posterior compartment consists of all the structures that include the posterior vaginal wall and structures posterior to it. During the process of vaginal delivery, fascia, muscles, and nerves may be stretched or disrupted. However, while these changes could be attributed to the physiological process of childbirth, in some women they can lead to pathological events with long-term consequences. Obstetric trauma to the posterior compartment has been implicated in the development of rectoceles, perineoceles, and fecal incontinence. However, as many women who develop these conditions tend to present many years after childbirth, either a direct link to its causation is not considered or it is attributed to the effects of ageing or the menopause. As much of this is already covered in the previous chapter, we will concentrate on the pathological effects of childbirth on the posterior compartment.

13.2 Rectoceles

The definition, etiology, and pathophysiology of rectoceles are not fully understood. A rectocele is an outpocketing of the anterior rectal wall into the lumen of the vagina [1]. Although obstetric trauma and defecatory disorders have been implicated, a rectocele has been identified in both asymptomatic and nulliparous women [2]. Women may present only when they become symptomatic, which could be many years after childbirth.

A rectocele may be the result of overdistensibility of an intact rectovaginal septum, disruption of the perineal membrane and detachment from the perineal body (Fig. 13.1), perineal hypermobility, or protrusion as a result of a deficient perineum. Dietz and Steensma [3] conducted a prospective study of 68 nulliparous

A.H. Sultan
Department of Obstetrics and Gynaecology,
Mayday University Hospital, Croydon, Surrey, UK

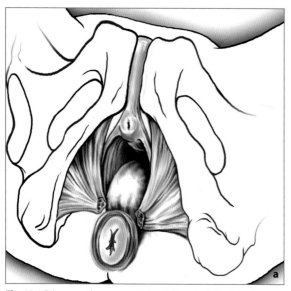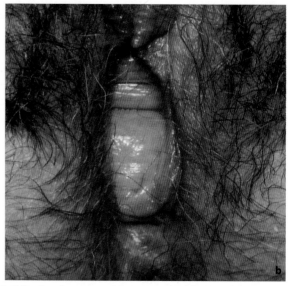

Fig. 13.1 Diagramatic representation (**a**) and photo (**b**) of a rectocele following disruption of the rectovaginal fascia and detachment from the perineal body with widening of the genital hiatus and herniation of the rectum

pregnant women, and performed translabial ultrasound during pregnancy, repeating it between two and six months postpartum. A defect of the rectovaginal septum was diagnosed if there was a discontinuity in the anterior anorectal muscularis of ≥10 mm in depth. Sonographic defects were identified in 2 of the 68 women before and in 8 of the 52 after childbirth. However, 4 of the 58 women were asymptomatic. The authors concluded that childbirth does play a role, as there were some de novo defects while other defects enlarged after delivery. This would suggest that vaginal delivery can cause disruption of the rectovaginal fascia. However, larger clinical studies are awaited that may identify obstetric risk factors such as baby weight, episiotomy, instrumental delivery, etc. It remains to be established whether modification of obstetric practice, and in particular meticulous restoration of the perineal and vaginal anatomy when repairing episiotomies and genital lacerations, may minimize the development of rectoceles. Surgical repair techniques for rectoceles are described in Chapter 44.

13.3 Obstetric Anal Sphincter Injuries (OASIS)

Obstetric anal sphincter injuries (OASIS) are reported to occur in 1.7% (2.9% in primiparae) of woman in centers where mediolateral episiotomies are practiced [4],

compared to 12% [5] (19% in primiparae) [6] in centers practicing midline episiotomy. However, rates as high as 7.5% have recently been reported in centers practicing mediolateral episiotomy, suggesting improvements in recognition of OASIS [7, 8]. However, despite recognition and primary repair of acute OASIS, 39% of those diagnosed have symptoms of anal incontinence and 34–91% have persistent anal sphincter defects on ultrasound within 3 months of delivery [9].

Pudendal neuropathy following vaginal delivery has also been implicated as a cause of incontinence, but prospective studies have shown that the vast majority of women suffer some degree of neuropraxia that recovers with time [10], or reinnervation occurs [11].

In order to standardize the classification of perineal trauma, Sultan [12] proposed the following classification that has been adopted by the Royal College of Obstetricians and Gynaecologists and also recommended by the International Consultation on Incontinence [13–15] (Fig. 13.2).

13.3.1 Applied Anatomy and Physiology

The anal canal measures about 3.5 cm in length, but in the female is shorter in its anterior aspect by 0.5 to 1 cm. The external anal sphincter (EAS) is made up of striated muscle that is subdivided into subcutaneous, superficial, and deep, and is responsible for voluntary

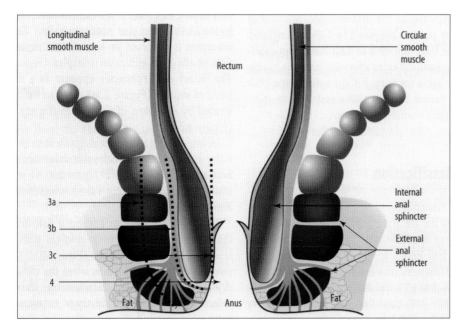

Fig. 13.2 Diagrammatic representation of the anal sphincters demonstrating the classification of major degrees of perineal tears (*3a–c* and *4*). Reproduced from [9], with permission

squeeze and reflex contraction pressure (Fig. 13.2). It is innervated by the pudendal nerve, which is a mixed sensory and motor nerve. The internal anal sphincter (IAS) is a thickened continuation of the circular smooth muscle of the bowel. It contributes about 70% of the resting pressure and is under autonomic control. It is separated from the EAS by the conjoint longitudinal muscle that is a continuation of the longitudinal smooth muscle of the bowel. As shown in Fig. 13.2, the subcutaneous EAS lies at a lower level than the IAS, but during regional or general anesthesia the paralyzed EAS lies almost at the same level as the IAS.

Damage to the EAS results in fecal incontinence, which is usually associated with urgency, and damage to the IAS is usually associated with flatus incontinence and passive soiling. However, damage to both sphincters can occur, giving rise to mixed symptoms.

13.3.2 Diagnosis of OASIS

A careful vaginal and rectal examination must be performed in all women who have undergone a vaginal delivery. In order to do this, there must be adequate exposure, good lighting, and analgesia. OASIS cannot be excluded without performing a proper rectal and vaginal examination (Fig. 13.3), as third/fourth-degree tears can occur despite an apparent intact perineum [15]. The IAS is thinner and paler than the striated

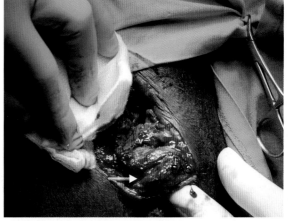

Fig. 13.3 A partial tear along the length of the external anal sphincter (*arrow*) that could be missed without a rectal examination. Reproduced from [9], with permission

EAS. The appearance of the IAS can be described as being analogous to the flesh of raw fish, as opposed to the red meat appearance of the EAS. The EAS is demarcated laterally by the perianal fat, an important landmark in identification of the EAS.

13.3.3 Repair of OASIS

In 1930, Royston described a commonly practiced technique in which the ends of the torn sphincter were approximated by inserting a deep catgut suture through the inner third of the sphincter muscle, and a second set through the outer third of the sphincter [16]. In 1948, Kaltreider and Dixon described their series of women since 1935 in whom one mattress or figure-of-eight suture was used [17]. Fulsher and Fearl described a technique in which sutures were inserted in the fascial sheath or capsule of the anal sphincter, and no sutures were allowed to pass through the sphincter muscle [18]. More specifically, Cunningham and Pilkington described inserting four interrupted sutures in the capsule of the EAS at the anterior, posterior, superior, and inferior points [19]. The end-to-end approximation type of repair has been the standard and is still used widely. However, in 1999, Sultan et al [20] explored the overlap technique of primary repair of the EAS (as described by Parks and McPartlin for secondary sphincter repair [21]). In addition, Sultan et al highlighted the importance of recognition and separate repair of the freshly torn IAS, which is largely responsible for maintaining the resting tone of the anal sphincter, as persistent IAS injury is associated with incontinence of flatus and passive soiling [20].

The morbidity associated with perineal trauma depends on the extent of perineal damage, technique and materials used for suturing, and the skill of the operator. Practitioners should therefore be adequately trained and adopt evidence-based techniques during perineal repair.

Repair should be conducted in the operating theatre where there is access to good lighting, appropriate equipment, and aseptic conditions. A specially prepared instrument tray containing a Weislander self-retaining retractor, four Allis tissue forceps, McIndoe dissecting scissors, tooth forceps, two artery forceps, stitch-cutting scissors, and a needle holder is useful (www.perineum.net).

A general or regional (spinal, epidural, caudal) anesthetic will provide analgesia as well as muscle relaxation, which is an important prerequisite to enable proper evaluation of the full extent of the injury. As the EAS is a striated muscle ring, under tonic contraction the torn muscle ends are prone to retract within its capsular sheath. Adequate muscle relaxation allows the torn ends of the EAS to be grasped and retrieved. This would enable repair of the torn muscles without tension, especially if the intention is to overlap the EAS.

Repair of OASIS should only be conducted by a doctor who has been formally trained (or under supervision) in primary anal sphincter repair. In view of the observed suboptimal outcome associated with primary anal sphincter repair when performed by obstetricians with varying degrees of experience, it has been suggested that perhaps a repair performed by colorectal surgeons may be associated with a better outcome [22–24]. Kairaluoma et al reported on 31 consecutive women who sustained OASIS (third and fourth degree) [25]. All had an EAS overlap repair immediately after delivery, performed by two colorectal surgeons. In addition to end-to-end repair of the IAS, they also performed a levatorplasty, to approximate the levator ani muscle in the midline, with two sutures. At a median follow-up of 2 years, 23% complained of anal incontinence, 23% developed wound infection, 27% complained of dyspareunia, and one developed a rectovaginal fistula. Thus, the outcome was no better when the repair was conducted by colorectal surgeons. Furthermore, in a survey of colorectal practice in the UK, only 6.7% of colorectal surgeons reported that they performed more than 10 acute repairs per year; 60% had never performed an acute sphincter repair; and 30% performed less than five per year [26]. It is therefore not surprising that only 19% of colorectal surgeons believed that they should be involved in the acute management of OASIS [26]. Therefore, the repair should be carried out by the most experienced obstetrician on the labor ward, who encounters this problem more frequently and is skilled in suturing the extensive vaginal tears that can often accompany OASIS. However, in a recent survey of candidates (mainly obstetricians) attending a hands-on workshop on repair of OASIS, only 13% were satisfied with their level of experience prior to performing their first unsupervised repair [27]. This suggests that there is an urgent need for structured and focused training in this area.

13.3.4 Timing of Repair

Nordenstam et al conducted a randomized study in which they found no difference in anal incontinence 12 months after primary repair when women who had repair immediately after the tear were compared to those whose repair was delayed for 8–12 h [7]. They concluded that there is no justification for delaying suturing. However, a delay in repair may be justified in exceptional circumstances when an experienced obstetrician is not available.

13.3.5 Technique of Repair

In the presence of a fourth-degree tear, the torn anal epithelium is repaired with interrupted sutures with the knots tied in the anal lumen using Vicryl (polyglactin) or Vicryl rapide 3-0 (Fig. 13.4). This technique has been widely described, and proponents of the technique argue that by tying the knots outside, the quantity of foreign material within the tissues would be reduced and hence reduce the risk of infection. However, this concern probably applies to the use of catgut that dissolves by phagocytosis, as opposed to the newer synthetic material such as Vicryl that dissolves by hydrolysis. A subcuticular repair of the anal epithelium via the transvaginal approach has also been described, and could be equally effective provided the terminal knots are secure [28].

The IAS should be identified and, if torn, repaired separately from the EAS. An end-to-end repair should be performed with interrupted mattress sutures [9] (Fig. 13.5). An association between IAS defects and severe symptoms of fecal incontinence 3 months after sustaining OASIS has been demonstrated [29]. Furthermore, the size of the IAS defect on ultrasound after primary repair of OASIS appears to be related to the severity of symptoms [30]. However, during secondary sphincter repair, the ends of the torn IAS are difficult to identify as they retract at the time of injury and the gap is replaced by scar tissue. Consequently, repair is invariably inadequate or impossible, highlighting the importance of recognition and primary repair of the IAS at the time of delivery.

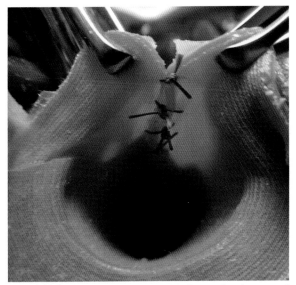

Fig. 13.4 Repair of the torn anal epithelium using interrupted Vicryl sutures

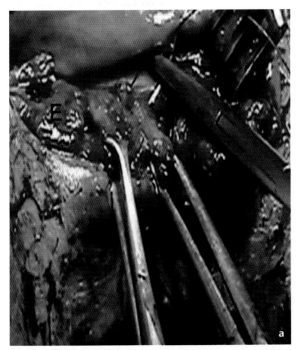

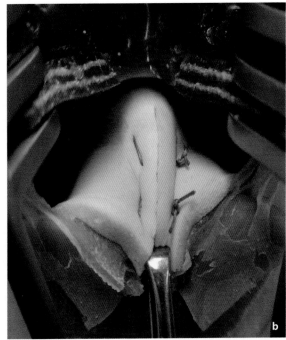

Fig. 13.5 a The torn ends of the internal sphincter being held by Allis forceps (*E* = external sphincter) and **b** repaired using mattress PDS 3-0 sutures. Reproduced from [9], with permission

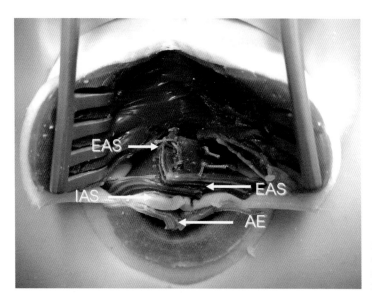

Fig. 13.6 Overlap of the external anal sphincter (*EAS*, repair; *AE*, anal epithelium; *IAS*, internal anal sphincter). Reproduced from [9], with permission

When the EAS is only partially torn (grade 3a and some 3b), an end-to-end repair should be performed using two or three mattress sutures instead of hemostatic "figure-of-eight" sutures. If there is a full-thickness EAS tear (some 3b, 3c, or fourth degree), either an overlapping (Fig. 13.6) or end-to-end method can be used [13]. A true overlap can only be performed if the two ends of the EAS are completely torn, along its full length and thickness, otherwise the residual fibers may need to be divided before an overlap repair. A recent Cochrane review [31] including three randomized studies [32–34] showed that, compared to immediate primary end-to-end repair of OASIS, early primary overlap repair appears to be associated with lower risks of fecal urgency and anal incontinence symptoms and deterioration of anal incontinence over time. Four women need to be treated with the overlap technique, to prevent one woman developing fecal incontinence. However, as the experience of the surgeon was addressed in only one of the three studies reviewed, it remains to be established if one technique is superior to the other in day-to-day practice [31].

However, two subsequent studies have reported excellent results using the overlap technique [35, 36] but long-term follow-up is required. The single most important predictor of incontinence following secondary repair is postoperative anal canal length [37], and it has been shown that a shorter anal canal length after primary repair is associated with a poorer outcome [38]. After repair of the sphincter, the perineal muscles should be sutured to reconstruct the perineal body, in order to provide support to the repaired anal sphincter. Finally, the vaginal skin should be sutured and the perineal skin approximated with a subcutaneous suture [9].

13.3.6 Suture Material

The anal epithelium is repaired using Vicryl 3-0. The sphincter muscles are repaired with either monofilament fine sutures such as 3-0 PDS (polydioxanone) or modern braided sutures such as 2-0 Vicryl (polyglactin), as these may cause less irritation and discomfort with equivalent outcome. Complete absorption of PDS takes longer than Vicryl, with 50% tensile strength lasting more than 3 months compared to 3 weeks respectively [34]. To minimize suture migration, care should be taken to cut the suture ends short and ensure that they are covered by the overlying superficial perineal muscles. Williams et al performed a factorial randomized controlled trial (n = 112), in which women were randomized into four groups: overlap with polyglactin (Vicryl; Ethicon, Edinburgh, UK); end-to-end repair with Vicryl; overlap repair with polydiaxanone (PDS; Ethicon, Edinburgh, UK); and end-to-end repair with PDS [34]. This trial was specifically designed to test a hypothesis regarding suture-related morbidity (need for suture removal due to pain, suture migration, or dyspareunia) using the two techniques. At six weeks there were no differences in suture-related morbidity between the different groups.

13.3.7 Role of Antibiotics

In a prospective, randomized placebo controlled study of patients who had sustained OASIS (n = 147), it has been shown that patients who received a single dose of intravenous second-generation cephalosporin had a significantly lower risk of perineal complications (8% compared to 24%) compared to placebo by 2 weeks after the repair [39]. We prescribe intravenous broad-spectrum antibiotics such as cefuroxime 1.5 g and metronidazole 1 g intraoperatively and continue this antibiotic regime orally for up to 5 days.

13.3.8 Stool Softeners

Constipation should be avoided, as passage of constipated stool, or indeed fecal impaction requiring manual evacuation, may disrupt the repair, and the majority consensus in the literature is that stool softeners should be prescribed [28]. Mahony et al performed a randomized trial (n = 105) of constipating versus laxative regimens and found that the use of laxatives was associated with a significantly earlier and less painful first bowel motion, as well as earlier discharge from hospital [40]. Nineteen per cent in the constipated regimen group experienced troublesome constipation (two required hospital admission for fecal impaction) compared to 5% in the laxative regimen group. There were no significant differences in continence scores, anal manometry, or endoanal scan findings.

A recent randomized study [41] has indicated that stool bulking agents such as ispaghula husk (Fybogel) should be avoided, as the authors found that incontinence occurred significantly more often (33% vs. 18%) when lactulose and Fybogel were consumed compared to lactulose only. We recommend lactulose 15 mL twice a day for 10 days but the dose could be modified according to the stool consistency.

13.3.9 Postoperative Catheterization

Severe perineal discomfort, particularly following instrumental delivery, is a known cause of urinary retention, and following regional anesthesia it can take up to 12 h before full bladder sensation returns. A Foley catheter should be inserted for up to 24 h unless medical staff can ensure that spontaneous voiding occurs at least every 3–4 h without undue bladder overdistension.

13.3.10 Postoperative Analgesia

The degree of pain following perineal trauma is related to the extent of the injury, and OASIS are frequently associated with other more extensive injuries such as paravaginal tears. In a systematic review, Hedayati et al found that rectal analgesia such as diclofenac is effective in reducing pain from perineal trauma within the first 24 h after birth [42]. In women who had a repair of a fourth-degree tear, diclofenac should be administered orally, as insertion of suppositories may be uncomfortable and there is a theoretical risk of poor healing associated with local anti-inflammatory agents. Codeine-based preparations are best avoided as they may cause constipation leading to excessive straining and possible disruption of the repair.

13.3.11 Follow-up

Ideally, these women should be under the care of a specialist team, e.g. a perineal clinic, and follow-up should be about 8–12 weeks after delivery. The perineal clinic is viewed as a supportive environment and women feel confident about the information provided by the team [43]. An information booklet should be given to these women to ensure that they understand the implications of sustaining OASIS and also to provide information as to where and when to seek help if symptoms of infection or incontinence develop. There is no consensus of opinion on when pelvic floor and anal sphincter exercises are best initiated but we recommend that they should be commenced when the discomfort resolves and the woman feels comfortable.

13.3.12 Management of Subsequent Pregnancies

There are no randomized studies to determine the most appropriate mode of delivery following a third/fourth-degree tear. At the first postpartum visit, a careful vaginal and rectal examination should be performed to check for complete healing, scar tenderness, and sphincter tone. In order to counsel women

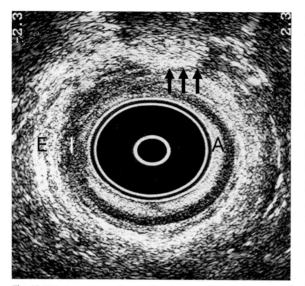

Fig. 13.7 Endoanal scan image showing overlap (*arrows*) of the external anal sphincter (*E*). *I*, internal anal sphincter; *A*, anal epithelium. Reproduced from [9], with permission

with previous third/fourth-degree tears appropriately, we find it useful to have a symptom questionnaire along with anal ultrasound (Fig. 13.7) and manometry results. If vaginal delivery is contemplated, then these tests should be performed during the current pregnancy. Fig. 13.8 presents a simple flow diagram demonstrating the management of subsequent delivery after OASIS that we follow in our unit. One study has shown that if a large sonographic defect (more than one quadrant) is present, or if the squeeze pressure increment (above resting pressure) is less than 20 mmHg, then the risk of impaired continence dramatically increases after a subsequent delivery [44]. We conducted a prospective study over a five-year period and found that if there is no evidence of significant compromise of anal sphincter function, a subsequent vaginal delivery is not associated with subsequent deterioration in function or symptoms [45]. We were therefore able to encourage asymptomatic women who

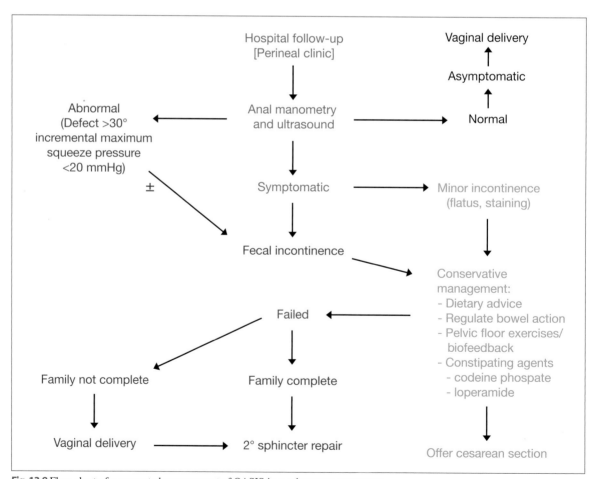

Fig. 13.8 Flow chart of a suggested management of OASIS in a subsequent pregnancy

have minimal compromise of their anal sphincter function to have a vaginal delivery.

These women should be counseled that they have an 88% [6] (in centers practicing midline episiotomy) to 95% [4] (in centers practicing mediolateral episiotomy) chance of not sustaining recurrent OASIS. If an episiotomy is considered necessary, e.g. because of a thick inelastic or scarred perineum, a mediolateral episiotomy should be performed. There is no evidence that routinely performed episiotomies prevent recurrence of OASIS. The threshold at which these women may be considered for a cesarean section may be lowered if a traumatic delivery is anticipated, e.g. in the presence of one or more additional relative risk factors, such as a large baby, shoulder dystocia, prolonged labor, or difficult instrumental delivery. However, in deciding the mode of delivery, counseling (and its clear documentation) is extremely important. Some of these women who have sustained OASIS may be scarred both physically and emotionally and may find it difficult to cope with the thought of another vaginal delivery. These women will require sympathy, psychological support, and serious consideration of their request for cesarean section.

Women who have minor degrees of incontinence (fecal urgency or flatus incontinence) may be controlled with dietary advice, constipating agents (loperamide or codeine phosphate), physiotherapy, or biofeedback. These women who have some degree of anal sphincter compromise (Fig. 13.8) but whose symptoms are controlled should be counseled and recommended a cesarean section.

Women who sustained a previous third/fourth-degree tear with subsequent severe incontinence and have failed conservative management should be offered secondary sphincter repair by a colorectal surgeon (or a urogynecologist with expertise in secondary sphincter repair), and all subsequent deliveries should be by cesarean section. Some women with fecal incontinence may choose to complete their family before embarking on anal sphincter surgery. It remains to be established whether these women should be allowed a vaginal delivery but it is likely that the damage has already occurred and the risk of further damage is minimal and possibly insignificant in terms of the outcome of surgery. The benefit, if any, should be weighed against the risks associated with cesarean section for all subsequent pregnancies. Women who have had a previous successful secondary sphincter repair for fecal incontinence should be delivered by cesarean section [46]. Clearly there are going to be women who do not entirely fit into any of the above categories, e.g. those who have isolated internal sphincter defects or those who have irritable bowel syndrome. The management of these women should be individualized, and a mutual decision should be made taking into account the symptoms, examination findings, and results of the investigations.

If there are no facilities for anal manometry and endosonography, then the management will depend on symptoms and clinical evaluation. Asymptomatic women without any clinical evidence of sphincter compromise as determined by assessment of anal tone could be allowed a vaginal delivery. All women who are symptomatic should be referred to a center with facilities for anorectal assessment and should be counseled for cesarean section.

13.3.13 Training Issues

It has been shown that up to half of OASIS are not recognized by the obstetrician or midwife [47, 48]. Inadequate training of doctors and midwives in perineal and anal sphincter anatomy [26] is believed to be a major contributing factor. In a survey of 75 doctors and 75 midwives in the UK, Sultan et al demonstrated inconsistencies in the classification of perineal trauma, as one-third of doctors were classifying third-degree tears as second-degree [26]. Most trainee doctors admitted that their training in recognizing (84%) and repairing (94%) OASIS was poor. Furthermore, in another study, 64% of consultants reported unsatisfactory or no training in the management of OASIS [49]. OASIS that were previously believed to be occult injuries [10] have now been proven to be undiagnosed injuries that could have been diagnosed clinically by a trained clinician [47]. McLennan et al also raised concern about training in the USA [50]. They surveyed 1,177 fourth-year residents and found that the majority had received no formal training in pelvic floor anatomy, episiotomy, or perineal repair, and supervision during perineal repair was limited.

A recent survey of candidates attending a hands-on training course using a latex model and fresh animal tissue has shown that training in this fashion was useful in diagnosis and repair of OASIS [27]. Siddighi et al demonstrated that residents in obstetrics and gynecology who underwent a structured training workshop improved their surgical ability with respect to managing OASIS [51]. As the occurrence of OASIS is unpredictable and unplanned, and opportunities for trainees to repair these injuries under authentic circumstances are few, a hands-on workshop in conjunction with competency-based training appears to be the best way forward (www.perineum.net).

13.4 Conclusions

Obstetric trauma to the posterior compartment can result in pelvic floor denervation, disruption of the fascial supports, and injury to the anal sphincter. Injuries to the anal sphincter can give rise to anal incontinence, and therefore accurate detection and diagnosis of the full extent of the injury is mandatory at delivery. Repair should be conducted by a trained clinician and the aim should be to restore the normal high-pressure zone of the anal canal represented by the anal length. Failure to identify and repair the internal sphincter at the time of the acute injury will increase the risk of fecal incontinence and jeopardize the ability to repair at a later date. Attention needs to be focused on training of doctors and midwives internationally in the identification and repair of OASIS.

References

1   Mellgren A, Anzen B, Nilsson BY et al. Results of rectocele repair. A prospective study. Dis Colon Rectum 1995;38:7–13.
2.   Shorvon PJ, McHugh S, Diamant NE et al. Defecography in normal volunteers: results and implications. Gut 1989;30:1737–1749.
3.   Dietz HP, Steensma AB. The role of childbirth in the aetiology of rectocele. BJOG 2006;113:264–267.
4.   Harkin R, Fitzpatrick M, O'Connell PR, O'Herlihy C. Anal sphincter disruption at vaginal delivery: is recurrence predictable? Eur J Obstet Gynecol Reprod Biol 2003; 109:149–152.
5.   Coats PM, Chan KK, Wilkins M, Beard RJ. A comparison between midline and mediolateral episiotomies. BJOG 1980;87:408–412.
6.   Peleg D, Kennedy CM, Merrill D, Zlatnik FJ. Risk of repetition of a severe perineal laceration. Obstet Gynecol 1999;93:1021–1024.
7.   Nordenstam J, Mellgren A, Altman D et al. Immediate or delayed repair of obstetric anal sphincter tears–a randomised controlled trial. BJOG 2008;115:857–865.
8.   Ekeus C, Nilsson E, Gottvall K. Increasing incidence of anal sphincter tears among primiparas in Sweden: a popu-

lation-based register study. Acta Obstet Gynecol Scand 2008;87:564–573.
9.   Sultan AH, Thakar R. Third and fourth degree tears. In: Sultan AH, Thakar R, Fenner D (eds) Perineal and anal sphincter trauma. Springer-Verlag, London, 2007, pp 33–51.
10.   Sultan AH, Kamm MA, Hudson CN et al. Anal sphincter disruption during vaginal delivery. N Engl J Med 1993; 329:1905–1911.
11.   Allen RE, Hosker GL, Smith ARB, Warrell DW. Pelvic floor damage and childbirth: a neurophysiological study. BJOG 1990;97:770–779.
12.   Sultan A H. Obstetric perineal injury and anal incontinence. Clin Risk 1999;5:193–196.
13.   Royal College of Obstetricians and Gynaecologists. Management of third and fourth degree perineal tears following vaginal delivery. Guideline No 29. London, RCOG Press, 2007.
14.   Norton C, Christensen J, Butler U et al. Anal Incontinenc, 2 edn. Health Publication Ltd, Plymouth, 2005, pp 985–1044.
15.   Sultan AH, Kettle C. Diagnosis of perineal trauma. In: Sultan AH, Thakar R, Fenner D (eds) Perineal and anal sphincter trauma. Springer-Verlag, London, 2007, pp13–19.
16.   Royston GD. Repair of complete perineal laceration. Am J Obstet Gynecol 1930;19:185–195.
17.   Kaltreider DF, Dixon DM. A study of 710 complete lacerations following central episiotomy. Southern Med J 1948;41:814–820.
18.   Fulsher RW, Fearl CL. The third-degree laceration in modern obstetrics. Am J Obstet Gynecol 1955;69:786–793.
19.   Cunningham CB, Pilkington JW. Complete perineotomy. Am J Obstet Gynecol 1955;70:1225–1231.
20.   Sultan AH, Monga AK, Kumar D, Stanton SL. Primary repair of obstetric anal sphincter rupture using the overlap technique. Br J Obstet Gynaecol 1999;106:318–323.
21.   Parks AG, McPartlin JF. Late repair of injuries of the anal sphincter. Proc R Soc Med 1971;64:1187–1189.
22.   Walsh CJ, Mooney EF, Upton GJ, Motson RW. Incidence of third-degree perineal tears in labour and outcome after primary repair. Br J Surg 1996;83:218–221.
23.   Sultan AH, Kamm MA. Faecal incontinence after childbirth. Br J Obstet Gynaecol 1997;104:979–982.
24.   Cook TA, Mortensen NJ. Management of faecal incontinence following obstetric injury. Br J Surg 1998;85:293–299.
25.   Kairaluoma MV, Raivio P, Aarnio MT, Kellokumpu IH. Immediate repair of obstetric anal sphincter rupture: medium-term outcome of the overlap technique. Dis Colon Rectum 2004;47:1358–1363.
26.   Sultan AH, Kamm MA, Hudson CN. Obstetric perineal tears: an audit of training. J Obstet Gynaecol 1995;15:19–23.
27.   Andrews V, Thakar R, Sultan AH. Structured hands-on training in repair of obstetric anal sphincter injuries (OASIS): an audit of clinical practice. Int Urogynecol J Pelvic Floor Dysfunct 2009;20:193–199.
28.   Sultan AH, Thakar R. Lower genital tract and anal sphincter trauma. Best Pract Res Clin Obstet Gynaecol 2002;16:99–116.
29.   Mahony R, Behan M, Daly L et al. Internal anal sphincter defect influences continence outcome following obstetric anal sphincter injury. Am J Obstet Gynecol 2007; 196:217.e1–5.
30.   Vaccaro C, Clemons JL. Anal sphincter defects and anal in-

continence symptoms after repair of obstetric anal sphincter lacerations in primiparous women. Int Urogynecol J Pelvic Floor Dysfunct 2008;19:1503–1508.

31. Fernando R, Sultan AH, Kettle C et al. Methods of repair for obstetric anal sphincter injury. Cochrane Database Syst Rev 2006;(3):CD002866.

32. Fernando R, Sultan AH, Kettle C et al. A randomised trial of overlap versus end-to-end primary repair of the anal sphincter. Neurourol Urodyn 2004;23:411–412.

33. Fitzpatrick M, Behan M, O'Connell R, O'Herlihy C. A randomized clinical trial comparing primary overlap with approximation repair of third-degree obstetric tears. Am J Obstet Gynecol 2000;183:1220–1224.

34. Williams A, Adams EJ, Tincello DG et al. How to repair an anal sphincter injury after vaginal delivery: results of a randomised controlled trial. BJOG 2006;113:201–207.

35. Molander P, Vayrynen T, Paavonen J et al. Outcome of primary repair of obstetric anal sphincter rupture using the overlap technique. Acta Obstet Gynecol Scand 2007; 86:1458–1462.

36. Lepisto A, Pinta T, Kylanpaa ML et al. Overlap technique improves results of primary surgery after obstetric anal sphincter tear. Dis Colon Rectum 2008;51:421–425.

37. Hool GR, Lieber ML, Church JM. Postoperative anal canal length predicts outcome in patients having sphincter repair for fecal incontinence. Dis Colon Rectum 1999;42:313–318.

38. Norderval S, Oian P, Revhaug A, Vonen B. Anal incontinence after obstetric sphincter tears: outcome of anatomic primary repairs. Dis Colon Rectum 2005;48:1055–1061.

39. Duggal N, Mercado C, Daniels K et al. Antibiotic prophylaxis for prevention of postpartum perineal wound complications: a randomized controlled trial. Obstet Gynecol 2008;111:1268–1273.

40. Mahony R, Behan M, O'Herlihy C, O'Connell PR. Randomized, clinical trial of bowel confinement vs. laxative use after primary repair of a third-degree obstetric anal sphincter tear. Dis Colon Rectum 2004;47:12–17.

41. Eogan M, Daly L, Behan M et al. Randomised clinical trial of a laxative alone versus a laxative and a bulking agent after primary repair of obstetric anal sphincter injury. BJOG 2007;114:736–740.

42. Hedayati H, Parsons J, Crowther CA. Rectal analgesia for pain from perineal trauma following childbirth. Cochrane Database Syst Rev 2003;(3):CD003931.

43. Williams A, Lavender T, Richmond DH, Tincello DG. Women's experiences after a third-degree obstetric anal sphincter tear: a qualitative study. Birth 2005; 32:129–136.

44. Fynes M, Donnelly V, Behan M et al. Effect of second vaginal delivery on anorectal physiology and faecal continence: a prospective study [see comments]. Lancet 1999; 18;354:983–986.

45. Scheer I, Thakar R, Sultan AH. Mode of delivery after previous obstetric anal sphincter injuries (OASIS) – a reappraisal? Int Urogynecol J Pelvic Floor Dysfunct 2009; 20:1095–1101.

46. Sultan AH, Stanton SL. Preserving the pelvic floor and perineum during childbirth-- elective caesarean section? BJOG 1996;103:731–734.

47. Andrews V, Thakar R, Sultan AH. Occult anal sphincter injuries – myth or reality? BJOG 2006;113:195–200.

48. Groom KM, Paterson-Brown S. Can we improve on the diagnosis of third degree tears? Eur J Obstet Gynecol Reprod Biol 2002 10;101:19–21.

49. Fernando RJ, Sultan AH, Radley S et al. Management of obstetric anal sphincter injury: a systematic review & national practice survey. BMC Health Serv Res 2002;2:9.

50. McLennan MT, Melick CF, Clancy SL, Artal R. Episiotomy and perineal repair. An evaluation of resident education and experience. J Reprod Med 2002;47:1025–1030.

51. Siddighi S, Kleeman SD, Baggish MS et al. Effects of an educational workshop on performance of fourth-degree perineal laceration repair. Obstet Gynecol 2007; 109:289–294.

Prevention of Perineal Trauma

14

Ranee Thakar and Abdul H. Sultan

Abstract Perineal trauma is a highly prevalent condition. The short- and long-term morbidity associated with perineal repair can lead to major physical, psychological, and social problems. Although it would be impossible to completely prevent perineal trauma, it could be minimized. Proven strategies include the practice of perineal massage in the antenatal period, delayed pushing in the second stage of labor with an epidural in situ, restrictive use of episiotomy, preference of a mediolateral over a midline episiotomy, and the use of a vacuum extractor instead of forceps for instrumental delivery. Other strategies have been suggested but remain unproven in randomized controlled trials. Further research in this area is required.

Keywords Anal sphincter • Birth positions • Episiotomy • Instrumental deliveries • Perineal massage • Perineal support • Perineum • Prevention • Second stage • Trauma

14.1 Introduction

Perineal trauma may occur spontaneously during vaginal birth or when a surgical incision (episiotomy) is intentionally made to enlarge the diameter of the vaginal outlet. The classification of perineal trauma is described in Chapter 13 [1, 2].

Perineal repair after childbirth affects millions of women worldwide. Approximately 85% of women sustain some form of perineal trauma during vaginal delivery [3, 4]. The prevalence of perineal trauma is dependent on variations in obstetric practice, including rates and types of episiotomy, which vary not only between countries but also between individual practitioners within hospitals. In the Netherlands the episiotomy rate is 8% compared to 14% in England, 50% in the US, and 99% in Eastern European countries. Rates also vary between hospitals in the same country, for example in the US the rates of episiotomy vary between 20% and 70% in individual units [5]. However, in recent years significant decreases in episiotomy rates have been observed after attention was drawn to the negative outcomes associated with the routine use of episiotomy [6]. In centers where mediolateral episiotomies are practised, the rate of obstetric anal sphincter injuries (OASIS) is 1.7% (2.9% in primiparae) compared to 12% (19% in primiparae) in centers practising midline episiotomy [7]. The incidence of OASIS is increasing, probably due to improved identification and classification of tears at the time of delivery.

The majority of women experience some form of short-term discomfort or pain following perineal repair, and up to 20% will continue to have long-term problems such as superficial dyspareunia [8]. Short- and long-term morbidity associated with perineal re-

R. Thakar
Department of Obstetrics and Gynaecology, Mayday
University Hospital, Croydon, Surrey, UK

pair can lead to major physical, psychological, and social problems affecting the woman's ability to care for her newborn baby and other members of the family [9]. Therefore, preventing perineal trauma in even a modest proportion of childbearing women would benefit large numbers of women. It would also reduce the cost of childbirth (with fewer sutures and less suturing time required) and the need for medical care. Identifying and modifying risk factors may be one way of reducing perineal trauma. However, certain antenatal risk factors such as maternal nutritional status, body mass index, ethnicity, infant birthweight, race, length of the perineal body, previous perineal trauma, and age cannot be altered at the time of delivery, but awareness of these factors might prompt modifications in the care pathway.

In this chapter we first discuss interventions with evidence from randomized controlled trials (RCTs), presented in the order in which a decision is taken about whether an intervention might have to be made in the course of patient care, i.e. starting in the antenatal period through to delivery of the fetus. We then mention other interventions for which evidence is weaker or lacking. The outcomes presented include perineal and anal sphincter trauma.

14.2 Interventions with Evidence from Randomized Controlled Trials

14.2.1 Antenatal Perineal Massage

It has been proposed that perineal massage (Fig. 14.1) during the last month of pregnancy may increase the flexibility of the perineal muscles, leading to a reduction in muscular resistance. This would allow the perineum to stretch at delivery without tearing, thereby avoiding the need for an episiotomy. A recent Cochrane review [10] that included four trials showed that, compared to controls, perineal massage undertaken by the woman or her partner (as little as once or twice a week from 35 weeks) reduced the likelihood of perineal trauma requiring suturing and episiotomy, in women who had not previously given birth vaginally. However, there was no difference in the incidence of all types of perineal trauma, instrumental deliveries, sexual satisfaction, or urinary and anal incontinence. Furthermore, the authors found that for every 15 women who practice

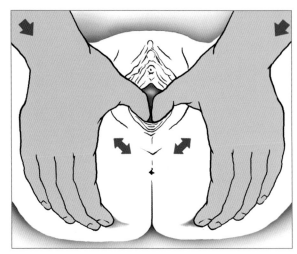

Fig. 14.1 Diagram demonstrating the technique of perineal massage

perineal massage in the antenatal period, one less woman would receive perineal suturing following the birth. Although perineal massage causes some transient discomfort in the first few weeks, it is generally well accepted by women. The majority (79%) report that they would massage again, and 87% would recommend it to another pregnant woman [11]. Therefore, women should be informed about the benefits of antenatal perineal massage and provided with information on the technique.

14.2.2 Water Birth

A recent Cochrane review of 11 RCTs of women laboring in water baths [12] showed no significant difference in second-, third- or fourth-degree tears, instrumental delivery, or cesarean section. The use of any analgesia also made no difference.

14.2.3 Position During Labour and Birth

It is controversial whether being upright or lying down has advantages for women delivering their babies. Several physiological advantages have been claimed for non-recumbent or upright labor, such as the effects of gravity, lessened risk of aortocaval compression, improved acid–base outcomes in the newborns, stronger and more efficient uterine contractions, improved alignment of the fetus for passage through the pelvis, and radiological evidence of larger pelvic outlet diameters with an increase in the total outlet area in the squatting and kneeling positions. The supine or semi-recumbent position for birth is widely used in modern obstetrics due to the medicalization of childbirth. The main advantage cited is easy access of the caregiver to the woman's abdomen to monitor the fetal heart rate. In addition, caregivers are comfortable with the dorsal position as it is the position in which they have usually been trained to conduct deliveries and is the conventional reference position for textbook descriptions of the mechanisms of vaginal delivery [13]. During labor and delivery, the woman may be placed in the lithotomy, lateral recumbent, kneeling, squatting, or standing position. A recent Cochrane review [13] which included 20 trials, showed that the use of any upright or lateral position, compared with supine or lithotomy positions, was associated with: reduced duration of the second stage of labor (largely due to a considerable reduction in women allocated to the use of the birth cushion), a reduction in assisted deliveries and episiotomies, an increase in second-degree perineal tears, and estimated blood loss greater than 500 mL with fewer abnormal fetal heart rate patterns. Due to the heterogenic nature of the trials included, the authors concluded that women should be encouraged to give birth in the position they find most comfortable. Further research is needed in this area.

14.2.4 Second-stage Pushing Advice

Two pushing techniques, the "Valsalva maneuver" (closed glottis pushing while holding the breath) and "spontaneous pushing" (open glottis pushing while breathing out) are approaches used to manage the second stage of labour. In a recent study, one hundred low-risk primiparous women between 38 and 42 weeks' gestation, who expected a spontaneous vaginal delivery, were randomized into the two groups. Although spontaneous pushing resulted in a shorter second stage without interventions and in improved newborn outcomes, there was no significant difference in perineal trauma [14]. In another recent RCT of coached (standardized instruction of closed glottis pushing with proper ventilation encouraged between contractions) versus uncoached (no coaching, to ensure that any expulsive efforts are voluntary) maternal pushing during the second stage of labour [15], Bloom et al showed that although coached maternal pushing is associated with a slightly shorter second stage, it confers no advantage in terms of perineal trauma.

Once the second stage is reached and the fetal head descends, women without epidural block generally feel a strong urge to push. In women with epidural block, the urge to push is often absent, and different strategies are undertaken to manage the second stage of labor. A recent meta-analysis, which included seven randomized studies to determine which method of pushing – passive descent or early pushing – most benefits women with epidurals during the second stage of labor [16], suggested that passive descent increases a woman's chance of having a spontaneous vaginal birth, decreases the risk of having instrumental delivery, and shortens the pushing time. No differences were found in rates of cesarean births, lacerations, or episiotomies.

14.2.5 Application of Obstetric Gel in the Second Stage of Labor

If friction force exerted at the time of vaginal delivery could cause perineal trauma, a simple way to reduce this would be to use a lubricant in the second stage of labor. To investigate the effects of a specially designed obstetric gel, Dianatal® (MPC International S.A., Luxembourg) on labor outcomes, Schaub et al [17] randomized 251 nulliparous women with singleton low-risk pregnancy to no obstetric gel use and obstetric gel use (intermittent application into the birth canal during vaginal examinations, starting prior to 4 cm dilatation until delivery). Systematic vaginal application of obstetric gel showed a significant reduction in second-stage duration and a significant increase in perineal integrity, without any adverse effects.

14.2.6 Application of Perineal Warm Packs in the Second Stage of Labor

Perineal warm packs are warm compressors that have been advocated for many years in the belief that they reduce perineal trauma and increase comfort during the late second stage of labor. Physiological studies support the potential beneficial effects of warm packs in dilating blood vessels, and increasing blood flow, the transmission of blood by reducing the level of nociceptive stimulation, and collagen extensibility [18]. In a large RCT [18], nulliparous women were randomly allocated to have warm packs (n = 360) applied to their perineum or to receive standard care (n = 357) in the late second stage of labor. The difference in the number of women who required suturing after birth was not significant. Women in the warm pack group had significantly fewer third- and fourth-degree tears (although this was not the primary outcome) and had significantly lower pain scores at birth and two days after birth compared with the standard care group. On questioning women and midwives about the effects of warm packs on pain, perineal trauma, comfort, feeling of control, satisfaction, and intentions of views during future pregnancies, the authors found that warm packs were highly acceptable as a means of relieving pain during the late second stage of labor. Eighty per cent of women and midwives felt that warm packs reduced perineal pain during birth. The majority of women (86%) said they would like to use perineal warm packs again for their next birth and would recommend them to friends (86%). Likewise, 91% of midwives were positive about using warm packs, with 93% considering using them in future as part of routine care in the second stage of labor [19]. Based on this, the authors recommended that this simple inexpensive practice should be incorporated into second-stage labor care.

14.2.7 Perineal Support

Practitioners have strongly advocated "support" to the perineum instead of stretching massage during delivery to reduce perineal trauma. In a large RCT of "hands on or poised" ("HOOP") methods of delivery, McCandlish et al [3] allocated women at the end of the second stage to either "hands on" (the midwife applies digital pressure on the baby's head and supports the perineum followed by lateral flexion to facilitate delivery of the shoulders) or "hands poised" (the midwife keeps her hands poised, not touching the head or perineum except if light pressure on the head is needed to prevent rapid expulsion, and allowing spontaneous delivery of the shoulders). Unfortunately, about 30% of the "hands-poised" group was actually delivered "hands on" because the midwife feared impending perineal trauma. There was significantly less pain at 10 days after giving birth in the

"hands-on" group, but no difference in anal sphincter tears or sutured perineal trauma. At 3 months postpartum, no differences were identified in terms of dyspareunia, or urinary or bowel problems.

In a retrospective study, Pirhonen et al [20] showed that the rate of sphincter tears was much lower in Turku, Finland (0.4%), than in Malmo, Sweden (2.9%). They suggested that the difference in Turku may be due to the practice of a procedure similar to Ritgen's maneuver (the fetal chin is reached for between the anus and the coccyx and pulled anteriorly, while using the fingers of the other hand on the fetal occiput to control the speed of delivery and keep traction of the fetal head). Ritgen recommended extracting the fetal head by this maneuver between contractions to protect the perineum. However, in a more recent Swedish study [21], in which more than 1,400 nulliparous women were randomized to the Ritgen's maneuver at the beginning of the second stage of labor, no significant difference in OASIS was observed. In this study, the Ritgen's maneuver was modified so that it was carried out during a contraction as opposed to the original description wherein it was performed between contractions.

14.2.8 Second-stage Perineal Massage

A popular technique in the second stage is a stretching massage or "stripping" of the perineum to ease it back over the head as it crowns. Stamp et al [22] performed a RCT of perineal sweeping massage with two lubricated fingers in the vagina during each uterine contraction in the second stage of labor. While there were clearly problems with randomization in this trial (708 in massage group vs. 632 in control group), massage did not decrease perineal trauma, postpartum pain, or urinary or anal incontinence assessed three months later.

14.2.9 Episiotomy

Episiotomy is still performed routinely in many parts of the world, in the belief that it protects the pelvic floor. However, evidence from RCTs suggests that routine episiotomy does not prevent severe posterior perineal tears. A systematic review that included eight RCTs to determine the possible benefits and risks of restrictive episiotomy versus routine episiotomy [23] revealed that compared with routine use, restrictive use of episiotomy resulted in less severe perineal trauma, less suturing, and fewer healing complications. There were no significant differences in severe vaginal/perineal trauma, dyspareunia, urinary incontinence, or measures of severe pain. The only disadvantage shown in restrictive use of episiotomy was an increased risk of anterior perineal trauma. However, this has no long-term implications [4]. This systematic review concluded that there is adequate evidence to support the restrictive rather than routine use of episiotomy, irrespective of the type of episiotomy performed.

Midline episiotomies are more popular in North America, as it is believed that they are more comfortable. However a quasi-randomised study by Coats in 407 nulliparous women, of mediolateral versus midline episiotomy when episiotomy was needed [24] showed that OASIS occurred with 24% of midline and 9% of mediolateral episiotomies. In this study, analysis was not performed according to "intention to treat", as subjects not receiving their assigned treatment were excluded. However, despite randomization, fewer women had a midline episiotomy, suggesting that the OASIS rate could have been higher. Pain and dyspareunia were similar in both groups, and more women resumed sexual intercourse in the first month in the midline episiotomy group.

Therefore, an episiotomy should only be performed when clinically indicated, and a mediolateral episiotomy is preferable to a midline episiotomy [23]. It is recommended that mediolateral episiotomies should be between 40 and 60 degrees from the midline. However, in a prospective study of women having their first vaginal delivery, Andrews et al [25] demonstrated that no midwives and only 13 (22%) doctors performed a truly mediolateral episiotomy and that the majority of the incisions were in fact directed closer to the midline. Furthermore, episiotomies angled closer to the midlines were associated with a higher incidence of OASIS [26]. Eogan et al [27] demonstrated that there was a 50% reduction in OASIS for every 6 degrees away from the midline. The current recommendation in the UK is that all relevant healthcare professionals should attend mandatory, multidisciplinary training in perineal/genital assessment and repair, and ensure that they maintain these skills [28].

14.2.10 Instrumental Delivery

In the early decades of the 20th century, forceps delivery (usually in association with a generous episiotomy) was promoted to protect the maternal pelvic floor and the fetal head. Yancey et al compared spontaneous delivery to elective outlet forceps in a RCT [29], and showed that forceps did not improve neonatal outcomes but did increase maternal trauma. In the nulliparous population, significant differences were found in the use of episiotomy (93 vs. 78%) and the incidence of deep perineal lacerations (24 vs. 10%) with forceps compared to spontaneous delivery (Fig. 14.2). However,

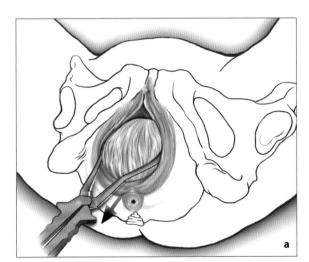 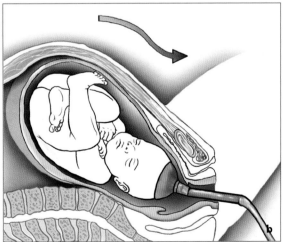

Fig. 14.2 Perineal trauma is more likely to occur with forceps delivery as the blades of the forceps applied around the fetus's head occupies part of the pelvic outlet (**a**), while this does not occur with the vacuum extractor (**b**)

these significant differences were not found in multiparous women.

In a meta-analysis of nine RCTs comparing vacuum extraction to forceps delivery, Thakar and Eason found that with vacuum extraction significantly fewer women sustain OASIS. One anal sphincter tear is avoided for every 18 women delivered by vacuum extraction instead of forceps [30]. The Royal College of Obstetricians and Gynaecologists recommends that the vacuum extractor should be the instrument of choice for operative vaginal birth [31]. A Cochrane review of forceps versus vacuum-assisted delivery [32] also noted that the vacuum extractor was associated with more vaginal births and less general and regional anesthesia. Perineal trauma is more likely to occur with forceps delivery, as the blades of the forceps applied around the fetus' head occupy part of the pelvic outlet, while this does not occur with the vacuum extractor (Fig. 14.2). In addition, forceps delivery is more likely to be associated with an episiotomy.

14.3 Proposed Techniques to Reduce Perineal Trauma

Various techniques have been suggested to reduce perineal trauma and are discussed next.

14.3.1 Antenatal Pelvic Floor Muscle Training

Evidence from RCTs has shown that antenatal pelvic floor muscle training can prevent and treat urinary incontinence during pregnancy and in the immediate postpartum period [33, 34]. However, the effect on perineal trauma is not known. A large cohort study (Norwegian mother and child cohort study) conducted to estimate whether women doing pelvic floor muscle training before and during pregnancy were at increased risk of perineal lacerations [35], episiotomy, instrumental delivery, or emergency cesarean section found no association between regular pelvic floor muscle training and any of the outcome measures.

14.3.2 Epidural Analgesia

Epidural analgesia has become popular in modern obstetric practice because of its excellent pain relief

in labor. Albers et al [36] found that epidural analgesia use in labor was associated with a higher incidence of sutured perineal trauma and this was attributed to factors such as nulliparity, a prolonged second stage, being non-hispanic white, and having an infant birthweight greater than 4000 g. Similarly, Robinson et al demonstrated an association between epidural use and increased OASIS because of more frequent use of operative vaginal delivery and episiotomy [37]. Epidural placement after engagement of the fetal head has been shown to be associated with a lower incidence of malposition, which in turn could reduce of the need for instrumental delivery and associated perineal trauma [38].

14.3.3 Head Flexion

The smallest cephalic diameter presents when the fetal head is in an occiput anterior position and well flexed. Various techniques recommended to maintain head flexion during birth include pressing the baby's chin towards its chest through the posterior perineum, restraint of the sinciput just anterior to the perineum, and downwards (posterior) pressure on the occiput between contractions when the perineum is less tense [30].

14.3.4 Active Restraint of Delivery of the Head

Myles' Textbook for midwives [39] recommends that active pushing should be discouraged once the perineum is tense, as rapid delivery of the fetal head could cause it to tear.

Yet a prevalent approach is to encourage the mother to push vigorously while the head delivers. A recent intervention study showed that slowing the delivery of the fetal head and instructing the mother not to push while the head is being delivered reduced OASIS from 4.03% to 1.17% [40].

14.3.5 Delivery of the Shoulders

Perineal trauma can occur during delivery of the head and/or during delivery of the shoulders. However, there has been no rigorous study of advantages in relation to whether the anterior or posterior shoulder should be delivered first. The optimal technique for delivering the posterior shoulder, in terms of direction and support, has not been studied.

14.3.6 *Interventions to Correct or Deliver with an Occipito-posterior Position*

Persistent occipito-posterior (OP) positioning of the fetal head is a risk factor for prolonged labor, instrumental delivery, and perineal trauma in primiparous and multiparous women, probably due to the greater presenting cephalic diameters [41]. In a case-control study, Fitzpatrick et al [42] compared 246 cases with persistent OP position in labour to 13,543 controls delivered with an occipito-anterior position, and found that anal sphincter trauma was significantly more common in the OP group (7% vs. 1%), irrespective of parity. Various methods of preventing an OP position during labor and delivery have been proposed, including positioning the laboring woman on hands and knees, oxytocin stimulation of labor, and manual or instrumental rotation of the head to occipito-anterior. A recent Cochrane review [43] comparing the hands-and-knees maternal position in late pregnancy and during labor when the fetus is in a lateral or posterior position, to no intervention, did not suggest any benefit in the use of this technique. None of the other proposed techniques have been subjected to RCTs.

14.4 Conclusions

Obstetric perineal trauma can have a devastating effect on a woman's social life, with associated psychological sequelae. Consequently, every attempt should be made to prevent such trauma leading to short-term effects such as pain and dyspareunia, or longer-term effects such as prolapse and incontinence. This chapter has highlighted interventions that may be used to minimize perineal trauma. However, it is equally important to recognize and repair trauma appropriately, and therefore a focused and intensive training program for doctors and midwives is essential. While cesarean section may eradicate perineal trauma, it is associated with an increased risk of mortality and morbidity and therefore should only be offered selectively.

References

1. Royal College of Obstetricians and Gynaecologists. Management of third and fourth degree perineal tears following vaginal delivery. Guideline no 29. RCOG Press, London, 2007.
2. Norton C, Christensen J, Butler U et al. Anal incontinence, 3rd International Consultation on Incontinence. Health Publication Ltd, Plymouth, 2005, pp 985–1044.
3. McCandlish R, Bowler U, van Asten H et al. A randomised controlled trial of care of the perineum during second stage of normal labour. BJOG 1998;105:1262–1272.
4. Rogers RG, Leeman LM, Migliaccio L, Albers LL. Does the severity of spontaneous genital tract trauma affect postpartum pelvic floor function? Int Urogynecol J Pelvic Floor Dysfunct 2008;19:429–435.
5. Royal College of Obstetricians and Gynaecologists. Methods and materials used in perineal repair. Guideline no. 23, RCOG Press, London, 2004.
6. Frankman EA, Wang L, Bunker CH, Lowder JL. Episiotomy in the United States: has anything changed? Am J Obstet Gynecol 2009;200:573–577.
7. Sultan AH, Thakar R. Third and fourth degree tears. In: Sultan AH, Thakar R, Fenner D (eds) Perineal and anal sphincter trauma, Springer-Verlag, London, 2007, pp33–51.
8. Barrett G, Pendry E, Peacock J, Victor CR. Sexual function after childbirth: women's experiences, persistent morbidity and lack of professional recognition. BJOG 1998;105:242–244.
9. Kettle C, Hills RK, Ismail KMK. Continuous versus interrupted sutures for repair of episiotomy or second degree tears. Cochrane Database Syst Rev 2007;(4):CD000947.
10. Beckmann MM, Garrett AJ. Antenatal perineal massage for reducing perineal trauma. Cochrane Database Syst Rev 2007;(1):CD005123.
11. Labrecque M, Eason E, Marcoux S. Women's views on the practice of prenatal perineal massage. BJOG 2001;108:499–504.
12. Cluett ER, Nikodem CVC, McCandlish RE, Burns E. Immersion in water in pregnancy, labour and birth. Cochrane Database Syst Rev 2002;(2):CD000111.
13. Gupta JK, Hofmeyr G J, Smyth RMD. Position in the second stage of labour for women without epidural anaesthesia. Cochrane Database Syst Rev 2004;(4):CD002006.
14. Yildirim G, Beji NK. Effects of pushing techniques in birth on mother and fetus: a randomized study. Birth 2008;35:25–30.
15. Bloom SL, Casey BM, Schaffer JI et al. A randomized trial of coached versus uncoached maternal pushing during the second stage of labor. Am J Obstet Gynecol 2006;194:10–13.
16. Brancato RM, Church S, Stone PW. A meta-analysis of passive descent versus immediate pushing in nulliparous women with epidural analgesia in the second stage of labor. J Obstet Gynecol Neonatal Nurs 2008;37:4–12.
17. Schaub AF, Litschgi M, Hoesli I et al. Obstetric gel shortens second stage of labor and prevents perineal trauma in nulliparous women: a randomized controlled trial on labor facilitation. J Perinat Med 2008;36:129–135.
18. Dahlen HG, Homer CS, Cooke M et al. Perineal outcomes and maternal comfort related to the application of perineal

warm packs in the second stage of labor: a randomized controlled trial. Birth 2007;34:282–290.

19. Dahlen HG, Homer CS, Cooke M et al. 'Soothing the ring of fire': Australian women's and midwives' experiences of using perineal warm packs in the second stage of labour. Midwifery 2009;25:e39–e48.

20. Pirhonen JP, Grenman SE, Haadem K et al. Frequency of anal sphincter rupture at delivery in Sweden and Finland – result of difference in manual help to the baby's head. Acta Obstet Gynecol Scand 1998;77:974–977.

21. Jonsson ER, Elfaghi I, Rydhstrom H, Herbst A. Modified Ritgen's maneuver for anal sphincter injury at delivery: a randomized controlled trial. Obstet Gynecol 2008;112:212–217.

22. Stamp G, Kruzins G, Crowther C. Perineal massage in labour and prevention of perineal trauma: randomised controlled trial. BMJ 2001;322:1277–1280.

23. Carroli G, Mignini L. Episiotomy for vaginal birth. Cochrane Database Syst Rev 2009;(1):CD000081.

24. Coats PM, Chan KK, Wilkins M, Beard RJ. A comparison between midline and mediolateral episiotomies. BJOG 1980;87:408–412.

25. Andrews V, Thakar R, Sultan AH, Jones PW. Are mediolateral episiotomies actually mediolateral? BJOG 2006; 113:245–246.

26. Andrews V, Sultan AH, Thakar R, Jones PW. Risk factors for obstetric anal sphincter injury: a prospective study. Birth 2006;33:117–122.

27. Eogan M, Daly L, O'Cconnell P, O'Herlihy C. Does the angle of episiotomy affect the incidence of anal sphincter injury? BJOG 2006;113:190–194.

28. Andrews V, Thakar R, Sultan AH. Structured hands-on training in repair of obstetric anal sphincter injuries (OASIS): an audit of clinical practice. Int Urogynecol J Pelvic Floor Dysfunct 2009;20:193–199.

29. Yancey MK, Herpolsheimer A, Jordan GD et al. Maternal and neonatal effects of outlet forceps delivery compared with spontaneous vaginal delivery in term pregnancies. Obstet Gynecol 1991;78:646–650.

30. Thakar R, Eason E. Prevention of perineal trauma. In: Sultan AH, Thakar R, Fenner D (eds) Perineal and anal sphincter trauma, Springer-Verlag, London, 2007, pp 52–64.

31. RCOG Audit Committee. Effective procedures in obstetrics suitable for audit. RCOG Audit Committee, Manchester, 1993.

32. Johanson R, Menon V. Vacuum extraction versus forceps for assisted vaginal delivery. Cochrane Database Syst Rev 1999;(2):CD000224.

33. Morkved S, Bo K, Schei B, Salvesen KA. Pelvic floor muscle training during pregnancy to prevent urinary incontinence: a single-blind randomized controlled trial. Obstet Gynecol 2003;101:313–319.

34. Sampselle CM, Miller JM, Mims BL et al. Effect of pelvic muscle exercise on transient incontinence during pregnancy and after birth. Obstet Gynecol 1998;91:406–412.

35. Bo K, Fleten C, Nystad W. Effect of antenatal pelvic floor muscle training on labor and birth. Obstet Gynecol 2009; 113:1279–1284.

36. Albers LL, Migliaccio L, Bedrick EJ et al. Does epidural analgesia affect the rate of spontaneous obstetric lacerations in normal births? J Midwifery Womens Health 2007; 52:31–36.

37. Robinson JN, Norwitz ER, Cohen AP et al. Epidural analgesia and third- or fourth-degree lacerations in nulliparas. Obstet Gynecol 1999;94:262.

38. Robinson CA, Macones GA, Roth WN, Morgan MA. Does station of the fetal head at epidural placement affect the position of the fetal vertex at delivery? Am J Obstet Gynecol 1996;175:991–994.

39. Myles MF. Textbook for midwives, 9 edn. Churchill Livingstone, Edinburgh, 1981.

40. Laine K, Pirhonen T, Rolland R, Pirhonen J. Decreasing the incidence of anal sphincter tears during delivery Obstet Gynecol 2008;111:1053–1057.

41. Sultan AH, Kamm MA, Hudson CN, Bartram CI. Third degree obstetric anal sphincter tears: risk factors and outcome of primary repair. BMJ 1994;308:887–891.

42. Fitzpatrick M, Mcquillan K, O'Herlihy C. Influence of persistent occiput posterior position on delivery outcome. Obstet Gynecol 2001;98:1027–1031.

43. Hunter S, Hofmeyr GJ, Kulier R. Hands and knees posture in late pregnancy or labour for fetal malposition (lateral or posterior). Cochrane Database Syst Rev 2007; (4): CD001063.

Invited Commentary

John O. L. DeLancey

The chapters contained in this section on the perineal body and posterior vagina during vaginal birth show the great progress that has been made in understanding birth-related injury. This section focuses on the full spectrum, from management of anal sphincter injury and the recognition and repair of acute trauma to the mechanism of injury by which this trauma arises, and, finally, to the important area of injury prevention. The pioneering work by Mr Sultan during the 1990s, utilizing recently developed techniques of endoanal ultrasound to reveal previously unsuspected anal sphincter injury, has led to tremendous improvements in our care of obstetric patients.

The primary focus of these efforts is the more careful evaluation of acute obstetric injuries at the time of delivery, and anatomically precise repair of each structure in the perineal body that has been injured. It should be emphasized here that there are excellent data about the effectiveness of different repair techniques and that obstetric units should make proactive efforts to assure that all physicians who repair these injuries know the latest data about proper suture and strategies. Mr Sultan and Ms Thakar have made great progress in describing improvements in training in perineal repair and should be credited for significantly reducing morbidity from vaginal delivery, on a worldwide basis.

Prevention is, of course, the best form of treatment. Although each person who is responsible for assisting with vaginal deliveries has their own personal feeling about how best to avoid perineal trauma, there are many conflicts between these opinions. Some think, for example that "ironing" the perineum is good, while others think the perineum should not be touched. Recently, well-conducted randomized trials have become available to provide information about which practices are most effective. The excellent review of these studies in Ms Thakar's section on prevention helps to shed light on which practices actually have proven efficacy and which, although they may provide comfort during birth, may not reduce the actual occurrence of injury during the delivery process, and so do not reduce the percentage lengthening that occurs within the tissues.

There are new opportunities on the horizon. For example, one can imagine a time in the future where "vaginal ripening" is practiced with pharmacologic agents in a similar way to mehtods currently used for cervical ripening. It seems logical that the same process of connective tissue reorganization that occurs in the cervix occurs in the perineal body, and increasing the pliability of these tissues would go a long way to reducing rupture and the need for repair. By making the birth canal dilate more easily, the downward traction on the connective tissues, muscles, and nerves might be lessened and injuries prevented. Similarly, techniques for antenatal stretching are becoming available and may also prove to be effective in lessening the injuries that occur.

Both prevention and appropriate treatment can only be developed if we have a complete and accurate understanding of the injury mechanism during birth. Dr Minini and his colleagues have provided an excellent review of the theories proposed to understand mechanisms of pelvic floor trauma. Knowing the exact mechanism of injury is critically important to reducing injury. For example, if prolonged compression is presumed to be a mechanism of injury, then shortening the second stage of labor would lessen the injury rate. In this instance, a forceps delivery to shorten the second stage

J.O.L. DeLancey
Department of Obstetrics and Gynecology, University of Michigan Medical School, Ann Arbor, MI, USA

would be a logical preventative strategy. On the other hand, if rapid dilatation of the tissues is responsible, then a longer second stage might actually be favorable. Dr Minini nicely summarizes many of the hypotheses that are currently in active debate. There has been a longstanding discussion of injury to the pelvic nerves as a potential mechanism of injury. There are also more recent data that look at avulsion of the levator ani, which has been detected with magnetic resonance imaging and ultrasonography. Further studies looking at both electromygraphic evaluation and muscle injury should help to shed light on what the primary and secondary processes are. Progress in this regard is occurring rapidly now that there are scientific techniques to study each of these issues.

Where should we go from here? It seems unlikely that it will be possible to avoid all injuries that happen in the pelvic floor at the time of vaginal delivery. However, reducing the rate of injury can save tens of thousands of women, if not hundreds of thousands of women, from subsequent problems. It is not necessary to completely eliminate a problem to still make great strides in preventing the suffering that many women experience. There has been great progress over the last centuries in reducing maternal mortality from childbirth and also reducing maternal morbidity. Although it has been typical in the recent past to focus on cesarian section to prevent pelvic floor injury, this would probably subject nine women to a major surgical procedure for every one woman who might receive protection. This seems like an illogical approach and the approaches outlined in the chapters in this section that focus on understanding the mechanism of injury, preventing injury, and optimizing repair when injury does occur should prove beneficial to many women.

Dr DeLancey gratefully acknowledges partial salary support from the NIH Office of Research on Women's Health Special Center of Research on Sex and Gender Factors Affecting Women's Health and National Institute for Child Health and Human Development Grant P50 HD 044406.

Invited Commentary

Rebecca G. Rogers

The accurate assessment, recognition, and treatment of pelvic floor trauma during pregnancy and following birth has gained increasing importance over the last decade. Formerly viewed as unavoidable sequelae of vaginal birth, pelvic floor changes following birth are common, and in some cases carry adverse long-term problems including pain, sexual dysfunction, bowel and bladder incontinence, and pelvic organ prolapse. On the other hand, the majority of women give birth without the development of serious pelvic floor problems. The challenge for practitioners is to both identify women at risk for problems and implement preventive practices that decrease the incidence of these disorders, without subjecting the many women not at risk for pelvic floor disorders to unnecessary interventions.

The Chapters in this section focus on three areas of interest regarding perineal outcomes. The first describes the global effects of birth on perineal and pelvic floor health. The second two articles focus more closely on genital tract trauma at delivery. Sultan discusses the incidence, recognition, and repair of third- and fourth-degree lacerations and Thaker discusses the prevention of these severe lacerations as well as more common but lesser trauma. In total, these three Chapters give a broad review of common problems facing women following birth, and how to recognize and prevent them.

Pregnancy and childbirth change anatomy and function. Anyone who provides gynecologic care to women knows this because they can easily distinguish a multiparous from a nulliparous woman on pelvic exam. Multiparous women typically have a widened genital hiatus, and decreased muscle tone, and may have minor "pelvic relaxation". Are these changes harbingers of future disability including symptomatic prolapse and incontinence, and should we intervene at birth with increased rates of cesarean section to avoid them? Why do some women deliver multiple times without problems, while others develop problems after a single delivery? Are all changes in vaginal anatomy pathologic?

Determination of the mechanism of changes that occur to the pelvic floor following pregnancy and childbirth is still in its infancy. In addition to observable trauma, other neurological and muscular alterations may not be readily apparent. Minini et al provide an overview of the current literature on observed damage to nerves, muscle, and fascia of the pelvic floor. We know that women with postpartum urinary incontinence and prolapse are more likely to have damage to the levator ani, including evulsion of the pubovisceralis from the symphysis pubis [1]. Nerve damage, whether it occurs from nerve stretching or compression, has also been documented [2]. What is less well understood are issues such as when in the birthing process damage occurs and whether or not the damage occurs with the first vaginal birth, or is cumulative over multiple deliveries. The tipping point where stretch injuries to the muscle, fascia, and nerves of the pelvic floor become critical is unclear, and has been explored with modelling [3]. In addition, we are just beginning to elucidate the complex interrelationships between various risk factors for urinary and anal incontinence and prolapse that are remote from delivery.

Part of the problem is that the majority of women present with incontinence and/or prolapse in mid-life, yet many of the exposures that place women at risk occur much earlier. Epidemiological studies have shown that by looking back to the histories of women who develop incontinence and prolapse, women who deliver

R.G. Rogers
Department of Obstetrics and Gynecology,
University of New Mexico, Albuquerque, NM, USA

G.A. Santoro, A.P. Wieczorek, C.I. Bartram (eds.) *Pelvic Floor Disorders*
© Springer-Verlag Italia 2010

vaginally are more likely to be incontinent and have prolapse than women who deliver by cesarean [4, 5]. Nearly all these data are retrospective and can only establish association, not causality. More prospective studies are needed to determine whether or not cesarean is protective of the pelvic floor in the majority of low-risk women giving birth or simply will prevent serious trouble in those at higher risk for problems. Minini's conclusion that cesarean delivery is protective overstates the complexity of this problem as well as its broad public health implications. Challenges to future researchers include ascertaining how these anatomical changes predict future functional disorders and identifying preventive measures other than cesarean delivery.

Sultan and Thaker focus our attention on observable trauma at the time of vaginal delivery. While the contribution of childbirth to posterior compartment prolapse or rectocele is unclear, vaginal birth clearly places women at risk for perineal laceration. Third- and fourth-degree lacerations that directly damage the external sphincter carry with them, for some, long-term sequelae including anal incontinence. Thankfully, preventive strategies including avoidance of forceps delivery or episiotomy have already been identified, and when implemented greatly decrease the incidence of third- and fourth-degree lacerations [6]. Newer data support careful examination of the perineum at the time of delivery to appropriately identify and repair lacerations. It seems that lacerations that were previously thought to be "occult" or hidden, may have been previously missed with inexpert examination. The careful description by Sultan of how to identify and repair these severe lacerations is a testimony to the extensive work in this area that his group has done on the comparative effectiveness of different repair methodologies and improvements in diagnosis.

Thankfully, not all genital tract trauma is severe.

Thakar thoughtfully reviews the data describing prevention of both severe and less severe lacerations, including perineal massage, pushing instructions, and delivery positions. The caveat that less perineal trauma equals improved birth outcomes makes common sense, although other groups, including ours, have noted that minor trauma has little impact on postpartum pain and an array of other pelvic floor functional outcomes [7]. More investigation is needed to further examine the role of these interventions in prevention of long-term dysfunction; these three chapters offer a springboard to beginning to understand the links between birth and pelvic floor function.

References

1   DeLancey JOL, Morgan DM, Fenner DE et al. Comparison of levator ani muscle defects and function in women with and without pelvic organ prolapse. Obstet Gynecol 2007;109:295–302.

2. Snooks SJ, Swash M, Henry MM et al. Risk factors in childbirth causing damage to the pelvic floor innervation. Int J Colorectal Dis 1986;1:20–24.

3. Ashton-Miller JA, DeLancey JO. On the biomechanics of vaginal birth and common sequelae. Annu Rev Biomed Eng 2009;11:163–176.

4. Mant J, Painter R, Vessey M. Epidemiology of genital prolapse: observations from the Oxford Family planning Association Study. Br J Obstet Gynaecol 1997;104:579–585.

5. Roitviet G, Hunskaar S. Urinary incontinence and age at the first and last delivery: the Norwegian HUNT/EPICONT study. Am J Obstet Gynecol 2006;195:433–438.

6. Albers LL, Sedler KD, Bedrick EJ et al. Midwifery care measures in the second stage of labor and reduction of genital tract trauma at birth: a randomized trial. J Midwifery Womens Health 2005;50:365–372.

7. Rogers RG, Leeman LM, Migliaccio L et al. Does the severity of spontaneous genital tract trauma affect postpartum pelvic floor function? Int Urogynecol J Pelvic Floor Dysfunct 2008;19:429–435.

Section IV
Urinary Incontinence and Voiding Dysfunction

Urinary Incontinence and Voiding Dysfunction: Introduction

Dmitry Pushkar

Urinary incontinence is one of the most important problems recognized by specialists in female health around the world. The International Continence Society (ICS) defines urinary incontinence as "the complaint of any involuntary leakage of urine" [1]. An evaluation of the epidemiology of this condition leads to better understanding of the impact of the problem on female health.

The prevalence of urinary incontinence in women has been the subject of many epidemiologic studies [2]. The reported prevalence has varied considerably in different studies. Possible explanations for this bias are that different populations of women were involved in the studies. In addition, different terminology and definitions for urinary incontinence have been used. Some investigators count the prevalence data according to such criteria as daily, weekly, monthly, or annual frequency of involuntary urinary leakage. In other cases, self-reported questionnaires are used for determination of the prevalence of urine loss. Thus, it is not always fair to compare the results of different population studies.

However, urinary incontinence appears to be related to female age, parity, body mass index, and other demographic factors. The influence of various factors on the prevalence of urinary incontinence was evaluated by means of a postal questionnaire in women aged 46–86 years resident in the city of Gothenburg, Sweden [3]. Age, parity, and a history of hysterectomy were all correlated with the prevalence of urinary incontinence, which increased in a linear fashion from 12.1% in women aged 46 years, to 24.6% in women aged 86 years. The prevalence of urinary incontinence was greater in parous women compared to nulliparous women, and increased with increasing parity. Urinary incontinence was more prevalent in women who had undergone a hysterectomy. The prevalence of urinary incontinence was unaffected by the duration of previous oral contraceptive usage and there was no evidence to suggest that the prevalence increased at the time of the last menstrual period.

Age

In the Norwegian EPINCONT (Epidemiology of Urinary Incontinence in Nord-Trøndelag) cross-sectional study on incontinence, 11,397 women were evaluated [4]. Twenty-five per cent of the women reported that they had involuntary loss of urine. The prevalence of incontinence increased with increasing age. The lowest prevalence was observed in the younger age groups (12% for women < 30 years), the highest was observed among the eldest (40% for women > 90 years). However, there was also a peak around middle age, with a prevalence of 30% among women aged 50–54 years.

According to results of the EPINCONT study, half of incontinent women were experiencing symptoms of stress incontinence alone.

Symptoms of urge incontinence alone affected only one in ten, while mixed incontinence was reported by one in three. The fraction of stress incontinence symptoms was highest among the women aged between 25 and 49 years; thereafter, there was a relative decrease with increasing age. Symptoms of urge incontinence were most frequent among the youngest (< 35 years) and oldest (> 65 years) women. Mixed incontinence increased with increasing age, except for a relatively high proportion (33%) in women aged 20–24 years.

D. Pushkar
Department of Urology, MSMSU, Moscow, Russia

G.A. Santoro, A.P. Wieczorek, C.I. Bartram (eds.) *Pelvic Floor Disorders*
© Springer-Verlag Italia 2010

The severity of incontinence varied between the different types. The fraction of severe incontinence was 17%, 28%, and 38% in the stress, urge, and mixed groups, respectively.

For all types, incontinence of moderate degree was present in almost 30% of the cases. Slight incontinence was found in 53% in the stress group, 39% in the urge group, and 31% in the mixed group. The differences between groups were statistically significant (P < 0.001).

Within each type of incontinence, severity increased with increasing age. In the stress group, 10% of women aged 25–44 years had severe incontinence compared with 15% in the age group 45–59 years, and 33% in the age group older than 60 years. In the urge group, the corresponding figures were 8%, 18%, and 45%, and in the mixed group 19%, 33%, and 53%.

Two-thirds of the incontinent women stated that their leakage was no problem or just a small nuisance, while about 10% were much bothered or experienced their incontinence as a great problem.

Among women with slight incontinence, only 10% answered that they were bothered by their symptoms. In comparison, 34% of those with moderate incontinence and 73% of those with severe incontinence were bothered.

The impact of urinary leakage differed between the incontinence types. Among the women who stated that they had symptoms of mixed incontinence, 47% were bothered.

The corresponding figures for urge and stress incontinence were 36% and 24%, respectively, with a statistically significant difference between the groups.

A total of 26% of the women had consulted a doctor about their urinary leakage. However, 54% of those with severe incontinence had consulted. Among those who were bothered or more severely affected by their incontinence, 64% had consulted.

Urinary incontinence has traditionally been viewed as a chronic and progressive disease. However, recent findings show that within three-year follow-up most women (60%) with urinary incontinence did not experience a significant change in their symptoms; only 13% worsened and 27% improved. Some degree of remission of urinary incontinence was found in 6% to 38% of young and middle-aged women, versus 10% of older women [5]. Incontinence due to transient causes such as infection, drug use, and delirium often regresses after treatment.

Race

Racial differences in development of urinary incontinence have been reported, although it is not yet clear whether the differences are biological, social, or both, or due to other factors. There could be several factors associated to lifestyle, diet, physical activities, or genetic anatomic attributes and tolerance to symptoms. In a study of the epidemiology and pathophysiology of pelvic floor dysfunction, Kim et al performed a nonsystematic review of the literature about current knowledge of the etiology of pelvic floor dysfunction [6]. The current literature suggests that white women are at increased risk for stress urinary incontinence compared to black women. Indeed, there is insufficient evidence to draw any conclusions regarding the role of racial differences in pelvic dysfunction. It is possible that differences in prevalence rates for both stress urinary incontinence and pelvic organ prolapse may be attributed to inherent anatomical and physiological differences among racial groups.

Pregnancy and Childbirth

The relationship between urinary incontinence and childbirth was an issue for discussion in the last century [7]. Many epidemiological investigations have identified correlation between childbirth, pregnancy, and development of urinary incontinence. It is well known that some women may experience involuntary leakage of urine during pregnancy, which resolves in the majority of cases within 6 to 12 months after delivery. Within 4 months after vaginal delivery, the incidence of urinary incontinence may reach 23% for stress incontinence and 12% for urge incontinence. About 4% of females developed fecal incontinence during that postpartum period [8]. In univariate analysis, post-delivery stress urinary incontinence was found to be increased in patients older that 30 years (26.2%) compared with younger patients (19.3%). Urge incontinence was increased in patients who had a forceps delivery (21%) compared with no forceps delivery (9%), an episiotomy (32.4%) compared with no episiotomy (18.7%), and a longer second stage of labor (108 min vs. 77 min, P = 0.01). Multivariate analysis showed that the two variables that remained significant for any urinary incontinence were maternal age ≥ 30 years and forceps delivery. There were no identified risk factors for fecal incontinence.

Mode of Delivery

The Norwegian Mother and Child Cohort Study [9] aimed to investigate the prevalence of urinary incontinence at 6 months postpartum and to study how continence status during pregnancy and mode of delivery influence urinary incontinence at 6 months postpartum in primiparous women. The study included 12,679 primigravidas who were continent before pregnancy. Urinary incontinence was reported by 31% of the women 6 months after delivery. Compared with women who were continent during pregnancy, incontinence was more prevalent 6 months after delivery among women who experienced incontinence during pregnancy. The association between incontinence postpartum and mode of delivery was not substantially influenced by incontinence status in pregnancy.

Another population-based survey evaluated the effect of mode of delivery on the incidence of urinary incontinence in primiparous women [10]. A total of 5,599 primiparous women who did not have incontinence before pregnancy completed the survey and submitted information on their urinary continence; 17.1% of responders reported leakage of urine. Women who had vaginal deliveries were more likely to have urinary incontinence than women who had cesarean deliveries. This risk increased with assisted delivery and perineal laceration. No statistical difference in the incidence of urinary incontinence was found among women who had elective cesarean deliveries (6.1%), women who had cesarean deliveries after laboring (5.7%), and women who had cesarean deliveries after laboring and pushing (6.4%). Although vaginal delivery increases the risk of urinary incontinence, labor and pushing alone without vaginal delivery do not appear to increase this risk significantly.

Obesity

The relationship between urinary incontinence and obesity has been confirmed in several studies. Hunskaar published a systematic review of literature on obesity as a risk factor for urinary incontinence in women [11]. Epidemiological literature of urinary incontinence with respect to overweight and obesity as a risk factor was evaluated. At the same time, the author reviewed all interventional studies assessing the effect of weight reduction on incontinence. There is level 3 evidence

and some level 2 evidence data to support that in addition to body mass index (BMI), waist–hip ratio and thus abdominal obesity may be an independent risk factor for incontinence in women. Only a few interventional studies have been carried out to assess the effect of weight reduction on incontinence. There is some evidence that weight-reduction procedures have an effect on incontinence after surgical weight reduction, and one study showed an effect after a weight-reduction program, thus giving some level 2 documentation. There are three randomized controlled trials (RCTs) which all show reduction of incontinence by weight loss (level of evidence 1). According to this study, epidemiological investigations document overweight and obesity as an important risk factor for urinary incontinence.

Classification and Diagnosis of Urinary Incontinence

The ICS divides lower urinary tract symptoms into three groups: storage symptoms, voiding, and post-micturition symptoms. Storage symptoms are experienced during the storage phase of the bladder and include increased daytime frequency, nocturia, urgency, and urinary incontinence. In each specific circumstance, urinary incontinence should be further described by specifying relevant factors such as type, frequency, severity, precipitating factors, social impact, effect on hygiene and quality of life, the measures used to contain the leakage, and whether or not the individual seeks or desires help because of urinary incontinence.

Continuous urinary incontinence may be due to extraurethral causes such as vesicovaginal, ureterovaginal, or urethrovaginal fistulas. Vaginal ectopy of the ureteral orifice is a rare condition, which may lead to permanent and involuntary loss of urine (Box IV.1).

Bladder abnormalities such as detrusor overactivity may be a reason for development of urge urinary incontinence. This is defined as a complaint of involuntary leakage accompanied by or immediately preceded by urgency. Urge incontinence can present as frequent small leaks of urine between voidings or as involuntary complete bladder emptying.

Stress urinary incontinence is the complaint of involuntary leakage on effort or exertion, or on sneezing or coughing. At present, there is no accepted classifi-

Box IV.1 Classification of urinary incontinence

Extraurethral leakage of urine
- Fistula (vesicovaginal, ureterovaginal, urethrovaginal)
- Ectopic ureter

Urethral leakage of urine
- Functional:
  - because of physical disability
  - because of lack of awareness or concern
- Bladder abnormalities:
  - overactivity:
    □ involuntary contractions
    □ decreased compliance
    □ hypersensitivity with incontinence
- Outlet abnormalities:
  - genuine stress incontinence
  - intrinsic sphincter deficiency
  - urethral instability
  - post-void dribbling
    □ urethral diverticulum
    □ vaginal pooing of urine
  - overflow incontinence

---

cation of stress urinary incontinence in clinical practice. In 1967, McGuire et al proposed a classification system for stress urinary incontinence based on the fluoroscopic images of the vesical neck and intrinsic sphincteric mechanism at rest and with straining [12]. This was a modification of a previous system proposed by Green [13]. McGuire's modification was unique in its

inclusion of type III stress incontinence, characterized by a proximal urethra that no longer functions as a sphincter. Blaivas and Olsson modified this classification system by adding a type 0 stress incontinence and dividing type II stress incontinence into two categories [14] (Box IV.2).

The symptoms of stress urinary incontinence may be evaluated through different diagnostic tools. A systematic review and evaluation of methods of assessing urinary incontinence showed that the gold-standard diagnostic test for urinary incontinence with which each reference test was compared is multichannel urodynamics [16]. A clinical history for diagnosing urodynamic stress incontinence in women was found to have a sensitivity of 0.92 and specificity of 0.56.

A cough stress test with a naturally filled bladder is effective in the diagnosis of stress urinary incontinence. A questionnaire such as the Urogenital Distress Inventory has shown a sensitivity of 0.88 and specificity of 0.60 [16]. Comparison of a pad test with multichannel urodynamics found it difficult to draw any conclusions about the diagnostic accuracy of the method. On the matter of primary diagnosis, in addition to clinical history the bladder diary appears to be the most cost-effective test when comparing the three primary care tests (diary, pad test, and questionnaire). Summarizing all the above, the basic evaluation of women with stress urinary incontinence includes a history, physical examination, cough stress test, voiding diary, post-void residual urine volume, and uri-

Box IV.2 Classification of stress urinary incontinence, adapted from [15]

Type 0
At rest: the bladder base above the symphysis pubis
At strain: rotational descend of urethra and bladder base, no leakage

Type I
At rest: the bladder base above the symphysis pubis
At strain: bladder base descends, vesical neck and urethra open with leakage

Type IIA
At rest: the bladder base above symphysis pubis
At strain: marked descend, vesical neck and urethra open with leakage

Type IIB
At rest: flat bladder base below pubis
At strain: further descent and rotation of bladder and urethra below pubis; urethra opens widely with leakage

Type III
At rest: bladder base above pubis; vesical neck and urethra are open
At strain: bladder base above pubis; vesical neck and urethra are open

nalysis. Urodynamics may be helpful in specialized secondary settings, but it is not yet clear whether urodynamics improve or predict the outcome of incontinence treatment [17].

References

1. Abrams P, Cardozo L, Fall M et al. The standardisation of terminology of lower urinary tract function: report from the standardisation sub-committee of the International Continence Society. Neurourol Urodynam 2002; 21:167–78.
2. Hunskaar S, Burgio K, Diokno AC et al. Epidemiology and natural history of urinary incontinence (UI). In: Abrams P, Cardozo L, Khoury S, Wein A (eds) International consultation on incontinence, 2 edn. Health Publication Ltd, Plymouth, 2002, pp 165–201.
3. Milsom I, Ekelund P, Molander U et al. The influence of age, parity, oral contraception, hysterectomy and the menopause on the prevalence of urinary incontinence in women. J Urol 1993;149:1459–1462.
4. Hannestad YS, Rortveit G, Sandvik H, Hunskaar S. A community-based epidemiological survey of female urinary incontinence: The Norwegian EPINCONT Study. J Clin Epidemiol 2000;53:1150–1157.
5. Waetjen LE, Brown JS, Modelska K. Effect of raloxifene on urinary incontinence: a randomized controlled trial. Obstet Gynecol 2004;103:261–266.
6. Kim S, Harvey MA, Johnston S. A review of the epidemiology and pathophysiology of pelvic floor dysfunction: do racial differences matter? J Obstet Gynaecol Can 2005;27:251–259.
7. Kelly HA, Dunn WM. Urinary incontinence in women without manifest injury of the bladder. Sur Gynecol Obstet 1914;18:444–450.
8. Baydock SA, Flood C, Schulz JA et al. Prevalence and risk factors for urinary and fecal incontinence four months after vaginal delivery. J Obstet Gynaecol Can 2009;31:36–41.
9. Wesnes SL, Hunskaar S, Bo K, Rortveit G. The effect of urinary incontinence status during pregnancy and delivery mode on incontinence postpartum. A cohort study. BJOG 2009;116:700–7.
10. Boyles SH, Li H, Mori T et al. Effect of mode of delivery on the incidence of urinary incontinence in primiparous women. Obstet Gynecol 2009;113:134–141.
11. Hunskaar S. A systematic review of overweight and obesity as risk factors and targets for clinical intervention for urinary incontinence in women. Neurourol Urodyn 2008;27:749–757.
12. McGuire EJ, Lytton B, Pepe V, Kohorn EI. Stress urinary incontinence. Obstet Gynecol 1976;47:255–264.
13. Green TH Jr. Classification of stress urinary incontinence in the female: an appraisal of its current status. Obstet Gynecol Survey 1968;23:632–634.
14. Blaivas JG, Olsson CA. Stress incontinence: classification and surgical approach. J Urol 1988;139:727–731.
15. Cundiff GW. The pathophysiology of stress urinary incontinence: a historical perspective. Rev Urol 2004;6(suppl 3):S10–18.
16. Martin JL, Williams KS, Abrams KR et al. Systematic review and evaluation of methods of assessing urinary incontinence. Health Technol Assess 2006;10:1–132, iii–iv.
17. Nygaard IE, Heit M. Stress urinary incontinence. Obstet Gynecol 2004;104:607–620.

Ultrasonography

15

Andrzej Paweł Wieczorek, Magdalena Maria Woźniak
and Aleksandra Stankiewicz

Abstract The complex anatomy and function of the pelvic floor is not yet fully understood. Understanding how muscles, nerves, ligaments, and fasciae interact and relate to pelvic organs is fundamental to establish what disease processes are involved in urinary incontinence and voiding dysfunctions. In the last two decades, growing attention has been paid to both increasing understanding of pelvic floor anatomy and improving technologies for diagnosis. Transperineal ultrasonography (TPUS) has become a valuable tool in the diagnostic workup of patients with urinary incontinence and voiding dysfunctions. The advent of high-resolution three-dimensional endovaginal ultrasonography (3D-EVUS) promises to further improve the imaging of pelvic floor anatomy; however, at present, the absence of standardization of the procedure limits its usefulness. The lack of uniformity frequently leads to confusion in the assessment of an image by the interpreting ultrasonographer. The equipment used, patient position, technique of examination, and manner of performing measurements may differ from one examiner to another and may influence the correct identification of pelvic floor structures. The aim of this chapter is to review basic information about techniques, equipment advantages, limitations, clinical usefulness, and the literature concerning ultrasound assessment in the diagnostics and monitoring of treatment of urinary incontinence and voiding dysfunctions with reference to two-dimensional (2D) and 3D-TPUS techniques, as well as 2D and 3D-EVUS.

Keywords Endovaginal ultrasound • Pelvic floor ultrasound • Three-dimensional ultrasound • Transperineal ultrasound • Urinary incontinence

15.1 Introduction

Female urinary incontinence and voiding dysfunctions are reported in the literature to range from 6% to 37.7% of the general population [1, 2]. The key to under-standing these disturbances is first a better comprehension of the anatomy and physiology of the lower urinary tract [3]. Despite huge progress in imaging techniques, there are still many controversies concerning the detailed morphology and function of pelvic floor structures taking part in maintaining continence [4]. Ultrasonography has currently replaced other diagnostic modalities for the assessment of these conditions. The primary role of this procedure is to detect

A.P. Wieczorek
Department of Pediatric Radiology, Children's Teaching
Hospital, Medical University of Lublin, Poland

G.A. Santoro, A.P. Wieczorek, C.I. Bartram (eds.) *Pelvic Floor Disorders*
© Springer-Verlag Italia 2010

what damage to the pelvic structures is responsible for the functional disturbances, in order to guide appropriate and selective management. In addition, another relevant role is evaluation of results after treatment, and an understanding of the causes of failure.

It is important to note that the main issue governing the range and quality of information obtained is the type of ultrasound equipment and the method used for scanning. In this chapter, in addition to a review of the literature, we describe the advantages and limitations of the various techniques of pelvic floor ultrasonography, which differ according to the access (abdominal, transperineal, translabial, endovaginal, endoanal, and endourethral ultrasound) and type of transducer (rotational, endfire, biplane, convex, and linear probe) used [5, 6].

15.2   External Ultrasound

Transabdominal ultrasonography has limited usefulness in the assessment of urinary incontinence and voiding dysfunction. Due to the wide distance between the transducer and the examined organs, and to the low

frequencies used, this modality provides low-resolution images of the urethra and pelvic floor structures [7]. Its role is reserved for the evaluation of bladder wall thickness, calculation of post-voiding bladder volume, and assessment of the upper urinary tract.

Transperineal (TPUS), translabial (TLUS), and introital ultrasound differ regarding the positioning of the transducer on the perineum (Fig. 15.1) (see also Chapter 7). For TPUS the transducer is placed in the perineum between the vaginal orifice and the anal margin. For TLUS the probe is positioned on the right or left labia, whereas for the introital approach, the transducer is placed between the labia. The general term TPUS is often used to refer to all the approaches described, as the quality of the ultrasonographic images and the amount of anatomical/functional information obtained is similar. Moreover, all techniques give the opportunity to obtain sagittal, coronal, and oblique sections, although the most commonly used approach is the midsagittal plane, which allows overall assessment of all anatomical structures (bladder, urethra, vaginal walls, anal canal, and rectum) located between the posterior surface of the symphysis pubis and the ventral part of the sacral bone.

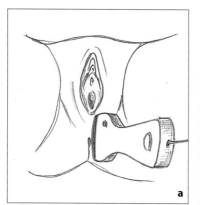 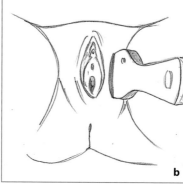 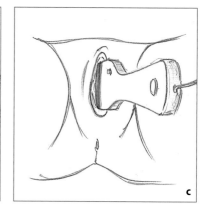

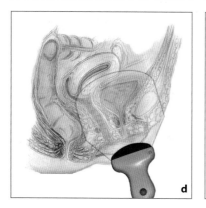 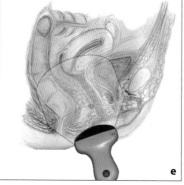

Fig. 15.1 Scheme of transducer placement on the perineum for perineal/transperineal (**a**), translabial (**b**), and introital (**c**) approach. The field of view depends on the placement of the transducer and may focus on either the anterior compartment (**d**) or the posterior compartment (**e**)

15.2.1 Examination Technique

No patient preparation or micturition are required before the examination and no rectal or vaginal contrast is used. Patients are recommended to feel comfortable with the amount of the urine in their bladder. Standardization of bladder filling is not possible in patients with urinary incontinence as most are not able to hold urine. However, the amount of the urine in the bladder can influence the results of measurements, with a full bladder resulting in a reduced mobility of the urethra [8]. The patient is placed in a supine position but, if necessary, can be asked to stand during the examination.

Different types of probe can be utilized: convex transducers are normally reserved for abdominal or obstetric examinations, at a frequency of 4-6 MHz, and endfire transducers are routinely used for gynecological or urological purposes, at higher frequencies (7–12 MHz), but with a smaller insonation angle resulting in a smaller field of view. Both types of probe allow the application of color Doppler for evaluation of urethral vascularity [9, 10] or assessment of the passage of urine due to bladder neck funneling [5].

Two-dimensional (2D), three-dimensional (3D) and four-dimensional (4D) TPUS imaging may also be carried out (see Chapter 7). Two-dimensional TPUS enables imaging in coronal, sagittal, and oblique sections, providing a flat image of the visualized anatomy. The main advantage of 2D TPUS is the simplicity of the technique and ready availability of equipment. It can be performed with almost every ultrasound scanner, which makes this method broadly accessible. A limitation of this modality is, however, represented by the low frequencies used and by the distance between the transducer and the scanned organs.

The following measurements, performed at rest or during functional tests (coughing, Valsalva maneuver, maximal pelvic floor contraction), can be taken in the midsagittal plane:

- Bladder wall thickness: normal value up to 5 mm; abnormal over 5 mm.
- Post-voiding residual bladder volume: for the assessment of bladder outlet or obstruction; post-voiding residual bladder volume should not exceed 50 mL [11].
- Bladder–symphysis distance (BSD): the distance between the bladder neck and the lower margin of the symphysis pubis. The value of BSD should be equal to approximately two-thirds of the length of the urethra, and differs individually, normally ranging between 20 mm and 30 mm (Fig. 15.2). The BSD value enables assessment of the position and mobility of the urethra and the bladder neck. There is no definition of "normal" for bladder neck descent, although a cut-off of 20 mm has been proposed to define hypermobility [5] and reported to

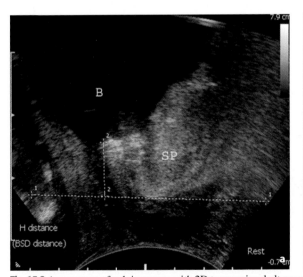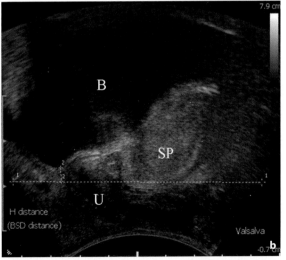

Fig. 15.2 Assessment of pelvic organs with 2D transperineal ultrasound, **a** at rest and **b** during Valsalva maneuver. Bladder–symphysis distance is the distance (*vertical line*) between the bladder neck and the lower margin of the symphysis pubis. The *horizontal line* indicates the lower margin of the symphysis pubis, and is a reference point for the measurements of bladder neck movement. *B*, bladder; *SP*, symphysis pubis; *U*, urethra

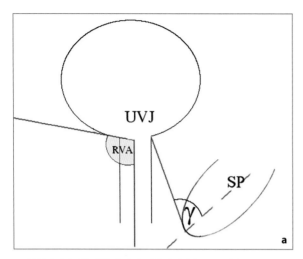

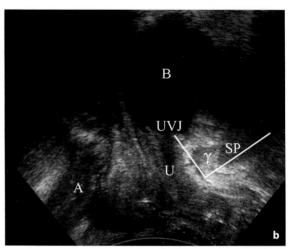

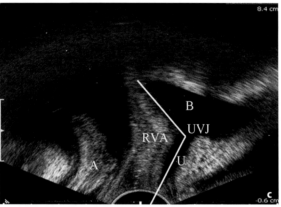

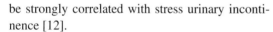

Fig. 15.3 Scheme of the ultrasound parameters in transperineal ultrasound: γ angle, between the inferior edge of the symphysis pubis (*SP*) and the urethrovesical junction (*UVJ*). Retrovesical angle (*RVA*), between proximal urethra (*U*) and trigonal surface of the bladder (*B*) (**a**). 2D transperineal ultrasound at rest; γ angle (**b**). Retrovesical angle (**c**). *A*, anal canal

be strongly correlated with stress urinary incontinence [12].

- Urethral length (taken as the distance from the bladder neck to the visible end of the external urethral orifice) and width. Normal values vary individually, ranging between 30 mm and 45 mm.
- γ angle: i.e., angle between the inferior edge of the symphysis pubis and the urethrovesical junction, at rest (Fig. 15.3) and on Valsalva [13].
- Urethral rotation: i.e., rotation of the proximal urethra on Valsalva [13].
- Retrovesical angle (RVA): i.e., angle between proximal urethra and trigonal surface of the bladder (Fig. 15.3) [13].

Three-dimensional TPUS enriches 2D examination by adding a third dimension (depth) (see Chapter 7). An advantage of this technique, compared to 2D mode, is the possibility of obtaining reconstructed sections to precisely visualize the relevant pelvic floor structures along their proper planes and to measure their volume.

The reconstructed axial plane allows evaluation of the levator ani muscle and its attachment to the pubic rami, and measurement of the diameter, area, and volume of the urogenital hiatus [14–16]. Another advantage of the 3D technique is the possibility of recording data for subsequent off-line assessment.

Four-dimensional ultrasound is the mode with a fourth dimension of time. As a result we get live action images of the internal anatomy. This technique is particularly helpful in recording functional tests of the pelvic floor (coughing, Valsalva maneuver, maximal pelvic floor contraction).

15.3 Endoluminal Ultrasound

Endoluminal US includes endovaginal (EVUS), endorectal (ERUS), and transurethral (TUUS) ultrasound (see Chapters 6 and 8).

Endovaginal US can be performed with the following transducers (see Chapter 6): (1) endfire transducer, commonly used in gynecological and urological practice; this type of probe gives sector 2D images and allows visualization of sagittal and transverse sections of the urethra and surrounding tissues; (2) electronic biplane transducer, with linear and transverse arrays and perpendicular beam formation (type 8848, B-K Medical, Herlev, Denmark); (3) mechanical 360° degree rotational probe, with multifrequencies (6 to 16 MHz) and axial ultrasound beam formation (type 2050, B-K Medical, Herlev, Denmark). An advantage of high-frequency EVUS is the detailed evaluation of urethral complex morphology, due to the direct contact of the transducer.

The presence of the transducer in the vagina, however, has the limitation that in patients with pelvic organ prolapse it can prevent the descent during functional assessment.

Endorectal US is commonly performed with the rotational probe (see Chapter 8). Although ERUS provides images of the urethra that are comparable to those from EVUS, its usefulness in clinical practice is limited. The main reasons for this are artifacts due to bowel movements and the presence of feces or air in the small bowel or rectum; a wide distance of the transducer from the area of interest that reduces the resolution [16]; and low acceptance by patients due to embarrassment and discomfort during scanning.

Transurethral US, also a dynamic 3D-US, was performed in the past by using a 10 MHz transducer, diameter 23 F, allowing 360-degree transverse images of the urethra and surrounding tissues (type 1850, B-K Medical, Herlev, Denmark) [17–19]. The main advantage of TUUS is the lack of a compression effect and the absence of urethral displacement [16]. Direct contact of the transducer also gives a precise image of urethral morphology. Structures that are visible with TUUS are the striated and smooth urethral sphincter muscles, vagina, and blood vessels with diameters exceeding 0.2 mm. The longitudinal smooth muscle layer appears as a well-defined internal hypoechoic ring. The outer circular smooth muscle layers and the striated muscle layers are a more irregular and hyperechoic zone. The circular smooth muscle layers and the striated sphincter muscle layers cannot always be differentiated easily.

The limitation of the endourethral approach is its invasiveness. It is also very embarrassing for the patient, and often not accepted by examined women. Additionally, it carries the risk of transmitting urinary tract infection. Due to these limitations, together with the introduction of high-frequency EVUS, the role of TUUS has been largely limited.

15.3.1 Examination Technique

Technical aspects of EVUS have been reported in Chapter 6. The use of the rotational probe and 3D reconstruction provides an overall view of the pelvic structures in the axial section. This modality allows assessment of the relationship between the urethral complex and the structures located between the posterior surface of the symphysis pubis (SP) and the internal margin of the pubovisceral muscle. The following qualitative and quantitative assessments can be obtained [20] (see Chapter 6):

- evaluation of the symmetry between the urethra and the anal canal, in the axial plane
- evaluation of the symmetry between the left and right branches of the pubovisceral muscle and visualization of the attachment of the muscle to the pubic rami on both sides, in the axial plane
- measurements of biometric indices of the levator hiatus (anterior–posterior and transverse diameters and levator hiatus area), in the axial plane
- identification of the superficial transverse perinei, bulbospongiosus, and ischiocavernosus muscles and assessment of the urogenital hiatus, in the axial plane
- urethral position (omega angle), in the coronal plane
- urethral length and width and bladder–symphysis distance, in the midsagittal plane
- evaluation of the bladder neck and bladder trigone, in the midsagittal plane.

The use of a high-frequency (5–12 MHz) biplane transducer provides a more detailed evaluation of the urethral complex (see Chapter 6) [21]. Compared to the rotational probe, it allows a dynamic assessment of the anterior compartment and analyses of urethral vascularity. The following qualitative and quantitative assessments can be obtained [21] (see Chapter 6):

- measurement of urethral length, depth, width and volume, in the axial and midsagittal planes
- measurement of BSD at rest and during Valsalva maneuver, in the midsagittal plane

- measurement of rhabdosphincter muscle length, depth, width, and volume, in the axial and midsagittal planes
- evaluation of the integrity of the perineal body
- functional dynamic assessment of bladder and urethral mobility
- evaluation of urethra vascularity.

The vascular pattern of the urethra may be obtained using color Doppler. To allow further off-line assessment, the data should be registered and stored as video files. We recommend performing two video acquisitions: one in the longitudinal plane at the level of the urethral lumen, and the second in the axial plane at the level of the midurethra. Quantitative assessment of the urethral blood perfusion may be performed with PixelFlux software (Chameleon Software, Freiburg, Germany) [22, 23] (Figs 9.10–9.13) (see Chapter 9).

Three-dimensional data acquisition may be obtained with the use of an automatic electromagnetic mover during 180 degrees (from the 9 o'clock to the 3 o'clock position) rotation of the probe. The 3D data can be further post-processed using the B-K Medical 3D Viewer (B-K Medical, Herlev, Denmark) in order to perform vascular render mode and maximum inten-

sity projection (MIP). Volume render mode (VRM) is a technique for analysis of the information inside a 3D volume by digitally enhancing individual voxels. It is currently one of the most advanced and computer-intensive rendering algorithms available [24]. Vascular render mode refers to the application of render mode to 3D data volume with color Doppler acquisition to provide visualization of the spatial distribution of the vascular networks. Maximum intensity projection is a 3D visualization modality involving a large amount of computation. It can be defined as the aggregate exposure at each point, which tries to find the brightest or most significant color or intensity along an ultrasound beam. The application of MIP in a 3D color mode reduces the intensity of the grayscale voxels so that they appear as a light fog over color information, which is therefore highlighted. In a color volume the colors are mapped to a given value in the volume. We recommend performing VRM and MIP to analyze the 3D data volume with color Doppler acquisition (Figs. 9.4, 15.4).

15.4 Discussion

Transabdominal ultrasound is a reliable method for assessment of the urinary bladder to determine bladder wall thickness and bladder neck wall mass, in patients with voiding dysfunctions and outflow obstruction [25]. It allows measurement of post-voiding residual urine volume and can help to determine whether additional tests are needed. The efficiency and safety of bladder US makes its use beneficial in a wide variety of populations, including hospitalized patients, children, and the elderly. Abdominal US can also be used for suprapubic aspiration of collections and evaluation of intravesical masses. Its role in the evaluation of urinary incontinence is limited. Sugaya et al [7] used this modality to assess the bladder neck morphology in women with urethral syndrome or stress urinary incontinence, in order to determine the ultrasonographic findings of these conditions. They reported that this technique provides useful information and should be carried out as a routine examination in female patients with micturition disorders.

The usefulness of TPUS in the assessment of urinary incontinence and voiding dysfunction has been widely reported in the literature. Bai et al [26] performed TPUS to evaluate the differences between patients with or without urethrovesical junction hyper-

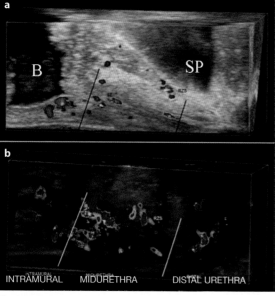

Fig. 15.4 Endovaginal ultrasound with transducer type 8848, B-K Medical. Vascular render mode reconstruction of a 3D Color Doppler dataset shows the spatial distribution of the vessels in the female urethra. *1*, intramural; *2*, midurethra; *3*, distal urethra. Scans obtained in two different patients show a poor (**a**) and rich (**b**) network of vessels. *B*, bladder; *SP*, symphysis pubis

mobility associated with stress urinary incontinence. They found the two groups differed in their bladder neck descent. Hypermobility of the bladder neck in nulliparous patients is not often seen. Harris et al [27] reported a bladder neck mobility of 31 degrees in nulliparous patients versus 38 degrees in parous patients.

In patients with stress incontinence, but also in asymptomatic women [28], urethral funneling (UF) may be observed on Valsalva maneuver and sometimes also at rest (Fig. 15.5). Its morphologic basis is unknown and its incidence is reported to range from 18.6% to 97.4%. Funneling is often associated with leakage, and occasionally weak grayscale echoes may be observed in the proximal urethra, suggesting urine flow and therefore incontinence during straining. However, funneling may also be observed in urge incontinence. Marked funneling has been shown to be associated with poor urethral closure pressures [5, 29]. Tunn et al [30] performed introital US in stress urinary incontinence, to distinguish patients with and without UF. The two groups were compared for clinical history, urodynamic results, and MRI findings. The results of this study, however, could not elucidate the pathogenesis of UF. The demonstration of UF crucially depends on the examination technique employed [30]. Schaer et al [28] evaluated the bladder neck in continent and stress-incontinent women, by TPUS (5 MHz curved linear array transducer) with the help of US contrast medium (galactose suspension-Echovist-300). This method allowed quantification of the depth and diameter of bladder neck dilation, showing that both incontinent and continent women may have bladder neck

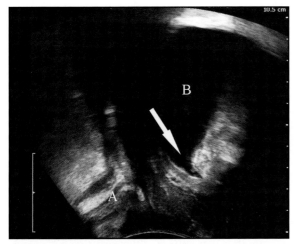

Fig. 15.5 2D transperineal ultrasound. Urethral funneling (*arrow*). *A*, anal canal; *B*, bladder

dilation and that urinary continence can be established at different locations along the urethra. Parity seemed to be a main prerequisite for a proximal urethral defect with bladder neck dilation.

Dietz et al [31] reported that bladder neck mobility and maximum urethral closure pressure are strong predictors of the diagnosis of urinary stress incontinence, provided that major confounders such as previous incontinence or prolapse surgery, pelvic radiotherapy, or urethral kinking on ultrasound are excluded. Bladder neck descent explains 29% and urethral closure pressure 12% of overall variability. Bladder neck mobility appears to be the stronger predictor. Hall et al [32] performed a comparison of periurethral blood flow resistive indices and maximum urethral closure pressure in women with stress urinary incontinence. They reported that TLUS and Doppler spectral waveform can confidently include assessment of morphology and urethral resistive indices.

Assessment of the urethral sphincter using a 3D-US scan predicts the outcome of continence surgery [33]. By performing 3D-TPUS with use of a sector endovaginal probe, Digesu et al [33] found that the rhabdosphincter volume was a predictive factor for surgical outcome. They reported that women whose continence surgery failed had significantly smaller preoperative urethral sphincter volumes (mean value 1.09 cm^3) than those who had an objective cure (3.79 cm^3) (P < 0.001). Ultrasonography plays a very important role in monitoring the results after treatment. It enables evaluation of the position of tapes and meshes, as improper positioning or dislodgement can cause unsuccessful surgery. Two-dimensional and 3D-TPUS were performed by Dietz et al [34] to assess the effectiveness of suburethral slings (tension-free vaginal tape: TVT, suprapubic arch sling: SPARC, and intravaginal sling: IVS). All three tapes could be visualized by ultrasound and showed comparable short-term clinical and anatomical outcomes. TVT and SPARC were highly echogenic, with SPARC being generally flatter and of wider weave. The IVS seemed narrower and less echogenic [34]. Three-dimensional ultrasound was also used by Ng et al [35], who found that the midurethral position of the TVT tape may not be essential in restoring continence and that the TVT tape, once inserted, may not always remain in the midurethral position.

In 1988, Quinn et al [36] performed a study where direct ultrasound images of the bladder neck and proximal urethra were obtained with use of an endovaginal transducer in women with a range of urinary symptoms. They found EVUS to be suitable for the assessment of many aspects of urinary incontinence. The 2D endovaginal technique was further developed into 3D mode. Umek et al [16] compared 3D-EVUS and 3D-ERUS in determining the morphology and measurements of the female urethra. They found that the ultrasound probe compressed and displaced the urethra when inserted vaginally, and therefore suggested that the endorectal approach should be used to investigate morphologic components of the female urethra [16]. In another study, the same authors used 3D-ERUS to evaluate the influence of pelvic floor contraction on the morphology of the components of the female urethra [37]. Sagittal and transverse urethral diameters decreased during voluntary pelvic floor contraction, which suggested compression of the urethra rather than contraction of the urethral sphincter muscle [37].

A key role in the diagnosis of urinary incontinence and voiding dysfunctions is assessment of the morphology and function of three pelvic floor structures, which are the endopelvic fascia, the levator ani muscle, and the perineal membrane. These structures provide support holding the pelvic organs in place, and contribute to maintaining urinary continence [3]. The feasibility of visualizing the endopelvic fascia by 3D-ERUS was reported by Reisinger et al [38]. These authors, however, found 3D-EVUS to be superior in the visualization of this fine structure. Three-dimensional EVUS with use of rotational or biplane transducers provides an accurate evaluation of the levator ani morphology and its attachment to the pubic rami and allows measurement of the biometric indices of the levator hiatus, as already reported with 3D-TPUS. In the presence of levator damage, this modality gives information about the location of the defect and assessment of its distribution. Additionally, the perineal membrane, a triangular fibrous layer that attaches the perineal body to the pubis, can be visualized. Endovaginal US also has a relevant role in detecting pelvic organ prolapse (POP) coexisting with urinary incontinence (see Chapter 24).

By performing 3D-EVUS with the use of a biplane transducer, we determined the rhabdosphincter volume that, according to Digesu et al [33], represents a predictive factor for surgical outcome. Our results (mean value 1.2 mL) were comparable to those obtained with 3D-ERUS by Athanasiou et al [39] and with the measurements performed with magnetic resonance imaging (MRI) by Tan et al [40], but differed from those reported by Umek et al [37] with transrectal scanning (mean value 0.6 mL). In patients with advanced degenerative changes of connective tissue (ageing), appearing on ultrasound as inhomogeneity of the urethral complex muscles, a worse therapeutic effect might be expected compared to patients with normal-appearing rhabdosphincter and smooth muscles. High-frequency EVUS also gives the opportunity to assess the urethral vascularity. The lumen of the urethra is surrounded by a prominent vascular plexus that is believed to contribute to continence [41]. The spatial distribution of urethral vessels with the different blood supply, their density and localization, and the intensity of perfusion of the blood flow play an important role in urethral function. It is possible that urinary incontinence and pelvic organ dysfunction may result in a change in urethral vasculature, possibly before the appearance of clinical signs [41]. Analyses of urethral vasculature could become a predictive parameter, which would allow implementation of prophylaxis or early treatment for patients before their symptoms become severe. In our study [23], performed in a group of 18 nulliparous females, we demonstrated that the urethral vasculature is different along its entire length. With the use of PixelFlux software, we found that the three regions of interest (ROI) defined in the longitudinal plane presented significant differences in the intensity of perfusion. The midurethra, which includes the rhabdosphincter muscle, showed the greatest intensity of perfusion (mean value 0.014 cm/s, $P < 0.05$), compared to the intramural part of the urethra (0.007 cm/s, $P < 0.05$) and to the distal urethra (0.005 cm/s, $P < 0.05$). However, the perfusion between the intramural and distal urethra was similar (0.57 cm/s, $P < 0.05$). No significant differences were found in the intensity of perfusion in the two ROIs defined in the axial section at the level of the midurethra. The parameters of perfusion appeared similar (0.76, $P < 0.05$) in the outer layer (rhabdosphincter) and inner layer of the urethra (circular smooth muscle, longitudinal smooth muscle, and submucosa) [22].

Transurethral US allows an accurate assessment of urethral morphology. Test–retest reliability of TUUS in measuring female urethral sphincter indices was performed by Heit [17]. The results showed that the urethral longitudinal smooth muscle layer was the only structure that could be measured reliably using US. Measurements of the rhabdosphincter were not reliable because the outer portion of that structure lies outside the depth of penetration of a 12.5 MHz transducer [17].

Dynamic TUUS and 3D reconstruction of the rhabdosphincter and urethra in continent and incontinent women was performed by Mitterberger et al [18]. Partial or complete loss of rhabdosphincter function was detected in patients with stress incontinence. The ultrasonographic findings were found to have a good correlation with the grade of incontinence. Furthermore, under contraction of the rhabdosphincter, an increase of the urethral length was observed. In incontinent patients, the urethral length did not increase significantly, due to reduced contractility of this muscle. They concluded that dynamic TUUS with 3D reconstructions allows the assessment of functional and morphological characteristics of the rhabdosphincter and urethra. Normal contraction of the rhabdosphincter results in an elongation of the urethra [18]. In another study, Schaer et al [19] correlated TUUS findings with histology.

Structures visible at TUUS were the striated and smooth urethral sphincter muscle layers, vagina, and blood vessels with diameters exceeding 0.2 mm. The longitudinal smooth muscle layer appeared as a well-defined internal hypoechoic ring. The outer circular smooth muscle layers and the striated muscle layers were more irregular, less definable hyperechoic structures. The circular smooth muscle layers and the striated sphincter muscle layers could not always be differentiated easily.

As already reported for TPUS, endocavitary US is particularly useful in choosing appropriate management and in postoperative follow-up. Endovaginal US may help to define the causes of unsuccessful surgery resulting from improper positioning of tapes and meshes [43], their elongation, too tight placement, folding, or asymmetry, most often seen in case of transobturator tapes (TOT) (Figs. 15.6, 15.7). The method is also very

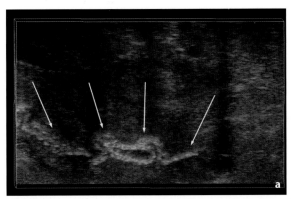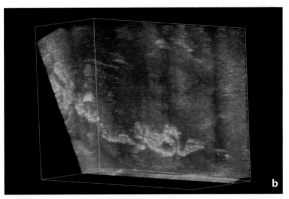

Fig. 15.6 Endovaginal ultrasound with biplane transducer (type 8848, B-K Medical). Visualization of folded tape (*arrows*) being a cause of unsuccessful surgery in B mode (**a**) and volume render mode (**b**)

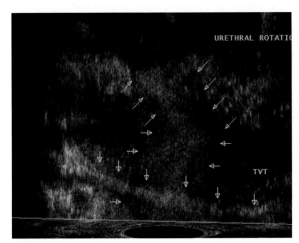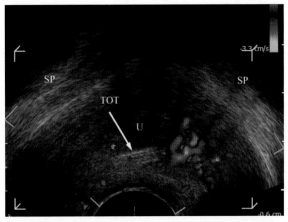

Fig. 15.7 3D endovaginal ultrasound with rotational transducer (type 2050, B-K Medical). Visualization in the coronal section of rotated tape (*TVT*) resulting in unsuccessful surgery (*arrows*)

Fig. 15.8 Endovaginal ultrasound with biplane transducer (type 8848, B-K Medical). Asymmetric distribution of color Doppler signal in patient with inflammatory complication after transobturator tape (*TOT*) insertion. *SP*, symphysis pubis; *U*, urethra

useful in the diagnosis of postoperative complications such as hematomas, fistulas, and small fluid collections, not visualized with abdominal ultrasound or TPUS. In case of inflammatory processes following insertion of tapes or meshes, color Doppler mode may confirm the presence of inflammation and locate the changes (Fig. 15.8). Defreitas et al [15] used endocavitary 3D-US to examine the distribution of periurethral collagen and to incorporate this technology into a practical treatment decision algorithm for women with stress urinary incontinence requiring collagen injection. They found that ultrasonographic evaluation of collagen volume and periurethral location was an affordable, non-invasive and objective technique to predict improvement after periurethral collagen injection [15].

The usefulness of EVUS in voiding dysfunctions has been reported in the literature. High-resolution multiplanar US allows comprehensive evaluation of abnor-

malities of the female urethra such as urethral diverticula, abscesses [43], tumors [44], and other urethral and paraurethral lesions [45, 46] (Figs. 15.9, 15.10). A number of diverticula and the location, size, configuration, and possible contents of the sac may be demonstrated (Fig. 15.11). Most important, the position of the neck of the diverticulum may be identified for the surgeon [47]. The method allows visualization of coexisting anatomical disturbances contributing to voiding dysfunctions, such as inborn abnormalities, as well as acquired conditions – most commonly changes connected to ageing, post-inflammatory changes, cystocele, rectocele, and others. Khullar et al [48] described a technique of measuring bladder wall thickness using EVUS. Ultrasonographic measurements showed a good intra- and interobserver reproducibility. Women with urinary symptoms and detrusor instability were found to have significantly thicker bladder walls than women with

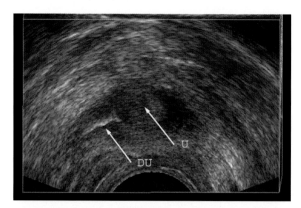

Fig. 15.9 Endovaginal ultrasound with biplane transducer (type 8848, B-K Medical). In the axial section a calcified dystopic insertion of the ureter to the urethra (*U*) is visualized. *DU*, dystopic ureter

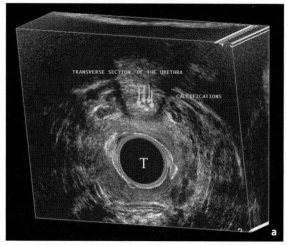

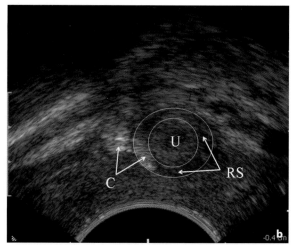

Fig. 15.10 Calcifications (*C*) in the urethral complex (*U*). **a** Endovaginal ultrasound with transducer type 2050 (*T*), B-K Medical. Axial section. Intraurethral localization of calcifications (*arrows*). **b** Endovaginal ultrasound with transducer type 8848, B-K Medical. Axial section. Calcifications localized within the rhabdosphincter and externally to the rhabdosphincter (*RS*)

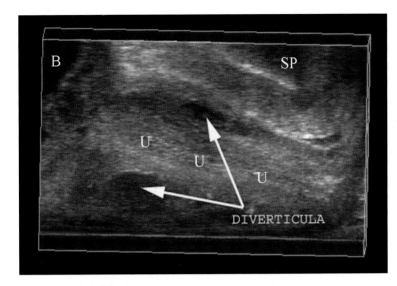

Fig. 15.11 Endovaginal ultrasound with transducer type 8848 B-K Medical. Diverticula of urethra are visualized in the sagittal section. *B*, bladder; *SP*, symphysis pubis; *U*, urethra

urodynamically diagnosed stress incontinence. This result was confirmed in another study by the same authors, who reported that a mean bladder wall thickness greater than 5 mm at EVUS is a sensitive screening method for diagnosing detrusor instability in symptomatic women without outflow obstruction [49].

The role of all types of US modalities (trans-abdominal, endovaginal, endorectal, transperineal, and intraurethral) in urogynecology was decribed by Rahmanou et al [50]. They suggested that transabdominal US is a useful technique to measure the bladder volume and to investigate bladder diverticula. Endorectal US has a role in visualization of the lower urinary tract in women with neurologically impaired anal sensation, while both TPUS and TUUS appear not to be clinically relevant for assessing the pelvic floor [50]. Interestingly, no specific use of EVUS was identified. Tunn et al [6], in updated recommendations on ultrasonography in urogynecology, conclude that ultrasonography is a supplementary, indispensable diagnostic procedure and that TPUS and ERUS are the most useful techniques. In patients undergoing diagnostic work-up for urge incontinence, US occasionally demonstrates urethral diverticula, leiomyomas, and cysts in the vaginal wall. These findings will lead to further diagnostic assessment. The same applies to the demonstration of bladder diverticula, foreign bodies in the bladder, and bullous edema. Moreover, this diagnostic procedure allows documentation of functional and morphologic findings, such as position and mobility of the bladder neck.

In conclusion, although TPUS is recognized as a gold standard technique in the diagnosis of urinary in-

continence and voiding dysfunctions, high-frequency EVUS offers a significant amount of additional information. This modality provides a detailed assessment of the morphology, vascularity, and functionality of the urethral complex and appears to play a relevant role in the management of these pathological conditions [4].

References

1. Boyles SH, Weber AM, Meyn L. Procedures for urinary incontinence in the United States, 1979–1997. Am J Obstet Gynecol 2003;189:70–75.
2. Olsen AL, Smith VJ, Bergstrom JO et al. Epidemiology of surgically managed pelvic organ prolapse and urinary incontinence. Obstet Gynecol 1997;89:501–506.
3. Sampselle CM, DeLancey JO. Anatomy of female continence. J Wound Ostomy Continence Nurs 1998; 25:63–64.
4. Haderer JM, Pannu HK, Genadry R, Hutchins GM. Controversies in female urethral anatomy and their significance for understanding urinary continence: observations and literature review. Int Urogynecol J Pelvic Floor Dysfunct 2002;13:236–252.
5. Dietz HP. Ultrasound imaging of the pelvic floor. Part I: two-dimensional aspects. Ultrasound Obstet Gynecol 2004;23:80–92.
6. Tunn R, Schaer G, Peschers U et al. Updated recommendations on ultrasonography in urogynecology. Int Urogynecol J Pelvic Floor Dysfunct 2005;16:236–241.
7. Sugaya K, Nishijima S, Oda M et al. Transabdominal vesical sonography of urethral syndrome and stress incontinence. Int J Urol 2003;10:36–42.
8. Dietz HP, Wilson PD. The influence of bladder volume on the position and mobility of the urethrovesical junction. Int Urogynecol J Pelvic Floor Dysfunct 1999;10:3–6.
9. Hall R, Kkhalsa S, Qualls C, Rogers RG. A comparison of

periurethral blood flow resistive indices and urethral closure pressure of incontinent women. Int Urogynecol J Pelvic Floor Dysfunct 2006;17:472–477.

10. Siracusano S, Bertolotto M, d'Aloia G et al. Colour Doppler ultrasonography of female urethral vascularization in normal young volunteers: a preliminary report. BJU Int 2001; 88:378–381.

11. Gehrich A, Stany MP, Fischer JR et al. Establishing a mean postvoid residual volume in asymptomatic perimenopausal and postmenopausal women. Obstet Gynecol 2007;110:827–832.

12. Dietz HP, Haylen BT, Vancaillie TG. Female pelvic organ prolapse and voiding function. Int Urogynecol J Pelvic Floor Dysfunct 2002;13:284–288.

13. Haylen BT, de Ridder D, Freeman RM et al. An International Urogynecological Association (IUGA)/International Continence Society (ICS) joint report on the terminology for female pelvic floor dysfunction. Int Urogynecol J 2010;21:5–26.

14. Dietz HP. Ultrasound imaging of the pelvic floor. Part II: three-dimensional or volume imaging. Ultrasound Obstet Gynecol 2004;23:615–625.

15. Defreitas GA, Wilson TS, Zimmern PE, Forte TB. Three-dimensional ultrasonography: an objective outcome tool to assess collagen distribution in women with stress urinary incontinence. Urology 2003;62:232–236.

16. Umek WH, Obermair A, Stutterecker D et al. Three-dimensional ultrasound of the female urethra: comparing transvaginal and transrectal scanning. Ultrasound Obstet Gynecol 2001;17:425–430.

17. Heit M. Intraurethral sonography and the test-retest reliability of urethral sphincter measurements in women. J Clin Ultrasound 2002;30:349–355.

18. Mitterberger M, Pinggera GM, Mueller T et al. Dynamic transurethral sonography and 3-dimensional reconstruction of the rhabdosphincter and urethra: initial experience in continent and incontinent women. J Ultrasound Med 2006;25:315–320.

19. Schaer GN, Schmid T, Peschers U, DeLancey JO. Intraurethral ultrasound correlated with urethral histology. Obstet Gynecol 1998;91:60–64.

20. Santoro GA, Wieczorek AP, Stankiewicz A. High-resolution three-dimensional endovaginal ultrasonography in the assessment of pelvic floor anatomy: a preliminary study. Int Urogynecol J Pelvic Floor Dysfunct 2009;20:1213–1222.

21. Stankiewicz A, Wieczorek AP, Woźniak MM et al. Comparison of accuracy of functional measurements of the urethra in transperineal vs. endovaginal ultrasound in incontinent women. Pelviperineology 2008;27:145–147.

22. Wieczorek AP, Woźniak MM, Stankiewicz A et al. The assessment of normal female urethral vascularity with Color Doppler endovaginal ultrasonography: preliminary report. Pelviperineology 2009;28:59–61.

23. Scholbach T, Girelli E, Scholbach J. Tissue pulsatility index: a new parameter to evaluate renal transplant perfusion. Transplantation 2006;81:751–755.

24. Santoro GA, Fortling B. The advantages of volume rendering in three-dimensional endosonography of the anorectum. Dis Colon Rectum 2007;50:359–368.

25. Kelly CE. Evaluation of voiding dysfunction and measurement of bladder volume. Rev Urol 2004;6(suppl 1):S32–S37.

26. Bai SW, Kwon JY, Chung Dj et al. Differences in urodynamic study, perineal sonography and treatment outcome according to urethrovesical junction hypermobility in stress urinary incontinence. J Obstet Gynaecol Res 2006;32:206–211.

27. Harris RL, Cundiff GW, Coates KW, Bump RC. Urinary incontinence and pelvic organ prolapse in nulliparous women. Obstet Gynecol 1998;92:951–954.

28. Schaer GN, Perucchini D, Munz E et al. Sonographic evaluation of the bladder neck in continent and stress-incontinent women. Obstet Gynecol 1999;93:412–416.

29. Huang WC, Yang JM. Bladder neck funneling on ultrasound cystourethrography in primary stress urinary incontinence: a sign associated with urethral hypermobility and intrinsic sphincter deficiency. Urology 2003;61:936–941.

30. Tunn R, Goldammer K, Gauruder-Burmester A et al. Pathogenesis of urethral funneling in women with stress urinary incontinence assessed by introital ultrasound. Ultrasound Obstet Gynecol 2005;26:287–292.

31. Dietz HP, Clarke B, Herbison P. Bladder neck mobility and urethral closure pressure as predictors of genuine stress incontinence. Int Urogynecol J Pelvic Floor Dysfunct 2002;13: 289–293.

32. Hall RJ, Rogers RG, Saiz L, Qualls C. Translabial ultrasound assessment of the anal sphincter complex: normal measurements of the internal and external anal sphincters at the proximal, mid-, and distal levels. Int Urogynecol J Pelvic Floor Dysfunct 2007;18:881–888.

33. Digesu GA, Robinson D, Cardozo L, Khullar V. Three-dimensional ultrasound of the urethral sphincter predicts continence surgery outcome. Neurourol Urodyn 2009;28:90–94.

34. Dietz HP, Barry C, Lim YN, Rane A. Two-dimensional and three-dimensional ultrasound imaging of suburethral slings. Ultrasound Obstet Gynecol 2005;26:175–179.

35. Ng CC, Lee LC, Han WH. Use of three-dimensional ultrasound scan to assess the clinical importance of midurethral placement of the tension-free vaginal tape (TVT) for treatment of incontinence. Int Urogynecol J Pelvic Floor Dysfunct 2005;16:220–225.

36. Quinn MJ, Beynon J, Mortensen NJ, Smith PJ. Transvaginal endosonography: a new method to study the anatomy of the lower urinary tract in urinary stress incontinence. Br J Urol 1988;62:414–418.

37. Umek WH, Laml T, Stutterecker D et al. The urethra during pelvic floor contraction: observations on three-dimensional ultrasound. Obstet Gynecol 2002;100:796–800.

38. Reisinger E, Stummvoll W. Visualization of the endopelvic fascia by transrectal three-dimensional ultrasound. Int Urogynecol J Pelvic Floor Dysfunct 2006;17:165–169.

39. Athanasiou S, Khullar V, Boos K et al. Imaging the urethral sphincter with three-dimensional ultrasound. Obstet Gynecol 1999;94:295–301.

40. Tan IL, Stoker J, Zwamborn AW, Entius KA et al. Female pelvic floor: endovaginal MR imaging of normal anatomy. Radiology 1998;206:777–783.

41. Ashton-Miller JA, DeLancey JO. Functional anatomy of the female pelvic floor. Ann N Y Acad Sci 2007; 1101:266–296.

42. Yang JM, Huang WC. Sonographic findings in a case of voiding dysfunction secondary to the tension-free vaginal tape (TVT) procedure. Ultrasound Obstet Gynecol 2004;23:302–304.

43. Huang WC, Yang SH, Yang SY et al. Vaginal abscess mimicking a cystocele and causing voiding dysfunction after Burch colposuspension. J Ultrasound Med 2009;28:63–66.

44. Yang JM, Yang SH, Huang WC. Two- and three-dimensional

sonographic findings in a case of distal urethral obstruction due to a paraurethral tumor. Ultrasound Obstet Gynecol 2005;25:519–521.

45. Yang JM, Huang WC, Yang SH. Transvaginal sonography in the diagnosis, management and follow-up of complex paraurethral abnormalities. Ultrasound Obstet Gynecol 2005;25:302–306.

46. Yang JM, Huang WC. Sonographic findings in acute urinary retention secondary to retroverted gravid uterus: pathophysiology and preventive measures. Ultrasound Obstet Gynecol 2004;23:490–495.

47. Prasad SR, Menias CO, Narra VR et al. Cross-sectional imaging of the female urethra: technique and results. Radiographics 2005;25:749–761.

48. Khullar V, Salvatore S, Cardozo L et al. A novel technique for measuring bladder wall thickness in women using transvaginal ultrasound. Ultrasound Obstet Gynecol 1994; 4:220–223.

49. Khullar V, Cardozo LD, Salvatore S, Hill S. Ultrasound: a noninvasive screening test for detrusor instability. Br J Obstet Gynaecol 1996;103:904–908.

50. Rahmanou P, Chaliha C, Khullar V. Role of imaging in urogynaecology. BJOG 2004;111(suppl 1):24–32.

Invited Commentary

Wiesław Jakubowski

Urinary incontinence and voiding dysfunctions are widespread clinical problems of multifactorial etiology. Despite huge progress in imaging diagnostics there are still many controversies concerning the detailed morphology and function of the organs involved in maintaining continence, which are the key to understand incontinence. The anatomy of the pelvic and perineal organs is that of a complex three-dimensional apparatus with very complex function. No consensus has yet been reached on which imaging tool would enable appropriate assessment of the pelvic floor, showing the causes of pelvic organ disturbances. The gold standard method is currently magnetic resonance; however, the most widely used diagnostic method for assessment of the statics and function of the female pelvic organs is ultrasonography. The advantages of this technique mean it has significantly replaced x-ray procedures. However, the majority of current international recommendations on ultrasonographic diagnostics of urinary incontinence suggest transperineal ultrasound as a method of choice, diminishing the role of other ultrasonographic techniques and approaches that are currently available.

Chapter 15 is a unique collection of descriptions about all the ultrasonographic techniques currently available that may be useful in the diagnostics of urinary incontinence and voiding dysfunctions. The authors claim that the role of ultrasonography is to define whether the pelvic floor organs taking part in the maintenance of continence remain normal or show any anatomical and/or functional disturbances. This simple categorization would allow significant shortening of the diagnostic and thera-

peutic process. However, it is underlined that the main issue conditioning the range and quality of obtained information is the type of ultrasound equipment and method used for scanning. It is important to realize that pelvic floor ultrasonography is a very wide field comprising a number of varied techniques, depending on the type of access and type of ultrasound transducers used. From this chapter we may learn about external ultrasound (transabdominal, perineal/transperineal, translabial, introital) and endoluminal ultrasound (endovaginal, endoanal, endourethral), the type of equipment needed for each approach, the advantages and limitations of each technique, and their clinical usefulness. The authors specify which techniques among all described methods are most suitable for various clinical applications, such as diagnosis of the causes of urinary incontinence and voiding dysfunctions and follow-up of surgical treatment, as well as diagnosis of the reasons for postoperative complications. In this chapter, the authors have managed to gather detailed information not only about techniques widely known but also about those that are still under research or exist as niche applications and are not used routinely nowadays, such as perfusion techniques enabling quantification of the vascular flow. Such a wide, multidisciplinary approach to imaging makes this chapter highly valuable for various specialties, not just radiologists, but also gynecologists, urologists, proctologists, and all those who deal with pelvic floor disorders. However, the authors highlight the special role of more sophisticated modalities such as novel 3D and 4D high-frequency endoluminal ultrasonography. They recommend high-frequency techniques as the ones that have the greatest impact on diagnostics and that will most probably, in the near future, become gold standard examinations in the diagnosis and monitoring of treatment of urinary incontinence and voiding dysfunctions.

W. Jakubowski
Department of Diagnostics Imaging, General Brodnowski Hospital, Medical University of Warsaw, Poland

G.A. Santoro, A.P. Wieczorek, C.I. Bartram (eds.) *Pelvic Floor Disorders*
© Springer-Verlag Italia 2010

Urodynamics

16

Edoardo Ostardo, Giuseppe Tuccitto, Francesco Beniamin
and Luigi Maccatrozzo

Abstract Urodynamic tests measure parameters related to the storage and voiding functions of the lower urinary tract. Investigations encompass a variety of tests, including cystometry, uroflow, urethral pressure profilometry, sphincter electromyography and radiological visualization of the bladder and urethra. The usefulness of urodynamics remains controversial, however it can provide a pathophysiological explanation of urinary dysfunction, guiding clinical management.

Keywords Cystomanometry • Electromyographic kinesiology • Pressure-flow study • Urethral profilometry • Urodynamics • Uroflowmetry • Valsalva leak point pressure test

16.1 Introduction

Urodynamics is the discipline that interprets the pathophysiology of the lower urinary tract. This term encompasses a variety of tests that investigate the function of the bladder and urethra and their component parts (bladder neck, urethral rhabdosphincter), and of the surrounding structures (muscular pelvic diaphragm). Urodynamics is the application of fluid physics and biomechanics for the comprehension of urinary tract dysfunction.

The most important investigation is represented by the voiding diary, which is completed by the patients at home in a specified period of time. This diary can be considered as a real urodynamic test, providing information on the hydration of the subject, frequency of voiding, urinary volumes voided, and associated symptoms (urgency, urinary incontinence, pain, use of pads etc). It is important, however, to recommend the patient to compile the diary without any modification of his normal lifestyle (e.g. water intake), and to discuss the results with him for a correct interpretation. The main indication is an objective evaluation of the reported symptoms and to obtain a baseline assessment against which to evaluate the effectiveness of treatment.

Urodynamic investigations include [1]:

- uroflowmetry
- cystometry
- pressure-flow studies
- urethral sphincter electromyography
- video-urodynamics
- urethral pressure profilometry
- Valsalva leak point pressure test.

16.2 Uroflowmetry

Uroflowmetry is a screening test that investigates the voiding pattern in order to identify conditions of bladder outlet obstruction. It records the micturition volume (mL) spontaneously emitted per unit time (s). It provides numerical parameters (maximum flow, average

E. Ostardo
Division of Urology, "Santa Maria degli Angeli" Hospital, Pordenone, Italy

flow, flow time, time to micturition, etc), and also allows analysis of urine flow against time curves for micturition. The results must be interpreted considering the voided volume, that should be comprised between 150 and 500 mL to consider the test reliable, and the post-void residual volume, estimated by ultrasonography. Uroflowmetry is performed with flowmeters to record the volume of urine flow in a unit of time. This examination is economical and easily repeatable, and allows a non-invasive evaluation of bladder emptying that can be represented with graphics. Its significance is limited in clinical situations not associated to outlet obstruction, however it is also valuable for an overall assessment of voiding function, expressed by the ratio between the total and post-void residual volumes estimated with ultrasound. The main parameters obtained from uroflowmetry are listed in Box 16.1 and illustrated in Fig. 16.1.

The maximum flow (Q_{max}) is the highest flow rate reached for a given curve. When urinary flow is continuous, the voiding time and flow time are the same. In case of intermittent flow, the voiding time (T_M) is longer than the flow time (T_Q), as the former is the sum of all the phases of urine flow and the intervals between them. The average flow (Q_{ave}) represents the ratio between voiding volume and flow time. The time to maximum flow (T_{Qmax}), indicates the symmetry of the curve corresponding to voiding flow against the maximum flow (Fig. 16.1). Some devices provide additional parameters such as pre-voiding time, which is the time from the command to urinate to the initial registration of flow on the transducer.

Typically, the pattern of the flow plot is a smooth bell-shaped curve in a normal flow, with the maximum flow rate in the first third of the curve. Various clinical conditions, however, result in an asymmetry of the ascending or descending tails. Detrusorial hypoactivity increases the upward phase, while an obstructive pathology increases the descending phase. Moreover, in the curve may be visualized some spikes that reflect the recruitment of additional abdominal pushing forces (straining) or incomplete urethral sphincter relaxation.

Interpretation of the uroflowmetry data should take account of a number of artefacts due to unsuitable environment, psychological factors, inadequate preparation or bladder filling, urge incontinence or presence of an urinary catheter, that may modify the signal and result in misleading values.

Uroflowmetry has been considered to be the most useful screening procedure for diagnosing bladder outlet obstruction, where the flow curve is flattened, with a prolonged flow and a reduced maximin flow rate. A pattern that is suggestive for the diagnosis of urethral stenosis, is a graph with Q_{max} and Q_{ave} having similar values. The presence of a two-phase flow plot is suggestive for

Box 16.1 Uroflowmetry parameters

Q_{max}	maximum flow rate (mL/s)
Q_{ave}	average flow rate (mL/s)
V_{ura}	voided volume (mL)
V_{res}	post-void residual volume (mL)
T_M	voiding time (s)
T_Q	flow time (s)
T_{Qmax}	time to maximum flow (s)

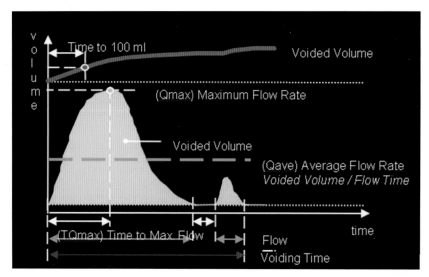

Fig. 16.1 Scheme of the uroflowmetry parameters

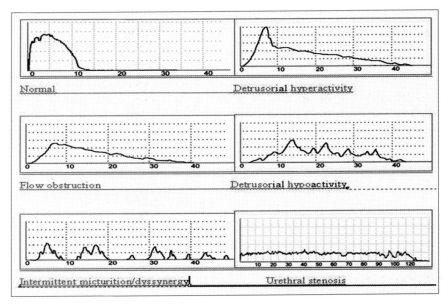

Normal

Detrusorial hyperactivity

Flow obstruction

Detrusorial hypoactivity

Intermittent micturition/dyssynergy

Urethral stenosis

Fig. 16.2 Morphology of urinary flow in various clinical conditions

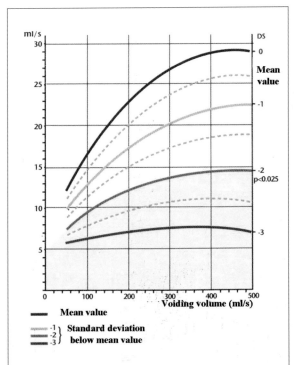

Fig. 16.3 Nomogram of Siroky

detrusorial overactivity and it is characterized by an initial high peak followed by a bell-shaped curve of lower amplitude. The peak reflects the high pressure in the volume of urine collected in the posterior urethra due to the phasic voluntary contraction of the striated urethral sphincter and to the pre-existing detrusor contraction at the time of call to void (Fig. 16.2).

The flow parameters obtained during the examination can be compared to published nomograms as reported by Siroky et al (Fig. 16.3) [2] in males aged over 50 years. Other nomograms (e.g. the Liverpool nomogram) (Fig. 16.4) express the maximum flow rates and voiding volume in areas of percentiles and can be applied for both males and females.

16.3 Cystometry and Pressure-Flow Study

Cystometry and the pressure-flow study describe the filling part of basic urodynamics study. It is performed by the use of pressure catheters (water-perfused, air-perfused or piezoelectric crystal) to assess bladder sensation, compliance, capacity and activity and the mechanics of micturition. Cystometry measures bladder filling and the pressure-flow study evaluates bladder emptying.

The study, shown schematically in Fig. 16.5, starts filling the bladder with normal saline through a biluminal catheter, for measurement of vesical pressure (P_{ves}) and for retrograde bladder filling. A rectal balloon catheter is inserted to measure abdominal pressure (P_{abd}). The activity of the detrusor muscle is assessed by measuring detrusor pressure (P_{det}), which is the difference between P_{ves} and P_{abd}.

Alternatively a three-channel catheter may be used for synchronous measurement of urethral pressure (P_{ura}). Although this method is particularly useful to evaluate

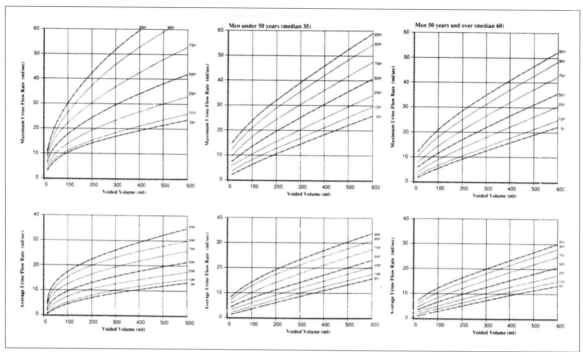

Fig. 16.4 Liverpool nomogram

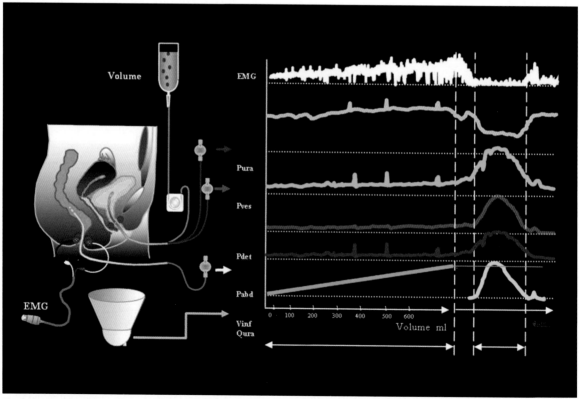

Fig. 16.5 Schematic representation of cystometry and pressure–flow study. Electromyography (*EMG*), *white*; urethral pressure (P_{ura}), *gray*; vesical pressure (P_{ves}), *light blue*; detrusor pressure (P_{det}), *violet*; abdominal pressure (P_{abd}), *red*; bladder volume (V_{inf}), *green*; urethra flow rate (Q_{ura}), *yellow*

the relaxation of the urethral wall during the emptying of the bladder, it can also explain urinary incontinence occurring during bladder filling due to a sudden deflection of the basal tone of smooth urethral muscle. However, the catheter frequently tends to be dislocated distally when the patient is asked to cough or jog.

The technique of examination (patient position, type and size of catheters, infusion rate and temperature of the medium infused) must always be indicated. The filling part provides information on the bladder compliance (sensations of bladder filling, bladder capacity, the relationship between the change in bladder volume and change in pressure).

The voiding phase assesses the detrusor contractility, the morphology of the pressure-flow curves, the voided volume against time and pressure and the residual volume. Analyses of these measurements will help to identify the bladder function.

To evaluate the synergy between detrusor contractility and sphincter relaxation during voiding, an electromyography (EMG) of the pelvic floor may be simultaneously performed using surface electrodes placed on the perineum or needle electrodes inserted in the external anal sphincter. Indications for neuro-physiological investigations include detrusor sphincter dyssynergy, neurogenic voiding dysfunction, not neuropathic pelvic muscle dyssynergy.

The test report should clearly indicate:

- position of the catheter (transurethral or transcystostomy)
- type of transducer (water or air-perfused; microtip with piezoelectric crystals)
- size of the catheter (usually 6 to 8 Fr.)
- medium infused (normal saline or iodate contrast)
- temperature of the medium infused (ambient/body/cold/frozen)
- infusion rate
- patient position (usually in standing position in men and sitting position in women).

During cystometry, some provocations may be necessary to elicit patient symptoms and should be annotated on the trace for future reference:

- asking the patient to cough or jog
- the sound of running water
- the patient has contact with cold water (e.g. hands)

- increasing the infusion rate
- postural changes
- pharmacological test
- suprapubic compression
- temperature of the medium infused (Lapides test of frozen water).

Cystometry provides the following measurements:

- sensitivity
- capacity
- compliance
- detrusor function
- continence.

Sensitivity is reported by the patient during the procedure and has the value of being a semi-objective parameter; in particular it is defined as:

- thermal sensation
- sensation of bladder filling
- first desire to void (mL)
- normal desire to void (mL)
- strong desire to void (mL)
- abnormal sensations (pain or urgency)
- non-specific bladder sensitivity:
  – sense of abdominal fullness or tension
  – symptoms of chills, hypotension, malaise.

The maximum cystometric capacity is related to:

- strong desire to void
- sensation of bladder filling or abnormal sensations such as pain
- detrusor contractility
- urinary incontinence
- the clinical condition of the subject.

The detrusor pressure (P_{det}) is measured at the maximum cystometric capacity. The maximum capacity usually varies between 400-600 ml in an adult male. The filling volume is guided by the patient sensation at the time, however, in pathological conditions, it should not exceed 600 mL. Bladder filling should be stopped in these circumstances:

- high filling volume in the absence of patient sensation
- bladder volume exceeding the value of strong desire to void

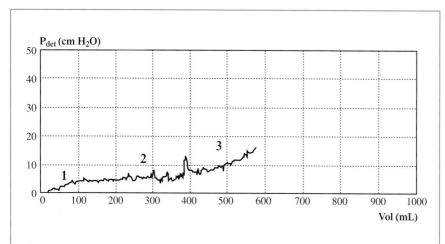

Fig. 16.6 Bladder compliance measures the relationship between the change in bladder volume (*Vol*) and change in detrusor pressure (P_{det}). P_{det} increases at the beginning of the filling phase due to a direct solicitation of muscle and stroma (1). During bladder filling, there is a little rise in P_{det} due to the passive (plasticity) and active (myogenic/neurogenic) adaptation of bladder wall (2). At the maximum cystometric capacity, there is a high rise in P_{det} (3)

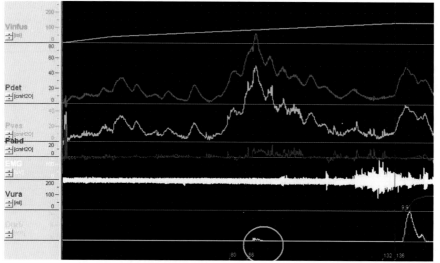

Fig. 16.7 Filling cystometry showing a detrusor overactivity incontinence (circle). During bladder filling, a voluntary contraction of the pelvic floor diaphragm is observed using electromyography (*EMG, white*). Detrusor pressure (P_{det}), *violet*; vesical pressure (P_{ves}), *light blue*; abdominal pressure (P_{abd}), *red*; voided volume (V_{URA}), *blue*; urethra flow rate (Q_{ura}), *yellow*

- occurrence of bladder/pelvic pain
- high detrusor pressure.

Bladder compliance measures the relationship between the change in bladder volume and change in pressure using the equation $\Delta V / \Delta P$ and it is expressed in mL/cmH$_2$O. During bladder filling, the bladder has the capacity to adapt to increasing volume due to the viscoelastic properties of the bladder wall and to the presence of neuroreceptors that induce relaxation of the detrusor muscle (Fig. 16.6).

During bladder filling, the detrusor muscle should remain relaxed despite provocation with little rise in pressure. Detrusor overactivity is characterised by an involuntary detrusor contraction that may be spontaneous or provoked and it is considered significant only if it replicates the patient's symptoms of urgency (Fig. 16.7). Detrusor contractions can be phasic or tonic, single or complex, short or prolonged and may also be associated with urinary leakage (detrusor overactive incontinence). The P_{det} at which the leak occurs is defined the detrusor leak point pressure [3].

Cystometry is essential to define causes of urinary incontinence. An involuntary leakage on increasing abdominal pressure (e.g., coughing, straining) in the absence of detrusor contraction is considered urodynamic stress incontinence. A leakage associated to involuntary detrusor contraction is considered urodynamic urge incontinence (Fig. 16.8).

Pressure-flow study measures the volume of bladder filling, the abdominal pressure and the detrusor pressure associated to the episodes of incontinence. It assesses the voiding function of the patient, who is asked to void into the flowmeter, and provides an evaluation of detrusor motor function as well as the resistance of the urethra.

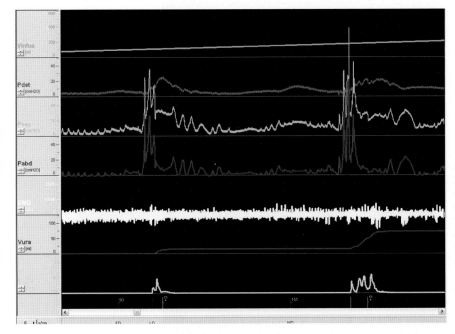

Fig. 16.8 Filling cystometry showing a mixed urinary incontinence (stress incontinence and idiopathic detrusor overactivity). Bladder volume (V_{INF}), *green*; detrusor pressure (P_{det}), *violet*; vesical pressure (P_{ves}), *light blue*; abdominal pressure (P_{abd}), *red*; electromyography (EMG), *white*; voided volume (V_{ura}), *blue*; urethra flow rate (Q_{ura}), *yellow*

In normal voiding there is a sustained detrusor contraction with continuous flow and complete emptying of the bladder. The main parameters influencing the urine flow rate are:

- detrusor contractility
- abdominal pressure
- bladder neck and urethral resistances.

In normal voiding, the urethra remains relaxed and this is associated to a little rise in intravesical pressure for a complete emptying of the bladder. Intravesical pressure increases in bladder outlet obstruction due to:

- urethral overactivity (functional or active obstruction occuring for increased contractility of the smooth or striated urethral muscles)
- anatomical factors (non-functional or passive obstruction occurring for a compression of urethral lumen, i.e. prostatic hypertrophy, or for urethral stenosis).

As consequences, the detrusor pressure is strictly related to the bladder neck-urethral resistance. High urethral closure pressure is associated to high P_{det} value and low resistance is associated to low P_{det} value.

In Fig. 16.9 is shown a pressure-flow study during normal voiding. The parameters that should be measured are the following:

- Q_{max} maximum flow rate
- $P_{det, ope}$ opening detrusor pressure
- $P_{det, max}$ maximum detrusor pressure
- $P_{det,Qmax}$ detrusor pressure at maximum rate
- V_{ura} voided volume
- V_{res} post-void residual volume.

The post-void residual volume must always be measured after voiding by emptying the bladder via the urethral catheter as its calculation by the subtraction of voided volume from filling volume may be inaccurate for several reasons, i.e. setting of the peristaltic pump, urinary leakage, etc.

Pressure-flow studies allow to identify the following conditions (Fig. 16.10):

- weak detrusor contractility: it is characterized by a diminished uroflow and a detrusor contraction of low magnitude, low duration or low speed, resulting in the inability to completely empty the bladder in an adequate period of time
- absent detrusor contractility: it is characterized by the absence of detrusor contraction during the study
- bladder outlet obstruction: it is associated with a diminished uroflow but with a sustained detrusor contraction of high magnitude.

Different nomograms (Abrams and Griffiths, Schafer, International Continence Society, URA, WF-max) have been developed for the quantification of obstruction and detrusor contractility from pressure-flow studies [3–5] (Figs. 16.11–16.14). They define the following parameters:

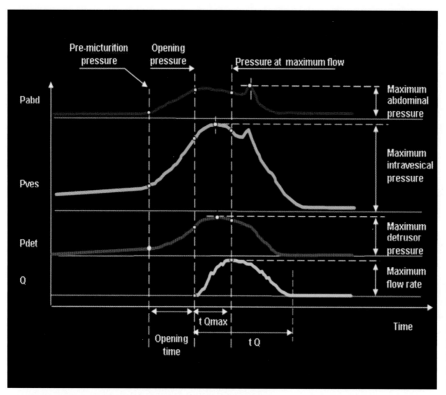

Fig. 16.9 Pressure-flow study during normal voiding showing vesical pressure (P_{ves}, *light blue*), abdominal pressure (P_{abd}, *red*), detrusor pressure (P_{det}, *violet*) and urine flow rate (Q, *yellow*). Q_{max}: maximum flow rate

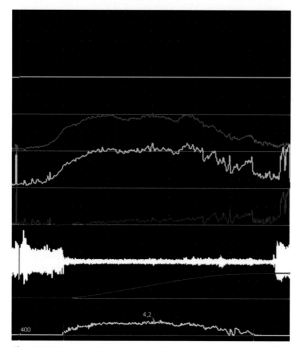

Fig. 16.10 Pressure-flow study in bladder outlet obstruction. The flow rate curve (Q_{ura}, *yellow*) is flattened and prolonged in presence of high detrusor (P_{det}, *violet*) and vesical (P_{ves}, *light blue*) pressures and normal abdominal pressure (P_{abd}, *red*). Electromyography (EMG), *white*; voided volume (V_{ura}), *blue*; bladder volume (V_{inf}), *green*

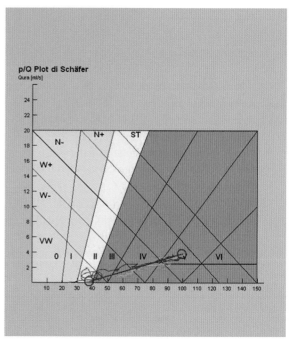

Fig. 16.11 Schafer nomogram groups voiding into obstructed (*red*), non-obstructed (*green*) or equivocal obstruction (*yellow*). (*ST*: strong detrusor contractility; *N*, normal detrusor contractility; *W*, weak detrusor contractility; *VW*, very weak detrusor contractility; $P_{detQmax}$, detrusor pressure at maximum flow rate, *x*, axis and Q_{max}, maximum flow rate; *y*, axis)

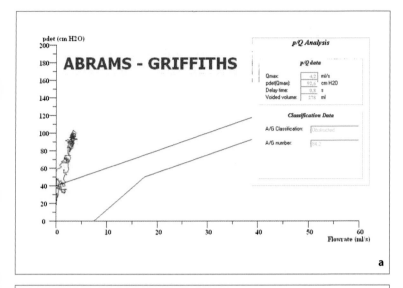

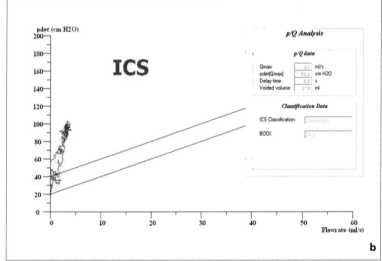

Fig. 16.12 Abrams-Griffiths (**a**) and ICS (**b**) nomograms group voiding into obstructed (superior area), non-obstructed (inferior area) or equivocal obstruction (intermediate area)

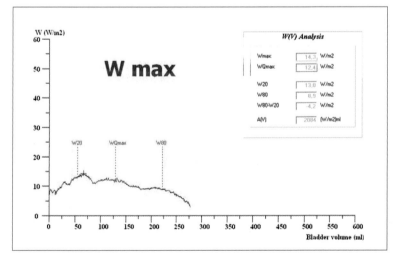

Fig. 16.13 *W max* nomogram evaluates the contractily power in relation to the void volume

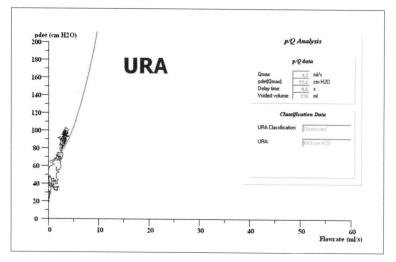

Fig. 16.14 *URA* nomogram measures the resistance of the urethra

bladder activity	=	bladder activity per unit time (proportional to the voiding volume, expressed in Joules)
vesical power	=	WF (Watts factor) → detrusor contractility
	=	PIP (projected isometric pressure) → degrees of contractility power
urethral resistance	=	PURR (passive urethral resistance relation) → urethral relaxation
	=	LPURR (linear passive urethral resistance relation) → urethral compression
	=	DAMPF (detrusor-adjusted mean PURR factor) → degrees of obstruction not influenced by the detrusor contractility. Differentiates the type of obstruction
	=	URA (urethral resistance) → P_{ope}/P_{det} α (related to the vesical power);
	=	OBI (obstruction index) → urethral relaxation.

Urodynamics is a minimal invasive investigation, well tolerated, repeatable, and reliable. It often has a prognostic value regarding the outcome of medical or surgical treatments (e.g. prior to surgery for stress urinary incontinence or before prostatectomy for benign prostatic obstruction) and enhances our understanding on the mechanisms of urinary incontinence and voiding dysfunction.

Clinical judgement, however, is essential in determining the significance of urodynamic data.

16.4 Electromyography

Electromyography provides objective documentation concerning the integrity of the innervation and the activity of the external urethral sphincter and pelvic floor muscles. Somatic innervation of the external sphincter derives from the second, third and fourth sacral spinal cord segments via the pudendal nerve. This sphincter is usually electrically silent at rest. There is a gradual increase in EMG activity during bladder filling, that reaches a maximum just prior to voiding. The initition of a voluntary detrusor contraction is associated to a complete relaxation of the external sphincter, that persists throughout micturition. At the end of voiding electromyographic activity resumes. An increase in EMG activity accompanies any sudden increase in abdominal pressure such as cough or movement.

The neuro-physiological assessment can be performed using two surface electrodes positioned in the perineal region or needle electrodes inserted in the urethral sphincter. Needle EMG, however, requires specific skills and artefacts may occur due to needle movement.

Three abnormal voiding patterns can be identified with EMG, as follows:

- Voiding dysfunction, characterized by intermittent flow and detrusor contractility due to involuntary contractions of the periurethral striated muscle in the absence of neurological injury
- Detrusor-urethral sphincter dyssynergy (Fig. 16.15), characterized by an involuntary contraction of the external sphincter during an involuntary detrusor con-

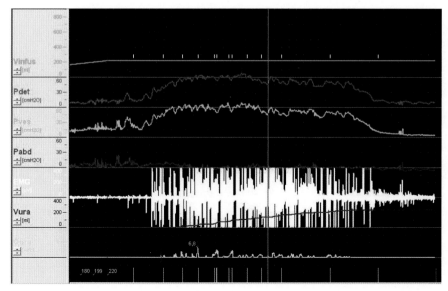

Fig. 16.15 Detrusor-external sphincter dyssynergy – type 3. Bladder volume (V_{inf}), *green*; detrusor pressure (P_{det}), *violet*; vesical pressure (P_{ves}), *light blue*; abdominal pressure (P_{abd}), *red*; electromyography (EMG), *white*; voided volume (V_{ura}), *blue*; urethra flow rate (Q_{ura}), *yellow*

traction [6]. In this pathological condition micturition is uncoordinated, usually due to neurological lesions between the brain stem (pontine micturition centre) and the sacral spinal cord (sacral micturition centre). These include traumatic spinal cord injury, multiple sclerosis, myelodisplasia and other forms of transverse myelitis. It has been classified into three main categories on the basis of the temporal relationship between the detrusor and external sphincter contraction:
Type 1: initial dyssynergy with a slow and gradual urethral sphincter relaxation
Type 2: intermittent dyssynergy, characterized by sporadic increases in EMG activity throughout the detrusor contraction
Type 3: continuous dyssynergy.

- Absent perineal muscles relaxation. Neurological lesions involve the sacral micturitional pathways as in myelodysplasia, tumours or injuries to the conus medullaris or cauda equina, herniated discs and anterior spinal artery occlusion. There is neither voluntary nor reflex activity of the involved muscles and sensation is lost (functional urethral obstruction). At EMG spontaneous potentials in the form of fibrillations and positive sharp waves can be seen.

16.5 Video-urodynamics

Video-urodynamics combines functional (cystometry, pressure-flow studies EMG) and morphological (radiographic visualization) assessment of the lower urinary tract for evaluating micturition disturbances.

The patient is catheterized with a triple-lumen urodynamic catheter for measuring intravesical and urethral pressure simultaneously. The third lumen is used for infusion of iodate contrast medium. With the patient in his usual voiding position (lying, sitting or standing), bladder filling is begun and continued until the patient feels a strong urge to void. At that point he is asked to try to urinate. A urethral pressure profile is obtained with simultaneous fluoroscopic control and representative events are recorded as video-files for off-line analyses.

During bladder filling, the following findings can be observed:

- Bladder shape. The normal bladder is round or elliptical in shape with a smooth outline and the bladder base is usually flat and located at or just above the symphysis pubis. Video features that can be seen are trabeculation of the bladder, fir tree-shaped bladder, presence of diverticulum, low bladder base position in the pelvic cavity. Trabeculation is usually seen in patient with detrusor overactivity where the detrusor contracts against a closed outlet.
- Vesicoureteric reflux during bladder filling (degree / site / type). In normal condition the ureteric valves prevent reflux into the upper system during both filling and voiding. If reflux occurs, the bladder volume and the P_{det} are measured.
- Bladder base movement on coughing, straining or other provocative maneuvers.

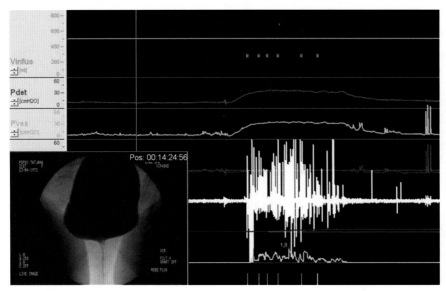

Fig. 16.16 Video-urodynamics showing detrusor-sphincter dyssynergy during bladder voiding (neurogenic bladder due to acute vascular brain damage). Bladder volume (V_{inf}), *green*; detrusor pressure (P_{det}), *violet*; vesical pressure (P_{ves}), *light blue*; abdominal pressure (P_{abd}), *red*; electromyography (EMG), *white*; voided volume (V_{ura}), *blue*; urethra flow rate (Q_{ura}), *yellow*

- Bladder neck integrity, position and function. A bladder neck position below the level of the upper third of symphysis pubis indicates the loss of pelvic floor support. Bladder neck hypermobility is a cause of stress urinary incontinence. An open bladder neck may be consequence of resection of the prostate for benign prostatic hyperplasia.

During bladder voiding, the following findings should be determined:

- Bladder neck opening. On voiding bladder neck should open widely. If it remains closed despite high detrusor pressure this is due to failure to relax.
- Urethral shape from the bladder neck to the external urethral meatus.
- Narrowing in urethra due to urethral stricture, benign prostatic obstruction, detrusor-sphincter dyssynergy (Fig. 16.16), urethral overactivity.
- Urethral diverticulum or ectasia of urethral segment.
- Vesicoureteric reflux during bladder voiding (degree / site / type).
- Post-void residual volume. Large diverticuli could impair bladder function significantly; the diverticulum fills up during voiding and later refills the bladder, causing a post-void residual volume.

To assess the integrity of the neuromuscular sphincteric system, the patient is asked to stop voiding voluntarily (stop test). There is an abrupt increase in EMG activity that represents a voluntary contraction of the external urethral sphincter (rhabdosphincter muscle). The mechanism of urethral closure subsequently involves the periurethral smooth muscle and the bladder neck. In this circumstance the pressure inside the bladder cavity rises due to detrusor contraction against a closed urethra (isovolumetric detrusor pressure: $P_{det, iso}$) (Fig. 16.17).

Pathological findings identified with the stop test include:

- failure of urethral closure (intrinsic sphincter deficiency, high voiding detrusor pressure)

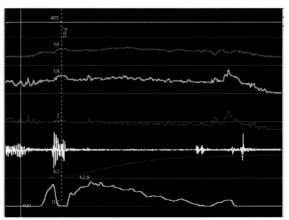

Fig. 16.17 If the patient is asked to stop voiding voluntarily (stop test), there is an abrupt increase in electromyographic (*EMG*, *white*) activity that represents the contraction of pelvic floor muscles. It is also observed a slight increase of the detrusor pressure (P_{det}, *violet*). Bladder volume (V_{inf}), *green*; vesical pressure (P_{ves}), *light blue*; abdominal pressure (P_{abd}), *red*; voided volume (V_{ura}), *blue*; urethra flow rate (Q_{ura}), *yellow*

- trapping of urine in the proximal urethra due to detrusor-external sphincter dyssynergy
- high urethral resistance with intra-prostatic reflux.

16.6 Urethral Pressure Profilometry

Urethral pressure profilometry is an useful technique to measure urethral function, particularly in females with symptoms of stress urinary incontinence and in males with complication after prostatic surgery.

Perfusion technique measures the total resistance to the escape of infused fluid from the catheter port into the urethra. The recorded pressure reflects the cumulative effect of the pressure exerted by the urethral walls against the catheter lumen and the resistance to flow from the perfusant hole. The urethral pressure is measured at 1 cm intervals from the bladder neck to the external meatus slowly withdrawing the catheter by a mechanical puller at a constant rate.

The urethral pressure profile is a graphic representation of intraluminal pressure along the length of the urethra and in female it is usually a bell-shaped curve. It begins to rise from the bladder neck and reaches the maximum pressure at the mid-urethral point, due at rest to the activity of the periurethral striated musculature. The pressure then decreases, and the curve has negative values at the level of the external meatus (Fig. 16.18). As it has been demonstrated a high degree variability when urethral profilometry is measured, it is recom-

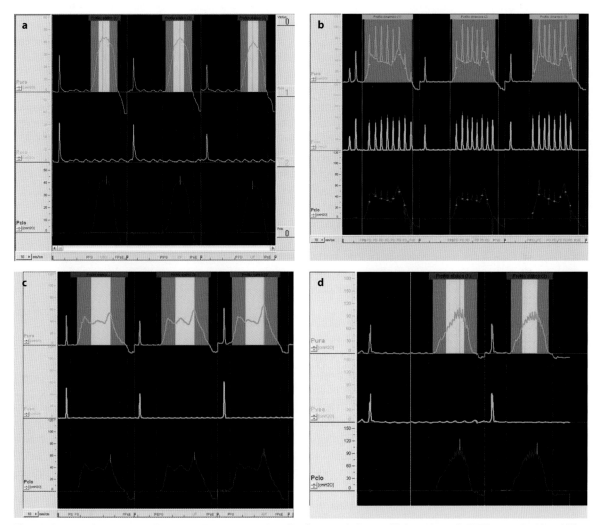

Fig. 16.18 Urethral pressure profilometry (UPP). **a** normal profile; **b** transmission coefficient (dynamic UPP); **c** urethral instability; **d** urethral pulsatility. Oscillations at the peak of the curve, synchronous with the heartbeat, are attributed to an increased pulsatility of the periurethral vascular plexus

mended to perform three profiles and use the lowest profile recorded [7] or averaging a series of profiles [8].

The two parameters of greatest importance are represented by:

- maximum urethral closure pressure ($P_{clo.\ max}$, cmH_2O), that corresponds to the maximum difference between the urethral pressure (P_{ura}) and the intravesical pressure (P_{ves}); a diminished $P_{clo,\ max}$ to 20 cmH_2O is pathognomonic for intrinsic urethral sphincter deficiency, or urethral defunctionalization; this condition, which can also be caused by neurogenic factors, is always associated with severe forms of urinary incontinence; a $P_{clo,\ max} \geq 100\ cmH_2O$ is suspected for urethral hyperactivity
- functional urethral length (FUL, mm). The FUL does not correspond to the anatomical urethral length, but it is the distance between the beginning and the end of the curve (area of continence) with positive urethral pressure.

The dynamic urethral pressure profilometry evaluates the functionality of extrinsic urethral support determined by the anatomical integrity of pubo-urethral and urethro-pelvic ligaments and the pubo-coccygeal muscle. During coughing, the coefficient of transmission of intra-abdominal pressure to the urethra (coefficient of urethral mobility) is determined. This technique, however, is limited to the assessment of female urethra, that is located in the pelvic area. In normal females, the urethra is not fixed, mainly in its proximal and intermediate parts. During micturition, the urethra rotates posteriorly, becoming co-axial with the bladder base and bladder neck to allow voiding.

The typical pressure profile in a male demonstrates the pressure exerted by the prostate as well as the sphincter pressure (biphasic profile). The profile starts with a prostatic rise in pressure to a prostatic plateau followed by a narrower and higher peak corresponding to membranous urethral segment where the striated urethral sphincter is situated. In males, resting urethral profilometry is limited to the evaluation of stress urinary incontinence, occurring after radical prostatectomy or for neurogenic lesions to the spinal cord.

The urethral profilometry has a limited role for the evaluation of urethral stricture or detrusor-sphincter dyssynergia, better assessed with video-urodynamics, pressure-flow study and EMG.

The increase in pressure above the maximum ure-thral pressure during voluntary pelvic floor contraction represents the strength of the pelvic floor muscles. This pelvic floor increment corresponds to the difference between the $P_{clo,\ max}$ during squeezing and the $P_{clo,\ max}$ at rest. The measurement of this index is useful for rehabilitation treatment.

16.7 Valsalva Leak Point Pressure Test

The Valsalva (or abdominal) leak point pressure is a measure of the ability of the bladder neck and urethral sphincter to maintain continence. It is the abdominal pressure at which leakage occurs when the patient is asked to do Valsalva manoeuvre with graduated increase in pressure and standardized conditions of bladder filling (300 mL) [9].

The examination can be performed with the patient in supine and orthostatic position, measuring the abdominal pressure (P_{abd}) with a rectal catheter and collecting any leakage of fluid in order to quantify the severity of incontinence. It is possible a synchronous EMG evaluation of the perineum using surface electrodes. The urinary leakage should replicates the patient's symptoms of incontinence.

Generally, three groups of leak point pressure can be identified (Fig. 16.19):

1. patients with stress incontinence due to reduced bladder neck support who leak at pressures more than 100 cmH_2O
2. patients with intrinsic sphincter deficiency who leak at pressure less than 60 cmH_2O
3. patients with intermediate situations who leak at pressure from 100 to 60 cmH_2O.

16.8 Conclusions

Urodynamic investigations encompass a variety of tests investigating both storage and voiding functions of the lower urinary tract. However, the significance of urodynamics should also involve the assessment of other pelvic floor disorders (e.g., obstructed defecation, chronic pelvic pain, etc.).

Main indications are represented by:

- detrusor overactivity with impaired contractility (DHIC)

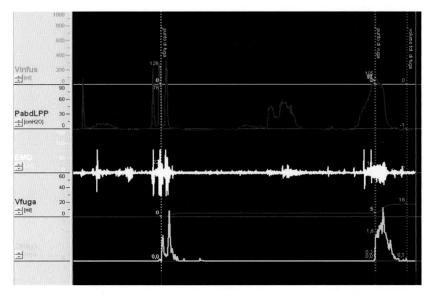

Fig. 16.19 Urinary leakage during coughing and Valsalva manoeuvre. The increment in electromyographic (EMG, *white*) activity represents the reflex contraction of pelvic floor muscles in an attempt to avoid leakage. Bladder volume (V_{inf}), *green*; abdominal pressure (P_{abd}), *red*; voided volume (V_{ura}), *blue*; urethra flow rate (Q_{ura}), *yellow*

- urinary incontinence and urinary retention
- urinary incontinence and bladder outlet obstruction
- double incontinence (urinary and fecal incontinence)
- urinary incontinence and obstructed defecation syndrome.

In a select group of these functional disorders, an useful adjunct to urodynamics is represented by the neuro-physiological study of the pelvic floor (sacral evoked potentials, external anal sphincter EMG or striated urethral sphincter EMG, pudendal nerve terminal motor latency).

References

1. Shafer W, Abrams P, Liao L et al. Good urodynamic practices: uroflowmetry, filling cystometry, and pressure-flow studies. Neurourol Urodyn 2002;21:261-274.
2. Siroky MB, Olsson CA, Krane RJ. The flow rate nomogram: I. Development. J Urol 1979; 122:665-668.
3. Abrams P, Cardozo L, Fall M et al. The standardisation of terminology of lower urinary tract function: report from the standardisation sub-committee of the International Continence Society. Neurourol Urodyn 2002; 21:167-178.
4. Abrams P, Griffiths D. The assessment of prostatic obstruction from urodynamic measurements and from residual urine. Br J Urol 1979;51:129-134.
5. Schafer W. Principles and clinical application of advanced urodynamic analysis of voiding function. Urol Clin North Am 1990;17:553-566.
6. Di Benedetto M, Yalla SV. Electro-diagnosis of striated urethral sphincter dysfunction. J Urol 1979;122:361.
7. Plane P, Susset J. Studies of female urethral pressure profile. I. The normal pressure profile. J Urol 1980;123:64.
8. Rud T. Urethral pressure profile in continent women from childhood to old age. Acta Obstet Gynecol Scand 1980; 59:331.
9. Chapple CR, MacDiarmid SA. Urodynamics made easy, 2nd edn. Churchill Livingstone, Edinburgh, 2000.

Invited Commentary

Paul Abrams

- ## Are urodynamics useful?
YES!

- ## What is the evidence?

Rather limited, chiefly constituting expert opinion. When the National Institute for Health and Clinical Excellence (NICE), the UK authority that develops guidelines for management and recommendations for new procedures, looked at female incontinence, it concluded that in "simple stress incontinence", urodynamics were not necessary as there was no evidence for their clinical effectiveness.

- ## Is absence of evidence, evidence of absence?

NO! The two relevant specialist organizations in the UK, the British Association of Urological Surgeons' Section of Female Urology and the British Society of Urogynaecology, both wrote to NICE opposing this conclusion.

This represented a very large body of professional expert opinion. Did they have competing interests of significance that led them to oppose NICE? Probably not, as urodynamics are not a significant source of private practice income in the UK, and no one is likely to be a part-owner of a urodynamics manufacturer or have invested in its stocks.

P. Abrams
Bristol Urological Institute, Southmead Hospital,
Bristol, UK

- ## Why is there so little evidence?

Those who see patients with lower urinary tract dysfunction see, on a daily basis, that the symptoms and signs of this dysfunction are not reliable enough to guide management, and believe that urodynamics offer great advantages to patients by selecting the appropriate care. The argument is similar to that which demands that we all physically examine patients even though there are no randomized controlled trials (RCTs) to prove that patient examination is useful!

- ## What are the principal messages?

The answer lies in the obvious! As with all clinical testing, its relevance is to set the test in the context of the patient's problems. Most patients with lower urinary tract dysfunction come because of symptoms that affect their quality of life, rather than having a dangerous condition.

The key to getting value from urodynamics is in the simple message:

"The primary aim of urodynamics is to reproduce the patient's symptoms"

The contribution of the International Continence Society (ICS) in setting the standard for urodynamics cannot be overestimated. The 2002 papers cited in the article, set out the modern terminology and the philosophy of urodynamics is described. Urodynamics are a test of "symptomatic verification". At the conclusion of the tests there should be one of three statements:

1. all the patient's symptoms were reproduced
2. some of the patient's symptoms were reproduced
3. none of the patient's symptoms were reproduced.

This requirement for one of the three simple statements reflects the need for urodynamics to be an interactive process between the patient and a clinician involved in that patient's management. To treat urodynamics in a similar way to an electrocardiogram is not appropriate.

• Why might urodynamics fail to reproduce the patient's symptoms?

There are a number of reasons for this:

- Biological variation: in the same way that a pulse or blood pressure measured in the morning is different from that measured in the evening, then repeated urodynamics are likely to vary to some degree. Nevertheless, good-quality studies that have looked at repeated urodynamics give good reliability, as the authors state.
- Technique: there are many issues around technique and some evidence that the ICS recommendations for urodynamics are not being followed, in terms of either clinician involvement, technical issues, such as size of catheters, or the need for tailored urodynamics for the individual patient's problems. Of particular interest is the methodology in relation to detection of detrusor overactivity thought to be responsible for a patient's symptoms of overactive bladder syndrome. Al-Hayek, in 2008, reviewed the literature and showed that between 30% and 100% of instances of detrusor overactivity will be missed if the patient is filled in the prone position [1]. It is counterintuitive to do urodynamics in the prone position as patients, by and large, suffer their symptoms when they are awake and up and about!

• How do we make urodynamics more acceptable to the doubters?

This can largely be accomplished by emphasising that, providing the philosophical and technical issues described above are dealt with, urodynamics are a relatively simple test with straightforward objectives. In addition to the statement on reproducing the patient's symptoms,

the urodynamicist should produce four statements in his or her report:

1. the detrusor activity during bladder filling
2. the urethral activity during bladder filling
3. the detrusor activity during voiding
4. the urethral activity during voiding.

These are termed the four diagnoses of urodynamics, although of course one would wish to have some information on bladder sensation and bladder capacity [2].

- Review of the existing evidence: although the value of urodynamics has not been determined by high-quality RCTs, where the quality of urodynamics has been assured, there are numerous case series in two particular clinical areas. The first shows how urodynamics predict outcome in women undergoing surgery for stress urinary incontinence. In this group of patients, detrusor overactivity during filling, more severe sphincter incompetence during filling, and poor detrusor contractility during voiding all predict worse outcome. Similarly, the objective demonstration of bladder outlet obstruction in men thought to have an enlarged prostate causing obstruction, improve the results of transurethral resection of the prostate. Similarly the demonstration of detrusor overactivity during filling, or detrusor underactivity during voiding, predicts less good postoperative outcome.
- Pressure flow analysis: Griffiths and colleagues [3] produced an excellent report for the ICS recommending the ICS nomogram for the diagnosis of benign prostatic obstruction. This supersedes all other nomograms, including the Abrams–Griffiths nomogram and the Schafer nomogram. There is no need to use any of the old nomograms, and use of the single ICS nomogram will allow comparisons between studies, which is vital in assessing new interventions.
- Using appropriate urodynamic tests for the individual patient: as the authors mention, there is a cascade of investigations from the screening test of urine flow studies and post-void residual estimation, through standard filling and voiding cystometry to video-urodynamics. To this should be added ambulatory urodynamics, best performed in regional centers where standard or video urodynamics have failed to show the abnormality in a patient whose quality of life is significantly compromised by their lower uri-

nary tract dysfunction. The issues around electromyography and urethral function studies are less clear but they have a well-established role in certain disorders, such as idiopathic voiding dysfunction in women and assessing urethral function in women with stress incontinence, respectively.

• *Urodynamics for the urodynamicist are a way of life!*

Questioning the significance of urodynamics is akin to questioning the depth of religious belief in a highly religious person. The urodynamicist may feel that RCTs to assess the value of urodynamics are unethical, as his or her lifetime's experience is full of multiple instances where urodynamics have changed patient management. Nevertheless, it may be necessary to accept the need for RCTs if there are persistent criticisms of urodynamics and their role in selecting patients for invasive management of lower urinary tract dysfunction.

References

1. Al-Hayek S, Belal M, Abrams P. Does the patient's position influence the detection of detrusor overactivity? Neurourol Urodyn 2008;27:279–286.
2. Abrams P. A simple method to teach about voiding disorders. BJU Int 2006;98:463.
3. Griffiths D, Hofner K, van Mastrigt R et al. Pressure flow studies of voiding, urethral resistance and urethral obstruction. Neurourol Urodyn 1997;16:521–532.

Tape Positioning

17

Michał Bogusiewicz and Tomasz Rechberger

Abstract According to current concepts, appropriate support of the urethra is crucial for female urinary continence. Reinforcement of suburethral structures by implantation of a non-absorbable tape under the midurethra is nowadays a first-choice treatment for stress urinary incontinence in women. The main mechanism of retropubic sling action relies on the angulation of the urethra on a fulcrum created by the tape. In the case of a transobturator sling, the urethral angulation occurs in only 24–50% of cured patients and continence is restored mainly as a result of urethral encroachment by the tape. Placement of the tape under the midurethra is associated with the best cure rate. However, a subset of patients may be also cured even if the tape is located outside this zone. Inappropriate positioning of the tape may increase the risk of postoperative complications. Development of voiding dysfunction or de novo urgency is more common if the tape is placed too tightly. Among several currently available techniques for tape placement, procedures utilizing a retropubic or transobturator approach are the most widely used. Regardless of the approach, tape location around the midurethra, creation of an adequate angle between the tape arms, and tension-free placement seem to be crucial for successful treatment outcome.

Keywords Midurethral sling • Stress urinary incontinence • Tape positioning • Ultrasonography

17.1 Theoretical Background of Midurethral Tape Action

Two pathophysiologic concepts of female stress urinary incontinence, namely the Integral Theory described by Petros and Ulmsten [1] and the hammock hypothesis proposed by DeLancey [2], set the background for midurethral sling functioning. According to the Integral Theory, continence is maintained due to an interplay between the pubourethral ligaments, vaginal wall, and pubococcygeus muscle. During effort, forward and backward forces produced by contraction of the pubococcygeus muscle and levator ani muscle, respectively, stretch the upper vagina enabling angulation ("kinking") of the urethra in a plane around the pubourethral ligaments. In this way the urethra is closed off. Thus, weakening of the pubourethral ligaments or laxity of the vaginal wall (the vaginal hammock) may result in stress incontinence [1].

The concept of the hammock hypothesis it that the urethra and vesical neck rest on a hammock-like supportive layer composed of the anterior vaginal wall

M. Bogusiewicz
2nd Department of Gynecology, Medical University of Lublin, Poland

G.A. Santoro, A.P. Wieczorek, C.I. Bartram (eds.) *Pelvic Floor Disorders*
© Springer-Verlag Italia 2010

and endopelvic fascia, which is laterally attached to the arcus tendineus fascia pelvis and levator ani muscle. During strain, pressure from above compresses the urethra against the hammock, closing its lumen. The instability of this supportive layer resulting from its damaged connections to the arcus tendineus fascia pelvis and levator ani muscle leads to stress urinary incontinence (SUI) [2].

Although other continence mechanisms such as contraction of the urethral sphincter and the "seal" provided by the urothelium and the submucosal vascular plexus play significant roles [3], it appears that reinforcement of the pubourethral ligaments and the suburethral hammock by implantation of a nonabsorbable tape under the midurethra is a highly effective way to surgically restore continence.

17.2 How Does the Midurethral Tape Work?

In 1995 Petros and Ulmsten [4], on the basis of the Integral Theory, developed a new minimally invasive anti-incontinence surgical technique, enabling suburethral tape positioning, which later led to development of the tension-free vaginal tape (TVT) technique [5]. Subsequently, numerous commercial kits using a polypropylene mesh sling following this principle have been marketed. According to the anatomical path taken by the tape they fall into two main categories: retropubic and transobturator. Moreover, several other procedures involving a prepubic approach or minislings (avoiding skin incision) have recently been introduced [6].

The mechanism of action of midurethral slings has been elucidated largely by means of real-time ultrasound. The retropubic tape (TVT) positioned under

the midurethra creates a fulcrum on which the urethra angulates (kinks). Several ultrasound studies have shown that this dynamic kinking and "knee angle" formation by the urethra is present in approximately 90% of cured patients [7–13] (Fig. 17.1).

Furthermore, during Valsalva maneuver the tape rotates towards the symphysis pubis, compressing the urethra and the surrounding tissue against it [7, 14, 15]. Placement of the tape does not change the mobility of the proximal urethra and, what is more interesting, the greater the preoperative urethral mobility, the higher the rate of TVT success [16]. Several studies indicate that TVT tends to transiently support the bladder neck, but the trend disappears over time [10, 14, 17–21]. It may be then speculated that restriction of the bladder mobility shortly after surgery results from the effect of healing or from less effective Valsalva maneuver due to pain or anxiety over "spoiling" the effect of the cure.

The mechanism of transobturator sling action is less obvious. Data relating to whether the transobturator tape (TOT) localizes to a more distal part of the urethra or in the same position as a TVT are contradictory [12, 13, 21, 22] (Fig. 17.1). Urethral kinking only occurs in 24–50% of patients who are continent after the transobturator procedure [12, 13, 23, 24]. According to Yang et al [23], the main anti-incontinence mechanism of this technique may be described as urethral encroachment by the tape. The phenomenon is seen on ultrasound study as a protrusion of the tape into the posterior wall of the urethra, with a transient narrowing of its lumen [23, 25]. Similarly to TVT, a temporary effect on bladder neck mobility occurs after TOT placement [21, 23, 25].

From a frontal view, the appearance of the retropubic and transobturator tapes is like a "V". The angle between the two arms of the tape at rest is smaller in

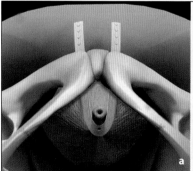 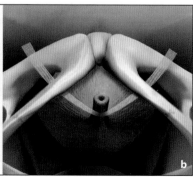

Fig. 17.1 Tape positioning with the suprapubic transvaginal (TVT) (**a**) and transobturator (TOT) (**b**) routes

a TVT (mean 116.3 degrees) than in a TOT, i.e an outside-in transobturator tape, and a TVT-O, i.e. an inside-out transobturator tape (mean 130.75 degrees and 137.84 degrees, respectively). However, on Valsalva maneuver, the angle between the two arms becomes flatter, averaging 138.9 degrees, and during retaining it closes to an average of 118.5 degrees, regardless of the mesh type [22].

If inserted correctly, the retropubic tape is located close to the high-pressure zone of the urethra [5]. Therefore, in the majority of cured patients, a positive pressure transmission in the middle portion of the urethra is observed during urethral pressure profilometry [10]. Moreover, the maximum urethral closure pressure and the urethral closure area appeared to increase after a TVT procedure [12]. No effect of TVT-O insertion on urethral pressure profile parameters was observed [12]. During cystometry, a postoperative increase of bladder volume at first sensation to void after TVT or TVT-O procedure was noted [12]. This finding may account for high rate of resolution of overactive bladder symptoms following a TVT procedure in women with mixed urinary incontinence [12, 26].

17.3 Does the Tape Position Affect Treatment Outcome?

From the theoretical point of view, placement of a tape precisely under the middle section of the urethra is essential for surgery to be effective. However, Dietz et al [27] reported that there is no association between tape position and subjective cure rate after TVT procedure. Correspondingly, in a series presented by Ng et al [28], among 31 cured women 9.7% had the TVT located in the proximal one-third and 22.6% in the distal one-third of the urethra. Furthermore, Lo et al [11] observed urethral kinking in five out of ten women with tapes implanted under the proximal urethra. It is probable that if the tape is situated relatively close to the midurethra, it may still work as a fulcrum. This explanation is supported by the fact that the pubourethral ligaments were discovered along the area between the 20th and 60th percentiles of the urethral length [29].

In some patients continence is restored even when a TVT is located close to the bladder neck and the urethra does not angulate during straining [11]. In these cases the tape is likely to work as a traditional pubovaginal sling by suspending the bladder neck and proximal urethra. In any case, in most cured patients the tape is positioned around the midurethra and this location produces the best outcome. Kociszewski et al [30] showed that when a TVT lays between the 50th and 80th percentile of the urethral length (measured from the bladder neck), the cure rate exceeds 90%, whereas location outside this zone is associated with treatment failure in more than one-third of patients. For proper functioning, the tape should remain at a certain distance from the urethral lumen. When this distance is greater than 5 mm, the risk of failure is increased five-fold, and when it is shorter than 3 mm, the risk of developing postoperative voiding dysfunctions or overactive bladder symptoms is significantly increased.

During straining, the TVT undergoes shape changes. Three variants of this dynamic shape change have been described. The first, when the tape is flat at rest and becomes curved (C-shaped) under straining, is associated with the highest success rate (98% of patients are cured and 2% improved). If the tape remains flat during an effort that suggests it is too far from the urethra, the cure rate is the lowest (50% cured, 25% improved, 25% failed). The third configuration, when the tape has a C-shape both at rest and during straining, suggests that it is placed too tightly, and the outcome is intermediate when compared to the other variants (75% cured, 15% improved, 10% failed) [30].

As in the case of TVT, the position of a TVT-O influences the cure rate. According to Yang et al [25], location of a tape under the proximal half of the urethra, a resting angle between the tape arms of less than 165 degrees, absent urethral encroachment at rest, and, further, persistent bladder neck funneling are independent risk factors for failure.

Unpublished observations from the authors' institution indicate that almost all failures of TOT procedure seen shortly after surgery are associated with placement of the tape close to the bladder neck.

Figs. 17.2 to 17.4 show different locations of tapes after outside-in transobturator sling. It is of great interest to know whether tapes change their position over time and, if this happens, whether this results in worse treatment outcome. It has been shown that TVT, together with surrounding tissues, migrates caudally in relation to the symphysis pubis, by about 1.8 mm

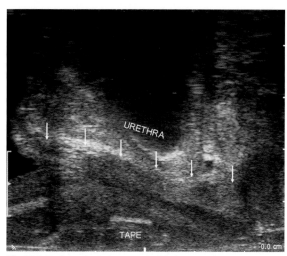

Fig. 17.2 Endovaginal ultrasound with linear probe. Longitudinal view. The transobturator tape was placed at the midurethra and the patient was continent after surgery

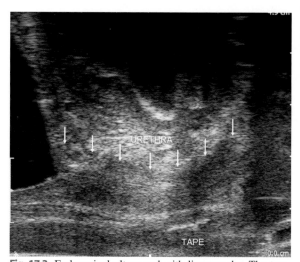

Fig. 17.3 Endovaginal ultrasound with linear probe. The transobturator tape was placed between the 50th and 80th percentile of the urethral length and the patient was continent after surgery

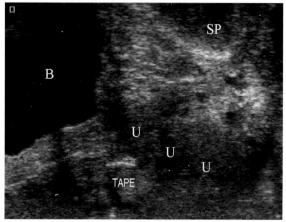

Fig. 17.4 Endovaginal ultrasound with linear probe. Longitudinal view. The transobturator tape was placed proximally (close to the bladder neck). Treatment failed

a year as reported by Dietz et al [19], or 1.7 mm over 3 years as found by Lo et al [11]. During Valsalva maneuver it tends to be pushed towards or even beneath the symphysis, together with the urethra and bladder, particularly in women who have undergone anterior colporrhaphy for prolapse concomitant with the TVT procedure [19]. However, the tape does not change its position in relation to the bladder neck, either at rest or on Valsalva maneuver [11, 21].

Hence, this tape descent may be attributed to worsening or recurrence of the prolapse rather then to real migration. As there is no evidence for shrinkage or alteration of TVT mobility over time [19], changes of tape location relative to the symphysis pubis are unlikely

to influence long-term treatment outcomes. One study concerning TOT showed that the tape remains in the same position over 2 years from the time of surgery [21]. On balance, although published data are based on a follow-up of 2–3 years, it seems that the tape position relative to the bladder neck and urethra is stable.

17.4 Tape Position and Postoperative Complications

A subset of patients develop voiding dysfunctions or de novo overactive bladder symptoms following midurethral sling procedures. Hypothetically, the risk of these complications is higher when the tape is positioned too close to the bladder neck, but it remains controversial if this really plays a role. Ducarme et al [31] showed that in patients with postoperative voiding dysfunctions the tape was located closer to the bladder neck; however, in cases of development of de novo urge incontinence it was closer to the urethral meatus than in patients without these complications. Nevertheless, these observations were not confirmed by others [21, 27]. It is much more likely that the risk of voiding dysfunctions and de novo urgency increases when the tape is inserted too tightly. In the study by Dietz et al [27], the incidence of these complications correlated with more cranial positioning of the tape. Kociszewski et al [30] only observed complications in patients with a distance of less than 3 mm between the tape and the urethral lumen. Furthermore, a

C-shaped appearance of the tape indicating that it was not placed in a tension-free manner was associated with six-fold higher risk of postoperative complications [30]. Similarly, after a TVT-O procedure, signs of tight tape placement, such as urethral encroachment at rest and a distance at rest of less than 12 mm between the tape and the symphysis pubis, were associated with development of voiding dysfunction [25].

Postoperative complications after TVT-O may also be related to inadequate repositioning of the tape arms. If, on Valsalva maneuver, the arms are too close to each other, the risk of voiding dysfunction substantially increases. Closer angulation at retaining is associated with de novo urge incontinence [22].

It is also apparent that voiding dysfunctions may develop in cases of intraoperatively unrecognized urinary tract perforation or urethral erosion by the tape [32, 33].

17.5 Techniques of Tape Positioning

Several different techniques for tape placement are currently available. Those that use a retropubic or transobturator approach are the most widely used. Although a number of retropubic and transobturator sling kits have been marketed, the procedures are all performed according to the rules described in the first reports. In recent years, mini-slings that avoid skin incisions, and the prepubic sling, have been introduced, but there is still not sufficient data on their long-term efficacy.

It is obvious that appropriate placement of the tape enables the highest success rate to be achieved. As there is no definitive intraoperative method of ensuring that the tape is positioned correctly, general principles such as midurethral tape location, creation of an adequate angle between the tape arms, and tension-free placement should be kept in mind while performing the sling procedure.

In all suprapubic and transobturator slings, the tape is introduced by means of specially designed needles or trocars (Figs. 17.5, 17.6). During the bottom-to-top retropubic technique, trocars are passed from a vaginal incision to a suprapubic exit site at the skin surface. The sagittal incision of the vaginal wall should start approximately 0.5–1.0 cm from the outer urethral meatus. The incision should be less than 1.5 cm long and should not extend over the bladder neck,

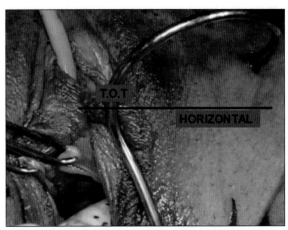

Fig. 17.5 Transobturator tape positioning (Outside-in technique)

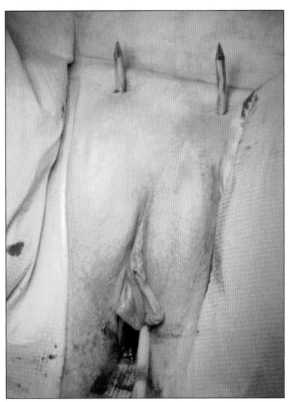

Fig. 17.6 Tension free vaginal tape positioning (Inside-out technique)

to avoid tethered vagina syndrome and/or voiding dysfunction. Laterally from the incision, a blunt paraurethral dissection 0.5–1.0 cm long is made on both sides, which enables identification of the inferior rim of the pubic bone. Then the tip of the needle is inserted into the prepared paraurethral incision and the needle passed through the retropubic space in close contact with the back of the pubic bone up to the skin incisions over the superior rim of the pubic bone. An accurate angle between the tape arms can be created when abdominal incisions are made approximately 4–6 cm apart (about 2–3 cm lateral to the midline on each side). When the procedure is performed on both sides, the tape creates a U-shaped sling around the urethra and can then be adjusted in a tension-free fashion. Starting the vaginal incision at the appropriate distance from the outer urethral meatus and introducing the needle in close contact with the back of the pubic bone maximizes the chance of appropriate midurethral tape placement. A straight probe can be introduced into the bladder to move the urethra and the bladder to the opposite side while the needle is inserted. It is widely accepted that cystoscopy is mandatory after placement of a retropubic sling [5, 43]. A top-to-bottom approach has been developed to get better control during passage of the needle through the retropubic space. The vaginal and skin incisions are performed in the same way as during the bottom-to-top procedure. The needle is passed from the skin incision towards the vaginal incision, with its tip in close contact with the posterior pubic bone [35].

The first transobturator procedure was described by Delorme [36]. As trocars are introduced through skin incisions lateral to the labium majus and inserted through the obturator foramen to a vaginal exit site at the midurethral position, this technique is termed 'outside-in'. In the transobturator techniques, appropriate tape location and angle between the tape arms depend mainly on identification of the correct point where the transobturator membrane should be perforated. Similarly to retropubic slings, the vaginal incision for the transobturator procedures starts 1 cm proximally to the urethral meatus and should extend to a distance of 1.5–2 cm. Then, the vagina is dissected laterally on either side of the urethra in a direction toward the ischiopubic ramus until the posterior part of the ischiopubic ramus and the internal obturator muscle can be palpated by a finger. By placing an index finger in the lateral vaginal fornix and a thumb in front of the obturator foramen, the lateral margin of the ischiopubic ramus can be identified. A skin incision should be made 15 mm lateral to the ischiopubic ramus on a horizontal line level with the preputium clitoridis. Insertion of the needle or trocar below this line may result in tape placement that is too proximal. The needle is first held vertically with the handle downwards

and, after crossing the obturator membrane, it is turned to a horizontal position, with the handle pointing medially. It is advised to use a finger to guide the tip of the needle into the vaginal incision, to avoid injury of the vagina or urethra.

The inside-out approach, described first by De Leval [37], uses specially designed needles called helical passers, and a steel winged guide which facilitates their passage through the dissection tract. The sagittal vaginal incision starts 1 cm proximally to the urethral meatus and is continued over a distance of 1 cm. The lateral dissection is carried out with scissors oriented on the horizontal plane with a 45 degree angle relative to the urethral sagittal plane, until it reaches the upper part of the ischiopubic ramus at the junction between the body of the pubic bones and the inferior pubic ramus. At this point the obturator membrane is perforated and the winged guide inserted into the dissected tract. The passers are pushed through the obturator membrane following the channel of the winged guide. Then, the handle of the device is rotated and simultaneously moved towards the midline until the handle is vertical to the floor.

The skin exit points are located 2 cm outside the thigh folds and 2 cm above the horizontal line traced at the level of the urethral meatus. With the transobturator approach, cystoscopy is not obligatory.

References

1. Petros P, Ulmsten U. An integral theory of female urinary incontinence. Experimental and clinical considerations. Acta Obstet Gynecol Scand 1990;69(suppl):153.
2. DeLancey JOL. Structural support to the urethra as it relates to stress urinary incontinence: the hammock hypothesis. Am J Obstet Gynecol 1994;170:1713–1723.
3. Ashton-Miller JA, DeLancey JOL. Functional anatomy of the female pelvic floor. Ann N Y Acad Sci 2007; 1101:266–296.
4. Ulmsten U, Petros P. Intravaginal slingplasty (IVS): an ambulatory surgical procedure for treatment of female urinary incontinence. Scand J Urol Nephrol 1995;29:75–82.
5. Ulmsten U, Henricksson L, Johnson P, Varhos G. An ambulatory surgical procedure under local anesthesia for treatment of female urinary incontinence. Int Urogynecol J 1996;7:81–86.
6. Rapp DE, Kobashi KC. The evolution of midurethral slings. Nat Clin Pract Urol 2008; 5:194–201.
7. Sarlos D, Kuronen M, Schaer GN. How does tension-free vaginal tape correct stress incontinence? Investigation by perineal ultrasound. Int Urogynecol J Pelvic Floor Dysfunct 2003;14:395–398.
8. Dietz HP, Wilson PD, Vancaille T. How does the TVT

achieve continence? Neurourol Urodyn 2000;19:393–394.

9. Masata J, Martan A, Kasikova E et al. Ultrasound study of effect of TVT operation on the mobility of the whole urethra. Neurourol Urodyn 2002;21:286–288.

10. Lo T-S, Wang AC, Horng S-G et al. Ultrasonographic and urodynamic evaluation after tension free vagina tape procedure (TVT). Acta Obstet Gynecol Scand 2001; 80:65–70.

11. Lo T-S, Horng S-G, Liang C-C et al. Ultrasound assessment of mid-urethra tape at three-year follow-up after tension-free vaginal tape procedure. Urology 2004;63:671–675.

12. Long CY, Hsu CS, Lo TS et al. Clinical and ultrasonographic comparison of tension-free vaginal tape and transobturator tape procedure for the treatment of stress urinary incontinence. J Minim Invasive Gynecol 2008;15:425–430.

13. Long CY, Hsu CS, Lo TS et al. Ultrasonographic assessment of tape location following tension-free vaginal tape and transobturator tape procedure. Acta Obstet Gynecol Scand 2008;87:116–121.

14. Masata J, Martan A, Svabik K et al. Ultrasound imaging of the lower urinary tract after successful tension-free vaginal tape (TVT) procedure. Ultrasound Obstet Gynecol 2006; 28:221–228.

15. Dietz HP and Wilson PD. The 'iris effect': how two-dimensional and three-dimensional ultrasound can help us understand anti-incontinence procedure. Ultrasound Obstet Gynecol 2004;23:267–271.

16. Fritel X, Zabak K, Pigne A et al. Predictive value of urethral mobility before suburethral tape procedure for urinary stress incontinence in women. J Urol 2002;168:2472–2475.

17. Viereck V, Nebel M, Bader W et al. Role of bladder neck mobility and urethral closure pressure in predicting outcome of tension-free vaginal tape (TVT) procedure. Ultrasound Obstet Gynecol 2006;28:214–220.

18. Harms L, Emons G, Bader W et al. Funneling before and after anti-incontinence surgery – a prognostic indicator? Part 2: tension-free vaginal tape. Int Urogynecol J Pelvic Floor Dysfunct 2007;18:289–294.

19. Dietz HP, Mouritsen L, Ellis G, Wilson PD. Does the tension-free vaginal tape stay where you put it? Am J Obstet Gynecol 2003;188:950–953.

20. Lukacz ES, Luber KM, Nager CW. The effects of the tension-free vaginal tape on proximal urethral position: a prospective, longitudinal evaluation. Int Urogynecol J Pelvic Floor Dysfunct 2003;14:179–184.

21. de Tayrac R, Deffieux X, Resten A et al. A transvaginal ultrasound study comparing transobturator tape and tension-free vaginal tape after surgical treatment of female stress urinary incontinence. Int Urogynecol J Pelvic Floor Dysfunct 2006;17:466–471.

22. Chene G, Cotte B, Tardieu A-S et al. Clinical and ultrasonographic correlations following three surgical anti-incontinence procedures (TOT, TVT and TVT-O). Int Urogynecol J 2008;19:1125–1131.

23. Yang J-M, Yang S-H, Huang W-C. Dynamic interaction involved in the tension-free vaginal tape obturator procedure. J Urol 2008;180:2081–2087.

24. Foulot H, Uzan I, Chopin N et al. Monarc transobturator sling system for the treatment of female urinary stress incontinence: results of a postoperative transvaginal ultrasonography. Int Urogynecol J Pelvic Floor Dysfunct 2007; 18:857–867.

25. Yang JM, Yang SH, Huang WC. Correlation of morphological alterations and functional impairment of the tension-free vaginal tape obturator procedure. J Urol 2009; 181:211–218.

26. Duckett JR, Tamilselvi A. Effect of tension-free vaginal tape in women with a urodynamic diagnosis of idiopathic detrusor overactivity and stress incontinence. BJOG 2006;113:30–33.

27. Dietz HP, Mouritsen L, Ellis G et al. How important is TVT location? Acta Obstet Gynecol Scand 2004;83:904–908.

28. Ng CCM, Lee C, Han WH et al. Use of three-dimensional ultrasound scan to assess the clinical importance of midurethral placement of the tension-free vaginal tape (TVT) for treatment of incontinence. Int Urogynecol J Pelvic Floor Dysfunct 2005;16:220–225.

29. Cruikshank S, Kovac R. The functional anatomy of the urethra: role of the pubourethral ligaments. Am J Obstet Gynecol 1997;176:1200–1205.

30. Kociszewski J, Rautenberg O, Perucchini D et al. Tape Functionality: Sonographic tape characteristics and outcome after TVT incontinence surgery. Neurourol Urodynam 2008;27:485–490.

31. Ducarme G, Rey D, Ménard Y, Staerman F. Échographie endovaginale et troubles mictionnels après TVT (tension-free vaginal tape). Gynecol Obstet Fertil 2004;2:18–22.

32. Tunn R, Gauruder-Burmester A, Kolle D. Ultrasound diagnosis of intra-urethral tension-free vaginal tape (TVT) position as a cause of postoperative voiding dysfunction and retropubic pain. Ultrasound Obstet Gynecol 2004; 23:298–301.

33. Vassallo BJ, Kleeman SD, Segal J, Karram MM. Urethral erosion of a tension-free vaginal tape. Obstet Gynecol 2003;101:1055–1058.

34. Ulmsten UJ, Johnson P, Rezaour M. A three-year follow up of tension-free vaginal tape for surgical treatment of female stress urinary incontinence. Br J Obstet Gynaecol 1999;106:345–350.

35. Deval B, Levardon M, Samain E et al. A French multicenter clinical trial of SPARC for stress urinary incontinence. Eur Urol 2003;44:254–258.

36. Delorme E. Transobturator urethral suspension: mini-invasive procedure in the treatment of stress urinary incontinence in women. Prog Urol 2001;11:1306–1313.

37. De Leval J. Novel surgical technique for the treatment of female stress urinary incontinence: transobturator vaginal tape inside-out. Eur Urol 2003;44:724–730.

Selection of Midurethral Slings for Women with Stress Urinary Incontinence

Joseph K.-S. Lee and Peter L. Dwyer

Abstract Midurethral sling procedures are currently the most commonly performed operations for stress urinary incontinence (SUI), and have proved to be effective and safe. Slings utilizing monofilament polypropylene mesh have the most favorable safety and efficacy results to date. Current data reflect concerns regarding the long-term efficacy of biological slings. Systematic reviews and meta-analyses of randomized controlled trials (RCTs) comparing a retropubic and a transobturator approach have demonstrated equivalence in early to midterm efficacy. The retropubic approach has a greater risk of bladder injury; the transobturator approach is associated with more vaginal perforations and groin pain, though fewer pelvic hematoma. For women with urodynamic stress incontinence (USI) and intrinsic sphincter deficiency (ISD), the transobturator route is less effective than the retropubic approach. Available RCT data are inadequate for definitive conclusions regarding the choice of slings in other important subgroups of patients, including those with recurrent incontinence, those undergoing concomitant prolapse surgery, the elderly, and the obese. The choice of stress incontinence procedure is based on the surgeon's experience as well as clinical grounds. The best results are often achieved with a procedure that works best in the individual surgeon's hands.

Keywords Intrinsic sphincter deficiency • Midurethral slings • Retropubic • Stress urinary incontinence • Transobturator

18.1 Introduction

There has been a significant shift in the focus of modern surgery for female stress urinary incontinence (SUI), from the proximal urethra and bladder neck, to providing additional support at the midurethra, without tension or significant compression, in order to improve continence without "fixing" the bladder neck. Petros and Ulmsten [1] based their proposed "Integral Theory" and sling position on Robert Zacharin's anatomical studies, showing the insertion of the pubourethral ligaments at the junction of the middle two-thirds and upper one-third of the anterior vaginal wall. Their sling placement used multifilament tapes which created a fibrotic reaction and were removed a few months later. However, because of the remodeling process, the ligaments were absorbed and failed to provide long-term success and support. Ulmsten et al, based on their earlier work with Petros, developed the tension-free midurethral sling [2]. Early

P.L. Dwyer
Department of Urogynaecology, Mercy Hospital for Women, Melbourne, VIC, Australia

results confirmed its ease of use as an ambulatory procedure [2], and subsequent long-term follow-up of up to 11 years has confirmed its long-term durability and relative safety [3].

Tension-free vaginal tape (TVT®; Gynecare, Somerville, NJ, USA) has rapidly gained worldwide acceptance due to low morbidity, decreased hospitalization, and equivalent success when compared to more traditional operations. Ward and Hilton reported the first randomized controlled trial (RCT) comparing 175 women having a TVT and 169 women having a Burch colposuspension [4]. Similar objective cure rates (defined as negative one-hour pad test) were reported at 2 years [5] (63% and 51% respectively, assuming those lost to follow-up were failures; 78% and 68%, respectively, carrying the last observed result forward), confirming the initial 6-month results. The equivalence of objective cure rates between TVT and Burch colposuspension was again confirmed at the 5-year follow-up [6] (33% and 26%, respectively, assuming women lost to follow-up were failures; 75% and 69%, respectively, carrying the last observed result forward).

Trends in surgical activity from the National Health Service (NHS) in the United Kingdom (UK) and Australia saw a rapid uptake of midurethral slings (MUSs) from 1998 and a corresponding decline in colposuspension [7]. The phenomenal success and popularity of TVT has perhaps itself led to the introduction of "clones" or "look-alike" slings with multiple modifications purported to appeal to a wide range of pelvic surgeons. However, the choice of surgery will vary according to the clinical situation and no one operation will suit all patients. For example, if infection is present, synthetic slings would be best avoided; or women having abdominal surgery for another indication may be better suited to a colposuspension or fascial sling.

18.2 Other Types of Retropubic Midurethral Slings

18.2.1 The Suprapubic Arch Sling (SPARC)

The Suprapubic Arch sling (SPARC®, American Medical Systems, Minnetonka, MN, USA) comes with a type 1 monofilament polypropylene mesh attached to a trocar designed to be inserted top-down

from abdominal wall, directing out towards a vaginal incision. SPARC's thinner trocar needle is to be passed under finger guidance top down, theoretically allowing the surgeon some control over the path of the needle, compared to the larger TVT trocars, which are passed from the vagina up to the suprapubic area, using the positioning of the instrument's handle for guidance.

Comparative studies between SPARC and TVT have yielded conflicting cure rates, although these appear to be lower in SPARC procedures [8–10] compared to TVT. Of the four reported RCTs [11–14], although two [12, 14] did not demonstrate a difference in bladder perforation rate, Tseng et al [13] and Lim et al [11] reported 4/31 and 4/61 perforations within the SPARC group compared to none and 1/61, respectively in the TVT group. Lord et al [14] reported the largest SPARC vs. TVT RCT, albeit with a short follow-up of 6–8 weeks, demonstrating higher incidence of urinary retention within the SPARC group, with more patients requiring a second operation to loosen the tape (6.5% vs. none). A meta-analysis confirmed that TVT outperforms SPARC in subjective cure rate (odds ratio (OR) 0.56 (95% confidence interval (CI) 0.35, 0.92); $P = 0.02$) and objective cure rate (OR 0.53 (95% CI 0.34, 0.82) $P = 0.005$) assessed by negative cough test and negative pad test [10].

18.2.2 Intravaginal Slingplasty (IVS)

Although designed as a bottom-up approach akin to TVT, the intravaginal slingplasty (IVS®,Tyco Healthcare, Mansfield, MA, USA) trocar comes with a blunt disposable tip and, more importantly, a multifilament polypropylene mesh with smaller pores of 55–65 μm and denser texture, consequently making it more stiff.

Meschia et al [15] reported the largest of the three RCTs [11, 15, 16] comparing TVT to IVS, totalling 190 patients with a two-year follow-up. Regardless of the definition of objective cure rates (any definition of continence, negative stress test, combining all three RCTs), TVT appears to have a higher rate of cure (OR = 0.51 (95% CI 0.3, 0.83); $P = 0.007$). A recent Danish report noted significant vaginal mesh exposure with the IVS tape, at a rate of 11.8% compared to none in a TVT group at 5-year follow-up. This comparative cohort study also demonstrated a significant decline in IVS cure rate compared to TVT over 5 years [17].

18.2.3 Self-made Slings

Several investigators [18, 19] have explored cutting and tailoring a piece of prepackaged off-the-shelf mesh and using it to perform a MUS, while adhering to the primary objective of achieving tension-free midurethral placement, sometimes using a Stamey needle carrier to facilitate sling placement. Such self-made suburethral slings have a financial advantage (reportedly only US $15) over more costly commercially packaged sling kits. A group from the University of California Los Angeles (UCLA) subsequently reported 5-year data from their cohort of 69 patients, confirming a reasonable subjective cure rate of 72%, with a further 16.4% who reported improvement [20]. Although some groups have reported good perioperative outcomes, including no bladder perforations or mesh exposure [19, 22], other groups have reported significant incidence of voiding difficulties (18%, [23]; 23% [21]) and mesh exposure (3% [21]). While further RCTs are needed to add maturity to the available data, these self-made slings can be made at low costs and therefore have an important place in the treatment of female SUI in developing countries.

18.2.4 Overview

Many other slings have been introduced, often faster than research could evaluate every modification. Further, long-term RCT data are generally not available, making it difficult to determine their relative efficacy and performance. Slings may well look alike, though they do have significant differences in design of trocars, mesh attachments, and mesh characteristics, and often come encumbered with a different learning curve. For polypropylene slings, differences in mesh variations include pore size, fibre size, tensile strength, and whether the material is bonded or knitted. An excess of vaginal mesh exposure and extrusions seen in the IVS tape, a multifilament microporous tape, has been described earlier. An excess of vaginal exposure/extrusions is also seen in Obtape (Obtape®, Mentor, Santa Barbara, CA, USA) [24, 25], a microporous unwoven thermally bonded tape.

The high risk of rejection or infection with the IVS and Obtape slings has shown that all slings are not equal. Careful evaluation of new slings or devices for safety and efficacy is needed before general intro-duction, as poor performance could be to the detriment of thousands of women.

18.3 Other Approaches for Sling Placement

18.3.1 The Transobturator Route

In an effort to decrease complications associated with passage of trocars through the retropubic space, the transobturator approach (TO) via the obturator foramina to deploy midurethral slings was developed in 2001 by Delorme [26]. In contrast to Delorme's outside-in approach, de Leval described an inside-out approach in 2003 [27]. Theoretically, these two approaches could reduce potential injury to the bladder, bowel, and other major vessels, compared to the retropubic approach (RP). Further, a wider vector of urethral support with a broad-based hammock could, in theory, minimise de novo urgency or postoperative voiding dysfunction.

18.3.2 Outside-in versus Inside-out

Although the outside-in technique requires more peri-urethral dissection, anatomical studies [28–31] suggest that the inside-out technique is associated with a more variable trajectory [30] and closer proximity to the deep external pudendal vasculature [19] and the obturator canal [28, 31], though the two methods share similar distances from the dorsal clitoral nerve [28].

Non-randomized cohort studies of 100 women comparing these two techniques have reported equivalence in efficacy rates at 12-months follow-up [32, 33] (86–92%). Three RCTs comparing both techniques reported similar efficacy at 3-months [34], 6-months [35] and 12-months follow-up [36]. Abdel-Fatah et al presented the 6-month results of their Evaluation of TransObturator Tape (E-TOT) study comparing 160 TVT-obturator (TVTO®,Gynecare, Somerville, NJ, USA), and 157 outside-in ARIS (ARIS®, Coloplast, Humlebaek, Denmark) procedures, demonstrating similar efficacy at 6 months (urodynamic stress incontinence (USI), 87.6% vs. 83.2%, P = 0.28) [35]. There appears to be more vaginal perforation within the outside-in group, of 5% versus 0% [34]. Data from a large Austrian transobturator tape (TOT) registry [37] reported an intraoperative bladder/urethral injury rate of 1%, the majority of which was in the outside-in group. Although the incidence of groin pain is reportedly up to 16% [38] for the inside-out technique, the RCT conducted by Liapsis et al [36] reported no difference in postoperative groin pain; however, But and Faganeli's RCT reported that the inside-out technique is more painful [34].

The jury remains out on whether the outside-in is better than inside-out technique.

18.3.3 Retropubic Versus Obturator

Comparison between the retropubic and transobturator approaches was evaluated in three meta-analyses [39–41], four updated RCTs [42–45], and nine further RCTs [46–54], though there are considerable variations in methodologies and outcome measures betweens these studies. RCTs are often powered for non-inferiority with a short- to medium-term follow-up. Nevertheless, meta analyses and subsequent RCTs [46–48, 50–54), with the exception of one [49], showed no significant difference in subjective and objective cure rates for SUI between the RP or TO approaches (Tables 18.1–18.3) [55–68]. Despite such equivalence, RCTs have short-term follow-up and are often not powered to examine important subgroups, such as patients with intrinsic sphincteric deficiency (ISD) who have the most severe form of SUI.

Analysis of randomized data comparing the RP and TO approaches confirmed that the TO approach comes with lower odds of bladder perforations (odds ratio (OR) 0.13 (95% CI 0.06, 0.27) [41]), pelvic hematoma (OR 0.25 (95% CI 0.05, 0.82) [69]), and symptoms of voiding dysfunction (OR 0.55 (95% CI 0.31, 0.98) [70]). Nevertheless the TO approach comes with a higher odds of vaginal perforations (OR 2.08 (95% CI 0.89, 4.95) [70]) and groin ache (OR 9.34 (95% CI 3.02, 28.9) [70]). Further, data also showed equivalence with regard to overall mesh exposure rate (0.8–4.8% vs. 1.5–5.9%) and de novo urgency rate (OR 0.89 (95% CI 0.54,1.86) [70]). It is important to note here that these recent RCTs were not powered to examine these subgroups specifically; hence conclusions, however suggestive, cannot be definitive at this stage.

In a recent large retrospective multivariate analysis of 1136 patients who underwent MUS [71], bladder perforations appear to be confined to inexperienced surgeons (< 50 slings). Other risk factors for bladder perforation include a history of previous cesarean section, colposuspension, body mass index (BMI) < 30 kg/m^2, use of local anesthesia, and presence of a rectocele. Combination of these risk factors gave good prediction (area under the curve (AUC) of 0.85 ± 0.06 from the receiver operator curve). Despite relatively low rates of bladder or urethral injuries [69], it remains prudent to confirm the integrity of the lower urinary tract by routine cystourethroscopy following any midurethral sling procedures. The presence of intravesical mesh in the long term can cause bladder pain, irritative urinary symptoms, recurrent urinary tract infections, and stone formation. Recognition of bladder perforation with trocar replacement appears to have no long-term sequelae.

The longest case series for the RP approach (TVT) is 11 years [72] and 2 years for the TO Obtape (Obtape®, Mentor, Santa Barbara, CA, USA) route [73], 3 years for TVTO [74], and between 2 [75] and 3 [76] years for Monarc (Monarc®, American Medical Systems, Minnetonka, MN, USA). It is prudent to obtain long-term data to confirm or refute these early findings from recent RCTs.

18.4 Predictors of Failure

Despite impressive cure rates for SUI, failure can occur, with re-operation rates that are similar for both the RP and TO approaches, ranging from 1.2% to 7% [41, 77]. It is unclear whether there are clinical factors that place a patient at higher risk for objective or subjective failure, since most RCTs are not powered for subgroup analyses. Combining data from heterogenous RCTs would also limit precision, reflecting inherent limitations of meta-analysis [78]. Nevertheless, it remains a clinical priority to ascertain clinical risk factors that could accurately predict surgical failures.

Identification of risk factors could facilitate preoperative counseling and potentially allow modification of the surgical approach to optimize patient outcomes.

Factors known to influence treatment success after surgery for SUI include ageing, medical comorbidities, incontinence severity, previous anti-incontinence surgery, recurrent SUI, concurrent prolapse

Table 18.1 RCTs of TVT vs. Monarc and SPARC vs. Monarc

Reference (first author)	Year	Cases	N	Follow-up (months)	Definition of cure	Objective cure (%)	Perforation (%) Bladder	Perforation (%) Vagina	Hematoma (%)	Groin thigh pain	Erosion Bladder	Erosion Vagina	Urinary tract infection	"Storage" LUT symptoms	"Voiding" LUT symptoms
Enzelsberger [55]	2005	TVT	52	15	Cough and USI	86.0	7.6	NR	5.7	NR	1.9	NR	5.7	9.6	7.6
		Monarc	53			84.0	0		0		1.8		5.6	11.2	5.6
Barry [46]	2008	TVT	107	3	Cough	78.0	8.5	NR	1.5	NR	1.2	NR	11.0	NR	11.0
		Monarc	80			82.8	0		0		5.4		9.0		10.3
Barber [48]	2008	TVT	88	12	Cough	92.4	7.0	1	NR	2.4	5.6	Not specified	NR	10.0	5.8
		Monarc	82			87.3	0	0		4.0	1.2			4.0	2.6
Schierlitz [49]	2008	TVT	67	6	USI	79.1	7.0	0	NR	0	NR	NR	21.0	NR	2.0
		Monarc	71			67.6	0	5		1			10.0		1.0
Freeman [52] (abstract)	2008	TVT	85	12	SUI ICIQFLUTs	37.6	NR	NR	NR	NR	NR	NR	NR	NR	NR
		Monarc	95			35.3	6.25								
Na [56] (abstract)	2005	SPARC	65	3	Overall	86.2	0.0	0	NR	NR	0	0	NR	NR	7.7
		Monarc	65			86.2	3.4	4.6			0	0			6.2
Wang [57]	2006	SPARC	29	9	Not defined	NR	0	0	3.4	NR	NR	3.4	NR	41.3	55.1
		Monarc	31				0	12.9	0		0	0		25.8	22.6

ICIQ FLUT, International Consultation on Incontinence modular questionnaire, female lower urinary tract symptoms; LUT, lower urinary tract; NR, not reported; SUI, stress urinary incontinence; USI, urodynamic stress incontinence

procedure, urethral mobility and function, and the presence or absence of concurrent urgency urinary incontinence (UUI) [79]. Retrospective analysis, using multiple logistic regression analysis, of over 1100 women who underwent MUS at our department has indicated that BMI > 25 kg/m^2, mixed urinary incontinence (MUI), previous continence surgery (ISD), and diabetes mellitus are independent risk factors for subjective failure, with concomitant prolapse operation conferring a protective effect [80]. While there may be significant inconsistency in the literature in this regard, with most studies being retrospective, poorly designed, and underpowered, and failing to control for confounding variables or lacking consistency in evaluation or follow-up [79, 81], data regarding some of these areas are emerging from randomized trials.

18.4.1 Intrinsic Sphincter Deficiency

Patients with significant urethral sphincteric impairment are recognized as a challenging population to treat, as they suffer from the severest form of SUI. Traditionally, ISD is defined as having Valsalva leak point pressure (VLPP) of less than 60 cmH$_2$O and/or maximum urethral closure pressure (MUCP) of less than 20 cmH$_2$O. Observational series of TVT [82] or TVTO [83] that stratified patients to VLPP < 60 cmH$_2$O or VLPP > 60 cmH$_2$O have shown lower cure rates (82% vs. 93.1%, P = 0.013) and higher risk of failure (OR 12.8 (95% CI 2.5, 60.8)).

In a non-randomized study comparing 97 and 39 patients who underwent SPARC and Monarc procedures respectively, Rapp et al [76] reported no differences in outcome, suggesting low VLPP < 60 cmH$_2$O may not be predictive of outcome. Data from three recent RCTs [44, 50, 77, 84, 85] designed to compare RP vs. TO, showed that VLPP was not predictive of outcome, although the total number of patients with low VLPP was only 50 [44, 84, 85], 30 [77, 85], and 32 [50]. Rechberger's [54] recent RCT reported a subanalysis of 85 patients with low VLPP < 60 cmH$_2$O (45 RP, 40 TO). More patients had failure after a TO approach compared to a RP approach (10/45 vs. 5/45). Concerns regarding the efficacy of TO MUS are also reflected in Abdel-Fatah's E-TOT RCT [35], with a subanalysis within their RCT of 43 patients with

MUCP < 30 cmH$_2$O. Irrespective of the route of TOT, women with low MUCP < 30 cmH$_2$O have a lower continence rate by urodynamic definition at 6 months compared to women with higher MUCP (58% vs. 90%, P < 0.01). The largest RCT to date examining the effectiveness of RP vs. TO specifically in ISD patients (VLPP < 60 cmH$_2$O and/or MUCP < 20 cmH$_2$O) studied at least 164 patients [49]. This RCT demonstrated a clear superiority in efficacy for the RP route in the treatment of female SUI with ISD, compared to the TO approach, as 1 in 16 women requested repeat surgery in the RP group compared to 1 in 6 within the TO group, with the risk ratio of repeat surgery being 2.6 (95% CI 0.9, 9.3).

The importance of urethral closure pressure was further highlighted in non-randomized studies that use a combination of VLPP and MUCP [86, 87]. These studies have shown higher failure rate (postoperative USI risk ratio (RR) 5.89; 95% CI 1.02–33.90) [86] and lower success (54.5% vs. 95.8%, P = 0.006) [87] when VLPP < 60 cmH$_2$O and MUCP < 42 cmH$_2$O were present in women undergoing the TO approach.

18.4.2 Effect of MUS on Lower Urinary Tract Function

Mixed urinary incontinence is common, with an estimated prevalence of 30% of all women with urinary incontinence, and is more bothersome than pure SUI [88]. Although MUS procedures are generally very effective in treating SUI, there is a concern these procedures might aggravate the urgency component or lead to de novo UUI, and consequent patient dissatisfaction.

Nevertheless, the effect of MUS on detrusor overactivity (DO) and MUI is emerging with favorable results. Rezapour and Ulmsten reported a subjective cure of 85% in women with MUI 4 years after TVT, although they excluded women with DO [89]. There are similar reports of substantial MUI resolution after TVT, although cure rates are typically lower than for pure SUI [90–93]. In a retrospective analysis of 276 women (99 TVT 52 SPARC, 125 Monarc) [94], those who underwent Monarc reported a lower de novo UUI rate of 8% at 9 months, compared to 17% for SPARC and 33% for TVT (P = 0.04). The authors also reported a higher rate of worsening of preoperative UUI for TVT or SPARC at 14–16%, compared to 6% for

Table 18.2 RCTs of retropubic vs. transobturator approach: I-STOP (CL Médical, Lyon, France), Obtape, IVS

Reference (first author)	Year	Cases	N	Follow-up (months)	Definition of cure	Objective cure (%)	Perforation (%) Bladder	Perforation (%) Vagina	Hematoma (%)	Groin thigh pain	Erosion Bladder	Erosion Vagina	Urinary tract infection	"Storage" LUT symptoms	"Voiding" LUT symptoms
Mansoor [58] (abstract)	2003	TVT	54	6	Overall	93.0	9.2	0	0	NR	NR	NR	NR	19	9.2
		TOT	44			96.0	0	0	0				NR	3	2.1
Riva [59] (abstract)	2006	TVT TOT	66	12	Overall	89.4	1.5	NR	0	0	1.5	Not specified	NR	22.7	1.5
			65			89.3	0	0	0	3.1	3.1			13.8	3.1
David-Montefiore [60]	2005	RP I-STOP	42	1	UDI	92.9	9.5	10.9	4.8	NR	NR	NR	NR	23.8	NR
		TO I-STOP	46			93.5	0	NR	0					19.6	
Daraï [42]	2006	RP I-STOP	42	10	UDI	88.5	NR		NR	NR	NR	NR	NR	20.8	NR
		TO I-STOP	46			86.5		NR						17.0	
Porena [61]	2005	TVT	47	13.4	Cough or patient report	93.6	2.1		4.2	NR	NR	0	NR	10.6	6.4
		Obtape	43			97.6	0		0			4.8		2.4	2.4
Constantini [62]	2007	TVT	73	31	SUI	71.4	2.7	0	1.4	NR	NR	0	0	14.0	9.0
		Obtape	75			77.3	1.3	5.3	0			4		11.0	6.7
Andonian [23]	2007	TVT	80	12	1-h pad < 2 g	86.0	13.8	NR	0	NR	NR	0	0	6.0	7.5
		Obtape	78			83.0	0		2.6			2.6	1.3	8.0	7.8
Rechberger [54]	2009	RP IVS 02	201	18	Cough	75.1	6.5	NR	2.0	NR	NR	2.0	7.5	8.6	5.0
		TO IVS 02	197			74.1	0		0			2.5	5.5	5.0	3.5

LUT, lower urinary tract; NR, not reported; RP, retropubic; SUI, stress urinary incontinence; UDI, urogenital distress inventory

Monarc (P = 0.02). The same group later reported a multivariate logistic regression model for 291 patients who underwent Monarc, bladder neck sling, SPARC, and TVT for prediction of DO [95]. Only sling type and maximum cystometric capacity on urodynamics are independent predictors of persistent DO post-operatively. TVT (OR 2.18 (95% CI 1.07, 4.44)) and SPARC (OR 1.51 (95% CI 0.61, 3.71)) are associated with higher odds of persistent postoperative DO compared to Monarc. This is consistent with results from meta-analysis of RCTs comparing RP to TO MUS, which showed a lower odds of de novo urgency (OR 0.89 (95% CI 0.54, 1.86)) [41] and overactive bladder (OAB) symptoms (0.55 (95% CI 0.35, 0.88)) [70]. Similarly, the TO approach also appears to have lower odds of voiding dysfunction compared to the RP approach (OR 0.55 (95% CI 0.31, 0.98) [41]; 0.43 (95% CI 0.25, 0.75) [70]). However, in a prospective randomised study of women with USI and ISD comparing the TVT sling to the TOT Monarc sling, the resolution and new development of OAB symptoms at 6 months postoperatively was not significantly different [96].

18.4.3 The Elderly

Ageing causes functional and anatomical changes in the lower urinary tract. The ageing lower urinary tract has a higher rate of detrusor overactivity, urgency incontinence, and ISD. Older women are also more likely to have had prior procedures for urinary incontinence and therefore may have higher rates of urethral fixation. Severe vaginal atrophy related to longstanding lack of estrogen support of the vaginal tissues in the older woman could potentially pose a greater risk of poor healing and erosion after vaginal incontinence surgery. It should come as no surprise that older age is associated with greater risks of post-sling surgery complications [97] and postoperative morbidity and mortality, with their higher incidence of medical comorbidities when subjected to more major open abdominal and vaginal surgical procedures in the past [98, 99].

Concerns regarding worse outcomes might have contributed to under-treatment of elderly woman in the past, with literature demonstrating under-representation of women aged over 70 years in SUI surgical trials [100], and elderly woman not receiving SUI surgery as often as younger woman [101]. A recent RCT demonstrated that at 6 months post-randomization, a group of

Table 18.3 RCTs of TVT vs. TVT-O

Reference (first author)	Year	Cases	N	Follow-up (months)	Defin of c
Ryu [63] (abstract)	2005	TVT	40	1	IQo
		TVTO	40		
Liapsis [36]	2006	TVT	46	12	Cough pa
		TVTO	43		
Meschia [43,64]	2006/ 2007	TVT	114	9	Cou
		TVTO	117		
Oliveira [65] (abstract)	2006	TVT	17	10	Over
		TVTO	28		
Zhu [66] (abstract)	2006	TVT	28	12.5	Subjec
		TVTO	27		
Zullo [67]	2007	TVT	35	16	Cou
		TVTO	37		
Laurikainen [38]	2007	TVT	134	3	Cou
		TVTO	131		
Rinne [45]	2008	TVT	134	12	Cou
		TVTO	131		
Palva [68] (abstract)	2009	TVT	131	36	Cou
		TVTO	125		
Araco [47]	2008	TVT	108	12	US
		TVTO	100		
Teo [51] (abstract)	2008	TVT	66	6	24-pa < 5
	2008	TVTO	61		
Tamussino [53] (abstract)	2009	TVT	171	3	Coug
		TVTO	178		
Karateke [50]	2009	TVT	81	12	Coug
		TVTO	83		

IQoL, Incontinence Quality of Life; LUT, lower urinary tract; NR reported; SP, suprapubic; USI, urodynamic stress incontinence

bjective cure (%)	Perforation (%)		Hematoma (%)	Groin or thigh pain unless otherwise specified	Erosion		Urinary tract infection	"Storage" LUT symptoms	"Voiding" LUT symptoms
	Bladder	Vagina			Bladder	Vagina			
94.8	0	0	NR	SP 7.5	NR	0	NR	NR	NR
100	0	0		12.5 thigh		0			
89	6.6	NR	0	NR	NR	2.1	6.5	10.8	NR
90	0		0			0	2.3	13.9	
92	4.0	NR	NR	0	NR	0	7.0	NR	10.5
89	0			5.1		0.8	4.3		6.0
100	NR	NR	NR	5.9	NR	5.9	11.8	21.4	17.6
85.7				14.3		3.6	17.8	17.6	3.6
92.6	NR	NR	NR	NR	NR	NR	NR	NR	NR
92.6									
91	11	11	2.8	0	0	0	6.6	9.0	2.8
89	0	0	0	2.5	0	0	2.5	0	0
98.5	0.7	0.7	0.7	1.5	NR	NR	8.0	2.2	NR
95.4	0	0	0	16.0			13.0	2.3	
95.5	NR	NR	NR	0	0	Not specified	14.2	1.5	0.7
93.1				0.8 abdominal pain	0.8		16.8	2.3	1.5
94.6									
89.5									
100	2.7	2.7	0	NR	NR	0.9	NR	7.4	13.9
83	0	0	5.6			3.0		6.0	17.0
78	0	0	NR	1.7 leg pain	5.3	Not specified	NR	5.1	4.5
83	0	0		26.4	2			11.3	1.6 clean intermittent catheterization
87	3.3	3.3	NR	NR	NR	NR	NR	NR	NR
80	0	0							
3.7	3.7	3.7	4.9	NR	4.9	Not specified	NR	7.4	9.9
0	0	0	2.4		2.4			6.0	7.2

elderly women over age of 70 who underwent immediate TVT surgery had significantly improved quality of life and patient satisfaction and fewer urinary problems compared to a control group waiting for the same surgery [102]. The rates of intraoperative and postoperative complications were similar to those observed in younger groups of women. Despite an age-related higher risk from surgery, invasive treatment of SUI in elderly women is better than no treatment.

Divergence in cure rates has been reported in comparative studies involving elderly woman who underwent TVT for SUI [103]. Cure rates ranged from 45% to 93% for elderly woman versus 73% to 95% for younger woman. Contributors to such differing results include considerable differences between the studies in length of follow-up, definition of cure, methodologies, and cut-offs, for ages ranging from 65 to 76 years. In an analysis of risk factors for failure, following a TVTO procedure involving 54 women with a mean follow-up of 9 months [104], age and previous incontinence surgery were identified as risk factors for surgical failure on univariate analysis, although their significance was lost following multivariate analysis. Studies analysing failure following TVT [105], or TVT and Monarc [106], have identified age as a risk factor for surgical failure. Larger studies with longer follow-up have not demonstrated age to be a risk factor following multiple logistic regressions [107].

A recent large retrospective study from our hospital reported outcomes involving 1225 woman (96 are more than 80 years of age) who underwent a midurethral sling procedure with a mean follow-up of 50 months [108] demonstrating an overall subjective cure rate of 85% (elderly 81%, younger 85%, P = 0.32), with no significant difference in cure rate between the retropubic and transobturator sling in the elderly group (82% vs. 79.3%, P = 0.75). The bladder perforation rate was similar between the two groups (3%). The hospitalization time was significantly longer in the elderly (1.6 ± 1.7 days vs. 0.7 ± 1.1 days, P < 0.001). It is our practice to routinely keep women over 80 years in hospital overnight, as opposed to using day surgery for MUS in younger women. Major perioperative complications were uncommon (1%). Of the patients who had an isolated sling procedure, 37% of the elderly and 9% of the young patients failed their first trial voiding (P < 0.001). However, the long-term rate of voiding difficulty was similar between the two groups (elderly 8% vs. young

6%, P = 0.21). The rate of de novo urge incontinence was similar between the two groups (7%).

Midurethral slings are effective in alleviating the burden of urinary incontinence in elderly woman. There are differences in reported cure rates following TVT in the elderly woman with SUI, with less data for TVTO or Monarc slings.

Older women undergoing midurethral sling surgery can expect continence rates that compare favorably to those of younger women.

18.4.4 The Obese

Women who are significantly overweight are more likely to have stress and urge urinary incontinence and failed stress incontinence surgery [109].

Two observational studies with short follow-up of 6 months [110, 111] have not identified BMI as a predictor of surgical failure following TVT. In contrast, a study of 760 women, with 5-year follow-up after TVT, has demonstrated a higher overall cure rate in women of normal weight compared to those with BMI > 35 kg/m² (81.2% vs. 52.1%, P = 0.0005) [112]. In a multivariate analysis of 138 women following TVT 5 years later [113], lower cure rates were also reported in women with BMI > 25 kg/m² (68.3% vs. 83.3%, P = 0.044). In our multivariate analysis of 1225 women, BMI > 25 kg/m² was again found to be an independent risk factor for surgical failure, confirming earlier reports, although there is no difference in failure rate between the type of slings for obese women [80].

18.5 Biological Slings and Exitless Slings

Suburethral autologous pubovaginal slings have been used since first described by Aldridge in 1942. The increasing popularity of minimally invasive midurethral slings has also led to the use of biological products in sling techniques. The purported advantages of using non-autologous xenografts include avoidance of harvesting, minimal dissection with lower perioperative morbidity, as well as possible lower rates of infection and erosion. Although reports are sparse, erosions do occur [114, 115].

Observational studies suggest Pelvicol (Pelvicol®, Bard CR, Covington, GA, USA) is inferior when compared with autologous fascial pubovaginal slings or TVT in the treatment of women with SUI. A comparative study reported 3-year outcomes of 48 women who underwent Pelvicol or autologous rectus fascial sling procedures, confirming an inferior cure rate (54% vs. 80.4%, P = 0.009) [116]. Women who underwent either autologous fascia pubovaginal sling or TVT reported lower scores for symptom severity, in a cross-sectional questionnaire survey of 173 women (81 autologous slings, 60 Pelvicol, 32 TVT) compared to those who had a Pelvicol pubovaginal sling [117].

The only RCT comparing retropubic Pelvicol to TVT studied 132 woman (74 Pelvicol, 68 TVT) with 3-year follow-up using a non-validated questionnaire. Assuming lost to follow-up data as failures (4 Pelvicol, 7 TVT), comparable cure rates were observed for Pelvicol (77.8%) and for TVT (79.1%) [118]. Similarly, there was no statistically significant difference in the rates of frequency, nocturia, de novo urgency, or dyspareunia between the two groups. A similar RCT comparing transobturator porcine dermis to transobturator synthetic polypropylene reported its 2-year outcomes (75 porcine dermis, 76 synthetic) in an abstract in 2008 [119]. Favorable results seen at 12 months (89.5% vs. 90.8%) were not replicated at 24 months, with the biological group reporting a higher failure rate 21.3% vs. 10.5%.

Another recent RCT comparing TVT, Pelvicol, and autologous fascial slings reported its interim results at the International Continence Society (ICS) meeting in 2008. Powered to have at least 76 women in each arm, using validated questionnaires, the authors reported a significant reduction in recruitment, possibly due to increasing popularity of TVT. In their interim analysis of 115 patients (30 TVT, 35 Pelvicol, 50 autologous) there was no detectable difference in clinical outcome (dry rate, improvement rate, re-operation rate, and self-catheterization rate) between TVT and autologous slings, although TVT utilized less operating time and postoperative in-hospital length of stay [120]. Pelvicol slings, however, had significantly lower improved and dry rates at 12 months (61% and 22%), compared to TVT (93% and 55%), or autologous slings (90% and 48%) (P < 0.0015). Not surprisingly, Pelvicol also had a significantly higher re-operation rate of 20% compared to 0% for TVT or autologous slings.

Reported data on the efficacy of Pelvicol slings for the treatment of female SUI, apart from one RCT, showed inferiority over existing suburethral slings. Data on other biological slings are too few to make a definitive clinical conclusion. The updated National Institute for Health and Clinical Excellence (NICE) Interventional Procedures Programme contains an overview of biological slings [121], echoing similar concerns about the long-term efficacy of the newer biological slings.

18.5.1 Exitless Mini-sling

The drive towards minimally invasive MUS has led to the development of "exitless mini-slings", the most popular of these being TVT-Secur (TVT-Secur®, Gynecare, Somerville, NJ, USA) [122] and MiniArc (MiniArc®, American Medical Systems, Minnetonka, MN, USA). The advantages claimed for these mini-slings over traditional RP or TO MUSs, mainly relate to avoiding the retropubic space, limiting the passage of materials through spaces containing known vessels, nerves, and viscera. Early studies of TVT-Secur and MiniArc reported short-term cure rates of 70.4–93.5% [123–125] and 75.7–90.2% respectively [125, 126]. A learning curve effect has been reported with TVT-Secur, together with a suggestion that it ought to be placed more tightly than usual TVT. The current immaturity of available data on long-term efficacy and complications precludes use of these devices outside of a clinical trial.

18.6 Surgeon-related Factors

Practice variations are often driven by surgical training, individual surgeon preferences, local norms, and potentially covert or overt manufacturers' influence. There is a paucity of data with regard to surgeon-related factors with regard to MUS selection. Large retrospective analysis has shown, not surprisingly, that surgeon experience has a direct influence on the rate of bladder perforation when using retropubic slings [71]. We suspect that this is true for other complications, e.g. pelvic hematomas, and probably also for success rates.

18.7 Summary

Midurethral sling procedures have become a routine urogynecological procedure and the cornerstone of anti-incontinence surgery, mainly because these procedures have proved to be durable, reproducible, safe, and effective. Not all slings have the same mesh or route of application. Slings utilizing macroporous monofilament polypropylene mesh have the most favorable safety and efficacy data to date. There are concerns regarding long-term efficacy with the use of biological slings. With follow-up to 12 months, systematic reviews and meta-analyses of RCTs comparing the retropubic or transobturator approach to midurethral slings have so far demonstrated equivalence in short-term efficacy. The retropubic approach attracts a greater risk of bladder injury, though if recognized and treated appropriately, this generally has no long-term consequences. The transobturator approach is associated with more vaginal perforations and groin pain, though less pelvic hematoma and voiding difficulty and possibly fewer overactive bladder symptoms.

There is emerging data that shows the transobturator route has less efficacy in women with intrinsic sphincter deficiency (VLPP < 60 cmH$_2$O, MUCP < 20 cmH$_2$O) compared to the retropubic route. The efficacy and safety of TVT are not compromised in the elderly or obese [109], based on observational data. There is less data available for the transobturator route for these subgroups and greater paucity of data for direct comparison between these slings. Retropubic slings may be preferable in young, physically active patients, the obese or those with ISD, as they have greater efficacy and their use is associated with less groin pain. A case could be made for using the trans-obturator sling in patients with previous retropubic operations or mixed urinary incontinence, and in elderly patients, to reduce the risk or difficulty of needle passage, as long as ISD is excluded. However, these patients may be found eventually to have improved cure rates with the retropubic MUS.

18.8 Conclusions

Women that respond best to midurethral sling surgery are those who have simple SUI, no ISD/MUI, no previous SUI or prolapse operations, and a mobile urethra.

The skill and experience of the surgeon, not only in performing the operation but in case selection, is an important factor in patient outcome.

References

1. Petros PE, Ulmsten UI. An integral theory of female urinary incontinence. Experimental and clinical considerations. Acta Obstet Gynecol Scand Suppl 1990;153:7–31.
2. Ulmsten U, Henriksson L, Johnson P, Varhos G. An ambulatory surgical procedure under local anaesthesia for treatment of female urinary incontinence. Int Urogynecol J Pelvic Floor Dysfunct 1996;7:81–85.
3. Nilsson CG, Palva K, Rezapour M, Falconer C. Eleven years prospective follow-up of the tension-free vaginal tape procedure for treatment of stress urinary incontinence. Int Urogynecol J Pelvic Floor Dysfunct 2008;19:1043–1047.
4. Ward K, Hilton P, United Kingdom and Ireland Tension-free Vaginal Tape Trial Group. Prospective multicentre randomised trial of tension-free vaginal tape and colposuspension as primary treatment for stress incontinence. BMJ 2002;325:67–70.
5. Ward KL, Hilton P on behalf of the UK and Ireland TVT Trial Group. A prospective multicenter randomized trial of tension-free vaginal tape and colposuspension for primary urodynamic stress incontinence: two-year follow-up. Am J Obstet Gynecol 2004;190:324–331.
6. Ward K, Hilton P on behalf of the UK and Ireland TVT Trial Group. Tension-free vaginal tape versus colposuspension for primary urodynamic stress incontinence: 5-year follow up. BJOG 2008;115:226–233.
7. Hilton P. Long-term follow-up studies in pelvic floor dysfunction: the Holy Grail or a realistic aim? BJOG 2008;115:135–143.
8. Gandhi S, Abramov Y, Kwon C et al. TVT versus SPARC: comparison of outcomes for two midurethral tape procedures. Int Urogynecol J Pelvic Floor Dysfunct 2006;17:125–130.
9. Paick JS, Oh SJ, Kim SW, Ku JH. Tension-free vaginal tape, suprapubic arc sling, and transobturator tape in the treatment of mixed urinary incontinence in women. Int Urogynecol J Pelvic Floor Dysfunct 2008;19:123–129.
10. Novara G, Ficarra V, Boscolo-Berto R et al. Tension-free midurethral slings in the treatment of female stress urinary incontinence: a systematic review and meta-analysis of randomized controlled trials of effectiveness. Eur Urol 2007;52:663–678.
11. Lim YN, Muller R, Corstiaans A et al. Suburethral slingplasty evaluation study in North Queensland, Australia: the SUSPEND trial. Aust N Z J Obstet Gynaecol 2005;45:52–9.
12. Andonian S, Chen T, St-Denis B, Corcos J. Randomized clinical trial comparing suprapubic arch sling (SPARC) and tension-free vaginal tape (TVT): one year results. Eur Urol 2005;47:537–541.
13. Tseng L, Wang A, Lin Y et al. Randomized comparison of the suprapubic arc sling procedure vs tension-free vaginal taping for stress incontinent women. Int Urogynecol J Pelvic Floor Dysfunct 2005;16:230–235.
14. Lord HE, Taylor JD, Finn JC at al. A randomized controlled equivalence trial of short-term complications and efficacy of tension-free vaginal tape and suprapubic urethral support sling for treating stress incontinence. BJU Int 2006;98:367–376.
15. Meschia M, Pifarotti P, Bernasconi F at al. Tension-free vaginal tape (TVT) and intravaginal slingplasty (IVS) for

stress urinary incontinence: a multicenter randomized trial. Am J Obstet Gynecol 2006;195:1338–1342.

16. Rechberger T, Rzeźniczuk K, Skorupski P et al. A randomized comparison between monofilament and multifilament tapes for stress incontinence surgery. Int Urogynecol J Pelvic Floor Dysfunct 2003;14:432–436.

17. Prien-Larsen JC, Hemmingsen L. Long term outcomes of TVT and IVS operations for treatment of female stress urinary incontinence: monofilament vs multifilament polypropylene tape. Int Urogynecol J Pelvic Floor Dysfunct 2009;20:703–709.

18. Rackley RR, Abdelmalak JB, Tchetgen MB et al. Tension-free vaginal tape and percutaneous vaginal tape sling procedures. Tech Urol 2001;7:90–100.

19. Rodríguez LV, Raz S. Polypropylene sling for the treatment of stress urinary incontinence. Urology 2001;58:783–785.

20. Rutman MW, Itano N, Deng D et al. Long-term durability of the distal urethral polypropylene sling procedure for stress urinary incontinence: minimum 5-year follow-up of surgical outcome and satisfaction determined by patient reported questionnaires. J Urol 2006;175:610–613.

21. Laurikainen E, Rosti J, Pitkäinen Y, Kilhoma P. The Rosti sling: a new, minimally invasive, tension-free technique for the surgical treatment of female urinary incontinence: the first 217 patients. J Urol 2004;171:1576–1580.

22. Lee JH, Kim KH, Lee HW et al. Distal urethral polypropylene sling surgical management for urodynamic stress incontinence in Korean women. Urol Int 2009;82:191–195.

23. Andonian S, St-Denis B, Lemieux M-C, Corcos J. Prospective clinical trial comparing ObtapeW and DUPS to TVT: one-year safety and efficacy results. Eur Urol 2007; 52:245–252.

24. Domingo S, Alama P, Ruiz N et al. Diagnosis, management and prognosis of vaginal erosion after transobturator suburethral tape procedure using a nonwoven thermally bonded polypropylene mesh. J Urol 2005;173:1627–1630.

25. Yamada BS, Govier FE, Stefanovic KB, Kobashi KC. High rate of vaginal erosions associated with the Mentor Obtape. J Urol 2006;176:651–654.

26. Delorme E. Transobturator urethral suspension: mini-invasive procedure in the treatment of stress urinary incontinence in women [French]. Prog Urol 2001;11:1306–1313.

27. DeLeval J. Novel surgical technique for the treatment of female stress urinary incontinence: transobturator vaginal tape inside-out. Eur Urol 2003;44:724–730.

28. Achtari C, McKenzie BJ, Hiscock R et al. Anatomical study of the obturator foramen and dorsal nerve of the clitoris and their relationship to minimally invasive slings. Int Urogynecol J Pelvic Floor Dysfunct 2006;17:330–334.

29. Spinosa JP, Dubuis PY, Riederer B. Transobturator surgery for female stress incontinence: a comparative anatomical study of outside-in vs inside-out techniques. BJU Int 2007;100:1097–1102.

30. Hinoul P, Vanormelingen L, Roovers JP et al. Anatomical variability in the trajectory of the inside-out transobturator vaginal tape technique (TVT-O). Int Urogynecol J Pelvic Floor Dysfunct 2007;18:1201–1206.

31. Zahn CM, Siddique S, Hernandez S, Lockrow EG. Anatomic comparison of two transobturator tape procedures. Obstet Gynecol 2007;109(3):701–706.

32. Debodinance P. Trans-obturator urethral sling for the surgical correction of female stress urinary incontinence: outside-in (Monarc) versus inside-out (TVT-O). Are the two ways reassuring? Eur J Obstet Gynecol Reprod Biol 2007; 133:232–238.

33. Lee KS, Choo MS, Lee YS. Prospective comparison of the 'inside–out' and 'outside–in' transobturator-tape procedures for the treatment of female stress urinary incontinence. Int Urogynecol J Pelvic Floor Dysfunct 2008;19:577–582.

34. But I, Faganelj M. Complications and short-term results of two different transobturator techniques for surgical treatment of women with urinary incontinence: a randomized study. Int Urogynecol J Pelvic Floor Dysfunct 2008;19:857–861.

35. Abdel-Fatah M, Ramsay I, Pringle S et al. (E-TOT) Study: a randomised prospective single-blinded study of two transobturator tapes in management of urodynamic stress incontinence: objective & patient reported outcomes. Int Urogynecol J Pelvic Floor Dysfunct 2008; 19(suppl 1):S2–S3.

36. Liapis A, Bakas P, Creatsas G. Monarc vs TVT-O for the treatment of primary stress incontinence: a randomized study Int Urogynecol J Pelvic Floor Dysfunct 2008;19:185–190.

37. Tamussino K, Hanzal, Kolle D. Transobturator tape for stress urinary incontinence: results of the Austrian registry. Am J Obstet Gynecol 2007;197:634e1–634e5.

38. Laurikainen E, Valpas A, Kivelä A et al. Retropubic compared with transobturator tape placement in treatment of urinary incontinence: a randomized controlled trial. Obstet Gynecol 2007;109:4–11.

39. Novara G, Ficarra V, Boscolo-Berto R et al. Tension-free midurethral slings in the treatment of female stress urinary incontinence: a systematic review and meta-analysis of randomized controlled trials of effectiveness. Eur Urol 2007;52:663–678.

40. Sung VW, Schleinitz MD, Rardin CR et al. Comparison of retropubic vs transobturator approach to midurethral slings: a systematic review and meta-analysis. Am J Obstet Gynecol 2007;197:3–11.

41. Latthe PM, Foon R, Toozs-Hobson P. Transobturator and retropubic tape procedures in stress urinary incontinence: a systematic review and meta-analysis of effectiveness and complications. BJOG 2007;114:522–531. Erratum in: BJOG 2007;114:1311.

42. Daraï E, Frobert J-L, Grisard-Anaf M et al. Functional results after the suburethral sling procedure for urinary stress incontinence: a prospective randomized multicentre study comparing the retropubic and transobturator routes. Eur Urol 2007;51:795–802.

43. Meschia M, Bertozzi R, Pifarotti P et al. Peri-operative morbidity and early results of a randomised trial comparing TVT and TVT-O. Int Urogynecol J Pelvic Floor Dysfunct 2007;18:1257–1261.

44. Porena M, Costantini E, Frea B et al. Tension-free vaginal tape versus transobturator tape as surgery for stress urinary incontinence: results of a multicentre randomised trial. Eur Urol 2007;52:1481–1491.

45. Rinne K, Laurikainen E, Kivelä A et al. A randomized trial comparing TVT with TVT-O: 12-month results. Int Urogynecol J Pelvic Floor Dysfunct 2008;19:1049–1054.

46. Barry C, Lim YN, Muller R et al. A multi-centre, randomised

clinical control trial comparing the retropubic (RP) approach versus the transobturator approach (TO) for tension-free, suburethral sling treatment of urodynamic stress incontinence: the TORP study. Int Urogynecol J Pelvic Floor Dysfunct 2008;19:171–178.

47. Araco F, Gravante G, Sorge R et al. TVT-O vs TVT: a randomized trial in patients with different degrees of stress incontinence. Int Urogynecol J Pelvic Floor Dysfunct 2008;19:917–926.

48. Barber MD, Kleeman S, Karram MM et al. Transobturator tape compared with tension-free vaginal tape for the treatment of stress urinary incontinence: a randomized controlled trial. Obstet Gynecol 2008;111:611–621.

49. Schierlitz L, Dwyer PL, Rosamillia A et al. Effectiveness of tension-free vaginal tape compared with transobturator tape in women with stress urinary incontinence and intrinsic sphincter deficiency. Obstet Gynecol 2008;112:1253–61.

50. Karateke A, Haliloglu B, Cam C, Sakalli M. Comparison of TVT and TVT-O in patients with stress urinary incontinence: Short-term cure rates and factors influencing the outcome. A prospective randomised study. Aust N Z J Obstet Gynaecol 2009;49:99–105.

51. Teo R, Moran P, Mayne C, Tincello D. Randomised trial of TVT and TVT-O for the treatment of urodynamic stress incontinence in women. Neurourol Urodyn 2008;27:572–573. https://www.icsoffice.org/ASPNET_Membership/Membership/Abstracts/Publish/46/000002.pdf (accessed 25 September 2009).

52. Freeman R, Holmes D, Smith P et al. Is trans-obturator tape (TOT) as effective as tension-free vaginal tape (TVT) in the treatment of women with urodynamic stress incontinence? Results of a multicentre RCT. Neurourol Urodyn 2008; 27:573–574. https://www.icsoffice.org/ASPNET_Membership/Membership/Abstracts/Publish/46/000003.pdf (accessed 25 September 2009).

53. Tamussino K, Tammaa A, Hanzal E et al. TVT vs TVT-O for primary stress incontinence: a randomized clinical trial. Int Urogynecol J Pelvic Floor Dysfunct 2008;19(suppl 1):S20–S21.

54. Rechberger T, Futyma K, Jankiewicz K et al. The clinical effectiveness of retropubic (IVS-02) and transobturator (IVS-04) midurethral slings: randomized trial. Eur Urol 2009;56:24–30.

55. Enzelsberger H, Schalupny J, Heider R et al. TVT versus TOT – a prospective randomised study for the treatment of stress urinary incontinence at a follow-up of 1 year. Geburtshilfe Frauenheilkd 2005;65:506–511.

56. Na YG, Roh AS, Youk SM et al. A prospective multicentre randomized study comparing transvaginal tapes (Sparc sling system) and transobturator suburethral tapes (Monarc sling system) for the surgical treatment of stress urinary incontinence. Eur Urol Suppl 2005;4:15.

57. Wang AC, Lin YH, Tseng LH et al. Prospective randomized comparison of transobturator suburethral sling (Monarc) vs suprapubic arc (Sparc) sling procedures for female urodynamic stress incontinence. Int Urogynecol J pelvic Floor Dysfunct 2006;17:439–443.

58. Mansoor A, Vedrine N, Darcq C. Surgery of female urinary incontinence using transobturator tape (TOT): a prospective randomized comparative study with TVT. Neurourol Urodyn

2003;22:488–489. https://www.icsoffice.org/publications/ 2003/pdf/088.pdf (accessed 27 October 2009).

59. Riva D, Sacca V, Tonta A et al. TVT versus TOT: a randomized study at 1 year follow up. Int Urogynecol J Pelvic Floor Dysfunct 2006;17(suppl 2):S93.

60. David-Montefiore E, Frobert J-L, Grisard-Anaf M, et al. Perioperative complications and pain after the suburethral sling procedure for urinary stress incontinence: a French prospective randomised multicentre study comparing the retropubic and transobturator routes. Eur Urol 2006;49:133–138.

61. Porena M, Kocjancic E, Costantini E et al. Tension free vaginal tape vs transobturator tape as surgery for stress urinary incontinence: results of a multicentre randomised trial. Neurourol Urodyn 2005;24:416–418. https://www.icsoffice.org/publications/2005/pdf/0008.pdf (accessed 27 October 2009).

62. Costantini E, Lazzeri M, Giannantoni A et al. Preoperative Valsalva leak point pressure may not predict outcome of mid-urethral slings. Analysis from a randomized controlled trial of retropubic versus transobturator mid-urethral slings. Int Braz J Urol 2008;34:73–81; discussion 81–83.

63. Ryu KH, Shin JS, Du JK et al. Randomized trial of tension-free vaginal tape (TVT) vs. tension-free vaginal, tape obturator (TVT-O) in the surgical treatment of stress urinary incontinence: comparison of operation related morbidity. Eur Urol Suppl 2005;4:15.

64. Meschia M, Pifarotti P, Bernasconi F et al. Multicenter randomized trial of TVT and TVT-O for the treatment of stress urinary incontinence. Int Urogynecol J Pelvic Floor Dysfunct 2006;17(suppl 2):S92–93.

65. Oliveira L, Girao M, Sartori M et al. Comparison of retropubic TVT, prepubic TVT and TVT transobturator in surgical treatment of women with stress urinary incontinence. Int Urogynecol J Pelvic Floor Dysfunct 2006;17(suppl 2):S253.

66. Zhu L, Lang J. A prospective randomized trial comparing TVT and TOT for surgical treatment of slight and moderate stress urinary incontinence. Int Urogynecol J Pelvic Floor Dysfunct 2006;17(suppl 2):S307.

67. Zullo M, Plotti F, Calcagno M et al. One-year follow-up of tension-free vaginal tape TVT and trans-obturator suburethral tape from inside to outside TVT-O for surgical treatment of female stress urinary incontinence: a prospective randomised trial. Eur Urol 2007; 51:1376–1384.

68. Palva K, Rinne K, Valpas A et al. Three years results of a RCT comparing TVT with TVT-O. Int Urogynecol J Pelvic Floor Dysfunct 2009;20(suppl 2):S74.

69. Morton H, Hilton P. Urethral injury associated with minimally invasive mid-urethral sling procedures for the treatment of stress urinary incontinence: a case series and systematic literature search. BJOG 2009;116:1120–1126.

70. Novara G, Galfano A, Boscolo-Berto R et al. Complication rates of tension-free midurethral slings in the treatment of female stress urinary incontinence: a systematic review and meta-analysis of randomized controlled trials comparing tension-free midurethral tapes to other surgical procedures and different devices. Eur Urol 2008;53:288–308.

71. Stav K, Dwyer PL, Rosamilia A et al. Risk factors for trocar injury to the bladder during mid urethral sling procedures. J Urol 2009;182:174–179.

72. Nilsson CG, Palva K, Rezapour M, Falconer C. Eleven years prospective follow-up of the tension-free vaginal tape

procedure for treatment of stress urinary incontinence. Int Urogynecol J Pelvic Floor Dysfunct 2008;19:1043–1047.

73. Juma S, Brito CG. Transobturator tape (TOT): two years follow-up. Neurourol Urodyn 2007;26:37–41.

74. Waltregny D, Gaspar Y, Reul O et al. TVT-O for the treatment of female stress urinary incontinence: results of a prospective study after a 3-year minimum follow-up. Eur Urol 2008;53:401–410.

75. Deridder D, Jacquetin B, Fischer A et al. Prospective multicentre trial of monarc transobturator sling for stress incontinence: 24 month functional data. Eur Urol 2006;5(2 suppl):267; abstract 978.

76. Rapp DE, Govier FE, Kobashi KC. Outcomes following mid-urethral sling placement in patients with intrinsic sphincteric deficiency: comparison of Sparc and Monarc slings. Int Braz J Urol 2009;35:68–75; discussion 75.

77. Barber MD, Kleeman S, Karram MM et al. Risk factors associated with failure 1 year after retropubic or transobturator midurethral slings. Am J Obstet Gynecol 2008;199:666.e1–7.

78. Shrier I, Platt RW, Steele RJ. Mega-trials vs. meta-analysis: precision vs. heterogeneity? Contemp Clin Trials 2007; 28:324–328.

79. Schafer W, Abrams P, Liao L et al. Good urodynamic practices: uroflowmetry, filling cystometry, and pressure-flow studies. Neurourol Urodyn 2002;21:261–274.

80. Stav K, Dwyer PL, Rosamilia A et al. Risk factors of treatment failure of midurethral sling procedures for women with urinary stress incontinence. Int Urogynecol J Pelvic Floor Dysfunct 2010;21:149-155.

81. Smith ARB, Daneshgari F, Dmochowski R et al. Surgery for urinary incontinence in women. In: Abrams P, Cordozo L, Koury S, Wein A (eds) 3rd Consultation on incontinence, 3 edn. Health Publication Ltd, Paris, 2005, pp 1297–1370.

82. Paick JS, Ku JH, Shin JW et al. Tension-free vaginal tape procedure for urinary incontinence with low Valsalva leak point pressure. J Urol 2004;172:1370–1373.

83. O'Connor RC, Nanigian DK, Lyon MB et al. Early outcomes of mid-urethral slings for female stress urinary incontinence stratified by Valsalva leak point pressure. Neurourol Urodyn 2006;25:685–688.

84. Costantini E, Lazzeri M, Giannantoni A et al. Preoperative Valsalva leak point pressure may not predict outcome of mid-urethral slings. Analysis from a randomized controlled trial of retropubic versus transobturator mid-urethral slings. Int Braz J Urol 2008;34(1):73–81; discussion 81–83.

85. Chen CC, Rooney CM, Paraiso MF et al. Leak point pressure does not correlate with incontinence severity or bother in women undergoing surgery for urodynamic stress incontinence. Int Urogynecol J Pelvic Floor Dysfunct 2008;19:1193–1198.

86. Miller JJ, Botros SM, Akl MN et al. Is transobturator tape as effective as tension-free vaginal tape in patients with borderline maximum urethral closure pressure? Am J Obstet Gynecol 2006;195:1799–1804.

87. Guerette NL, Bena JF, Davila GW. Transobturator slings for stress incontinence: using urodynamic parameters to predict outcomes. Int Urogynecol J Pelvic Floor Dysfunct 2008;19:97–102.

88. Dooley Y, Lowenstein L, Kenton K et al. Mixed incontinence is more bothersome than pure incontinence subtypes. Int Urogynecol J Pelvic Floor Dysfunct 2008;19:1359–1362.

89. Rezapour M, Ulmsten U. Tension-Free Vaginal Tape (TVT) in women with mixed urinary incontinence – a long-term follow-up. Int Urogynecol J Pelvic Floor Dysfunct 2001; 12(suppl 2):S15–S18.

90. Ankardal M, Heiwall B, Lausten-Thomsen N et al. Short- and long-term results of the tension-free vaginal tape procedure in the treatment of female urinary incontinence. Acta Obstet Gynecol Scand 2006;85:986–992.

91. Chene G, Amblard J, Tardieu AS et al. Long-term results of tension-free vaginal tape (TVT) for the treatment of female urinary stress incontinence. Eur J Obstet Gynecol Reprod Biol 2007;134:87–94.

92. Deffieux X, Donnadieu AC, Porcher R et al. Long-term results of tension-free vaginal tape for female urinary incontinence: follow up over 6 years. Int J Urol 2007;14:521–526.

93. Doo CK, Hong B, Chung BJ et al. Five-year outcomes of the tension-free vaginal tape procedure for treatment of female stress urinary incontinence. Eur Urol 2006;50:333–338.

94. Botros SM, Miller JJ, Goldberg RP et al. Detrusor overactivity and urge urinary incontinence following trans obturator versus midurethral slings. Neurourol Urodyn 2007; 26:42–45.

95. Gamble TL, Botros SM, Beaumont JL et al. Predictors of persistent detrusor overactivity after transvaginal sling procedures. Am J Obstet Gynecol 2008;199:696.e1–696.e7.

96. Schierlitz L, Dwyer PL, Rosamilia A et al. A prospective analysis of the effect of TVT retropubic and Monarc transobturator sling on lower urinary tract symptoms (LUTS) in women with urodynamics stress incontinence (USI) and intrinsic sphincter deficiency (ISD). Int Urogynecol J Pelvic Floor Dysfunct 2008;19:s43.

97. Anger JT, Litwin MS, Wang Q et al. The effect of age on outcomes of sling surgery for urinary incontinence. J Am Geriatr Soc 2007;55:1927–1931.

98. Sung VW, Weitzen S, Sokol ER et al. Effect of patient age on increasing morbidity and mortality following urogynecologic surgery. Am J Obstet Gynecol 2006;194:1411–1417.

99. Sultana CJ, Campbell JW, Pisanelli WS et al. Morbidity and mortality of incontinence surgery in elderly women: an analysis of medicare data. Am J Obstet Gynecol 1997; 176:344–348.

100. Morse AN, Labin LC, Young SB et al. Exclusion of elderly women from published randomized trials of stress incontinence surgery. Obstet Gynecol 2004;104:498–503.

101. Shah AD, Kohli N, Rajan SS, Hoyte L. The age distribution, rates, and types of surgery for stress urinary incontinence in the USA. Int Urogynecol J Pelvic Floor Dysfunct 2008;19:89–96.

102. Campeau L, Tu LM, Lemieux MC et al. A multicenter, prospective, randomized clinical trial comparing tension-free vaginal tape surgery and no treatment for the management of stress urinary incontinence in elderly women. Neurourol Urodyn 2007;26:990–994.

103. Gerten KA , Markland AD , Lloyd LK, Richter HE. Prolapse and incontinence surgery in older women. J Urol 2008;179:2111–2118.

104. Chen HY, Yeh LS, Chang WC, Ho M. Analysis of risk factors associated with surgical failure of inside-out transobturator vaginal tape for treating urodynamic stress inconti-

nence. Int Urogynecol J Pelvic Floor Dysfunct 2007; 18:443–447.

105. Cetinel B, Demirkesen O, Onal B et al. Are there any factors predicting the cure and complication rates of tension-free vaginal tape? Int Urogynecol J Pelvic Floor Dysfunct 2004;15:188–193.

106. Barber MD, Kleeman S, Karram MM et al. Risk factors associated with failure 1 year after retropubic or transobturator midurethral slings. Am J Obstet Gynecol 2008; 199:666.e1–7.

107. Koops SE, Bisseling TM, van Brummen HJ et al. What determines a successful tension-free vaginal tape? A prospective multicentre cohort study: results from the Netherlands TVT database. Am J Obstet Gynecol 2006;194:65–74.

108. Stav K, Dwyer PL, Rosamilia A et al. Mid urethral sling procedures for stress urinary incontinence are effective and safe in women over 80 years of age. Neurol Urodyn 2009; in press.

109. Dwyer PL, Lee ET, Hay DM. Obesity and urinary incontinence in women. Br J Obstet Gynecol 1988;95:91–96.

110. Rafii A, Darai E, Haab F et al. Body mass index and outcome of tension-free vaginal tape. Eur Urol 2003;43:288–292.

111. Ku JH, Oh JG, Shin JW et al. Outcome of mid-urethral sling procedures in Korean women with stress urinary incontinence according to body mass index. Int J Urol 2006;13:379–384.

112. Hellberg D, Holmgren C, Lanner L, Nilsson S. The very obese woman and the very old woman: tension-free vaginal tape for the treatment of stress urinary incontinence. Int Urogynecol J Pelvic Floor Dysfunct 2007;18:423–429.

113. Lee KS, Choo MS, Doo CK et al. The long term (5-years) objective TVT success rate does not depend on predictive factors at multivariate analysis: a multicentre retrospective study. Eur Urol 2008;53:176–182.

114. Webster TM, Gerridzen RG. Urethral erosion following autologous rectus fascial pubovaginal sling. Can J Urol 2003;10:2068–2069.

115. Rudnicki M. Biomesh (Pelvicol®) erosion following repair of anterior vaginal wall prolapse. J Pelvic Floor Dysfunct 2007;18:693–695.

116. Giri SK, Hickey JP, Sil D et al. Long-term results of pubovaginal sling surgery using acellular cross-linked porcine dermis in the treatment of urodynamic stress incontinence. J Urol 2006;175:1788–1792.

117. Morgan DM, Dunn RL, Fenner DE et al. Comparative analysis of urinary incontinence severity after autologous fascia pubovaginal sling, pubovaginal sling and tension-free vaginal tape. J Urol 2007;177:604–609.

118. Adbel-Fattah M, Barrington JW, Arunkalaivanan AS. Pelvicol pubovaginal sling versus tension-free vaginal tape for treatment of urodynamic stress incontinence: a prospective randomised 3-year follow-up study. Eur Urol 2004; 46:629–635.

119. Riva D, Baccichet R, Paparella L et al. Synthetic versus biological trans-obturator sling for stress urinary incontinence: a randomized study. Int Urogynecol J Pelvic Floor Dysfunct 2008;19(suppl 1):S1.

120. Guerrero K, Whareham K, Watkins A et al. A randomised control trial comparing TVT, pelvicol and autologous fascial slings for the management of stress urinary incontinence in women. Neurourol Urodyn 2008;27:571. https://www.icsoffice.org/ASPNET_Membership/Membership/Abstracts/Publish/46/000001.pdf (accessed 25 september 2009).

121. National Institute for Health and Clinical Excellence. Interventional Procedures Programme. Insertion of biological slings for stress urinary incontinence in women. National Institute for Health and Clinical Excellence, London, 2005. www.nice.org.uk/nicemedia/pdf/ip/IPG154guidance.pdf (accessed 25 September 2009).

122. Debodinance P, Lagrange E, Amblard J et al. TVT-Secur: more and more minimally invasive. Preliminary prospective study of 110 cases. J Gynecol Obstet Biol Reprod 2008;37:229–236.

123. Neuman M. Perioperative complications and early follow up with 100 TVT-Secur procedures. J Minim Invasive Gynecol 2008;15:480–484.

124. Meschia M, Barbacini P, Ambrogi V et al. TVT-Secur: a minimally invasive procedure for the treatment of primary stress incontinence. One year data from a multicentre prospective trial. Int Urogynecol J Pelvic Floor Dysfunct 2009;20:313–317.

125. Jiminez Calvo J, Hualde Alfaro A, Raigoso Ortega O et al. Our experience with mini tapes (TVT Secur and MiniArc) in the surgery for stress incontinence. Actas Urol Esp 2008; 32:1013–1018.

126. Debodinance P, Delporte P. MiniArc. Preliminary prospective study on 72 cases. J Gynecol Obstet Bio Reprod 2009;38:144–148.

Injectable Biomaterials

19

Pierpaolo Curti

Abstract Stress urinary incontinence (SUI) affects a large proportion of middle-aged and elderly women, considerably lowering their quality of life and causing major economic costs to society. Intra-urethral injections with bulking agents are used as an alternative to the traditional surgical procedures. Continuous advances in materials technology made available many urethral bulking agents.

In an attempt to improve the long-term outcome, newer and more durable substances have been investigated. The chapter describes different injection techniques performed under general, locoregional, or local anesthesia, according to the surgeon's preference. The complication rates of SUI injection therapy are acceptably low. The technique can be considered a useful option only for patients with comorbidity precluding anaesthesia. Regarding efficacy, most of the published studies analyzed a small number of patients with short follow-up periods.

Keywords Biocompatible materials • Bulking agent • Injectable Biomaterials • Stress urinary incontinence • Urethral sphincter

19.1 Introduction

Stress urinary incontinence (SUI) affects a large proportion of middle-aged and elderly women, considerably lowering their quality of life and causing major economic costs to society. When all conservative means are ineffective, surgical treatment is required; options include open or laparoscopic retropubic suspension, bladder neck needle suspension, suburethral sling procedures, or periurethral/transurethral injection of bulking agents. Tension-free tapes are considered minimally invasive procedures, yielding a lesser degree of discomfort and a faster return to normal daily activities for the patients, but they still require the use of the operating room, troncular anaesthesia, and an overnight hospital stay in most instances. Intra-urethral injections with bulking agents have been used as an alternative to the traditional surgical procedures, with results, due to the different characteristics of the bulking agents used varying (biocompatibility, systemic allergic reaction, and permanence in the tissue) [1].

19.2 Injectable Biomaterials

Continuous advances in materials technology made available many urethral bulking agents [1].

The first report concerning urethral injection, using sodium morrhuate, was in 1938 [2].

The 1980s saw the advent of polytetrafluoroethylene

P. Curti
Urology Clinic, Department of Surgery, A.O.U.I.,
Policlinic Hospital, Verona, Italy

(PFTE, Teflon – Polytef), produced by the pyrolysis of Teflon. The paste used for injection therapy was a mixture of PTFE, glycerin and polysorbate [3].

The agents more commonly used in the 1990s were glutaraldehyde cross-linked (GAX) bovine collagen, silicone, and autologous tissues, such as fat or cartilage.

GAX bovine collagen (Contigen®) is formed by cross-linking bovine dermal collagen with glutaraldehyde. The GAX-collagen contains at least 95% of type I collagen and 1–5% of type III collagen linked with glutaraldehyde and dispersed in phosphate-buffered physiological saline [4].

Silicon particles (Macroplastique®) is a soft tissue bulking agent, consisting of soft, flexible, highly-textured irregularly shaped implants of heat-vulcanized polydimethylsiloxane (a solid silicone elastomer) suspended in a bio-excretable carrier gel. The carrier gel is a pharmaceutical grade, water-soluble, low molecular weight polyvinylpyrrolidone (PVP or povidone) hydrogel, which is absorbed by the reticuloendothelial system and excreted unchanged in the urine. Polydimethylsiloxane elastomer and PVP have favorable biocompatibility properties. Polydimethylsiloxane is well tolerated by the cellular immune system and is non-genotoxic, non-carcinogenic, and non-teratogenic [5].

Porcine dermal implant (Permacol™), in contrast to GAX collagen, is porcine collagen rather being from a bovine source, so its biocompatibily is very high. Permacol™ has been licensed for permanent implantation into humans since March 1998. The material is maintained in its three-dimensional structure rather than being reconstituted. Its structural architecture is very similar to human dermis and it is readily colonized by host cells and blood vessels [2].

Autologous tissues such as fat and cartilage have also been used in the past for this purpose [6]. Autologous fat has been used for cosmetic and defect reconstruction since the 1890s but was first introduced in 1989 to treat urinary incontinence. It is an ideal bulking agent because it is biocompatible, easily accessible, and inexpensive [7].

The fat is harvested with a 60 mL syringe and a 16 gauge needle applied to the fatty subcutaneous space of the abdomen, while moved back and forth in a radial direction, exerting a negative pressure. Filling the syringe with saline and placing it in a vertical position, the fat floats to the top and the excess of saline is ejected.

Histological studies show that some fat integrates as a graft, while the remainder is reabsorbed and eventually replaced by connective tissue.

The ultimate long-term survival of autotransplanted adipose cells is unpredictable; therefore, the long-term success of this procedure varies in relation to fat reabsorption and the number of injections over time. Using magnetic resonance, some authors have demonstrated a 55% volume loss 6 months after fat injection, and no residual fat volume beyond 6 months. Other authors have reported a survival rate for transplanted fat cells of 20–30% after one year. The brief viability of the fat probably depends on an insufficient neovascularization that begins along the periphery of the graft but is never adequate at its center.

To improve graft survival, some authors have suggested mixing the harvested fat with Ringer's solution or insulin, but no method has been shown to consistently improve the outcome. For this reason, to maintain the desired volume, some surgeons have transplanted 50% more fat than they believe necessary [8].

Looking for the ideal substance for paraurethral injections, Atala and colleagues in 1993 published their experience regarding the effect of injectable chondrocytes in vivo [9].

Chondrocytes, isolated from biopsy of the external pinna of the patient's ear, are expanded in tissue culture media in vitro. The harvest of auricular cells is generally succesful, and culture of sufficient cells for transplant takes 7 weeks. Surplus cells, useful for additional injection in case of an incomplete result, are preserved by freezing.

Calcium alginate gel, a suspension of alginate, a natural polysaccharide in brown seaweed, and calcium solution have been used as a synthetic substrate to create an injectable material with chondrocytes and to mantain unaltered architecture of the cartilage. Alginate undergoes hydrolytic biodegradation over time, according to the concentration of each of the polysaccharides, leaving space for the cartilage matrix to replace alginate by growth of new cartilage, which maintains the volume of the original injection [10].

Chondrocyte formation was not noted in patients who had treatment failure, whereas patients who were cured had a biocompatible region of engineered autologous tissue present rather than foreign materials.

However, there have been no further reports on the use of autologous chondrocytes for SUI in recent years.

More recently, agents with new profiles have been introduced into clinical practice.

Coaptite consists of calcium hydroxylapatite (CaHA) spherical particles and an aqueous (carboxymethylcellulose) gel carrier. CaHA is a principal constituent of human bone and teeth. Exogenous CaHA has been used in orthopedic and dental applications, in addition to soft-tissue bulking, including vocal cord, and cosmetic facial and ureteral orifice augmentation. The synthetically produced CaHA particles range in diameter from 75 to 125 µm. CaHA particles placed in soft tissue favor fibroblast infiltration. The gel carrier suspends the CaHA particles and provides most of the initial augmentation bulking effect, then it is designed to degrade over some months, facilitating ingrowth of tissue around the particles. New tissue formation in the area previously occupied by the gel ensures long-term efficacy [11].

In an attempt to improve the long-term outcome, newer and more durable substances have been investigated.

Ethylene vinyl alcohol copolymer (EVOH – Tegress) is a substance that has been successfully used to treat cerebral aneurysms, carotid-cavernous fistulae, and esophagobronchial fistulae in man. It is a biocompatible polymer which is dissolved in an 8% dimethyl sulfoxide (DMSO) carrier to allow injection of a very low-viscosity fluid into tissue.

Once the material comes in contact with body tissue and fluid, dissipation of the DMSO from the polymer results in formation of a precipitate of a coherent solid mass. This material is durable, not biodegradable, and non-allergenic [12].

Carbon-coated zirconium oxide beads is another material that was approved by the Food and Drug Administration in 1999 for the treatment of women with SUI. The beads are suspended in a gel carrier. The carbon beads are not biodegradable and do not migrate owing to their large particle size, so they have a great degree of permanence in the tissues [13].

NASHA/Dx (Zuidex™) gel is a dextranomer/hyaluronic acid (Dx/HA) copolymer. Dextranomer (dextran 2,3-dihydropropyl-2-hydroxy-1,3 propanediethylether) is made by hydrophylic dextran polymer particles (microspheres 80–120 µm), configured as a network. It acts as a cell carrier, recruiting connective fibers from the surrounding tissues. It is non-allergenic, as it has no free dextran molecules. Hyaluronic acid (HA) is a 1% solution, highly viscous, high molecular weight polysaccharide. It is non-immugenic as it is not extracted from animals but from bacteria [2].

The most recent substance introduced into clinical practice is polyacrylamide hydrogel (PAHG), commercially known as Bulkamid. This is a non-toxic, non-reabsorbable sterile gel consisting of approximately 2.5% cross-linked polyacrylamide and 97.5% water. It is homogeneous, stable, not biodegradable, and has tissue-like viscosity and elasticity. One of the main properties of Bulkamid is continuous water exchange between the PAHG and the surrounding tissues. The gel is highly biocompatible and is being used in many medical fields such as plastic, esthetic surgery and ophthalmic surgery. PAHG is also used in the production of soft contact lenses.

Cross-linked polyacrylamides are very stable due to their large molecular size and inability to pass through biological membranes. Moreover, they are resistant to physical and chemical degradation. Many clinical studies report excellent biocompatibility and longevity of the product [14].

19.3 Safety

The complication rates of SUI injection therapy are acceptably low: they can be divided into those that are generic to all substances or agent-specific complications [2].

Urinary tract infections (UTIs) and short-term voiding dysfunction including urinary retention and hematuria are common with all of the injectable agents and are frequently self-limiting.

The most-reported agent-specific complications concern particle migration, granulomatous reaction, and hypersensitivity.

Particle migration locally and systemically has been reported for several agents including Teflon, silicone, and carcon-coated zirconium beads. Migration has been attibuted to small particles within the injectable agent, so it may be due to technical problems rather than the property of the agent.

Another very annoying complication is a granulomatous reaction, locally or at distant migration sites. The risk of a granuloma seems to be related to the injection of non-biodegradable agents, like Teflon, carbon-coated zirconium beads, or silicone, but there are many reports in the literature regarding granuloma using NASHA/Dx gel so that this agent has now been abandoned like Teflon, which, in addition to migration and granuloma formation, seems to have another serious side-effect – carcinogenesis.

PAHG is well accepted by human tissue, and foreign-body reaction is minimal. A urethral implantation study in pigs showed that gel deposits in urethrovesical tissue stayed soft and elastic for more than 13 months, with little or no foreign-body reaction of the surrounding tissue.

Also for Tegress injection, a lack of a significant fibrotic response has been demonstrated in animal studies.

Another very dangerous agent-specific complication is a systemic allergic reaction due to previous exposure to the substance injected. Because of the potential antigenicity, which affects approximately 3% of patients, GAX collagen application requires a skin test in all patients, 30 days before treatment [15].

Porcine collagen, unlike GAX collagen, is not from a bovine source, so patients do not have to undergo a skin test preoperatively [16].

In the literature there are similar reports of vaginal erosion associated with CaHA injection. This seems unlikely to be the result of direct tissue toxicity of the CaHA and carrier gel, but it is more likely to be a result of CaHA having a greater particle density, which may potentially cause increased and prolonged local tissue pressure effects [11].

19.4   Injection Technique

In the literature, different injection techniques are described since there is no standardized procedure. The points to be focused upon are the anesthetic technique, the site of the injection, and guidance for correct positioning of the material [1].

The anesthetic techniques employed during injection of bulking agents are not well documented in the literature. Most authors do not pay much attention to the anesthetic technique during this maneuver, stating that it may be performed under either general, locoregional or local anesthesia, according to the surgeon's preference. There are no studies comparing the different types of anesthetic techniques.

The administration of general and/or local anesthesia usually depends exclusively on the investigator's preference, and often it is not clear if different anesthetic techniques have been used in the same report.

The use of local anesthesia could certainly make it possible to perform this minimally invasive procedure in an office setting, reducing costs.

When the operator chooses local anesthesia, after placing the female patient in the lithotomy position, the introitus and urethra may be anesthetized with topical 2% lidocaine gel or 2.5% lidocaine – 2.5% prilocaine cream (Emla™) for 10 minutes. Following this, a 1% lidocaine solution may be injected periurethrally or transurethrally, as additional anesthesia, in different sites of the urethra.

The bulking materials may be injected in a retrograde (more common) or antegrade fashion.

Whether one route of injection is better than another is not well documented in the literature. Schulz et al [17] compared the transurethral injection route with a paraurethral one. The authors showed a trend towards better subjective and objective outcomes in favour of transurethral injection, although this did not reach statistical significance. Although there is no evidence that a transurethral route is better than a paraurethral one, the argument in favor of the former is supported by the finding of more complications following paraurethral injection [18].

Technically, EVOH is slightly more difficult to apply than other agents because the injection rate should be very slow to allow the substance to have adequate contact with the tissue and establish the spongy mass [12].

The ideal location for injection is not accurately defined, so that the site of injection may vary from the bladder neck, usually chosen, to the midurethra. The procedures also differ in terms of number of implants, volume of material injected for a single session, and needle size.

One of the most useful technical improvements is represented by the "non-endoscopic" injection. This procedure is most comfortable for the patient but does not allow visualization of the bolus of material and the urethral coaptation; nevertheless, some published data suggest that the endoscopic visualization does not necessarily correlate with its efficacy [19].

19.5   Cost

For patients affected by SUI, pads represent a major source of cost, so a treatment that reduces pad usage is likely to be extremely beneficial. Cost analyses for

SUI therapy should compare the different type of treatment (pharmacological therapy, urethral injection, surgery), include long-term follow-up, utilize health-economics models, and consider actual cost data [4].

Current cost constraints for SUI injection therapy are limited because this analysis is influenced by the different type of agents used, the number of injections, the post-surgery hospital stay, and the costs of secondary interventions (retreatment or treatment of complications).

19.6 Efficacy

A great number of contributions are published in literature regarding this topic. Despite careful selection, the International Consultation on Incontinence and a recent review by Keegan et al [4] published for the Cochrane Library stated that, considering the lack of long-term follow-up and health-economic data, injection therapy cannot be recommended at present as an alternative therapy for women who are fit for other surgical procedures. It is a useful option only for patients with comorbidity precluding anaesthesia.

Most published studies analyze a small number of patients, with short follow-up periods. At present, there are no papers comparing injection therapy with conservative treatment and no data suggesting that any one substance is superior to the others with respect to efficacy, durability, or safety. On the contrary, the finding of a similar response to injection of autologous fat and placebo (saline solution) does not support the hypothesis of the usefulness of injection therapy as a first-line option [20]. Certainly, it is an option for women who do not desire surgery or who wish to have future pregnancies, but patients and physicians should know that a single injection session is unlikely to achieve a good result. Assuming that only 17% of patients with lower urinary tract symptoms expect a complete cure from their treatment [21], injection therapy appears to have the profile required to meet the patient's goal, although measurement of quality of life strictly depends on the instrument used and does not always correspond to the patient's satisfaction [2, 22].

19.7 Conclusions

As bulking materials develop, understanding of the preferred injection technique is also being gained, as well as knowledge about the best delivery method and injection site. Both periurethral and transurethral injections are equally efficacious, but there is evidence to suggest that the transurethral route results in fewer complications. Injection therapy is less effective than surgery, but has a better safety profile. Every effort should be taken to make these devices safer and easier to manage.

References

1. Appell RA, Dmochowski RR, Herschorn S. Urethral injections for female stress incontinence. BJU Int 2006;98(suppl 1):27–30.
2. Chapple CR, Wein AJ, Brubacker L et al. Stress incontinence injection therapy: what is best for our patients? Eur Urol 2005;48:552–565.
3. Chaliha C, Williams G. Periurethral injection therapy for treatment of urinary incontinence. Br J Urol 1995; 76:151–155.
4. Keegan PE, Atiemo K, Cody JD et al. Periurethral injection therapy for urinary incontinence in women. Cochrane Database Syst Rev 2007;(3):CD003881.
5. Meulen PH, Berghmans LCM, van Kerrebroeck P. Systematic review: efficacy of silicone microimplants (Macroplastique®) Therapy for stress urinary incontinence. Eur Urol 2003;44:573–582.
6. Smith ARB, Daneshgari F, Dmochowski R et al. Surgery for urinary incontinence in women. In: Abrams P, Cardozo L, Khoury S, Wein A. Incontinence, 3rd International Consultation on Incontinence, 2005, pp 1297–1370.
7. Santarosa RP, Blaivas JG. Periurethral injection of autologous fat for the treatment of sphincteric incontinence. J Urol 1994;151:607–611.
8. Haab F, Zimmern PE, Leach GE. Urinary stress incontinence due to intrinsic sphinteric deficiency: experience with fat and collagen periurethral injections. J Urol 1997; 157:1283–1286.
9. Atala A, Cima LG, Kim W et al. Injectable alginate seeded with chondrocytes as a potential treatment for vesicoureteral reflux. J Urol 1993;150:745–747.
10. Bent AE, Tutrone RT, McLennan MT et al. treatment of intrinsic sphincter deficiency using autologous ear chondrocytes as a bulking agent. Neurourol Urodyn 2001; 20:157–165.
11. Mayer RD, Dmochowski RR, Appell RA et al. Multicenter prospective randomized 52-week trial of calcium hydroxylapatite versus bovine dermal collagen for treatment of stress urinary incontinence. Urology 2007; 69:876–880.
12. Kuhn A, Stadlmayr W, Sohail A, Monga A. Long-term results and patients' satisfaction after transurethral ethylene vinyl alcohol (Tegress®) injections: a two-centre study. Int Urogynecol J 2008;19:503–507.
13. McCrery RJ, Appell RA. Safety of carbon bead injection for incontinence in patients taking warfarin. J Urol 2006; 67:97–99.
14. Lose G, Mouritsen L, Nielsen JB. A new bulking agent

(polyacrylamide hydrogel) for treating stress urinary incontinence in women. BJU Int 2006;98:100–104.

15. Winters JC, Appell R. Periurethral injection of collagen in the treatment of intrinsic sphincter deficiency in the female patient. Urol Clin North Am 1995;22:673–678.

16. Bano F, Barrington JW, Dyer R. Comparison between porcine dermal implant (Permacol) and silicone injection (Macroplastique) for urodynamic stress incontinence. Int Urogynecol J 2005;16:147–150.

17. Schulz JA, Nager CW, Stanton SL, Baessler K. Bulking agents for stress urinary incontinence: short-term results and complications in a randomized comparison of periurethral and transurethral injections. Int Urogynecol J Pelvic Floor Dysfunct 2004;15:261–265.

18. Pickard R, Reaper J, Wyness L et al. Periurethral injection therapy for urinary incontinence in women. Cochrane Database Syst Rev 2003;(2):003881.

19. von Kerrebroeck P, ter Meulen P, Larsson G et al. Efficacy and safety of a novel system (NASHA/Dx copolymer using the implacer device) for treatment of stress urinary incontinence. Urology 2001;58:12–15.

20. Lee EP, Kung RC, Drutz HP. Periurethral autologous fat injection as treatment for female stress urinary incontinence: a randomized double-blind controlled trial. J Urol 2001;165:153–158.

21. Robinson D, Anders K, Cardozo L et al. What do women want? Interpretation of the concept of cure. J Pelvic Med Surg 2003;9:273–277.

22. Groutz A, Blaivas JG, Kesler SS et al. Outcome results of transurethral collagen injection for female stress incontinence: assessment by urinary incontinenc score. J Urol 2000;164:2006–2009.

Artificial Urinary Sphincter in Women

20

Amrith Raj Rao and Philippe Grange

Abstract Artificial urinary sphincter provides an option to restore continence when other methods have failed. Patient selection, details and workings of the artificial urinary sphincter, open and laparoscopic insertion of these devices are described with postoperative management and early/late complications discussed.

Keywords Urinary sphincter • Artificial urinary sphincter • Urinary incontinence • Surgical procedure • Laparoscopic procedure

20.1 Introduction

Artificial urinary sphincter (AUS) is a surgical device that is implanted to restore continence control in men, women, and children. In women, AUS is usually considered as the last resort to restore continence after failure of other anti-incontinence procedures; albeit, there are indications for the primary insertion of AUS. The procedure requires appropriate patient selection with proper counseling, and operative insertion by a surgeon well versed with the anatomy of the pelvis and possessing sound knowledge of reconstructive techniques.

The patient should be followed up to detect any possible complications and manage them accordingly. In this chapter we outline the device, indications, contraindications, operative technique, and a brief review of the current literature on the laparoscopic approach to the insertion of AUS.

20.2 Artificial Urinary Sphincter

The most commonly used device AMS 800™ (American Medical Systems) consists of three main parts: an inflatable urethral cuff, a pressure-regulating balloon reservoir, and a control pump. These are connected to each other with non-kink connecting tubing.

20.2.1 Inflatable Cuff

The cuff (Fig. 20.1) surrounds the urethra/bladder neck circumferentially. Cuffs range in size from 4 cm to 11 cm, at intervals of 0.5 cm. In women and children, the cuff is placed around the bladder neck. In men, the cuff is placed around the bulbar urethra.

20.2.2 Pressure-regulating Balloon Reservoir

The balloon (Fig. 20.2) is placed usually in the suprapubic region. It acts as both a reservoir and a pressure-

P. Grange
Laparoscopic Urology,
Department of Urology, Kings College Hospital,
London, UK

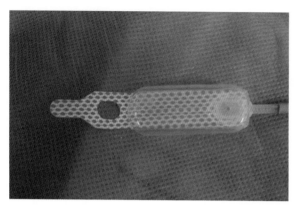

Fig. 20.1 AMS 800™ inflatable cuff

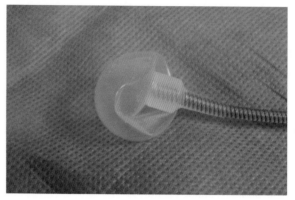

Fig. 20.2 AMS 800™ pressure regulating balloon reservoir

regulating system. Different pressure preset balloon reservoirs are available (41–50, 51–60, 61–70, 71–80, 81–90 cm water).

The balloon with the lowest pressure required to occlude the bladder neck is selected. This can vary from patient to patient.

20.2.3 Control Pump

The control pump (Fig. 20.3) is placed below the labia majora in women. The pump has a unidirectional valve, refill-delay resistor, and deactivation button. Squeezing and releasing the soft part of the pump releases the pressure in the cuff by pushing the fluid to the balloon reservoir, allowing the patient to void. The refill-delay resistor slowly allows the fluid from the reservoir to fill into the cuff (3 to 5 minutes) through the pump, thus occluding the urethra. Activation of the deactivation button situated on the hard upper part of the pump stops the fluid from being transferred between the components.

20.2.4 Connecting Tubing

The AMS 800™ comes with two sets of colour-coded tubing. The clear tubing connects to the pump from the cuff and the dark tubing connects the pump to the balloon reservoir. Each tubing is connected to its counterpart using quick-connect sutureless window connectors and a connecting assembly tool.

The filling solution for the device should be iso-osmotic, as the silicone elastomer can over time allow the fluid to shift across an osmotic gradient. Therefore,

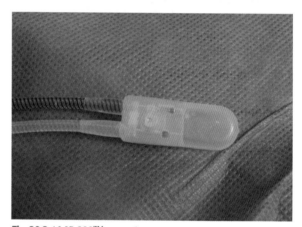

Fig. 20.3 AMS 800™ control pump

the manufacturers recommend using isotonic saline to fill the components of the AUS. Certain centers prefer to use contrast media to identify radiologically the site of failure if the device malfunctions in the future.

The manufacturer's recommendations must be followed, as not all contrast media are iso-osmotic, and failure to do so may lead to fluid leakage and to mechanical failure. More information can be obtained from the manufacturer's website [1].

20.2.5 Indications

- Primary implantation for severe genuine type III stress incontinence (intrinsic sphincter deficiency)
- secondary implantation after previous failed anti-incontinence procedures
  - salvage implantation for persistent incontinence
  - in association with urethrolysis on an obstructed scarred urethra.

20.2.6 Contraindications

- Previous pelvic radiotherapy
- any active perineal or pelvic infections.

20.3 Operation

20.3.1 Preoperative Counseling and Preparation

The patient should be thoroughly evaluated before undertaking the procedure. Good manual dexterity is necessary both to recycle the pump that is placed in the labia majora and also to be able to self-catheterize if necessary in the immediate postoperative period. Proper counseling should be provided on how the device works, the preoperative work-up, the operative procedure, and possible complications with their implications. Therefore, the patient needs to have a reasonable mental aptitude to make an informed decision about undergoing the procedure.

Investigations such as urine culture, video-urodynamic evaluation with urethral pressure profilometry, and urethrocystoscopy (especially in patients with previous failed anti-incontinence procedure) should have been carried out. Any focus of infection should be treated appropriately, as this carries a higher risk of prosthetic infection.

20.3.2 Open Procedure for Insertion of AUS

20.3.2.1 Abdominal Approach

Access to the bladder neck can be by either a transperitoneal or pre-peritoneal route, using a lower midline or a Pfannenstiel incision. The pelvic anatomy is first defined and dissection is then carried out to free the bladder neck from the underlying vaginal wall. The operation can be difficult in women who have had previous pelvic operations or have had anti-incontinence procedures, as the scar tissue can be quite dense and adherent. Careful dissection with control of hemostasis is essential to avoid injuring the urethra, bladder, or indeed the vagina. The risk of infection and erosion is higher if the vaginal wall or the urethra is injured. A combined transvaginal and transabdominal approach has also been described for difficult cases.

20.3.2.2 Vaginal Approach

The transvaginal route for implantation of AUS has been reported by a few authors, suggesting the advantage of avoiding the scar secondary to previous surgery on the bladder neck. In this approach, the balloon reservoir is placed in the suprapubic region and the pump is placed in the labia majora through a separate suprapubic incision. Although the number of patients treated in this manner is not as high as for the open abdominal approach, the results are encouraging, with one series of 34 patients showing a 100% success rate with no cases of erosion or extrusion [2].

20.3.2.3 Laparoscopic Extraperitoneal Approach

The patient is placed in a supine position, preferably on an anti-slip gel mattress. Deep vein thrombosis prophylaxis includes TEDS® stockings and the Flowtron® pump during the procedure and in the immediate postoperative period. Unless contraindicated, we routinely administer low molecular weight heparin in the postoperative period. The pressure areas of the body are protected with gel pads.

The abdominal wall, genitals, and perineum are cleaned thoroughly with iodine-based solution. Sterile access to the vagina is also required during surgery. A combination of antibiotics (depending on the local microbiological resistance) to cover gram-positive, gram-negative and anaerobic organisms is administered at induction and continued for 48 hours after the operation.

A 16 Fr Foley catheter with 10 mL in the balloon is inserted through the urethra into the bladder and emptied completely. The patient is in a moderately head-down position with arms alongside the body (Fig. 20.4). The burden for an assistant of holding a camera is eased by using a robotic camera holder: Freehand® (Prosurgics Ltd), which maintains a stable picture throughout the operation (Fig. 20.5) [3]. An 11 mm clear vision port (e.g. Visiport™) is inserted with a 10 mm telescope in the midline, about five fingers' breadth above the upper border of the symphysis pubis. Once the soft connective tissue of the space of Retzius is identified, CO_2 gas insufflation is started. In our experience a pressure of 9 mmHg is sufficient to give adequate space to carry out the procedure. This space is developed using smooth movements of the 10 mm zero degree telescope, initially following the contour of the upper border of the symphysis pubis and the pubic rami. There is an advantage of clarity with the newer high-definition stacks and a deflectable-tip video-endoscope. We do not feel the need for a balloon dilatation technique, which remains an alternative option. Once the space is created, the useful landmarks to identify are the pubic symphysis; pectineal ligaments; pelvic diaphragm – endopelvic fascia and levator ani; external iliac veins, with their characteristic

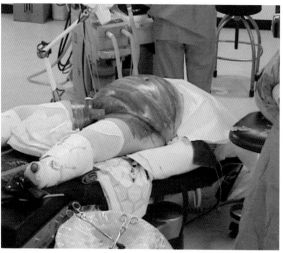

Fig. 20.4 The patient position with a slight head down position

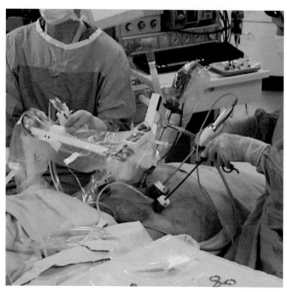

Fig. 20.5 Laparoscopic approach using the Freehand® robotic camera holder

respiratory movements; and inferior epigastric vessels (Fig. 20.6). Two additional left ports are inserted for the operator sitting on the left: one 12 mm port medial to the left inferior epigastric vessel and one 5 mm lateral to the inferior epigastric vessels. The moderate triangulation obtained may seem limited to surgeons used to more conventional broad triangulation. However, this allows an ergonomic and comfortable position preventing tiredness in the long run. An additional 5 mm port is placed on the assistant's side.

The key to success is identification of the bladder neck. The catheter balloon helps identification of the anterior wall of the bladder. The incision of the endopelvic fascia will give access to the para-urethral vaginal wall. As in open surgery, a bi-digital intravaginal palpation will enable assessment of the thickness of the vaginal tissue via the tip of a smooth instrument introduced through one of the ports. In some cases the pubo-urethral (anterior part of the pubococcygeus) ligament can be divided; however, it is important in any case to preserve the lateral urethral ligaments.

In secondary implantation, the principles remain the same, but the difficulty is as expected related to the type and number of prior procedures, which could include use of various non-absorbable materials. The key is to follow the pelvic bone and then the pelvic wall. In the most challenging cases, deliberately opening the anterior wall of the bladder is a safe option if away from the bladder neck itself.

The real difficulty in such circumstances is to create a plane between the bladder neck and vagina, which often is replaced by strong fibrotic scar tissue.

During the surgery, the three most helpful things

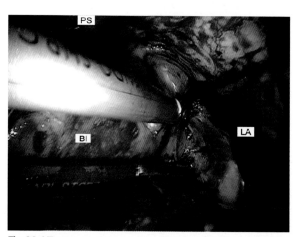

Fig. 20.6 Exposure of the vagina and the anatomical landmarks. *Bl*, bladder; *PS*, pubic symphysis; *LA*, levator ani

are patience, patience, and patience. A lack of one of these will inevitably end up in perforation of either the vagina or the urethra, and a lack of two of them will invariably lead to perforation of both! By successively using the suction device and right-angled instrument, the bladder neck is slowly freed from the underlying vaginal wall by alternating the dissection from either side. The extent of separation should be long enough to be able to safely accommodate insertion of the cuff (Fig. 20.7). An approximate guide would be a free movement of the measurement tape in the space. The guide tape from the manufacturer is used to measure the circumference of the bladder neck to select the size of the cuff (as it comes in different sizes). The components of the AMS 800™ AUS are then prepared according to the manufacturer's recommendation. It is vital to remove all the air bubbles from the cuff and both the tubes before occluding them to be inserted inside the abdomen. The vacuumed cuff is then inserted through the 12 mm port, placed around the bladder neck, and locked (Fig. 20.8).

The pump is prepared according to the manufacturer's manual and the tubing is clamped. The pump is placed in the fat of the labia majora. Access to the labia is performed laparoscopically, going anterior to the superior pubic ramus just lateral to the insertion of the rectus muscle. This dissection is also aided by manually feeling from outside on the labia when performing blunt

dissection by the laparoscopic suction device (Fig. 20.9).

Finally, the vacuumed balloon (reservoir) is introduced through the 12 mm port and placed in the space of Retzius just lateral to the bladder (Fig. 20.10). Each tubing – of the cuff, pump, and balloon – is exteriorized through the 12 mm port and they are connected to each other after filling the chambers according to the manufacturer's recommendation (Fig. 20.11). The connecting tubes are then internalized. Hemostasis is controlled at low gas pressure. The port incisions are closed.

Drains are avoided to minimize prosthetic infection. The pump is then squeezed and released several times to remove all the fluid from the cuff (deflate the cuff) and then the deactivation button is activated (Fig. 20.12). In addition to other advantages of the laparoscopic approach, the cosmetic result is quite obvious (Fig. 20.13). Reactivation is carried out usually around 4 to 6 weeks later.

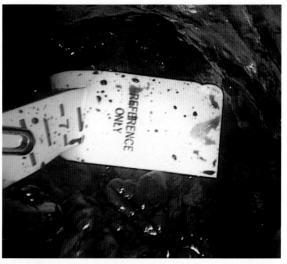

Fig. 20.8 Measuring the bladder neck

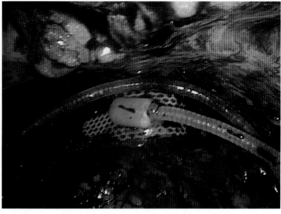

Fig. 20.9 Passing the cuff around the bladder neck

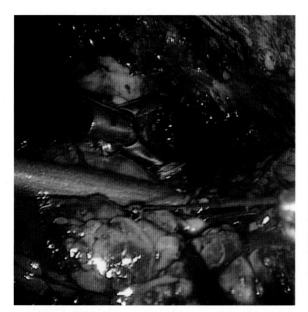

Fig. 20.7 Disseting the bladder neck with a rigth angled instrument and the sucker

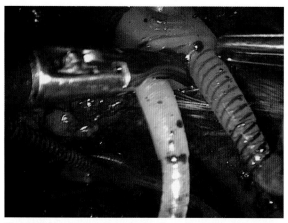

Fig. 20.10 Creation of the space for the pump in the labia majora

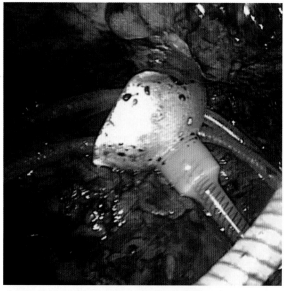

Fig. 20.11 Internalization of the balloon reservoir

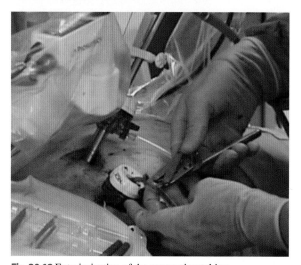

Fig. 20.12 Exteriorization of the connecting tubing

20.4 Complications

20.4.1 Perioperative Complications

20.4.1.1 Injury During Trocar Placement

Injury to the intra-abdominal organs can occur with placement of the trocar. This can be minimized by the use of Visiport™, which allows trocar placement under observation. Injury can also be avoided by performing this procedure by the extra-peritoneal approach. Injury to the bladder, urethra, and vagina may occur, especially in a patient who has undergone previous pelvic surgery.

20.4.2 Early Postoperative Complications

20.4.2.1 Urinary Retention

Urinary retention is usually due to the edema surrounding the bladder neck, as a result of surgery. If there is failure to void after removal of the catheter, the patient may be taught to perform self catheterisation until the edema settles down.

20.4.2.2 Infection and Extrusion of the Prosthesis

Staphylococcus epididermis is the most common cause of prosthetic infection, although other organisms are also implicated. Infection invariably leads to extrusion of the prosthesis. Initial conservative management with high-dose intravenous antibiotics can be attempted. However, if the infection persists, the entire device needs to be removed and re-implanted a few months later.

The risk of early erosion or extrusion is higher if there has been urethral injury during the time of implantation. The reported incidence is around 1–3%, which has decreased with the introduction of delayed activation [4–6]. Erosion is also common if AUS is implanted in women who have received pelvic irradiation [7].

20.4.3 Late Postoperative Complications

20.4.3.1 Urethral Atrophy, Erosion or Extrusion

Constant extrinsic pressure on the urethra by the cuff may lead to thinning of the wall and ultimately to erosion of the prosthesis into the urethra. Another un-common but reported cause of urethral injury is an attempt at urethral catheterization by medical staff who do not understand the functioning of the AUS cuff. Erosion or extrusion requires removal of all the components of the AUS and, if suitable, a delayed implantation may be considered.

20.4.3.2 Mechanical Failure

The life of an AMS 800™ is around 10 years. Device failure has been reported to occur in 7.6–21% of pa-tients [5, 8]. The most common cause of failure is leakage of fluid, with the cuff being the most common site. If the leakage occurs early, only the defective component may be replaced. However, if it is a de-layed failure, it is better to replace the entire system due to the high probability of other components failing subsequently [5].

20.4.3.3 Recurrent/Persistent Urinary Incontinence

Various factors can contribute to incontinence follow-ing the implantation of AUS. Video-urodynamic eval-uation should be carried out to rule out detrusor over-activity, and the screening would indicate the position of the cuff, and the emptying and filling of the cuff (if contrast-based solution was used to fill the components at the time of implantation). Urethrocystoscopy should be carried to rule out cuff erosion.

20.5 Brief Review of the Literature on AUS Implantation in Women

20.5.1 Open Procedure

The transabdominal approach has been considered the gold standard in the insertion of AUS. This can be done either transperitoneally or by a pre-peritoneal approach.
The success rate of open insertion of AUS is quoted to be around 61–90% [9–11].

The disadvantages of the open approach are the length of incision, longer hospital stay, and poor visu-alization in the pelvis, especially in women with a very large body habitus, problems which could poten-tially be overcome by a laparoscopic approach.

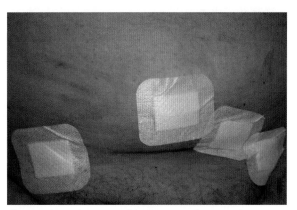

Fig. 20.13 Four tiny scars of the laparoscopic approach

20.5.2 Laparoscopic Procedure

There are only a few case reports and case series re-porting the laparoscopic implantation of AUS [12–14]. This reflects the dramatic change in the manage-ment of stress urinary incontinence using the tape procedure in the last decade. However, for a subset of patients who fail after these procedures, AUS may be a suitable option.

Recently two series have published their outcome of the laparoscopic approach to the implantation of AUS. Rouprêt et al reported on the outcome of 12 women who had laparoscopic insertion of AUS [13]. Eleven out of the 12 had undergone previous anti-incontinence procedures. Incontinence was resolved in eight women at a mean follow-up of about 12 ± 8 months. Conversion to an open procedure was neces-sary in three cases, due to vaginal and bladder injuries. Urinary retention was observed in five cases but these patients voided successfully at a later date. The mean operative time was 181 ± 39 minutes. The authors concluded that a laparoscopic approach was feasible, but larger studies with longer follow-up are required to evaluate it further [13].

Mandron et al reported on a larger series of 25 pa-tients, all of whom had had previous urogynecological procedures [14]. Six patients had concomitant surgery for urogenital prolapse. No conversion to open proce-dure was reported, and all 25 patients had AUS im-planted. Only one vaginal perforation occurred, which was repaired laparoscopically with no further com-plications. Two patients had vaginal erosion and the AUS was removed. Five patients developed urinary retention but subsequently voided.

The mean operative time for AUS insertion was 71 minutes, and at a follow-up of around 26 months, 19 had complete continence and the remaining four had social continence. The authors concluded that the procedure was safe and demonstrated similar results to open surgery but with the advantages of laparoscopic approach [14].

20.6 Conclusions

AUS is an option to restore continence in women, usually following a failed anti-incontinence procedure. The success rate of achieving continence is quite high, although patient selection is of paramount importance to avoid disappointment. Insertion of AUS should be performed by surgeons who have adequate experience, as the procedure can be difficult due to previous surgeries and can carry a significant morbidity. Postoperative follow-up should be rigorous to pick up complications and manage them accordingly. Traditionally, an open abdominal approach has been used to implant the AUS; however, recently laparoscopic insertion is gaining popularity with the advantages attributed to minimally invasive surgery.

References

1 American Medical Systems. www.AmericanMedicalSystems.com (accessed 14 May 2010).
2. Appell R. Technique and results in the implantation of the artificial urinary sphincter in women with Type III stress urinary incontinence by a vaginal approach. Neurourol Urodyn 1988;7:613–619.
3. Sharma D, Brown C, Kouriefs C et al. Initial experience with The FreeHand robotic camera holder in laparoscopic urology. J Endourol 2009;23(1):A249.
4. Hussain M, Greenwell TJ, Venn SN, Mundy AR. The current role of the artificial urinary sphincter for the treatment of urinary incontinence. J Urol 2005;174:418–424.
5. Ratan HL, Summerton DJ, Wilon SK, Terry TR. Development and current status of the AMS 800 artificial urinary sphincter. EAU-EBU Update Series 2006;4:117–128.
6. Webster GD, Perez LM, Khoury JM, Timmons SL. Management of type III stress urinary incontinence using artificial urinary sphincter. Urology 1992;39(6):499–503.
7. Thomas K, Venn SN, Mundy AR. Outcome of the artificial urinary sphincter in female patients. J Urol 2002; 167(4):1720–1722
8. Light JK. Abdominal approach for implantation of the A.S. 800 artificial urinary sphincter in females. Neurourol Urodyn 2005;7(6):603–611.
9. Costa P, Mottet N, Rabut B et al. The use of an artificial urinary sphincter in women with type III incontinence and a negative Marshall test. J Urol 2001;165(4):1172–1176.
10. Petero Jr VG, Diokno AC. Comparison of the long-term outcomes between incontinent men and women treated with artificial urinary sphincter. J Urol 2006;175:605–609.
11. Diokno AC, Hollander JB, Alderson TP. Artificial urinary sphincter for recurrent female urinary incontinence: indications and results. J Urol 1987;138:778–780.
12. Grange P, Mignot H. Laparoscopic artificial sphincter implantation in multioperated women. 2nd International Consultation on Incontinence, 2nd edn. Health Publications, Plymouth, 2002.
13. Rouprêt M, Misraï V, Vaessen C et al. Laparoscopic approach for artificial urinary sphincter implantation in women with intrinsic sphincter deficiency incontinence: a single-centre preliminary experience. Eur Urol 2010; 57(3):499–504.
14. Mandron E, Bryckaert PE, Papatsoris AG. Laparoscopic artificial urinary sphincter implantation for female genuine stress urinary incontinence: technique and 4-year experience in 25 patients. BJU Int 2010; 2 February, epub ahead of print.

Sacral Nerve Stimulation

21

Giuseppe Tuccitto, Francesco Beniamin,
Edoardo Ostardo and Luigi Maccatrozzo

Abstract Female voiding dysfunctions as urge-frequency syndrome, urge incontinence and non-obstructive urinary retention, are often refractary to conservative management. Sacral neuromodulation is an established treatment in case of non-neurogenic patients. Recent reports have shown that sacral neuromodulation has a sustained efficacy and acceptable safety profile in the long term. The most common adverse events such as lead migration, infection, and pain at the implantation site are transient and can be treated effectively. There are no permanent sequelae following adverse events and the procedure is completely reversible.

The major frontiers for sacral neuromodulation in adults are interstitial cystitis and chronic pain syndromes, neurogenic bladder from spinal cord injury, fecal incontinence, constipation and erectile dysfunction.

Keywords Sacral neuromodulation • Urinary dysfunction • Urinary incontinence

21.1 Historical Overview

The use of electric currents to treat urological pathology has a long history. In 1878, Saxtorph [1] reported intravesical electrostimulation in patients with an acontractile bladder and complete urinary retention Later, Katona [2] applied intravescical electro-stimulation in patients with chronic neurogenic retention and neurogenic overactivity. The most important electrical stimulation was applied in the spinal cord and in the sacral root. In the late 1960s, Nashold [3] began experiments with spinal cord stimulation; he subsequently transferred the experience gained to humans, and in 1972 reported on the first four patients with stimulator implants. In 1975, Jonas et al [4] examined the parameters for most effective stimulation of the spinal cord. In 1972, Brindley et al [5] began electrical stimulation of the sacral ventral roots in baboons and from 1976 [6] started implanting sacral anterior root stimulators in paraplegic patients with incontinence, presenting their experience with the first 50 cases in 1986.

Tanagho used the canine model for sacral root stimulation because the anatomy of the sacral nerves is similar to that in humans. In 1982, Tanagho and Schmidt [7] presented the first results of sacral root stimulation in paraplegic dogs. After many experimental studies of the parameters of nerve stimulation performed by Thuroff, Tanagho started the first human clinical trials in 1982.

The best model to achieve continence and promote bladder evacuation was a combination of stimulation of the ventral root of S3 or S4, with extensive dorsal rhizotomy and selective peripheral neurotomy. The observation made by Tanagho and Schmidt [8] that

G. Tuccitto
Division of Urology, Regional Hospital, Treviso, Italy

sphincteric contraction suppresses detrusor activity and stabilizes the entire micturition reflex mechanism in cases where the sensory pathways are intact is the basis of neuromodulation.

In 1988, Schmidt [9] described the three stages of electrode placement.

First a needle was placed into the sacral foramina near the sacral roots for test stimulation; then in cases of root integrity, the needle was replaced by temporary percutaneous stimulation. If the patient demonstrated a significant improvement, a permanent neural prosthesis was implanted.

21.2 Mode of Action

The precise mode of action of neuromodulation is unknown. The stimulation of afferent nerve fibers modulates reflex pathways involved in the filling and evacuation phase of the micturition cycle, through spinal circuits mediating somato-visceral interactions within the sacral spinal cord [10]. Two mechanisms are important:

1. activation of efferent fibers to the striated urethral sphincter reflexively causes detrusor relaxation
2. activation of afferent fibers causes inhibition at a spinal and/or supraspinal level.

The S3 spinal nerve is the preferential site of lead implantation because it is the site of 60.5% of the overall pudendal afferent activity [11]. We know that supraspinal pathways are also involved.

Positron emission tomography (PET) and functional magnetic resonance imaging (MRI) have been used to study brain activity in patients with detrusor hyperactivity or urinary retention. Detrusor hyperactivity was associated most prominently with differences in activity in the orbifrontal cortex [12] and cerebellum [13]. Furthermore, neuromodulation in women with urinary retention changed activity in the midbrain, cerebellum, cingulate gyrus, and prefrontal cortex [14].

Brain activity has been investigated in patients with urge incontinence during acute and chronic sacral neuromodulation (SN), and it is possible that some of the beneficial effects observed originate from supraspinal brain areas, which are inhibited or activated via the caudal spinal cord.

21.3 Indications

The US Food and Drug Administration (FDA) approved SN for intractable urge incontinence in 1997, and for urgency–frequency and non-obstructive urinary retention in 1999.

The classical indications for SN are unsuccessful attempts at conservative treatments for overactive bladder (including urinary urgency–frequency and urge incontinence) and non-obstructive urinary retention or idiopathic retention.

The use of SN in patients with partial cord injury, multiple sclerosis (MS), peripheral neuropathy, parkinsonism, or myelodysplasia is controversial. SN in MS may be effective but it is important to remember that bladder symptoms in individuals with MS can change over time.

SN is not approved by the FDA for the pain that is a prevalent component of interstitial cystitis (IC), but some symptoms of IC such as urinary urgency and frequency, and nocturia, are indications for neuromodulation.

SN has been used in conditions of chronic genitourinary pain; the results have shown a dramatic reduction in visual-analog pain scores but evidence is only available from small series or case reports.

21.4 Selection Criteria

Patient selection begins with a history, physical examination, urinalysis and urine culture, voiding diaries, and other simple diagnostic tests such as pelvic ultrasound and cystoscopy.

Urodynamic examination is used to detect detrusor overactivity with or without urge incontinence or detrusor acontractility.

It is also very important to identify abnormal pelvic floor muscle function during physical examination or urodynamic examination (electromyographic activity).

The most important indicator for patient selection is a successful trial stimulation. This test is performed with placement of a temporary or permanent (two-stage implant technique) electrode under local anesthesia.

The patient is tested over either 7 or 30 days, and if their symptoms improve by at least 50%, then they are a candidate for implantation of a permanent implantable pulse generator.

21.5 Implant Technique

The traditional technique of SN is a two-step procedure. During the first step, percutaneous nerve evaluation (PNE), the physician evaluates the bladder symptoms for 7–14 days. A test needle is inserted into the third sacral foramen to stimulate the sacral root. Lead migration is the most important complication of this test; other complications are technical failures or pain. This procedure is used during an acute phase to test neural integrity. A typical S3 motor response is movement of the pelvic floor, plantar flexion of the big toe, and paresthesia in the rectum, perineum, scrotum, or vagina. Fluoroscopy can be used for S3 localization in anterior/posterior and lateral imaging.

If the patient's symptoms improve by at least 50%, then they are a candidate to undergo step two, in which a permanent implantable pulse generator is implanted into the soft tissue of the patient's buttock.

Some patients who fail a PNE test are still good candidates for SN therapy; for this reason a two-step implant technique was developed.

Under local anesthesia, a permanent electrode is implanted and connected to an external stimulator. The thin lead has four sets of self-anchoring tines, allowing minimally invasive percutaneous placement; this technique is widely used in Europe and the US. Chronic stimulation is performed for 4 weeks, and if there is a good clinical response a permanent implantable pulse generator will be implanted.

The traditional technique is unilateral stimulation, but many authors think that bilateral stimulation may be more effective for voiding dysfunction. There is only one prospective randomized crossover trial [15] to compare the unilateral approach with bilateral sacral nerve stimulation; this study did not find any significant differences when comparing the results of unilateral with bilateral stimulation. Bilateral stimulation might be indicated when a unilateral test fails [16]. It is possible that there will be a group of patients in which bilateral stimulation will be indicated.

21.6 Results

In 1999, Schimdt et al [17] published a prospective randomized study in which the results of NS therapy for urge incontinence were evaluated. Overall, 76 patients were treated in a multicenter trial: 34 patients were implanted and 42 patients were treated with standard conservative therapy. After 6 months of treatment, there was a significant difference in results between two groups: in the first group, 47% of patients were completely dry and 29% showed a greater than 50% reduction in incontinence episodes. In the control group, the results were significantly worse. During evaluation of therapy after 6 months, the stimulation group returned to baseline symptoms when stimulation was stopped.

In 2001, Jonas et al [18] published a multicenter trial which enrolled 177 patients with urinary retention refractory to conservative therapy; 37 patients were assigned to the treatment group and 31: to the control group. After 6 months in the stimulation group, 69% of patients had had their catheterization removed, and 14% showed more than 50% reduction in voiding volume per catheterization. The effectiveness of SN therapy was sustained for 18 months after implantation. A recent study published from van Kerrebroek [19] reported on a total of 172 patients implanted – for urge incontinence (103), urgency–frequency (28), and urinary retention (31): 84% of implanted patients with urge incontinence, 71% with urgency–frequency, and 78% with urinary retention went on to have a successful outcome at 5-year follow-up, if they had shown a successful outcome after one year [20–24].

21.7 Complications

Of 914 stimulation test procedures carried out [20], 181 adverse events occurred (19.8%): lead migration (11.8% of procedures), technical problems (2.6%), and pain (2.1%) represent the main adverse events.

For 219 patients who underwent implantation of the permanent system, adverse events were: pain at the stimulator site (15.3%), new pain (9%), suspected lead migration (8.4%), transient electric shock (5.5%), pain at the lead site (5.4%), and adverse change in bowel function (3%). Surgical revision of the implanted neurostimulator was performed in 2.2% of cases [20].

Hijaz et al [25] described the complications of 161 patients implanted with tined lead . He reported eight explants due to infection and seven due to loss of effect; in 26 patients, a revision was performed due to a decrease in clinical response.

In 2006, van Voskuilen et al [22] described 194 adverse events in 149 patients undergoing NS: 129 reoperations were performed (repositioning of the implanted pulse generator, revision of electrode, reoperation parameter changes in patients implanted with 7th ITRELL-I IPG), and 21 patients had their system explanted. van Voskuilen reported data on complications in 39 patients implanted with tined lead: there were seven severe adverse events, of which three needed reoperation. Three patients had a reoperation to reposition the IPG after they complained of pain [26].

It is clear from the literature and the authors' experience with the tined lead implantation that there is a decrease in reoperation rate.

21.8   Conclusions

Sacral nerve modulation procedures prolong subjective benefit in patients with urinary dysfunction. In a group of patients with highly therapy-resistant lower urinary tract symptoms, SN using stimulating therapy is safe, minimally invasive, and reversible. The new minimally invasive approach for SN is easier to perform than the classic open method. The complication rate using the tined lead is low. It does not carry the risk of systemic side-effects encountered in pharmacologic therapy, or the potential morbidity that open surgical procedures may carry. Sacral nerve modulation should be considered before using a more invasive procedure.

References

1   Madersbacher H. Konservative therapie der neurogenen blasendydisfuktion. Urologe A 1999;38:24–29.
2.   Katona F. Stages of vegetative afferentation in reorganization of bladder control during intravesical electrotherapy. Urol Int 1975;30:192–203.
3.   Nashold BS Jr, Friedman H, Boyarsky S. Electrical activation of micturition by spinal cord stimulation. J Surg Res 1971;11:144–147.
4.   Jonas U, Heine JP, Tanagho EA. Studies on the feasibility of urinary bladder evacuation by direct spinal cord stimulation. I. Parameters of most effective stimulation. Invest Urol 1975;13:142–150.
5.   Brindley GS. Electrode-arrays for making long-lasting electrical connexion to spinal roots. J Physiol 1972;222:135P–136P.
6.   Brindley GS, Polkey CE, Rushton DN et al. Sacral anterior root stimulators for bladder control in paraplegia: the first 50 cases. J Neurol Neurosurg Psychiatry 1986;49:1104–1114.
7.   Tanagho EA, Schmidt RA. Bladder pacemaker: scientific basis and clinical future. Urology 1982;20:614–619.
8.   Tanagho EA, Schmidt RA. Electrical stimulation in the cli-

nical management of the neurogenic bladder. J Urol 1988;140:1331–1339.
9.   Schmidt RA. Application of neurostimulation in urology. Neurourol Urodyn 1988;7:585–592.
10.   Thon WF, Baskin LS, Jonas U et al. Surgical principles of sacral foramen electrode implantation. World J Urol 1991;9:133.
11.   Huang JC, Deletis V, Vodusek DB, Abbott R. Preservation of pudendal afferents in sacral rhizotomies. Neurosurgery 1997;41:411–415.
12.   Athwal BS, Berkley KJ, Hussain I et al. Brain responses to changes in bladder volume and urge to void in healthy men. Brain 2001;124:369.
13.   Matsuura S, Kakizaki H, Mitsui T et al. Human brain region response to distention or cold stimulation of the bladder: a positron emission tomography study. J Urol 2002;168:2035.
14.   Blok BF, Willemsen AT and Holstege G. A PET study on brain control of micturition in women. Brain 1998;121:2033.
15.   Scheepens WA, de Bie RA, Wiel EH et al. Unilateral versus bilateral sacral neuromodulation in patients with chronic voiding dysfunction. J Urol 2002;168:2046–2050.
16.   van Kerrebroek PE, Scheepens W, de Bie R et al. European experience with bilateral sacral neuromodulation in patients with chronic lower urinarytract dysfunction. Urol Clin North Am 2005;32:51–57.
17.   Schmidt RA, Jonas U, Oleson KA et al. Sacral nerve stimulation for treatment of refractory urinary urge incontinence. Sacral Nerve Stimulation Study Group. J Urol 1999; 162:352–357.
18.   Jonas U, Fowler CJ, Chancellor MB et al. Efficacy of sacral nerve stimulation for urinary retention: Result 18 month after implantation. J Urol 2001;165:15–19.
19.   van Kerrebroek PE, van Voskuilen AC, Heesakkers JPFA et al. Results of sacral neuromodulation therapy for urinary voiding dysfunction: outomes of prospective, worldwide clinical study. J Urol 2007;178:2029–2034.
20.   Siegel SW, Catanzaro F, Dijkema HE et al. Long-term results of a multicenter study on sacral nerve stimulation for treatment of urinary urge incontinence, urgency–frequency and retention. Urology 2000;56:87–91.
21.   Oerlemans DJ, van Kerrebroeck PEV. Long-term results of sacral nerve stimulation for neuromodulation of the lower urinary tract. Neurourol Urodyn 2008;27:28–33.
22.   van Voskuilen AC, Oerlemans DJ, Weil EH et al. Long-term results of neuromodulation by sacral nerve stimulation for lower urinary tract symptoms: A retrospective single center study. Eur Urol 2006;49:366–372.
23.   Hassouna MM, Siegel SW, Nyeholt AA et al. Sacral neuromodulation in the treatment of urgency–frequency symptoms: a multicenter study on efficacy and safety. J Urol 2000;163:1849–1854.
24.   Dasgupta R, Wiseman OJ, Kitchen N et al. Long-term results of sacral neuromodulation for women with urinary retention. BJU Int 2004;94:335–337.
25.   Hijaz A, Vasavada SP, Daneshgari F et al. Complications and troubleshooting of two-stage sacral neuromodulationtherapy: A single institution experience. Urology 2006; 68:533–537.
26.   van Voskuilen AC, Oerlemans DJ, Weil EH et al. Medium-term experience of sacral neuromodulation by tined lead implantation. BJU Int 2007;99:107–110.

Invited Commentary

Dmitry Pushkar

It was great pleasure for us to be asked to comment on Section IV.

Notwithstanding the success achieved in the treatment of stress urinary incontinence in female patients, this section remains rather controversial and there is a separate chapter on sacral neuromodulation, a rather new type of treatment that has become popular for several types of voiding functions.

I am glad the authors included a special chapter on tape positioning, as this is one of the crucial points in the "cookbook" of synthetic tape procedures. Some authors say that tape positioning may change with insignificant movements of the tape. I believe that these movements cannot be properly measured. We also recall that these procedures are performed in a supine position. As a result, when the patient gets up and moves, the tape will change its position slightly. At the same time, tape position affects treatment outcome and we all understand that proper intraoperative tape placement is the best way to minimize any subsequent functional complications.

The authors have presented a comprehensive analysis of tape positioning, which is very important, as many consider synthetic tape procedures well established, and do not concern themselves with the details of these procedures. Taking into consideration that there are increasing numbers of patients with concomitant stress urinary incontinence and pelvic organ prolapse, the issue of proper tape positioning is becoming even more important. It is still controversial whether we should perform prolapse repair simultaneously with synthetic tape placement. Proper tape positioning has become more challenging for these types of patients, and is a separate issue.

Selecting an appropriate midurethral sling, unfortunately, remains surgeon dependent. What we do know for sure in 2010 is that the only material that should be used for midurethral tape is microporous knitted prolene. With several dozen specially prepared kits available for the treatment of stress urinary incontinence in females, we still have very few randomized controlled trials (RCTs) comparing these tapes. Often the selection of midurethral slings is dependent on the availability of these various kits. Some data show that transobturator slings have less efficacy than retropubic slings in women with reduced maximal urethral closure pressure. Again, these data should be re-evaluated with a larger patient population. Recurrent stress urinary incontinence is of tremendous importance both for procedure selection and tape positioning. These patients should be treated in dedicated centers where a large number of surgical procedures are performed each year.

For several years there have been several so-called mini-slings available, which are thought to lead to fewer complications with the same efficacy as mid-urethral slings. Unfortunately, no RCTs have been conducted for these types of procedures. We believe that mini-slings are still experimental, and should be used within the framework of clinical trials.

Separate attention is focused on injectable biomaterials for patients with stress urinary incontinence. This treatment has been attracting specialists for over 100 years. We used to believe that continence could be provided by obstruction and narrowing of the urethral lumen. However, negative results in the use of periurethral injections made specialists understand the complexity of continence. The main attraction of injectable materials is still safety, and the fact that they do not require general anesthesia. This type of treatment is used

D. Pushkar
Department of Urology, MSMSU, Moscow, Russia

G.A. Santoro, A.P. Wieczorek, C.I. Bartram (eds.) *Pelvic Floor Disorders*
© Springer-Verlag Italia 2010

less and less, and when it is used, the patient should be informed that several treatment sessions are likely to be necessary in a majority of cases. Finally, mini-slings requiring only local anesthesia are enjoying more popularity. These procedures could potentially serve patients scheduled for periurethral injections. The search for a perfect injectable biomaterial continues, even though the concept itself does not seem solid.

An artificial urinary sphincter (AUS) has never been a primary option for patients with stress urinary incontinence. At the same time, AUSs may be reserved for selected groups of patients, especially for those with a non-mobile, well-supported urethra, and a history of several unsuccessful anti-incontinence procedures. Unfortunately, many patients may require revision surgery due to malfunction, erosion, or infection of the device. For this particular group of patients, spiral sling procedures were introduced some years ago. This type of procedure, which may lead to better func-

tional results with fewer of the complications typical of AUS, would be a last resort for this difficult subset of females.

Regarding sacral nerve stimulation (SNS) and difficult-to-cure patients with lower urinary tract symptoms, we think mainly of overactive bladders. SNS has emerged as a standard of care for patients with overactive bladders, and I believe it should be considered an appropriate next step if drugs, behavioral interventions, and pelvic floor rehabilitation have provided insufficient relief. The exact mechanism of SNS remains unknown. However, modulation of afferent nerves at several levels, and manipulation of the guarding reflex, are key elements in restoring a more normal urinary tract function. Recently this therapy was tried in neurogenic patients with good preliminary results. I believe that new devices and alternative stimulation targets will emerge soon, which may result in SNS becoming an easier and more first-line treatment.

Biofeedback

22

Kari Bø and Paolo Di Benedetto

Abstract Biofeedback has been defined as "a group of experimental procedures where an external sensor is used to give an indication on bodily processes, usually for the purpose of changing the measured quality". Pelvic floor muscle training (PFMT) can be conducted with and without biofeedback. The aim of this chapter is to give an overview of randomized controlled trials (RCTs) comparing the results of PFMT with and without biofeedback on stress and mixed incontinence. Fifteen RCTs were found using the reference lists of the UK National Institute for Health and Clinical Excellence (NICE) guidelines and the International Consultation on Incontinence (ICI). The studies are flawed by the use of different training dosage in the PFMT alone and PFMT with biofeedback groups, and sample sizes of the groups are generally small. While a few studies showed improved pelvic floor muscle function in favor of using biofeedback, none of the trials showed statistically significant improvement of urinary incontinence when biofeedback was added to the training. Based on the existing evidence from RCTs, PFMT is effective when used alone, and biofeedback is not necessary to achieve efficacy. However, some patients may be motivated to adhere to a training program and work harder using biofeedback. If available, interested and cooperative patients should be given the option of using biofeedback.

Keywords Biofeedback • Exercise • Feedback • Pelvic floor muscle training

22.1 Introduction

Shumway-Cook and Wollacott [1] have described feedback as all the sensory information that is available as the result of a movement that a person has produced. Feedback can be intrinsic (coming from the person her/himself), or extrinsic (coming from the outside, e.g. from a therapist telling how the person performs a given task). It can be given during a move-ment/maneuver such as during a pelvic floor muscle (PFM) contraction, or be expressed or explained after the action, e.g. the therapist explains a record of PFM contractions to the patient. Figures 22.1 and 22.2 show the first attempt to contract the PFM in young nullipara women without and with SUI, respectively. In pelvic floor rehabilitation, verbal feedback is usually given to all patients during instruction to make a contraction, using vaginal palpation or visual observation of movement of the perineum.

Biofeedback, on the other hand, has been defined as "a group of experimental procedures where an external sensor is used to give an indication on bodily

Kari Bø
Department of Sports Medicine, Norwegian School of Sport Sciences, Oslo, Norway

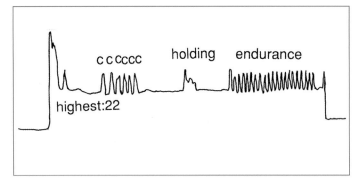

Fig. 22.1 Recordings of vaginal squeeze pressure measured by fiberoptic microtup transducer connected to an airfilled balloon (Camtach AS, Sandvika, Norway); first attempts of pelvic floor muscle contraction of a 19-year-old female student with no pelvic floor symptoms. *C*, PFM contraction (highest 22 cmH$_2$O from resting pressure to peak). The woman attempts to hold, but she is not able to do so for a long time, which is very common at the first attempts to do a PFM contraction. She is, however, able to do several repetitions of coordinated contractions

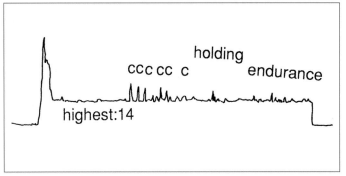

Fig. 22.2 Recordings of vaginal squeeze pressure measured by fiberoptic microtup transducer connected to an airfilled balloon (Camtach AS, Sandvika, Norway. First attempts of pelvic floor muscle contraction of an 18-year-old female student with proven stress incontinence with urodynamic assessment and 43 g of leakage on ambulatory pad test. She can contract correctly, assessed by vaginal palpation, but her voluntary contractions are weak and uncoordinated and she fatigues rapidly. She cannot hold and she is not able to repeat contractions

processes, usually with the purpose of changing the measured quality" [2]. Biofeedback equipment was developed within the area of psychology, mainly for measurement of sweating, heart rate, and blood pressure during different forms of stress. In the western world, Kegel [3] was the first to report results of pelvic floor muscle training (PFMT) on urinary incontinence (UI) and pelvic organ prolapse. He based his training protocol on thorough instruction of correct contraction, using vaginal palpation and clinical observation for direct feedback of ability to perform a correct contraction. In addition, he used a manometer to measure vaginal squeeze pressure as biofeedback of strength of the contraction during the training program. Today, a variety of biofeedback apparatus is commonly used in clinical practice to assist with PFMT, and the biofeedback can be visual, auditory, or both.

22.2   Purpose of Using Biofeedback

In urology or urogynecology textbooks, the term "biofeedback" is often used to classify a method that is different from PFMT. However, biofeedback is not a treatment by itself. It is an adjunct to training, measuring the response from a single PFM contraction.

Hence the correct terminology should be PFMT with or without biofeedback.

In the area of PFMT, both vaginal and anal surface electromyography (EMG), and urethral and vaginal squeeze pressure measurements have been utilized with the purpose of making the patients more aware of muscle function, and to enhance and motivate patients' effort during training [4, 5]. Today ultrasound and magnetic resonance imaging (MRI) can also be used as biofeedback during a PFM contraction. These methods have the advantage of being able to show both the lift (sagittal plane) and the squeeze (constriction of the hiatus in the axial plane) [6, 7].

As several research groups have found that more than 30% of women may not be able to perform a correct PFM contraction at their first consultation [8–11], some authors have suggested that biofeedback can be used to teach a correct contraction. A correct PFM contraction is described as a squeeze around the urethra, vagina, and rectum, with an inward and forward lift of the perineum [8, 12]. The most common errors during attempts to contract the PFM are to use outer pelvic muscles (e.g. the hip adductors, abdominal and gluteal muscles) [9]. In addition, Bump et al [11] found that as many as 25% were straining/pressing down instead of lifting inwards.

This is important, as straining/Valsalva opens the levator hiatus, and such maneuvers may weaken the muscles. It is imperative to be aware that erroneous attempts at PFM contractions (e.g. straining) may be registered by both manometers and dynamometers [13, 14], and contractions of other muscles than the PFM may affect surface EMG activity [15]. It takes a person to explain and instruct how to do a correct contraction, and manometers, dynamometers, or surface EMG cannot distinguish between correct and incorrect contractions. To date, vaginal palpation or ultrasound/MRI are the most valid methods for feedback/biofeedback of correct contraction and relaxation of the PFM.

Given that the patients are able to perform a correct PFM contraction, the different biofeedback apparatuses can measure the following:

- maximal voluntary contraction (MVC)
- length of the contraction (local muscular endurance)
- coordination of the contraction
- ability to repeat contractions (local muscle endurance)
- ability to relax after voluntary contraction.

Hence, the indications for use of PFMT with and without biofeedback are: UI, fecal incontinence, pelvic organ prolapse, sexual disorders, voiding difficulties, constipation, and pain.

22.3 Effect of Biofeedback Training

Since Kegel first presented his results on PFMT [3], several randomized controlled trials (RCTs) have shown that PFMT without biofeedback is more effective for stress urinary incontinence (SUI) than no treatment [16]. The recent International Consultation on Incontinence (ICI) report concluded that there did not appear to be any benefit of adding clinic-based (grade of recommendation, A) or home-based biofeedback (grade of recommendation, B) to a PFMT program [5]. National Institute for Health and Clinical Excellence (NICE) guidelines [17] found that cure rates reported after PFMT ranged between 16% and 69%, and cure rates after PFMT with biofeedback ranged from 15% to 73%. They concluded that a trial of supervised PFMT of at least 3-months duration

should be offered as first-line treatment to women with stress or mixed UI and that perineometry or pelvic floor EMG as biofeedback should not be used as a routine part of PFMT.

Table 22.1 shows the protocols and results of published RCTs comparing PFMT with and without biofeedback for SUI or mixed urinary incontinence (MUI) [18–32]. There are differences between studies in the probes used, the feedback provided, and whether biofeedback was undertaken at home or in the clinic. Treatment duration varied from 4 weeks to 6 months and the total number of participants ranged from 12 [20] to 135 [22]. When participants are randomized, some of the groups become very small. Although Berghmans et al [23] demonstrated faster progress in the biofeedback group, there is no convincing evidence that PFMT with biofeedback adds any additional benefit to PFMT alone. Four studies found a significant increase in PFM function in the PFMT + biofeedback group compared to PFMT alone, measured with either EMG [22, 32] or vaginal pressure transducers [30, 31]. Wong et al [26] found a significant subjective improvement in PFMT alone over PFMT + biofeedback in one study, and the opposite in another trial [29]. No statistically significant differences were found in objective measures of UI in any of the studies.

Unfortunately, most of the trials are flawed, with different training dosages in the two arms of the studies. The study of Glavind et al [24] was confounded by a difference in training frequency, and the effect might be due to a double training dosage in the biofeedback group, the use of biofeedback, or both. Pages et al [30] compared 60 min of group training 5 days a week with 15 min of individual biofeedback training 5 days a week, and found that the individualized biofeedback training protocol was more effective as assessed by women's report and measurement of PFM strength.

Also, the adherence to training with and without biofeedback differed [32]. When the two groups under comparison receive different dosage of training in addition to biofeedback, it is impossible to conclude what is causing a possible effect.

Other factors may also bias the results of studies comparing PFMT with and without biofeedback. Since PFMT is effective without biofeedback, a large sample size may be needed to show any additional effect over PFMT alone. In most of the published studies comparing PFMT with PFMT combined with biofeedback, the

Table 22.1 Randomized controlled trials comparing pelvic floor muscle training with or without biofeedback in women with stress and mixed urinary incontinence

Author (year)	Population and diagnosis	Design and groups	Intervention/training protocol	Adherence
Shepherd et al (1983) [18]	$n = 22$ with SUI (mean age 48 years, range 23–67 years), urodynamic assessment	RCT: (1) PFMT with biofeedback ($n = 11$); (2) PFMT ($n = 11$)	Both groups: home exercise with weekly clinic visits; (1) PFMT with BF; (2) PFMT. Duration: 3 months	Not stated; 3/11 in group 2 performed only 2 exercise sessions
Castleden et al (1984) [19]	$n = 19$ with SUI (mean age 55 years, range 23-85 years), urodynamic assessment	Crossover RCT: (1) PFMT with BF ($n = 19$); (2) PFMT ($n = 19$)	Supervised exercise with 4–5 contractions every hour; (1) PFMT with BF: measurement of MVC > 1/day; (2) PFMT. Duration: 2 weeks in each treatment; no wash-out period between treatments	Not stated
Taylor and Henderson (1986) [20]	$n = 12$ postmenopausal women with SUI (age 55–79 years); self-report of urine loss	RCT: (1) PFMT with daily biofeedback; (2) PFMT with vaginal sensor; (3) PFMT with weekly biofeedback; (4) PFMT	All groups had weekly clinic visits and home exercise with 100 repetitions/day. (1) PFMT with BF; (2) PFMT with vaginal sensor: used the vaginal sensor detached from BF-machine during exercise; (3) PFMT with weekly BF at clinic; (4) PFMT. Duration: 8 weeks	All subjects participated at all nine weekly visits at the clinic
Ferguson et al (1990) [21]	$n = 20$ (group 1, mean age 37.1 ± 6.4 years; group 2, mean age 35.8 ± 4.6 years) with SUI, urodynamic assessment	RCT: (1) PFMT with BF ($n = 10$); (2) PFMT ($n = 10$)	Both groups did home exercise, strength and endurance. Duration: 6 weeks. (1) PFMT with BF; (2) PFMT	Not stated (participants contacted weekly to document adherence; result not reported)

Outcome measure	Result (mean ± SD)		Follow-up
	Before	After	
Frequency of micturition/day	(1) 8.6; (2) 8.0	(1) 6.1; (2) 7.8	No follow-up
Incontinence episodes/week	(1) 6.5; (2) 5.5	(1) 1.1; (2) 4.1	
Vaginal squeeze pressure (cmH$_2$O)	(1) 6.4; (2) 7.1	(1) 19.3; (2) 11.2	
	Before – after: NS; between groups: NS		
VAS (completely dry to wet all the time)	(1) +23.9; (2) +6.7; significant (P < 0.05) improvement after 4 weeks; between groups: NS		No follow-up
Vaginal squeeze pressure (cm H$_2$O)	(1) +2.0, (2) +1.5; significant (P < 0.001) improvement after 4 weeks; between groups: NS		
Continence rate		(1) 100%; (2) not stated; (3) not stated; (4) 67 %. Overall the experimental groups (1–3) had a continence rate of 67%	No follow-up
MUCP (cmH$_2$O)	(1) 45.6 ± 10.6; (2) 42.7 ± 15.2	1) 50.0 ±13.7; ((2) 46.8 ± 6.9	12–24 months' follow-up
	NS		
Functional urethral length (cm)	(1) 2.5 ± 0.2; (2) 2.7 ± 0.3	(1) 2.6 ± 0.3; (2) 2.8 ± 0.3	3/20 underwent surgery
	NS		
Vaginal squeeze pressure (cmH$_2$O)	(1) 23.2 ± 10.1; (2) 38.3 ± 15.8	(1)33.4 ± 15.1; (2) 46.5 ± 20.7	8/20 discontinued exercising and reported unchanged (n = 4) or improved condition (n = 4)
	Significant (P < 0.05) improvement in both groups; between groups: NS		
Pressure area (cmH$_2$O/s)	(1) 146.5 ± 79.1; (2) 239.6 ± 98.8	(1) 234.4 ± 124.0; (2) 328.5 ± 139.7	7/20 continued exercise and reported unchanged (n = 1) or improved (n = 6) condition
	Significant (P < 0.05) improvement in both groups; between groups: NS		

(cont →)

Table 22.1 (continued)

Author (year)	Population and diagnosis	Design and groups	Intervention/training protocol	Adherence
Ferguson et al (1990) [21]				
Burns et al (1990) [22]	$n = 135$ with SUI (or mixed incontinence $n = 12$) (mean age 62 years, > 55 years), urodynamic assessment	RCT: (1) PFMT with BF ($n = 40$); (2) PFMT ($n = 43$); (3) control ($n = 38$)	(1) PFMT with BF: weekly 20 min sessions using BF with PT; (2) PFMT: daily home exercise 4 times/day; (3) control group. Duration: 8 weeks	Not stated
Berghmans et al (1993) [23]	$n = 40$ with mild to moderate SUI (group 1, mean age 46.40 ± 12.12 years, group 2, mean age 50.25 ± 10.50 years), pad test	RCT: stratified on severity of incontinence; (1) PFMT with BF ($n = 20$); (2) PFMT ($n = 20$)	Both groups had three training sessions/week at clinic; contractions varied from 3–30 s, with 10–30 repetitions in different positions (25–35 min). (1) PFMT with BF; (2) PFMT. Both groups received a home-based program to practice 3 times/day. Duration: 4 weeks	Not stated
Glavind et al (1996) [24]	$n = 34$ with SUI (median age 45 years, range 40–48 years), urodynamic assessment	RCT: (1) PFMT with BF ($n = 19$); (2) PFMT ($n = 15$)	(1) PMFT with BF: 4, weekly, + 2–3 sessions with PT using BF, instructed to do exercise at 3/day at home; (2) PFMT: 2–3 sessions with PT, instructed to do exercise at 3/day at home. Duration: 3 months	17/19 in group 1 and 7/14 in group 2 reported doing regular PFMT
Sherman et al (1997) [25]	$n = 39$ with SUI or mixed incontinence (mean age 32.9 ± 7.8 years), urodynamic assessment	RCT: stratified on diagnosis, (1) PFMT with BF ($n = 23$); (2) PFMT ($n = 16$)	Both groups had supervised sessions with 2 weeks' intervals and home exercise. Home exercise consisted of 10 s contraction/10 s relaxation for 20 min 2/day. (1) PFMT with BF; (2) PMFT. Duration: 2 months	Participants reported how much they felt they practiced their exercise on scale 1–2–3: (1) 1/15/6; (2) 5/9/1; between groups ($P = 0.01$)
Wong et al (1997) [26]	$n = 17$ with SUI (mean age 48.2 ± 7.3 years), urodynamic assessment	RCT: (1) PFMT with BF ($n = 10$); (2) PFMT ($n = 7$)	8 treatment sessions 2/weekly at clinic; (1) PFMT with BF; (2) PFMT. Duration: 8 weeks	Not stated

Outcome measure	Result (mean ± SD)		Follow-up
	Before	After	
30-min pad test (g)	(1) 4.8 ± 5.5; (2) 10.3 ± 8.1	(1) 1.4 ± 1.7; (2) 3.4 ± 4.7	
	Significant (P < 0.05) improvement in both groups; between groups: NS		
24-h pad test (g)	(1)10.6 ± 8.6; (2) 14.9 ± 15.9	(1) 5.6 ± 4.7; (2) 5.8 ± 5.6	
	Significant (P < 0.05) improvement in group 2, between groups NS		
Incontinence episodes (%)		(1) –54%; (2) –61%; (3) +9%	No follow-up
48-h pad test (g)	(1) 26.6 ± 24.5; (2) 29.0 ± 31.7	(1) 12.2 ± 15.4; (2) 12.5 ± 12.0	No follow-up
	Significant (P < 0.01) improvement in both groups; between groups: NS		
Urine loss – pad test (g)	(1) 9.0; (2) 12.8	(1) 0.8; (2) 10.0	2–3 year follow- up using questionnaire; cured: group 1: 5/19, group 2: 0/14; improved: group 1: 8/19; group 2: 4/14; regular exercise: group 1: 17/19; group 2: 7/14
	Significant improvement in group 1; significantly (P = 0.02) more improvement in group 1 compared to group 2		
Cured		(1) 11/19; (2) 3/15	
	Between groups: NS (P = 0.06)		
MUCP (cmH$_2$O)	(1) 9.68 ± 16.50; (2) 51.46 ± 23.73	(1) 80.16 ± 27.50; (2) 77.18 ± 38.41	No follow-up
Changes in 1 hour pad test (g)		(1) 7.4 ± 6.1; (2) 18.7 ± 24.8	No follow-up

(cont →)

Table 22.1 (continued)

Author (year)	Population and diagnosis	Design and groups	Intervention/training protocol	Adherence
Wong et al (1997) [26]				
Laycock et al (2001) [27]	$n = 101$ with SUI (age 20–64 years), frequency–volume chart history	RCT: (1) PFMT with BF ($n = 40$); (2) PFMT with cones ($n = 41$); (3) PFMT ($n = 20$)	All groups had 6 visits with PT during the intervention period, and home exercise 10 min/day with or without equipment. (1) PFMT with BF; (2) PFMT with cones; (3) PFMT. Duration 3 months	Compliance: (1) 79%; (2) 77%; (3) 81%
Mørkved et al (2002) [28]	$n = 94$ with SUI or mixed incontinence (group 1: age 47.8 ± 8.2 years, group 2: age 45.4 ± 8.1 years), urodynamic assessment, history and pad test.	RCT: stratified on pad test results; (1) PFMT with BF ($n = 53$); (2) PFMT ($n = 50$)	Both groups had exercise supervised by a PT 1/week for 2 months, and every second week for 4 months; 3 sets of 10 repetitions. Participants were encouraged to do the sets at home once/day. (1) PFMT with BF; (2) PFMT. Duration: 6 months.	PFMT >3/week: (1) 88.9%; (2) 85.3%

Outcome measure	Result (mean ± SD)		Follow-up
	Before	After	
	Significant improvement in both groups, between groups: NS		
Changes in incontinence episodes/week		(1) 2.0 ± 3.5; (2) 9.1 ± 12.3	
	NS, between groups: NS		
Changes in IIQ score		(1) 8.5 ± 19.9; (2) 24.5 ± 10.8	
	Significant ($P < 0.05$) more improvement in group 2 compared with group 1		
Incontinence episodes/day	(1) 2.04; (2) 2.00; (3) 1.71	(1) 1.77; (2) 1.05; (3) 0.47	No follow-up
Objective cure (≤ 2 g urine loss in standardized pad test)		(1) 28/48; (2) 21/46	No follow-up
	Between groups: NS		
Standardized pad test (g)	(1) 25.7; (2) 29.0	(1) 6.1; (2) 10.6	
	Significant improvement in both groups ($P < 0.01$); between groups: NS		
48-h pad test (g)	(1) 40.6; (2) 44.6	(1) 6.5; (2) 6.0	
	Significant improvement in both groups ($P < 0.01$); between groups: NS		
Incontinence episodes	(1) 2.8; (2) 2.8	(1) 1.9; (2) 1.9	
	Significant improvement in both groups ($P < 0.01$); between groups: NS		
SAI	(1) 9.1; (2) 9.2	(1) 9.5; (2) 9.4	
	Significant improvement in group 1 ($P = 0.01$) and group 2 ($P = 0.04$); between groups: NS		
Vaginal squeeze pressure (cmH$_2$O)	(1) 13.6; (2) 14.4	(1) 22.5; (2) 22.0	
	Significant improvement in both groups ($P < 0.01$); between groups: NS		

(cont →)

Table 22.1 (continued)

Author (year)	Population and diagnosis	Design and groups	Intervention/training protocol	Adherence
Wong et al (2001) [29]	$n = 38$ with SUI (mean age 46 years, range 30–62 years), urodynamic assessment	RCT: (1) PFMT with BF ($n = 19$); (2) PFMT with BF and EMG from abdominal muscle ($n = 19$)	4 biweekly sessions supervised by a PT, each training consisted of 5 sets including 3 fast and 2 slow contractions. (1) PFMT with BF; (2) PFMT with BF and measurement of EMG from abdominal muscle	Not stated
Pages et al (2001) [30]	$n = 40$ with SUI (age 51.1 years, range 27–80 years), physical examination and history.	RCT: (1) PFMT with BF ($n = 13$); (2) PFMT ($n = 27$)	Both groups had 90 min introduction to PFMT; (1) PFMT with BF: additional 20 min introduction to BF. PT 5/week for 4 weeks. 4 sets with 10 repetitions; (2) PFMT: 60 min group therapy 5/week for 4 weeks and home exercise. Clinic exercise in different positions and during normal activities. At home, participants of both groups were told to contract 100 times/day. Pool training twice/week. After 4 weeks, all participants continued the same exercise at home, without BF device.	Not stated

Outcome measure	Result (mean ± SD)		Follow-up
	Before	After	
MVC (cmH$_2$O)	(1) 12.9 ± 10.2; (2) 11.4 ± 7.2	(1) 21.7 ± 14.0; (2) 16.8 ± 8.1	No follow-up
	Significant improvement in group 1 (P = 0.003) and group 2 (P = 0.015); between groups: NS		
Incontinence episodes/week	(1) 9.1 ± 14.6; (2) 3.5 ± 5.6	(1) 4.1 ± 10.7; (2) 1.5 ± 3.0	
	Significant improvement in group 2 (P = 0.04); between groups: NS		
1-h pad test (g).	(1) 9.1 ± 14.6; (2) 12.5 ± 12.7	(1) 23.0 ± 69.0; (2) 3.9 ± 3.9	
	Significant improvement in group 2 (P = 0.008); between groups: NS.		
PFM endurance (s)	(1) 5.8 ± 8.5; (2) 5.0 ± 7.8	(1) 6.7 ± 3.0; (2) 6.3 ± 2.9	
	No significant improvement; between groups: NS		
IIQ-7 score	(1) 28.57; (2) 19.05	(1) 14.29; (2) 14.29	
	Significant improvement in group1 (P = 0.02); significantly more improvement (P = 0.04) in group 1 compared to group 2		
UDI-6 score	(1) 50.00; (2) 35.70	(1) 16.67; (2) 27.8	
	Significant improvement in group 1 (P = 0.01) and group 2 (P = 0.04); significantly more improvement in group 1 (P = 0.04) compared to group 2		
No incontinence episodes and symptoms (%)		(1) 28; (2) 22	3-months follow-up: (1) 62%; (2) 69%

(cont →)

Table 22.1 (continued)

Author (year)	Population and diagnosis	Design and groups	Intervention/training protocol	Adherence
Pages et al (2001) [30]				
Aksac et al (2003) [31]	$n = 50$ with SUI (mean age group 1: 51.6 ± 5.8 years, group 2: 52.5 ± 7.9 years, group 3: 54.7 ± 7.8 years), urodynamic assessment	RCT: (1) PFMT with BF ($n = 20$); (2) PFMT ($n = 20$); (3) control ($n = 20$)	(1) PFMT with BF: 20 min sessions 3 times/week. Weekly follow up with PT for 8 weeks; (2) PFMT: 10 contractions 3 times/day home exercise. Weekly follow up sessions for 8 weeks; (3) control: hormone replacement therapy (estradiol hemihydrate 2 mg/day and norethisterone acetate 1 mg/day)	Not stated

Outcome measure	Result (mean ± SD)		Follow-up
	Before	After	
	Between groups: NS		
Fewer incontinence episodes (−50%) and symptoms (%)		(1) 68; (2) 74	(1) 38%; (2) 31%
	Between groups: NS		
Vaginal squeeze pressure (cmH$_2$O) (median)	(1) 25 ± 8; (2) 25 ± 15	(1) 75 ± 21; (2) 38 ± 22	(1) 73 ± 20; (2) 36 ± 25
	Significant improvement in both groups (P < 0.01); significantly more improvement in group 1 compared with group 2 (P < 0.05)		
1-h pad test (g) (median)	(1) 20.5 ± 1.7; (2) 19.9 ± 2.5; (3) 29.1 ± 3.2	1) 1.2 ± 0.2; (2) 2.1 ± 0.4; (3) 28.2 ± 3.7	No follow-up
	Significant improvement in group 1 and 2 (P < 0.001), group 3: NS; between group 1 and 2: NS; significant difference between group 1 and 2 compared with group 3 (P < 0.001)		
Vaginal squeeze pressure (cmH$_2$O) (median)	(1) 19.1 ± 4.8; (2) 20.3 ± 6.2; (3) 18.7 ± 4.9	(1) 50.5 ± 11.5; (2) 37.5 ± 8.7; (3) 20.0 ± 3.9	
	Significant improvement in group 1 and 2 (P < 0.001), group 3: NS; significant difference between group 1 and 2 compared with group 3 (P < 0.001); significant difference between group 1 and 2 (P < 0.001)		
PFM strength via digital palpation (median)	(1) 3.3 ± 0.4; (2) 3.5 ± 0.5; (3) 3.3 ± 0.4	(1) 4.9 ± 0.2; (2) 4.8 ± 0.4; (3) 3.3 ± 0.6	
	Significant improvement in group 1 and 2 (P < 0.001), group 3: NS; significant difference between group 1 and 2 compared with group 3 (P < 0.001); between group 1 and 2: NS		
Incontinence frequency (median)	(1) 2.3 ± 0.7; (2) 2.3 ± 0.6; (3) 2.1 ± 0.9	(1) 3.5 ± 0.5; (2) 3.5 ± 0.5; (3) 2.4 ± 0.9	
	Significant improvement in group 1 and 2 (P < 0.001), group 3: NS; significant difference between group 1 and 2 compared with group 3 (P < 0.001); between group 1 and 2: NS		
SAI (median)	(1) 3.5 ± 0.4; (2) 4.5 ± 0.3; (3) 3.6 ± 0.7	(1) 8.1 ± 0.8; (2) 7.5 ± 1.2; (3) 3.6 ± 0.6	
	Significant improvement in group 1 and 2 (P < 0.001), group 3: NS; significant difference between group 1 and 2 compared with group 3 (P < 0.001); between group 1 and 2: NS		

(cont →)

Table 22.1 (continued)

Author (year)	Population and diagnosis	Design and groups	Intervention/training protocol	Adherence
Aksac et al (2003) [31]				
Aukee et al (2002) [32]	$n = 30$ (age range 31–69 years, mean age group 1: 50.8 years and group 2: 51.8 years), urodynamic assessment.	RCT: (1) PFMT with BF ($n = 15$); (2) PFMT ($n = 15$)	Both groups performed exercise at home 5 times/week, 20 min sessions; (1) PFMT with BF: +5 clinic visits with PT; (2) PFMT. Duration: 12 weeks	(1) mean 68 home sessions with BF (range 9–130) + 47.5 training days without BF (range 6–93); (2) mean training days 56.2 (range 21–87)

BF, biofeedback; EMG, electromyogram; IIQ, Incontinence Impact Questionnaire Short Form; MUCP, maximum urethral closure pressure; NS, no significant difference; PFM, pelvic floor muscle; PFMT, pelvic floor muscle training; PT, physiotherapist; SAI, Social Activity Index; SUI, stress urinary incontinence; UDI, Urogenital Inventory Short Form; VAS, visual-analog scale

sample sizes are small, and type II error may have been the reason for not finding an additional effect [5]. However, in the three largest RCTs, no significant additional effect on UI of adding biofeedback was demonstrated [22, 27, 28].

Only one RCT was found evaluating the effect of PFMT with and without biofeedback for overactive bladder (OAB). Wang et al [33] randomized 120 women, mean age 52.7 years (standard deviation (SD) 13.7 years), with symptoms of OAB to 12 weeks of PFMT, PFMT with biofeedback, or electrical stimulation.

The results showed that the groups receiving PFMT with and without biofeedback were better than the electrical stimulation group, but there were no statistically significant differences between training with and without biofeedback.

The use of home-based biofeedback requires patients to undress, go to a private room, and insert a vaginal or rectal device in order to exercise, and many patients may not like this [34]. On the other hand, some may find it motivating to use biofeedback to control and enhance the strength of the contractions when training.

Some of the new apparatus has built in registration of adherence to the training program. Any factor that may stimulate high adherence and intensive training should be recommended for the purpose of enhancing the effect of a training program. Hence, when available and the patient is motivated to use it, biofeedback can be suggested as an option for home training.

At office follow-ups, in order to record improvement, detect non-improvement at an early stage, and motivate the patient, the physiotherapist should use a responsive, reliable, and valid assessment tool to measure the response to training [14].

Outcome measure	Result (mean ± SD)		Follow-up
	Before	After	
VAS (median)		(1) 8.1 ± 0.8; (2) 7.5 ± 1.2; (3) 3.6 ± 0.6	
	Significant difference between group 1 and 2 compared with group 3 (P < 0.001); between group 1 and 2: NS		
EMG (µV), supine	(1) 15.3 ± 4.4; (2) 17.8 ± 6.8	(1) 25.8 ± 10.0; (2) 20.1 ± 8.6	No follow-up
	Significant improvement in both groups (P < 0.001); significant difference between group 1 and group 2 (P = 0.02)		
EMG (µV), standing	(1) 13.5 ± 4.7; (2) 14.7 ± 7.2	(1) 21.4 ± 10.3; (2) 20.9 ± 8.6	
	Significant improvement in both groups (P < 0.001); between groups: NS		
Leakage index	(1) 45.5 ± 10.1; (2) 38.5 ± 11.0	(1) 34.9 ± 10.4; (2) 38.1 ± 10.5	
	NS		
24-h pad test	(1) 28.1 ± 29.4; (2) 47.1 ± 34.6	(1) 19.0 ± 19.7; (2) 22.5 ± 19.6	
	Significant improvement in both groups; between groups: NS		

22.4 Clinical Recommendations for the Use of Biofeedback

1. Instruct in correct PFM contraction using vaginal palpation, visual observation, ultrasound, or MRI to give feedback of the contraction.
2. If a home biofeedback tool is available at an acceptable cost, ask if the woman is motivated to use it in her training program.
3. If the patient is cooperative and motivated, give thorough instruction on how to use and clean the apparatus.
4. Follow general strength training recommendations with three sets of 8–12 close-to-maximum contractions per day. The sets can be done separately or put together at one time-point, fitting into the individual patient's time schedule. As the use of biofeedback requires the patient to undress, we suggest that the training is done in one session.
5. Follow-up visits with the physiotherapist at least weekly or bi-weekly are recommended, to follow up improvement/non-improvement.

References

1. Shumway-Cook A, Wollacott MH (eds). Motor control: theory and practical applications, 2 edn. Williams &Wilkins, Baltimore, 1995.
2. Schwartz G, Beatty J (eds). Biofeedback: theory and research. Academic Press, New York, 1977.
3. Kegel AH. Progressive resistance exercise in the functional restoration of the perineal muscles. Am J Obstet Gynecol 1948;56:238–249.
4. Bø K (2007) Pelvic floor muscle training for stress urinary incontinence. In: Bø K, Berghmans B, Mørkved S, Van Kampen M (eds). Evidence based physical therapy for the pelvic floor: bridging science and clinical practice. Elsevier Ltd, Churchill Livingstone, Kidlington, 2007, pp 171–187.

5. Hay-Smith J, Berghmans B, Burgio K et al. Adult Conservative management. In: Abrams P, Cardozo L, Khoury S, Wein A (eds) Incontinence. 4th International Consultation on Incontinence, Paris, 5–8 July 2008. Health Publications Ltd, Portsmouth, 2009.

6. Brækken IH, Majida M, Engh ME et al. Test–retest and intra-tester reliability of two-, three- and four-dimensional perineal ultrasound of pelvic floor muscle anatomy and function. Int Urogynecol J Pelvic Floor Dysfunct 2008; 19:227–235.

7. Brækken IH, Majida M, Engh ME et al. Test–retest reliability of pelvic floor muscle contraction measured by 4D ultrasound. Neurourol Urodyn 2009;28:68–73.

8. Kegel AH. Stress incontinence and genital relaxation: a non-surgical method of increasing the tone of sphincters and their supporting structures. Ciba Clin Symp 1952;4:35–51.

9. Bø K, Larsen S, Oseid S et al. Knowledge about and ability to correct pelvic floor muscle exercises in women with urinary stress incontinence. Neurourol Urodyn 1988;7:261–262.

10. Benvenuti F, Caputo GM, Bandinelli S et al. Reeducative treatment of female genuine stress incontinence. Am J Phys Med 1987;66:155–168.

11. Bump R, Hurt WG, Fantl JA, Wyman JF. Assessment of Kegel exercise performance after brief verbal instruction. Am J Obstet Gynecol 1991;165:322–329.

12. DeLancey JO. The anatomy of the pelvic floor. Curr Opin Obstet Gynecol 1994;6:313–316.

13. Bø K, Kvarstein B, Hagen R, Larsen S. Pelvic floor muscle exercise for the treatment of female stress urinary incontinence: II. Validity of vaginal pressure measurements of pelvic floor muscle strength and the necessity of supplementary methods for control of correct contraction. Neurourol Urodyn 1990;9:479–487.

14. Bø K, Sherburn M. Evaluation of pelvic floor muscle function and strength. Phys Ther 2005;85:269–282.

15. Turker KS. Electromyography: some methodological problems and issues. Phys Ther 1993;73:698–710.

16. Hay-Smith EJC, Dumoulin C. Pelvic floor muscle training versus no treatment, or inactive control treatments, for urinary incontinence in women. Cochrane Database Syst Rev 2006;(1):CD005654.

17. Welsh A. Urinary incontinence – the management of urinary incontinence in women. National Collaborating Centre for Women's and Children's Health. The National Institute for Health and Clinical Excellence. RCOG Press, Royal College of Obstetricians and Gynaecologists, London, 2006.

18. Shepherd A, Montgomery E, Anderson RS. A pilot study of a pelvic exerciser in women with stress incontinence. Obstet Gynecol 1983;3:201–202.

19. Castleden CM, Duffin HM, Mitchell EP. The effect of physiotherapy on stress incontinence. Age Ageing 1984; 13:235–237.

20. Taylor K, Henderson J. Effects of biofeedback and urinary stress incontinence in older women. J Gerontol Nurs 1986; 12:25–30.

21. Ferguson KL, McKey PL, Bishop KR et al. Stress urinary incontinence: effect of pelvic muscle exercise. Obstet Gynecol 1990;75:671–675.

22. Burns PA, Pranikoff K, Nochajski T et al. Treatment of stress incontinence with pelvic floor exercises and biofeedback. J Am Geriatr Soc 1990;38:341–344.

23. Berghmans LC, Frederiks CM, de Bie RA et al. Efficacy of biofeedback, when included with pelvic floor muscle exercise treatment, for genuine stress incontinence. Neurourol Urodyn 1996;15:37–52.

24. Glavind K, Nøhr SB, Walter SB. Biofeedback and physiotherapy versus physiotherapy alone in the treatment of genuine stress urinary incontinence. Int Urogynecol J Pelvic Floor Dysfunct 1996;7:339–343.

25. Sherman RA, Davis GD, Wong MF. Behavioral treatment of exercise- induced urinary incontinence among female soldiers. Mil Med 1997;162:690–694.

26. Wong K, Fung B, Fung LCW, Ma S. Pelvic floor exercises in the treatment of stress urinary incontinence in Hong Kong Chinese women. Papers to be read by title, ICS 27th annual Meeting, Yokohama, Japan, 1997, pp 62–63.

27. Laycock J, Brown J, Cusack C et al. Pelvic floor reeducation for stress incontinence: comparing three methods. Br J Community Nurs 2001;6:230–237.

28. Mørkved S, Bø K, Fjørtoft T. Effect of adding biofeedback to pelvic floor muscle training to treat urodynamic stress incontinence. Obstet Gynecol 2002;100:730–739.

29. Wong K, Fung K, Fung S et al. Biofeedback of pelvic floor muscles in the management of genuine stress incontinence in Chinese women. Physiotherapy 2001;87:644–648.

30. Pages IH, Jahr S, Schaufele MK, Conradi E. Comparative analysis of biofeedback and physical therapy for treatment of urinary stress incontinence in women. Am J Phys Med Rehabil 2001;80:494–502.

31. Aksac B, Aki S, Karan A et al. Biofeedback and pelvic floor exercises for the rehabilitation of urinary stress incontinence. Gynecol Obstet Invest 2003;56:23–27.

32. Aukee P, Immonen P, Penttinen J et al. Increase in pelvic floor muscle activity after 12 weeks' training: a randomized prospective pilot study. Urology 2002;60:1020–1024.

33. Wang AC, Wang YY, Chen MC. Single blind, randomized trial of pelvic floor muscle training, biofeedback assisted pelvic floor muscle training, and electrical stimulation in the management of overactive bladder. Urology 2004; 63:61–66.

34. Prashar S, Simons A, Bryant C et al. Attitudes to vaginal/urethral touching and device placement in women with urinary incontinence. Int Urogynecol J Pelvic Floor Dysfunct 2000;11:4–8.

Medical Treatment of Urinary Incontinence, Urinary Retention, and Overactive Bladder

23

Francesco Pesce and Maria Angela Cerruto

Abstract The management of patients with lower urinary tract dysfunction is a challenge. Antimuscarinic drugs represent the first-line treatment in cases of overactive bladder syndrome (OAB). Over the past 10 years, the use of botulinum neurotoxin has revolutionized the treatment of intractable symptoms associated with OAB. All the other drugs used in the treatment of OAB (i.e. α-adrenoceptor (AR) antagonists, β-AR antagonists, prostaglandin synthesis inhibitors, vanilloid agents, cannabinoids) are investigational, and their use is either not recommended or indicated only in specific situations. In the management of stress urinary incontinence, dual serotonin and norepinephrine (noradrenalin) reuptake inhibitors (such as imipramine and duloxetine), bridging the gap between conservative treatment strategies and surgical procedures, would enhance the strength of contraction of the striated urethral sphincter, through a central effect. The pharmacological treatment of chronic urinary retention with and without urinary incontinence (UI) has the purpose of preventing damage to the upper urinary tract by normalizing bladder emptying and endourethral pressures. The drugs employed for this aim are: α-AR antagonists, acetylcholine analogs, cholinesterase inhibitors with their parasympathomimetic effect, endovesical prostaglandins, baclofen, benzodiazepines, and dantrolene. The development of pharmacologic treatment for UI is slow, and the use of some drugs that are currently marketed and prescribed is often based on tradition rather than evidence-based medicine and patient's expectation.

Keywords Overactive bladder • Pharmacotherapy • Treatment • Urinary incontinence • Urinary retention • Urgency

23.1 Introduction

The management strategy for patients with urinary incontinence is an interesting matter for discussion. The term "strategy" is usually used in medicine to describe the journey from the symptoms to the cure, but whatever situation we consider, there is still an understated meaning of "strategy" being part and parcel of the "art of the war". To plan a treatment strategy it is mandatory to know the enemy – in this context, urinary incontinence (UI). UI is "the complaint of any involuntary leakage of urine", and "in each specific circumstance it should be further described by specifying relevant factors, social impact, effect on hygiene and quality of life, the measures used to contain the

F. Pesce
Neuro-Urology Unit, CPO Hospital, Roma, Italy

G.A. Santoro, A.P. Wieczorek, C.I. Bartram (eds.) *Pelvic Floor Disorders*
© Springer-Verlag Italia 2010

leakage and whether or not the patient seeks or desires help because of it" [1]. In such a way, using language of war, it is possible to map out the "campaign" against incontinence, modifying the plans according to circumstances.

To define a treatment strategy, it is important to improve knowledge of the pathophysiology of UI and its management by means of a thorough review of relevant literature, leading to definition of levels of evidence and grades of recommendation for improved counseling of patients (so-called "evidence-based medicine" – EBM) (Box 23.1).

Box 23.1 Levels of evidence and grades of recommendation according to Oxford guidelines (modified from [2])

Levels of evidence (LE)
- *Level 1:* systematic reviews, meta-analyses, good-quality randomized controlled clinical trials (RCTs)
- *Level 2:* RCTs, good-quality prospective cohort studies
- *Level 3:* case-control studies, case series
- *Level 4:* expert opinion

Grades of recommendation (GR)
- *Grade A:* based on level 1 evidence (highly recommended)
- *Grade B:* consistent level 2 or 3 evidence (recommended)
- *Grade C:* level 4 studies or "majority evidence" (optional)
- *Grade D:* evidence inconsistent/inconclusive (no recommendation possible)

During our lifetime we spend about 98% of time collecting urine inside the bladder, and, when the correct amount of urine has been reached, the anatomic–functional unit of the lower urinary tract (LUT) makes complete and rapid bladder emptying possible.

When growing up, both humans and animals learn to voluntarily control micturition, in order to void only under suitable social and hygienic conditions. The physiological succession of the storage and voiding phases is assured by a baseline neurological mechanism that interacts with a complex neuroanatomic system, through a sequence of related and associated activities, which are modifiable by environmental, social, and behavioral factors. Micturition, as a final product of this complex mechanism, entails careful neurological control involving both the central and peripheral (somatic and autonomic) nervous systems [3, 4]. Ageing, pelvic floor disorders, hypersensitivity disorders, morphologic bladder changes, neurological diseases, local inflammations, infections, and tumors, and bladder outlet obstruction may alter the normal voluntary control of micturition, leading to UI. The main aim of pharmacotherapy for UI is to restore normal control of micturition, inhibiting the emerging pathological involuntary reflex mechanism.

23.2 Types of Urinary Incontinence

When the functional and anatomic unit of the LUT (characterized by the bladder, bladder neck, urethra, and pelvic floor) does not work properly, or in the case of an imbalance within the nervous control mechanisms, a micturition disorder occurs. This LUT dysfunction (LUTD) may be described as an alteration involving either the storage or the voiding phase, or both. Urinary incontinence may be considered as a storage symptom or a sign suggestive of LUTD, and the condition is defined by the presence of specific urodynamic observations, associated with its characteristic symptoms and signs. UI as a symptom may be classified as follows:

- urge urinary incontinence (UUI) is the complaint of involuntary leakage accompanied by or immediately preceded by urgency; urgency, with or without UUI, usually with frequency and nocturia, can be described as overactive bladder syndrome, urge syndrome, or urgency-frequency syndrome
- stress urinary incontinence (SUI) is the complaint of involuntary leakage on effort or exertion, or on sneezing or coughing
- mixed urinary incontinence (MUI) is the complaint of involuntary leakage associated with urgency and also with exertion, effort, sneezing, or coughing
- enuresis, continuous UI, and other types of UI.

According to the International Continence Society (ICS) Standardization of Terminology, the term "overflow incontinence" is no longer recommended [1]. If used, a precise definition and any associated pathophysiology should be stated. Patients with chronic retention of urine may be incontinent and have this kind of UI.

23.3 Pharmacotherapy

Pharmacotherapy should aim at: clearing up infections (antibiotics), inhibiting detrusor overactivity (antimuscarinics), relaxing the pelvic floor (alpha-blockers), reducing urinary volume, or increasing urethral closure pressure.

23.3.1 Pharmacotherapy of Urge Urinary Incontinence and Overactive Bladder

Antimuscarinic drugs represent the first-line treatment in cases of overactive bladder syndrome (OAB). OAB is a syndrome characterized by "urgency, with or without urge incontinence, usually with frequency and nocturia [...] if there is no proven infection or other obvious pathology" [1]. This combination of symptoms is suggestive of urodynamically demonstrable detrusor overactivity (DO), defined as "an urodynamic observation characterised by involuntary detrusor contractions during the filling phase" [1]. OAB is not synonym of DO, and vice versa. Actually, DO is only detected by conventional techniques in about half of patients with OAB and, on the other hand, up to 50% of patients with DO did not complain of relevant clinical symptoms. The only currently available tool to link the two disorders is urodynamics. Nevertheless, the two disorders would seem to only partially share a common underlying pathophysiological mechanism and treatment strategies. The rationale for antimuscarinic treatment is based on blockade of muscarinic receptors at both detrusor and non-detrusor sites, which prevents OAB symptoms and DO without suppressing detrusor contraction during bladder emptying; decreases urgency and leakage episodes; increases bladder capacity; reduces the number of voids per day; and improves patient quality of life.

Because most antimuscarinic drugs lack selectivity for bladder receptors, they may cause a number of adverse effects that some patients find intolerable. The occurrence of systemic side-effects is due to the wide distribution of muscarinic receptors in several parts of the body (Table 23.1).

Table 23.1 Muscarinic receptors and tissue distribution

Receptor subtype	Localization
M1	Brain; glands; sympathetic ganglia
M2	Heart; smooth muscle; midbrain
M3	Smooth muscle; glands; brain
M4	Forebrain; striated nucleus
M5	Substantia nigra

Table 23.2 Antimuscarinic side-effects

Target	Receptor	Antimuscarinic effect
Iris/ciliary body	M2	Blurred vision
Lacrimal glands	M3	Xerophthalmia
Salivary glands	M3	Xerostomia
Heart	M2	Tachycardia
Stomach/esophagus	M2	Dyspepsia
Colon	M2	Constipation
Central nervous system	M1, M2, M4, M5	Dizziness, somnolence, impaired memory

Table 23.2 lists some of the most common antimuscarinic side-effects according to muscarinic receptors and tissue targets.

The recent introduction of more selective agents (such as darifenacin and solifenacin) should allow a further reduction in the incidence of adverse events and patient withdrawal. When antimuscarinic therapy fails, other drugs may be employed.

Other drugs used in the treatment of UUI are:

- drugs with "mixed" action
- drugs acting on membrane channels
- α-adrenoceptor (AR) antagonists
- β-adrenoceptor (AR) agonists
- prostaglandin synthesis inhibitors
- other drugs.

The use of botulinum neurotoxin (BoNT) in the LUT was pioneered as early as 20 years ago, with injections into the urethral sphincter in patients with spinal cord injury and external sphincter dyssynergia, to reduce bladder-voiding pressures, urethral pressures, and post-void residual urine. Over the past 10 years, the use of botulinum neurotoxin type A (BoNTA) has revolutionized the treatment of intractable symptoms associated with OAB. According to the recent recommendations on the use of BoNTA in the treatment of LUT and pelvic floor disorders, the use of BoNTA is highly recommended in order to treat both refractory neurogenic and idiopathic DO in patients willing to use (clean)intermittent self-catheterization (grade of recommendation A) [5].

Taking into account the Oxford system [2] to give a more suitable reading key to all data available in the literature for the treatment of UUI and OAB, tolterodine, fesoterodine, oxybutynin, propiverine, darifenacin, trospium and solifenacin show the highest

Table 23.3 Levels of evidence and grades of recommendation of drugs with antimuscarinic action

Drug	Level of evidence	Grade of recommendation
Antimuscarinic drugs		
Tolterodine	1	A
Fesoterodine	1	A
Trospium	1	A
Darifenacin	1	A
Solifenacin	1	A
Propantheline	2	B
Atropine	3	C
Drugs with mixed action		
Oxybutynin	1	A
Propiverine	1	A
Dicycloverine	4	C
Flavoxate	4	D

Table 23.4 Levels of evidence and grades of recommendation of non-antimuscarinic drugs

Drug	Level of evidence	Grade of recommendation
Antidepressants		
Imipramine	3	C
α-AR antagonists		
Alfuzosin	3	C
Doxazosin	3	C
Prazosin	3	C
Terazosin	3	C
Tamsulosin	3	C
β-AR agonists		
Terbutaline	3	C
Salbutamol	3	C
COX-inhibitors		
Indometacin	2	C
Flurbiprofen	2	C
Other drugs		
Baclofen	3	C
Capsaicin	2	C
Resiniferatoxin	2	C
Botulinum toxin	1	A
Estrogens	2	C
Desmopressin	1	A

COX, cyclo-oxygenase

level of evidence (level 1) with a grade of recommendation A (Table 23.3).

From two recent systematic reviews and meta-analyses of RCTs with antimuscarinic drugs for OAB, it emerged that antimuscarinics are efficacious, safe, and well-tolerated treatments that improve health-related quality of life [6, 7]. Profiles of each drug and dosage differ and should be considered in making treatment choices. Due to the large number of drugs available on the market, the selection of the most appropriate one for every individual patient might be quite a complex task. The choice of the first drug to be used, the selection of the most appropriate dosage, formulation, and route of administration, the criteria for selection of a second anticholinergic drug in case of insufficient efficacy or intolerable adverse events, and, finally, costs are some of the most important issues that should be evaluated. Currently it is possible to state that extended-release (ER) formulations should be preferred to the immediate-release (IR) formulations due to the more favorable profile of efficacy and adverse events. With regard to IR formulations, dose escalation might yield some improvements in efficacy, but at the cost of a significant increase in the rate of adverse events. More clinical studies are needed to determine which of the available drugs should be used as first-, second-, and third-line treatments [7].

All the other drugs used in the treatment of OAB (i.e. α-AR antagonists, β-AR antagonists, prostaglandin synthesis inhibitors, vanilloid agents, cannabi-noids) are investigational, and their use is either not recommended (grade D) or indicated only in specific situation (grade C) (Tables 23.3, 23.4).

23.3.2 Pharmacotherapy of Stress Urinary Incontinence

Specific causes of female SUI include problems of urethral weakness and vaginal relaxation; the role of childbirth and possible related pelvic muscle tears; urethral and vaginal support; and ageing effects.

The aim of the pharmacological treatment of SUI is to increase the endourethral pressure acting either on the urethral smooth and striated muscles or on the pelvic floor. Several drugs are proposed with this purpose, such as estrogens, α-AR agonists, β-AR antagonists, clenbuterol, serotonin and norephinephrine (noradrenalin) reuptake inhibitors (imipramine and duloxetine).

In women, estrogen-sensitive tissues of the bladder, urethra, and pelvic floor play an important role in the urinary continence mechanisms. The urethra has four functional estrogen-sensitive layers that contribute to maintaining positive urethral pressure, and thus urinary continence: the urothelium, vascularization, connective tissue, and muscular tissue. Estrogens appear to be able to increase urethral closure pressure, improve the transmission of abdominal pressure to the proximal urethra, and increase the sensitivity threshold of the bladder.

The role of estrogens in the treatment of female SUI is controversial. When administered as a monotherapy, estrogens do not seem to be an effective treatment; however they may play a role in combination with other drugs such as α-agonists.

α-AR agonists may increase urethral resistance, thereby modifying the urethral pressure. They are used in combination with estrogens or other non-surgical therapeutic options, with interesting results. Nevertheless, because of unacceptable cardiovascular side-effects, there is currently no α-AR agonist that is effective in monotherapy, or in combination with other drugs, for SUI treatment.

The rationale for the use of β-AR antagonists in the treatment of SUI is that blocking urethral β-ARs may amplify the effect of noradrenalin on α-adrenoceptors. Although the use of propanolol showed positive effects on SUI, currently there are no RCTs supporting its administration. Clenbuterol is a β2-AR agonist that is able to increase maximal urethral closure pressure, improving continence in women with SUI. Further well-designed RCTs on the effectiveness of this drug are needed in order to define its mechanism of action and its clinical potential in the treatment of SUI [8].

In the management of SUI, dual serotonin and noradrenalin reuptake inhibitors (such as imipramine and duloxetine), bridging the gap between conservative treatment strategies and surgical procedures, would enhance the strength of contraction of the striated urethral sphincter, through a central effect on Onuf's nucleus, at the sacral spinal level.

Duloxetine has been shown to give 54% reduction of UI episodes. Nausea is the most common side-effect, occurring in up to 23–28% of cases, and causing therapy withdrawal in up to 5.7% of patients. According to the Oxford System, duloxetine has a grade of recommendation A (Table 23.5). Although the benefits of duloxetine seem to be maintained for up to 30 months in patients who continued treatment, these fa-

Table 23.5 Drugs used in the treatment of stress urinary incontinence

Drug	Level of evidence	Grade of recommendation
Duloxetine	1	A
Imipramine	3	D
Methoxamine	2	D
Midodrine	2	C
Ephedrine	3	D
Norephedrine	3	D
Estrogens	2	D

vorable results need to be interpreted cautiously, as many patients discontinued treatment and those with better responses are more likely to continue taking medication (level of evidence 3) [9].

23.3.3 Pharmacotherapy in Patients with Chronic Retention of Urine with and without Urinary Incontinence

The pharmacological treatment of chronic urinary retention with and without UI has the purpose of preventing damage to the upper urinary tract by normalizing bladder emptying and endourethral pressures.

The drugs employed for this aim are: α-AR antagonists, acetylcholine analogues, cholinesterase inhibitors with their parasympathomimetic effect, endovesical prostaglandins, baclofen, benzodiazepines, and dantrolene (Table 23.6).

Acetylcholine analogues such as bethanechol and carbachol, cholinesterase inhibitors, and β-AR antagonists have not been documented to have beneficial effects that significantly increase endovesical pressures improving bladder voiding.

Stimulation of detrusor activity by intravescical instillation of prostaglandins has been reported to be successful; however, the effect is controversial and no RCTs are available.

α-AR antagonists could have a role in reducing urethral resistance, but RCTs are lacking and the currently available evidence is inconsistent. Phenoxybenzamine is no longer used because of uncertainties about its carcinogenic effects and its side-effects.

Baclofen, benzodiazepines, and dantrolene sodium

Table 23.6 Drugs used in the treatment of chronic retention of urine with and without urinary incontinence

Drug	Level of evidence	Grade of recommendation
α-AR antagonists		
Alfuzosin	4	C
Doxazosin	4	C
Prazosin	4	C
Terazosin	4	C
Tamsulosin	4	C
Phenoxybenzamine	4	Not recommended
Acetylcholine analogues		
Bethanecol	4	D
Carbachol	4	D
Cholinesterase inhibitors		
Distigmine	4	D
Other drugs		
Baclofen	4	C
Benzodiazepines	4	C
Dantrolene	4	C

play a role in decreasing outflow resistance, particularly in patients with associated pelvic floor spasticity [8].

23.4   Conclusions

Many drugs have been proposed for a range of possible central and peripheral pharmacologic targets in UI, but often with disappointing results because of poor efficacy and side-effects. The development of pharmacologic treatment for UI is slow, and the use of some drugs that are currently marketed and prescribed is based on tradition rather than EBM. All treatment strategies in the management of UI come from a combination of knowledge, diagnostic devices, and therapeutic options, but strategies cannot be planned without attention to what patients want. The

majority of women have realistic expectations regarding treatment outcomes and cure. A process of consultation between the patient and healthcare advisor is mandatory, and should be based on an appropriate explanation of the patient's problem and expectations, alternative lines of management, indications, and risks of treatment.

References

1. Abrams PA, Cardozo L, Fall M et al. The standardisation of terminology of lower urinary tract function: report from the standardisation sub-committee of the International Continence Society. Neurourol Urodyn 2002;21:167–178.
2. Oxford Centre for Evidence-based Medicine. Levels of evidence (March 2009). http://www.cebm.net/levels_of_evidence.asp (accessed 26 November 2009).
3. Morrison J, Birder L, Craggs M et al. Neural control. In: Abrams P, Cardozo L, Khoury S, Wein A (eds) Incontinence. Health Publication Ltd, Paris, 2005, pp 363–422.
4. Mostwin J, Bourcier A, Haab F et al. Pathophysiology and urinary incontinence, fecal incontinence and pelvic organ prolapse. In: Abrams P, Cardozo L, Khoury S, Wein A (eds) Incontinence. Health Publication Ltd, Paris, 2005, pp 423–484.
5. Apostolidis A, Dasgupta P, Denys P et al. Recommendations on the use of botulinum toxin in the treatment of lower urinary tract disorders and pelvic floor dysfunctions: a European Consensus Report. Eur Urol 2009;55:100–120.
6. Chapple CR, Khullar V, Gabriel Z et al. The effects of antimuscarinic treatments in overactive bladder: an update of a systematic review and meta-analysis. Eur Urol 2008; 54:543–562.
7. Novara G, Galfano A, Secco S et al. A systematic review and meta-analysis of randomised controlled trials with antimuscarinic drugs for overactive bladder. Eur Urol 2008; 54:740–764.
8. Andersson KE, Appell R, Cardozo L et al. Pharmacological treatment of urinary incontinence. In: Abrams P, Cardozo L, Khoury S, Wein A (eds) Incontinence. Health Publication Ltd, Paris, 2005, pp 809–854.
9. Bump RC, Voss S, Beardsworth A et al. Long-term efficacy of duloxetine in women with stress urinary incontinence. BJU Int 2008;102:214–218.

Invited Commentary

G. Willy Davila

Disorders of bladder control are primarily of neuromuscular origin. This can be expanded to a statement that all pelvic floor dysfunctions have at least a component of neuromuscular dysfunction contributing to the pathophysiology of the condition – at least at its initiation. The application of rehabilitative therapy to pelvic floor conditions is well accepted and recognized as a valuable treatment option for the vast majority of patients with urinary and fecal incontinence. The use of this approach for other pelvic floor conditions such as pain and prolapse is less well recognized and accepted. In Chapter 22, Bø and Di Benedetto review their experience in the management of pelvic organ prolapse (POP) with biofeedback and physiotherapy. Therapy for POP has been limited, until now, to the use of pessaries or reconstructive surgery, but interest in physiotherapy for POP has been increasing, primarily due to patients' interest in less invasive options. In the realm of self-help options for POP, it is important to educate patients about the importance of early detection of POP, as initiation of physiotherapy once the vaginal mucosa is exteriorized is rather ineffective. If initiated early in the course of prolapse progression, and associated with other behavioral modification interventions such as avoidance of heavy lifting, smoking cessation, and weight loss, physiotherapy may indeed be very useful in surgery avoidance. Data are limited, but this chapter allows the clinician to present outcome data from well-designed studies to his/her patients who wish to consider physiotherapy for POP.

Medical therapy (pharmacotherapy) for the various forms of voiding dysfunction, including urinary incontinence, has represented the mainstay of therapy, at least in the US and many parts of Europe. A growing understanding of the biochemistry and physiology of lower urinary tract (LUT) function – focused mainly on the role of cholinergic and adrenergic receptors – has led to the development of pharmacologic agents with specific LUT targets. This has led to improved efficacy as well as safety and reduced side-effects (read this as improved compliance with prescribed therapy) associated with new agents. The future holds promise for newer, even more LUT-specific agents for patients with urinary incontinence and voiding dysfunction. Chapter 23, by Pesce and Cerruto, addresses LUT dysfunction as "the enemy" in a war to improve patients' bladder symptoms and quality of life. It is a comprehensive "tour" through the various pharmacotherapeutic agents and conditions they are intended to treat. This Chapter does not stop to address each agent in detail, so it is more what in the US is called a "whistle stop tour", leaving the reader with a generalized review of LUT pharmacotherapy. However, the focus is firmly on evidence-based medicine and scientific reports. The reader can readily perform a literature search for each agent for more details.

G.W. Davila
Department of Gynecology, Urogynecology and Reconstructive
Pelvic Surgery, Cleveland Clinic Florida, Weston, FL, USA

G.A. Santoro, A.P. Wieczorek, C.I. Bartram (eds.) *Pelvic Floor Disorders*
© Springer-Verlag Italia 2010

Section V
Fecal Incontinence

Fecal Incontinence: Introduction

Giuseppe Di Falco and Giulio Aniello Santoro

Continence depends on a number of factors that include stool consistency, the capacity of the sigmoid colon to retard progress of stool, the compliance and sensation of urgency of the rectum, phasic contractions of the puborectalis muscle to form a normal anorectal angle, a normal internal (IAS) and external anal sphincter (EAS) function, and normal sensation in the anal canal [1–3].

Fecal incontinence (FI) is the inability to control the release of bowel contents. The etiology of FI can be subdivided into three main groups: (1) functional, (2) sphincter weakness, and (3) sensory loss (Table V.1) [1–3]. The majority of patients with incontinence are women with an obstetric injury, and symptoms can occur even in an elderly population who had experienced vaginal deliveries earlier in life [4]. It is important to differentiate between minor levels of functional loss and the clinical state in which there is a serious disruption of normal life. Minor degrees of FI are defined as the occasional fecal staining of underwear (fecal leakage or soiling or seepage), incontinence of flatus, incontinence in the presence of loose stool only, or rectal urgency. Major incontinence is defined as the frequent and inadvertent voiding per anum of formed stool, and represents the most severe form of FI [1–3]. Several incontinence severity scales have been described in the last ten years [5–9]. The most popular grading scale is the Parks' system (Table V.2) [5]. However, this grading scale has the disadvantages of not taking into consideration the frequency of leakage episodes. The Cleveland Clinic Florida Fecal Incontinence Score (CCF-FIS) considers the kind of content and frequency of leakage and, in addition, includes questions on the use of pads or lifestyle alteration (Table V.3) [1].

Diagnosing the cause and assessing the severity of FI precede any treatment [10–12]. The physiology of defecation and continence has been traditionally studied with anorectal manometry and neurophysiologic investigations (pudendal nerve terminal motor latency, mucosal electrosensitivity, electromyography) [12–15]. Anorectal manometry provides a number of useful clinical data; however, it can only offer indirect and not very reliable information on the integrity of anal sphincters, based on registration of the resting pressure, squeeze pressure, and rectoanal inhibitory reflex [13, 14]. The importance of endoanal (EAUS) and transperineal (TPUS) ultrasound in delineating the different structures of the anal canal and the pelvic floor has been confirmed in numerous studies [16–20]. The ultrasonographic images of the anal sphincters are realistic, and their modifications are well correlated to anorectal function [19, 20]. EAUS has better diagnostic specificity and sensitivity when compared with digital examination and computerized tomography. Magnetic resonance imaging (MRI) has been suggested as a better diagnostic procedure [21–23]. However, differences in definition of anal canal anatomy have been described in relation to the technique used. The endoanal coil has been used for a long time; however, it could distort the anatomy and, recently, a phased-array technique has been preferred [21–23]. With this procedure, all the main features of the anal canal morphology shown with EAUS are similarly confirmed: good resolution of the IAS; shorter EAS at the anterior anal canal in females; no precise subdivision of the EAS into two or three parts; and difficulty measuring the perineal body. The only significant advantage of phased-array

G.A. Santoro
Pelvic Floor Unit and Colorectal Service, 1st Department
of General Surgery, Regional Hospital, Treviso, Italy

G.A. Santoro, A.P. Wieczorek, C.I. Bartram (eds.) *Pelvic Floor Disorders*
© Springer-Verlag Italia 2010

Table V.1 Etiology of fecal incontinence

Category	Mechanism	Common causes
Functional	Rapid transit	Irritable bowel syndrome, inflammatory bowel disease, tumors
	Pelvic floor dyssynergia	Idiopathic, spinal cord injury
	Psychological	Dementia, psychosis, behavioral
Sphincter weakness	Sphincter muscle injury	Obstetrical trauma, accidental trauma, surgical trauma
	Pudendal nerve injury	Obstetrical trauma, idiopathic, peripheral neuropathy
	Central nervous system injury	Spina bifida, spinal cord injury, cerebrovascular accident
Sensory loss	Afferent nerve injury	Diabetic neuropathy, spinal cord injury

Table V.2 Grading of fecal incontinence according to Parks [5]

Grade	Description
Parks I	Fully continent
Parks II	Soiling or incontinence to gas
Parks III	Incontinence to liquid stool
Parks IV	Incontinence to solid stool

Table V.3 Cleveland Clinic Florida Fecal Incontinence Score (CCF-FIS) [1]

Type of incontinence	Frequency				
	Never	Rarely	Sometimes	Usually	Always
Incontinence to solid stool	0	1	2	3	4
Incontinence to liquid stool	0	1	2	3	4
Incontinence to gas	0	1	2	3	4
Need to wear a pad	0	1	2	3	4
Lifestyle alteration	0	1	2	3	4

Never: 0; rarely: < 1 month; sometimes: < 1 week to ≥ 1 month; usually: < 1 day to ≥1 week; always: ≥ 1 day

MRI over endoanal MRI and EAUS is the imaging of a wider field of view [24, 25]. Considering technical characteristics, time consumption, costs, and availability of instruments in the hospitals, in our opinion MRI should be used in cases of clinical complexity when EAUS is unable to give reliable information.

The treatment of FI remains somewhat empirical despite considerable advances in understanding the pathophysiology of this condition. Most patients have acquired anal incontinence, secondary to obstetric laceration [1, 2, 4], previous anorectal surgery (such as fistulotomy or hemorrhoidectomy) [26–29], or trauma (such as impalement). These injuries are the most amenable to surgical management, specifically anal sphincteroplasty [30–33]. Other causes of incontinence, such as longstanding prolapse or third- to fourth-degree hemorrhoids, often respond to treatment of the primary disorder alone. More difficult to treat are the neurogenic injuries, such as those resulting from massive neuromuscular trauma, myelomeningocele, or demyelinating diseases of the spinal cord, and diabetic neuropathy. A procedure suited to injuries of this type is to create a neosphincter with transposition of the gracilis muscle [34–38], or an artificial bowel sphincter [39]. Inflammatory conditions, such as ulcerative colitis, Crohn's colitis, amebic colitis, or radiation-induced proctitis, can cause incontinence by diarrhea or because of decreased compliance of the rectum secondary to inflammation or scarring, and treatment should be aimed at the primary problem. Sacral nerve stimulation represents a new therapeutic approach for the specific group of patients with idiopathic FI, in which traditional pelvic repair would not be effective [40–42]. An innovative treatment is radiofrequency energy delivered to the anal sphincter, creating precise submucosal thermal lesions. Over time, these lesions are resorbed, and the tissue contracts [43, 44]. In patients in whom there is no functioning sphincter muscle at all and in whom it is impractical to create a neosphincter, a defunctioning stoma is often the best option.

In these section, the accuracy and reliability of EAUS, TPUS and MRI in the evaluation of anal sphincter injury will be discussed and compared. The usefulness of anorectal manometry and neurophysiologic investigations will also be described. A critical appraisal of the numerous procedures available for the treatment of the different forms of FI will be presented.

References

1. Jorge JM, Wexner SD. Etiology and management of fecal incontinence. Dis Colon Rectum 1993;36:77–97.
2. Santoro GA, Bartolo DCC. Incontinence surgery. In: Beynon J, Carr ND (eds) Recent advances in coloproctology. Springer-Verlag, London, 2000, pp 123–134.
3. Rudolph W, Galandiuk S. A practical guide to the diagnosis and management of fecal incontinence. Mayo Clin Proc 2002;77:271–275.
4. Oberwalder M, Dinnewitzer A, Baig K et al. The association between late-onset fecal incontinence and obstetric anal sphincter defects. Arch Surg 2004;139:429–432.
5. Parks AG. Anorectal incontinence. J R Soc Med 1975; 68:21–30.
6. Pescatori M, Anastasio G, Bottini C, Mentasti A. New grading and scoring for anal incontinence. Evaluation of 335 patients. Dis Colon Rectum 1992;35:482–487.
7. Vaizey CJ, Carapeti E, Cahill JA, Kamm MA. Prospective comparison of fecal incontinence grading systems. Gut 1999;44:77–80.
8. Rockwood TH, Church JM, Fleshman JW. Patient and surgeon ranking of the severity of symptoms associated with fecal incontinence. Dis Colon Rectum 1999;42:1525–1532.
9. Rockwood TH, Church JM, Fleshman JW. Fecal incontinence quality of life scale: quality of life instrument for patients with fecal incontinence. Dis Colon Rectum 2000;43:9–17.
10. Whitehead WE, Wald A, Norton NJ. Treatment options for fecal incontinence. Dis Colon Rectum 2001;44:131–144.
11. Keighley MRB, Fielding JWL. Management of faecal incontinence and results of surgical treatment. Br J Surg 1983;70:463–468.
12. Liberman H, Faria J, Ternent CA et al. A prospective evaluation of the value of anorectal physiology in the management of fecal incontinence. Dis Colon Rectum 2001; 44:1567–1574.
13. Simpson RR, Kennedy ML, Hung Nguyen M et al. Anal manometry: a comparison of techniques. Dis Colon Rectum 2006;49:1033–1038.
14. Perry RE, Blatchford GJ, Christensen MA et al. Manometric diagnosis of anal sphincter injuries. Am J Surg 1990;159:112–117.
15. Fleshman JW. Determination of pudendal nerve terminal motor latency. In: Smith LE (ed) Practical guide to anorectal testing. Igaku-Shoin, New-York, 1995, pp 221–226.
16. Thakar R, Sultan A. Anal endosonography and its role in assessing the incontinent patient. Best Pract Res Clinic Obstet Gynaecol 2004;18:157–173.
17. Gold DM, Bartram CI, Halligan S et al. Three-dimensional endoanal sonography in assessing anal canal injury. Br J Surg 1999;86:365–370.
18. Christensen AF, Nyhuus B, Nielsen MB, Christensen H. Three-dimensional anal endosonography may improve diagnostic confidence of detecting damage to the anal sphincter complex. Br J Radiol 2005;78:308–311.
19. Sentovich SM, Blatchford GJ, Rivela LJ et al. Diagnosing anal sphincter injury with transanal ultrasound and manometry. Dis Colon Rectum 1997;40:1430–1434.
20. Tjandra JJ, Milsom JW, Schroeder T, Fazio VW. Endoluminal ultrasound is preferable to electromyography in mapping anal sphincter defects. Dis Colon Rectum 1993; 36:689–692.
21. Stoker J, Rociu E, Zwamborn AW et al. Endoluminal MR imaging of the rectum and anus: technique, applications and pitfalls. Radiographics 1999;19:383–398.
22. Williams AB, Malouf AJ, Bartram CI et al. Assessment of external anal sphincter morphology in idiopathic fecal incontinence with endocoil magnetic resonance imaging. Dig Dis Sci 2001;46:1466–1471.
23. Morren GL, Beets-Tan GH, van Engelshoven MA. Anatomy of the anal canal and perianal structures as defined by phased-array magnetic resonance imaging. Br J Surg 2001;88:1506–1512.
24. Rociu E, Stoker J, Eijkemans MJC et al. Fecal incontinence: endoanal US versus endoanal MR imaging. Radiology 1999;212:453–458.
25. Beets-Tan RGH, Morren GL, Betts GL et al. Measurement of anal sphincter muscles: endoanal US, endoanal MR imaging, or phased-array MR imaging? A study with healthy volunteers. Radiology 2001;220:81–89.
26. Bennett RC, Friedman MHW, Goligher JC. Late results of haemorrhoidectomy by ligature and excision. BMJ 1963;2:216–219.
27. Speakman CT, Burnett SJ, Kamm MA, Bartram CI. Sphincter injury after anal dilatation demonstrated by anal endosonography. Br J Surg 1991;78:1429–1430.
28. Khubchandani IT, Reed JF. Sequelae of internal sphincterotomy for chronic fissure in ano. Br J Surg 1989; 76:431–434.
29. Kennedy HL, Zegarra JP. Fistulotomy without external sphincter division for high anal fistula. Br J Surg 1990; 77:898–901.
30. Fang DT, Nivatvongs S, Vermeulen FD et al. Overlapping sphincteroplasty for acquired anal incontinence. Dis Colon Rectum 1984;27:720–722.
31. Ctercteko GH, Fazio VW, Jagelman DG et al. Anal sphincter repair: a report of 60 cases and review of the literature. Aust N Z J Surg 1988;58:703–710.
32. Miller R, Orrom WJ, Cornes H et al. Anterior sphincter pli-

cation and levatorplasty in the treatment of faecal incontinence. Br J Surg 1989;76:1058–1060.

33. Zorcolo L, Covotta L, Bartolo DCC. Outcome of anterior
sphincter repair for obstetric injury: comparison of early
and late results. Dis Colon Rectum 2005;48:524–531.

34. Faucheron JL, Hannoun L, Thome C, Parc R. Is fecal continence improved by nonstimulated gracilis muscle transposition? Dis Colon Rectum 1994;37:979–983.

35. Konsten J, Baeten CGMI, Havenith MG, Soeters PB. Morphology of dynamic graciloplasty compared with the anal
sphincter. Dis Colon Rectum 1993;35:559–563.

36. Seccia M, Menconi C, Balestri R, Cavina E. Study protocols
and functional results in 86 electrostimulated graciloplasties.
Dis Colon Rectum 1994;37:897–904.

37. Baeten CGMI, Geerdes BP, Adang EMM et al. Anal dynamic
graciloplasty in the treatment of intractable faecal incontinence. N Engl J Med 1995;332:1600–1605.

38. Wexner SD, Gonzalez-Padron A, Rius J et al. Stimulated
gracilis neosphincter operation. Dis Colon Rectum 1996;
39:957–964.

39. Wong WD, Jensen LL, Bartolo DCC, Rothenberger DA.

Artificial anal sphincter. Dis Colon Rectum 1996;39:1345–
1351.

40. Malouf AJ, Vaizey CJ, Nicholls RJ, Kamm M. Permanent
sacral nerve stimulation for fecal incontinence. Ann Surg
2000;232:143–148.

41. Ganio E, Ratto C, Masin A et al. Neuromodulation for fecal
incontinence: outcome in 16 patients with definitive implant.
The initial Italian Sacral Neurostimulation Group (GINS)
experience. Dis Colon Rectum 2001;44:965–970.

42. Matzel KE, Kamm MA, Stosser M et al. Sacral spinal nerve
stimulation for faecal incontinence: multicentre study. Lancet
2004;363:1270–1276.

43. Takahashi T, Garcia-Osogobio S, Valdovinos MA et al. Radio-frequency energy delivery to the anal canal for the treatment of fecal incontinence. Dis Colon Rectum 2002;
45:915–922.

44. Efron JE, Corman ML, Fleshman J et al. Safety and effectiveness of temperature-controlled radio-frequency energy
delivery to the anal canal (Secca procedure) for the treatment of fecal incontinence. Dis Colon Rectum 2003;
46:1606–1618.

Giulio Aniello Santoro and Giuseppe Di Falco

Abstract Endoanal ultrasonography (EAUS) is important in patients with fecal incontinence (FI) to differentiate between incontinent patients with intact anal sphincters
and those with sphincter lesions (defects, scarring, thinning, thickening, and atrophy).
High-resolution multiplanar reconstructions and rendering techniques further enhance
the accuracy of EAUS. Ultrasonographic findings may lead to appropriate therapy
(sphincteroplasty, graciloplasty, injection of bulking agents, sacral nerve stimulation),
and the technique also serves as a surveillance tool to monitor results following
surgical treatment. In addition, detection of occult tears after vaginal delivery may
have a role in the prevention of FI, with a recommendation that women at increased
risk have an elective cesarean section.

Keywords Anal sphincters lesion • Endoanal ultrasonography • External sphincter
atrophy • Fecal incontinence • Three-dimensional ultrasonography

24.1 Introduction

Fecal incontinence (FI) is a complex problem of diverse causes. Childbirth and anorectal surgery (hemorrhoidectomy, lateral sphincterotomy, fistulotomy,
and transanal stapling) are the main causes because
the anal sphincters and the pudendal nerve may be
damaged [1–4]. A systematic evaluation is fundamental to reveal the underlying pathophysiology and lead
to appropriate therapy. As previously reported in Chapter 8, with endoanal ultrasonography (EAUS) the
anatomy and pathology of the sphincter complex can
be visualized in detail [5–7]. Features shown by EAUS
can help to differentiate between incontinent patients
with intact anal sphincters and those with sphincter

lesions (defects, scarring, thinning, thickening, and
atrophy) [8–10]. In addition, a major impact of EAUS
has been to image tears of the sphincters that are not
apparent on clinical examinations, so-called "occult
tears", initially reported in 35% of first-time vaginal
deliveries [4, 11, 12]. Diagnosis of undetected defects
may have a role in the prevention of FI, enabling a
recommendation that women at increased risk have
an elective cesarean section.

Specific scores have been reported to define the severity of the sphincter damage [13–15]. Starck et al [13]
used a score from 0 to 16 to describe the extent of the
endosonographic defects, with a score of 0 indicating
no defect, and a score of 16 a defect > 180 degrees involving the whole length and depth of the sphincter
(Table 24.1). Tears are defined by an interruption of the
fibrillar echo texture. Scarring is characterized by loss
of normal architecture, with an area of amorphous texture
that usually has low reflectiveness. The operator should

G.A. Santoro
Pelvic Floor Unit and Colorectal Service, 1st Department
of General Surgery, Regional Hospital, Treviso, Italy

identify if there is a combined lesion of the internal (IAS) and external (EAS) anal sphincters, and of the puborectalis muscle (PR), or if the lesion involves just one muscle. The number, circumferential (radial angle in degrees or in hours of the clock site) and longitudinal (proximal, distal or full length) extension of the defect, presence of scarring, differences in echogenicity and thickness of the sphincters, and other local alteration should be carefully assessed and should always be described. However, finding a sphincter defect does not necessarily mean that it is the cause of FI, as many people have sphincter lesions without having symptoms of incontinence [16]. On the other hand, patients with FI and an apparent intact sphincter can have muscle degeneration or atrophy, or pudendal neuropathy [3, 17]. The size of the defects appears to correlate with the severity of FI, as reported by Thakar and Sultan [8]; however, Voyvodic et al [18] failed to demonstrate a relationship between muscle injuries and the severity of

clinical symptoms. Ultrasonography should, therefore, be complementary to anorectal manometry, neurophysiologic tests, or other imaging modalities [19, 20].

24.2 Internal Anal Sphincter Abnormalities

The majority of lesions of the IAS are due to obstetric or iatrogenic injuries, often in combination with injuries to the EAS. Minor degrees of FI (soiling) due to IAS injuries have been reported in 29% of patients after hemorrhoidectomy or mucoprolapsectomy [21]. Manual anal dilatation [22] or lateral internal sphincterotomy [23] for the treatment of anal fissure have been associated with FI in 27% and 50% of patients, respectively. Up to 60% of patients can become incontinent following fistula surgery [24].

Defects of the IAS are easily recognized given the

Table 24.1 Ultrasonographic scoring system to define the severity of sphincter lesion (13)

Defect characteristic	Score 0	Score 1	Score 2	Score 3
Internal sphincter defect				
Length	None	Half or less	More than half	Whole
Depth	None	Partial	Total	–
Size	None	≤ 90°	91–180°	> 180°
External sphincter defect				
Length	None	Half or less	More than half	Whole
Depth	None	Partial	Total	–
Size	None	≤ 90°	91–180°	> 180°

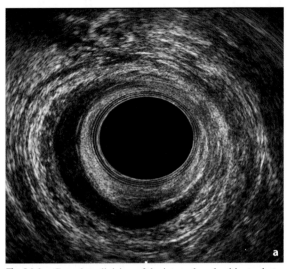 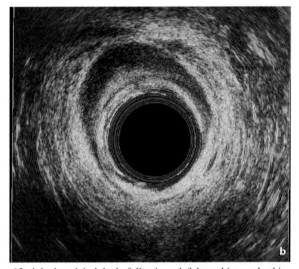

Fig. 24.1 a Complete division of the internal anal sphincter between 12 o'clock and 4 o'clock following a left lateral internal sphincterotomy for fissure. The remaining muscle appears slightly thicker for a retraction phenomenon. **b** Internal sphincter lesions between 3 o'clock and 9 o'clock

prominent appearance of the IAS in the mid-anal canal, and they appear as hyperechoic breaks in the normally hypoechoic ring. The pattern of sphincter disruption is related to the type of surgery. Patients who are incontinent after sphincterotomy have a single defect in the IAS associated with a thickening of the remaining muscle for a retraction phenomenon (Fig. 24.1). Patients who are incontinent following manual dilatation exhibit a diffuse thinning of the IAS, or disruption of the IAS at more than one site (Fig. 24.2) [25]. Patients who become incontinent following hemorrhoidectomy have defects in the site of the hemorrhoidal cushions (Fig. 24.3) [26]. Fistula surgery or obstetric trauma is associated with combined IAS and EAS injuries (Fig. 24.4) [13, 15]. A thinning of the IAS of less than 2 mm in a patient more than 50 years old is abnormal, and the term "primary degeneration of the IAS" has been used to describe this. Vaizey et al [17] reviewed the EAUS examinations of 38 patients with passive FI and intact anal sphincter. The IAS appeared thinner than normal and hyperechoic, and these conditions were combined with reduced resting pressure and normal squeeze pressure, rectal sensitivity, and pudendal latency. Incontinent patients with IAS degeneration were found to be older than those with obstetric trauma. An apparently opposite EAUS condition is an abnormal thickness of the IAS (Fig. 24.5). This seems typical of older ages and presents without differences of anal canal levels [6].

Ultrasonographic imaging may help to follow up clinical results after treatment [27] (Fig. 24.6). In a study by de la Portilla et al [28], 3D-EAUS evaluation of injectable silicone biomaterial (PTQ) implants to treat fecal incontinence due to IAS damage demonstrated that all the implants were properly located at 3 months. At 24 months, 75% (33/37) of implants were still properly located. The authors found that the continence deterioration suffered by most patients after the first year from the injection was not related to the localization and number of the implants the patient had.

24.3 External Anal Sphincter Abnormalities

One of the most important contributions of EAUS has been in the correct imaging of the EAS [5, 6], which is of major importance for continence. The most frequent cause of FI is an obstetric injury to the EAS. All

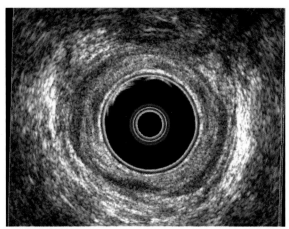

Fig. 24.2 Fragmentation of the internal anal sphincter following manual dilatation

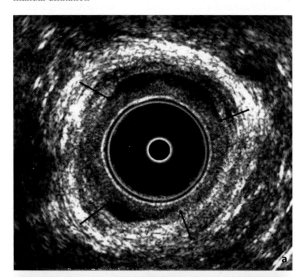

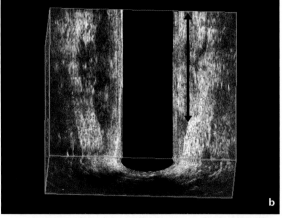

Fig. 24.3 Internal anal sphincter lesions following hemorrhoidectomy. **a** Two defects can be demonstrated between 2 o'clock and 6 o'clock (90°) and between 7 o'clock and 10 o'clock (90°) (*arrows*). **b** Three-dimensional reconstruction in the coronal plane allows the length of the defect to be measured (2.2 cm) (*arrow*)

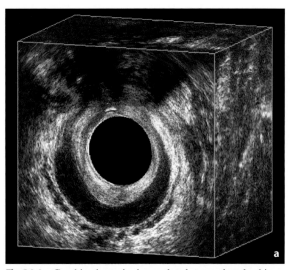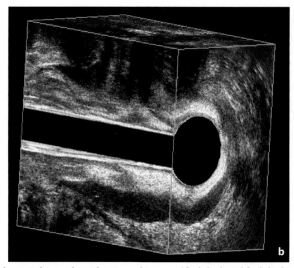

Fig. 24.4 **a** Combined anterior internal and external anal sphincter damage due to obstetric trauma between 10 o'clock and 2 o'clock. **b** Reconstruction in the longitudinal plane shows the complete loss of both sphincters anteriorly and the presence of scar

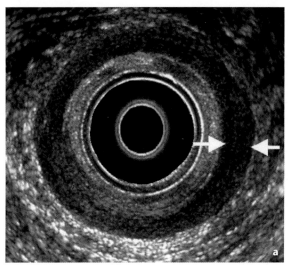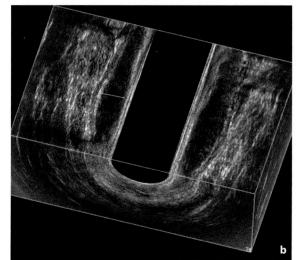

Fig. 24.5 Abnormal thickness of the internal anal sphincter (4.1 mm) (*arrows*) in a 42-year-old female with intra-anal prolapse. Axial plane (**a**), coronal plane (**b**)

obstetric trauma affects the sphincters anterior to a horizontal line through the mid-canal. Any tear of the anal sphincters posterior to this line is due to some other etiology. External sphincter tears from obstetric trauma always involve the upper sphincter, and may extend down throughout the length of the sphincter [4, 8–10]. The appearance of an EAS defect is a break in the circumferential integrity of the mixed hyperechoic band (Fig. 24.7). A defect can have either a hypoechoic or hyperechoic density pattern. This corresponds to replacement of the normal striated muscle with granulation tissue, and fibrosis. The majority of obstetric injuries are associated with a single, large defect in the EAS anterior to the anal canal that can be linked to an additional division of the IAS (Fig. 24.4). In examining a female subject, it is important to remember the ultrasonographic differences between the natural gaps (hypoechoic areas with smooth, regular edges, occurring in the upper part of the anal canal) and the sphincter ruptures (mixed echogenicity due to scarring, with irregular edges and loss of symmetry) occurring at the upper anterior part of the anal canal. Surgery for a fistula can also be responsible for damage to the EAS. This is more likely to occur during treatment of complex, high

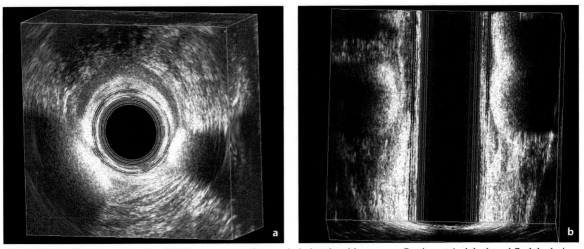

Fig. 24.6 a Bulking agent injection (PTQ), seen as two hyperechoic bands with strong reflection at 4 o'clock and 7 o'clock, in a female with fecal incontinence due to internal sphincter lesion after sphincterotomy for fissure. **b** Reconstruction in the coronal plane allows evaluation of the correct position and extent of the material injected

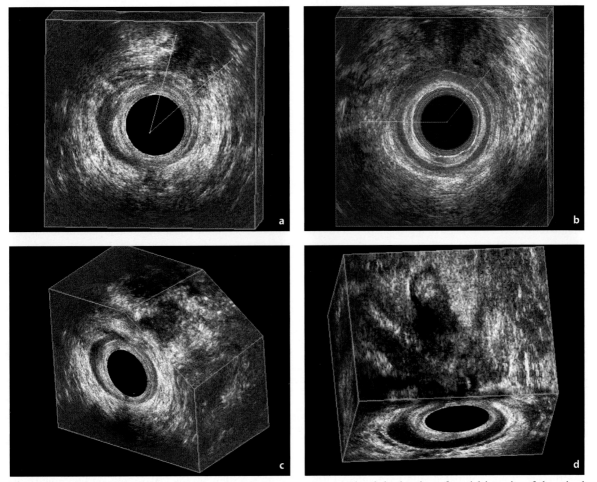

Fig. 24.7 External sphincter defects following obstetric trauma appear as a break in the circumferential integrity of the mixed hyperechoic muscle. The extent of the defect is measured in the axial plane as an angle: **a** = 33°; **b** = 130°. Three-dimensional reconstructions allow maesurement of the length of the lesions in the oblique plane (**c**) or coronal plane (**d**)

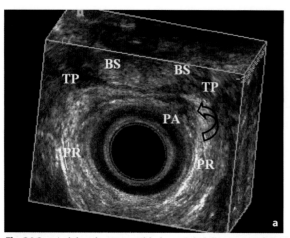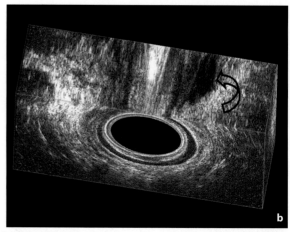

Fig. 24.8 **a** Axial endosonographic image showing a tear of the left puboanalis (*PA*) appearing as a scar in the medial aspect of the puborectalis (*PR*). *BS*, bulbospongiosus; *TP*, transverse perinei. **b** Three-dimensional reconstruction in the coronal plane in the same patient. The *arrow* indicates the PA damage

fistulas or in patients who have undergone multiple operations for a recurrent or persistent fistula.

Endoanal US has an important role in detecting clinically occult anal sphincter injuries after a vaginal delivery [4, 8, 9, 11, 12]. Using EAUS, Donnelly et al [29] found anal sphincter injury in 35% of primiparous vaginal deliveries. Sultan et al [4] reviewed EAUS findings in 79 primiparous women before and after vaginal delivery, and identified anal sphincter defects in 28 (35%), of whom nine (32%) reported altered continence to stool. Sphincter defects were not identified in those women who delivered by caesarean section. Deen et al [30] studied 46 patients with postpartum FI and found that 87% had a recognizable anal sphincter defect on EAUS. In a prospective study, de Parades et al [12] did not confirm previous observations that anal sphincter injury is common after forceps delivery. In a large population of 93 healthy females, anal sphincter injury was identified by ultrasonography in < 13% of cases after forceps delivery, and the development of FI was not related to these defects. The only factor with significant predictive value for anal sphincter injury was perineal tear. Pinta et al [31] analyzed possible risks factors associated with sphincter rupture during vaginal delivery. A total of 52 females with a third- or fourth-degree perineal laceration were compared with 51 primiparous females with no clinically detectable perineal laceration. EAUS found a persistent defect of the EAS in 39 females (75%) in the rupture group, compared with ten females (20%) in the control group (P < 0.001). An abnormal presentation was the only risk factor for anal sphincter rupture

during vaginal delivery. Fecal incontinence related to anal sphincter defects is likely to occur even in an elderly population of women who experienced vaginal deliveries earlier in life [9]. Oberwalder et al [32] reported that 71% of women with late-onset FI had occult sphincter defects on EAUS results. The onset of FI was at a median age of 61.5 years.

Distinguishing isolated tears of the EAS from those involving the support structures is often difficult, as these structures are an integral part of the sphincter [33]. Tears of the puboanalis create asymmetry of the low reflective triangular area just inside the PR that extends down into the longitudinal layer (Fig. 24.8). Tears of the transverse perinei are seen as asymmetrical to these structures just below and lateral to the PR (Fig. 24.9).

A limitation of EAUS is the definition of EAS atrophy in patients with idiopathic FI because of the vague contours of the muscle ring [34]. The reason for this is that fat replacement and loss of muscle fibers reduce the clarity of the outer interface reflection, so that the outer border of the EAS is not visible and therefore it is impossible to measure its thickness. Endoanal magnetic resonance imaging (MRI) is more accurate in detecting atrophy as there is a thinner EAS, with replacement of muscle by fat [34–36].

High-resolution multiplanar ultrasonography may help to detect sphincter damage [37–41]. Three-dimensional reconstruction offers the possibility of measuring EAS length, thickness, area, and volume (Figs. 24.3, 24.4, 24.7). The relationship between the radial angle and the longitudinal extent of a sphincter tear

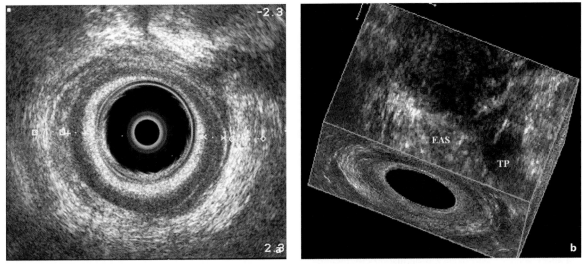

Fig. 24.9 a Axial endosonographic image showing a tear of the left transverse perinei. **b** In the coronal plane the lesion of the transverse perinei (*TP*) appears as a hypoechoic band lateral to the external sphincter ring (*EAS*)

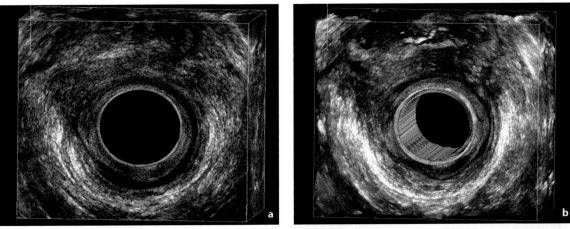

Fig. 24.10 Fifty-seven-year-old female with a large anterior external anal sphincter tear between the 9 o'clock and 3 o'clock position, combined with an internal sphincter defect between the 7 o'clock and 11 o'clock position as a consequence of an obstetric trauma. Comparing with normal mode (**a**), volume render mode with high-opacity, normal-thickness and high-luminance setting provides a better visualization of the anterior defect of the external sphincter, and the presence of mixed echogenicity scar tissue (**b**)

can be assessed and graded. The length of the remaining intact sphincter muscle can also be evaluated, improving the selection of patients for surgical repair of the anal sphincter complex and helping the surgeon to judge how far the repair should extend. A rendering technique can be particularly useful in evaluating anal sphincter lesions [38]. By using a combination of the different postprocessing display parameters, the rendered image provides better visualization performance when there are minor degrees of difference of echogenicity between the lesion and the surrounding tissues. Compared with normal mode, a rupture of the EAS in the anal canal can be better visualized by setting the render mode with high-opacity, normal-thickness, and high-luminance parameters (Fig. 24.10). An external sphincter tear will appear as a low-intensity defect in the context of the brightest segments of this striated muscle. It is also possible to detect EAS atrophy by using render mode with a normal-opacity, high-thickness and high-luminance setting, in order to separate the color and the intensity data of muscular fibers and fat tissue replacement. As a consequence, the outer border of the EAS can be better delineated and the muscle thickness measured (Fig. 24.11) [38]. In addition, thinning of the anterior part of the EAS can be precisely assessed in the coronal plane (Fig. 24.12).

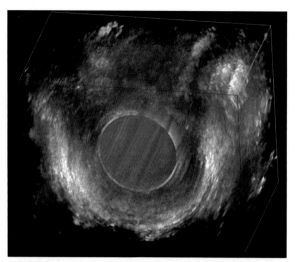

Fig. 24.11 Volume render mode with normal-opacity, high-thickness and high-luminance setting provides a better visualization of the outer border of the external sphincter and allows assessment of the presence of external sphincter atrophy

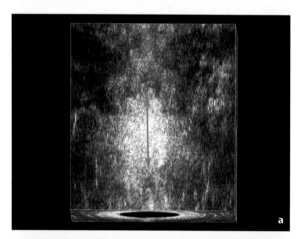

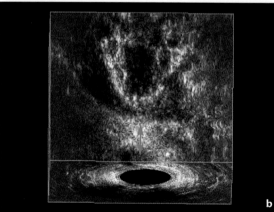

Fig. 24.12 Measurement of the longitudinal anterior length of the external sphincter in the coronal plane in female. **a** Normal (17.7 mm, *arrow*) and **b** reduced length (7.8 mm, *arrow*)

EAUS also serves as a surveillance tool to monitor results following sphincteroplasty or graciloplasty (Figs. 24.13, 24.14) [42–44]. Savoye-Collet et al [42] noted improvement in FI in 18/21 (86%) patients in whom EAUS documented closure of the EAS defect after overlapping anterior sphincter repair. In contrast, eight of the ten patients who had a persistent defect in the EAS still had significant FI. Dobben et al [43] also found that patients with a persistent ultrasonographic EAS defect had a worse clinical outcome than those without an EAS defect (P = 0.003). Starck et al [44] reported that the extent of endosonographic EAS defects after primary repair of obstetric sphincter tears increased over time and was related to anal incontinence.

24.4 Puborectalis Muscle Abnormalities

Defects of the PR are related to childbirth or to anorectal surgery. At EAUS, a shorter length or complete loss of one or both branches of the PR can be detected (Fig. 24.15).

It is not possible, however, to identify the detachment of the branches from the pubic rami, as these cannot be seen with EAUS. For this reason, endovaginal or transperineal ultrasonography represent the best modalities for assessing PR abnormalities (see Chapters 37, 38).

24.5 Accuracy and Reliability

The main indication for EAUS in patients with FI is to detect anal sphincter defects and damage to the pelvic floor muscles. Dobben et al [45] found anal inspection and digital rectal examination not an appropriate tool to depict IAS defects and inaccurate (true positive rate 36%) for determining EAS defects < 90 degrees. Therefore, in daily clinical practice, a sufficient diagnostic work-up in evaluating FI should comprise EAUS. The accuracy of EAUS in the assessment of FI has been supported by surgical findings. Gold et al [7] reported that sensitivity and specificity in locating the defect were 100%, and accuracy in the topographic detection of the defect was 90%. Deen et al [46] investigated 44 incontinent patients with EAUS. All sonographically detected EAS defects were confirmed at operation, and

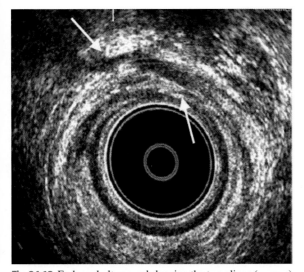

Fig. 24.13 Endoanal ultrasound showing the two slings (*arrows*) of an anterior overlapping external sphincter repair

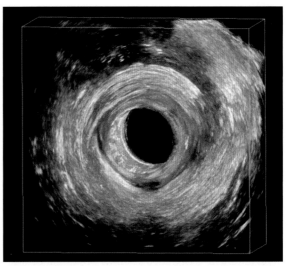

Fig. 24.14 Endoanal ultrasound showing a graciloplasty. The muscle encircles the whole circumference of the anal canal

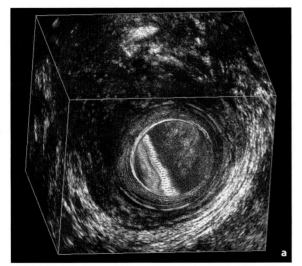

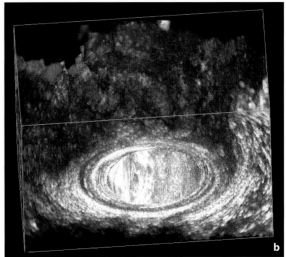

Fig. 24.15 3D-EAUS with volume rendering. Puborectalis muscle damage. **a** Partial lesion of the right branch of the puborectalis. **b** Complete loss of the right branch of the puborectalis

21 of 22 IAS defects were also confirmed at surgery. The sensitivity and specificity of EAUS were 100% for EAS defects and 100% and 95.5%, respectively, for IAS lesions. Sultan et al [9] compared preoperative ultrasonographic findings with intraoperative results in 12 consecutive patients who underwent surgical repair for FI. Endoanal ultrasound correctly identified all sphincter defects at the time of surgery. Sentovich et al [47] examined the accuracy and reliability of EAUS. In 22 incontinent women with known anal sphincter injury, the accuracy was 100%. However, in nulliparous women, EAUS falsely identified sphincter injury in 5–25% of normal anal sphincters. In this group, an intact IAS was more accurately predicted than an intact EAS (95% vs. 85%). Overall clinical agreement in the interpretation of the ultrasound results between experienced ultrasonographers (interobserver reliability) was good (81% agreement). Agreement was significantly better for the IAS (74%, fair) than the EAS (61%, poor; P = 0.0002) and in evaluating the distal anal canal (0–1.5cm) (78%) than the proximal anal canal (2.0–2.5 cm from the anal verge) (48% agreement; P < 0.0001). However, Gold et al [7] found a very good (kappa = 0.80) interobserver agreement for diagnosis of sphincter

disruption. There was no disagreement with respect to combined or isolated IAS tears, although there was some disagreement regarding isolated EAS tears. Abramowitz et al [48] demonstrated interobserver concordance in 98.9% of cases.

Benefits of three-dimensional (3D)-EAUS in the evaluation of FI have been reported [38–41]. Christensen et al [39] investigated the differences between 3D and 2D-EAUS in visualizing damage to the anal sphincter complex. The overall agreement between two observers was 98.2% using 3D and 87.9% using 2D methods. We assessed the differences between 2D- and 3D-EAUS in defining the longitudinal extent of a sphincter defect in a personal series of 33 patients with FI due to obstetrical injury [38]. The longitudinal extent of an EAS tear was graded as either proximal, central, or distal only, or a combination of two levels, or full-length involvement. Two-dimensional EAUS localized the defect in the mid-anal canal in 94% of patients. After 3D reconstruction, the defects were localized in the upper plus mid-anal canal in four patients (12%), limited to the mid-anal canal in 22 patients (67%), and in the mid plus distal anal canal in six patients (18%). The overall agreement between 2D- and 3D-EAUS was moderate (kappa = 0.25) for EAS tears in the upper plus mid-anal canal, good (kappa = 0.71) for mid-anal canal only lesions, and poor (kappa = 0.14) for defects extending to the mid plus distal anal canal. West et al [40] examined whether 3D-EAUS measurements (EAS length, thickness, area, and volume) can be used to detect EAS atrophy, and compared the results with MRI measurements. Agreement between 3D-EAUS and endoanal MRI was 61% for IAS defects and 88% for EAS defects. However, correlation was poor for EAS atrophy, suggesting that 3D-EAUS measurements are not suitable parameters for assessing EAS atrophy. In another study, the same authors [49] found that FI in parous females was not associated with loss of sphincter volume. Williams et al [50] assessed changes to anal canal morphology in the absence of sphincter trauma. After delivery, there was significant shortening of the length of the anterior portion of the EAS, which could only be demonstrated with 3D reconstructions on longitudinal and coronal planes. This change did not correlate with any functional symptoms. The authors reported that only 68% of females with third-degree tears had 3D-EAUS evidence of sphincter damage. In another series of 45 women who had had vaginal delivery, the same authors [41] found evidence

of postpartum trauma in 29% of cases. Damage involved the EAS in 11% of patients, the puboanalis in 11% of cases, and the transverse perinei in 7% of cases. External sphincter defects were associated with a significant decrease in squeeze pressure and an increase in incontinence score, and represented the only functionally significant component. Tears to the puboanalis or transverse perinei did not affect pressure or incontinence score.

Endoanal ultrasonography is the anorectal physiology modality most likely to change a patient's management plan. Liberman et al [19] reported that 11% of patients within a medical group were treated surgically after EAUS findings of sphincter lesions and 7% of patients were changed from surgical to medical therapy because of normal-appearing sphincters at EAUS. A recent study from Groenendijk et al [51] demonstrated a considerable diagnostic value of EAUS in directing therapy of patients with fecal incontinence

24.6   EAUS versus MRI

Several studies have compared the diagnostic accuracy of EAUS and endoanal or external phased array MRI in assessing anal sphincter integrity [34, 52]. The reported results of these studies vary, with some of the variability attributable to differences in study design, patient population, and the level of experience of readers [34, 52]. Dobben et al [53] found fair agreement (kappa = 0.24) between both imaging techniques in a multicenter study with a large cohort of patients with FI. Malouf et al [54] evaluated 2D-EAUS and endoanal MRI prospectively in 52 patients with FI, and reported that both techniques are comparable in diagnosing EAS defects. However, 2D-EAUS appeared to be superior in demonstrating IAS lesions. Rociu et al [55] retrospectively compared 2D-EAUS and endoanal MRI to surgery in 22 patients with FI and found MRI to be the most accurate technique for depicting IAS and EAS defects. They also found that EAS atrophy can only be accurately depicted at endoanal MRI and not at 2D-EAUS. Williams et al [36] found that patients with a thin IAS (< 2 mm) and/or a poorly defined EAS at EAUS were more likely to have EAS atrophy, and endoanal MRI should be considered to determine whether the sphincter is grossly atrophic. West el al [40] evaluated whether 3D-EAUS could be used to detect EAS atrophy in 18 females with FI. They reported that, despite the multiplanar capability, 3D-EAUS was not able to demonstrate EAS atrophy.

The current consensus is that both techniques can be used for demonstrating defects of the anal sphincter complex and can be considered useful in the selection of patients for surgery [53].

References

1. Jorge JM, Wexner SD. Etiology and management of fecal incontinence. Dis Colon Rectum 1993;36:77–97.
2. Nichols CM, Gill EJ, Nguyen T et al. Anal sphincter injury in women with pelvic floor disorders. Obstet Gynecol 2004;104:690–696.
3. Snooks SJ, Setchell M, Swash M, Henry MM. Injury to innervation of pelvic floor sphincter musculature in childbirth. Lancet 1984;2:546–550.
4. Sultan AH, Kamm MA, Hudson CN et al. Anal sphincter disruption during vaginal delivery. N Engl J Med 1993;329:1905–1911.
5. Stoker J, Halligan S, Bartram CI. Pelvic floor imaging. Radiology 2001;218:621–641.
6. Frudinger A, Halligan S, Bartram CI et al. Female anal sphincter: age-related differences in asymptomatic volunteers with high-frequency endoanal US. Radiology 2002; 224:417–423.
7. Gold DM, Halligan S, Kmiot WA, Bartram CI. Intraobserver and interobserver agreement in anal endosonography. Br J Surg 1999;86:371–375.
8. Thakar R, Sultan A. Anal endosonography and its role in assessing the incontinent patient. Best Pract Res Clinic Obstet Gynaec 2004;18:157–173.
9. Sultan AH, Kamm MA, Talbot IC et al. Anal endosonography for identifying external sphincter defects confirmed histologically. Br J Surg 1994;81:463–465.
10. Nielsen MB, Hauge C, Pedersen JF, Christiansen J. Endosonographic evaluation of patients with anal incontinence: findings and influence on surgical management. AJR Am J Roentgenol 1993;160:771–775.
11. Abramowitz L, Sobhani I, Ganansia R et al. Are sphincter defects the cause of anal incontinence after vaginal delivery? Results of a prospective study. Dis Colon Rectum 2000;43:590–598.
12. de Parades V, Etienney I, Thabut D et al. Anal sphincter injury after forceps delivery: myth or reality? A prospective ultrasound study of 93 females. Dis Colon Rectum 2004;47:24–34.
13. Starck M, Bohe M, Valentin L. Results of endosonographic imaging of the anal sphincter 2–7 days after primary repair of third or fourth-degree obstetric sphincter tears. Ultrasound Obstet Gynecol 2003;22:609–615.
14. Fowler GE, Adams EJ, Bolderson J et al. Liverpool ultrasound pictorial chart: the development of a new method of documenting anal sphincter injury diagnosed by endoanal ultrasound. BJOG 2008;115:767–772.
15. Norderval S, Markskog A, Rossaak K, Vonen B. Correlation between anal sphincter defects and anal incontinence following obstetric sphincter tears: assessment using scoring systems for sonographic classification of defects. Ultrasound Obstet Gynecol 2008;31:78–84.
16. Felta-Bersma RJ, van Baren R, Koorevaar M et al. Unsuspected sphincter defects shown by anal endosonography after anorectal surgery. Dis Colon Rectum 1995;38:249–253.
17. Vaizey CJ, Kamm MA, Bartram CI. Primary degeneration of the internal anal sphincter as a cause of passive faecal incontinence. Lancet 1997;349:612–615.
18. Voyvodic F, Rieger NA, Skinner S et al. Endosonographic imaging of anal sphincter injury. Does the size of the tear correlate with the degree of dysfunction? Dis Colon Rectum 2003;46:735–741.
19. Liberman H, Faria J, Ternent CA et al. A prospective evaluation of the value of anorectal physiology in the management of fecal incontinence. Dis Colon Rectum 2001; 44:1567–1574.
20. Reddymasu SC, Singh S, Waheed S et al. Comparison of anorectal manometry to endoanal ultrasound in the evaluation of fecal incontinence. Am J Med Sci 2009;337:336–339.
21. Bennett RC, Friedman MHW, Goligher JC. Late results of haemorrhoidectomy by ligature and excision. BMJ 1963;2:216–219.
22. Snooks S, Henry MM, Swash M. Faecal incontinence after anal dilatation. Br J Surg 1984;71:617–618.
23. Khubchandani IT, Reed JF. Sequelae of internal sphincterotomy for chronic fissure in ano. Br J Surg 1989; 76:431–434.
24. Kennedy HL, Zegarra JP. Fistulotomy without external sphincter division for high anal fistula. Br J Surg 1990;77:898–901.
25 Speakman CT, Burnett SJ, Kamm MA, Bartram CI. Sphincter injury after anal dilatation demonstrated by anal endosonography. Br J Surg 1991;78:1429–1430.
26. Abbasakoor F, Nelson M, Beynon J et al. Anal endosonography in patients with anorectal symptoms after haemorrhoidectomy. Br J Surg 1998;85:1522–1524.
27. Soerensen MM, Lundby L, Buntzen S, Laurberg S. Intersphincteric injected silicone biomaterial implants: a treatment for fecal incontinence. Colorectal Dis 2009;11:73–76.
28. de la Portilla F, Vega J, Rada R et al. Evaluation by three-dimensional anal endosonography of injectable silicone biomaterial (PTQ) implants to treat fecal incontinence: long-term localization and relation with the deterioration of the continence. Tech Coloproctol 2009;13:195–199.
29. Donnelly V, Fynes M, Campbell D et al. Obstetric events leading to anal sphincter damage. Obstet Gynecol 1998; 92:955-61.
30. Deen KJ, Kumar D, Williams JG et al. The prevalence of anal sphincter defects in fecal incontinence. A prospective endosonic study. Gut 1993;34:685–688.
31. Pinta TM, Kylanpaa ML, Salmi TK. Primary sphincter repair: are the results of the operation good enough? Dis Colon Rectum 2004;47:18–23.
32. Oberwalder M, Dinnewitzer A, Baig MK et al. The association between late-onset fecal incontinence and obstetric anal sphincter defects. Arch Surg 2004;139:429–432.
33. Williams AB, Bartram CI, Halligan S et al. Anal sphincter

damage after vaginal delivery using three-dimensional anal endosonography. Obstet Gynecol 2001;97:770–775.

34. Cazemier M, Terra MP, Stoker J et al. Atrophy and defects detection of the external anal sphincter: comparison between three-dimensional anal endosonography and endoanal magnetic resonance imaging. Dis Colon Rectum 2006;49:20–27.

35. Stoker J, Rociu E, Zwamborn AW et al. Endoluminal MR imaging of the rectum and anus: technique, applications and pitfalls. Radiographics 1999;19:383–398.

36. Williams AB, Bartram CI, Modhwadia D et al. Endocoil magnetic resonance imaging quantification of external anal sphincter atrophy. Br J Surg 2001;88:853–859.

37. Williams AB, Bartram CI, Halligan S et al. Multiplanar anal endosonography - normal anal canal anatomy. Colorectal Dis 2001;3:169–174.

38. Santoro GA, Fortling B. The advantages of volume rendering in three-dimensional endosonography of the anorectum. Dis Colon Rectum 2007;50:359–368.

39. Christensen AF, Nyhuus B, Nielsen MB, Christensen H. Three-dimensional anal endosonography may improve diagnostic confidence of detecting damage to the anal sphincter complex. Br J Rad 2005;78:308–311.

40. West RL, Dwarkasing S, Briel JW et al. Can three-dimensional endoanal ultrasonography detect external anal sphincter atrophy? A comparison with endoanal magnetic resonance imaging. Int J Colorect Dis 2005;20:328–333.

41. Williams AB, Spencer JD, Bartram CI. Assessment of third degree tears using three-dimensional anal endosonography with combined anal manometry: a novel technique. BJOG 2002;109:833–835.

42. Savoye-Collet C, Savoye G, Koning E et al. Anal endosonography after sphincter repair: specific patterns related to clinical outcome. Abdom Imaging 1999;24:569–573.

43. Dobben AC, Terra MP, Deutekom M. The role of endoluminal imaging in clinical outcome of overlapping anterior anal sphincter repair in patients with fecal incontinence. AJR Am J Roentgenol 2007;189:W70–W77.

44. Starck M, Bohe M, Valentin L. The extent of endosonographic anal sphincter defects after primary repair of obstetric sphincter tear increases over time and is related to anal incontinence. Ultrasound Obstet Gynecol 2006; 27:188–197.

45. Dobben AC, Terra MP, Deutekom M et al. Anal inspection and digital rectal examination compared to anorectal physiology tests and endoanal ultrasonography in evaluating fecal incontinence. Int J Colorectal Dis 2007; 22:783-790.

46. Deen KI, Kumar D, Williams JG et al. Anal sphincter defects: correlation between endoanal ultrasound and surgery. Ann Surg 1993;218:201–205.

47. Sentovich SM, Wong WD, Blatchford GJ. Accuracy and reliability of transanal ultrasound for anterior anal sphincter injury. Dis Colon Rectum 1998;41:1000–1004.

48. Abramowitz L, Sobhani I, Ganansia R et al. Are sphincter defects the cause of anal incontinence after vaginal delivery? Results of a prospective study. Dis Colon Rectum 2000;43:590–598.

49. West RL, Felt-Bersma RJF, Hansen BE et al. Volume measurement of the anal sphincter complex in healthy controls and fecal-incontinent patients with a three-dimensional reconstruction of endoanal ultrasonography images. Dis Colon Rectum 2005;48:540–548.

50. Williams AB, Bartram CI, Halligan S. Alteration of anal sphincter morphology following vaginal delivery revealed by multiplanar anal endosonography. BJOG 2002; 109:942–946.

51. Groenendijk AG, Birnie E, de Blok S et al. Clinical-decision taking in primary pelvic organ prolapse; the effects of diagnostic tests on treatment selection in comparison with a consensus meeting. Int Urogynecol J 2009; 20:711-19.

52. deSouza NM, Hall AS, Puni R et al. High resolution magnetic resonance imaging of the anal sphincter using a dedicated endoanal coil. Comparison of magnetic resonance imaging with surgical findings. Dis Colon Rectum 1996;39:926–934.

53. Dobben AC, Terra MP, Slors JFM et al. External anal sphincter defects in patients with fecal incontinence: comparison of endoanal MR imaging and endoanal US. Radiology 2007;242:463–471.

54. Malouf AJ, Williams AB, Halligan S et al. Prospective assessment of accuracy of endoanal MR imaging and endosonography in patients with fecal incontinence. AJR Am J Roentgenol 2000;175:741–745.

55. Rociu E, Stoker J, Eijkemans MJC et al. Fecal incontinence: endoanal US versus endoanal MR imaging. Radiology 1999;212:453–458.

Transperineal Ultrasonography

25

Bruno Roche, Guillaume Zufferey and Joan Robert-Yap

Abstract Transperineal ultrasonography is an imaging technique that is not often used; however, in the specialty of coloproctology, it has its place. In this age of economic health reforms, this test, which is relatively cheap and accessible, is very useful in identifying and assessing rectoceles, intussusceptions, evacuatory apparatus lesions, and perineal muscle movement. Lesions and asynchronous movement of these muscles can lead to evacuatory dysfunction, particularly chronic constipation. One can assess this disorder quickly and accurately with transperineal ultrasound and prescribe the appropriate biofeedback or physiotherapy as necessary. The most cost-effective and practical use is in the prediction of sphincter repair outcome as a treatment of fecal incontinence. We have been able to demonstrate that this prediction is possible when displacement of the puborectal sling is measured. The degree of displacement can infer neurological integrity to the puborectalis and/or sphincter muscles. The measurement of this displacement correlates accurately with postoperative sphincter repair outcome. This allows the surgeon to give a prognosis to patients preoperatively, so that they can decide on the best treatment options and know what to expect. The reproducibility of the test is rather good, and the technical training period quite short. Transperineal ultrasonography is often readily available, as it requires no special ultrasound probe. It is easily performed with little inconvenience to the patient. It is not time consuming or painful, and thus is well tolerated by patients. It has the advantage of giving a dynamic visualization and assessment of the perineal muscles, while being a very cost-effective investigation when compared with magnetic resonance imaging or other imaging techniques

Keywords Fecal incontinence • Puborectalis muscle • Sphincter repair • Transperineal ultrasonography

25.1 Introduction

Anal endosonography with a rotating axial or multiplanar probe inserted into the anal canal is a well-described method for visualization of the anal sphincter [1, 2]. This technique has permitted significant advances in the diagnosis and management of patients with fecal incontinence [3, 4] and the detection of sphincter damage [5]. It has also been found to be useful in the assessment of perianal abscess and fistula-in-ano [6, 7], staging of anal carcinoma [8], and detection of myopathic hypertrophy

B. Roche
Proctology Unit, University Hospital, Geneva, Switzerland

G.A. Santoro, A.P. Wieczorek, C.I. Bartram (eds.) *Pelvic Floor Disorders*
© Springer-Verlag Italia 2010

of the internal anal sphincter giving rise to pain and constipation [9].

However, the technique is not widely available and requires expensive equipment. The very nature of anal endosonography, with the introduction of a rigid object into the anal canal, may alter the physiology. Another drawback is that there is no dynamic evaluation of the perineum.

Since the pelvic anatomy permits the use of standard external ultrasound probes, perineal ultrasonography is an excellent additional test to endoanal ultrasonography.

25.2 Perineal Ultrasonography

Recent studies suggest that pelvic floor disorders and the mobility of the perineum can be assessed by dynamic perineal sonography [10, 11]. Perineal sonography allows easy identification of the puborectalis muscle and a reliable assessment of its mobility [12, 13].

Nevertheless, this technique is not widely used to investigate patients before surgical sphincter repair, possibly because its predictive ability is not well documented.

25.2.1 The Technique of Transverse External Sonography

Perineal sonography is performed in the dorsal gynecologic position. Transverse images are obtained by placing the probe on the perineum, between the anus and the introitus. The probe is progressively inclined until the concentric muscular layers of the anal sphincter are visible. The entire anal canal can be scanned by changing the application pressure and probe inclination [11, 12].

Transverse and longitudinal images of the puborectalis muscle, and internal (IAS) and external (EAS) anal sphincters are recorded with a 6 MHz linear probe and printed.

In the transverse plane, the IAS is seen as the prolongation of the muscular layer of the rectal wall. The IAS is visible as a hypoechogenic homogenous ring. The EAS is visible as an echogenic inhomogeneous ring. The mean EAS thickness is 4.7 mm (range 3.5–6.1 mm). In the upper part of the anal canal (Fig. 25.1a), the EAS is absent anteriorly, and posteriorly is in close contact with the puborectalis muscle sling running posteriorly around the rectum at the ano-rectal junction. At the middle level (Fig. 25.1b), the EAS appears as a homogenous echogenic circular ring, the outer limits of which are not clearly defined. At the lower part of the anal canal, subcutaneously, only the EAS is visible and it appears as an oval echogenic structure (Fig. 25.1c).

The procedure is well tolerated by participants who judged the discomfort engendered by examination to be only minor [11].

The patients appreciated the dorsal position because it allowed them to follow the examination on the screen. With perineal sonography, the best-quality images of the anal sphincter were obtained using the 6 MHz probe [11].

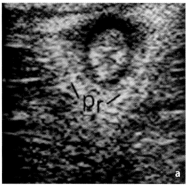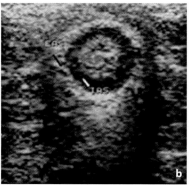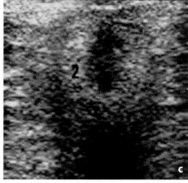

Fig. 25.1 Perineal sonograms of the anal sphincter. Transverse images (up is anterior). **a** Upper anal canal. **b** Middle anal canal. **c** Lower anal canal. The internal anal sphincter (*IAS*) forms a hypoechogenic homogenous ring seen in **b**. The mucosa and submucosa are indistinguishable from one another and are seen immediately internal to the IAS. The external anal sphincter (*EAS*) is seen as a circular echogenic layer at the middle level (**b**) and as an ovoid echogenic layer (2) at the lower level (**c**). The puborectalis muscle (*Pr*) is seen at the ano-rectal junction (**a**) as a V-shaped sling

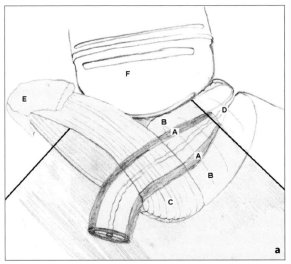 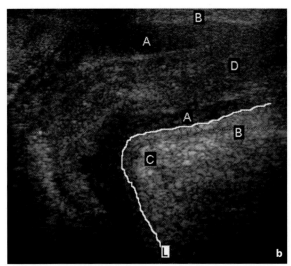

Fig. 25.2 View of the perineum, centered on the puborectal and sphincter muscle in the sagittal plane, with the same orientation as in echography. **a** Representation of the anatomy. **b** View of the echography. *A*, internal sphincter; *B*, external sphincter; *C*, puborectalis muscle; *D* anal canal; *E*, pubic bone; *F*, ultrasound probe; *L*, white line, underlining the inner border of the external sphincter and the puborectal sling

25.2.2 The Technique of Sagittal External Sonography

With the sphincter visible, the scanning plane is rotated through 90 degrees to obtain a longitudinal section, permitting visualization of the entire anal canal and the puborectal sling (Fig. 25.2a) behind the rectum at the ano-rectal junction [12].

To determine movement of the puborectal sling, the first caliper is fixed on the anterior border of the pubo-rectalis, with the patient in the resting position. Holding the probe in a constant position, the patient is then asked to either strain or squeeze. The image is then frozen in the position of maximum puborectal displacement and the second caliper placed on the anterior border of the puborectalis in its new position. The distance between the two calipers can then be measured. The puborectalis is identified in the transverse plane, and is seen in the upper anal canal as a U-shaped sling running posteriorly to the rectum at the ano-rectal junction (Fig. 25.1a). On longitudinal images, the muscular sling behind the rectum is easily visible at the ano-rectal junction as an echogenic, poorly demarcated area (Fig. 25.2b). However, the movements of the sling in relation to the anal canal and distal rectum can be followed very precisely during squeezing and straining (Fig. 25.3).

25.2.3 Clinical Applications

The clinical applications of perineal ultrasound can be quite useful and practical, but are limited.

- In centers where endoanal ultrasound is not available, this technique can be used to visualize the perineal structures. Therefore, visualization of suspected lesions and tumors can benefit from this ultrasound technique.
- Assessment of abscesses and fistulae is possible but not ideal.
- In the evaluation of anal incontinence, one can also visualize the anal sphincter and defaecatory apparatus.
- In cases of chronic constipation or evacuatory obstruction disorders, this dynamic ultrasound method can offer an evaluation of the integrity of the defaecatory apparatus and the mobility of the perineal muscles. This gives a good indication of the integrity of the nervous supply in this region. One can also easily determine if there is asynchronous movement during evacuation and retention efforts, thus confirming a clinical diagnosis and selecting good treatment options, such as physiotherapy.
- One can also confirm the presence of a rectocele or intussusceptions and evaluate their size and dynamic progression (Fig. 25.3c).

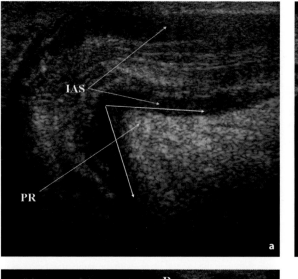

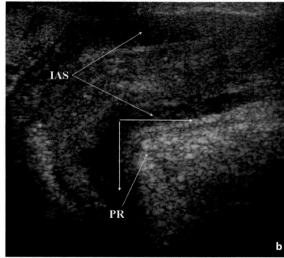

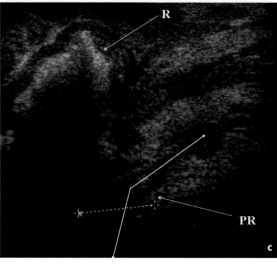

Fig. 25.3 Perineal anal sphincter sonograms, longitudinal images. **a** Contraction of the puborectalis muscle (*PR*) and narrowing of the anorectal angle (*ARA*) (*white arrows*) during squeezing; *IAS*, internal anal sphincter. **b** Resting position with 90° ARA (*white arrows*). **c** Relaxation of *PR* with posterior displacement during straining opening of the ARA (*white arrows*); *R*, rectocele

Although perineal ultrasonography can be useful in these clinical indications, there are certainly other diagnostic tools that are superior in this area, such as endoanal ultrasound and magnetic resonance imaging. Depending upon the clinical findings, each case should be evaluated individually, according to the availability of resources and access to diagnostic imaging techniques.

In our institution, the most useful clinical indication we have found for perineal ultrasonography is in determining the state of the puborectalis muscle sling. We have found a way to measure and quantify the movement range of the puborectalis muscle and thus indirectly infer the integrity of the musculo-nervous supply to it and the anal sphincter apparatus. This information is useful in predicting the success of a sphincter repair in patients suffering from incontinence due to sphincter rupture.

In a first prospective study [13], we compared the displacement of the puborectal sling in a group of normal volunteers and patients with pelvic floor disorders. During squeezing, the sling moves anteriorly by a mean of 15.5 mm ± 2.2 mm (standard error of the mean (SEM)). All normal volunteers had an anterior displacement of more than 7 mm. In the patients, anterior displacement was 7.4 ± 2.0 mm (SEM), significantly less than in the normal volunteers (P = 0.001).

On straining, the puborectal sling moves posteriorly. The mean posterior displacement in normal volunteers was 16.5 ± 1.4 mm (SEM). The displacement was greater than 6 mm in all these subjects. In the patients, the mean posterior displacement was 2.1 ± 1.6 mm (SEM). The difference between the volunteers and patients was significant (P < 0.001).

We conducted a prospective study of a consecutive sample of patients with anal incontinence and a documented rupture of the anal sphincter, who underwent an overlapping sphincter repair between 1999 and 2005 at the University of Geneva Hospital (Geneva, Switzerland) [14]. The main independent variable was the amplitude of the voluntary contraction of the puborectal sling, measured by sonography before surgery.

During the preoperative visit, every patient with sphincter rupture was investigated clinically and by standard endoanal echography. A complementary perineal ultrasound was performed and the voluntary contraction of the sling was measured. All sphincteroplasties were performed by the same experienced senior surgeon. All patients with demonstrated sphincter rupture were surgically corrected by reconstruction in the first instance, independently of the presence of a residual anal sphincter contraction, as recommended generally in the literature [15, 16].

The average preoperative Miller score was 13.3 (standard deviation (SD) 4.2, range 3–18). None of the patients were asymptomatic: 2 (1.8%) of the 109 patients had a score between 1 and 3 (flatus incontinence only), 37 (33.9%) had a score between 4 and 9, and 70 (64.2%) had scores of 10 or more. In contrast, 3 months after the operation, the average Miller score was 2.6 (SD 4.3, range 0–18, difference P < 0.001), 60 (55.0%) patients were completely asymptomatic, 29 (26.7%) had a score between 1 and 3, 12 (11.0%) had scores between 4 and 9, and 8 (7.3%) had scores of 10 or more. The mean score improvement was 10.7 (SD 5.2, range 0–18): 6 (5.6%) patients did not improve at all, 8 (7.4%) improved by 1–3 points, 39 (36.1%) improved by 4–9 points, and 55 (50.9%) improved by 10 points or more.

25.2.4 Associations Between Preoperative Assessments and Clinical Outcomes

The voluntary contraction of the puborectal sling, measured preoperatively, was not associated with concurrent symptom scores. The correlation between the voluntary contraction and the preoperative Miller score was weak (– 0.07) and statistically non-significant (P = 0.47) (Fig. 25.4). In contrast, the voluntary contraction was markedly associated with the postoperative Miller score (Fig. 25.5). The correlation coeffi-

cient was strong (0.63) and significant (P < 0.001).

Based on the previous analyses, we selected ≤ 8 mm to define an abnormal voluntary contraction. The sensitivity of this test to identify any symptoms after surgical repair was moderate (0.61), but the specificity was excellent (0.95), meaning that most patients who eventually become asymptomatic are correctly identified by a voluntary contraction greater than 8 mm.

The positive predictive value was also above 0.90, meaning that among those who have a voluntary

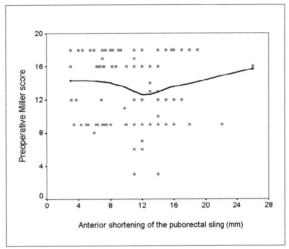

Fig. 25.4 Associations between the anterior displacement of the puborectal sling and the preoperative Miller score in 109 women who underwent surgical repair for anal incontinence. Non-parametric regression lines are superimposed

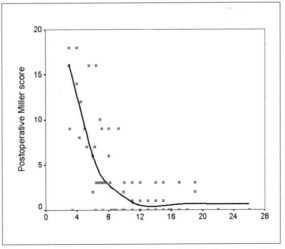

Fig. 25.5 Associations between the anterior displacement of the puborectal sling and the postoperative Miller score in 109 women who underwent surgical repair for anal incontinence. In contrast, the voluntary contraction was markedly associated with the postoperative Miller score

contraction of 8 mm or less, the majority will have symptoms after surgery.

The sensitivity and specificity were both excellent, and the negative predictive value was very accurate, meaning that among those with a voluntary contraction > 8 mm, almost all will become asymptomatic or will suffer from flatus incontinence only [14].

The test we used requires minimum time and is relatively inexpensive to perform compared to magnetic resonance imaging or other imaging tests. After performing the mandatory endoanal ultrasound, it is very easy to take the standard plane or curved linear probe of 6 MHz and to obtain perineal images in the same session. The patients tolerate the test very well as it is performed quickly and painlessly. The limitations of this study include a fairly small sample size, and the unknown applicability of the results in other settings. In particular, the results we obtained may be related to the surgical technique used at our hospital, namely the overlapping anterior sphincteroplasty, and to the skills and experience of the surgeon. Finally, measurement of the voluntary contraction of the puborectal sling requires ultrasound equipment and appropriate skills.

The proportions of asymptomatic patients and those of patients with only flatus symptoms increased as the voluntary contraction increased (Fig. 25.6). The voluntary contraction of the puborectal sling, maintained as a continuous variable, discriminated very well between patients with a favorable and unfavorable outcome.

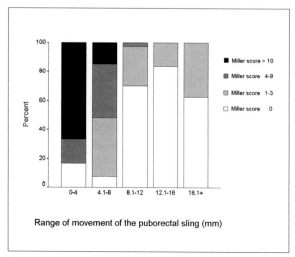

Fig. 25.6 Association between the anterior displacement of the puborectal sling (categorized) and clinical outcome after surgical repair for anal incontinence. Clinical outcome is categorized as asymptomatic (Miller score 0, *white bars*), flatus incontinence (Miller score 1–3, *light grey bars*), symptomatic (Miller score 4–9, *dark grey bars*), and severely symptomatic (Miller score 10 or higher, *black bars*)

may not be fully relieved by surgery and that other treatment modalities could be warranted later, such as physiotherapy or sacral nerve stimulation. As a result of these findings, we are convinced that measurement of voluntary contraction of the puborectal sling is a very useful tool, and these results are systematically discussed in every preoperative consultation in our establishment.

25.3 Discussion

Based on our results, we suggest that the value of 8 mm discriminates best between a normal and an abnormal voluntary puborectalis contraction [12–14]. Among women with a normal voluntary contraction, almost all went on to become asymptomatic or minimally symptomatic following surgical repair, in contrast to less than half of the women who had an abnormal voluntary contraction. We suggest that the results of the preoperative assessment of voluntary contraction of the puborectal sling be used in discussion with the patient about the best course of action. Those with a good result can be reassured about the high probability of a favorable outcome. Those with a worse result, especially if the voluntary contraction is less than 4 mm, should be warned of the possibility that symptoms

25.4 Conclusions

Perineal sonography is a technique that is easy to perform with standard ultrasound probes. It allows a dynamic evaluation of anterior and posterior movements of the puborectalis muscle. The availability and excellent tolerance of this method suggest a potential application as a screening test in the population with defecation disorders, and that it is a good predictor for functional outcome after surgical sphincter repair for postobstetric incontinence.

References

1. St Ville EW, Jafri SZH, Madrazo BL et al. Endorectal sonography in the evaluation of rectal and perirectal diseases. AJR Am J Roentgenol 1991;157:503–508.

2. Bachman-Nielsen MB, Pedersen JF, Hauge C et al. Endosonography of anal sphincter: findings in healthy volunteers. AJR Am J Roentgenol 1991;157:1191–1202.

3. Bachmann-Nielsen MB, Hauge C, Pedersen JF, Christiansen J. Endosonographic evaluation of patients with anal incontinence: finding and influence on surgical management. AJR Am J Roentgenol 1993;160:771–775.

4. Kamm MA. Obstetric damage and faecal incontinence. Lancet 1994;344:730–733.

5. Sultan AH, Kamm MA, Hudson CN et al. Anal sphincter disruption during vaginal delivery. N Engl J Med 1993;329:1905–1911.

6. Mulder CJ, Tio TL, Tytgat GN. Transrectal ultrasonography in the assessment of perianorectal fistula and/or abscess in Crohn disease. Gastroenterology 1988;94:A313.

7. Law PJ, Talbot RW, Northover JM. Anal endosonography in the evaluation of perianal sepsis and fistula in ano. Br J Surg 1989;76:752–755.

8. Goldman S, Glimelius B, Norming U et al. Transanorectal ultrasonography in anal carcinoma. Acta Radiol 1988; 29:337–341.

9. Kamm MA, Hoyle CH, Burleigh DE et al. Hereditary internal anal aphincter myopathy causing proctalgia fugax and constipation. Gastroenterology 1991; 100:805–810.

10. Beer-Gabel M, Teshler M, Schechtman E, Zbar AP. Dynamic transperineal ultrasound vs. defecography in patients with evacuatory difficulty: a pilot study. Int J Colorectal Dis 2004;19:60–67.

11. Roche B, Deleaval J, Fransioli A, Marti MC. Comparison of transanal and external perineal ultrasonography. Eur Radiol 2001;11:1165–1170.

12. Roche B. Endorectal and anal sonography. In: Marti MC, Givel JC (eds) Surgical management of anorectal and colonic diseases, 2 edn. Springer-Verlag, Berlin, 1998, pp 71–84.

13. Fransioli A, Weber B, Cunningham M et al. Dynamic evaluation of puborectalis muscle function by external perineal sonography. Tech Coloproctol 1996;3:125–129.

14. Zufferey G, Perneger T, Robert-Yap J et al. Measure of the voluntary contraction of the puborectal sling as a predictor of successful sphincter repair in the treatment of anal incontinence. Dis Colon Rectum 2009;52:704–710.

15. Gilliland R, Altomare DF, Moreira H Jr et al. Pudendal neuropathy is predictive of failure following anterior overlapping sphincteroplasty. Dis Colon Rectum 1998;41:1516–1522.

16. Chen AS, Luchtefeld MA, Senagore AJ et al. Pudendal nerve latency. Does it predict outcome of anal sphincter repair? Dis Colon Rectum 1998;41:1005–1009.

Abstract Imaging is an integral part of the workup of patients with fecal incontinence. Endoanal ultrasound (EAUS) and endoanal magnetic resonance imaging (MRI) have been demonstrated to be comparable in the detection of external sphincter defects. Given the availability and costs, EAUS can be considered as an initial imaging test for detecting external sphincter defects in patients with fecal incontinence. Endoluminal MRI can be used as an alternative. Endoanal MRI is advantageous as compared to EAUS in demonstrating and grading external sphincter atrophy. External sphincter atrophy at endoanal MRI has been demonstrated to be a negative predictor of the outcome of anterior anal repair. In candidates for anterior anal repair, endoluminal MRI should be considered, to identify patients with external sphincter atrophy. External phased array coil MRI can replace endoluminal MRI in experienced hands.

Keywords Atrophy • Anal sphincter • Fecal incontinence • Magnetic resonance imaging

26.1 Introduction

The workup of patients with fecal incontinence primarily comprises clinical history, physical examination, anofunctional tests (e.g. manometry), and endoanal ultrasound (EAUS). Magnetic resonance imaging (MRI) was introduced in the 1990s as an alternative for EAUS. The primary reason was the difficult delineation of the external sphincter at EAUS. MRI has a high intrinsic contrast resolution, which has proved to be beneficial for delineating the external sphincter. In this chapter the role of MRI in patients with fecal incontinence is described. As treatment is primarily aimed at the external sphincter, the emphasis is on evaluation of the external sphincter.

26.2 Technique

26.2.1 MRI Coil

In patients with fecal incontinence, MRI has primarily been studied using an endoluminal coil. The advantage of a dedicated coil is the high signal to noise ratio (SNR) close to the coil. This high SNR can be used for obtaining images with high spatial resolution. As the anal sphincter muscles are only a few millimeters thick, optimal spatial resolution is advantageous. The distension caused by the coil could be considered a disadvantage, as the anal sphincter components are stretched. Although some thinning will occur, the high spatial resolution will more than compensate for this. Subtle changes in the architecture of anal sphincter components and in signal intensity are visible. It is possible that some distension might be beneficial to

J. Stoker
Department of Radiology, Academic Medical Center,
University of Amsterdam, The Netherlands

visualize a sphincter defect. This will occur as overlapping torn sphincter parts are displaced, which may help in identifying the defect.

We use a 17 mm cylindrical coil with a length of 8 cm. The coil is protected by a 19 mm outer diameter coil holder, which has a length of 10 cm [1]. The diameter of the endoanal coil is comparable to the diameter of an endosonography transducer, facilitating comparison of findings.

26.2.2 Preparation

The coil we use is a multiple-use coil (we use the coil in hundreds of examinations), and appropriate hygienic measures are taken (including disinfectant) for each procedure. The coil is covered by a condom and some lubricant is applied. It is introduced in the left lateral position. After careful positioning of the coil, the patient turns to a supine position, and prior to imaging the coil position is checked.

To prevent artifacts of peristalsis, we ask patients not to eat or drink for four hours prior to the examination and we use a bowel relaxant (butylscopolamine bromide, Buscopan, Boehringer, Ingelheim, Germany). When butylscopolamine bromide is not approved for this application (such as in the USA), glucagon can be used as an alternative. However, glucagon is more effective for reducing small bowel peristalsis than large bowel contractions. For further reduction of artifacts we ask patients not to squeeze their anal sphincter, pelvic floor muscles, or gluteal muscles during the examination.

26.2.3 Imaging Protocol

A practical imaging approach comprises an axial oblique and coronal oblique moderately T2-weighted turbo spin-echo sequences (TSE) (at 1.5T TR 2,500 ms; TE 70 ms). These imaging sequences are angulated for optimized visualization of the anal sphincter muscles.

In patients with fecal incontinence, the endoanal MRI procedure is well tolerated and probably comparable to that at EAUS [2]. Endoanal MRI is more time consuming than EAUS (approximately 30 minutes versus 10 minutes room time).

When visualization of the complete pelvic floor is needed, or dynamic information about the pelvic floor, additional sequences with an external coil are mandatory.

Although experience is limited, the anal sphincter can also be studied with external phased array coils. Experienced readers achieve comparable results to endoanal MRI for external sphincter defects and external sphincter atrophy [3, 4]. When further studies confirm these initial findings, external coil MRI could be a valuable alternative. This is especially advantageous as it can be performed with almost any MRI machine and in only 15 minutes.

26.3 MRI Findings

External sphincter lesions primarily concern local defects and scarring. A defect is demonstrated as a discontinuity of the external sphincter, often with some scar tissue (Fig. 26.1). More frequently, no conspicuous defect is visible, but normal sphincter tissue is replaced by scar tissue. Scar tissue can be recognized as tissue with low signal intensity (relative black) and disturbed architecture. Normal anal sphincter tissue has a multilayered appearance, which is distorted by the scar tissue. Identification of subtle scar tissue is facilitated by scar tissue in the fat-

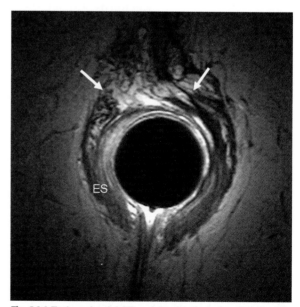

Fig. 26.1 Endoanal axial T2-weighted turbo spin-echo in a 50-year old female patient with severe fecal incontinence. She had a history of a complete rupture and episiotomy with primary repair. MRI shows an anterior external sphincter defect (*arrows*). The edges and adjacent parts of the torn external sphincter are fibrous (scar tissue) with distorted architecture and low signal intensity (compare to posterior part of external sphincter (*ES*))

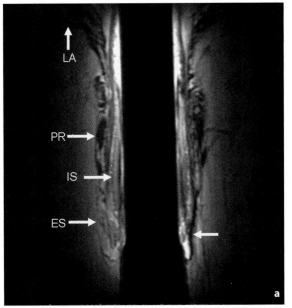 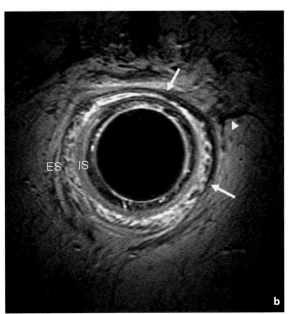

Fig. 26.2 Endoanal coronal (**a**) and axial (**b**) T2-weighted turbo spin-echo in a 56-year-old female patient with fecal incontinence show severe atrophy of the external sphincter (*ES*) and scar tissue of the left anterolateral external sphincter (*arrows*) with adjacent scar tissue in the ischioanal space (*arrowhead*). There is also atrophy of the internal sphincter (*IS*) and moderate atrophy of the puborectal muscle (*PR*) and levator ani (*LA*). Compare to Fig. 26.3

containing ischioanal space, directly adjacent to the external sphincter (Fig. 26.2). The external sphincter can either be thickened, thinned, or of approximately normal thickness at the area of scar tissue. Internal sphincter defects have a similar appearance, although scar tissue can be somewhat less hypointense (Fig. 26.3). However, the normal internal sphincter has high signal intensity and therefore there is considerable contrast between scar tissue and normal internal sphincter.

Interobserver agreement of endoanal MRI for sphincter defects is best when the sphincters are either both intact or both disrupted [5]. For individual sphincters, interobserver agreement for defects was fair (external anal sphincter) and moderate (internal anal sphincter) [5]. A study in 30 patients reported moderate to good interobserver agreement for external sphincter defects [3]. Intraobserver agreement was fair to very good and depended upon experience.

Generalized atrophy of the external sphincter can present as either thinning, fatty replacement, or – most frequently – both. Measuring the external sphincter thickness is helpful. However, visual evaluation of the presence of fat is important, as in some patients fascial borders remain intact while the muscle bulk is greatly reduced (Fig. 26.2).

With ageing, there is a physiological thinning of the external sphincter. At endoanal MRI, the external sphincter is 4.32 mm in women aged 35 years or younger and 3.9 mm in women older than 65 year [6]. In men the values are 5.21 mm and 3.45 mm, respectively. Internal sphincter atrophy is visible as thinning of the internal sphincter. With ageing, there is a physiological thickening of the internal sphincter. These physiological changes of the external and internal sphincter were also demonstrated at EAUS [7]. An internal sphincter with a thickness less than 2 mm, in a middle-aged or elderly individual, is considered atrophied (Fig. 26.2).

26.4 Accuracy for Sphincter Defects

In the 15 years since the introduction of endoanal MRI, several studies have been published on the accuracy of endoanal MRI in detecting anal sphincter defects. Initial studies concerned rather small series, demonstrating that accuracy is good (up to 95%) for demonstrating external sphincter defects [8, 9]. As EAUS is the standard technique for demonstration of anal sphincter defects, a comparison of endoanal MRI and EAUS is important. Two single-center studies and one larger multicenter comparative study have been performed.

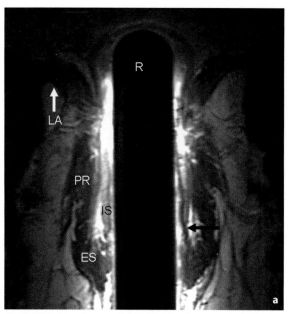 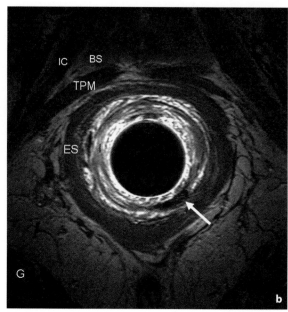

Fig. 26.3 Endoanal coronal (**a**) and axial (**b**) T$_2$-weighted turbo spin-echo in a 46-year-old male patient with anal pain demonstrate normal anatomy of the external sphincter (*ES*) and puborectalis muscle (*PR*) at the right side. The inferior part of the internal sphincter (*IS*) is abnormal (best seen in the axial plane (**a**); compare to Fig. 10.6), with disturbed architecture of the complete inferior internal sphincter ring and scar tissue of the internal sphincter left posterolateral (*black arrow in* **a***; white arrow in* **b**) after previous surgery. *BS*, bulbospongiosus muscle; *G*, gluteus musculature; *IC*, ischiocavernous muscle; *LA*, levator ani (*white arrow in* **b**); *TPM*, transverse perineal muscle; *R,* coil with tip in distal rectum

The first comparative study retrospectively compared both techniques to findings at surgery. The study concerned 22 patients with fecal incontinence undergoing anterior anal sphincter repair [10]. There was better agreement of endoanal MRI with surgical results for external sphincter defects compared to findings at EAUS for diagnosing lesions of the external anal sphincter (κ MRI 0.85 vs. EAUS 0.53) and internal anal sphincter (κ MRI 0.64 vs. EUS 0.49).

These findings were not confirmed in a prospective study in a larger number of patients. In this study, findings at EAUS and endoanal MRI in 52 patients were compared to the final diagnosis made by an expert panel, based on all available information [11]. Complete agreement between endoanal MRI and EAUS and the final diagnosis was found in 62%. Findings at EAUS were more frequently confirmed by the expert panel than findings at endoanal MRI. Discordant findings primarily concerned internal sphincter lesions. The authors concluded that MRI is inferior in diagnosing internal anal sphincter injury. The differences between both studies are probably related to differences in experience with either technique and differences in the disease spectrum and reference standard.

The third study compared EAUS and endoanal MRI for detection of external sphincter defects [12]. This multicenter study concerned 237 patients (214 women). There was agreement between endoanal MRI and EAUS in 146 patients (61%; κ = 0.24: fair agreement). A selection of patients (n = 36) underwent anterior anal sphincter repair. In these patients there was no significant difference in the detection of external anal sphincter defects between endoanal MRI and EAUS (P = 0.23). The sensitivity and positive predictive value of endoanal MRI were 81% and 89% respectively, and 90% and 85% respectively for EAUS). Based on these three studies, one can conclude that EUS and endoanal MRI are comparable in the detection of external sphincter defects.

Obstetric trauma is considered to be a major cause of sphincter defects. These sphincter defects may coincide with defects of other pelvic floor muscles, which may also result from obstetric trauma. In a study of 105 severe fecal-incontinent patients, defects of the puborectal muscle or levator ani were identified [13]. These defects were rarely solitary findings but associated with internal or external sphincter defects in these patients presenting with fecal incontinence. Atrophy

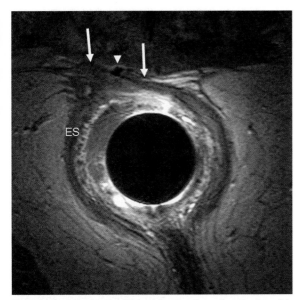

Fig. 26.4 Endoanal axial T2-weighted turbo spin-echo in a 34-year-old female patient with fecal incontinence. She had a complete rupture 4 years earlier and underwent anterior anal repair for an anterior external defect at EAUS. Fecal incontinence had not improved after anterior anal repair. At endoanal MRI there is reasonable left-over-right overlap of the external sphincter parts (*arrows*). There is some atrophy of the external sphincter. Susceptibility artifact (*arrowhead*) anterior. *ES*, external anal sphincter

of the puborectal muscle or levator ani muscle almost always coincided with external sphincter atrophy.

In patients who have experienced unsuccessful anterior anal repair, imaging can be performed to identify the cause of the failure. A study with 30 patients with fecal incontinence has shown that at endoanal MRI, patients with a visible overlap and less than 20% fat tissue had a better clinical outcome (Fig. 26.4) [14]. Further, preserved external sphincter thickness correlated significantly with better surgical outcome (see 26.5 on sphincter atrophy). Residual external sphincter defects were better demonstrated at EAUS, which might be related to the rather limited experience with post-surgical endoanal MRI. To my knowledge, MRI has not been studied in evaluating other surgical treatments.

26.5 Accuracy for Sphincter Atrophy

External sphincter atrophy was a finding known from electromyography. This entity had become somewhat neglected following the widespread replacement of electromyography by EAUS.

As the external sphincter is very well delineated at endoanal MRI, detection of atrophy was an easy task (Fig. 26.2). A study with histopathological verification in 25 patients demonstrated that endoanal MRI is accurate in detecting external sphincter atrophy [15]. Endoanal MRI had a sensitivity of 89%, specificity 94%, positive predictive value 89%, and negative predictive value 94% for external sphincter atrophy.

External sphincter atrophy is a finding related to sphincter function. In a prospective series of 200 patients, external anal sphincter atrophy was present in 123 patients (62%) at endoanal MRI [16]. The atrophy was severe in 44 patients (22%) and mild in 79 (40%). Maximal squeeze pressure and squeeze increment pressure were significantly decreased in individuals with external sphincter atrophy. Patients with severe atrophy had a significantly lower maximal squeeze and squeeze increment pressure than patients with mild atrophy. This is concordant with an earlier study in which 16 patients with fecal incontinence and decreased squeeze pressure, and nine controls with normal squeeze pressures, were studied [17]. Anal squeeze pressure correlated with external sphincter volume and fat content.

Two studies have evaluated the role of endoanal MRI in predicting the outcome of anterior anal repair. One study performed endoanal MRI in 20 female patients scheduled for anterior anal repair. Eight of these patients had external sphincter atrophy. The outcome was significantly better in those patients without external sphincter atrophy [18]. A further study in 30 patients demonstrated that baseline measurement of preserved external anal sphincter bulk correlated with a better outcome [14]. These studies demonstrate that external sphincter atrophy at endoanal MRI is a negative predictor of outcome of anterior sphincter repair.

Studies on EAUS and detection of external sphincter atrophy are sparse, and have limited patient numbers and conflicting results. In a comparative study of 20 female patients, external sphincter atrophy was identified in eight patients at endoanal MRI and in no patients with EAUS [18]. In a study of 18 patients, three-dimensional (3D) EAUS and endoanal MRI showed no difference in the assessment of external anal sphincter atrophy, but there was a substantial difference in grading [19]. However, another study with 18 fecal-incontinent patients showed that correlation between EAUS and endoanal MRI for external anal sphincter thickness, length, and area was poor [20]. The decreased delineation of the external anal sphincter border in external sphincter atrophy probably impairs accurate evaluation.

Abnormal thinning (< 2 mm) of the internal anal sphincter can be found in patients with idiopathic degeneration [21]. Atrophy of the internal anal sphincter is most easily appreciated at an axial image, and a cut-off of 2 mm thickness is used to identify internal sphincter atrophy in older individuals. Internal sphincter atrophy is nicely demonstrated at both endoanal MRI (Fig. 26.2) and EAUS.

26.6   MRI in the Management of Fecal-incontinent Patients

The results of EAUS and endoanal MRI in the detection of external sphincter defects are comparable. The widespread experience and availability, and lower costs and time efficiency, favor EAUS as the first-choice technique for detecting external sphincter defects. Endoanal MRI can be used as an alternative. In experienced hands, external phased array MRI can replace endoanal MRI. This is a time-efficient alternative, which lacks the discomfort associated with the introduction of an endoanal device, a drawback of both endoanal MRI and EUS.

The principal role of endoanal MRI is in demonstrating and grading external sphincter atrophy. This finding is a negative predictor of the outcome of anterior anal repair. With current knowledge, MRI is the preferred method to demonstrate external sphincter atrophy. Data on EAUS are sparse and conflicting. Therefore, in patients considered for anterior anal repair, MRI should be performed to identify individuals with external sphincter atrophy. The use of external phased array MRI is a valuable alternative in experienced hands.

Neither EAUS nor endoanal MRI play a role in selecting patients for pelvic floor rehabilitation. In a series of 250 fecal-incontinent patients, neither technique had substantial predictive value for the outcome of pelvic floor rehabilitation [22].

26.7   Conclusions

The evidence on the role of endoanal MRI in fecal incontinence is considerable but not extensive. Endoanal MRI can be used as an alternative to EAUS for detecting external sphincter defects. Current evidence indicates that endoanal MRI should be used in patients considered for anterior anal repair. The role of MRI in other surgical treatment options has not been studied and is an obvious topic for future research. One can speculate that external sphincter atrophy at MRI could be an important finding for sacral neuromodulation. Technical developments in MRI, such as diffusion and diffusion tensor imaging, could be of value in patients with fecal incontinence.

References

1. Stoker J, Rociu E, Zwamborn AW, Laméris JS. Endoluminal MR imaging of the rectum and anus: technique, applications, and pitfalls. Radiographics 1999;19:383–398.
2. Deutekom M, Terra MP, Dijkgraaf MG et al. Patients' perception of tests in the assessment of faecal incontinence. Br J Radiol 2006;79:94–100.
3. Terra MP, Beets-Tan RG, van der Hulst et al. Evaluating anal sphincter defects in patients with fecal incontinence: Endoanal MR imaging versus external phased array MR imaging. Radiology 2005;236:886–895.
4. Terra MP, Beets-Tan RG, van der Hulst VPM et al. MR imaging in evaluating atrophy of the external anal sphincter in patients with fecal incontinence. Am J Roentgenol 2006;187:991–999.
5. Malouf AJ, Halligan S, Williams AB et al. Prospective assessment of interobserver agreement for endoanal MRI in fecal incontinence. Abdom Imaging 2001;26:76–78.
6. Rociu E, Stoker J, Eijkemans MJC, Laméris JS. Normal anal sphincter anatomy and age- and sex-related variations at high-spatial-resolution endoanal MR imaging. Radiology 2000;217:395–401.
7. Frudinger A, Halligan S, Bartram CI, Price et al. Female anal sphincter: age-related differences in asymptomatic volunteers with high-frequency endoanal US. Radiology 2002;224:417–423.
8. deSouza NM, Puni FR, Zbar A et al. MR imaging of the anal sphincter in multiparous women using an endoanal coil: correlation with in vitro anatomy and appearances in fecal incontinence. AJR Am J Roentgenol 1996;167:1465–1471.
9. deSouza NM, Hall AS, Puni R et al. High resolution magnetic resonance imaging of the anal sphincter using a dedicated endoanal coil. Comparison of magnetic resonance imaging with surgical findings. Dis Colon Rectum 1996;39:926–934.
10. Rociu E, Stoker J, Eijkemans MJ et al. Fecal incontinence: endoanal US versus endoanal MR imaging. Radiology 1999;212:453–458.
11. Malouf AJ, Williams AB, Halligan S et al. Prospective assessment of accuracy of endoanal MR imaging and endosonography in patients with fecal incontinence. AJR Am J Roentgenol 2000;175:741–745.
12. Dobben AC, Terra MP, Slors JFM et al. External anal sphincter defects in patients with fecal incontinence. Comparison of endoanal MR imaging and endoanal US. Radiology 2007; 242:463–471.
13. Terra MP, Beets-Tan RGH, Vervoorn I et al. Pelvic floor muscle lesions at endoanal MR imaging in female patients with faecal incontinence. Eur Radiol 2008;18:1892–1901.

14. Dobben AC, Terra MP, Deutekom M et al. The role of endo-luminal imaging in clinical outcome of overlapping anterior anal sphincter repair in patients with fecal incontinence. AJR Am J Roentgenol 2007;189:W70–77.

15. Briel JW, Zimmerman DDE, Stoker J et al. Relationship between sphincter morphology on endoanal MRI and histo-pathological aspects of the external anal sphincter. Int J Co-lorectal Dis 2000;15:87–90.

16. Terra MP, Deutekom M, Beets-Tan RG et al. Relationship between external anal sphincter atrophy at endoanal magnetic resonance imaging and clinical, functional, and anatomic characteristics in patients with fecal incontinence. Dis Colon Rectum 2006;49:1149–1159.

17. Williams AB, Bartram CI, Modhwadia D et al. Endocoil magnetic resonance imaging quantification of external anal sphincter atrophy. Br J Surg 2001;88:853–859.

18. Briel JW, Stoker J, Rociu E et al. External anal sphincter

atrophy on endoanal magnetic resonance imaging adversely affects continence after sphincteroplasty. Br J Surg 1999;86: 1322–1327.

19. Cazemier M, Terra MP, Stoker J et al. Atrophy and defects detection of the external anal sphincter: comparison between three-dimensional anal endosonography and endoanal magne-tic resonance imaging. Dis Colon Rectum 2006;49:20–27.

20. West RL, Dwarkasing S, Briel JW et al. Can three-dimen-sional endoanal ultrasonography detect external anal sphin-cter atrophy? A comparison with endoanal magnetic reso-nance imaging. Int J Colorectal Dis 2005;20:328–333.

21. Vaizey CJ, Kamm MA, Bartram CI. Primary degeneration of the internal anal sphincter as a cause of passive faecal in-continence. Lancet 1997;349:612–615.

22. Terra MP, Deutekom M, Dobben AC et al. Can the outcome of pelvic-floor rehabilitation in patients with fecal inconti-nence be predicted? Int J Colorectal Dis 2008;23:503–511.

Invited Commentary

Clive I. Bartram

Surgery for fecal incontinence started with the Parks' postanal repair and has now diversified into a variety of measures to improve anorectal function. However, two questions for imaging to answer remain: is the sphincter intact and what is the quality of the sphincteric muscle?

Endoanal ultrasound has proved particularly useful in determining sphincter integrity. This has led to a greater awareness of occult sphincter tears after childbirth, and how inadvertent damage to the internal sphincter may result from procedures such as anal dilatation or lateral internal anal sphincterotomy.

In the arguments for endoanal ultrasound versus magnetic resonance imaging (MRI), visualization of the internal sphincter is certainly easier on sonography. The signal differences between scar tissue and normal external sphincter on MRI and their grayscale counterparts on ultrasound may be comparable, but it is perhaps a matter of personal experience as to which procedure one is more familiar with, that determines which one uses. Scarring extending into adjacent fat is a very helpful secondary feature to confirm a tear on MRI. Some studies have not shown a good correlation of external anal sphincter (EAS) measurement between three-dimensional (3D) endosonography and endoanal MRI. It is important in making measurements from ultrasound to measure from the inner border of the interface reflection. These reflections are generated at the tissue interface, and extend down into the layer further away from the probe to a depth that corresponds to the axial resolution of the transducer. Using the outer border of one and the inner border of another to measure thickness can make quite a difference. Using the inner borders of both, there is a good correlation between endoanal ultrasound and MRI.

Where MR really excels is in determining external sphincter atrophy. There is a very marked difference in signal between external sphincter muscle fibers and fat in the ischioanal fossae and fat or connective tissue in the longitudinal layer. The inner and outer borders of the external sphincter are therefore defined precisely, and both muscle thinning, and the area and proportion of fat content can be estimated and give a reliable estimation of atrophy compared to single-fiber electromyography (EMG) readings.

The significance of a thin internal sphincter in fecal incontinence remains slightly uncertain. A correlation with passive incontinence has been found, but in the study, external sphincter atrophy was excluded by pudendal motor nerve latencies, which may be challenged as these become abnormal relatively late in denervation [1]. No ultrasound criteria for EAS atrophy were available at that time, but in a later study, loss of the outer interface reflection was shown to have a 70% predictive value for atrophy, increasing to 74% if abnormal thinning of the internal sphincter was found [2]. Whether internal sphincter thinning is just part of atrophy of a separate entity really requires further study.

Perineal ultrasound may have some limitations in assessing the anal sphincters, but has the advantage of allowing movement, particularly of the puborectalis sling, to be estimated. There is evidence that 8 mm movement of the sling during voluntary contraction differentiates between normal (more than) and abnormal (less than), and that abnormal movement has a significant influence on the outcome after sphincter repair. This may therefore be a simple method to detect neuropathy and puborectalis atrophy. Actual tears of the puborectalis are more common than routinely diagnosed, and could be a cause

C.I. Bartram
Diagnostic Imaging, Princess Grace Hospital, London, UK

G.A. Santoro, A.P. Wieczorek, C.I. Bartram (eds.) *Pelvic Floor Disorders*
© Springer-Verlag Italia 2010

of impaired movement, which needs to be considered. However, without MRI to determine muscle bulk, this is a promising addition to the current imprecise sonographic assessment of atrophy.

Imaging remains central to the preoperative assessment of fecal incontinence to answer the fundamental questions of sphincter integrity and atrophy.

References

1. Vaizey CJ, Kamm MA, Gold DM et al. Clinical, physiological, and radiological study of a new purpose-designed artificial bowel sphincter. Lancet 1998;352:105–109.
2. Williams AB, Bartram CI, Modhwadia D et al. Endocoil magnetic resonance imaging quantification of external anal sphincter atrophy. Br J Surg 2001;88:853–859.

Abstract Anorectal manometry is considered a valuable test for the diagnosis and management of fecal incontinence. It is used to identify functional sphincter weakness, poor rectal compliance, and rectal sensation impairment. Anal resting pressure may be reduced in fecal incontinence, and dysfunction of the internal anal sphincter may be suspected in these patients. Maximal voluntary contraction is frequently impaired in incontinent patients and this sign is related to external anal sphincter dysfunction. A significant decrease or loss of rectal sensation may contribute to fecal incontinence by impairing the recognition of impending defecation, and substantial decreases in rectal compliance are associated with urge fecal incontinence. The rehabilitative treatment of fecal incontinence is guided by anorectal manometry, and the algorithm for multimodal rehabilitation is based on manometric reports. Furthermore, anorectal manometry can help to select candidates for overlapping sphincteroplasty, and identifies those patients with rectal prolapse who are at high risk for postoperative incontinence, modifying the surgical strategy of simple correction of prolapse. In conclusion, anorectal manometry offers decisive data for understanding the pathophysiology of fecal incontinence and can modify the therapeutic strategy.

Keywords Anorectal manometry • Anal sphincters • Biofeedback • Fecal incontinence • Multimodal rehabilitation • Rectal reservoir • Rectal sensation • Sacral neuromodulation • Sphincteroplasty • Sphincter-saving operations

27.1 Introduction

Fecal incontinence is defined as failure to control the elimination of stool and/or flatus [1]. The cause may be multifactorial, because the incontinence is often a consequence of concurrent disruption of several mechanisms that maintain continence (anal sphincters, rectal reservoir, rectal sensation, pelvic floor integrity, nerve supply to the pelvic floor, cortical awareness, stool volume and consistency). Diagnostic workup of fecal incontinence is based on imaging techniques, to discover abnormalities of structural integrity involving the sphincter muscles, and on functional instrumental studies, to evaluate the neuromuscular function of the anorectum. Anorectal manometry is used to identify functional sphincter weakness, poor rectal compliance, and impairment of rectal sensation. In fact, the clinical utility of anorectal manometry is limited by the relative absence of standardization of test protocols and normative data from a large number of healthy individuals

F. Pucciani
Department of Medical and Surgical Critical Care,
University of Firenze, Italy

[2]. Nevertheless, it is considered a valuable test for the diagnosis and management of fecal incontinence [3].

27.2   Anorectal Manometry

Routine diagnostic manometry entails the following.

- Exploration of the anal sphincter apparatus, including smooth and striated components. Anal resting pressure (ARP) reflects the tonic activities of both the internal anal sphincter (IAS) and the external anal sphincter (EAS); several studies attribute approximately 55% of ARP to the IAS, 15% to the vascular anal cushions, and the remaining 30% to the EAS [4, 5]. Maximal voluntary contraction (MVC) is the squeeze pressure obtained by asking the patient to maximally contract the anus; it reflects the contractile activity of the external anal sphincter.
- Evaluation of the rectoanal inhibitory reflex (RAIR); this is the reflex inhibition of IAS tone that is elicited by distending a rectal balloon with different volumes of air. It is part of the sampling reflex responsible for triggering the impulse to defecate [6, 7]. Transient relaxation of the IAS allows the stool contents from the rectum to come into contact with specialized sensory organs in the upper anal canal; the sensation of rectal content alerts the patient to discharge flatus or to defecate.
- Detection of rectal sensation. Volumetric perception of fecal mass is reproduced by distending a rectal balloon with increasing volumes [3]. The conscious rectal sensitivity threshold (CRST) is the lowest volume of air that evokes the first sensation; constant sensation (CS) is the volume that communicates a need to stool; maximum tolerated volume (MTV) measures the threshold volume for urgency to defecate and for pain.
- Monitoring of rectal compliance. Rectal compliance, as determined by the pressure/volume ratio at several different distending volumes, reflects tonic adaptation of the rectal wall (rectum distensibility) to the incoming fecal load [8].

27.3   Anorectal Manometry and Fecal Incontinence

As a result of these intrinsic features, anorectal manometry is capable of providing objective information about the mechanisms of fecal continence. When used in incontinent patients, manometric data suggest which continence mechanisms may be malfunctioning. However, manometric findings in incontinent patients are aspecific and must be completed with data obtained using other diagnostic techniques, both morphologic (magnetic resonance imaging (MRI), endoanal ultrasound) and functional (anal neurophysiologic tests), to obtain a correct pathophysiological profile of incontinence.

Anal resting pressure may be reduced in fecal incontinence [9]. Dysfunction of the IAS may be suspected in these patients, especially if they have passive fecal incontinence [10], and endoanal ultrasound will confirm the suspicion. A recent study by Bordeianou et al observed a positive correlation between ARP and the presence of sphincter defects on endoanal ultrasound [11]. Incontinent patients with sphincter defects had significantly lower mean ARP than those without sphincter defects. It should be noted that the discriminative power of ARP data between continent and incontinent patients is poor, with low sensitivity and specificity [12], because of the wide range of normal pressures. However, manometry is more precise than a digital examination for the evaluation of anal tone [13].

Maximal voluntary contraction is frequently impaired in patients who are affected by fecal incontinence. The amplitude and duration of squeeze tone are lower than in healthy controls, with high sensitivity (92%) and specificity (97%) [14]. This sign is related to external anal sphincter dysfunction, and patients often have urge incontinence with loss of stool because of inability to suppress defecation [10]. Endoanal ultrasound will be able to detect EAS lesions, and neurophysiologic anal tests (electromyography (EMG), pudendoanal reflex) could be useful in diagnosing pudendal nerve injury [3, 15].

The RAIR, the transient decrease in resting anal pressure in response to rapid inflation of a rectal balloon, often cannot be elicited when anal pressures are very low (< 10 mmHg). Therefore, in some incontinent patients with low ARP, it is not possible to judge if the reflex is present or absent, if normal or not. However, there are some reports on RAIR modifications in patients affected by fecal incontinence. Eyers and Thomson observed that RAIR was of longer duration in patients with fecal soiling and pruritus ani than in controls [16]. An ambulatory manometric study confirmed that abnormal transient IAS relaxation may lead to fecal soiling and pruritus ani [17]. The duration of RAIR is also longer in patients affected by idiopathic fecal incontinence than in controls; a prolonged contraction time (CT), with a slow return to the prestimulation values, is the typical sign [18]. A longer RAIR impairs the fecal continence mechanism. When small amounts of stool elicit RAIR with a prolonged CT in patients with poor external anal sphincter recruitment, and in the presence of a CRST that is higher than that of the RAIR threshold, fecal passive incontinence may occur.

A significant decrease or loss of rectal sensation (raised CRST, raised CS) may contribute to fecal incontinence by impairing the recognition of impending defecation. When stool enters the rectum, the perception of rectal distension gives the conscious stimulus to contract the anal sphincter for the preservation of continence; if stool is not perceived, the contractive voluntary response is not elicited, and fecal incontinence may occur. Diabetes mellitus [19] and multiple sclerosis [20] may exhibit this pathophysiological mechanism of incontinence but some other types of patients have the same dysfunction. Some studies suggest that biofeedback training improves sensory thresholds [21, 22]. Normalization or reduction of the first detectable sensation (CRST) correlates with therapeutic success, and is considered of value in the biofeedback training of patients with fecal incontinence [3].

The compliance of the rectum, as with the MTV, may contribute to fecal incontinence. A reduction of rectum distensibility decreases rectal capacity, as testified by simultaneous impairment of MTV, and substantial decreases in compliance are associated with an increased frequency of stool, rapid transit of stool through the rectum, and urge fecal incontinence [3]. Rectal inflammation, fibrosis of the rectum, radiotherapy, and replacement of the rectum, as with sphincter-saving operations, are all factors that decrease rectal compliance.

27.4 Anorectal Manometry and Treatment of Fecal Incontinence

Anorectal manometry is a diagnostic test but it may provide information that guides management of fecal incontinence. Rehabilitative treatment is the first-line conservative therapy for incontinence after failure of medical treatment. A systematic review has shown that rehabilitation cures up to half and improves up to two-thirds of patients [23]. Multimodal rehabilitation may be used as rehabilitative protocol [24]. The algorithm for this rehabilitation management is based on manometric reports. Biofeedback and pelviperineal kinesitherapy are indicated by low anal resting pressures or weak maximal voluntary contraction. Volumetric rehabilitation (sensory retraining) is indicated for disordered rectal sensation or impaired rectal compliance. Electrostimulation is only a preliminary step when patients need to feel the anoperineal plane. The usual procedural sequence is: (1) volumetric rehabilitation; (2) electrostimulation; (3) pelviperineal kinesitherapy; and (4) biofeedback. Their combination is suggested by manometric data. The same protocol of multimodal rehabilitation has also been used in patients who are incontinent after sphincter-saving operations [25]. Very low anal pressure (mean pressure < 17 mmHg) and impairment of both compliance and MTV were associated with bad post-rehabilitative results. Furthermore, anorectal manometry can help to select candidates for surgical therapy of fecal incontinence. Low anal resting pressures (< 10 mmHg) and low maximal voluntary contraction (< 40 mmHg) are considered cut-off values for overlapping sphincteroplasty [26]. The same cut-off values identify those patients with rectal prolapse who are at high risk for postoperative incontinence, modifying the surgical strategy of simple correction of prolapse [27]. Finally, the therapeutic success of sacral nerve stimulation applied to fecal incontinence seems to be related to a significant increase of both desire to defecate and maximal tolerated volume [28].

27.5 Conclusions

In conclusion, anorectal manometry may be considered an important tool in the diagnostic workup of fecal incontinence. It offers decisive data for understanding the pathophysiology of fecal incontinence, and can modify the therapeutic strategy.

References

1. Miner PB. Economic and personal impact of fecal and urinary incontinence. Gastroenterology 2004;126:S8–S13.
2. Azpiroz F, Enck P, Whitehead WE. Anorectal functional testing: review of collective experience. Am J Gastroenterol 2002;97:232–240.
3. American Gastroenterological Association (AGA). American Gastroenterological Association medical position statement

on anorectal testing techniques. Gastroenterology 1999; 116:732–760.

4. Lestar B, Penninckx F, Kerreman R. The composition of anal basal pressure: an in vivo and in vitro study in man. Int J Colorectal Dis 1989;4:118–122.

5. Andromanakos N, Filippou D, Skandalakis P et al. Anorectal incontinence. Pathogenesis and choice of treatment. J Gastrointest Liver Dis 2006;15:41–49.

6. Nothmann BJ, Schuster MM. Internal anal sphincter derangement with anal fissures. Gastroenterology 1974;67:216–220.

7. Kumar D, Waldron D, Williams NS et al. Prolonged anorectal manometry and external anal sphincter electromyography in ambulant human subjects. Dig Dis Sci 1990;35:641–648.

8. Madoff RD, Orrom WJ, Rothenberger DA et al. Rectal compliance: a critical reappraisal. Int J Colorectal Dis 1990;5:37–40.

9. Bharucha AE, Fletcher JG, Harper CM et al. Relationship between symptoms and disordered continence mechanisms in women with idiopathic fecal incontinence. Gut 2005; 54:546–555.

10. Engel AF, Kamm MA, Bartram CI et al. Relationship of symptoms in fecal incontinence to specific sphincter abnormalities. Int J Colorectal Dis 1995;10:152–155.

11. Bordeianou L, Kil Yeon L, Rockwood T et al. Anal resting pressures at manometry correlate with the fecal incontinence severity index and with presence of sphincter defects on ultrasound. Dis Colon Rectum 2008;51:1010–1014.

12. Raza N, Bielefeldt K. Discriminative value of anorectal manometry in clinical practice. Dig Dis Sci 2009;54:2503–2511.

13. Hallan RI, Marzouk DE, Waldron DJ et al. Comparison of digital and manometric assessment of anal sphincter function. Br J Surg 1989;76:973–975.

14. Sun WM, Donnelly TC, Read NW. Utility of a combined test of anorectal manometry, electromyography and sensation in determining the mechanism of "idiopathic" fecal incontinence. Gut 31992;3:807–813.

15. Uher EA, Swash M. Sacral reflexes. Physiology and clinical application. Dis Colon Rectum 1998;41:1165–1177.

16. Eyers AA, Thomson JP. Pruritus ani: is anal sphincter dysfunction important in aetiology? BMJ 1979;2:1549–1551.

17. Farouk R, Duthie GS, Pryde A et al. Abnormal transient internal sphincter relaxation in idiopathic pruritus ani: physiological evidence from ambulatory monitoring. Br J Surg 1994;81:603–606.

18. Pucciani F, Bologna A, Rottoli ML et al. Idiopathic faecal incontinence and internal anal sphincter dysfunction: role of the rectoanal inhibitory reflex. Tech Coloproctol 1997;5:14–18.

19. Wald A, Tunuguntia AK. Anorectal sensory motor dysfunction in fecal incontinence and diabetes mellitus. Modification with biofeedback therapy. N Engl J Med 1984;10:1282–1287.

20. Caruana BJ, Wald A, Hinds JP et al. Anorectal sensory and motor function in neurogenic fecal incontinence. Comparison between multiple sclerosis and diabetes mellitus. Gastroenterology 1991;100:465–470.

21. Miner PB, Donnelly TC et al. Investigation of mode of action of biofeedback in treatment of fecal incontinence. Dig Dis Sci 1990;35:1291–1298.

22. Ozturk R, Niazi S, Stessman M et al. Long-term outcome and objective changes of anorectal function after biofeedback therapy for fecal incontinence. Aliment Pharmacol Ther 2004;20:667–674.

23. Norton C, Kamm MA. Anal sphincter biofeedback and pelvic floor exercises for faecal incontinence in adults – a systematic review. Aliment Pharmacol Ther 2001;15:1147–1154.

24. Pucciani F, Iozzi L, Masi A et al. Multimodal rehabilitation for faecal incontinence: experience of an Italian centre devoted to faecal disorder rehabilitation. Tech Coloproctol 2003;7:139–147.

25. Pucciani F, Ringressi MN, Redditi S et al. Rehabilitation of fecal incontinence after sphincter-saving surgery for rectal cancer: encouraging results. Dis Colon Rectum 2008; 51:1552–1558.

26. Ternent CA, Shahidaran M, Blatchford GJ et al. Transanal ultrasound and anorectal physiology findings affecting continence after sphincteroplasty. Dis Colon Rectum 1997; 40:462–467.

27. Yoshioka K, Hyland G, Keighley MRB. Anorectal function after abdominal rectopexy: parameters of predictive value in identifying return of continence. Br J Surg 1989;76:64–68.

28. Michelsen HB, Buntzen S, Krog K et al. Rectal volume tolerability and anal pressures in patients with fecal incontinence treated with sacral nerve stimulation. Dis Colon Rectum 2006;49:1039–1044.

Invited Commentary

Anton Emmanuel

There is no doubt that anorectal physiological assessment is potentially helpful in some patients with fecal incontinence. However, the lack of uniformity of performance and interpretation of the investigations has compromised a definitive role for such testing across the board. As such, symptoms and appearances on endoanal ultrasound have come to be regarded by many practitioners as more valuable definers of treatment and clinical outcome.

One controversial issue is whether anal sphincter manometry can really provide objective information about fecal incontinence. One of the points raised in this review is that correlations between manometry and appearances on endoanal ultrasound are not surprising and do not differentiate cause from effect. While it is helpful in an individual situation if there is agreement between manometry and structure, in most circumstances the doctor will defer to the findings of the ultrasound if there is discord between the investigations. It is certainly true, for example, that outcome after anterior sphincter repair is more closely related to sonographic integrity than to sphincter pressures.

The poor relationship between treatment and physiology extends even to conservative therapies. Biofeedback outcome does not relate to baseline anal manometry or rectal sensitivity. Considerable discrepancy exists in the literature about whether anal squeeze pressure or rectal distension sensitivity can be used as biological foci for behavioral biofeedback therapy. While some studies have shown minor changes in these parameters, others have failed to, and none have shown any predictive value from these measures. Equally, many centres do not use any true sensory

biofeedback in treating fecally incontinent patients, and report success rates that are the equal of those centers that do. All in all, it is reasonable to conclude that existing anorectal physiological parameters do not provide uniform correlation with clinical presentations or with treatment outcomes.

However, it is clear that there are potentially fruitful areas where physiological measurement can complement symptom and structural assessment. Broadly speaking, anorectal physiology tests can be subdivided into:

- measuring anal sphincter pressures
- determining anorectal sensitivity thresholds
- identifying rectal compliance (distension–pressure relationship)
- assessing anorectal reflexes.

The measurement of pudendal nerve terminal motor latencies has fallen out of favor. This relates in part to the neurophysiological invalidity and poor reproducibility of the test. However, most importantly to the clinician, pudendal nerve terminal motor latency does not correlate with maximum squeeze pressure, and normal latencies do not exclude weakness of the anal sphincters and puborectalis.

More promising physiological targets, however, are beginning to emerge. Recent publications have investigated the phases of the rectoanal inhibitory reflex (RAIR). The excitation latency and durations of latency and recovery have been shown to reflect specific fecal incontinence symptoms. Understanding this and other anorectal reflexes may both help the understanding of the pathophysiology of urgency and fecal soiling, and lead to novel treatment targets for electrical neuromodulation.

A. Emmanuel
GI Physiology Unit, University College Hospital, London, UK

G.A. Santoro, A.P. Wieczorek, C.I. Bartram (eds.) *Pelvic Floor Disorders*
© Springer-Verlag Italia 2010

A further assessment of even more direct potential clinical relevance is the so-called "porridge enema" test. In brief, a cereal and water paste is mixed up to the consistency of a semi-formed stool and instilled into the rectum. Patients are asked to walk around the unit for 10 to 15 minutes to assess their functional capacity to retain the content without soiling or urge incontinence. Recent publications have shown this assessment to have clinical utility in predicting outcome after stoma reversal.

Sphincter Repair and Postanal Repair

28

Johann Pfeifer

Abstract Several factors are responsible for continence, and treatment options vary. We distinguish between morphological defects of the sphincter mechanism and functional incontinence disorders. Possible candidates for sphincter repair should have a clinical and physiological workup. If a distinct defect is localized, sphincter repair can be done either as a direct repair or as an overlapping sphincteroplasty. No protective stoma is needed. For idiopathic fecal incontinence, the method of postanal repair has been described. Short-term results for overlapping sphincter repair (< 5 years) are successful in about 75% of patients. In the long run (>10 years), the success rate decreases significantly. Success rates for postanal repair are in the range of about 20–30%. Despite poor long-term results, sphincteroplasty is the best surgical treatment option for isolated, preferably anterior sphincter defects. Physiological tests are useful for planning an operation. At present, postanal repair is not a first-line treatment in idiopathic fecal incontinence.

Keywords Anal sphincter defect • Fecal incontinence • Obstetric injury • Overlapping sphincter repair • Postanal repair

28.1 Introduction

Several mechanisms, either alone or in combination, produce symptoms of fecal incontinence: (a) consistency and amount of stool (e.g. diarrhea), (b) damage to the mucosa of the colon and rectum (e.g. colitis), (c) neurologic factors (e.g. diabetes, Parkinson's disease), (d) miscellaneous (congenital disorders, rectocele, etc), and (e) injuries to the anal sphincter and pelvic floor muscles. The latter are the most interesting for surgeons. Trauma as well as previous operative procedures such as fistula surgery [1], hemorrhoidectomy [2],

manual dilatation (Lord's procedure) [3], or internal sphincterotomy due to anal fissure [4] have all been described as causes of fecal incontinence. Anal sphincter damage sustained during childbirth is one of the most common causes in middle-aged woman [5]. Occult sphincter defects have been diagnosed by anal ultrasound in 35% of primiparous women [6]. Newer prospective studies confirm the high rate of injuries in vaginal deliveries [7]. Damon et al reported that if signs of clinical fecal incontinence and a history of vaginal delivery were present, an anal sphincter defect could be seen upon endoanal ultrasound (EAUS) in 62% of patients [8]. With midline episiotomies and/or operative vaginal delivery, the incidence of sphincter defects can reach 50% [9]. Looking into the gynecological literature, the incidence of a third-degree sphincter rupture

J. Pfeifer
Department of General Surgery,
Medical University of Graz, Austria

G.A. Santoro, A.P. Wieczorek, C.I. Bartram (eds.) *Pelvic Floor Disorders*
© Springer-Verlag Italia 2010

during vaginal delivery in the normal population is about 2% [10].

28.2 Workup

The first step in evaluating patients suffering from fecal incontinence is always a careful history. Questions should focus on type and degree of incontinence as well as on changes in the patient's lifestyle. A scoring system (Williams, Pescatori, Wexner, AMS Score, etc) is often used to rate incontinence more accurately. A distinct sphincter disruption can often be palpated upon dynamic digital-rectal examination. Clinical evaluation and endoscopy should exclude structural disorders (polyps, tumors, etc) and pseudoincontinence. If basic investigation fails to show any evidence of fecal incontinence, or an operation is planned, a more sophisticated physiological workup is necessary. Our basic physiology testing includes anal manometry, EAUS, and neurophysiologic assessment. An interesting, recently published study from Geneva, Switzerland, showed that voluntary contraction of the puborectal sling before sphincter repair for anal incontinence is a good prognostic tool. A movement of more than 8 mm as seen on perineal ultrasound had a postoperative success rate of 98.7% [11]. As electromyography (EMG) of the pelvic floor with concentric needles or a single fiber is painful, it should only be done in selected patients [12]. Pudendal nerve terminal motor latency measurement (PNTML) is useful, as this test may influence the prognosis after surgical corrections of sphincter defects [13, 14]. In selected cases, special investigations may be added as necessary (incontinence test, defecography, etc).

28.3 Indication

If conservative treatment options fail, patients may be considered for surgery. The operative technique of sphincteroplasty is only suitable for isolated disruption of the sphincter muscle. Patients best suited for surgical corrections are those in whom incontinence is secondary to an (obstetrical) anterior sphincter defect [14]. Patients with an isolated defect used to be scheduled for immediate surgery, but now sacral nerve modulation is the recommended first-line treatment in some centers, even in the presence of sphincter defects [15–19]. A pre-existing internal anal sphincter (IAS) defect, in contrast

to an isolated external anal sphincter (EAS) defect, does not preclude successful sphincteroplasty [20]. Due to the disappointing long-term results, postponement of the operation may be the best option. Before considering an operative approach, pelvic floor training such as a biofeedback may merit a trial [21].

28.4 Technique

The patient receives full bowel preparation, perioperative antibiotics, and a Foley catheter. In most circumstances the operation is performed under general anesthesia with the patient in the lithotomy or prone jackknife position. The operation starts with a semicircular incision around the anus. After the ischiorectal fossae are entered, the sphincter muscles are identified and freed. The next step is to transect the scarred tissue. When necessary, an additional levatorplasty can be performed [22]. The internal sphincter muscle can then be sutured as a special distinct layer [13], but a significant improvement with the internal imbrication has not been demonstrated [23]. Then the external sphincter muscles are repaired with mattress sutures. After the muscle repair, a simple wound closure is done with the midportion left open for drainage. Postoperatively, daily showers or sitz baths are recommended. The wound usually closes within 4–6 weeks.

28.5 Special Technical Remarks

- Overlapping or apposition: in 1940, the collective results of the American Proctological Society on end-to-end repair reported failure rates as high as 40% [24]. That is why the overlapping repair, which was suggested in 1971 by Sir Allan Parks, was accepted immediately [25]. Thereafter, although it was modified several times, many centers including ours preferred the overlapping sphincter repair [23, 26, 27] to a simple apposition of the sphincter muscles [28]. In a recent Cochrane review, meta-analyses showed that there was no statistically significant difference in perineal pain, dyspareunia, flatus, and fecal incontinence between the two repair techniques at 12 months, but showed a statistically significant lower incidence in fecal urgency and lower anal incontinence scores in the overlap group. The overlap technique was also associated with a statistically significant lower risk that anal incontinence symptoms will worsen over a 12-month period. There was no significant difference in quality of life [29]. However, recent publications have reported far from perfect results with the overlapping technique. Some patients even developed new evacuation disorders [30]. In a recent prospective randomized study, Tjandra et al found no significant difference in functional outcome of overlapping versus apposition of the sphincter ends [31]. But in principle the sphincter defect should not exceed more than "three hours" or 90° in EAUS, as overlapping may thus become technically impossible. A direct relationship between the size of the tear and the degree of dysfunction could not, however, be confirmed [32].

- Scar: scar tissue can be nicely quantified with EAUS. In a prospective study correlating clinical signs with the postoperative EAUS picture, there seems to be a benefit for the patient if the scar is used for overlapping and not resected. However, excessive scarring itself may make overlap impossible [33].
- Suture material: a number of different suture materials have been suggested by various authors – monofilament nylon, pull-out wire, catgut, silk, PDS. My own preference is 2/0 absorbable suture material (e.g. Vicryl®) for the repair. However, some recommend much stronger sutures such as 0 or 1. I myself have found that it is important to use a soft suture material, as stiffer sutures tend to lead to discomfort to the patient and, with time, may cut through the (sometimes atrophic) muscles.
- Diverting stoma: in patients with a severe trauma to the perineum other than after delivery, a proximal colostomy is often constructed to avoid septic complications and to facilitate nursing management [34].
- A diverting stoma for a secondary obstetrical repair is usually not needed if the central portion of the wound is left open for drainage [13, 26, 35]. Some colorectal surgeons prefer to close the wound and insert a drain [36]. It is my experience that even if the wound is closed carefully, it will very likely not heal well. This was supported recently by Martinez et al, who saw a spontaneous skin disruption after wound closure in 43.7% of patients [37]. The presence of a stoma itself does not improve the rate of wound healing by primary intention [38]. Furthermore, stoma-related complications are reported in more than 50% of these patients [39].

28.6 Special Problems

In recent decades, there have been numerous publications on sphincteroplasty indications, technique, and results. There are a few points that should be highlighted.

- Primary versus secondary repair: in the acute, emergency trauma situation, initial treatment consists of debridement of non-viable tissue, removal of foreign material, open drainage, and often proximal colostomy with distal washout. Depending on the extent of injury and the associated trauma, reconstructive surgery may be deferred.
- The approach in patients with obstetrical trauma is somewhat different. A third- or fourth-degree perineal tear must be repaired immediately, although defects after repair are reported in up to 66% [40, 41]. As about 40% of these women eventually have clinical signs of incontinence [41, 42], it must be stressed that a specialist should do the repair, to minimize late complications. For secondary repair after obstetric injury, a delay of at least 6 months to 1 year had been recommended to allow the tissue to return to normal [38]. Soerensen et al from Denmark, however, looked prospectively at sphincter repairs done as a delayed primary (within 72 hours post partum) or as an early secondary reconstruction (within 14 days after delivery) without a covering stoma in women who had sustained a third-degree or fourth-degree obstetric tear. They found equal results with acceptable long-term functional outcome in both groups [35].
- Failed primary repair: there seems to be no difference in outcome in patients who had an unsuccessful primary repair and those who had no previous repair. In about 62%, a repeated repair can be expected to be successful, although patients who had undergone more than two previous repairs had poorer clinical results [43].
- Age: sphincteroplasty can be done even in elderly patients [38], and success can be expected in about 75% of them. Simmang et al found no difference in outcome in patients with a mean age of 66 years (range 55–81 years) compared to younger ones [44]. This was confirmed by our group in patients over the age of 60 years [45], and in a recent study by Evans et al [46]. However, Nikiteas et al reported poorer results in patients older than 50

years, especially with concomitant obesity and perineal descent [47].

- Pudendal neuropathy: if a patient has a uni- or bilateral pudendal neuropathy preoperatively, it is important to explain to the patient that the outcome of the sphincteroplasty may be disappointing [12, 14, 48]. Nonetheless, this should not deter the colorectal surgeon from attempting the repair if a distinct sphincter defect is seen on EAUS.

- Biofeedback: in a one-year follow-up study of 48 patients after a third- or fourth-degree sphincter laceration, after one month ten patients (21%) complained of anal incontinence, eight of flatus only. After one year, none complained of fecal incontinence and three (7%) of gas incontinence [49]. The authors concluded that pelvic floor exercises seem to suffice as first-line treatment. In the light of poor long-term results with the overlapping sphincteroplasty, pelvic floor exercises seem to be an appropriate first-line approach. It is of utmost importance that after successful repair patients be referred for pelvic floor exercises and biofeedback [50]. Long-term results of EMG biofeedback training are promising [51].

- Combination with other perineal operations: sometimes a sphincter defect can be diagnosed in combination with other perineal pathologies. Combining the sphincteroplasty with levatorplasty, procedures for urinary incontinence and/or pelvic organ prolapse [22] provide good outcome and are cost-effective [52]. Sphincteroplasty can also be part of a more extensive perineal reconstruction of the pelvic floor for cloaca-like deformities [22, 53, 54].

- Costs: sphincteroplasty is a relatively inexpensive operation compared to more sophisticated procedures such as artificial bowel sphincter, dynamic graciloplasty, and sacral nerve modulation [55]. Successful primary repair compared to secondary repair substantially improves quality of life and reduces the overall cost of treatment [56].

28.7 Short-term Results of Sphincteroplasty

In the short term (< 5 years), the results of the sphincteroplasty are usually quite good, with success rates of about 75% (Table 28.1) [57-65], although it is well known that a persistent defect after repair is associated with a poor immediate outcome [66]. Technically, this can happen if the suture material cuts through the muscle, allowing the sphincter ends to retract [5]. Furthermore, isolated internal anal sphincter defects often present as persistent fecal incontinence [5].

28.8 Long-term Results of Sphincteroplasty

Unfortunately, the long-term results of sphincteroplasty are not so promising (Table 28.2) [67-70]. Only about one-third of patients are totally continent, and about half of the patients are satisfied with their results if they are not incontinent for feces [67].

Table 28.1 Results for overlapping sphincteroplasty: short term (< 5 years)

Author	Year	N	Age in years, mean (range)	Success (%)
Fang et al [57]	1984	79	? (17–68)	89
Lauberg et al [58]	1988	19	? (23–64)	47
Yoshioka and Keighley [59]	1989	27	34 (17–81)	74
Fleshman et al [60]	1991	28	38 (22–75)	75
Engel et al [61]	1994	55	32 (26–52)	76
Oliveira et al [26]	1996	55	48 (27–72)	71
Morren et al [62]	2001	55	39 (24–73)	56
Elton and Stoodley [63]	2002	20	n.a.	80
Tjandra et al [31]	2003	23	45 (31–68)	74
Pfeifer [64]	2004	41	34 (19–71)	73
Martinez et al [37]	2006	16	n.a.	87
Barisic et al [65]	2006	65	n.a.	74

n.a. not available

Table 28.2 Results for overlapping sphincteroplasty: long term (> 5 years)

Author	Year	N	Age in years, mean (range)	Success (%)
Gilliland et al [12]	1998	77	47 (25–80)	60
Malouf et al [30]	2000	55	43 (26–67)	50
Karoui et al [67]	2000	86	n.a.	49
Halverson and Hull [68]	2001	71	38.5 (22–80)	46
Buie et al [69]	2001	191	37 (20–74)	62
Barisic et al [65]	2006	65	n.a.	48
Maslekar et al [70]	2007	64	n.a.	80
Soerensen et al [35]	2008	22	31 (22–38)	50

n.a. not available

28.9 Quality of Life

28.9.1 Literature

Despite the large number of tests, questionnaires, and scores, measuring quality of life is difficult. Essentially, three techniques are available for measuring quality of life, and each has advantages and disadvantages. Recent publications on the outcome of sphincteroplasty for each technique may be summarized as follows.

- Descriptive measures: these questionnaires do not provide summary scores (e.g. Mayo Clinic Fecal Incontinence Questionnaire). Malouf et al recently reported long-term results (> 5 years) for patients after sphincteroplasty [30]. Forty-seven patients could be contacted. One had a proctectomy and end ileostomy due to Crohn's disease, seven had undergone further incontinence surgery, and one patient had not had a covering stoma closed. Thus, 38 patients answered the questionnaire and were available for follow-up. None of these patients was fully continent (stool and gas); only four were continent for liquid and stool, six had no fecal urgency, and eight had no passive soiling. Twenty (52%) were still wearing a pad, and 25 (66%) reported lifestyle restriction [30].
- Severity measures: this kind of measurement usually rates the type and frequency of incontinence, with either grading systems (e.g. Parks, Williams) or summary scales (e.g. Wexner, Vaizey). The latter are mostly used to assess pre- and postoperative results after sphincteroplasty (Tables 28.1 and 28.2). Hull et al recently published another incontinence questionnaire for outcome after sphincteroplasty [71].The disadvantages of all these measurements

are that impact on quality-of-life changes is not directly addressed, though it is clear that a higher frequency of incontinence episodes after sphincteroplasty leads to a lower quality of life [72]. A Wexner score of 9 or higher indicates a significant impairment of quality of life [73].

- Halverson and Hull used the Fecal Incontinence Severity Index (FISI), as proposed by Rockwood et al [74], and the Fecal Incontinence Quality of Life Scale (FIQLS) to assess long-term results after sphincteroplasty [68]. The mean follow-up of the 71 patients was 69 months (range 48–141 months). Twenty-four patients (54%) were incontinent for liquid or solid stool, and only six patients (14%) were fully continent. However, 15 patients (34%) achieved the best possible FIQLS of 16. The median FISI as rated by patients and surgeons was 20, with a closed relation between the two raters in the regression analysis (r = 0.98). In principle, the FISI is recommended when incontinence occurs frequently; however, the lack of assessment of urgency in this index may limit its applicability [72].
- Impact measures: although it is important to know the severity of fecal incontinence, it is also important to understand and measure the impact of fecal incontinence on patients, or rather the effect on quality of life. General questionnaires have a long history of use, with established reliability, validity, and population norms (e.g. the Short Form-36 (SF-36)). One of the newest measurement tools is the FIQLS, which is very sensitive and appears to be useful. Halverson and Hull nicely demonstrated the mismatch of full continence (14%) and excellent quality of life (34%), which cannot be detected with other measurement tools [68].
- Another excellent tool to measure quality of life is

a so-called Direct Questioning of Objectives (DQO). Questions of this kind have been used for quality-of-life assessment in patients with inflammatory bowel disease [75] and neuropathic fecal incontinence [76]. The advantage is that each patient spontaneously lists issues that are important to him/herself. Then he/she rates the ability to perform a particular activity (e.g. going shopping) on an objective scale. To my knowledge, this kind of quality-of-life measurement has not yet been used for patients after sphincter repair.

Recent publications have addressed the issue of sexuality and sphincter repair. Interestingly, sexual activity and function were similar following anal sphincteroplasty, compared with controls, despite more pronounced symptoms of fecal incontinence [77, 78]. However, fecal incontinence of solid stool and depression related to fecal incontinence were correlated with poorer sexual function [77]. Similar results have been reported by Trowsbridge et al [78]. Anal continence rates 5 years after anal sphincteroplasty are disappointing and adversely impact quality of life, yet do not appear to relate to sexual function [78].

28.9.2 Third-degree Sphincter Tears without Secondary Repair

In a recent study at our hospital, 30 primiparous patients who had had a third-degree sphincter tear were identified from the charts from January 1993 to June 2000. All these women were at home and had "no problems". Patients were asked to fill in a quality-of-life questionnaire and were then evaluated by clinical assessment, proctology, EAUS, anal manometry, and PNTML. Demographic data as well as the results of the physiological investigations are listed in Tables 28.3 and 28.4. Interestingly, the physiological results are poor but life quality seems to be better than expected according to the tests. Our explanation in this young age group is that this might be, at least in part, due to denial of symptoms and the fact that young mothers focus their life on the newborn child. Furthermore, urgency as a symptom of external sphincter laceration can be easily dealt with when a patient is at home near to a toilet and not in the workplace. The Austrian government provides financial support that allows mothers in Austria to stay at home for the first 30 months after delivery.

Table 28.3 Third-degree sphincter tears without secondary repair: demographic data and history

Characteristic	Values (range)
Number of patients	30
Age, years	31 (23–46)
Follow-up months (range)	31 (3–88)
Incontinence for solid stool, n	0
Incontinence for liquid stool, n	2
Incontinence for gas, n	8
Satisfied with their situation, n	27

Table 28.4 Third-degree sphincter tears without secondary repair: physiological results

Test and parameters	Results ($\pm$ standard deviation)
Anal manometry	
Mean resting pressure (mmHg)	47.9 ($\pm$ 20.9)
Maximal resting pressure (mmHg)	70.6 ($\pm$ 14.6)
Mean squeeze pressure (mmHg)	33.6 ($\pm$ 14.6)
Maximal squeeze pressure (mmHg)	68.5 ($\pm$ 23.6)
Length of the high-pressure zone (cm)	2.1 ($\pm$ 0.8)
PNTML (ms)	
Left	1.9 ($\pm$ 0.2)
Right	1.9 ($\pm$ 0.2)
EAUS (number of patients)	
Upper anal canal:	
Rupture/scar	3
Normal	27
Mid-anal canal:	
EAS thinning/scar	3
EAS defect (incomplete)	27 (total 19; partial 8)
IAS defect	6
IAS shape altered	4
IAS + EAS	6
Lower anal canal:	
Intact EAS	20
Thinning EAS	10

28.10 Postanal Repair

Before the advent of EAUS, incontinence patients were often categorized as having idiopathic or neurologic fecal incontinence [79]. One of the most often used surgical options was the postanal repair as described by Sir Allan Parks to restore the anorectal angle, increase anal pressure, and lengthen the anal canal [80]. The short- and long-term results are not especially good (Tables 28.5 and 28.6) [81-91] compared to sphinctero-

Table 28.5 Results of postanal repair: short term (< 5 years)

Author	Year	N	Success (%)
Womack et al [81]	1988	16	68
Miller et al [82]	1988	17	59
Braun et al [83]	1991	31	84
Briel and Schouten [84]	1995	37	46
Athanasiadis et al [85]	1995	31	52
Matsuoka et al [86]	2000	21	35

Table 28.6 Results of postanal repair: long term (> 5 years)

Author	Year	N	Success (%)
Yoshioka and Keighley [87]	1989	116	24
Setti Carraro et al [88]	1994	54	52
Rieger et al [89]	1997	22	58
Abbas et al [90]	2005	47	68
Mackey et al [91]	2009	57	52

plasty. Some studies could confirm that some patients had an occult sphincter defect [88]. The problem of patient selection is of utmost importance. Patients with excessive posterior pelvic floor mobility are poor candidates for postanal repair [92], and it has been suggested that they could be excluded with preoperative dynamic magnetic resonance imaging (MRI). The final function of the postanal repair is unclear. Some speculate that success appears to be related more to improved sphincter pressure and anal sensation [93, 94]; others believe that the efficacy of postanal repair is due more to local scarring and anal stenosis than restoration of the anorectal angle [95]. Despite the low success rate, the absence of any mortality and the low morbidity suggest that postanal repair may be a valid therapeutic approach, especially as a second surgical approach after failed primary surgery [96]. It should, however, be offered only to selected patients with persistent, severe fecal incontinence despite an anatomically intact EAS, who are not candidates for or refuse all other operative modalities. Interestingly, in a recent published series of 57 patients, although 48% complained of severe fecal incontinence, in the long run (9.1 years, range 2.2–18.7 years), 79% (n = 45) were satisfied with the outcome [91].

28.11 Conclusions

Sphincteroplasty, despite poor long-term results, is currently the best and cheapest surgical treatment option

for isolated, preferably anterior sphincter defects. Physiological tests are useful for planning an operation, but they do not necessarily reflect the quality-of-life outcome in these patients. Today, postanal repair is not a first-line treatment in idiopathic fecal incontinence.

References

1. Chang SC, Lin JK. Change in anal continence after surgery for intersphincteral anal fistula: a functional and manometric study. Int J Colorectal Dis 2003;18:111–115.
2. Zbar AP, Beer-Gabel M, Chiappa AC, Aslam M. Fecal incontinence after minor anorectal surgery. Dis Colon Rectum 2001;44:1610–1619.
3. Anscombe AR, Hancock BD, Humphreys WV. A clinical trial of the treatment of haemorrhoids by operation and the Lord procedure. Lancet 1974;2:250–253.
4. Garcea G, Sutton C, Mansoori S et al. Results following conservative lateral sphincteromy for the treatment of chronic anal fissures. Colorectal Dis 2003;5:311–314.
5. Jorge JM, Wexner SD. Etiology and management of fecal incontinence. Dis Colon Rectum 1993;36:77–97.
6. Sultan AH, Kamm MA, Hudson CN et al. Anal-sphincter disruption during vaginal delivery. N Engl J Med 1993;329:1905–11.
7. Zetterstrom J, Mellgren A, Jensen LL et al. Effect of delivery on anal sphincter morphology and function. Dis Colon Rectum 1999;42:1253–1260.
8. Damon H, Henry L, Barth X, Mion F. Fecal incontinence in females with a past history of vaginal delivery: significance of anal sphincter defects detected by ultrasound. Dis Colon Rectum 2002;45:1445–1451.
9. Belmonte-Montes C, Hagerman G, Vega-Yepez PA et al. Anal sphincter injury after vaginal delivery in primiparous females. Dis Colon Rectum 2001;44:1244–1248.
10. de Leeuw JW, Struijk PC, Vierhout ME, Wallenburg HC. Risk factors for third degree perineal ruptures during delivery. BJOG 2001;108:383–387.
11. Zufferey G, Perneger T, Robert-Yap J et al. Measure of the voluntary contraction of the puborectal sling as a predictor of successful sphincter repair in the treatment of anal incontinence. Dis Colon Rectum 2009;52:704–710.
12. Gilliland R, Altomare DF, Moreira H Jr et al. Pudendal neuropathy is predictive of failure following anterior overlapping sphincteroplasty. Dis Colon Rectum 1998;41:1516–1522.
13. Pfeifer J, Oliveira L, Wexner SD. Die Sphinkterplastik zur Behandlung der fäkalen Inkontinenz – Technik und Ergebnisse. Akt Chir 1996;31:1–5.
14. Pla-Martí V, Moro-Valdezate D, Alos-Company R et al. The effect of surgery on quality of life in patients with faecal incontinence of obstetric origin. Colorectal Dis 2007;9:90–95.
15. Conaghan P, Farouk R. Sacral nerve stimulation can be successful in patients with ultrasound evidence of external anal sphincter disruption. Dis Colon Rectum 2005;48:1610–1614.
16. Jarrett ME, Dudding TC, Nicholls RJ et al. Sacral nerve stimulation for fecal incontinence related to obstetric anal

sphincter damage. Dis Colon Rectum 2008;51:531–537.

17. Vitton V, Gigout J, Grimaud JC et al. Sacral nerve stimulation can improve continence in patients with Crohn's disease with internal and external anal sphincter disruption. Dis Colon Rectum 2008;51:924–927.

18. Chan MK, Tjandra JJ. Sacral nerve stimulation for fecal incontinence: external anal sphincter defect vs. intact anal sphincter. Dis Colon Rectum 2008;51:1015–1024.

19. Melenhorst J, Koch SM, Uludag O et al. Is a morphologically intact anal sphincter necessary for success with sacral nerve modulation in patients with faecal incontinence? Colorectal Dis 2008;10:257–262.

20 Oberwalder M, Dinnewitzer A, Baig M et al. Do internal anal sphincter defects decrease the success rate of anal sphincter repair? Tech Coloproctol 2006;10:94–97.

21. Jorge JM, Habra-Gama A, Wexner SD. Biofeedback therapy in colon and rectal practice. Appl Psychophysiol Biofeedback 2003;28:47–61.

22. Steele SR, Lee P, Mullenix PS et al. Is there a role for concomitant pelvic floor repair in patients with sphincter defects in the treatment of fecal incontinence? Int J Colorectal Dis 2006;21:508–514.

23. Briel JW, de Boer LM, Hop WC, Schouten WR. Clinical outcome of anterior overlapping external anal sphincter repair with internal anal sphincter imbrication. Dis Colon Rectum 1998;41:209–214.

24. Blaisdell PC. Repair of the incontinent sphincter ani. Surg Gynecol Obstet 1940;70:692–697.

25. Parks AG, McPartlin JF. Late repair of injuries of the anal sphincter. Proc R Soc Med 1971;64:1187–1189.

26. Oliveira L, Pfeifer J, Wexner SD. Physiological and clinical outcome of anterior sphincteroplasty. B J Surg 1996;83:502–505.

27. Abramov Y, Feiner B, Rosen T et al. Primary repair of advanced obstetric anal sphincter tears: should it be performed by the overlapping sphincteroplasty technique? Int Urogynecol J Pelvic Floor Dysfunct 2008;19:1071–1074.

28. Arnaud A, Sarles JC, Sielezneff I et al. Sphincter repair without overlapping for fecal incontinence. Dis Colon Rectum 1991;34:744–747.

29. Fernando R, Sultan AH, Kettle C et al. Methods of repair for obstetric anal sphincter injury. Cochrane Database Syst Rev 2006;3:CD002866.

30. Malouf AJ, Norton CS, Engel AF et al. Long term results of overlapping anterior anal-sphincter repair for obstetric trauma. Lancet 2000;355:260–265.

31. Tjandra JJ, Han WR, Goh J et al. Direct repair vs. overlapping sphincter repair: A randomized, controlled trial. Dis Colon Rectum 2003;46:937–942.

32. Voyvodic F, Rieger NA, Skinner S et al. Endosonographic imaging of anal sphincter injury: does size of the tear correlate with the degree of dysfunction? Dis Colon Rectum 2003;46:735–741.

33. Moscovitz I, Rotholtz NA, Baig MK et al. Overlapping sphincteroplasty: does preservation of the scar influence immediate outcome? Colorectal Dis 2002;4:275–279.

34. Pfeifer J, Kronberger L, Uranüs S. Injuries to hollow visceral organs. Acta Chir Austrica 1998;6:338–340.

35. Soerensen MM, Bek KM, Buntzen S et al. Long-term outcome of delayed primary or early secondary reconstruction of the anal sphincter after obstetrical injury. Dis Colon Rectum 2008;51:312–317.

36. Gangi S, Prosperini U, Costanzo MP et al. Technic of overlapping sphincter anal repair in the treatment of traumatic anal incontinence Ann Ital Chir 1995;66:393–396.

37. Martínez Hernández Magro P, Godínez Guerrero MA, Rivas Larrauri E et al. Anal incontinence caused by an obstetric trauma. Experience with the technique of overlapping sphincteroplasty. Ginecol Obstet Mex 2006;74:418–423.

38. Young CJ, Mathur MN, Eyers AA, Solomon MJ. Successful overlapping anal sphincter repair: relationship to patient age, neuropathy, and colostomy formation. Dis Colon Rectum 1998;41:344–349.

39. Hasegawa H, Yoshioka K, Keighley MRB. Randomized trial of fecal diversion for sphincter repair. Dis Colon Rectum 2000;43:961–965.

40. Fitzpatrick M, Behan M, O'Connell PR, O'Herlihy C. A randomized clinical trial comparing primary overlap with approximation repair of third-degree obstetric tears. Am J Obstet Gynecol 2000;183:1220–1224.

41. Hayes J, Shatari T, Toozs-Hobson P et al. Early results of immediate repair of obstetric third-degree tears: 65% are completely asymptomatic despite persistent sphincter defects in 61%. Colorectal Dis 2007;9:332–336.

42. Poen AC, Felt–Bersma RJ, Strijers RL et al. Third-degree obstetric perineal tear: long-term clinical and functional results after primary repair. Br J Surg 1998;85:1433–1438.

43. Giordano P, Renzi A, Efron J et al. Previous sphincter repair does not affect outcome of repeat repair. Dis Colon Rectum 2002;45:635–640.

44. Simmang C, Birnbaum EH, Kodner IJ et al. Anal sphincter reconstruction in the elderly: does advancing age affect outcome? Dis Colon Rectum 1994;37:1065–1069.

45. Pfeifer J, Rabl H, Uranüs S, Wexner SD. Ist die Sphinkterplastik zur Behandlung der Fäkalen Inkontinenz bei Patienten älter als 60 Jahre gerechtfertigt? Langenbecks Arch Chir Suppl II 1996;474–476.

46. Evans C, Davis K, Kumar D. Overlapping anal sphincter repair and anterior levatorplasty: effect of patient's age and duration of follow-up. Int J Colorectal Dis 2006;21:795–801.

47. Nikiteas N, Korsgen S, Kumar D, Keighley MRB. Audit of sphincter repair: factors associated with poor outcome. Dis Colon Rectum 1996;39:1164–1170.

48. Chen AS, Luchtefeld MA, Senagore AJ et al. Pudendal nerve latency. Does it predict outcome of anal sphincter repair? Dis CoLon Rectum 1998;41:1005–1009.

49. Sander P, Bjarnesen J, Mouritsen L, Fuglsang-Frederiksen A. Anal incontinence after obstetric third-/fourth-degree laceration. One-year follow-up after pelvic floor exercises. Int Urogynecol J 1999;10:177–181.

50. Jensen LL, Lowry AC. Biofeedback improves functional outcome after sphincteroplasty. Dis Colon Rectum 1997;40:197–200.

51. Ryn AK, Morren GL, Hallbook O, Sjodahl R. Long–term results of electromyographic biofeedback training for fecal incontinence. Dis Colon Rectum 2000;43:1261–1266.

52. Halverson AL, Hull TL, Paraiso MF, Floruta C. Outcome of sphincteroplasty combined with surgery for urinary incontinence and pelvic organ prolapse. Dis Colon Rectum 2001; 44:1421–1426.

53. Novi JM, Mulvihill BH, Morgan MA. Combined anal sphincteroplasty and perineal reconstruction for fecal incontinence in women. J Am Osteopath Assoc 2009;109:234–236.

54. Kaiser AM. Cloaca-like deformity with faecal incontinence after severe obstetric injury—technique and functional outcome of ano-vaginal and perineal reconstruction with X-flaps and sphincteroplasty. Colorectal Dis 2008; 10:827–832.

55. Hetzer FH, Bieler A, Hahnloser D et al. Outcome and cost analysis of sacral nerve stimulation for faecal incontinence. Br J Surg 2006;93:1411–1417.

56. Tan EK, Jacovides M, Khullar V et al. A cost-effectiveness analysis of delayed sphincteroplasty for anal sphincter injury. Colorectal Dis 2008;10:653–662.

57. Fang DT, Nivatvongs S, Vermeulen FD et al. Overlapping sphincteroplasty for acquired anal incontinence. Dis Colon Rectum 1984;27:720–722.

58. Laurberg S, Swash M, Henry MM. Delayed external sphincter repair for obstetric tear. Br J Surg 1988;75:786–788.

59. Yoshioka K, Keighley MR. Sphincter repair for fecal incontinence. Dis Colon Rectum 1989;32:39–42.

60. Fleshman JW, Dreznik Z, Fry RD, Kodner IJ. Anal sphincter repair for obstetric injury: manometric evaluation of functional results. Dis Colon Rectum 1991; 34:1061–1067.

61. Engel AF, Kamm MA, Sultan AH et al. Anterior anal sphincter repair in patients with obstetric trauma. Br J Surg 1994; 81:1231–1234.

62. Morren GL, Hallbook O, Nystrom PO et al. Audit of anal sphincter repair. Colorectal Dis 2001;3:17–22.

63. Elton C, Stoodley BJ. Anterior anal sphincter repair: results in a district general hospital. Ann R Coll Surg Engl 2002;84:321–324.

64. Pfeifer J. Quality of life after sphincteroplasty. Acta Chir Iugosl 2004;51:73–75.

65. Barisic GI, Krivokapic ZV, Markovic VA, Popovic MA. Outcome of overlapping anal sphincter repair after 3 months and after a mean of 80 months. Int J Colorect Dis 2006;21:52–56.

66. Ternent C, Shashidharan M, Blatchford GL et al. Transanal ultrasound and anorectal physiology findings affecting continency after sphincteroplasty. Dis Colon Rectum 1997; 40:462–467.

67. Karoui S, Leroi AM, Koning E et al. Results of sphincteroplasty in 86 patients with anal incontinence. Dis Colon Rectum 2000;43:813–820.

68. Halverson AL, Hull TL. Long-term outcome of overlapping anal sphincter repair. Dis Colon Rectum 2002;45:345–348.

69. Buie WD, Lowry AC, Rothenberger DA, Madoff RD. Clinical rather than laboratory assessment predicts continence after anterior sphincteroplasty. Dis Colon Rectum 2001;44:1255–1260.

70. Maslekar S, Gardiner AB, Duthie GS. Anterior anal sphincter repair for fecal incontinence: Good longterm results are possible. J Am Coll Surg 2007;204:40–46.

71. Hull TL, Floruta C, Piedmonte M. Preliminary results of an outcome tool used for evaluation of surgical treatment for fecal incontinence. Dis Colon Rectum 2001; 44:799–805.

72. Baxter NN, Rothenberger DA, Lowry AC. Measuring fecal incontinence. Dis Colon Rectum 2003;46:1591–1605.

73. Rothbarth J, Bemelman WA, Meijerink WJHJ et al. What is the impact of fecal incontinence on quality of life? Dis Colon Rectum 2001;44:67–71.

74. Rockwood TH, Church JM, Fleshman JW et al. Fecal Incontinence Quality of Life Scale: quality of life instrument for patients with fecal incontinence. Dis Colon Rectum 2000; 43:9–16.

75. Maunder RG, Cohen Z, McLeod RS, Greenberg GR. Effect of intervention in inflammatory bowel disease on health-related quality of life: a critical review. Dis Colon Rectum 1995;38:1147–1161.

76. Pager CK, Solomon MJ, Rex J, Roberts RA. Long-term outcomes of pelvic floor exercise and biofeedback treatment for patients with fecal incontinence. Dis Colon Rectum 2002;45:997–1003.

77. Pauls RN, Silva WA, Rooney CM et al. Sexual function following anal sphincteroplasty for fecal incontinence. Am J Obstet Gynecol 2007;197:618.e1–6.

78. Trowbridge ER, Morgan D, Trowbridge MJ et al. Sexual function, quality of life, and severity of anal incontinence after anal sphincteroplasty. Am J Obstet Gynecol 2006;195:1753–1757.

79. Browning GG, Parks AG. Postanal repair for neuropathic faecal incontinence: correlation of clinical result and anal canal pressures. Br J Surg 1983;70:101–104.

80. Parks AG. Anorectal incontinence. Proc R Soc Med 1975; 68:681–690.

81. Womack NR, Morrison JF, Williams NS. Prospective study of the effects of postanal repair in neurogenic faecal incontinence. Br J Surg 1988;75:48–52.

82. Miller R, Bartolo DC, Locke-Edmunds JC, Mortensen NJ. Prospective study of conservative and operative treatment for faecal incontinence. Br J Surg 1988; 75:101–105.

83. Braun J, Töns C, Schippers E et al. Results of Parks postanal repair in idiopathic anal insufficiency. Chirurg 1991;62:206–210.

84. Briel JW, Schouten WR. Disappointing results of postanal repair in the treatment of fecal incontinence. Ned Tijdschr Geneeskd 1995;139:23–26.

85. Athanasiadis S, Sanchez M, Kuprian A. Long-term follow-up of Parks posterior repair. An electromyographic, manometric and radiologic study of 31 patients. Langenbecks Arch Chir 1995;380:22–30.

86. Matsuoka H, Mavrantonis C, Wexner SD et al. Postanal repair for fecal incontinence – is it worthwhile? Dis Colon Rectum 2000;43:1561–1567.

87. Yoshioka K, Keighley MR. Critical assessment of the quality of continence after postanal repair for faecal incontinence. Br J Surg 1989;76:1054–1057.

88. Setti-Carraro P, Kamm MA, Nicholls RJ. Long-term results of postanal repair for neurogenic faecal incontinence. Br J Surg 1994;81:140–144.

89. Rieger NA, Sarre RG, Saccone GT et al. Postanal repair for faecal incontinence: long-term follow-up. Aust N Z J Surg 1997;67:566–570.

90. Abbas SM, Bissett IP, Neill ME, Parry BR. Long-term outcome of postanal repair in the treatment of faecal incontinence. A N Z J Surg 2005;75:783–786.

91. Mackey P, Mackey L, Kennedy M et al. Postanal repair–

Do the long-term results justify the procedure? Colorectal Dis 2010;4:367–372.

92. Healy JC, Halligan S, Bartram CI et al. Dynamic magnetic resonance imaging evaluation of the structural and functional results of postanal repair for neuropathic fecal incontinence. Dis Colon Rectum 2002;45:1629–1634.

93. Miller R, Orrom WJ, Cornes H et al. Anterior sphincter plication and levatorplasty in the treatment of faecal incontinence. Br J Surg 1989;76:1058–1060.

94. Orrom WJ, Miller R, Cornes H et al. Comparison of anterior sphincteroplasty and postanal repair in the treatment of idiopathic fecal incontinence. Dis Colon Rectum 1991;34:305–10.

95. van Tets WF, Kuijpers JH. Pelvic floor procedures produce no consistent changes in anatomy or physiology. Dis Colon Rectum 1998;41:365–369.

96. Engel AF, Brummelkamp WH. Secondary surgery after failed postanal or anterior sphincter repair. Int J Colorectal Dis 1994;9:187–190.

Dynamic Gracioplasty

29

Carlo Ratto

Abstract The purpose of dynamic gracioplasty (DG) is to substitute sphincters that are affected by a very wide or multiple lesion or severe functional impairments causing fecal incontinence (FI). DG is based on transposition of the gracilis muscle around the anal canal; moreover, electrical stimulation of the gracilis nerve pedicle is usually added to guarantee the functional "dynamicity" of this correction. The most common clinical indications for DG is FI secondary to congenital malformations, multiple sclerosis, or cauda equina neurinoma, and severe lesion(s) of the external anal sphincter. However, a neuropathic but intact native sphincter, previously treated with DG, is now mostly treated with sacral nerve stimulation. Additonally, DG has been used in total ano-rectal reconstruction following an abdomino-perineal resection. The results of DG have been variable. Continence rates range from 35% to 85%, with the best results being obtained in centers with higher surgical volume. Mortality rates range from 0% to 13%, and morbidity has occurred in more than 50% of patients.

Keywords Congenital malformations • Dynamic gracioplasty • Electrical stimulation • Fecal incontinence • Neuropathic sphincter • Total ano-rectal reconstruction

29.1 Introduction

Fecal incontinence (FI) is a distressing condition [1] with consequent limitation in daily activity due to the social stigma and embarrassment of being incontinent of feces. Incontinence of stool or flatus occurs at least weekly in 2.2% of adults [2], and is higher in women with obstetric-related structural sphincter damage [3, 4], and elderly people [5], possibly due to degeneration of the sphincter mechanism over time [6]. Consequently, patients' quality of life (QoL) is negatively affected; loss of self-esteem, and limitations in traveling or working

C. Ratto
Department of Surgical Sciences, Catholic University, Roma, Italy

and maintaining personal relationships may adversely affect patients and their families, with economic consequences [1].

Numerous treatment modalities are available today, but the correct indications are not yet established. Nonsurgical options (dietary and medical therapies, and biofeedback [4, 7]) can be useful in selected cases with mild FI. Surgical strategies include sacral nerve stimulation (SNS), sphincteroplasty (overlapping sphincter repair), dynamic gracioplasty (DG), artificial anal sphincter implantation (artificial bowel sphincter, ABS) and, as the final option, end colostomy [8, 9]. While SNS is directed to improve functional disorders of continence mechanisms, even severe ones, the aim of sphincteroplasty is to restore external sphincter continuity, and the purpose of DG and ABS is to substitute

G.A. Santoro, A.P. Wieczorek, C.I. Bartram (eds.) *Pelvic Floor Disorders*
© Springer-Verlag Italia 2010

sphincters that are affected by a very wide or multiple lesion or severe functional impairments.

In particular, DG is based on transposition of the gracilis muscle around the anal canal; because encirclement of just the anus with a voluntary muscle is unlikely to be enough to ensure continence to feces in all conditions, electrical stimulation of the gracilis nerve pedicle is usually added to guarantee the functional "dynamicity" of this correction.

29.2 Background

The anatomical characteristics of the gracilis muscle make it ideal for anal encirclement: it is very close to the anal region because the proximal part is attached to the pubic bone, and it is long enough to be transposed around the anal canal. Finally, the vasculonervous pedicle can be preserved because it is very proximal, and this ensures the vitality and function of the muscle. Because this muscle is originally only auxiliary for adduction, flexion, and exorotation in the hip and the knee, its transposition should not cause any disorder of leg functions. However, because the gracilis muscle is mainly composed of fast twitch and forceful muscle fibers but is quickly fatigued (type II fibers), it is not suitable for maintaining continual continence of the anal canal. The additional use of neurostimulation with a gracilis muscle wrap was first reported by Baeten et al [10] in 1988; the purpose of electrical stimulation is to induce the type II muscle fibers of the gracilis muscle to change into type I muscle fibers that resemble those of the internal anal sphincter. The implantable pulse generator lasts seven to eight years [11, 12]. Under electrical stimulation, the transposed gracilis muscle can develop a dynamic function; if the patient feels the urge to defecate, the stimulator can be switched off (using an external remote control carried by the patient), interrupting any stimulus reaching the muscle, and the muscle will relax, making stool passage possible. At the end of defecation, the stimulator can be switched on, and the gracilis will contract. With this technique, continence can be restored.

29.3 Preoperative Assessment

A complete patient history needs to be taken in order to identify both the possible causes of FI and reasons to contraindicate DG (see below). An accurate investigation of FI frequency and characteristics, the modality of normal evacuation, and acquired habits due to FI (wearing a pad, limitations of daily activities) can give an adequate assessment of FI severity. Specific scores (i.e. Cleveland Clinic score, St Mark's incontinence score) can be constructed based on these data. Assessment of the patient's QoL, using specific questionnaires (Fecal Incontinence Quality of Life [FIQL], Short Form-36 [SF-36]), should be considered useful parameters of this functional affliction. Thereafter, physical examination will evaluate the sphincter function during rest, squeeze, and strain. The sensitivity of the anal region should be evaluated for touch, pain, or temperature, or with electrical stimuli in the anus. Rectal sensitivity can be tested with an inflatable balloon. This assessment is worthwhile to select patients with altered sensation who would not be able to empty the bowel even after the DG procedure.

The structure of sphincters can be imaged with endoanal sonography or magnetic resonance to identify lesions and determine the extent of the defect or possible absence of the external sphincter. Sphincter function can be evaluated with anal manometry, in particular resting and squeeze pressures. The innervation of the sphincters can be assessed with electromyography (EMG) and a pudendal nerve terminal motor latency (PNTML) test. Defecography can exclude concomitant dysfunctions (rectal prolapse, rectocele, enterocele, intussusception).

29.4 Indications

The best indications for DG include an absent native sphincter, or a severely defective native sphincter that cannot be repaired. The most common clinical conditions causing such severe FI are congenital malformations (anal atresia and spina bifida), multiple sclerosis, or cauda equina neurinoma, and trauma of the external anal sphincter (very often due to iatrogenic injury – surgical or obstetrical).

Prior to the introduction of SNS, a neuropathic but intact native sphincter was also considered a main indication for this operation; but now this condition is mostly treated with SNS. Additonally, DG has been used in total ano-rectal reconstruction following an abdomino-perineal resection.

However, this approach seems contraindicated in

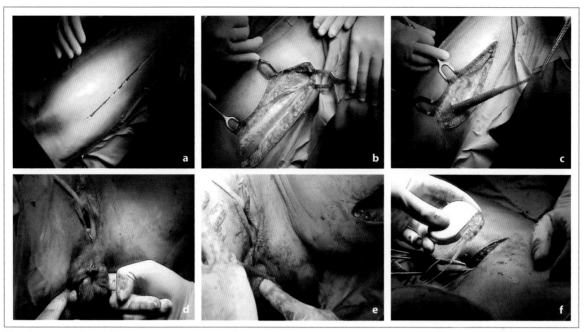

Fig. 29.1 Dynamic graciloplasty: **a**) skin incision; **b**) gracilis muscle is exposed and **c**) isolated; **d**) perianal tunnel is prepared; **e**) gracilis muscle has been transposed in perianal space and a "gamma" loop is repared; **f**) the electrostimulator (connected to the electrodes implanted close to the nerve pedicle of the gracilis muscle) is placed in a subfascial pocket at level of rectum abdominis muscle

cases of inflammatory bowel disease, physical or mental incapacity or poor motivation, pelvic or perineal sepsis, chronic diarrhea, pregnancy, or receptive anal intercourse.

29.5   Technique

One or two incisions are made in the upper thigh, and the gracilis muscle is identified (Fig. 29.1a,b). This is mobilized towards its insertion into the medial aspect of the tibia, ligating the peripheral vessels but preserving its proximal neurovascular bundle. Next (Fig. 29.1c), the distal tendon is cut (a small incision below the knee can be used). Two incisions are made on the right and left lateral sides to the anus, and, from these, a circumferential tunnel is created around the anal canal structures (Fig. 29.1d); another tunnel is made from one of the perianal incisions to that in the leg, passing the strong Scarpa's fascia. Thereafter, the gracilis is wrapped around the anal canal (Fig. 29.1e), usually according to one of three configurations based on the anatomical situation: a gamma loop (the most used), an epsilon loop, or an alpha loop (Fig. 29.2). The modified alpha or split-sling loop was developed to make a perfect circular loop, with a hole in the mid-part of the

muscle, where the distal part is pulled through. Finally, the distal tendon is sutured to the ischial spine, or (less frequently) to the skin. In selected cases, a protective colostomy is chosen.

The electrodes and the electrostimulator can be placed during the same operation or 4–6 weeks after the transposition. The first electrode needs to be distal to the nerve entrance (about 4 cm). The position of the cathode is determined under electrical stimulation, as close as possible to the intramuscular branches of the nerve (Fig. 29.3). Both the electrodes are pulled through the muscle, perpendicularly to the muscle fibers, and anchored to the epimysium. Thereafter, they are tunneled subcutaneously to reach a pocket made in the lower abdominal wall, under the rectus abdominis fascia, and connected to an electrostimulator (Fig. 29.1f).

After the operation, patients are encouraged to start walking the next day and to wear elastic stockings for 4–6 weeks. The electrostimulator is switched on 3–7 days after the operation for the "training period", using a pulse width of 210 μs, and programming the stimulator to a low frequency of 2.1 Hz for 2 weeks, increased to 5.2 Hz for 2 weeks more, and then increased to 10 Hz for another 2 weeks; finally, the stimulator is programmed to 15 Hz. The "training period" is completed

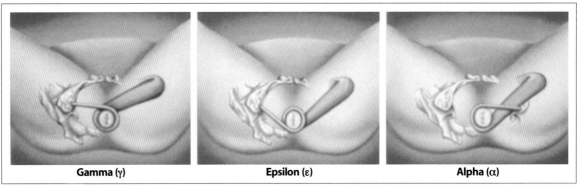

| Gamma (γ) | Epsilon (ε) | Alpha (α) |

Fig. 29.2 Scheme of dynamic graciloplasty: three different modalities to transpose the gracilis muscle around the anal canal

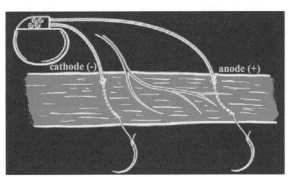

Fig. 29.3 Scheme of position of electrodes for electrostimulation in dynamic graciloplasty

and the stimulator can be switched off only for defecation. When the battery life ends, the stimulator must be replaced under local anesthesia.

29.6 Results

The results of dynamic graciloplasty have been variable. Continence rates range from 35% to 85% [13–31]. The best results have been obtained in centers with higher surgical volume. Mortality rates range from 0% to 13%, and morbidity has occurred in more than 50% of patients [32, 33]. Most patients develop complications from the procedure, and a few suffer from multiple complications. The most common morbidity is infection [33]. Infections can be minor (skin infections or infections around the anus), and amenable to antibiotic treatment. However, more severe infections can involve the implanted device and make explantation necessary. Constipation can be due to a too-tight encirclement around the anus (in about 15% of cases); the use of laxatives or enemas is often necessary; obstructed defecation is responsible for half of the conversions to

colostomy. Insufficient contraction of the gracilis can be due to electrical or muscular problems. Other complications include problems with the stimulator and leads, and pain, swelling, and parasthesia in the donor leg. Because this procedure has a high mortality and morbidity rate, dynamic graciloplasty is unlikely to have a wide application. Practice in experienced or well-trained centers should be recommended.

Patients with incontinence based on muscular deficiencies will have the greatest benefit – up to complete continence; maintained sensory function of the rectal ampulla and the pelvic floor is essential for a good result. On the other hand, patients with congenital malformations tend to have a worse outcome than those with acquired ano-rectal dysfunction [16, 20, 33]. With the advent of other newer treatment modalities, such as SNS, patients with extensive sphincter loss or congenital ano-rectal abnormalities are the only groups suitable for DG.

Evaluation of DG outcome, in terms of clinical improvement of FI and patients' QoL after this operation, is still debatable. It seems clear that functional outcome is strictly correlated with QoL scores. Moreover, the final results are conditioned by the adverse events related to development of postoperative complications. Patient mental health and physical limitations are factors that negatively affect the outcome.

References

1. Damon H, Guye O, Seigneurin A et al. Prevalence of anal incontinence in adults and impact on quality-of-life. Gastroenterol Clin Biol 2006;30:37–43.
2. Nelson R, Norton N, Cautley E, Furner S. Community based prevalence of anal incontinence. JAMA 1995; 274:559–561.
3. Mellgren A, Jensen LL, Zetterstrom JP et al. Long-term cost

of fecal incontinence secondary to obstetric injuries. Dis Colon Rectum 1999;42:857–865; discussion 865–867.

4. Kamm MA. Diagnostic, pharmacological, surgical and behavioural developments in benign anorectal disease. Eur J Surg Suppl 1998;582:119–123.

5. Campbell AJ, Reinken J, McCosh L. Incontinence in the elderly: prevalence and prognosis. Age Ageing 1985;14:65–70.

6. Laurberg S, Swash M. Effects of aging on the anorectal sphincters and their innervation. Dis Colon Rectum 1989;32:737–742.

7. Parker SC, Thorsen A. Fecal incontinence. Surg Clin North Am 2002;82:1273–1290.

8. Vaizey CJ, Kamm MA, Nicholls RJ. Recent advances in the surgical treatment of faecal incontinence. Br J Surg 1998; 85:596–603.

9. Madoff RD. Surgical treatment options for fecal incontinence. Gastroenterology 2004;1(suppl 1):S48–54.

10. Bacten C, Spaans F, Fluks A. An implanted neuromuscular stimulator for fecal continence following previously implanted gracilis muscle: report of a case. Dis Colon Rectum 1988; 31:134–137.

11. Madoff RD, Parker SC, Varma MG, Lowry AC. Faecal incontinence in adults. Lancet 2004;364:621–632.

12. Chapman AE, Geerdes B, Hewett P et al. Systematic review of dynamic gracioloplasty in the treatment of faecal incontinence. Br J Surg 2002;89:138–153.

13. Ho KS, Seow-Choen F. Dynamic gracioloplasty for total anorectal reconstruction after abdominoperineal resection for rectal tumour. Int J Colorectal Dis 2005;20:38–41.

14. Rosen HR, Urbarz C, Novi G et al. Long-term results of modified gracioloplasty for sphincter replacement after rectal excision. Colorectal Dis 2002;4:266–269.

15. Baeten CG, Geerdes BP, Adang EM et al. Anal dynamic gracioloplasty in the treatment of intractable fecal incontinence. N Engl J Med 1995;332:1600–1605.

16. Baeten CG, Bailey HR, Bakka A et al. Safety and efficacy of dynamic gracioloplasty for fecal incontinence: report of a prospective, multicenter trial. Dynamic gracioloplasty therapy study group. Dis Colon Rectum 2000;43:743–751.

17. Bresler L, Reibel N, Brunard L et al. Dynamic gracioloplasty in the treatment of severe fecal incontinence. French multicentric retrospective study. Ann Chir 2002;127:520–526.

18. Cavina E, Seccia M, Banti P, Zocco G. Anorectal reconstruction after abdominoperineal resection. Experience with double-wrap gracioloplasty supported by low-frequency electrostimulation. Dis Colon Rectum 1998;41:1010–1016.

19. Geerdes BP, Zoetmulder FA, Heineman E et al. Total anorectal reconstruction with a double dynamic gracioloplasty

after abdominoperineal reconstruction for low rectal cancer. Dis Colon Rectum 1997;40:698–705.

20. Koch SM, Uluda O, Rongen M et al. Dynamic gracioloplasty in patients born with an anorectal malformation. Dis Colon Rectum 2004;47:1711–1719.

21. Mander BJ, Abercrombie JF, George BD, Williams NS. The electrically stimulated gracilis neosphincter incorporated as part of total anorectal reconstruction after abdominoperineal excision of the rectum. Ann Surg 1996; 224:702–711.

22. Mander BJ, Wexner SD, Williams NS et al. Preliminary results of a multicenter trial of the electrically stimulated gracilis neoanal sphincter. Br J Surg 1999;86:543–1548.

23. Penninckx F. Belgian experience with dynamic gracioloplasty for faecal incontinence. Br J Surg 2004;91:872–878.

24. Rongen MJ, Uludag O, Naggar KEL et al. Long-term follow-up of dynamic gracioloplasty for fecal incontinence. Dis Colon Rectum 2003;46:716–721.

25. Rouanet P, Senesse P, Bouamrirene D et al. Anal sphincter reconstruction by dynamic gracioloplasty after abdominoperineal resection for cancer. Dis Colon Rectum 1999; 42:451–456.

26. Rullier E, Zerbib F, Laurent C et al. Morbidity and functional outcome after double dynamic gracioloplasty for anorectal reconstruction. Br J Surg 2000;87:909–913.

27. Thornton MJ, Kennedy ML, Lubowski DZ, King DW. Long-term follow-up of dynamic gracioloplasty for faecal incontinence. Colorectal Dis 2004;6:470–476.

28. Wexner SD, Baeten C, Bailey R et al. Long-term efficacy of dynamic gracioloplasty for fecal incontinence. Dis Colon Rectum 2002;45:809–818.

29. Williams NS, Patel J, George BD et al. Development of an electrically stimulated neoanal sphincter. Lancet 1991; 338:1166–1169.

30. Edden Y, Wexner SD. Therapeutic devices for fecal incontinence: dynamic gracioloplasty, artificial bowel sphincter and sacral nerve stimulation. Expert Rev Med Devices 2009; 6:307–312.

31. Tan EK, Vaizey C, Cornish J et al. Surgical strategies for faecal incontinence--a decision analysis between dynamic gracioloplasty, artificial bowel sphincter and end stoma. Colorectal Dis 2008;10:577–586.

32. Muller C, Belyaev O, Deska T et al. Fecal incontinence: an up-to-date critical overview of surgical treatment options. Langenbecks Arch Surg 2005;390:544–552.

33. Chapman AE, Geerdes B, Hewett P et al. Systematic review of dynamic gracioloplasty in the treatment of faecal incontinence. Br J Surg 2002;89:138–153.

Radiofrequency Energy and Injectable Biomaterials

30

Mario Trompetto and Maurizio Roveroni

Abstract The use of radiofrequency and injection of different types of biomaterials for the treatment of fecal incontinence have gained attention from coloproctologists because of their safety and feasibility. The initial functional results of these treatments have been encouraging, although more recently their effectiveness in the long term has been questioned. The possibility of performing the treatment as a day case operation is a great advantage both for surgeons and patients.

Keywords Bulking agents • Fecal incontinence • Secca procedure

30.1 Introduction

Fecal incontinence is a debilitating disorder and its treatment is a very demanding problem for all those interested in its solution, particularly colorectal surgeons. Surgical options are considered when conservative treatments have failed, and must be tailored to the specific cause of the incontinence.

Long-term results of sphincteroplasty are often unsatisfactory, while more demanding operations such as graciloplasty and the use of an artificial bowel sphincter are plagued by an unacceptable percentage of complications and negative side-effects. The only treatment that seems promising in long-term functional results is sacral nerve modulation, but the problem of selecting the right patients for its use has not yet been resolved.

For all these reasons, in the last 5–10 years the attention of coloproctologists has moved to some new less invasive treatments that seem to combine safety

and feasibility to give acceptable functional results in the short and medium term.

These options can be a good alternative in cases of minor fecal incontinence, when a sphincter defect is minimal or absent, or when previous surgery to treat the functional disorder has failed. A further good option for these minimally invasive treatments can be a keyhole deformity of the anal canal after previous anal surgery.

These new treatments have been gaining popularity in recent years, particularly the local injection of bulking agents and the use of radiofrequency energy.

30.2 Radiofrequency Energy Delivery (Secca® Procedure)

This procedure has been used for many years for several non-colorectal disorders, particularly in the field of gastroesophageal reflux disease, but also in orthopedics (laxity of the joint capsule) and urology (benign prostatic hyperplasia).

The heat released by the radiofrequency energy can generate an anatomically advantageous modification of the anal canal. The result of the treatment is a

M. Trompetto
Colorectal Eporediensis Centre, "Santa Rita" Clinic, Vercelli,
Policlinic of Monza, Italy

G.A. Santoro, A.P. Wieczorek, C.I. Bartram (eds.) *Pelvic Floor Disorders*
© Springer-Verlag Italia 2010

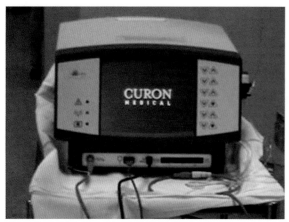

Fig. 30.1 Secca® device

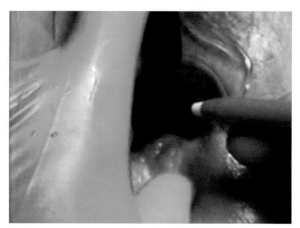

Fig. 30.2 Secca® procedure

very rapid contraction of the collagenous tissue of the anal canal followed by wound healing. The consequent tightening of the anal canal seems to give satisfactory functional results.

The Secca® device comprises an anoscopic barrel with four nickel-titanium curved needle electrodes (22 gauge, 6 mm in length; Curon Medical, USA) (Fig. 30.1). Thermocouples are present at the base and within the tip of each needle to monitor tissue and mucosal temperature at any time during radiofrequency delivery. On deployment, there is a reduction in electrical impedance, indicating proper contact of the electrode with the submucosal layer.

30.2.1 Technique

The treatment can be easily and safely performed as an outpatient procedure. Antibiotic prophylaxis (ciprofloxacin

and metronidazole) is advisable, although there is no need for bowel preparation. Patients can be positioned in the classic jack-knife or gynecologic position, depending on the preference of the surgeon, and local anesthesia is administered.

After a digital examination and anoscopy, the device is positioned under direct visualization of the anal canal. Penetration of the needles starts 1 cm below the dentate line.

When the needles are correctly placed in the tissue, the generator delivers radiofrequency energy to the needles for 90 s at a preselected temperature of 85°C (Fig. 30.2). Continuous delivery of cooling water (45°C) to the base of each needle avoids possible thermal lesion of the mucosa.

A series of three or four similar procedures is performed proximally up to 15 mm from the dentate line, for a total of 16–20 lesion sets (Fig. 30.3).

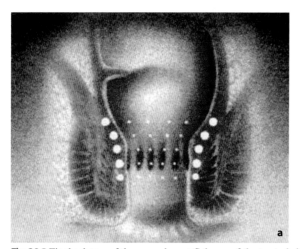

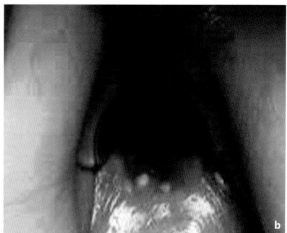

Fig. 30.3 Final scheme of the procedure. **a** Scheme of the treated sites. **b** Thermal lesions

30.2.2 Results

To date, few papers have been published about the safety and feasibility of the technique [1–3]. While some studies have confirmed good short-term functional results, some more controversial papers have been published very recently. Felts-Berma et al [4] treated 11 patients; in six there was an improvement in fecal incontinence with a change in Vaizey score from 18.3 to 11.5 (P = 0.03) but without any modification of the parameters of anal manometry and rectal compliance. Takahashi-Monroy et al [5] found a significant and sustained improvement in fecal incontinence symptoms and quality of life in 19 patients treated and followed for up to 5 years. A prospective study by Lefebure et al [6] confirmed the safety of the procedure but failed to demonstrate a significant functional result because most of the 15 treated patients remained in the moderate incontinence category and their quality of life did not improve. Kim et al [7] did not find any advantages in the treatment of eight patients with the Secca procedure, which was also associated with considerable complications such as anoderm ulcerations, anal bleeding, anal pain, and anal mucosal discharge.

Failure of the procedure does not preclude any other more invasive treatments, although if there is scarring of the anal canal, which is probably the main factor involved in improvement of continence, this can make any subsequent procedure more demanding from a technical point of view.

30.3 Injectable Biomaterials

Urologists have obtained good results in enhancing the function of the vesical neck using local injections of autologous fat, collagen, and polytetrafluoroethylene. However, it has not been possible for coloproctologists to achieve similar functional results using the same materials to treat patients complaining of fecal incontinence.

Recently, new types of bulking agents, as calcium hydroxylapatite, silicone-based biomaterials, and carbon-coated microbeads, have been used for the treatment of fecal incontinence with encouraging results. To date no significant differences in functional results have been found when comparing these materials with each other or with other new bulking agents [8].

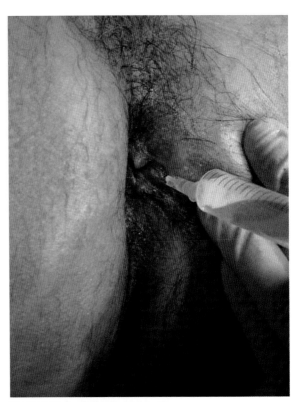

Fig. 30.4 Perianal anesthetic injection

30.3.1 Technique

The treatment can be performed as an outpatient case using ordinary local anesthesia (Fig. 30.4); antibiotic prophylaxis (ciprofloxacine and metronidazole) is mandatory. Injection of the bulking agent must be done by inserting the needle into the skin at 2.5 cm from the anal margin and pushing it forward to reach the intersphincteric space, which is checked by a finger placed in the anal canal. The injection must be slow, allowing visible formation of a small, elastic ball in the anal canal (Fig. 30.5). Three or four injections in different parts of the anal circumference are needed to tighten the anal canal. The number of injections and the volume of the injected bulking agent can vary from case to case, depending on the size and location of the sphincter defect or generalized sphincteric dysfunction.

30.3.2 Results

The results of the first published papers were very satisfactory with a subjective improvement in almost all patients in a short time period [9–12], although Maeda

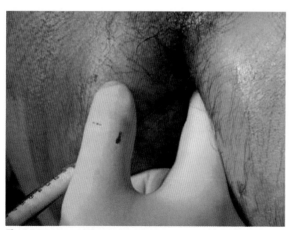

Fig. 30.5 Intersphincteric injection under assessment by a finger inserted in the anal canal

et al [13] reported unsatisfactory results in six patients treated with silicone biomaterial (PTQ™; Uroplasty BV, Geleen, The Netherlands) followed up at 61 months.

Altomare et al [14] found an increase in anal pressure but no improvement in the quality of life of 33 unselected patients who underwent anal submucosal injections with carbon-coated microbeads (Durasphere®, Carbon Medical Technologies, St Paul, MN, USA).

We treated a group of ten patients using calcium hydroxylapatite ceramic microsphere. They were assessed at 3, 6, and 12 months, and results showed a marked improvement in 80%, with a significant reduction in Fecal Incontinence Scoring System (FISS) score from 85.6 ± 9.4 to 28.0 ± 29.0 (P = 0,008) at 12 months [15].

A systematic review on the use of injectable bulking agents for fecal incontinence by Luo et al [16] confirmed their safety but failed to demonstrate clear evidence for their effectiveness in managing passive fecal incontinence.

References

1. Takahashi T, Garcia-Osogobio S, Valdovinos MA et al. Radio-frequency energy delivery to the anal canal for the treatment of fecal incontinence. Dis Colon Rectum 2002; 45:915–922.

2. Efron JE, Corman MI, Fleshman J et al. Safety and effectiveness of temperature-controlled radio-frequency energy delivery to the anal canal (the SECCA procedure) for the treatment of fecal incontinence. Dis Colon Rectum 2003; 43:1606–1618.

3. Takahashi T, Garcia-Osogobio S, Valdovinos MA et al. Extended two-years results of radio-frequency energy delivery for the treatment of fecal incontinence. Dis Colon Rectum 2003;46:711–715.

4. Felt-Bersma RJ, Szojda MM, Mulder CJ. Temperature-controlled radiofrequency energy (SECCA) to the anal canal for the treatment of faecal incontinence offers moderate improvement. Eur J Gastroenterol Hepatol 2007;19:575–580.

5. Takahashi-Monroy T, Morales M, Garcia-Osogobio S et al. SECCA procedure for the treatment of fecal incontinence: results of five-year follow-up. Dis Colon Rectum 2008; 51:355–359.

6. Lefebure B, Tuech JJ, Bridoux V et al. Temperature-controlled radio frequency energy delivery (SECCA procedure) for the treatment of fecal incontinence: results of a prospective study. Int J Colorect 2008;23:993–997.

7. Kim DW, Yoon HM, Park JS. Radiofrequency energy delivery to the anal canal: is it a promising new approach to the treatment of fecal incontinence? Am J Surg 2009;197:14–18.

8. Maeda Y, Vaizey CJ, Kamm MA. Pilot study of two new injectable bulking agents for the treatment of fecal incontinence. Colorectal Dis 2008;10:268–272.

9. Malouf AJ, Vaizey CJ, Norton CS, Kamm MA. Internal anal sphincter augmentation for fecal incontinence using injectable silicone biomaterial. Dis Colon Rectum 2001;44:595–600.

10. Kenefick NJ, Vaizey CJ, Malouf Aj et al. Injectable silicone biomaterial for fecal incontinence due to anal sphincter dysfunction. Gut 2002;51:225–228.

11. Davis K, Kumar D, Poloniecki J. Preliminary evaluation of a injectable anal sphincter bulking agent (Durasphere) in the management of fecal incontinence. Aliment Pharmacol Ther 2003;18:237–243.

12. Tjandra JJ, Lim JF, Hiscock R, Rajendra P. Injectable silicone biomaterial for fecal incontinence caused by internal anal sphincter dysfunction is effective. Dis Colon Rectum 2004;47:2138–2146.

13. Maeda Y, Vaizey CJ, Kamm MA. Long-term results of perianal silicone injection for fecal incontinence. Colorectal Dis 2007;9:357–361.

14. Altomare DF, La Torre F, Rinaldi M et al. Carbon-coated microbeads anal injection in outpatient treatment of minor fecal incontinence. Dis Colon Rectum 2008;51:432–435.

15. Ganio E, Marino F, Trompetto M et al. Injectable synthetic calcium hydroxylapatite ceramic microspheres (Coaptite) for passive fecal incontinence. Tech Coloproctol 2008; 12:99–102.

16. Luo C, Samaranayake CB, Plank LD, Bisset JP. Systematic review on the efficacy and safety of injectable bulking agents for passive fecal incontinence. Colorectal Dis; 2009;6 March epub ahead of print.

Artificial Bowel Sphincter

31

Giovanni Romano, Francesco Bianco and Luisa Caggiano

Abstract Fecal incontinence is a socially devastating problem. The treatment algorithm depends on the etiology of the disease. Large anal sphincter defects can be treated by sphincter replacement procedures: the dynamic graciloplasty and the artificial bowel sphincter (ABS). The best indications for the ABS are lesions of the anal sphincters that are inaccessible to local repair and not responsive to sacral nerve stimulation test or not indicated for such a test. A recent article that published experiences with the ABS showed that this technique had a high rate of morbidity, surgical reinterventions, and explants. Complications leading to explantation included perioperative infections, failure of wound healing, erosion of part of the device throughout the skin or the anal canal, late infection, and mechanical malfunction of the device due to cuff or balloon rupture. The ABS is suitable for well-motivated, selected patients with fecal incontinence of more than one year's duration and whose condition is affected by an important personal, familial, and/or social disability.

Keywords Anal sphincter • Artificial bowel sphincter • Fecal incontinence

31.1 Introduction

Fecal incontinence (FI) is a distressing condition. The social stigma and embarrassment of being incontinent of feces can lead people to severely limit their activity. Incontinence of stool or flatus occurs at least weekly in 2.2% of adults [1]. This rate may be higher in women, especially in those with obstetric-related structural sphincter damage. With increasing age, the prevalence of FI also rises, which may reflect degenerative changes of the sphincter mechanism over time. The consequences of FI on patients' quality of life (QoL)

may be substantial. Loss of self-esteem, difficulty traveling or maintaining employment, and strain on personal relationships may adversely affect patients and their families, with economic consequences borne by the individual and state.

The treatment of severe FI is surgery (Fig. 31.1). The surgical options include sacral nerve stimulation (SNS), overlapping sphincter repair (sphincteroplasty), dynamic graciloplasty (DG), artificial bowel sphincter (ABS), and, failing that, end colostomy [1].

The best indications for the ABS are lesions of the anal sphincters that are inaccessible to local repair and not responsive to SNS test or not indicated for such a test.

The ABS is suitable for well-motivated, selected patients with FI of more than a year's duration and whose condition is regarded as an important personal, familial, and/or social disability.

F. Bianco
Division of Colon and Rectal Surgery,
Department of Oncologic Surgery,
National Cancer Institute "G. Pascale", Napoli, Italy

G.A. Santoro, A.P. Wieczorek, C.I. Bartram (eds.) *Pelvic Floor Disorders*
© Springer-Verlag Italia 2010

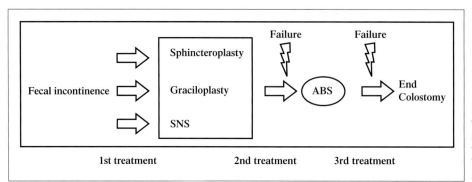

Fig. 31.1 Surgical treatment in severe fecal incontinence: decision tree. *ABS*, artificial bowel sphincter; *SNS*, sacral nerve stimulation

31.2 Artificial Bowel Sphincter

The current device used for FI consists of three silastic components: the occlusive cuff in different models with respect to length (8–14 cm) and height (2.0 cm or 2.9 cm), a control pump with a septum and a pressure-regulating balloon with avalaible pressures that range from 80 cmH$_2$O to 120 cmH$_2$O in 10 cm gradations.

The occlusive cuff is implanted around the anus and is connected by silastic tubing to the control pump placed in the scrotum of males or in the major labium of females. The control pump is also connected to the pressure-regulating balloon implanted in the space of Retzius. When activated, the cuff is distended and the anus is occluded. The pressure-regulating balloon maintains the cuff pressure. To defecate, the patient compresses the control pump several times, and the fluid is displaced out of the cuff and into the regulating balloon (Fig. 31.2). The

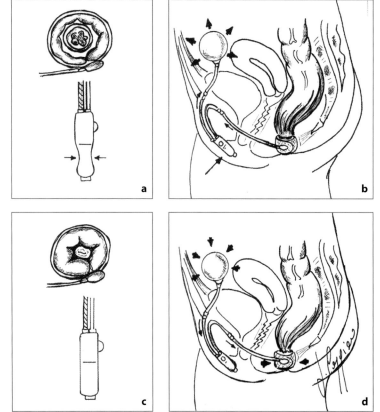

Fig. 31.2 a, b Anal opening: manipulation of the control pump transfers the fluid from the cuff to the balloon. **c, d** Progressive anal closure: after defecation the fluid is moved from the balloon to the cuff

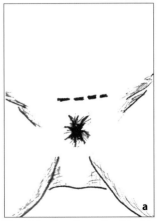
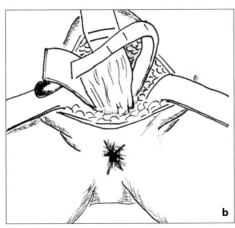
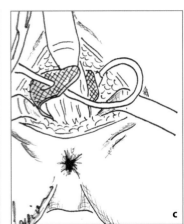

Fig. 31.3 a Anterior perianal incision. **b** Sizer use. **c** Position of the cuff

artificial sphincter is placed with the patient under general anesthesia in the lithotomy position after having undergone a mechanical and antibiotic bowel preparation and rectal irrigation with betadine solution. Either through an anterior perianal incision or bilateral perianal incisions, blunt dissection is used to create a circumferential tunnel around the anal

canal (Fig. 31.3) several centimeters deep in the ischiorectal fossa. The occlusive cuff is appropriately sized and placed with the connection tubing on the same side as the patient's dominant hand. A suprapubic incision is made and the pressure-regulating balloon placed in the space of Retzius (Fig. 31.4).

Blunt dissection creates a dependent pouch in the

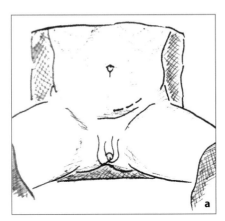
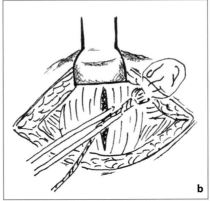
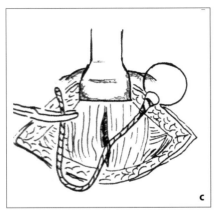
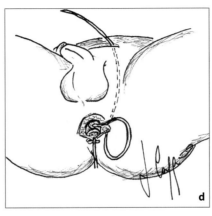

Fig. 31.4 a Suprapubic incision. **b, c** Placement of regulating balloon. **d** Connection tubing

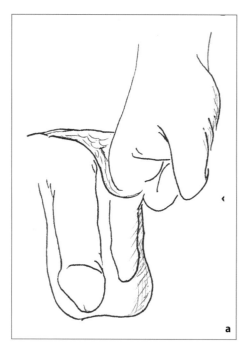 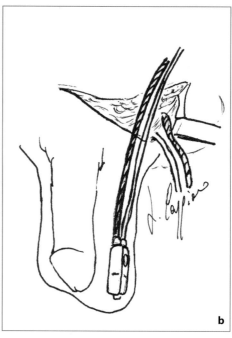

Fig. 31.5 a The pouch in the scrotum. **b** The control pump is placed

scrotum or labia, into which the control pump is placed (Fig. 31.5). The tubings are connected but the device is left deactivated for the first 6–8 weeks postoperatively.

Two months of deactivation are desirable after implantation to ensure tissue integration of the device. The system can then be activated simply by firmly squeezing the pump, a procedure that does not require anesthesia and that can be performed during an office visit. Deactivation of the cuff in the open position is also necessary for transanal endoscopic procedures in order to avoid any tearing or damage to the cuff during passage of the endoscope.

Postoperative clinical evaluation checks the proper positioning of the control pump and its accessibility, the efficacy of anal closure by digital rectal examination, and the quality of anal opening after manipulation of the pump by the patient. It is important during the first postoperative months to detect any migration of the cuff. If it is too close to the anal margin, there is risk of skin damage and erosion, leading to contamination of the material and explantation. Postimplantation monitoring is also possible with x-rays (in the ABS there is a radio-opaque fluid), endoanal ultrasonography, and anal manometry for determination of three manometric parameters (basal pressure with closed ABS, basal pressure with opened ABS, and time required for the ABS to close again after being opened).

31.3 Results

Analysis of recent studies on the ABS demonstrated that this technique has a high rate of morbidity, surgical reinterventions, and explants. Complications leading to explantation included perioperative infection, failure of wound healing, erosion of part of the device throughout the skin or the anal canal, late infection, and mechanical malfunction of the device due to cuff or balloon rupture. An Italian multicenter retrospective analysis [2] showed the outcome of artificial anal sphincter implantation for severe FI in 28 patients. Early infections occurred in four patients, requiring removal of the device in three. Dehiscence of the perineal wound occurred in nine patients. After activation of the device, the cuff had to be removed in further four patients (for rectal erosion in two, anal pain in one, and late infection in one). The cuff was accidentally broken in one patient. A new anal cuff was successfully repositioned in two patients. Overall, five patients had complete removal of the device and two had removal of the cuff only. Twenty-one patients available for long-term evaluation had a major improvement in fecal continence. The median American Medical System incontinence score decreased significantly from 98.5 to 5.5 (P < 0.001). Similar figures were observed using the Continence Grading Scale (from 14.9 to 2.6; P < 0.001). Twelve patients developed symptoms of obstructed defecation, while two complained of anal pain.

Results from a multicenter cohort study conducted under US Food and Drug Administration supervision showed an 85% functional success rate in patients who retained their ABS. Out of 112 patients included in the trial, 51 (46%) required revision operation because of infection, and 41 (37%) required complete explantation [3–7]. Accordingly, the overall success rate was 53%, but for most included centers, this was their first experience with the device. Parker et al [4–7] reported data from the University of Minnesota, one of the leader groups in the use of the ABS. They identified two patient groups: those who received implants between 1989 and 1992 (n = 10; mean follow-up, 91 months) and those who received implants between 1995 and 2001 (n = 37; mean follow-up, 39 months). The overall success rate in the former group was 60% (4/10 explants). The latter group had an overall success rate of 49%, with revision and infection rates of 37% and 34%, respectively. Those patients who had a successful implant achieved a 100% functional success rate at two years.

In 2008, Melenhorst et al published a prospective single-center study [5]. This study included 34 patients (25 female and 9 male) with persisting or recurrent end-stage FI, who were observed between 1997 and 2006. The majority of patients had large (> 33% of circumference) anal sphincter defects. One patient had a rectum perforation during the initial surgery, and placement of the ABS was abandoned. She awaits a second implant attempt. Thirty-three patients were implanted. Thirteen patients (39%) complained of a rectal evacuation problem, and in 12 patients, this could be managed conservatively. One patient had a revision of the system with placement of a wider anal cuff. Seven patients (21.2%) had an infection of the system, which led to seven explantations. One of these patients was successfully implanted with a new ABS. In one patient, the ABS was successfully converted to a dynamic graciloplasty. In two patients, a colostomy was performed. The other three patients had no other interventions. One patient was explanted due to persisting perianal pain without an infection. She received a colostomy. Twenty-six reinterventions (including explantations) had to be performed.

Carmona et al reported their experience with 17 consecutive patients (14 female, 3 male; median age 46) who underwent sphincter implantation between 1996 and 2002 [6]. Clinical evaluation, incontinence severity, and quality of life were assessed. Anorectal manometry, endoanal ultrasound, and pudendal nerve latency were performed preoperatively and at several stages of follow-up. The study was completed in December 2007 and the mean follow-up was 68 months (range 3–133 months). Morbidity occurred in 100% of patients, of whom 65% required at least one reoperation. After the first implant, 11 devices had to be removed (65%) and seven patients had a new implant. Finally, the ABS was activated in nine cases (53%). Fecal continence improved from a median of 17.5 (Wexner score) preoperatively to 9 (P = 0.005), 5.5 (P = 0.005) and 10 (P = 0.092) at 6 months, 12 months, and at the end of follow-up, respectively. There was a significant improvement in quality of life in all postoperative controls (P < 0.05). Severity of the FI did not show a correlation with the quality of life in the preoperative period but did at 6 months, 12 months, and at the end of follow-up.

Early results of ABS use showed that this technique was feasible, with 75% of patients retaining a functioning device after a mean of 20–58 months [6]. The high explantation rate and the frequency of adverse events decreased with appropriate surgical and perioperative management after an initial learning curve for the surgical team. Evaluation of the effectiveness of the technique was based on significant improvement in continence and quality of life in patients who retained a functioning device. However, in some patients, FI remains or is only partially improved by ABS. Outlet-type constipation and/or colonic slow-transit constipation are frequent after ABS and may interfere with the functional outcome of the device. Michot et al evaluated the functional outcome of ABS based on post-implant constipation, with or without obstructed defecation (OD), and assessed pre-implantation data to help predict post-implantation constipation in a cohort of 44 implanted patients.

From 1996 to 2005, 44 patients (31 women and 13 men; mean age, 50 ± 14 years) were implanted for severe FI. Before implantation of the ABS, a rectal prolapse was treated with rectopexy in four patients, and a Delorme procedure in one patient, while one patient underwent a Sullivan procedure for rectocele. In two cases, a rectopexy was performed after implantation of the ABS. During follow-up, nine patients (20.4%) had constipation with no OD, and 16 patients (36.4%) had constipation with OD. The remaining 19 patients

(43.2%) were not constipated. Eighteen of the 25 patients (72%) with postoperative constipation were still incontinent at the end of follow-up, but only four patients out of 19 (21%) without postoperative constipation (P = 0.003) were incontinent. Although osmotic laxatives improved constipation in patients with post-implant constipation without OD, liquid stools induced by laxatives worsen the continence. In patients with post-implant OD, chronic rectal fecal impaction resulted in an overflow pseudo-incontinence. Daily rectal enemas were effective in emptying the rectal ampulla and preventing incontinence in these patients, but the compliance to treatment was very poor, resulting in eight colostomies and one Malone procedure in this group. In the group of patients with no post-implant constipation, anal incontinence was explained in four cases by diarrhea (21%). In two cases (10.5%), the patients had had diarrhea that could not be managed by medical treatment before surgery. In the two other cases (10.5%), patients experienced leakage during intermittent diarrhea episodes, which severely affected their quality of life. Although the duration of follow-up was shorter in patients with OD, a revision of the ABS was more frequently necessary in this group than in the others (P = 0.04). However, despite the replacement of all or part of the ABS, evacuation difficulties persisted in six patients [8].

In cases of incontinence resulting from sequelae of anal agenesis, there is a lower chance of success. The lack of anal sensitivity and a rectal reservoir, and the existence of associated colonic motor disorders make all the techniques of sphincteric substitution more uncertain.

Indications for use of the ABS are broadening and have reached the complex field of anorectal reconstruction following abdominoperineal excision. Between 1999 and 2003 we carried out a total anorectal reconstruction in 12 patients (1 male and 11 female, mean age 54 years) previously operated on with an abdominal perineal resection by performing a perineal colostomy and placing an artificial bowel sphincter around the perineal stoma. Ten patients had been operated on for rectal cancer (T1–T2, N0, M0), one had had a colostomy in childhood for rectal agenesia, and one patient had been treated with a Miles operation 10 years before for a giant benign tumor (leiomyoma) of the pelvis. None of the patients operated on for rectal cancer developed local or distant recurrences. Three patients had the cuff explanted for skin erosion, and in one patient the device was totally removed as a consequence of the radiotherapy. The patient with total anal resection for rectal agenesia developed diarrhea that influenced the continence score, but it was successfully controlled with drugs and dietary measures. All the others patients achieved an objective good grade of continence [9].

31.4 Discussion

Many attempts have been made to develop an ABS to treat FI, but up to date these devices have been associated with many complications, such as infection, obstructed defecation, and skin erosion, and their effectiveness is still debated. Erosion is recognized as one of the most serious complications of alloplastic implants placed around the bowel. This may be the result of ischemia after the use of the artificial anal sphincter, because the cuff may produce a heterogeneous application of pressure with localized high-pressure zones, which may damage the bowel wall embedded in these areas. The use of circumferential occlusive devices has been limited by the development of intestinal ischemia and ulceration in animal models and humans.

A novel ABS has been developed from the School of Electronics, Information and Electrical Engineering of Shanghai, Jiao Tong University, to simulate the normal physiology of the human anorectum. With the aim of engineering a safe and reliable device, a model of the human colonic blood flow has been built, and a relation between the colonic blood flow rate and the operating occlusive pressure of the anorectum is achieved.

Tissue ischemia is analyzed based on constitutive relations of the human anorectum. The results showed that at the planned operating occlusion pressure of < 4 kPa, the ABS should not risk the vascularity of the human colon [10].

More recently, promising results in the management of severe, refractory FI have been achieved with SNS. Multicenter studies have demonstrated that SNS produces marked improvement of symptoms in patients suffering from this debilitating condition. These studies report an objective evaluation of two surgical options proposed for severe FI using standardized questionnaires, and contribute to answering the question of the capacity of SNS to offer the same results to patients that would previously have been treated with ABS.

As compared with the more aggressive sphincter surgery, one of the main advantage of SNS is the possibility to predict the outcome by a test period using a temporary external stimulator. This pre-therapeutic test should contribute to consideration of SNS as a valid option to treat FI, either alone, or in conjunction with other surgical approaches [11].

31.5 Conclusions

The implantation procedure for an ABS is very easy and quick (60–90 min) but the risk of system malfunctioning, infection, and explantation remains high. Although morbidity and the need for revision surgery is high following implantation of the ABS, the outcome in terms of continence and quality of life is significantly improved, so that the ABS may be considered an effective treatment option for severe FI. Patients should be well informed and their skill to manage the device evaluated. When all the other treatment options have failed, the ABS procedure should be proposed, particularly in young and motivated patients, as it remains the only alternative to a definitive colostomy.

References

1. Tan EK, Vaizey C, Cornish J, Darzi A, Tekkis PP. Surgical strategies for faecal incontinence – a decision analysis between dynamic graciloplasty, artificial bowel sphincter and end stoma. Colorectal Dis 2007;10:577–586.

2. Altomare DF, Dodi G, La Torre F et al. Multicentre retrospective analysis of the out come of the artificial anal sphyncter implantation for severe fecal incontinence. Br J Surg 2001;88:1481–1486.

3. Wong WD, Congilosi S, Spencer M et al. The safety and efficacy of the artificial bowel sphincter for faecal incontinence: results from a multicentre cohort study. Dis Colon Rectum 2002;45:1139–1153.

4. Parker SC, Spencer MP, Madoff RD. Artificial bowel sphincter: long term experience at a single institution. Dis Colon Rectum 2003;46:722–729.

5. Melenhorst J, Koch SM, van Gemert WG, Baeten CG. The artificial bowel sphincter for faecal incontinence: a single centre study. Int J Colorectal Dis 2008;23:107–111.

6. Carmona R, Alós Company R, Vila JR et al. Long term results of artificial bowel sphincter for treatment of severe fecal incontinence. Are they what we hoped? Colorectal Dis 2009;11:831–837.

7. Lehur PA, Meurette G. The artificial bowel sphincter in the treatment of severe fecal incontinence in adults. In: Ratto C and Doglietto GB (eds) Fecal incontinence. Springer-Verlag, Milan, 2007, pp 193–200.

8. Gallas S, Leroi AM, Bridoux V et al. Constipation in 44 patients implanted with an artificial bowel sphincter. Int J Colorectal Dis 2009;24:969–974.

9. Romano G, Bianco F, Ciorra G. Total anorectal reconstruction with an artificial bowel sphyncter. In: Delaini GG (ed) Rectal cancer. Springer-Verlag, Milan, 2005, pp 176–182.

10. Zan P, Yan G, Liu H. Modeling of human colonic blood flow for a novel artificial anal sphincter system. J Zhejiang Univ Sci 2008;B9(9):734–738.

11. Meurette G, La Torre M, Regenet N et al. Value of sacral nerve stimulation in the treatment of severe faecal incontinence: a comparison to the artificial bowel sphincter. Colorectal Dis 2009;11:631–635.

Sacral Neuromodulation

Donato F. Altomare, Marcella Rinaldi and Filippa Cuccia

Abstract Sacral nerve stimulation (SNS) is a new minimally invasive treatment available in the armamentarium for the treatment of pelvic floor dysfunctions, particularly fecal incontinence, and involves electrostimulation of the sacral nerves by means of an implantable pulse generator. Despite the fact that the exact mechanisms of action and neural pathways involved are still incompletely known, SNS has gained wide acceptance among colorectal surgeons for its ability to influence several factors responsible for continence, and as a reliable pre-implantation test, with very low surgical risk and a wide range of indications. In fact, fecal incontinence of any etiology (except complete spinal cord injury) and severity has been tested, although with variable success rates. About 15 years since its introduction in coloproctology, studies on the long-term outcome have confirmed its reliability and effectiveness, not only in symptom control but also in improving quality of life. Finally, evaluation of the cost-effectiveness ratio compared with other treatments for fecal incontinence confirms the advantages of SNS, making this technique the first option in the management algorithm of this disabling disease.

Keywords Fecal incontinence • Neuromodulation • Sacral nerve stimulation

32.1 Introduction

Sacral nerve modulation (SNM) or sacral nerve stimulation (SNS) therapy is an innovative, minimally invasive technique for treating patients with functional disorders of the pelvic floor, particularly urinary and fecal incontinence, by affecting central and peripheral nervous control of these functions and recruiting residual anorectal function by stimulation of the pelvic nerves.

Before its introduction into clinical practice in coloproctology [1], any attempt to correct fecal incontinence aimed to narrow the anal canal or to reinforce the anal sphincters, and there was no possibility of influencing other factors involved in the continence mechanism, such as anorectal sensitivity and motility.

Despite its recent introduction in coloproctology and the fact that the mechanism of action is still incompletely known, this procedure is progressively replacing most of the older ones and is currently at the top of the list of management options in an ideal algorithm for the treatment of patients with fecal incontinence. The SNS technique has the unique advantage over other techniques that it is possible to conduct a

D.F. Altomare
Colorectal Unit, Department of Emergency and Organ
Transplantation, University of Bari, Italy

predictive test, which can be used to select patients who will respond to the therapy, before implanting the pulse generator. In fact the technique usually includes a first step during which the S3 root is checked and stimulated electrically to evoke a motor and sensory response of the anus and perineum, a tined lead (Interstim® 3889–28 cm, Medtronic Inc., Minneapolis, MN, USA) is then percutaneously implanted and connected to an external screener (Mod. 3625 Medtronic Inc., Minneapolis, MN, USA) for a temporary two-week stimulation period during which the patient fills in a diary of defecation and a quality-of-life questionnaire. Patients responding favorably will then be submitted to a permanent implant of a subcutaneous electrostimulator (Interstim® II, 3058, Medtronic Inc., Minneapolis, MN, USA) (Fig. 32.1).

32.2   Technical Improvements

Technically, the procedure has evolved very rapidly in the last ten years. The original technique, in which a wide presacral incision was necessary to identify the sacral foramen for the electrode implant and to suture it at the periostium under general anesthesia, has been abandoned in favor of a percutaneous Seldinger-like positioning of the electrode under fluoroscopy and local anesthesia.

The use of a monopolar percutaneous test for the nerve evaluation test (PNE), using an easily displaceable electrode (Medtronic Interstim 3057–6SC, Inc., Minneapolis, MN, USA), has been replaced by use of a quadripolar tined lead [2], which gives better performance and cannot be displaced accidentally [3].

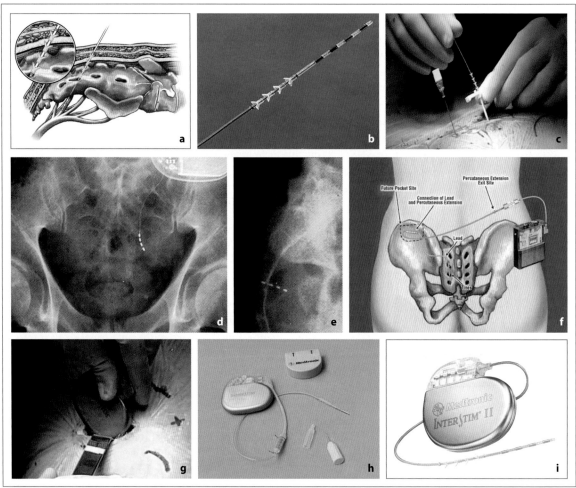

Fig. 32.1 Technique of SNM. **a** S3 root is checked and stimulated electrically; **b** the quadripolar tined lead; **c** percutaneous implant of the electrode; **d-e** radiological control of the electrode position; **f** connection of the electrode to an external screener; **g** permanent implant of the electrostimulator; **h** Interstim; **i** Interstim II

The size and performance of the implantable pulse generator has also improved, resulting in greater patient comfort and further allowing safe implantation in patients who are underweight and have thin subcutaneous tissue. Furthermore, the patients' programmer has also improved in usability and performance.

32.3 Mechanisms of Action

The exact working mechanism of SNS remains unknown, despite intensive research. The original idea that it could work by improving anal sphincter function [4] has not been confirmed [5], although a sphincter contraction can be induced by SNS. This contraction has been shown to be the result of a polysynaptic reflex rather than a direct activation of the alpha-motoneurons [6] and, when present, is not sufficient to explain the restored continence. Improved anorectal sensation, instead, seems to play a major role in the control of continence. This mechanism also needs an intact ascending neural pathway to the central nervous system (CNS), so one of the contraindication for SNS is complete spinal cord injury. The effects of SNS stimulation on the CNS have been investigated mostly in patients with urinary incontinence: positron emission tomography (PET) studies [7] have demonstrated that, via the spinal cord, SNS influences some brain areas involved in alertness and awareness, leading to a reduced excitability of some areas of the cortex [8].

Several other mechanisms have been suggested, such as activation of the autonomic nervous system [9] and an effect on colorectal motility [10]. Animal experiments have also demonstrated that SNS can inhibit colonic activity and enhance activity of the internal anal sphincter (IAS), via a somatosympathetic reflex [11]. Finally, a normalization of enhanced levels of rectal mucosal tachykinins (substance P) has been demonstrated after SNS in incontinent patients [12]. At present, it is reasonable to suppose that several SNS-activated mechanisms act together.

32.4 Indications

Uncertainties concerning the true mechanism of action of SNS are inevitably reflected in its clinical indications. Initially, SNS was indicated in cases of fecal incontinence of mild severity, after failure of other minor procedures, and in the presence of intact neural pathways and target organs. Consequently there was a long list of contraindications to the procedure, including congenital anorectal malformations, previous rectal surgery, prolapse, chronic diarrhea, irritable bowel disease, various neuropathies, partial spinal cord injury, ulcerative colitis, anal fistulas, pregnancy, and mental or physical inability to adhere to treatment. However, a progressive widening of the indications has occurred after positive individual case reports, and the procedure itself has been extended favorably even to the opposite complaint of constipation in its different forms [13].

A pragmatic trial and error philosophy has demonstrated that SNS may be effective in cases of fecal incontinence caused by external anal sphincter damage [14–16], radiation [17], rectal prolapse [18], Crohn's disease [19], partial spinal lesions [20] and cauda equina [21], some neurological diseases (like muscular dystrophy and systemic sclerosis) [22, 23], and even in cases of incontinence after rectal resection for cancer [24, 25]. The association with other pelvic floor dysfunctions like urinary incontinence or retention is a further motivation to test SNS in these patients due to the possibility of sorting out both problems simultaneously [26, 27].

A placebo effect has also been excluded by a double blind randomized crossover trial [28], so that the procedure has been certified as effective and safe by the National Institute for Health and Clinical Excellence (NICE) [29]. Even a recent Cochrane review [13] and the American Society of Colon and Rectal Surgeons (ASCRS) guidelines [30] have confirmed this statement.

The International Consultation on Incontinence (ICI) guidelines produced in 2008 suggest sphincter repair only in cases of wide anal sphincter defect or major perineal abnormalities (cloaca, rectovaginal fistulas, rectal prolapse), while the PNE test for SNS has already been introduced as a first option in patient with an intact anal sphincter or minor sphincter lesions.

32.5 Prognostic Factors

Since the device is very expensive and about 30–40% of the cases tested do not respond favorably, any attempt to identify factors that are statistically related to a successful outcome after temporary nerve stimulation is advisable to save money for the national health system and prevent unnecessary surgery; however, at present no clinical (patients' features, etiology of incontinence, motor or sensory response to nerve stimulation test) or laboratory preoperative investigations (anal manometry, electrophysiological tests, etc) have been shown to be prognostic factors [31–34]. Similar negative findings were reported in relation to prediction of success after positive temporary test [35].

32.6 Long-term Outcome and Quality of Life

The true Achilles' heel for any therapy of fecal incontinence is the maintenance of its efficacy in the long term [36]. Although SNS was only introduced in coloproctology disorders in 1995 [1], there are already several reports on its long-term efficacy [37–39]. Most patients implanted for SNS (between 70% and 85%) still maintain their improvements after 5 to 10 years. In the experience of the Italian Sacral Neuromodulation Group (GINS) from 52 patients with at least 5-years follow-up, 74% achieved at least a 50% improvement of continence and 50% had at least 70% improvement. Although these data are less impressive than the 91% success rate as a short-term outcome in a review of the European Centers performing SNS, reported at the First Joint meeting of the European Council of Coloproctology and European Association of Coloproctology in Geneva in 2004, the results are still encouraging when compared with the long-term outcome of other surgical techniques such as postanal repair, sphincteroplasty, or artificial sphincters.

However, the results of treatment of functional diseases like fecal incontinence must be measured mainly in terms of improvement in patients' quality of life, and a significant improvement of this parameter has been demonstrated in both early and long-term outcome in several studies using general health questionnaires (SF-36) and disease-specific questionnaires like the Fecal Incontinence Quality of Life Scale (FIQLS) [38, 40, 41].

32.7 Cost-effectiveness of Sacral Nerve Stimulation for Fecal Incontinence

Some studies [42, 43] have also addressed the economic matter of the cost-effectiveness of this relatively expensive procedure. Of course each analysis must be carried out within each national health system to be reliable,

and at present, reassuring information is available only in the UK and Spain. In both countries the incremental cost-effectiveness ratio (ICER) for SNS has been demonstrated to be within the cost per quality-adjusted life year (QALY) gained recommended by their national health systems.

References

1. Matzel KE, Stadelmaier U, Hohenfellner M, Gall FP. Electrical stimulation of sacral spinal nerves for treatment of faecal incontinence. Lancet 1995;346:1124–1127.
2. Spinelli M, Malaguti S, Giardiello G et al. A new minimally invasive procedure for pudendal nerve stimulation to treat neurogenic bladder: description of the method and preliminary data. Neurourol Urodyn 2005;24:305–309.
3. Ratto C, Morelli U, Paparo S et al. Minimally invasive sacral neuromodulation implant technique: modifications to the conventional procedure. Dis Colon Rectum 2003;46:414–417.
4. Rosen HR, Urbarz C, Holzer B et al. Sacral nerve stimulation as a treatment for fecal incontinence. Gastroenterology 2001;121:536–541.
5. Michelsen HB, Buntzen S, Krogh K, Laurberg S. Rectal volume tolerability and anal pressures in patients with fecal incontinence treated with sacral nerve stimulation. Dis Colon Rectum 2006;49:1039–1044.
6. Fowler CJ, Swinn MJ, Goodwin RJ et al. Studies of the latency of pelvic floor contraction during peripheral nerve evaluation show that the muscle response is reflexly mediated. J Urol 2000;163:881–883.
7. Blok BF, Groen J, Bosch JL et al. Different brain effects during chronic and acute sacral neuromodulation in urge incontinent patients with implanted neurostimulators. BJU Int 2006;98:1238–1243.
8. Sheldon R, Kiff ES, Clarke A et al. Sacral nerve stimulation reduces corticoanal excitability in patients with faecal incontinence. Br J Surg 2005;92:1423–1431.
9. Kenefick NJ, Emmanuel A, Nicholls RJ, Kamm MA. Effect of sacral nerve stimulation on autonomic nerve function. Br J Surg 2003;90:1256–1260.
10. Uludag O, Morren GL, Dejong CH, Baeten CG. Effect of sacral neuromodulation on the rectum. Br J Surg 2005; 92:1017–1023.
11. Vitton V, Abysique A, Gaigé S et al. Colonosphincteric electromyographic responses to sacral root stimulation: evidence for a somatosympathetic reflex. Neurogastroenterol Motil 2008;20:407–416.
12. Gooneratne ML, Facer P, Knowles CH et al. Normalization of substance P levels in rectal mucosa of patients with faecal incontinence treated successfully by sacral nerve stimulation. Br J Surg 2008;95:477–483.
13. Mowatt G, Glazener C, Jarrett M. Sacral nerve stimulation for fecal incontinence and constipation in adults: a short version Cochrane review. Neurourol Urodyn 2008;27:155–161.
14. Conaghan P, Farouk R. Sacral nerve stimulation can be suc-

cessful in patients with ultrasound evidence of external anal sphincter disruption. Dis Colon Rectum 2005;48:1610–1614.

15. Melenhorst J, Koch SM, Uludag O et al. Is a morphologically intact anal sphincter necessary for success with sacral nerve modulation in patients with faecal incontinence? Colorectal Dis 2008;10:257–262.

16. Jarrett ME, Dudding TC, Nicholls RJ et al. Sacral nerve stimulation for fecal incontinence related to obstetric anal sphincter damage. Dis Colon Rectum 2008;51:531–537.

17. di Visconte MS, Munegato G. The value of sacral nerve stimulation in the treatment of faecal incontinence after pelvic radiotherapy. Int J Colorectal Dis 2009;24:1111–1112.

18. Jarrett ME, Matzel KE, Stösser M et al. Sacral nerve stimulation for fecal incontinence following surgery for rectal prolapse repair: a multicenter study. Dis Colon Rectum 2005; 48:1243–1248.

19. Vitton V, Gigout J, Grimaud JC et al. Sacral nerve stimulation can improve continence in patients with Crohn's disease with internal and external anal sphincter disruption. Dis Colon Rectum 2008;51:924–927.

20. Jarrett ME, Matzel KE, Christiansen J et al. Sacral nerve stimulation for faecal incontinence in patients with previous partial spinal injury including disc prolapse.Br J Surg 2005;92:734–739.

21. Gstaltner K, Rosen H, Hufgard J et al. Sacral nerve stimulation as an option for the treatment of faecal incontinence in patients suffering from cauda equina syndrome. Spinal Cord 2008;46:644–647.

22. Kenefick NJ, Vaizey CJ, Nicholls RJ et al. Sacral nerve stimulation for faecal incontinence due to systemic sclerosis. Gut 2002;51:881–883.

23. Buntzen S, Rasmussen OO, Ryhammer AM et al. Sacral nerve stimulation for treatment of fecal incontinence in a patient with muscular dystrophy: report of a case. Dis Colon Rectum 2004;47:1409–1411.

24. Ratto C, Grillo E, Parello A et al. Sacral neuromodulation in treatment of fecal incontinence following anterior resection and chemoradiation for rectal cancer. Dis Colon Rectum 2005;48:1027–1036.

25. Jarrett ME, Matzel KE, Stösser M et al. Sacral nerve stimulation for faecal incontinence following a rectosigmoid resection for colorectal cancer. Int J Colorectal Dis 2005; 20:446–451.

26. Altomare DF, Rinaldi M, Petrolino M et al. Permanent sacral nerve modulation for fecal incontinence and associated urinary disturbances. Int J Colorectal Dis 2004;19:203–209.

27. Leroi AM, Michot F, Grise P, Denis P. Effect of sacral nerve stimulation in patients with fecal and urinary incontinence. Dis Colon Rectum 2001; 44:779–789.

28. Leroi AM, Parc Y, Lehur PA et al. Efficacy of sacral nerve stimulation for fecal incontinence: results of a multicenter double-blind crossover study. Ann Surg 2005;242:662–669.

29. National Institute for Health and Clinical Excellence. Sacral nerve stimulation for faecal incontinence. Interventional Pro-

cedure Guidance No 99. National Institute for Health and Clinical Excellence, London, 2004.

30. Tjandra JJ, Dykes SL, Kumar RR et al; Standards Practice Task Force of The American Society of Colon and Rectal Surgeons. Practice parameters for the treatment of fecal incontinence. Dis Colon Rectum 2007;50:1497–1507.

31. Gourcerol G, Gallas S, Michot F et al. Sacral nerve stimulation in fecal incontinence: are there factors associated with success? Dis Colon Rectum 2007;50:3–12.

32. Altomare DF, Rinaldi M, Lobascio PL et al. Factors affecting the outcome of temporary sacralnerve stimulation for faecal incontinence. The value of the new tined lead electrode. Colorectal Dis 2009; in press.

33. Govaert B, Melenhorst J, van Gemert WG, Baeten CG. Can sensory and/or motor reactions during percutaneous nerve evaluation predict outcome of sacral nerve modulation? Dis Colon Rectum 2009;52:1423–1426.

34. Vallet C, Parc Y, Lupinacci R et al. Sacral nerve stimulation for faecal incontinence: response rate, satisfaction and the value of preoperative investigation in patient selection. Colorectal Dis 2009; 13 Apr 13, epub ahead of print.

35. Dudding TC, Parés D, Vaizey CJ, Kamm MA. Predictive factors for successful sacral nerve stimulation in the treatment of faecal incontinence: a 10-year cohort analysis. Colorectal Dis 2008;10:249–256.

36. Müller C, Belyaev O, Deska T et al. Fecal incontinence: an up-to-date critical overview of surgical treatment options. Langenbecks Arch Surg 2005;390:544–552.

37. Matzel KE, Lux P, Heuer S et al. Sacral nerve stimulation for fecal incontinence: long term outcome. Colorectal Dis 2009;11:636–641.

38. Altomare DF, Ratto C, Ganio E et al. Long-term outcome of sacral nerve stimulation for fecal incontinence. Dis Colon Rectum 2009;52:11–17.

39. El-Gazzaz G, Zutshi M, Salcedo L et al. Sacral neuromodulation for the treatment of fecal incontinence and urinary incontinence in female patients: long-term follow-up. Int J Colorectal Dis 2009; 2 June, epub ahead of print.

40. Hetzer FH, Hahnloser D, Clavien PA, Demartines N. Quality of life and morbidity after permanent sacral nerve stimulation for fecal incontinence. Arch Surg 2007;142:8–13.

41. Ripetti V, Caputo D, Ausania F et al. Sacral nerve neuromodulation improves physical, psychological and social quality of life in patients with fecal incontinence. Tech Coloproctol 2002;6:147–152.

42. Dudding TC, Meng Lee E, Faiz O et al. Economic evaluation of sacral nerve stimulation for faecal incontinence. Br J Surg 2008;95:1155–1163.

43. Brosa M, Muñoz-Duyos A, Navarro-Luna A et al. Cost effectiveness analysis of sacral neuromodulation (SNM) with Interstim for faecal incontinence in Spain. Curr Med Res Opin 2008;24:907–917.

Future Treatment

Bruno Roche, Guillaume Zufferey and Joan Robert-Yap

Abstract The future of incontinence treatment will be guided by the increasing risk of the ever-aging population. Prevention of risk factors such as more conservative delivery techniques or less aggressive anal surgery will reduce the number of incontinent patients. Concerning therapy, new imaging will be helpful to plan surgical treatment and reduce organ injuries. There still remains a huge discrepancy between the incidence of incontinence that is actually reported and the amount of money put into research. These issues must be addressed in the near future. The area of nerve stimulation will continue to play a large role, and the development of direct pudendal nerve stimulation has yet to reveal its long-term effectiveness. Finally, the substitution of old and degenerative tissue by new tissue derived from stem cells is a promising way to treat general tissue degeneration.

Keywords Anal incontinence • Future • Nerve stimulation • Stem cells

33.1 Introduction

The future of incontinence treatment will be guided by the increasing risk of the ever-aging population. New applications of imaging and new therapeutic developments will permit the treatment of a larger patient population. Technologic developments have brought great advances in the therapeutic areas; however, there is still much to develop in terms of understanding the pathophysiology of this disorder and focusing more on the reporting of this problem. There still remains a huge discrepancy between the incidence of incontinence that is actually reported and the amount of money put into research. These issues must be addressed in the near future.

33.2 Pathophysiological and Behavioral Aspect

An accurate measurement of the incidence of fecal incontinence can only be made with new and improved epidemiological studies. This will be of increasing importance because of clinical conditions arising as a result of the increasing geriatric population. Patient education for risk factors should be developed and may have a positive social impact on perineal diseases and also play a role in diminishing the burden and cost to society.

This improvement can only be realized with greater access for the general population to information, through the media and internet. Patients' groups, doctors, and politicians should be made aware of this problem and the impact it has on society, in relation not only to the costs but also to individuals' quality of life and economic factors.

B. Roche
Proctology Unit, University Hospital, Geneva, Switzerland

G.A. Santoro, A.P. Wieczorek, C.I. Bartram (eds.) *Pelvic Floor Disorders*
© Springer-Verlag Italia 2010

33.3 Diagnostic Problems

33.3.1 Prevention of Incontinence

One rarely speaks about incontinence prevention with patients; however, it is something we should address when we discuss certain treatments and options for anal surgery or delivery. We should also deal with postpartum problems more aggressively and ensure that women begin early physiotherapy after childbirth. As women age we tend to investigate the problem of incontinence after it has long been established; however, premenopausal women should be educated to already begin physiotherapy and home exercises routinely to prevent the problem from even starting.

This approach needs to be studied in order to see if there is any positive result. Bowel habits should also be discussed routinely with the patient, to avoid long-term problems in the future such as rectocele or a descending pelvic floor.

33.3.2 Diagnostic Tests and Normal Values

Over the past 10 years, there have been new developments in the fields of diagnostic imaging and testing for fecal incontinence and pelvic floor disorders. However, there are still discrepancies in the correlation of test results with clinical findings and symptoms.

This may result from the fact that we cannot image certain anatomical areas accurately or may be because we are misinterpreting these images. We still need to discover where the aberrations are and find ways to measure these abnormalities. With the development of nuclear magnetic resonance imaging we have much more accurate pictures of anatomy, but in order to use these in the evaluation of incontinence, we have to know what we are searching for and how we can better obtain these images. Routine post-obstetric complications should focus not only on sphincter damage but also on pelvic floor stability and imaging for ruptures and muscle damage such as in the levator ani muscles. This will improve understanding of the damage that contributes to post-obstetric incontinence.

33.3.3 Standardization of Quality of Life

In this area there must be a focus on preparing a quality-of-life questionnaire that is standard for most cultures and societal norms. It should gauge and measure the severity of disruption of the normal daily activities of life, based upon the symptoms of fecal incontinence. If there were a more homogeneous and concise method applied to this measurement, data collection would be more accurate. However, there remains the ever-present problem of detecting incontinence. This is where we have failed; not only is it important to measure the burden on the patient and on society, but it is essential to begin to discuss it and allow patients to bring the subject forward without fear of shame and ridicule. As fecal incontinence is under-reported and under-diagnosed, there is a mismatch between the amount of research done for diagnosis and treatment and the incidence of this problem.

33.3.4 Study of Pathophysiological Mechanisms

When we start an evaluation of an incontinent patient, we must think of physiology and anatomy in order to discover the mechanisms that have failed, resulting in the presenting symptoms. It is here where we can progress in our understanding of this disorder and thus improve our methods for detecting early problems so we can image or measure them. Progress in imaging methods has resulted in great advances in the understanding of incontinence, but the fine regulation of rectal sensation, storage, and anal pressure are still poorly correlated with function, and this area needs more research and development. Another important contributor to continence is the bowel habit of the patient and one must try to understand and begin to look into childhood bowel habits and tendencies in order to understand future problems for adults.

33.4 Research Priorities

In areas of relatively new technology, there is still room for development. When we started to measure pudendal nerve terminal motor latency, we assumed that our measurements would remain consistent and yield a true correlation with the damage that caused the incontinence. However, as time passed, we saw this was not necessarily the case. The usefulness of this test has decreased and it is not often performed now. However, we all learned that the pudendal nerve plays a large role in incontinence. Our center has detected a way to indirectly measure the contribution of the pudendal nerve to continence, thus guiding us to correct treatment choices (see Chapter 25). In anal incontinence, a sphincter rupture is often the cause; however, when we repair the sphincter not every patient recovers well. Many have tried to predict the outcome of sphincter repair with little success, but we have found that measuring the movement of the puborectal sling can predict this very well. The better the movement, the better the result of the sphincter repair long term. Therefore, we feel that those with poor movement of the puborectal sling likely have poor innervation to this muscle and will likely benefit from other treatment such as sacral nerve modulation. This treatment has a good and well-proven success rate in carefully selected cases; however, in those cases that fail, we propose a direct stimulation of the pudendal nerve. This procedure is now becoming more common but is still in development. It should not be excluded for those who had a failed sacral nerve modulation with a neurological component contributing to incontinence. As more procedures are performed and more data collected, we will have better answers about the success of this treatment procedure.

33.5 Development of Novel Imaging with Treatment Applications

Surgical navigation, which utilizes virtual reality (VR) for assisting surgical procedures, similar to the concept of automobile navigation, is attracting much attention. However, when a surgeon consults an image displayed on a monitor, there is a mismatch with the actual visual field of the patient's operative field; hence, a technology for dynamic three-dimensional (3D) images that fuse together the actual and the virtual space has become necessary. Augmented reality (AR) is the superimposition of VR reconstructions onto a real patient's images, in real time [1]. This results in the visualization of internal structures through overlying tissues, providing a virtual transparent vision of surgical anatomy

[2]. Although its application is in a preliminary stage, convincing evidence has been found showing that it is an effective teaching tool for training residents, according to Shuhaiber's report [3]. Its widespread use and the universal transfer of such technology remain limited until there is a better understanding of registration and ergonomics. Mixed reality (MR) was defined by Milgram and Kishino [4] in 1994, as anywhere between the extremes of the virtuality continuum (VC) where the VC extends from the completely real through to the completely virtual environment, with AR and augmented virtuality ranging in between. MR refers to the merging of real and virtual fields to produce new environments and visualizations where physical and digital objects coexist and interact in real time.

A new concept of "image overlay surgery" consists of the integration of VR, AR, and MR technology, in which computer-generated dynamic 3D images of a video are superimposed on the actual space in front of the surgeon, on the patient's operative field. Such a system allows surgical navigation using OsiriX Software (OsiriX Foundation, Switzerland) [5, 6].

The skin of the image is transparent, and the display shows the patient's intraperitoneal anatomy (Fig. 33.1).

The surgeon is able to minimize gaze movement and can utilize the image assistance without interfering with operation of the forceps, reducing the gap of the VR.

The presented method provides an easy way to determine safety margins related to patient set-up errors upon registration of bony anatomy. Unexpected organ injury could be avoided. A significant reduction of operation time by improved planning and intraoperative support is anticipated, as well as significantly fewer intraoperative injuries and less bleeding.

Therefore, a simple image overlay system by OsiriX that takes into consideration the technological and cost aspects, and the installation setting, has the potential to contribute greatly to the reproduction of surgical plans prepared before surgery and to reduce the frequency of unexpected events during surgery [7]. Further research is needed to evaluate its long-term clinical impact on patients, surgeons, and hospital administrators. We anticipate that this system will continue to further evolve for the application of medical care in the near future, reducing invasiveness and improving quality of life for the patients and enhancing medical education, among other uses.

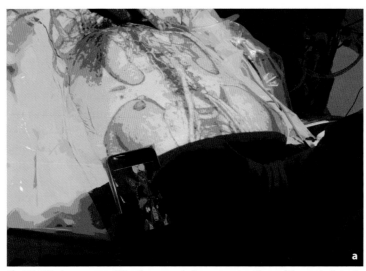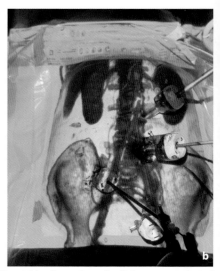

Fig. 33.1 During surgery, 3D volume-rendering reconstructions of the gastrointestinal tract, blood vessels, and soft tissue are projected on the patient's abdomen

33.6 Development of Novel Treatments

Fecal and/or urinary incontinence is a common condition in the elderly as well as among women, especially after childbirth. Although a few alleviating treatments are available, surgical therapies are perhaps the best option to achieve long-term continence. However, medical and/or surgical treatments are still unsatisfactory. Physical, psychic, and moral repercussions of incontinence thus require the development of new therapeutic approaches.

Tissue engineering using muscle progenitor cells or embryonic stem cells (ESC) holds great promise for reconstructive surgery and is currently a hot area of active research. Recent insights in stem cell biology and biomaterials enable us to achieve, in vitro, organized 3D cell cultures that are close to natural tissues. In this context, natural biopolymers like collagen and

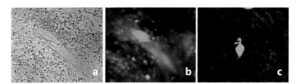

Fig. 33.2 Cell culture of myoblasts transduced with a lentivector carrying the green fluorescent protein (GFP) transgene. **a** Phase contrast image of cultured myoblasts fused into myotubes. **b** Fluorescent microscopy of GFP-transduced myoblasts which can differentiate into myotubes (same field as in **a**). **c** 3D fibrin gels labeled with Alexa-647 enabling visualization of the fiber network

fibrin are among the best candidates for such cellular constructs (Fig. 33.2).

33.6.1 Physiopathology and Molecular Mechanisms of Incontinence

It is likely that sphincter muscles are prone to similar degenerative processes as other muscles. The pathophysiology of incontinence is frequently described as damage at the cellular level. Little is known about the physiopathological basis of sphincter dysfunction at the molecular level. Most hypotheses point to the potential roles of both ageing and mechanical stress. In the external urethral sphincter of aged multiparous rabbits, a selective decrease in the volume of type 2 (fast) muscle fibers and/or conversion of type 2 to type 1 (slow) muscle fibers has been described [8]. Ageing may alter the expression of structural genes and affect cellular growth and death. An age-dependent increase of apoptosis of the striated muscle fibers of the urethral sphincter has been associated with a decrease in the number of striated muscle cells [9]. Ischemia–reperfusion injury, which occurs in ageing tissues, may also affect mitochondrial function in the urinary tract [10]. In guinea pigs subjected to ischemia, the expression of p53, Bax, c-Jun, c-Fos, and Caspase-3 is upregulated [11]. Tissue stretching and stress may also induce growth and muscle hypertrophy. This stretch-induced signal-transduction mechanism exists in the bladder when outlet obstruction (e.g. by the prostate) is present, and involves several molecular cascades including growth factors, cytoskeletal structures, and protein kinases. Intrinsic satellite cells are found in the urethral sphincter. After an acute injury by notexin, these intrinsic satellite cells have been shown to be activated and were postulated to be involved in sphincter regeneration [12, 13].

33.6.2 Potential Cell-based Strategies to Restore the Urinary or Anal Sphincter Function

Sphincter dysfunction is a multifactorial process. Several aspects of sphincter dysfunction may represent targets for regenerative therapy. Three main strategies can be combined: restoring the sphincter itself, restoring pelvic floor support including the sphincters, and restoring sphincter innervations.

The first objective for regenerative therapy will consist of restoring the sphincter itself. The concept of stem cell therapy and tissue engineering is thus a promising approach in order to replace, repair, or enhance the biological functions of a damaged sphincter by injection of new cells.

Cell transplantation for pelvic reconstructive procedure is under development. Stem cells have recently been employed to engineer new functional urogynecologic structures in animal models. Early results showed that the creation of a functional and anatomical bladder is feasible in vivo [14]. Tissue engineering techniques have also been used to attempt urethral reconstruction in animals [12, 13, 15]. The results obtained on the animal models are promising but require a greater depth of physiopathological, cellular, and molecular knowledge, with an awareness that the differentiation of these cells is not optimized yet.

The second strategic approach for regenerative therapies of sphincter dysfunction will target restoring pelvic floor support. Synthetic or biologic prostheses are developed as "meshes" of various shape and surgically implanted to anatomically restore the integrity of the pelvic floor. Enriching this prosthesis with progenitor cells will allow insertion of potentially "active" meshes, which will give enhanced tolerability and elasticity to the tissues. This extension of the technique of extracellular matrices as 3D prostheses will help to restore not only the anatomy but, more importantly, the function of the pelvic floor.

Finally, in order to restore a properly functional sphincter, the issue of tissue denervation will need to be addressed. Peripheral nerve regeneration by cellular therapy has been developed. Co-injection of myogenic and neurogenic progenitor cells into the urethra has been reported. Transplanting neurogenic stem cells will not only allow regeneration of damaged axons, but also promote regeneration of a functional sphincter [16–18].

This growth-promoting signaling is probably bidirectional. In a rat model of urethral sphincter deficiency, muscular progenitor cells isolated from limb muscles of an older animal regenerated a myogenic program when injected into an irreversibly injured sphincter. The maturation of muscular progenitor cells activated nerve regeneration and restored functional motor units [13].

33.7 Conclusions

The future of incontinence treatment is crucial, in the face of the evolution of the ever-aging population. Prevention of risk factors such as more conservative delivery techniques or less aggressive anal surgery will reduce the number of incontinent patients. Concerning therapy, new imaging will be helpful to plan surgical treatment and reduce organ injuries. The area of nerve stimulation will continue to play a large role, and the development of direct pudendal nerve stimulation has yet to reveal its long-term effectiveness. Finally, the substitution of old and degenerative tissue by new tissue derived from stem cells is a promising way to treat general tissue degeneration.

References

1. Tang SL, Kwoh CK, Teo MY et al. Augmented reality systems for medical applications. IEEE Eng Med Biol Mag 1998;17:49–58.
2. Marescaux J, Rubino F, Arenas M et al. Augmented-reality-assisted laparoscopic adrenalectomy. JAMA 2004;292:2214–2215.
3. Shuhaiber JH. Augmented reality in surgery. Arch Surg 2004;139:170–174.
4. Milgram P, Kishino AF. Taxonomy of mixed reality visual displays. IEICE Trans Inform Syst 1994;E77-D:1321–1329.
5. Rosset A, Spadola L, Ratib O. OsiriX. An open-source soft-

ware for navigating in multidimensional DICOM images. J Digit Imaging 2004;17:205–216.

6. Rosset C, Rosset A, Ratib O. General consumer communication tools for improved image management and communication in medicine. J Digit Imaging 2005;18:270–279.

7. Rosset A, Spadola L, Pysher L, Ratib O. Informatics in radiology (infoRAD): navigating the fifth dimension: innovative interface for multidimensional multimodality image navigation. Radiographics 2006;26:299–308.

8. Tokunaka S, Fujii H, Hashimoto H, Yachiku S. Proportions of fiber types in the external urethral sphincter of young nulliparous and old multiparous rabbits. Urol Res 1993;21:121–124.

9. Strasser H, Tiefenthaler M, Steinlechner M et al. Age dependent apoptosis and loss of rhabdosphincter cells. J Urol 2000;164:1781–1785.

10. Fry CH, Ikeda Y, Harvey R et al. Control of bladder function by peripheral nerves: avenues for novel drug targets. Urology 2004;63(3 suppl 1):24–31.

11. Thiruchelvam N, Nyirady P, Peebles DM et al. Urinary outflow obstruction increases apoptosis and deregulates Bcl-2 and Bax expression in the fetal ovine bladder. Am J Pathol 2003;162:1271–1282.

12. Yiou R, Lefaucheur JP, Atala A. The regeneration process of the striated urethral sphincter involves activation of intrinsic satellite cells. Anat Embryol 2003;206:429–435.

13. Yiou R, Yoo JJ, Atala A. Restoration of functional motor units in a rat model of sphincter injury by muscle precursor cell autografts. Transplantation 2003;76:1053–1060.

14. Atala A. Experimental and clinical experience with tissue engineering techniques for urethral reconstruction. Urol Clin North Am 2002;29:485–492, ix.

15. Lee JY, Paik SY, Yuk SH et al. The effects of periurethral muscle-derived stem cell injection on leak point pressure in a rat model of stress urinary incontinence. Int Urogynecol J Pelvic Floor Dysfunct 2003;1431–37; discussion 37.

16. Imitola J, Park KI, Teng YD et al. Stem cells: cross-talk and developmental programs. Philos Trans R Soc Lond B Biol Sci 2004;359:823–837.

17. Hall H, Baechi T, Hubbell JA. Molecular properties of fibrin-based matrices for promotion of angiogenesis in vitro. Microvasc Res 2001;62:315–326.

18. Kang SB, Lee HN, Lee JY et al. Sphincter contractility after muscle-derived stem cells autograft into the cryoinjured anal sphincters of rats. Dis Colon Rectum 2008;51:1367–1373.

Invited Commentary

Steven D. Wexner

Dr Pfeifer has clearly and expertly outlined the methods, techniques, results, and morbidity of sphincter repair and postanal repair in Chapter 28. Although the initial reported success rates with sphincter repair were in excess of 90%, several long-term studies have revealed those success rates are in the vicinity of 15% to 30% [1–4]. There are certain factors that may be predictive of failure, including pudendal neuropathy. However, prior sphincter repair does not appear to auger for failure of subsequent sphincter repair [5]. Because of the unfortunately poor long-term efficacy of this operation, it is certainly not a panacea. Current debate centers around whether the anal sphincters should be repaired, as, although the procedure may improve incontinence, it may also induce significant scarring. If scarring is produced and the result is suboptimal, then subsequent procedures such as stimulated graciloplasty, artificial bowel sphincter, and even sacral nerve stimulation may not be as successful. Therefore, a discussion must be held with the patients as to whether a sphincter defect should be addressed by overlapping repair or whether the patient should directly proceed to one of the newer alternatives. This discussion is especially important in light of the fact that several recent studies have found sacral nerve stimulation to be successful even in sphincter defect of up to 120 degrees [6].

In Chapter 30, Drs Trompetto and Roveroni have quite expertly addressed the issues surrounding the results of using radiofrequency energy and injectable biomaterials. They have also touched upon most of the literature surrounding the use of injectable materials.

Several other injectable agents exist, ranging from autologous fat, as described by Shafik [7] and Bernardi et al [8], to polytetrafluoroethylene (PTFE) [9], silicone [10], carbon beads [11], and other agents [12–14]. We have performed an outpatient open-label pilot study of ten patients in whom carbon beads were injected [15]. The only morbidity was extravasation of the beads in one patient. We noted that 80% of patients demonstrated an initial significant improvement in Cleveland Clinic Florida (Wexner) incontinence scores [16] as well as improvements in the fecal incontinence quality of life scores in all scales. We reported our experience with radiofrequency in a five-center open-label prospective trial [17] including 43 females and 7 males with a mean age of 61 years (range 30–80 years) and a mean duration of fecal incontinence of 14.9 years. Twenty-two per cent of patients had had prior surgery for fecal incontinence, and at 6 months' follow-up the Cleveland Clinic Florida (Wexner) incontinence scores [16] had significantly decreased from 14.9 to 11.1. In addition, significant improvements were noted in all four scales in the American Society of Colorectal Surgeons' fecal incontinence quality of life (Rockwood) scores, along with SF-36 improvements noted in both social functioning and mental health. The results seem to have been sustained, as supported by Takahashi et al, at both one year and two years [18, 19]. Clearly, radiofrequency does have a role in the armamentarium for the treatment of fecal incontinence [17, 20].

Chapter 31 quite expertly delves into the method of placement, results, and potential problems associated with the artificial bowel sphincter. We recently reported our experience at Cleveland Clinic Florida with over 50 patients in whom these sphincters have been implanted, in some cases also explanted, and

S.D. Wexner
Division of Colon and Rectal Surgery,
Cleveland Clinic Florida, Weston, FL, USA

occasionally even reimplantated [21]. Although the operation is technically easy, it is associated with an exceptionally high morbidity, and accordingly requires a resolute patient and an expert dedicated surgical team. Many of the inherent problems associated with the artificial bowel sphincter may be due to the fact that the operation entails implantation of a foreign body in close proximity to the anus. Our recent series reveals that the only predictable adverse prognosticators for infection and subsequent explantation were a prior perianal infection and an early bowel movement after sphincter implantation [21]. Other variables that may inherently have seemed to be associated with infection and subsequent explantation, such as obesity, diabetes, and a history of trauma, did not prove to be associated. Our success rate was certainly within the realm of expectation, despite the potential problems associated with the artificial bowel sphincter; patients who have suffered significant muscle loss may still be candidates for this operation although it is my personal preference to occasionally augment the perianal muscle with a gracilis transposition prior to implantation of the artificial bowel sphincter. Although there is no proof that the addition of healthy muscle bulk in any way prevents infection or explantation inherently, it seems an appropriate methodology.

In our recent study, we reported the results of 51 artificial bowel sphincter implantations in 47 patients, 43 of whom were female. Our mean patient age was 48.8 ± 12.5 years (range 79 years), and they had a mean Cleveland Clinic Florida (Wexner) incontinence score of 18 ± 1.4 range (0–20). The etiology of incontinence was imperforate anus in 47% of patients, obstetric injury or other prior iatrogenic injury in 29%, and other causes in 24%. Multivariate analysis was undertaken to try to determine any factors associated with failures of the artificial bowel sphincter. Overall, there was a 41.2% incidence of infection – 35.3% early-stage and 5.9% late-stage infection. No significance was found on univariate analysis for age, body mass index (BMI), etiology of incontinence, history of perianal infection or prior perianal surgery, gender, diabetes, or presence of a stoma. Multivariate analysis did reveal that the only independent factors were the time between artificial bowel sphincter implantation and first postoperative bowel movement and a history of perianal sepsis. Late-stage failures are more often due to device malfunction, indicating the need more

for mechanical refinement than for different surgical methodology.

The method by which sacral neuromodulation works remains completely unclear, as reported in Chapter 32. Despite the lack of a defined mechanism of action, it certainly has significant appeal based upon the high success rate coupled with the very low morbidity. We recently published two studies, one on the efficacy [22] and one on the morbidity [23] of sacral nerve stimulation. One hundred and twenty patients underwent successful implantation, with an overall success rate at one year of 83%. Our primary parameter for measuring success was a reduction of 50% or more in the frequency of episodes of incontinence. Secondary parameters included the American Society of Colon and Rectal Surgeons quality of life (Rockwood) scale; significant improvements were also noted using this instrument. These results have continued for up to five years in the implanted population. As compared to the very high rates for morbidity associated with the artificial bowel sphincter and stimulated graciloplasty, our study revealed a rate of significant complications in only 10% of patients. None of these complications were related to perianal sepsis as would have been seen with other methods of perianal encirclement with either autologous tissues, such as a transposed gracilis muscle, or an artificial device, such as the artificial bowel sphincter.

Drs Roche, Zufferey, and Robert-Yap have beautifully presented a very challenging theme predicting the future. They note that treatment needs to become more focused, and that in order for this to happen, we need to develop a better understanding of the etiology and mechanism of fecal incontinence so that we can hopefully more appropriately address them in a meaningful way. This chapter emphasizes that, although there are clearly a plethora of both traditional and more recent treatments of fecal incontinence, including many new modalities, there is also significant room remaining for improvement [24].

References

1. Matsuoka H, Mavrantonis C, Wexner SD et al. Postanal repair for fecal incontinence – is it worthwhile? Dis Colon Rectum 2000;43:1561–1567.
2. Halverson AL, Hull TL. Long-term outcome of overlapping anal sphincter repair. Dis Colon Rectum 2002;45:345–348.
3. Bravo Gutierrez A, Madoff RD, Lowry AC et al. Long-term

results of anterior sphincteroplasty. Dis Colon Rectum 2004;47:727–731; discussion 731–732.

4. Zorcolo L, Covotta L, Bartolo DC. Outcome of anterior sphincter repair for obstetric injury: comparison of early and late results. Dis Colon Rectum 2005;48:524 –531.

5. Oberwalder M, Dinnewitzer A, Baig MK et al. Do internal anal sphincter defects decrease the success rate of anal sphincter repair? Tech Coloproctol 2006;10:94–97; discussion 97.

6. Chan MK, Tjandra JJ. Sacral nerve stimulation for fecal incontinence. Dis Colon Rectum 2008;51:1015–1025.

7. Shafik A. Perianal injection of autologous fat for treatment of sphincteric incontinence. Dis Colon Rectum 1995;38:583–587.

8. Bernardi C, Favetta U, Peascatori M. Autologous fat injection for treatment of fecal incontinence: manometric and echographic assessment. Plast Reconstr Surg 1998; 102:1626–1628.

9. Shafik A. Polytetrafluoroethylene injection for the treatment of partial fecal incontinence. Int Surg 1993;78:159–161.

10. Tjandra JJ, Lim JF, Hiscock R et al. Injectable silicone biomaterial for fecal incontinence caused by internal anal sphincter dysfunction is effective. Dis Colon Rectum 2004;47: 2138–2146.

11. Altomare DF, La Torre F, Rinaldi M et al. Carbon-coated microbeads anal injection in outpatient treatment of minor fecal incontinence. Dis Colon Rectum 2008;51:432–435.

12. Ganio E, Marino F, Giani I et al. Injectable synthetic calcium hydroxylapatite ceramic microspheres (Coaptite) for passive fecal incontinence. Tech Coloproctol 2008;12:99–102.

13. Siproudhis L, Morcet J, Laine F. Elastomer implants in faecal incontinence: a blind, randomized placebo-controlled study. Aliment Pharmacol Ther 2007;25:1125–1132.

14 Stojkovic SG, Lim M, Burke D et al. Intra-anal collagen injection for the treatment of faecal incontinence. Br J Surg 2006;93:1514–1518.

15. Weiss EG, Efron JE, Nogueras JJ. Submucosal injection of carbon coated beads is a successful and safe office based treatment for fecal incontinence. Dis Colon Rectum 2002;45:a46–47.

16. Jorge JM, Wexner SD. Etiology and management of fecal incontinence. Dis Colon Rectum 1993;36:77–97.

17. Efron JE, Corman ML, Fleshman J et al. Safety and effectiveness of temperature-controlled radio-frequency energy delivery to the anal canal (Secca procedure) for the treatment of fecal incontinence. Dis Colon Rectum 2003;46:1606–1616; discussion 1616–1618.

18. Takahashi T, Garcia-Osogobio S, Valdovinos MA et al. Radio-frequency energy delivery to the anal canal for the treatment of fecal incontinence. Dis Colon Rectum 2002;45:915–922.

19. Takahashi T, Garcia-Osogobio S, Valdovinos MA et al. Extended two-year results of radio-frequency energy delivery for the treatment of fecal incontinence (the Secca procedure). Dis Colon Rectum 2003;46:711–715.

20. Shawki S, Wexner SD. Newer concepts in fecal incontinence: injectables and sacral nerve stimulation. Semin Colon Rectal Surg 2010;1:30-36.

21. Wexner SD, Jin HY, Weiss EG et al. Factors associated with failure of the artificial bowel sphincter: a study of over 50 cases from Cleveland Clinic Florida. Dis Colon Rectum 2009;52:1550–1557.

22. Wexner SD, Coller JA, Devroede G et al. Sacral nerve stimulation for fecal incontinence: results of a 120-patient prospective multicenter study. Ann Surg 2010;251:441–449.

23. Wexner SD, Hull T, Edden Y et al. Infection rates in a large investigational trial of sacral nerve stimulation for fecal incontinence. JOGS; pub online March 31, 2010.

24. Edden Y, Wexner SD. Therapeutic devices for fecal incontinence: dynamic graciloplasty, artificial bowel sphincter and sacral nerve stimulation. Expert Rev Med Devices 2009;6:307–312.

Biofeedback

34

Beatrice Salvioli and Luciano Pellegrini

Abstract Biofeedback is a conservative treatment that is widely recognized to be, along with lifestyle modifications and pharmaceutical support, one of the first-line approaches in fecal incontinence. Although data in the literature are controversial with regard to its real benefit, and studies lack standardized protocols, this technique is relatively easy, readily accepted by patients, has no side-effects, and is of great help for patients' physical and psychological well-being. Compliance, cognitive capacities, and major sphincteric lesions are the limiting steps of successful therapy. So far, little is known about predictive factors of good outcome in patients with fecal incontinence. Future placebo-controlled randomized studies are needed to better evaluate pelvic floor retraining in individuals who do not respond to advice/education alone, and to evaluate sensory retraining in incontinent patients. Outcomes should include standardized measures, validated quality-of-life questionnaires, and long-term assessment of therapeutic success.

Keywords Anal sphincters • Biofeedback • Fecal incontinence

34.1 Introduction

For many years, international experts have been promoting biofeedback therapy as the gold standard treatment of fecal incontinence [1, 2]. Studies report overall good outcome in more than 70% of patients [3, 4]. The main modalities used consist of measures of voluntary contraction, and modification of anorectal perception and coordination.

34.2 Technique

Biofeedback is a strategy that is based on operating conditions derived from psychological learning theory, and is an effective therapy in patients with fecal incontinence associated with impaired functioning of the puborectalis and external anal sphincter muscles [5, 6]. Continence is a complex mechanism, in which different anatomical and functional parts interplay, and any condition that alters this equilibrium can theoretically cause defecation disorders [7]. The puborectalis muscle and external anal sphincter complex are striated muscles under conscious control, and so individuals can be taught to voluntarily strengthen and relax them [7].

Biofeedback training in fecal incontinence aims to instruct patients how to recognize and achieve control

B. Salvioli
Department of Clinical Medicine, S. Orsola-Malpighi Hospital, University of Bologna, Italy

of their striated muscle sphincter apparatus, by means of techniques that are directed to modification of rectal perception and increasing external anal sphincter responsiveness [8].

Modes of therapeutic action presume that the patient is able to comprehend and willing to cooperate with the therapist. Different devices can be utilized and methods used include visual, verbal, or auditory feedback. Patients with fecal incontinence are taught to squeeze the anal muscles without increasing intra-abdominal pressure or inappropriately contracting the thigh or gluteal muscles [9]. Essentially, three modalities of treatment are employed to teach patients to exercise the anal muscles.

The first method consists of anal manometric catheter, intra-anal electromyography (EMG) electrodes, or perianal external EMG electrodes.

Ultrasound has also been used to monitor sphincter contraction [10]. Pressures or EMG signals are displayed on a monitor or chart recorder [11] to illustrate to the patient how the sphincter functions and to teach them how to isolate anal sphincter contraction from buttock movement and abdominal effort. Portable devices are available to customize home treatment and to monitor progress.

The second mode consists of a three-balloon system to facilitate sensory–motor coordination, by correctly identifying rectal distention and responding by immediate contraction to compensate inhibition of the internal anal sphincter [6].

The third approach implies sensory impairment retraining, and the patient is taught to discriminate a smaller volume of balloon distention, by gradually reducing rectal volume inflation [8].

The goals of biofeedback therapy in fecal incontinence are basically targeted to improving sphincter strength and endurance, improving rectal sensation and yielding sensory–motor coordination.

Muscle strength [11] and duration of squeeze are important in preserving continence [12], and some authors have focused biofeedback treatment on improving force and endurance [11, 12]. Patients are taught to isolate the pelvic muscles and to perform maximal voluntary contraction, concentrating on both the amplitude and duration of squeeze. Moreover, repeated contractions and relaxations are recommended at the beginning and end of home exercises. These quick contract and relax exercises improve the strength and function of fast twitch muscle fibers, in order to prevent accidents caused by increased intra-abdominal pressure, which are exacerbated during coughing, pulling, and lifting. To build up endurance, in patients with an adequate maximal contraction, submaximal squeeze is requested.

Other authors have focused on increasing the responsiveness of the external sphincter to rectal distention [8], while others have tried to modify both [3, 13].

External anal sphincter defect following obstetric trauma does not always lead to incontinence, and this could be explained by counterbalanced strengthening of the puborectalis muscle. In fact, levator ani contraction has been demonstrated to be an independent variable with the strongest correlation to severity of incontinence and the strongest predictive value of response to treatment [14]. The unresponsiveness of the external sphincter to retraining [8, 15] could be due to perineal muscular damage or, alternatively, to short, instead of more prolonged, treatment [16].

Amelioration of rectal sensitivity and sensory–motor coordination are believed to be important factors related to improvement [17, 18]. The enhanced ability to contract the anal sphincters with biofeedback training is likely to modify urgency by reducing large bowel peristalsis and inducing retrograde peristalsis. Patients with a hypersensitive rectum (e.g. urge incontinence) are trained to encourage relaxation and suppression of "urgency" in response to increasing-volume rectal balloon distention. The mechanisms by which training augments rectal perception are probably based on recruitment of sensory neurons adjacent to damaged afferent pathways. In those who are insensitive to distention, the aim is to lower the threshold for first sensation, using progressively reduced balloon rectal volumes.

By coordination training, patients learn how to promptly contract the pelvic floor muscles as balloon rectal distention is perceived, without increasing intra-abdominal pressure.

In patients with fecal seepage, a small amount of stool matter may seep out during sampling reflex or spontaneously [19], and during assessment and management these patients are conventionally grouped together with passive or urge-incontinent patients [20]. It has recently been found that these patients show fairly distinctive manometric and defecation patterns compared to incontinent patients, revealing that a combination of impaired rectal perception and incomplete evacuation (i.e. dyssinergic defecation) are at the basis of the development of fecal seepage. Biofeedback strengthening exercises could thus be ineffective, suggesting that correction of the underlying mechanism by improving sensation and rectoanal coordination facilitates a more complete evacuation [21].

Success is highly dependent on the motivation of the patient and that of the therapeutic team, in physical medicine, behavioral medicine, dietetics, and gastroenterology.

A multimodal biofeedback training (i.e. enhancing strength, rectal sensory perception, and sensory–motor coordination) is the approach of choice [8], but since the pathophysiology of fecal incontinence is multifactorial [22], customized treatment is preferable.

34.3 Biofeedback in Fecal Incontinence: Evidence-based Medicine

There is an abundant literature on biofeedback therapy in fecal incontinence and, overall, success is reported to be around 70% [3, 23–25] and is sustained even at long-term follow-up [26]. It has been suggested that the efficacy of biofeedback therapy diminishes with time [27], but a recent study showed that therapy produces persistent clinical and anorectal function improvement at 12 months of follow-up [28].

A Cochrane review identified only five out of 109 studies that met the criteria included in their analysis, and concluded that there is not enough evidence suggesting the utility of biofeedback as treatment in fecal incontinence, or about which aspects are the most helpful or which patients are most likely to be helped [13]. Lack of uniformity in methodologies, lack of randomized controlled study, heterogeneous patient populations, small sample sizes, short follow-up periods, and lack of validated outcome measures, are all variables that limit evaluation of the success rate of this technique [29].

The mechanism of improvement of biofeedback has yet to be elucidated. Progress in patients with intact sphincters may be related to an enhanced ability to contract the external sphincter thereby reducing large bowel movements and inducing retrograde peristalsis [30]. In patients with sphincteric damage, biofeedback could increase the residual functional capacity [31]. An effect on the internal anal sphincter is debatable and could be the result of modification of autonomic function, as demonstrated in patients with constipation, using laser Doppler rectal mucosal blood flow [32].

It is questionable whether biofeedback has a specific effect above and beyond an interactive educational intervention alone [23, 24, 33], and a study conducted to compare education/verbal instruction plus biofeedback versus education/verbal instruction alone, concluded that incontinent patients had a good response to both [33]. Patients receiving biofeedback, unlike a control group, showed increases of manometric parameters (resting and squeeze pressures), and complete response to treatment was present, respectively, in 86% versus 46% of patients, hence questioning whether the authors' conclusion about lack of differences was due to a type II error. However, the results of this study are confirmed by a large randomized study comparing different modalities of treatment (i.e. standard medical/nurse advice, advice plus verbal instruction on sphincter exercise, hospital-based computer-assisted sphincter pressure biofeedback, hospital biofeedback plus home EMG device), showing an overall improvement in 50% of patients, sustained at one year of follow-up, in all four groups [34]. These conclusions suggest that patient coping strategies and interaction with a therapist seem to play a key role in improvement of continence.

Predictors of outcome are not well established. Biofeedback can increase both rectal sensation and external anal sphincter contraction [35], but this improvement is not always associated with significant changes in any of the objective indices of sphincter function, or with symptom improvement [36]. Success has been correlated to structurally intact sphincters [30], while other studies did not find such correlation [37, 38]. Sphincter squeeze duration may be more important than strength [12, 39]. Success seems to correlate more with improvement in rectal sensation than with sphincteric strengthening [8, 40] and also with an increased feeling of control and self-confidence.

Poor prognostic factors for biofeedback outcome are dementia, cognitive impairment, anus deformity, megarectum [41], and total absence of rectal sensitivity [42]. Pudendal neuropathy seems to be a negative factor for biofeedback success [36, 43] even though in another study, symptomatic improvement was not precluded by neurological damage [36].

More recently, evidence has demonstrated that impaired defecatory maneuvers and younger age [44] are poor predictive factors of biofeedback outcome. The paradoxical coexistence of defecatory difficulties in incontinent patients is one worsening factor that has to be taken into account. Pre-existent dyssynergic defecation and excessive straining may lead to perineal damage [45, 46] that can eventually lead to frank fecal incontinence.

References

1. Chiarioni G, Ferri B, Morelli A et al. Biofeedback treatment of fecal incontinence: where are we, and where are we going? World J Gastroenterol 2005;11:4771–4775.
2. Whitehead WE, Wald A, Norton N. Treatment options for fecal incontinence: consensus conference report. Dis Colon Rectum 2001;44:131–144.
3. Heymen S, Jones KR, Ringel Y et al. Biofeedback treatment of fecal incontinence: a critical review. Dis Colon Rectum 2001;44:728–736.
4. Norton C, Kamm MA. Anal sphincter biofeedback and pelvic floor exercises for faecal incontinence in adults: a systematic review. Aliment Pharmacol Ther 2001;15:1147–1154.
5. Engel BT, Nikoomanesh P, Schuster MM. Operant conditioning of rectosphincteric responses in the treatment of fecal incontinence. N Engl J Med 1974;290:646–649.
6. Buser WD, Miner PB. Delayed rectal sensation with fecal incontinence. Successful treatment using anorectal manometry. Gastroenterology 1986;91:1186–1191.
7. Rao SS. Pathophysiology of adult fecal incontinence. Gastroenterology 2004;126:S14-S22.
8. Miner PB, Donnelly TC, Read NW. Investigation of mode of action of biofeedback in treatment of fecal incontinence. Dig Dis Sci 1990;35:1291–1298.
9. Solomon MJ, Rex J, Eyers AA et al. Biofeedback for fecal incontinence using transanal ultrasonography: novel approach. Dis Colon Rectum 2000;43:788–792.
10. Diamant NE, Kamm MA, Wald A et al. AGA technical review on anorectal testing techniques. Gastroenterology 1999;116:735–760.
11. MacLeod JH. Management of anal incontinence by biofeedback. Gastroenterology 1987;93:291–294.
12. Chiarioni G, Scattolini C, Bonfante F et al. Liquid stool incontinence with severe urgency: anorectal function and effective biofeedback treatment. Gut 1993;34:1576–1580.
13. Norton C, Hosker G, Brazzelli M. Effectiveness of biofeedback and/or sphincter exercises for the treatment of fecal incontinence in adults. Cochrane Database Syst Rev 2000;(2):CD002111.
14. Fernandez-Fraga X, Azpiroz F, Malagelada JR. Significance of pelvic floor muscles in anal incontinence. Gastroenterology 2002;123:1441–1450.
15. Loening-Baucke V. Efficacy of biofeedback training in improving faecal incontinence and anorectal physiologic function. Gut 1990;31:690–695.
16. Aziporz F, Fernandex-Fraga X, Merletti R et al. The puborectalis muscle. Neurogastroenterol Motil 2005;17(suppl 1):68–72.
17. Bharucha AE. Fecal incontinence. Gastroenterology 2003;124:1672–1685.
18. Whitehead WE, Wald A, Norton NJ. Treatment options for fecal incontinence. Dis Colon Rectum 2001;44:131–144.
19. Miller R, Bartolo DC, Cerbero F, Mortensen NJ. Anorectal sampling: a comparison of normal and incontinent patients. Br J Surg 1988;75:44–47.
20. Hoffmann BA, Timmcke AE, Gathright JB Jr et al. Fecal seepage and soiling: a problem of rectal sensation. Dis Colon Rectum 1995;38:746–748.
21. Rao SSC, Stessman M, Kempf J. Is biofeedback therapy (BT) useful in patients with anal seepage? Gastroenterology 1999;116:G4636.
22. Rao SSC, Patel RS. How useful are manometric tests of anorectal function in the management of defecation disorders? Am J Gastroenterol 1997;92:469–475.
23. Rao SSC, Welcher KD, Happel J. Can biofeedback therapy improve anorectal function in fecal incontinence? Am J Gastroenterol 1996;91:2360–2366.
24. Enck P. Biofeedback training in disordered defecation. A critical review. Dig Dis Sci 1993;38:1953–1960.
25. Rao SSC. The technical aspects of biofeedback therapy for defecation disorders. Gastroenterologist 1998;6:96–103.
26. Enck P, Daublin G, Lubke HJ et al. Long-term efficacy of biofeedback training for fecal incontinence. Dis Colon Rectum 1994;37:997–1001.
27. Ferrara A, De Jesus A, Gallagher JT et al. Time-related decay of the benefits of biofeedback therapy. Tech Coloproctol 2001;5:131–135.
28. Ozturk R, Niazi S, Stessman M et al. Long-term outcome and objective changes of anorectal function after biofeedback therapy for fecal incontinence. Aliment Pharmacol Ther 2004;20:667–674.
29. Norton C. Behavioral management of fecal incontinence in adults. Gastroenterology 2004;126:S64-S70.
30. Herbst F, Kamm MA, Morris GP et al. Gastrointestinal transit and prolonged ambulatory colonic motility in health and fecal incontinence. Gut 1997;41:381–389.
31. Norton C, Kamm MA. Outcome of biofeedback for fecal incontinence. Br J Surg 1999;86:1159–1163.
32. Emmanuel AV, Kamm MA. Successful response to biofeedback for constipation is associated with specifically improved extrinsic autonomic innervation to the large bowel. Gastroenterology 1997;112(suppl):A729.
33. Ilnyckyj A, Fachnie E, Tougas G. A randomized-controlled trial comparing an educational intervention alone vs education and biofeedback in the management of faecal incontinence in women. Neurogastroenterol Motil 2005; 17:58–63.
34. Norton C, Chelvanayregam S, Wilson-Barnett J et al. Randomized controlled trial of biofeedback for fecal incontinence. Gastroenterology 2003;125:1320–1329.
35. Berti Riboli E, Frascio M, Pitto G et al. Biofeedback conditioning for fecal incontinence. Arch Phys Med Rehabil 1988;69:29–31.
36. Bharucha AE. Outcome measures for fecal incontinence: anorectal structure and function. Gastroenterology 2004; 126:S90-S98.
37. Leroi AM, Dorival MP, Lecouturier MF et al. Pudendal neuropathy and severity of incontinence but not presence of an anal sphincter defect may determine the response to biofeedback therapy in fecal incontinence. Dis Colon Rectum 1999;42:762–769.

38. Rieger NA, Wattchow DA, Sarre RG et al. Prospective trial of pelvic floor retraining in patients with fecal incontinence. Dis Colon Rectum 1997;40:821–826.

39. Patankar SK, Ferrara A, Levy JR et al. Biofeedback in colorectal practice. Dis Colon Rectum 1997;40:827–831.

40. Wald A. Biofeedback for neurogenic fecal incontinence: rectal sensation is a determinant of outcome. J Pedriatr Gastroenterol Nutr 1983;2:302–306.

41. Whitehead WE, Thompson WG. Motility as a therapeutic modality. In: Schuster MM (ed) Atlas of gastrointestinal motility in health and disease. Williams & Wilkins, Baltimore, 1993, pp 300–316.

42. Cerulli MA, Nikoomanesh P, Schuster MM. Progress in bio-

feedback conditioning for fecal incontinence. Gastroenterology 1979;76:742–746.

43. Van Tets WF, Kuijpers JH, Bleijenberg G. Biofeedback treatment is ineffective in neurogenic fecal incontinence. Dis Colon Rectum 1996;39:992–994.

44. Fernandez-Fraga X, Azpiroz F, Aprici A et al. Predictors of response to biofeedback treatment in anal incontinence. Dis Colon Rectum 2003;46:1218–1225.

45. Kiff ES, Barnes PR, Swash M. Evidence of pudendal neuropathy in patients with perineal descent and chronic straining at stool. Gut 1984;25:1279–1282.

46. Snooks SJ, Barnes PR, Swash M et al. Damage to the innervation of the pelvic floor musculature in chronic constipation. Gastroenterology 1985;89:977–981.

Medical Treatment

35

Pier Francesco Almerigi, Valentina Ciaroni
and Gabriele Bazzocchi

Abstract Fecal incontinence is a common dysfunction whose prevalence is underestimated and increases with age. A conservative approach with changing of bowel habits, dietary modifications, and medical treatment may be considered for minor degrees of incontinence. The best choice of medical treatment can be reached through an accurate integration of clinical features and instrumental diagnostic results. The main goal of conservative treatment should be not the complete resolution of dysfunction but the improvement of symptoms and quality of life.

Keywords Alosetron • Amitryptiline • Bowel habits • Diarrhea • Fecal incontinence • Fiber implementation • Hygienic measures • Loperamide • Phenylephrine gel • Urgency

35.1 Introduction

Conservative treatment should always be the first approach in the management of fecal incontinence. In patients with minor degrees of incontinence this kind of therapy can avoid surgical intervention. Other indications for non-operative options are surgical failure and neuropathic incontinence. An accurate integration of clinical features and instrumental diagnostic results, in order to recognize the underlying causes, leads to the best management. Non-operative treatment includes bowel habit training, hygienic measures, dietary modification, and drug therapy (oral or topical).

35.2 Hygienic Measures

Patients affected by fecal incontinence deserve careful and accurate hygienic measures; in particular, institutionalized patients need to be followed by qualified personnel. These measures include cleaning the perianal skin after each soiling episode, avoiding skin excoriation, using appropriate soaps, and application of zinc oxide cream or calamine lotion [1], using disposable incontinence pads to protect the skin [2].

35.3 Bowel Habits

The use of laxatives may play a role in the treatment of overflow incontinence in patients with fecal impaction. These patients may benefit from a regular habit of rectal emptying with bisacodyl or glycerol enemas or suppositories, which has a demonstrated success rate in 60–80% of cases [3]. The daily use of osmotic laxative (lactulose 10 ml twice daily) in

P.F. Almerigi
Unit of General Surgery, Department of General Surgery
and Organ Transplantation, S. Orsola-Malpighi Hospital,
University of Bologna, Italy

association with a weekly enema has been shown to be effective in elderly patients with dementia [4]. Enemas are also useful to induce bowel movements and leave the rectum empty between evacuations.

35.4 Dietary Modification

Changes in dietary habits are effective in different conditions. First of all they are helpful in cases of lactose or fructose intolerance, in which dietary modifications can avoid diarrhea stools [5]. The use of fiber implementation is contraindicated in patients with fecal impaction [6], but psyllium and gum agar have been shown to be effective in reducing incontinence episodes and increasing stool consistency [7]. The intake of coffee should be reduced or avoided, since it has been shown that it tends to trigger the gastrocolonic reflex and to increase colonic motility [8].

35.5 Medical Treatment

The first goal of the medical treatment of fecal incontinence is to obtain solid stools. For this reason, any medical conditions predisposing to diarrhea have to be excluded and treated. These may include malabsorptive states, diabetes mellitus, dietary indiscretions, or all conditions of pseudo-obstruction. Adequate doses of antidiarrheals have to be used, and can also be employed for prophylactic use prior to a period of stress in patients with severe urgency, to achieve the aim of firmer stools.

Loperamide 4 mg, diphenoxylate 5 mg, or codeine sulfate 60 mg can be used regularly, up to four times daily. Loperamide increases colonic transit time [9], reduces stool weight [10], increases internal sphincter tone [11], and improves continence after proctectomy [12]. Diphenoxylate/atropine and codeine phosphate may be an alternative treatment with similar effectiveness [13].

In female patients with diarrhea-predominant irritable bowel syndrome (IBS-D), the use of serotonin axis agents (alosetron, ramosetron, piboserod) can be considered. These agents have been shown to be effective in slowing colonic transit, increasing colonic compliance to distension, and decreasing colonic hypersensitivity. These effects may be very useful in incontinent patients even if there are no data suggesting that they can improve fecal continence [14–16].

Amitryptiline (a tricyclic antidepressant) has been shown to be effective in the treatment of fecal incontinence [17]. It leads to the formation of firmer stool by increasing colonic transit time and decreasing the amplitude and frequency of the rectal motor complex [18].

Topical application of phenylephrine gel has been considered for patients with fecal incontinence due to internal anal sphincter weakness. This $\alpha 1$ agonist agent has been shown to be effective in increasing resting anal pressure in healthy subjects and in patients with fecal incontinence [19], although randomized trials are still disappointing [20].

References

1. Leung F, Rao SSC. Treatment of fecal incontinence in the elderly. In: Mezey MD, Callahan CM, Berkman BJ (eds) The encyclopedia of elder care: the comprhensive resource on geriatric and social care. Springer-Verlag, New York, 2001, p 2614.
2. Shirran E, Brazzelli M. Absorbent products for containing urinary and/or faecal incontinence in adults. Cochrane Database Syst Rev 2000;(2):CD001406.
3. Lowery SP, Srour JW, Whitehead WE et al. Habit training as treatment of encopresis secondary to chronic constipation. J Pediatric Gastroenterol Nutr 1985;4:397–401.
4. Tobin GW, Brocklehurst JC. Fecal incontinence in residential homes for the elderly: prevalence, aetiology and management. Age Ageing 1986;15:41–46.
5. Choi YK, Johlin FC Jr, Summers RW et al. Fructose intolerance: an under-recognized problem. Am J Gastroenterol 2003;98:1348–1353.
6. Voderholzer WA, Schatke W, Muhldorfer BE et al. Clinical response to dietary fiber treatment of chronic constipation. Am J Gastroenterol 1997;92:95–98.
7. Bliss DZ, Jung HJ, Savik K et al. Supplementation with dietary fiber improves fecal incontinence. Nurs Res 2001;50:203–213.
8. Rao SSC, Welcher K, Zimmerman B et al. Is coffee a colonic stimulant? Eur J Gastroenterol Hepatol 1998;10:113–118.
9. Sun WM, Read NW, Verlinden M. Effects of loperamide oxyde on gastrointestinal transit time and anorectal function in patients with chronic diarrhea and faecal incontinence. Scand J Gastroenterol 1997;32:34–38.
10. Herbst F, Kamm MA, Nicholls RJ. Effects of loperamide on ileoanal-pouch function. Br J Surg 1998;85:1428–1432.
11. Read M, Read NW, Barber DC et al. Effects of loperamide on anal sphincter function in patients complaining of chronic diarrhea with fecal incontinence and urgency. Dig Dis Sci 1982;27:807–814.
12. Hollgren T, Fasth S, Delbro DS et al. Loperamide improves anal sphincter function and continence after restorative proctocolectomy. Dig Dis Sci 1994;39:2612–2618.
13. Palmer KR, Corbett CL, Holdsworth CD. Double blind crossover study comparing loperamide, codeine and di-

phenoxylate in the treatment of chronic diarrhea. Gastro-enterology 1980;79:1272–1275.

14. Mayer EA, Berman S, Derbyshire SW et al. The effect of the 5-HT3 receptor antagonist, alosetron, on brain responses to visceral stimulation in irritable bowel syndrome patients. Aliment Pharmacol Ther 200216:1357–1366.

15. Andresen V, Hollerbach S. Reassessing the benefits and risks of alosetron: what is its place in the treatment of irritable bowel syndrome? Drug Saf 2004;27:283–292.

16. Bharuca AE, Camilleri M, Haydock S et al. Effects of a serotonin 5-HT receptor antagonist SB-207266 on gastrointestinal motor and sensory function in humans. Gut 2000;47:667–674.

17. Farrar JT. The effects of drugs on intestinal motility. Clin Gastroenterol 1982;11:673–681.

18. Santoro GA, Eitan BZ, Pryde A et al. Open study of low dose amitriptyline in the treatment of patients with idiopathic fecal incontinence. Dis Colon Rectum 2000; 43:1676–1681.

19. Cheetham MJ, Kamm MA, Phillips RK. Topical phenylephrine increases anal canal resting pressure in patients with faecal incontinence. Gut 2001;48:356–369.

20. Carapeti EA, Kamm MA, Phillips RK. Randomized controlled trial of topical phenylephrine in the treatment of faecal incontinence. Br J Surg 2000;87:38–42.

Fecal incontinence (FI) is a source of considerable stress for the individual affected and is a condition that causes a loss of self-esteem and a sense of social alienation.

The prevalence of FI approaches 1.3% in women aged 65 years or more, and has an incidence of 10.3% in residential homes for the elderly.

The main causes of major FI are disruption of the external anal sphincter (third-degree perineal tear and anal fistula surgery), pudendal neuropathy (diabetes), central nervous system pathologies (spinal cord lesions, tumors, multiple sclerosis), congenital malformations (ano-rectal atresias, and spinal dysraphism), severe chronic constipation, bowel inflammation (ulcerative colitis or radiation), and being frail elderly.

Minor FI can be the consequence of anal pathologies (hemorrhoids or rectal prolapse), other factors (including anxiety, medications, diet, alcohol, and caffeine), and weakness of the internal and/or external anal sphincters.

The committee of the International Consultation on Incontinence (ICI) recommends a trial of conservative and drug management [1] in the vast majority of patients before considering surgical treatment, because conservative management is comparatively inexpensive and involves no significant morbidity. Furthermore, this type of treatment can be employed by community-based healthcare providers for both primary and secondary prevention.

The management of FI will depend on the cause as well as whether the individual is an adult or a child. In adults it is obviously different in various types of pathologies (neurogenic and non-neurogenic), and requires a dedicated team.

In non-neurogenic patients, the initial assessment (history and examination) has the goal to primarily distinguish between urgency FI and passive loss of stool (passive FI). In all patients with FI, digital examination of the pelvic floor muscles shows weak or absent external anal sphincter activity.

The basic management includes patient information and education, diet and fluid advice, regular bowel habit, medical treatment (as reported by Almerigi et al, Chapter 35) and simple exercises (pelvic floor muscle training or PFMT) to enhance awareness and strengthening of the external anal sphincter and levator ani muscles.

PFMT is indicated as an early and low-cost intervention in the treatment of FI, being easier and more compliant for the patients: the program includes strengthening of phasic and tonic fibers of the levator ani and external anal sphincter in order to control fecal urgency, and deferring defecation during a bowel-retraining program. Unfortunately there is only weak evidence suggesting the efficacy of pelvic floor muscle exercises in FI.

This initial management can often be performed in primary care; in the case of failure after 8–12 weeks of treatment, further investigations and specialized management are needed. Biofeedback techniques and functional electrical stimulation are considered as specialized approaches. Biofeedback training is the focus of Chapter 34 by Salvioli and Pellegrini: it is indicated as a specialized implementation of a training program enabling "feedback" of the biological signal of the patient. The responses that are reinforced with a biofeedback training protocol include:

- the sensory perception associated with rectal distension and potential loss of stool

P. Di Benedetto
Department of Rehabilitation Medicine, Institute of Physical Medicine and Rehabilitation, University of Udine, Italy

G.A. Santoro, A.P. Wieczorek, C.I. Bartram (eds.) *Pelvic Floor Disorders*
© Springer-Verlag Italia 2010

- a short-latency contraction of the external anal sphincter
- an inhibition of abdominal activity that would increase rectal pressure.

Generally, biofeedback training protocols are applicable to patients with loss of coordination between rectal sensation and contraction of the external anal sphincter, which generally happens automatically with the urge to defecate. Biofeedback training can also be used to re-educate rectal sensation and improve patient awareness of rectal filling. Some patients are more motivated if they have some form of feedback to inform on correct muscle activity [2].

Regarding functional electrical stimulation, at present there are insufficient data to allow reliable conclusions to be drawn on its effects in the management of FI. Theoretically, functional electrical stimulation reduces urge FI (by activation of the pudendo-anal reflex), improves the body schema and the sensory function of the rectal ampulla, and (in association with PFMT) strengthens the pelvic floor muscles [3].

In the case of severe FI that fails to respond to this treatment, it is mandatory to take into consideration sphincteroplasty, gracilis transposition (with a low-frequency stimulator implanted), sacral nerve stimulation, artificial sphincter, or colostomy formation [1].

In neurogenic patients (notably in patients with spinal cord injury), effective management of the bowel is important not only to prevent gastrointestinal complications, but mainly for the psychosocial implications of the successful reintegration of the patients to their home and community, and for their quality of life. In these patients an effective bowel-management regimen must take into consideration:

- diet and nutritional factors
- use of pharmachological agents
- an appropriate program that is consistent with the neurological condition and needs of the individual

- other factors (availability of a caregiver, home accessibility, return to work and school).

A bowel program is a scheduled, regularly performed routine aimed at effectively evacuating the bowel in a timely and predictable manner, so that unplanned evacuations and the development of other gastrointestinal complications are avoided or minimized. The bowel program should be initiated early during the acute care period following the spinal cord lesion. The procedures obviously depend upon the level, the extent and completeness of the medullary lesion [4, 5].

There is no doubt that FI worsens the quality of life, and the results of the management and treatment are often frustrating, but sometimes they are definitely successful. For this reason and because of the importance of primary and secondary prevention of FI, more public awareness and major professional interest are needed in this neglected area in order to improve management of this embarrassing condition.

References

1. Norton C, Whitehead WE, Bliss DZ et al. Conservative and pharmachological management of faecal incontinence in adults. In: Abrams P, Cardozo L, Khoury S, Wein A (eds) Incontinence, Vol 2. Health Publication Ltd, Paris, 2005, pp 1523–1563.
2. Laycock J. Faecal incontinence: treatment. In: Laycock J, Haslam J (eds) Therapeutic management of incontinence and pelvic pain. Springer-Verlag, London Berlin Heidelberg, 2002, pp 136–137.
3. Sahlin Y, Berner E. Fecal Incontinence. In: Bø K, Berghmans B, Mørkved S, Van Kampen M (eds) Evidence-based physical therapy for the pelvic floor. Elsevier, Edinburgh London New York, 2007, pp 304–308.
4. Maynard F, Ardner M, Karunas B. Evaluation of a bowel program success in SCI. J Am Paraplegia Soc 1991;14:69.
5. Chen D, Nussbaum SB. The gastrointestinal system and bowel management following spinal cord injury. In: Hammond MC (ed) Topics in spinal cord injury medicine. Physical Medicine and Rehabilitation Clinics of North America. Saunders, Philadelphia London Toronto, 2000, pp 45–56.

Section VI
Pelvic Organ Prolapse

Pelvic Organ Prolapse: Introduction

Tomasz Rechberger

Pelvic organ prolapse (POP) represents a significant health as well as economic problem worldwide and may have a deleterious impact on a woman's quality of life; however, it rarely has significant morbidity or mortality. It is estimated that 25% of women older than 60 years suffer from some degree of POP, and more than 300,000 operations for POP are performed annually in the US alone [1, 2].

Pelvic organ prolapse among women, which is manifested by protrusion of the vagina or uterus out of the introitus, is caused by damage of the muscles, fascias, and ligaments that stabilize organs located in the pelvis [3]. Current understanding of this disorder is based on the assumption that support to the pelvic organs (urethra, bladder, uterus, and rectum) is provided directly by the vagina and indirectly by the structures involved in vaginal support [4, 5]. Therefore, it is generally accepted that any damage to components involved in the support mechanism can result in loss of vaginal stability and prolapse of the pelvic organs. The unique structure of the pelvic floor could be considered in terms of the complex interaction between the vagina and its supportive ligaments and fascias that are designed to withstand the downward descent of the pelvic organs in response to an increase in abdominal pressure. The etiology of POP is complex, involving a potential injury to the ligaments, muscles, connective tissue, and innervation of the pelvis. The incidence of POP is associated with several other factors including age, parity, abdominal circumference, and body mass index. Vaginal support defects may include a cystocele (a weakening of the vesicovaginal

musculo-connective tissue), a rectocele (a weakening of the rectovaginal musculo-connective tissue), a paravaginal defect (a defect in the level II support of the vagina at the level of the arcus tendinous fascia pelvis), or a defect in the level I apical support of the vagina (the cardinal-uterosacral ligament complex). Evaluation is typically performed with the patient in the dorsal lithotomy position. Clinical manifestation of these abnormalities, besides a subjective feeling of fullness in the introitus, is often accompanied by several functional disturbances such as stress and mixed urinary incontinence, difficulties in bladder emptying (especially in advanced prolapse), and various problems with bowel emptying. Stool incontinence, which occurs among 7% of patients with POP and as often as 31% among women with stress urinary incontinence (SUI), is usually not dependent on posterior vaginal wall prolapse [6, 7]. It is mainly a result of external anal sphincter damage caused by obstetric trauma; however, estrogen deprivation after menopause as well as aging itself are also considered causative factors [8, 9]. Advanced POP among sexually active women may cause avoidance behavior due to decreased self-esteem [10]. The most advanced prolapse could be even a causative factor for hydronephrosis and hydroureter; both of these anomalies almost always disappear after surgical correction of POP [11, 12].

The most common symptom which accompanies POP is the feeling of "something coming down" out of vagina [13]. Vaginal and low back pains are also symptoms that are relatively often reported by affected women, and the intensity of complaints parallels the clinical advancement of disease [14]. It has been shown that the number of patients suffering from common symptoms associated with POP increases rapidly with the advancement of the leading point below 1 cm of

T. Rechberger
2nd Department of Gynecology, Medical University of Lublin, Poland

the hymenal ring (Pelvic Organ Prolapse Quantification (POPQ) stage 2 and 3) [15]. In another study, investigators found that only 18% of patients reported symptoms of a vaginal bulge, and this increased up to 78% among women with stage 3 prolapse [16].

Epidemiological data concerning POP are relatively scarce and very often inconclusive, mainly due to the various definitions used by investigators. Few studies have attempted to describe and document the distribution of genital tract support abnormalities in female populations [17–19]. The main clinical message from all these studies is that a very large percentage of females had some relaxation of the pelvic floor, with 5–6% demonstrating prolapse beyond the introitus, which usually increased with the patient's age. Moreover, it is clear that racial and occupational factors are also important when studying the prevalence of POP [9, 20]. Estimated life risk for being operated due to POP is as high as 11%, and this risk is strictly age dependent [17]. The number of operations due to POP is 0.4 per 10,000 among the age group 20–29 years, and rises to 34 per 10,000 among women in their 70s. Brubaker et al reported that the risk for clinically important POP is 4% for the whole population, but of course numbers are much higher among patients seeking gynecological help [9].

According to the Oxford Family Planning Association, the most important risk factor for POP is vaginal delivery [21]. However, it should be stressed that fetal body weight > 4500 g, prolongation of the second stage of delivery, and use of forceps and vacuum extractor, which are established risk factors for SUI occurrence, do not markedly influence the progression of the disease [22]. Additional commonly cited risk factors for prolapse occurrence are obesity, stool impaction, occupational status, and lung diseases with protracted coughing [21–25]. Moreover, it has been suggested by Nguen et al that anatomical abnormalities of the bony pelvis, as well as abnormalities in the lumbosacral part of the vertebral column could also cause POP [26]. Menopause as a single risk factor for POP occurrence was reported by Swift [27]. However, other researchers have not confirmed this finding [28, 29].

Some congenital anomalies which predispose to POP are a decreased amount of type I collagen accompanied by an increased amount of type III collagen and fragmentation of elastin fibers, which causes increased elasticity of the extracellular matrix (ECM) components stabilizing the urogenital organs within the bony pelvis [4, 30, 31]. There is strong evidence that the quantity and quality of collagen in the pelvic support tissues of women with pelvic static disorders is inferior to that in women with normal support [32, 33]. Moreover, women affected by congenital connective tissue diseases such as Ehlers–Danlos syndrome and Marfan's syndrome have a higher risk of pelvic floor disorders, including pelvic organ prolapse and urinary incontinence, compared with unaffected individuals [34, 35]. It has also been shown that in genetically modified mice with a lack of elastin gene, POP was a normal occurrence due to interruption of the metabolic pathway of elastin synthesis and repair [36].

Therefore, Carley and Schaffer propose that POP should be considered a genetically caused disease [37]. Recently, Norton et al, using a linkage analysis, have presented significant evidence that a predisposition gene for pelvic floor disorders is located on chromosome 9 [38].

On the other hand, in a previously published study investigating the biomechanical properties of vaginal and systemic skin in women affected by POP, it was found that POP is a disease of vaginal, rather than systemic, supportive tissue [39].

Taking all these facts into account, we should consider POP as a multifactorial disease, with obstetric trauma as a main risk-predisposing factor [30].

From a clinical point of view, a proper classification system which enables physicians to objectively assess POP severity is of critical importance [40]. Lack of standardized terminology has meant that none of the previously used classification systems proposed by Porges (1963), Baden and Walker (1972), and Beecham (1980) were commonly used or accepted by various medical societies [3, 41–43] (Fig. VI.1).

There is currently only one genital tract prolapse classification system that has attained international acceptance and recognition: the POPQ, which has been developed by an international committee made up of members from the International Continence Society (ICS), the American Urogynecologic Society (AUGS), and the Society of Gynecologic Surgeons (SGS). This system has been formally recognized and adopted by these three societies [44]. It is a very precise system, which has shown good intra- as well as interexaminer reliability. This classification has been confirmed in recent IUGA/ISC joint report from 2010 [45]:

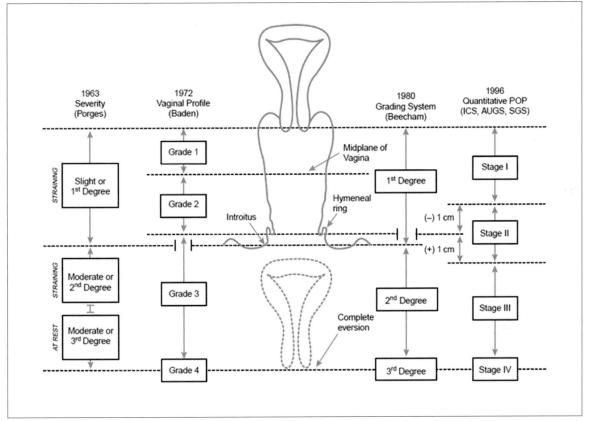

Fig. VI.1 Classification of pelvic organ prolapse according to various clinical classifications [43]. *AUGS*, American Urogynecologic Society; *ICS*, International Continence Society; *SGS*, Society of Gynecologic Surgeons. Modified from [43], with permission

Stage (0) No prolapse is demonstrated.

Stage (I) Most distal portion of the prolapse is more than 1 cm above the level of the hymen.

Stage (II) Most distal portion of the prolapse is 1 cm or less proximal to or distal to the plane of the hymen.

Stage (III) The most distam portion of the prolapse is more than 1 cm below the plane of the hymen.

Stage (IV) Complete eversion of the total lenght of the lower genital tract is demostrated.

However, some clinicians have claimed that it could be somewhat difficult to learn and use, and therefore the "half-way" vaginal profile proposed by Baden and Walker is more applicable to the clinical setting [46, 47] (Fig. VI.1).

At present, surgery is the only effective treatment for POP and can be performed by an abdominal or vaginal approach. The vaginal approach, while less invasive, is less efficient and still demands significant surgical skills as well as regional or general anesthesia and – in the majority of cases – hospitalization of at least 1–3 days [48]. Over the last ten years, many new, potentially more effective treatments have been developed, mainly based on introduction of artificial polypropylene as well as xenogenic prostheses in order to reinforce connective tissue support of the female pelvic organs [49].

Moreover, this new type of surgery, besides being less invasive, pays much more attention not only to the anatomical but also to the functional outcome of the procedure, especially in terms of bladder and bowel functions as well as vaginal coital capacity. It has been estimated that, due to demographic trends, the need for prolapse surgery may increase by as much as 45% in the near future [50]. This increase in demand will necessitate attempts to improve surgical outcomes, and this could be mainly achieved by a much better understanding of the real nature of POP [51, 52]. Therefore, it is imperative to develop animal models (although there is no perfect substitute for a human) that will enable better understanding of the mechanics of pelvic floor disorders.

References

1. Boyles SH, Weber AM, Men L. Procedures for pelvic organ prolapse in the United States, 1979–1997. Am J Obstet Gynecol 2003;188:108–115.
2. Boyles SH, Weber AM, Meyn L. Procedures for urinary incontinence in the United States, 1979–1997. Am J Obstet Gynecol 2003;189:70–75.
3. Tegerstedt G. Clinical and epidemiological aspects of pelvic floor dysfunction. Thesis. Stockholm: Department of Obstetrics and Gynaecology, Stockholm Söder Hospital Department of Medical Epidemiology and Biostatistics, Clinical Epidemiology Unit, Söder Hospital, 2004.
4. Norton PA. Pelvic floor disorders: the role of fascia and ligaments. Clin Obstet Gynecol 1993;36:926–938.
5. DeLancey JO. The anatomy of the pelvic floor. Curr Opin Obstet Gynecol 1994;6:313–316.
6. Jackson SL, Weber AM, Hull TL et al. Fecal incontinence in women with urinary incontinence and pelvic organ prolapse. Obstet Gynecol 1997;89:423–427.
7. Zetterstrom J, Lopez A, Holmstrom B et al. Obstetric sphincter tears and anal incontinence: an observational follow-up study. Acta Obstet Gynecol Scand 2003;82:921–928.
8. Johnston S. Urogenital health. J Obstet Gynecol Can 2001;23:973–977.
9. Brubaker L, Bump R, Jacquetin B et al. (2002) Pelvic organ prolapse. In: Abrams P, Cardozo L, Khoury A. Incontinence. 2 edn. Health Publication Ltd, Plymouth, pp 243–265.
10. Ellerkmann RM, Cundiff GW, Melick CF et al. Correlation of symptoms with location and severity of pelvic organ prolapse. Am J Obstet Gynecol 2001;185:1332–1337; discussion 1337–1338.
11. Barrington JW, Edwards G. Posthysterectomy vault prolapse. Int Urogynecol J Pelvic Floor Dysfunc 2000;11:241–224.
12. Yanik FF, Akpolat T, Kocak I. Acute renal failure- an unusual consequence of uterine prolapse. Nephrol Dial Transplant 1998;13:2648–2650.
13. Shaw W. The Manchester Operation for Genital Prolapse. J Obstet Gynaecol Brit Emp 1947;54:633–635.
14. Swift SE, Tate SB, Nicholas J. Correlation of symptoms with degree of pelvic organ support in a general population of women: what is pelvic organ prolapse? Am J Obstet Gynecol 2003;189:372–377; discussion 377–379.
15. Swift S, Pound T, Dias J. Case-control study of the etiology of severe pelvic organ prolapse. Int Urogynecol J 2001;12:176–192.
16. Otto L, Urankar R, Clark A. Correlation of symptoms of pelvic organ prolapse to clinical stage [Abstract]. Int Urogynecol J 1999;10(suppl 1):S25.
17. Samuelsson EU, Victor FTA, Tibblin G, Svardsudd KF. Signs of genital prolapse in a Swedish population of women 20 to 59 years of age and possible related factors. Am J Obstet Gynecol 1999;180:299–305.
18. Bland DR, Earle BB, Vitolins MZ, Burke G. Use of the pelvic organ prolapse staging system of the International Continence Society, American Urogynecologic Society, and the Society of Gynecologic Surgeons in perimenopausal women. Am J Obstet Gynecol 1999;181:1324–1328.
19. Versi E, Harvey M, Cardozo L et al. Urogenital prolapse and atrophy at menopause: a prevalence study. Int Urogynecol J 2001;12:107–110.
20. Muir TW, Stepp KJ, Barber MD. Adoption of the pelvic organ prolapse quantification system in peer-reviewed literature. Am J Obstet Gynecol 2003;189:1632–1635.
21. Mant J, Painter R, Vessey M. Epidemiology of genital prolapse: observation from the Oxford Family Planning Association study. Br J Obstet Gynaecol 1997;104:579–585.
22. Rinne KM, Kirkinen PP. What predisposes young women to genital prolapse? Eur J Obstet Gynaecol Reprod Biol 1999;84:23–25.
23. Davis GD. Uterine prolapse after laparoscopic uterosacral transection in nulliparous airborne trainees: a report of three cases. J Reprod Med 1996;41:279–282.
24. Jorgensen S, Hein HO, Gyntelberg F. Heavy lifting at work and risk of genital prolapse and herniated lumbar disc in assistant nurses. Occup Med 1994;44:47–49.
25. Lubowski DZ, Swash M, Nichols J, Henry MM. Increases in pudendal nerve terminal motor latency with defecation straining. Br J Surg 1988;75:1095–1097.
26. Nguyen JK, Lind LR, Choe JY et al. Lumbosacral spine and pelvic inlet changes associated with pelvic organ prolapse. Obstet Gynecol 2000;95:332–336.
27. Swift SE. The distribution of pelvic organ support in a population of female subjects seen for routine gynecologic health care. Am J Obstet Gynecol 2000; 183:L277–285.
28. Olsen AL, Smith VJ, Bergstrom JO et al. Epidemiology of surgically managed pelvic organ prolapse and urinary incontinence. Obstet Gynecol 1997;89:501–506.
29. Progetto Menopausa Italia Study Group. Risk factors for genital prolapse in non-hysterectomized women around menopause- results from a large cross-sectional study in menopausal clinics in Italy. Eur J Obstet Gynaecol Reprod Biol 2000;93:124–140.
30. Koduri S, Sand PK. Recent developments in pelvic organ prolapse. Cur Opin Obstet Gynecol 2000;12:399–404.
31. Norton PA, Baker JE, Sharp HC, Warenski JC. Genitourinary prolapse and joint hypermobility in women. Obstet Gynecol 1995;85:225–228.
32. Jackson SR, Avery NC, Tarlton JF et al. Changes in metabolism of collagen in genitourinary prolapse. Lancet 1996;347:1658–1661.
33. Makinen J, Soderstrom KO, Kiilholma P, Hirvonen T. Histological changes in the vaginal connective tissue of patients with and without uterine prolapse. Arch Gynecol 1986;239:17–20.
34. McIntosh LJ, Stanitski DF, Mallett VT et al. Ehlers–Danlos syndrome: relationship between joint hypermobility, urinary incontinence, and pelvic floor prolapse. Gynecol Obstet Invest 1996;41:135–139.
35. McIntosh LJ, Mallett VT, Frahm JD et al. Gynecologic di-

sorders in women with Ehlers-Danlos syndrome. J Soc Gynecol Investig 1995;2:559–564.

36. Liu X, Zhao Y, Gao J et al. Elastic fiber homeostasis requires lysyl oxidase-like 1 protein. Nat Genet 2004;36:178–182.

37. Carley ME, Schaffer J. Urinary incontinence and pelvic organ prolapse with Marfan or Ehlers-Danlos syndrome. Am J Obstet Gynecol 2000;182:1021–1023.

38. Allen-Brady K, Norton PA, Farnham JM et al. Significant evidence for a predisposition gene for pelvic floor disorders on chromosome 9. Am J Hum Genet 2009;84:678–682.

39. Epstein LB, Graham CA, Heit MH. Systemic and vaginal biomechanical properties of women with normal vaginal support and pelvic organ prolapse. Am J Obstet Gynecol 2007;197:165.e1–165.e6.

40. Emge LA, Durfee RB. Pelvic organ prolapse: four thousand years of treatment. Clin Obstet Gynecol 1966;9:997–1032.

41. Baden WF, Walker TA. Genesis of the vaginal profile: a correlated classification of vaginal relaxation. Clin Obstet Gynecol 1972;15:1048–1054.

42. Beecham CT. Classification of vaginal relaxation. Am J Obstet Gynecol 1980;136:957–958.

43. Theofrastous JP, Swift SE. The clinical evaluation of pelvic floor dysfunction. Obstet Gynecol Clin North Am 1998; 25:783–804.

44. Bump RC, Mattiasson A, Bo K et al. The standardization of terminology of female pelvic floor dysfunction. Am J Obstet Gynecol 1996;175:10–17.

45. Haylen BT, de Ridder D, Freeman RM et al. An International Urogynecological Association (IUGA)/ International Continence Society (ICS) joint report on the terminology for female pelvic floor dysfunction, Int Urogynecol J 2010;21:5-26

46. Hall AF, Theofrastous JP, Cundiff GC et al. Interobserver and intraobserver reliability of the proposed International Continence Society, Society of Gynecologic Surgeons, and American Urogynecologic Society pelvic organ prolapse classification system. Am J Obstet Gynecol 1996;175: 1467–1471.

47. Kobak WH, Rosenberger K, Walters MD. Interobserver variation in the assessment of pelvic organ prolapse. Int Urogynecol J 1996;7:121–124.

48. Davila GW, Guerette N. Current treatment options for female urinary incontinence – a review. Int J Fertil Womens Med 2004;49:102–112.

49. Birch C, Fynes MM. The role of synthetic and biological prostheses in reconstructive pelvic floor surgery. Curr Opin Obstet Gynecol 2002;14:527–535.

50. Luber KM, Boero S, Choe JY. The demographics of pelvic floor disorders: current observations and future projections. Am J Obstet Gynecol 2001;184:1496–1501.

51. DeLancey JOL. The hidden epidemic of pelvic floor dysfunction: achievable goals for improved prevention and treatment. Am J Obstet Gynecol 2005;192:1488–1495.

52. Abramowitch SD, Feola A, Jallah ZA, Moalli PA. Tissue mechanics, animal models, and pelvic organ prolapse: a review. Eur J Obstet Gynecol Reprod Biol 2009;144S:S146–S158.

Clive I. Bartram

Abstract Pelvic floor prolapse occurs with decompensation of the support mechanisms, notably the levator ani muscle and pelvic floor fascia, which may be secondary to local trauma, diffuse weakening from menopause or ageing, and, above all, muscle atrophy. Muscle weakness exposes the pelvic ligaments to persistent stretching, for which they are not designed, and once they give way organ prolapse results. The etiology of prolapse is therefore complex. Imaging, particularly with modalities giving an overview of the pelvis, such as magnetic resonance imaging (MRI), and to a lesser extent ultrasound, are ideally suited to establish the extent and severity of organ prolapse and specific damage to the support structures that may be more extensive than clinically apparent, and to show the underlying weakness of pelvic floor musculature. Imaging is therefore a key to our understanding and management of pelvic floor prolapse.

Keywords Cystocele • Defecography • Enterocele • Magnetic resonance imaging • Pelvic floor • Rectal prolapse • Ultrasonography • Uterine prolapse

In the 1970s, the application of neurophysiological techniques to the pelvic floor demonstrated a connection between nerve damage, muscle atrophy [1], and pelvic floor dysfunction. This illustrates how understanding of these disorders has been based on an accumulation of knowledge from various disciplines. In imaging, the establishment of diagnostic criteria draws heavily on detailed comparisons with clinical, histological, and neurophysiological findings. However, once achieved, an imaging study may reveal more than is suspected clinically, and the ease and safety of most examinations allows the incidence to be established in relatively large groups. Progress in the management and understanding of pelvic floor dysfunction has been based on innovation, with interaction and integration between clinical and radiological fields.

An excellent analogy of how the pelvic floor works is the "boat in a dry dock" by Norton [2]. The boat is normally supported by water – the levator ani muscles – and stabilized by its moorings – the pelvic floor ligaments. The boat needs its water support to function normally, and if the water is taken out, because the moorings are not made to withstand such stress, the boat will topple over. Likewise, if the levator ani is weakened for any reason, the endopelvic fascia will be put under continuous strain for which it is not designed, so the pelvic floor will decompensate, resulting in generalized descent and prolapse.

C.I. Bartram
Diagnostic Imaging, Princess Grace Hospital,
London, UK

G.A. Santoro, A.P. Wieczorek, C.I. Bartram (eds.) *Pelvic Floor Disorders*
© Springer-Verlag Italia 2010

The "dry dock" concept may be applied to a number of particular stresses: notably childbirth, menopause, and ageing. These can produce a variety of either diffuse or localized abnormalities. So, for example, vaginal delivery may seem on initial inspection to just affect the anal sphincter, but imaging may show that there are also tears in the levator ani and pubocervical fascia. There may also be damage to the pudendal nerve that will lead to muscle atrophy and summate with the focal tears to cause weakening of the pelvic floor structure, though perhaps initially not to the point where there is overt decompensation. However, when other factors come into play, such as the menopause and the effects of ageing, what started as a seemingly trivial injury may then present with extensive global dysfunction and problems such as pelvic organ prolapse.

Endoanal ultrasound first drew attention to the relatively high incidence of occult sphincter tears after vaginal delivery [3] and shows the sphincters in considerable detail. The striated muscle fascicles are contained in a complex connective tissue fascia that creates the typical acoustic pattern of this layer. The outer and inner boundaries of the external sphincter are demarcated by interface reflections. Loss of the outer interface reflection, and increased reflectivity of the external anal sphincter layer, provide good evidence of atrophy [4], but magnetic resonance imaging (MRI) is able to show this more directly as there is a clear distinction between the low signal from muscle and the high signal from fat, allowing the muscle volume and percentage of fat replacement to be calculated [5]. Most of the original work on atrophy used an MRI endocoil that is no longer available commercially. However, atrophy can be diagnosed on high-quality external phased array MRI [6], and developments using spectroscopy (Fig. 36.1) are promising, showing good correlation between an increased lipid peak and levator weakness on dynamometry [7]. The integration between clinical testing and imaging is again seen, with reduced vaginal closure force and levator defects [8], and distorted pelvic architecture on

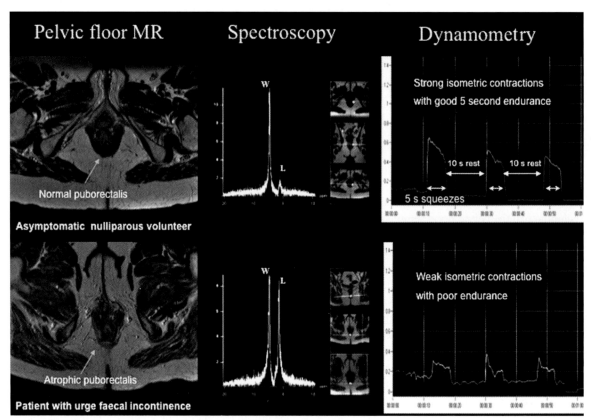

Fig. 36.1 Magnetic resonance spectroscopy of an atrophic puborectalis showing an increased lipid (*L*) peak (*W* = resonance peak for water) in a patient with fecal incontinence with corresponding weak contractions and increased fatiguability on dynamometry. Figure kindly supplied by Dr Chatoor, University College London Hospital

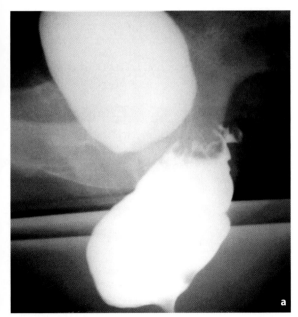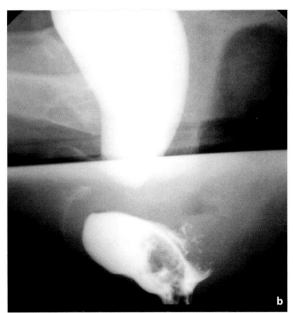

Fig. 36.2 a There is marked pelvic floor descent at rest, but with the rectum filled (**a**) no cystocele is apparent. However, when the rectum empties (except for trapping in a rectocele), in **b**, the vacated space in the pelvic outlet is filled by a large cystocele

MRI with prolapse [9]. Endoanal ultrasound has a limited window on the extent of atrophy, whereas with MRI the entire levator may be assessed. The morphology of the levator ani relates to the strength of the pelvic floor, and its susceptibility to prolapse.

The tone of the pelvic floor is reflected by the position of the anorectal junction at rest in relation to the pubococcygeal line, its strength by the lift on voluntary contraction, and sphincter function on urinary and rectal voiding. All these may be studied on dynamic fluoroscopy, which, although it has a radiation penalty, remains a simple and cost-effective method for studying evacuatory and prolapse problems. The main limitation is that only opacified structures are visualized, and lesions such as levator tears have to be inferred from relatively gross positional changes of opacified organs. The view also tends to be very compartmentalized, unless extended examinations with opacification of the bladder, rectum and vagina, and even the peritoneal cavity are undertaken to give a more global view. In one study, peritoneography was used to show that deep rectogenital pouches are common in constipation [10]. About half fill with bowel during evacuation but this did not impede rectal emptying, disproving an earlier concept of "defecation block". The "crowded pelvis" [11] was a term based on observations of combined bladder and rectal studies showing that cystoceles might only become apparent when the rectum empties

(Fig. 36.2), and enteroceles when both have emptied, owing to the space limitations within the bony pelvis. Dynamic MRI has recently shown that anorectal redundancy contributes to intrarectal intussusception in the solitary rectal ulcer syndrome [12]. Dynamic MRI may also find levator ani hernias [13] that are unsuspected on cystocolpoproctography, and this may alter surgical management.

MRI has many advantages: freedom from radiation hazard, excellent anatomical detail and soft tissue differentiation, dynamic information, and a global view that can easily relate organs to a fixed bony point such as the pubococcygeal line. Dynamic imaging was initially limited to studies during rest/stress maneuvers to show pelvic floor relaxation. Later evacuatory examinations [14] were developed to show voiding function and events that may occur only at the end of maximal pelvic floor straining and rectal emptying, such as intussusception, and trapping in rectoceles and enteroceles. Dynamic ultrasound examinations of the pelvic floor have been facilitated by developments in 3D imaging, and are now playing a growing investigative role [15], having many of the imaging advantages of magnetic resonance, with the added benefits of ease of examination and cost.

Patients may be inhibited in discussing pelvic floor problems, or in straining adequately during clinical examination for fear of inadvertent incontinence. Imaging is a powerful tool to allocate patients into treatment-defined groups, and in revealing important background problems related to prolapse, notably muscle tears and atrophy [16]. Most pelvic floor dysfunction is complex and multifactorial. Imaging is a key element in providing a global view of prolapse, its severity, and associated damage to pelvic floor structures. During the last decade there have been important advances in how these are imaged, and continued work as to their clinical relevance and impact in patient management.

References

1. Henry MM, Parks AG, Swash M. The pelvic floor musculature in the descending perineum syndrome. Br J Surg 1985;69:470–472.
2. Norton PA. Pelvic floor disorders: the role of fascia and ligaments. Clin Obstet Gynecol 1993;36:926–938.
3. Sultan AH, Kamm MA, Hudson CN et al. Anal-sphincter disruption during vaginal delivery. N Engl J Med 1993; 23:1905–1911.
4. Cazemeir M, Terra MP, Stoker J et al. Atrophy and defects detection of the external anal sphincter: comparison between three-dimensional anal endosonography and endoanal magnetic resonance imaging. Dis Colon Rectum 2006;49:20–27.
5. Williams AB, Bartram CI, Modwadia D. Endocoil magnetic resonance imaging quantification of external sphincter atrophy. Br J Surg 200188:853–859.
6. Terra MP, Betts-Tan RG, van der Hulst VPM et al. MRI in evaluation atrophy of the external sphincter in patients with fecal incontinence. AJR Am J Roentgenol 2006;187:991–999.
7. Chatoor DR, Emmanuel AV, De Vita E et al. Tissue characterisation and strength of the puborectalis muscle. Colorectal Dis 2008;10(suppl 1):39.
8. DeLancey JO, Morgan DM, Fenner DE et al. Comparison of levator ani muscle defects and function on women with and without pelvic organ prolapse. Obstet Gynecol 2007; 109:295–302.
9. Huebner M, Margulies RU, DeLancey JO. Pelvic architectural distortion is associated with pelvic organ prolapse. Int Urogynecol 2008;19:863–867.
10. Halligan S, Bartram C, Hall C, Wingate J. Enterocoele revealed by simultaneous evacuation proctography and peritoneography: does "defecation block" exist? AJR Am J Roentgenol 1996;167:461–466.
11. Kelvin FM, Maglinte DDT. Dynamic cystoproctography of the female pelvis and their interrelationships AJR Am J Roentgenol 1997;169:769–774.
12. Ortega AE, Klipfel N, Kelso R et al. Changing concepts in the pathogenesis, evaluation and management of solitary rectal ulcer syndrome. Am Surg 2008;74:967–972.
13. Kaufman HS, Buller JL, Thomson JR et al. Dynamic pelvic magnetic resonance imaging and cystocolpoproctography alter surgical management of pelvic floor disorders. Dis Colon Rectum 2001;44:1583–1584.
14. Colaiacomo MC, Masselli G, Polettini E et al. Dynamic MR imaging of the pelvic floor: a pictorial review. Radiographics 2009;29:e35, epub ahead of print.
15. Dietz HP, Simpson J. Levator trauma is associated with pelvic organ prolapse. Br J Obstet Gynecol 2008;115:979–984.
16. Bharucha AE, Fletcher JG, Harper CM et al. Relationship between symptoms and disordered continence mechanisms in women with idiopathic faecal incontinence. Gut 2005;54:546–555.

Endoluminal Ultrasonography

37

Giulio Aniello Santoro, Andrzej Paweł Wieczorek,
Magdalena Maria Woźniak and Aleksandra Stankiewicz

Abstract The pathophysiology of pelvic organ prolapse (POP) is complex. The most common mechanisms underlying pelvic floor disorders are represented by damages to the connective tissue supporting the pelvic organs and to the levator ani muscle occurring during childbirth. Management of POP still seems to be guided largely by personal preferences and experience rather than evidence-based medicine. Diagnostic tests frequently result in a revised initial management plan; however, no guidelines exist concerning their optimal use in a clinical practice setting, and their use as a routine strategy appears not to be an option. The advent of high-resolution three-dimensional ultrasonography and dynamic ultrasonography has improved our understanding of pelvic floor function. On the basis of ultrasonographic findings, additional tests may be performed in selected conditions to optimize treatment planning and to identify the reason for surgical failure.

Keywords Cystocele • Endoanal ultrasonography • Endovaginal ultrasonography • Enterocele • Intussusception • Levator ani • Pelvic organ prolapse • Pubovisceral muscle • Rectocele • Three-dimensional ultrasonography

37.1 Introduction

Pelvic organ prolapse (POP) is a very common clinical problem that affects more than 30% of women aged 50 years and older [1, 2]. In the United States, it is estimated that one in every ten women will require surgical therapy for pelvic organ dysfunction. Unfortunately, up to 30% of operations performed each year for POP are unsuccessful [2–4]. Once a female has undergone surgery for POP, her risk of developing a further prolapse is 500% greater than in the general population. This indicates the necessity for a precise

diagnosis of the nature and severity of the POP and of the interrelationships of the pelvic organs, to obtain an adequate correction of the underlying structural alterations that lead to prolapse. Moreover, little is known about those factors that prevent or promote recurrence of prolapse after repair. Most patients are selected for treatment on the basis of clinical history and physical examination with POP Quantification (POP-Q) scoring. The pelvic examination, however, does not provide adequate information on the fascial and muscular defects underlying a specific disease. For this reason, the use of additional diagnostic tests may be very helpful in the assessment of pelvic floor disorders to improve our approach to surgical repair of POP and to identify the reasons for the high rate of surgical failure. However, due to a lack of evidence for their clinical value,

G.A. Santoro
Pelvic Floor Unit and Colorectal service, 1st Department
of General Surgery, Regional Hospital, Treviso, Italy

G.A. Santoro, A.P. Wieczorek, C.I. Bartram (eds.) *Pelvic Floor Disorders*
© Springer-Verlag Italia 2010

no guidelines exist to date concerning the optimal use of these tests in a clinical practice setting.

Techniques for imaging of the pelvic floor, including evacuation proctography, cystocolpodefecography, voiding cystourethrography, dynamic magnetic resonance imaging (MRI), and ultrasonography, are valuable to quantify and define pelvic floor support [5].

Defecography represents a long-established diagnostic procedure for the investigation of posterior compartment disorders [6] (see Chapter 39). However, controversy still exists as to the interpretation and clinical utility of this modality, largely due to absent or imperfect reference standards for comparison. Furthermore, defecography is uncomfortable for the patient, requires exposure to ionizing radiation, and, when used without opacification of the bladder, lacks the ability to visualize the anterior and central compartments. Cystocolpodefecography is even more invasive, poorly tolerated, and requires an additional radiation dose.

Recently, more advanced imaging modalities have become available, such as MR defecography, and dynamic and three-dimensional (3D) ultrasonography. MR defecography is a much more comprehensive examination that allows assessment of coexisting bladder and uterocervical prolapse, which is fundamental when planning surgical treatment [7] (see Chapter 40). Moreover, MRI may determine the architectural distortion associated with pelvic prolapse [8]. However, this technique is very expensive, time consuming and limited to referral centers.

Ultrasonography has become an established procedure in the diagnostic evaluation of pelvic floor disorders [9]. Ultrasound examination has several important advantages over other imaging modalities: absence of ionizing radiation, relatively easy to perform, minimal discomfort, cost-effectiveness, reduced time requirement, and wide availability. Two-dimensional transperineal ultrasonography (2D-TPUS), and more recently 3D-TPUS, can define the presence of cystocele or recto/enterocele, hypermobility of the urethra, and levator ani damage [10] (see Chapter 38). However, TPUS is not able to evaluate precisely the disorders of the central and posterior compartment of the pelvic floor, as reported by Broekhuis et al [11]. These authors compared TPUS and dynamic MRI in patients with POP and found a good correlation in the assessment of the anterior compartment but no correlation regarding assessment of the posterior and central compartments. The recent advent of high-frequency 3D en-

dovaginal (3D-EVUS), 3D endoanal (3D-EAUS), and dynamic endovaginal ultrasonography provide us with a new alternative to visualize the pelvic floor structures and to evaluate all pelvic organ movements [12, 13].

This chapter reviews the indications, results, and limitations of endoluminal ultrasonography and illustrates morphologic and functional ultrasonographic features in patients with POP. The techniques of examination and normal pelvic floor anatomy were previously reported in detail in Chapters 6 and 8.

37.2   Levator Ani Damage

The levator ani muscle is thought to be of central importance for pelvic organ support, and levator trauma seems to be a major cause of POP in parous woman [14]. DeLancey et al [15] have found that women with POP have an odds ratio of 7.3 for having a major levator injury compared with asymptomatic women. Levator tears and avulsion are the most common consequence of hyperstretching of the levator ani during the second stage of labor [16] (see Chapter 12). Disconnection of the levator ani from its insertion on the inferior pubic ramus and the pelvic sidewall occurs in 15–36% of POP patients, according to many studies [2, 3, 17, 18]. Anatomically, the levator ani muscle and the connective supportive structures (uterosacral

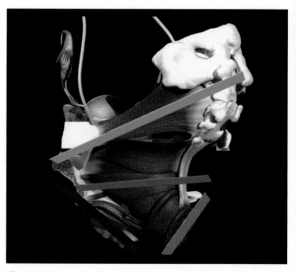

Fig. 37.1 Schematic illustration showing that the various pelvic floor structures are located in different planes (*gray plane*: pubococcygeous muscle; *green plane*: puborectalis muscle; *blue plane*: anal triangle of perineum; *violet plane*: urogenital triangle of perineum) (© Primal Pictures Ltd., with permission)

ligaments, endopelvic, pubocervical, and rectovaginal fascia) are partners in providing pelvic support. A healthy levator ani with normal tone prevents transmission of pressure to connective tissue. Once the muscle is damaged, the area of the levator hiatus through which the urethra, vagina, and anal canal traverse to enter into the perineum, increases. As a consequence, the ligaments are burdened to carry an increasing share of the load, which may, over time, result in connective tissue failure and development of prolapse. Huebner et al [8] reported an odds ratio of 8.3 for POP when both levator defect and architectural distortion to the connective structures were present. Levator ani defects

appeared to be a necessary condition for architectural distortion to occur. These authors found that women with anterior predominant prolapse were more likely than those with posterior or apical prolapse to have levator defects and architectural distortion [8].

Levator tear and damage to the connective tissues can be difficult to detect clinically, and bilateral or symmetric defects and thinning of the levator ani may be overestimated or underestimated by palpation of the muscle alone [19]. Modern imaging techniques enable visualization of the morphology of the levator ani, levator hiatus, and pelvic fascia and ligaments [6, 8–19]. As the defect itself is still not unequivocally defined, levator ani trauma can

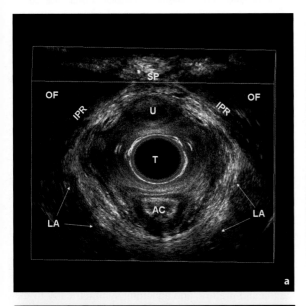

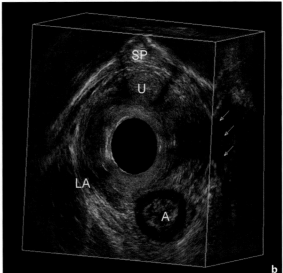

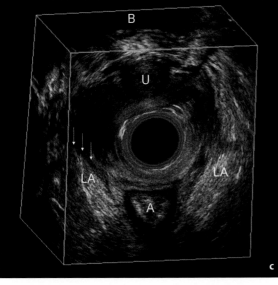

Fig. 37.2 Three-dimensional endovaginal ultrasonography with rotating transducer. **a** Normal female. Levator ani (*LA*) avulsion from the left (**b**) and right (**c**) pubic rami (*arrows*). *A*, anal canal; *B*, bladder; *IPR*, inferior pubic rami; *OF*, obturator foramen; *SP*, symphysis pubis; *T*, transducer; *U*, urethra

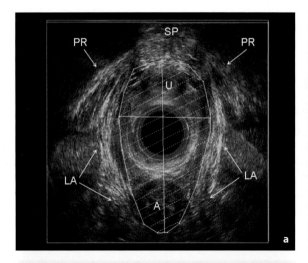

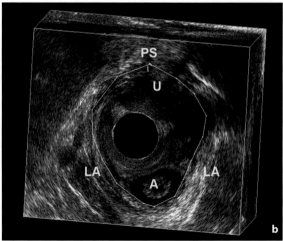

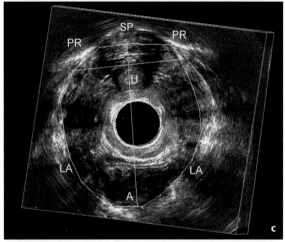

Fig. 37.3 Three-dimensional endovaginal ultrasonography with rotating transducer. The levator hiatal area, measured in the axial plane, increases with the POP-Q stage.
a Normal female: 12.4 cm^2. **b** POP-Q stage II: 17.5 cm^2.
c POP-Q stage III: 24 cm^2. *A*, anal canal; *LA*, levator ani muscle; *PR*, pubic rami; *SP*, symphysis pubis; *U*, urethra

be indirectly assessed by measurement of the levator hiatus by ultrasonograhpy. Athanasiou et al [20] reported that high-frequency 2D-EVUS allows assessment of levator function at rest and during contraction and Valsalva maneuver in the axial plane. They found that levator hiatal area was significantly larger in women with prolapse compared with those without (17.8 cm^2 vs. 13.5 cm^2). The authors demonstrated that the greater the prolapse staging the larger the hiatal area (P < 0.001), as assessed by the maximum descent of the leading organ.

High-resolution 3D-EVUS allows detailed visualization of the complex anatomy of the pelvic floor structures in their proper planes (axial, coronal, sagittal, and oblique), clarifying their spatial relationship (Figs. 6.13, 37.1). Compared to 3D-TPUS, the resolution of 3D-EVUS is theoretically better because the probe is closer to the pelvic floor structures. In healthy asymptomatic women, a normal levator ani appears as a well-defined horseshoe-shaped muscular structure surrounding the anus from its posterior part, localized laterally to the vagina and urethra, and attaching symmetrically to the pubic rami [15] (Fig. 6.15). Levator ani defects or avulsion can be precisely visualized and localized (Fig. 37.2). Moreover, the biometric indices of the levator hiatus can be determined in various POP-Q stages (Figs. 6.16, 37.3).

This technique also allows identification of defects in the connective tissue, such as detachment of the vaginal sulci from the lateral pelvic sidewall, with unilateral or bilateral widening of the paravaginal spaces, and asymmetry of the urethra and anus (Fig. 37.4).

37.3 Cystocele

Cystocele refers to prolapse of the bladder (Fig. 37.5). It is common in elderly women and may cause symptoms such as pelvic heaviness, dryness of the vagina, discomfort, and difficulties in emptying the bladder [21]. An isolated anterior vaginal wall prolapse is usually not difficult to diagnose at clinical examination. However, cystocele frequently coexists with other disorders involving the middle and the posterior compartments, such as uterine prolapse, rectocele, enterocele, and peritoneocele [22, 23]. In these cases it is sometimes difficult to establish a correct diagnosis at clinical examination only. Radiological examination is therefore used to complement the clinical assessment. Cystodefecoperitoneography is the most commonly used method, where contrast medium in the urinary bladder enables visualization of the bladder base. However, several studies [24, 25] have demonstrated a relatively poor correlation between clinical examination and radiological findings, suggesting that the contrast in the bladder is not useful in the routine preoperative assessment of patients with genital prolapse.

High-frequency 3D-EVUS and dynamic EVUS allow imaging of the anterior compartment (see Chapter 15) and represent useful modalities to detect defects of the connective supporting structures, subclinical cystoceles, or multicompartmental damage. At 3D-reconstruction, paravaginal defects or asymmetry of the urethral axis can be visualized in the axial plane, and rotation of urethra or the presence of small cystocele can be identified in the coronal plane (Fig. 37.6).

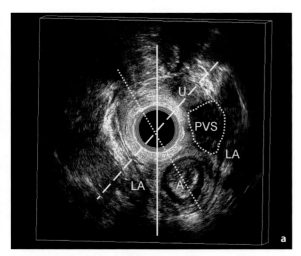
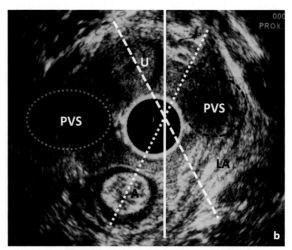

Fig. 37.4 Three-dimensional endovaginal ultrasonography with rotating transducer. Demonstration of paravaginal defects (**a**, left side; **b**, bilateral), asymmetry of the urethral and anal canal axis (**a**, **b**) and levator ani damage (**b**, avulsion of the right arm) in two females with pelvic organ prolapse. *A*, anal canal; *LA*, levator ani; *PVS*, paravaginal space; *U*, urethra

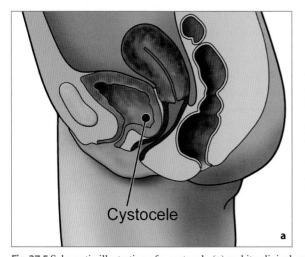
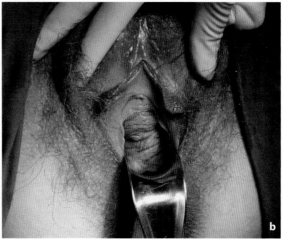

Fig. 37.5 Schematic illustration of a cystocele (**a**) and its clinical appearance (**b**)

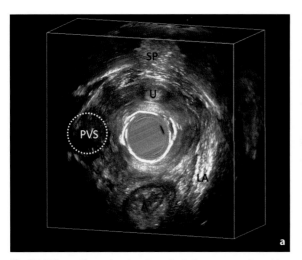
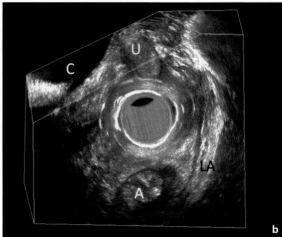

Fig. 37.6 Three-dimensional endovaginal ultrasonography with rotating transducer and volume render mode. **a** In the axial plane, the right arm of the levator ani (*LA*) is detached from the pubic rami and the right paravaginal space (*PVS*) is widened. **b** On the same side, using an oblique coronal plane, an early-stage cystocele (*C*) can be seen. *A*, anal canal; *SP*, symphysis pubis; *U*, urethra

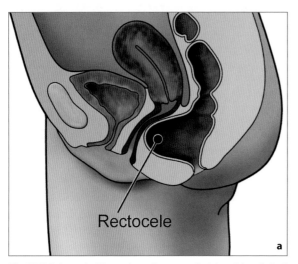
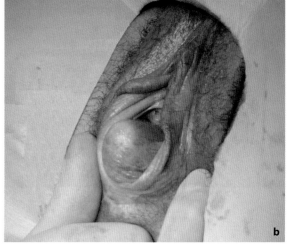

Fig. 37.7 Schematic illustration of a rectocele (**a**) and its clinical appearance (**b**)

37.4   Rectocele

Rectocele refers to an abnormal bulge of the anterior rectal wall, usually observed during defecation (Fig. 37.7). It is also defined as a posterior vaginal wall prolapse. This terminology, however, is not precise, as a posterior vaginal wall prolapse may also be due to the presence of an enterocele.

Rectocele is common in women after vaginal birth trauma (multiple or prolonged deliveries, forceps , perineal tears) and can also develop in women with chronic constipation. The underlying etiology is a weakening of the support structures of the pelvic floor and thinning or tear of the rectovaginal fascia. Symptoms related to the rectocele include: vaginal bulging, defecatory dysfunction, and a sensation of incomplete evacuation.

Several modalities to quantify the extend of rectocele have been reported. To date, defecography has been "the gold standard" for its evaluation. At evacuation proctography, a rectocele is measured as the depth of the wall protrusion beyond the expected margin of the normal anterior rectal wall. A depth of < 2 cm is considered within normal limits; rectocele should be considered moderate if its size is 2–4 cm, and large if it is > 4 cm. MRI is also used to assess rectocele during straining or defecation.

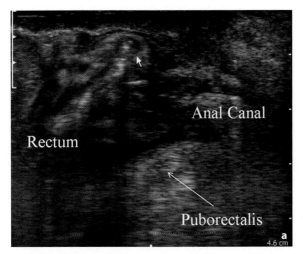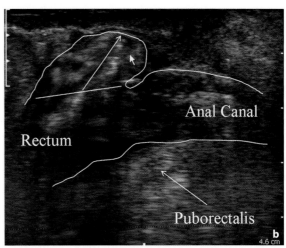

Fig. 37.8 Endovaginal ultrasonography with biplane probe. Longitudinal view of the posterior compartment using the linear array of the probe (positioned on the top of the image). **a** During Valsalva maneuver, a rectocele is demonstrated as bulging of the anterior rectal wall (*arrow*). **b** Rectocele depth is measured perpendicular to the expected contour of the anterior rectal wall (*arrow*)

More recently, TPUS has been shown to demonstrate rectocele, enterocele, and rectal intussusception. Perniola et al [26] performed a comparative clinical study to determine the agreement between defecation proctography and TPUS. They found a poor agreement between the two methods in the measurements of quantitative parameters. However, when ultrasound showed a rectocele or rectal intussusception, there was a high likelihood of this diagnosis being confirmed on proctography.

Dynamic EVUS performed with the use of a biplane probe (type 8848 – linear array, B-K Medical; see Chapter 6) seems to be an accurate modality to demonstrate a rectocele during straining and defecation (Fig. 6.12). This procedure is non-invasive and does not require any contrast medium. On ultrasound, the anorectal angle (ARA) at rest and during Valsalva maneuver is determined, as well as the presence/absence of a rectocele and its maximum depth. Rectocele depth, as on defecography, is measured perpendicular to the expected contour of the anterior rectal wall (Fig. 37.8). Similarly to TPUS [18], EVUS has the following limitations: it is operator dependent; it is performed in a supine position; Valsalva maneuver does not represent physiological defecation; it can prevent development of the prolapse due to the presence of the probe.

For these reasons, ultrasound may underevaluate rectocele. On the other hand, other studies have suggested that defecography overdiagnoses this abnormality [27]. We agree with Perniola et al [26] that ultrasonography cannot replace defecation proctography in

clinical practice, but it should be performed as an initial examination or screening method in patients with defecatory disorders. Positive findings on ultrasound may avoid more invasive tests, whereas negative findings require confirmation by defecography.

Murad Regadas [28] described a dynamic 3D anorectal ultrasonography (echodefecography) to assess patients with obstructed defecation. The technique consists of positioning a 360 degree rotational transducer (type 2050, B-K Medical; see Chapter 8; Fig. 8.2) into the rectum at 6–7 cm from the anal margin. Four automatic 3D acquisitions are performed to identify anatomical and functional changes induced by straining. The images are evaluated in the axial and longitudinal planes. This modality has been shown to represent an alternative tool to defecography.

37.5 Intussusception

Rectal intussusception is defined as an invagination of the rectal wall into the rectal lumen. It may be described as anterior, posterior, or circumferential. The intussusception may involve the full thickness of the rectal wall or only the mucosa. It can be classified as intra-rectal (if it remains in the rectum), intra-anal (if it extends into the anal canal), or external (if it forms a complete rectal prolapse).

There is often no identifiable cause in adults, although it is more common in multiparous women, suggesting it

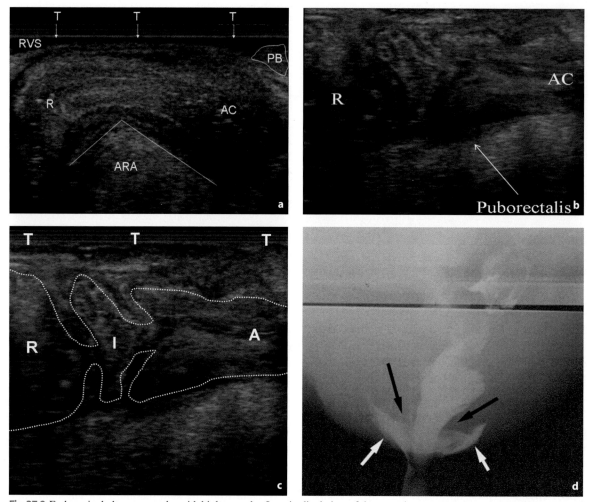

Fig. 37.9 Endovaginal ultrasonography with biplane probe. Longitudinal view of the posterior compartment using the linear array of the probe (positioned on the top of the image). **a** At rest. **b, c** During Valsalva maneuver, an intussusception (*I*) is demonstrated as wide invaginating rectal folds. **d** Intussusception at defecography. *AC*, anal canal; *PB*, perineal body; *R*, rectum; *RVS*, rectovaginal septum; *T*, transducer

may be a sign of more global pelvic floor damage. Small intrarectal intussusception may be detected in asymptomatic patients; however, if the invagination becomes intra-anal, the patient experiences a sensation of incomplete defecation due to outlet obstruction.

A defecographic study showed that most prolapse commences around 6–8 cm upstream of the anorectal junction [29]. However, proctographic diagnosis is often difficult because the intussusception may not be clearly distinguished from normal mucosal descent. A relatively useful indicator of true intussusception is the presence of abnormally wide invaginating rectal folds measuring more than 3 mm [30]. MR defecography has several advantages over evacuation proctography in the diagnosis of rectal intussusception: it allows differentiation between mucosal versus full-thickness descent and it provides additional information on movements of the whole pelvic floor.

Dynamic EVUS with the use of the linear array of the 8848 probe may detect rectal intussusception. Invagination may be seen as an infolding of the rectal wall into the rectal lumen while asking the patient to push, or during maximal Valsalva maneuver (Fig. 37.9). The intussusception may be observed to enter the anal canal or exteriorized beyond the anal canal. This technique is relatively easy to perform and provides adequate information comparable to MRI and proctography for the proper management of this disorder. Additionally, it may be used to evaluate whether a good functional outcome is achieved after treatment.

37.6 Mucosal Rectal Prolapse

Mucosal rectal prolapse creates a circular thickening of the mucosal layer of the anal canal that narrows the lumen (Fig. 37.10).

This condition is almost always associated with an anterior–posterior asymmetry and an increased thickness of the internal anal sphincter (IAS). Three-dimensional EAUS is an accurate modality to detect these abnormalities in mucosal prolapse (Figs. 8.2, 37.11). Any internal sphincter measuring more than 4 mm in thickness, regardless of the patient's age, is considered to be an indicator of an underlying mucosal prolapse or solitary

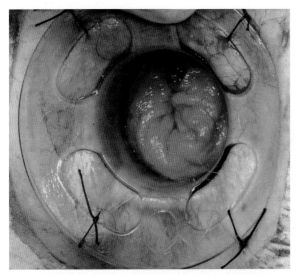

Fig. 37.10 Clinical appearance of a mucosal rectal prolapse as a circular thickening of the mucosal layer of the anal canal narrowing the lumen

rectal ulcer syndrome. It is interesting to note that the IAS thickness recovers after surgical treatment, as reported by Halligan et al [31].

37.7 Enterocele

An enterocele is diagnosed when small bowel loops enter the rectovaginal space (Fig. 37.12). Large enterocele may herniated into the vagina, resulting in a posterior vaginal wall prolapse that needs to be differentiated from rectocele. An enterocele may be symptomatic, causing a sense of fullness and incomplete evacuation. It occurs primarily in patients who have had a hysterectomy, due to separation of the pubocervical and rectovaginal fascia. There is an association with multiparity, age, and obesity. A redundant sigmoid may also prolapse into the rectovaginal space as a sigmoidocele. Diagnosis of an enterocele on proctography is only possible if oral contrast has been administered before the examination. Enteroceles are often apparent only when the rectum and bladder are emptied, as otherwise the limited space in the pelvis prevents small bowel descent. Alternatively, enteroceles are usually diagnosed at the end of the procedure when the rectovaginal space widens after evacuation, and pressure from the adjacent full rectum is reduced. The advent of MR defecography holds considerable promise in the diagnosis of enteroceles and other forms of pelvic herniation; however, this requires an open technique which is very expensive and not widely available.

Transperineal ultrasonography has also been used to demonstrate the presence of an enterocele [19]. Steensma

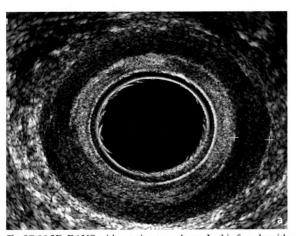
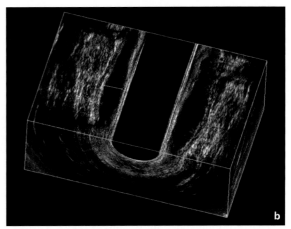

Fig. 37.11 3D-EAUS with rotating transducer. In this female with a mucosal rectal prolapse, the internal anal sphincter is thicker than 4 mm. **a** Axial view. **b** Coronal view

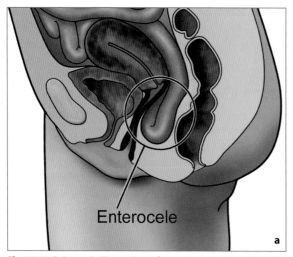
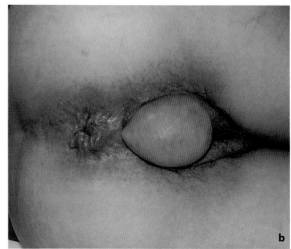

Fig. 37.12 Schematic illustration of an enterocele (**a**) and its clinical appearance (**b**)

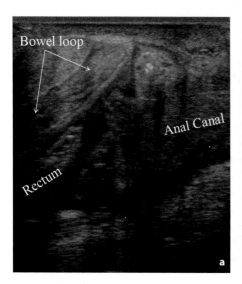
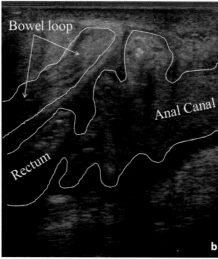

Fig. 37.13 Endovaginal ultrasonography with biplane probe. Longitudinal view of the posterior compartment using the linear array of the probe (positioned on the top of the image). **a, b** During Valsalva maneuver, an enterocele is demonstrated as a bowel loop entering into the rectovaginal space

et al [27] reported a good agreement between 3D-TPUS and defecography for detecting enterocele. Similarly to TPUS, dynamic EVUS with 8848 probe (linear array) may be used as an alternative to evacuation proctography. Enterocele is ultrasonographically diagnosed as a herniation of abdominal contents into the rectovaginal space (Fig. 37.13). It can be graded into small, when the most distal part descends into the upper third of the vagina; moderate, when the most distal part descends into the middle third of the vagina; and large, when the most distal part descends into the lower third of the vagina. Enterocele may also be concomitant with the presence of rectocele (Fig. 37.14). A limitation of EVUS is the difficulty of distinguishing an enterocele from a sigmoidocele.

Another limitation is the so-called "crowded pelvis", which refers to competition of the anatomic space in the pelvis. In some cases an enterocele that is visible during straining competes for the same anatomic space as a rectocele, which might prevent the true prolapse size from becoming visible.

37.8   Pelvic Floor Dyssynergy

Anismus, also known as spastic pelvic floor syndrome, or paradoxical puborectalis syndrome, is a phenomenon characterized by a lack of normal relaxation of the puborectalis muscle during defecation. The patient experiences constipation and incomplete evacuation. Although the diagnosis of anismus may be suggested by tests of anorectal physiology (electromyography and anorectal manometry), proctography and dynamic

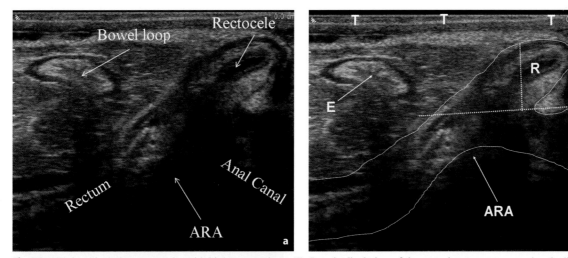

Fig. 37.14 Endovaginal ultrasonography with biplane transducer (*T*). Longitudinal view of the posterior compartment using the linear array of the probe (positioned on the top of the image). **a, b** During Valsalva maneuver, an enterocele (*E*) is demonstrated as a bowel loop entering into the rectovaginal space and a rectocele (*R*) as a bulging of the anterior rectal wall. *A*, anal canal; *ARA*, anorectal angle

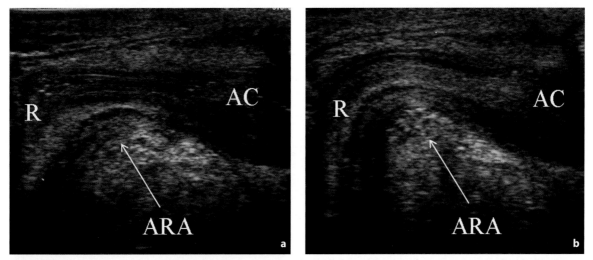

Fig. 37.15 Endovaginal ultrasonography with biplane probe. Longitudinal view of the posterior compartment using the linear array of the probe (positioned on the top of the image). **a** At rest. **b** During Valsalva maneuver, the anorectal angle (*ARA*) becomes narrower due to the contraction of the puborectalis muscle, indicating a pelvic floor dyssynergy. *AC*, anal canal; *R* rectum

MR defecography have an important diagnostic role. Various abnormalities have been described, including prominent puborectal impression and acute anorectal angulation during straining and defecation [32].

Dynamic EVUS with the linear array of the biplane probe may easily document pelvic floor dyssynergy. Images are acquired at rest, and during straining and Valsalva maneuver. The ARA, measured by placing lines through the hypoechoic band representing the posterior IAS and through the posterior wall of the distal rectum, becomes narrower, and the puborectalis muscle becomes thicker during Valsalva maneuver

(Fig. 37.15). These findings may guide the treating physician to use biofeedback therapy. Moreover, EVUS can be used to evaluate the results after treatment.

37.9   Uterovaginal Prolapse

Uterovaginal prolapse affects 50% of parous women, with 20% of these being symptomatic. It develops as a consequence of the uterosacral ligaments breaking. The uterus descends into the vagina and can fall outside the vaginal opening (complete uterine prolapse). Vaginal vault prolapse usually refers to an apical vaginal relaxation in a patient who has had a hysterectomy. Continued descent of the apex of the vagina results in complete eversion of the vagina. Dynamic MR defecography as well as TPUS may document these conditions. Endovaginal ultrasound, however, cannot be used in this disorder, as the presence of the probe in the vagina prevents development of the uterovaginal prolapse [13].

37.10   Postoperative Follow-up

Three-dimensional EVUS seems to be a very reliable and useful modality in the postoperative follow-up of prolapse surgery. This modality is particularly needed in cases when the expected correction of anatomy does not result in improve of the function. Post-processing techniques (render mode, multiplanar reconstruction, and tilting) allow precise evaluation of the positioning of meshes or tapes (Fig. 37.16), providing a number of items of information in a patient with complications (see Chapter 60). Dynamic EVUS may also be used to assess the function of these plastic elements to prevent POP during straining or Valsalva maneuver (Fig. 37.17).

37.11 Discussion

Surgical principles of reconstructive surgery are aimed at either restoring anatomy with a presumed restoration of function, or creating compensatory anatomical mechanisms [33]. So far, decision making in relation to operative treatment has been mainly on the basis of clinical assessment, which has a limited role in evaluating the pathomorphologic changes leading to POP.

Assessment of the anatomic alterations and evaluation of the function should both form part of a preoperative workup of the pelvic floor. However, the role of additional diagnostic testing in selecting treatment for primary POP has not been clarified [33]. Pelvic organ prolapse and symptoms of pelvic organ dysfunction are poorly correlated. Constipation, obstructed defecation, urinary and fecal incontinence, and voiding dysfunction are frequently reported in patients with POP, but it remains questionable whether these symptoms are directly related to the degree of anterior or posterior vaginal wall prolapse [34]. In other words, there are no specific symptoms related

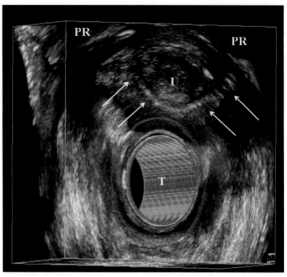

Fig. 37.16 Three-dimensional endovaginal ultrasonography with rotating transducer (*T*). In the axial plane, the transobturator sling (*arrows*) is visualized as a hyperechoic band. *PR*, pubic ramus; *U*, urethra

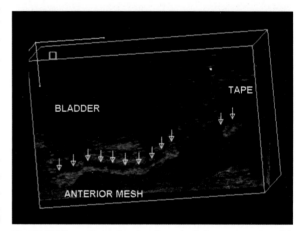

Fig. 37.17 Three-dimensional endovaginal ultrasonography with biplane probe. Longitudinal view of the anterior compartment. Visualization of an anterior mesh and transobturator tape as hyperechoic bands (*arrows*)

to the descent in the different compartments. In addition, diagnostic tests bear the risk of overestimating the severity of POP as compared to clinical examination, and also carry the risk of overtreatment. As consequence, no benefit in relation to symptoms can be expected from surgical correction of POP detected with diagnostic testing. Broekhuis et al [35] reported a low agreement between patients' symptoms as assessed with validated questionnaires and findings on dynamic MRI of the pelvic floor. In view of the low correlations, these authors suggested that dynamic

MRI is not likely to have an additional value in the prediction of symptoms. On the other hand, Hetzer et al [36] reported that MR defecography findings led to changes in the surgical approach in 67% of patients, and Kaufman et al [37] showed that dynamic MRI led to altered operative plans in 41% of cases. Groenendijk et al [38] reported that, on average, additional diagnostic tests resulted in a revised initial management plan in 38% of cases. Overall, defecography was regarded as most valuable (assigned diagnostic value 49%) compared with MRI, which was rated the least useful (assigned diagnostic value 20%). However, despite tests, consensus was not reached in one-quarter of cases. An interesting conclusion that can be drawn from this study is that to obtain more relevant information, diagnostic tests should be selected on the basis of specific pelvic floor disorders. The assigned value of defecography increased significantly in cases of posterior vaginal wall prolapse POP-Q stage > 2 (assigned diagnostic value 74% vs. overall value 49%), as well the value of EAUS in cases of fecal incontinence (assigned diagnostic value 68% vs. overall value 38%). The same authors [39] indicated that anorectal function testing (anorectal manometry, surface electromyography, pudendal nerve terminal motor latencies, EAUS) is not useful in the workup of patients with POP and constipation, because it fails to discriminate between symptomatic and asymptomatic patients. Broekhuis et al [11] reported that POP staging with the use of POP-Q, dynamic MRI, and TPUS only correlates in the anterior compartment, whereas correlation in the posterior compartment is poor. This study is in agreement with Dietz et al [40], who found good correlation between TPUS and POP-Q for the anterior and central compartment and poor correlation for the posterior compartment.

In the workup of patients with posterior vaginal wall prolapse, defecography is recommended as a helpful diagnostic tool, as physical examination overestimates the presence of posterior wall defects by mistaking enteroceles for rectoceles (high false-positive rate) but often misses occult defects like enteroceles, rectal prolapse, intussusception, and solitary ulcer syndrome or pelvic floor dyssynergia (high false-negative rate) [34].

Groenendijk et al [41] reported that defecography can be regarded as the best available diagnostic test for evaluation of the anorectum. Harvey et al [42] found that evacuation proctography altered the intended diagnosis and therapy in 18% and 28% of patients, respectively. In contrast, the routine postoperative use of colpocystodefecography is unjustified unless there is clinical evidence of surgical failure [43].

Dynamic ultrasonography (TPUS or EVUS) and 3D high-resolution ultrasonography (3D-TPUS, 3D-EVUS, 3D-EAUS) provide an accurate assessment of POP. The 3D reconstruction allows a spatial assessment of the pelvic floor, which facilitates visualization of the causative lesion of prolapse. However, ultrasonography does not seem to lead to a consequent improvement in prediction of prolapse symptoms as compared to POP-Q system [44].

Despite this, ultrasonography has other significant advantages, such as evaluation of the anatomy (fascia, ligaments, muscles) as well as of the function (at rest, during contraction, weak straining, and forceful straining) of the pelvic floor. Ultrasonographic techniques are able to define the presence and grade of cystocele, rectocele, and enterocele, and to detect levator trauma and connective tissue damage. More research will be needed to define the role of these modalities in the workup of POP and to classify morphologic subtypes of prolapse. The ultrasound findings of specific muscle or connective tissue damage may, in the future, affect surgical decision making.

37.12 Conclusions

The treatment decision in patients undergoing POP surgery is still based on history taking and pelvic examination. The routine use of a "battery" of diagnostic testing appears not to be an option. In view of the high correlations, imaging is not likely to have an additional value for the anterior compartment, and POP-Q can be regarded as the gold standard of POP staging in the anterior compartment. In assessment of the central and posterior compartments, clinical examination alone has not been proven adequate, and additional tests are needed. However, at this stage, the available evidence does not provide proof for the superiority of any one of the various imaging techniques. An optimal compromise could be to perform a multicompartmental ultrasonography of the pelvic floor (dynamic TPUS/EVUS and high-resolution 3D-ultrasonography) as the initial diagnostic test in all patients with POP. On the basis of ultrasonographic findings, additional tests may be further performed in selected cases, to direct therapy.

References

1. Kerkhof MH, Hendriks L, Brolmann HA. Changes in connective tissue in patients with pelvic organ prolapse – a review of the current literature. Int Urogynecol J Pelvic Floor Dysfunct 2009;20:461–474.

2. Hsu Y, Chen L, Huebner M et al. Quantification of levator ani cross-sectional area differences between women with and those without prolapse. Obstet Gynecol 2006; 108:879–883.

3. Dietz HP. The aetiology of prolapse. Int Urogynecol J Pelvic Floor Dysfunct 2008;19:1323–1329.

4. Whiteside JL, Weber AM, Meyn LA, Walters MD. Risk factors for prolapse recurrence after vaginal repair. Am J Obstet Gynecol 2004;191:1533–1538.

5. Stoker J, Halligan S, Bartram CI. Pelvic floor imaging. Radiology 2001;218:621–641.

6. Maglinte DDT, Bartram C. Dynamic imaging of posterior compartment pelvic floor dysfunction by evacuation proctography. Techniques, indications, results and limitations. Eur J Radiol 2007;61:454–461.

7. Mortele KJ, Fairhurst J. Dynamic MR defecography of the posterior compartment: Indications, techniques and MRI features. Eur J Radiol 2007;61:462–472.

8. Huebner M, Margulies RU, De Lancey JOL. Pelvic architectural distortion is associated with pelvic organ prolapse. Int Urogynecol J Pelvic Floor Dysfunct 2008;19:863–867.

9. Tunn R, Schaer G, Peschers U. Update recommendations on ultrasonography in urogynecology. Int Urogynecol J 2005;16:236–241.

10. Majida M, Brekken IH, Umek W et al. Interobserver repeability of three- and four-dimensional transperineal ultrasound assessment of pelvic floor muscle anatomy and function. Ultrasound Obstet Gynecol 2009;33:567–573.

11. Broekhuis SR, Kluivers KB, Hendriks JC et al. POP-Q, dynamic MR imaging, and perineal ultrasonography: do they agree in the quantification of female pelvic organ prolapse? Int Urogynecol J Pelvic Floor Dysfunct 2009;20:541-549.

12. Santoro GA, Wieczorek AP, Stankiewicz A et al. High-resolution three-dimensional endovaginal ultrasonography in the assessment of pelvic floor anatomy: a preliminary study. Int Urogynecol J Pelvic Floor Dysfunct 2009; 20:1213–1222.

13. Stankiewicz A, Wieczorek AP, Woźniak MM et al. Comparison of accuracy of functional measurements of the urethra in transperineal vs. endovaginal ultrasound in incontinent women. Pelviperineology 2008;27:145–147.

14. Singh K, Jakab M, Reid W et al. Three-dimensional magnetic resonance imaging assessment of levator ani morphologic features in different grades of prolapse. Am J Obstet Gynecol 2003;188:910–915.

15. DeLancey JO, Morgan DM, Fenner DE et al. Comparison of levator ani muscle defects and function in women with and without pelvic organ prolapse. Obstet Gynecol 2007; 109:295–302.

16. DeLancey JO, Kearney R, Chou Q et al. The appearance of levator ani muscle abnormalities in magnetic resonance images after vaginal delivery. Obstet Gynecol 2003;101:46–53.

17. Tunn R, DeLancey JO, Howard D et al. Anatomic variations in the levator ani muscle, endopelvic fascia, and urethra in nulliparas evaluated by magnetic resonance imaging. Am J Obstet Gynecol 2003;188:116–121.

18. Dietz HP, Steensma AB. The prevalence of major abnormalities of the levator ani in urogynaecological patients. BJOG 2006;113:225–230.

19. Dietz HP, Steensma AB. Posterior compartment prolapse on two-dimensional and three dimensional pelvic floor ultrasound: the distinction between true rectocele, perineal hypermobility and enterocele. Ultrasound Obstet Gynecol 2005;26:73–77.

20. Athanasiou S, Chaliha C, Toozs-Hobson P et al. Direct imaging of the pelvic floor muscles using two-dimensional ultrasound: a comparison of women with urogenital prolapse versus controls. BJOG 2007;114:882–888.

21. Olsen AL, Smith VJ, Bergstrom JO et al. Epidemiology of surgically managed pelvic organ prolapse and urinary incontinence. Obstet Gynecol 1997;89:501–506.

22. Mellgren A, Bremmer S, Johansson C et al. Defecography. Results of investigations in 2,816 patients. Dis Colon Rectum 1994;37:1133–1141.

23. Maglinte DD, Kelvin FM, Fitzgerald K et al. Association of compartment defects in pelvic floor dysfunction. Am J Roentgenol 1999;172:439–444.

24. Kelvin FM, Maglinte DD, Benson JT et al. Dynamic cystoproctography: a technique for assessing disorders of the pelvic floor in women. Am J Roentgenol 1994;163:368–370.

25. Kenton K, Shott S, Brubaker L. Vaginal topography does not correlate well with visceral position in women with pelvic organ prolapse. Int Urogynecol J 1997;8:336–339.

26. Perniola G., Shek C, Chong CCW et al. Defecation proctography and translabial ultrasound in the investigation of defecatory disorders. Ultrasound Obstet Gynecol 2008;31:567–571.

27. Steensma AB, Oom DMJ, Burger CW, Rudolph Schouten W. Assessment of posterior compartment prolapse; a comparison of evacuation proctography and 3D transperineal ultrasound. Colorectal Dis 2009; 29 April epub ahead of print.

28. Murad Regadas SM, Regadas FSP, Rodrigues LV et al. A novel three-dimensional dynamic anorectal ultrasonography technique (echodefecography) to assess obstructed defecation: a comparison with defecography. Surg Endoscopy 2008;22:974–979.

29. Broden B, Snellman B. Procidentia of the rectum studied with cineradiography. A contribution to the discussion of causative mechanism. Dis Colon Rectum 1968;11:330–347.

30. Shorvon PJ, McHugh S, Diamant NE et al. Defecography in normal volunteers: results and implications. Gut 1989;30:1737–1749.

31. Halligan S, Sultan A, Rottenberg G et al. Endosonography of the anal sphincters in solitary rectal ulcer syndrome. Int J Colorectal Dis 1995;10:79–82.

32. Kuijpers HC, Bleijenberg G. The spastic pelvic floor syndrome. Dis Colon Rectum 1985;28:669–672.

33. Vimplis S, Hooper P. Assessment and management of pelvic organ prolapse. Curr Obstet Gynecol 2005;15:387–393.

34. Altman D, Lopez A, Kierkegaard J et al. Assessment of posterior vaginal wall prolapse: comparison of physical findings to cystodefecoperitoneography. Int Urogynecol J 2005;16:96–103.

35. Broekhuis SR, Futterer JJ, Hendriks JCM et al. Symptoms of pelvic floor dysfunction are poorly correlated with findings on clinical examination and dynamic MR imaging of the pelvic floor. Int Urogynecol J 2009; 20:1169–1174.

36. Hetzer FH, Andreisek G, Tsagari C et al. MR defecography in patients with fecal incontinence and their effect on surgical management. Radiology 2006;240:449–457.

37. Kaufman HS, Buller JL, Thompson JR et al. Dynamic pelvic magnetic resonance imaging and cystocolpodefecography alter surgical management of pelvic floor disorders. Dis Colon Rectum 2001;44:1575–1584.

38. Groenendijk AG, Birnie E, de Blok S et al. Clinical-decision taking in primary pelvic organ prolapse; the effects of diagnostic tests on treatment selection in comparison with a consensus meeting. Int Urogynecol J 2009;20:711–719.

39. Groenendijk AG, Birnie E, Boeckxstaens GE et al. Anorectal function testing and anal endosonography in the diagnostic work-up of patients with primary pelvic organ prolapse. Gynecol Obstet Invest 2009;67:187–194.

40. Dietz HP, Haylen BT, Broome J. Ultrasound in the quantification of female pelvic organ prolapse. Ultrasound Obstet Gynecol 2001;18:511–514.

41. Groenendijk AG, van der Hulst VP, Birnie E, Bonsel GJ. Correlation between posterior vaginal wall defects assessed by clinical examination and by defecography. Int Urogynecol J 2008;19:1291–1297.

42. Harvey CJ, Halligan S, Bartram CI et al. Evacuation proctography: a prospective study of diagnostic and therapeutic effects. Radiology 1999;211:223–227.

43. Finco C, Savastano S, Luongo B et al. Colpocystodefecography in obstructed defecation: is it really useful to the surgeon? Correlating clinical and radiological findings in surgery for obstructed defecation. Colorectal Dis 2007;10:446–452.

44. Kluivers KB, Hendriks JCM, Shek C, Dietz HP. Pelvic organ prolapse symptoms in relation to POP-Q, ordinal stages and ultrasound prolapse assessment. Int Urogynecol J 2009; 19:1299–1302.

Translabial Ultrasonography

Hans Peter Dietz

Abstract Translabial ultrasound is the most commonly used imaging method in the investigation of women with lower urinary tract symptoms and female pelvic organ prolapse, due to its simplicity, low cost and non-invasive nature. This chapter will summarize practical applications and recent research findings in this field. Pelvic floor ultrasound is helpful in the evaluation of anatomical findings in women with lower urinary tract symptoms, prolapse, and obstructed defecation, and it has enabled us to identify pathologies that were virtually unknown until very recently. The widespread application of cross-sectional imaging in female urology and urogynecology will allow us to improve current therapeutic options and to develop entirely new approaches, targeting underlying pathology rather than symptoms.

Keywords 3D Ultrasound • Female pelvic organ prolapse • Lower urinary tract • Pelvic floor • Ultrasound • Urogynecology

38.1 Introduction

Translabial or transperineal/introital ultrasonography is currently the most commonly used imaging method in urogynecology due to its simplicity, limited cost, non-invasive nature, and patient acceptance. The methodology was summarized in Chapter 7. On the following pages I will give an overview of both clinical and research uses of this technique.

38.2 The Anterior Compartment

The original indication for pelvic floor ultrasound was (and still is) the assessment of bladder neck mobility and funneling of the bladder neck, both of which are considered important in women with urinary incontinence. Fig. 38.1 shows the standard orientation used to describe bladder neck mobility in a comparison of findings before and after childbirth. The position of the bladder neck is determined relative to the inferoposterior margin of the symphysis pubis, and comparative studies have shown good correlations with radiological methods previously used for this purpose (for an overview see [1]). The one remaining advantage of x-ray fluoroscopy may be the ease with which the voiding phase can be observed, although some investigators have used specially constructed equipment to document voiding with ultrasound [2].

H.P. Dietz
Department of Obstetrics, Gynecology and Neonatology,
Sidney Medical School-Nepean, University of Sydney,
Australia

G.A. Santoro, A.P. Wieczorek, C.I. Bartram (eds.) *Pelvic Floor Disorders*
© Springer-Verlag Italia 2010

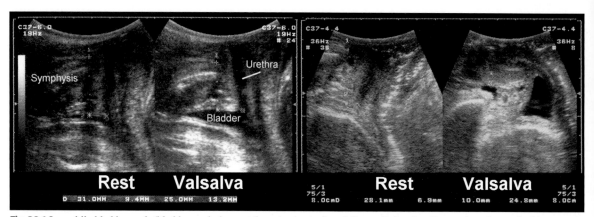

Fig. 38.1 Immobile bladder neck (bladder neck descent 6 mm) prior to first delivery (*left pair of images*), and a marked increase in bladder neck mobility (bladder neck descent 38.1 mm) after childbirth (*right pair of images*). From [4], with permission

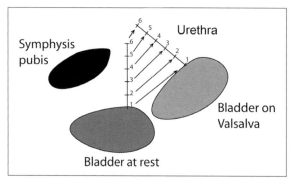

Fig. 38.2 Schematic representation of the determination of segmental urethral mobility (urethral motion profile, UMP). From [4], with permission

Recently, it has become clear that it is not so much bladder neck mobility that is important for stress urinary incontinence, but rather mobility of the midurethra [3], which can be assessed with a high degree of repeatability and in a semi-automatic fashion by obtaining a "urethral motion profile" [5] (Figs. 38.2, 38.3). Since further progress in research on the pathophysiology of stress urinary incontinence is unlikely unless we can combine spatial information on urethral mobility with pressure measurements at a high spatial and temporal resolution, this method is likely to be important in the future. The technique has already been used to determine normal values for urethral mobility

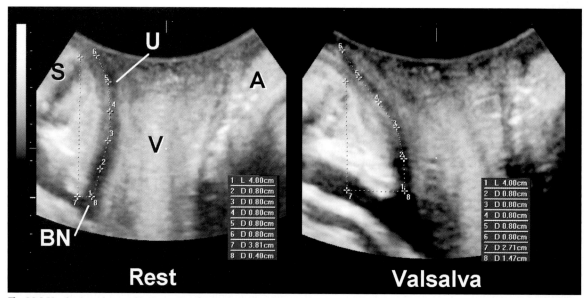

Fig. 38.3 Urethral motion profile determination in the midsagittal plane. After tracing of the urethra from external to internal meatus and division into five equal segments, the location of each of the resulting six points is determined relative to the inferoposterior symphyseal margin. *A*, anal canal; *BN*, bladder neck; *S*, symphysis pubis; *U*, urethra; *V*, vagina. From [5], with permission

in nulliparous women [5], to assess childbirth-related changes [5] and the effect of suburethral slings [6], and to show that stress urinary incontinence and urodynamic stress incontinence are related more to midurethral mobility than to mobility of the bladder neck [3].

38.2.1 Residual Urine

Translabial ultrasound can be used to determine residual urine, using a formula originally developed for transvaginal ultrasound [7] (Fig. 38.4). While it is reasonable to use this formula $((X * Y * 5.9) - 14.9 =$ residual in milliliters, where X and Y are the two largest diameters at right angles to each other), as it should matter little whether a midsagittal image is obtained with a vaginal or a perineal probe, the method is currently being validated for translabial ultrasound.

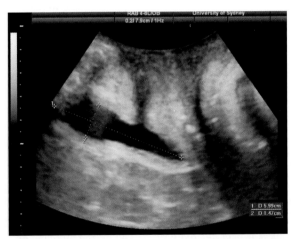

Fig. 38.4 Determination of residual urine by translabial ultrasound: the two largest diameters (X and Y), at right angles to each other, are measured. The volume in milliliters is obtained by multiplying the result by 5.9 and subtracting 14.9 mL

38.2.2 Bladder Neck Mobility

Bladder neck position and mobility can be assessed with a high degree of reliability. Points of reference are the central axis of the symphysis pubis [8] or its inferoposterior margin [9] (Fig. 38.1). The full bladder is less mobile [10] and may prevent complete development of pelvic organ prolapse. It is essential not to exert undue pressure on the perineum so as to allow full development of pelvic organ descent. Measurements of bladder neck position are performed at rest and on maximal

Valsalva maneuver, and the difference yields a numerical value for bladder neck descent. On Valsalva, the proximal urethra may be seen to rotate in a postero-inferior direction. The extent of rotation can be measured by comparing the angle of inclination between the proximal urethra and any other fixed axis. Some investigators measure the retrovesical angle (RVA) or posterior urethrovesical angle (PUV) between the proximal urethra and trigone; others determine the angle between the central axis of the symphysis pubis and a line from the inferior symphyseal margin to the bladder neck [11]. The reproducibility of bladder neck descent seems good, with intraclass correlations were between 0.75 and 0.98, indicating "excellent" agreement [12].

There is no definition of "normal" for bladder neck descent, although cut-offs of 20 and 25 mm have been proposed to define hypermobility. The latter seems to make more sense since it is closer to the 95th centile for bladder neck mobility in young asymptomatic nulliparae [12]. Bladder filling, patient position, and catheterization have all been shown to influence measurements (see [1] for an overview), and as mentioned above it can occasionally be quite difficult to obtain an effective Valsalva maneuver, especially in nulliparous women who routinely co-activate the levator muscle [13]. Perhaps not surprisingly, publications to date have presented widely differing reference measurements in nulliparous women. While two series documented mean or median bladder neck descent of only 5.1 mm [14] and 5.3 mm [15] in continent nulliparous women, another study on 39 continent nulliparous volunteers measured an average of 15 mm of bladder neck descent [16].

The author has obtained measurements of 1.2–40.2 mm (mean 17.3 mm) in a group of 106 stress-continent nulligravid young women aged 18–23 years [12]. It is likely that methodological differences account for those discrepancies, with all known confounders tending to reduce descent.

The etiology of increased bladder neck descent is likely to be multifactorial. The wide range of values obtained in young nulliparous women suggests a congenital component, which has been confirmed in a twin study [17]. Vaginal childbirth is probably the most significant environmental factor [4, 18], with a long second stage of labor and vaginal operative delivery being associated with increased postpartum descent. Fig. 38.1 shows markedly increased bladder neck mobility after a vacuum delivery at term. This association between increased bladder descent and vaginal parity is also evident in

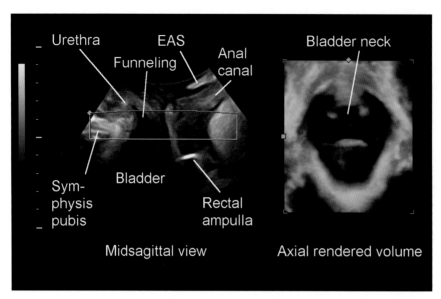

Fig. 38.5 Funneling of the bladder neck as shown in a patient with urodynamic stress incontinence. The most common findings in uncomplicated stress incontinence are as shown here: mild anterior compartment descent with a Green II rotatory descent of the bladder neck, an open retrovesical angle, funneling (as shown in the midsagittal plane on the left), and an intact puborectalis muscle, as shown in the rendered volume on the right

older women with symptoms of pelvic floor dysfunction [19], and it seems at least partly due to levator trauma (see below).

38.2.3 Funneling and Stress Incontinence

In patients with stress incontinence, but also in asymptomatic women, funneling of the internal urethral meatus may be observed on Valsalva maneuver (Fig. 38.5) and sometimes even at rest [20]. Funneling is often (but not necessarily) associated with leakage. Other indirect signs of urine leakage on B mode real-time imaging are weak grayscale echoes ("streaming") and the appearance of two linear ("specular") echoes defining the lumen of a fluid- filled urethra. However, funneling may very occasionally also be observed at the time of a detrusor contraction and cannot be used to prove urodynamic stress incontinence.

Its anatomical basis is unclear. Marked funneling has been shown to be associated with poor urethral closure pressures [21, 22]. In the past it has been held that funneling may explain why so many women with stress incontinence are also urge incontinent, since urine entering the proximal urethra is thought to trigger a voiding reflex.

However, funneling is commonly seen in women without urge incontinence, and even after suburethral slings that have cured both stress and urge incontinence.

38.2.4 Color Doppler Imaging of Stress Incontinence

Color Doppler ultrasound can demonstrate urine leakage on Valsalva maneuver or coughing [23] (Figs. 38.6, 38.7). Agreement between color Doppler and fluoroscopy was high in a controlled group with indwelling catheters and identical bladder volumes [24]. Both velocity and energy mapping were able to document leakage. Color Doppler ultrasound was slightly more likely to show a positive result, probably due to its better motion discrimination. Color Doppler imaging may also facilitate the documentation of leak point pressures [25]. Whether this is in fact desired will depend on the clinician and

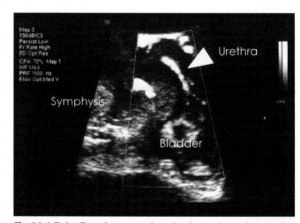

Fig. 38.6 Color Doppler energy imaging in urodynamic stress incontinence. The Doppler signal outlines most of the proximal urethra (*arrowhead*). From [1], with permission

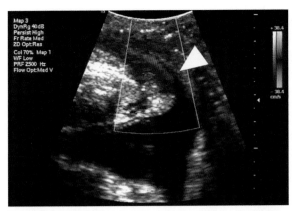

Fig. 38.7 Color Doppler ultrasound demonstrating urine leakage (*arrowhead*) through the urethra on Valsalva maneuver. From [1], with permission

his/her preferences, and one may well argue that urine leakage and leak point pressures can easily be determined clinically.

38.2.5 Cystocele

Clinical examination is limited to grading anterior compartment prolapse, which we call "cystocele". In fact, imaging will identify a number of anatomical situations that are difficult, if not impossible, to distinguish clinically. There are at least two types of cystoceles, with very different functional implications (Fig. 38.8). A cystourethrocele is associated with above-average flow rates and urodynamic stress incontinence (Figs. 38.5–38.7 and left image in 38.8), while a cystocele with intact retrovesical angle (right image in 38.8) is generally associated with voiding dysfunction and a

low likelihood of stress incontinence [26]. Even more interestingly, the latter is associated with levator trauma, while this is not the case for cystourethrocele [27]. Finally, a cystocele will occasionally prove to be due to a cystic mass such a Gartner duct cyst (Fig. 38.9), a urethral diverticulum (Fig. 38.10), or an anterior enterocele, all of which are likely to be missed on clinical examination, or even a leiomyoma [28].

38.2.6 Urethral and Paraurethral Pathology

Modern B mode systems allow a detailed assessment of the urethra. The true dimensions of the urethral rhabdosphincter have only recently become clear, as imaging in the midsagittal plane does not show the ventral aspect of the muscle well, and as transvaginal ultrasound results in artifacts due to the varying angle between incident beam and muscle fibers, leading to underestimates of sphincter area and volume. Fig. 38.11 shows a normal urethra and illustrates how much easier it is to identify the donut-shaped rhabdosphincter in the axial compared to the sagittal plane.

Paraurethral vessels are often rather prominent and occasionally require verification with Doppler in order to avoid misdiagnosis.

Urethral diverticula are often overlooked for years in women with recurrent bladder infections and symptoms of frequency, urgency, and pain or burning on voiding, until imaging is undertaken. Urethral structure and spatial relationships are much better appreciated in the axial plane (Fig. 38.10), which is particularly useful in the differential diagnosis of Gartner cyst and

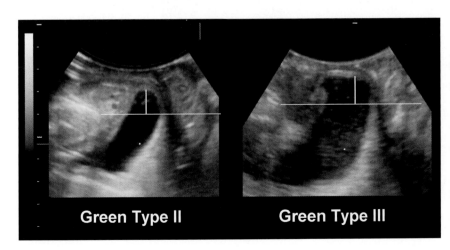

Green Type II   **Green Type III**

Fig. 38.8 The two commonest presentations of cystocele. The left image shows typical findings in a patient with mild stress urinary incontinence and anterior vaginal wall descent (clinically a cystourethrocele Grade II). The right image demonstrates appearances in a patient with a cystocele with intact retrovesical angle. Usually such women present with prolapse and are often continent

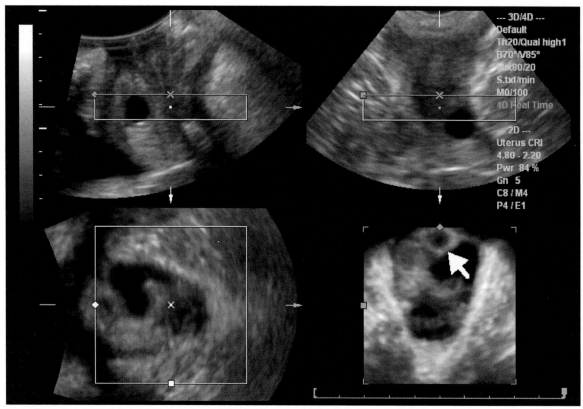

Fig. 38.9 Gartner duct cyst in orthogonal planes and in a rendered volume as seen with 3D translabial ultrasound. The rendered volume (bottom right) clearly shows that the cystic structure remains external to the urethral rhabdosphincter (*arrow*)

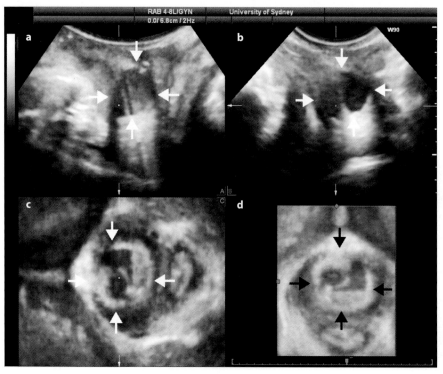

Fig. 38.10 Urethral diverticulum as seen on 3D translabial ultrasound, outlined by *arrows*. The extent of the diverticulum is clearly apparent, both in sectional planes (**a–c**) and in the rendered volume (**d**). It is typical in that it develops into the vagina and surrounds the urethra in a horseshoe-like pattern, in this case mostly towards the patient's left. The diverticular tract was identified cystoscopically at 5 o'clock

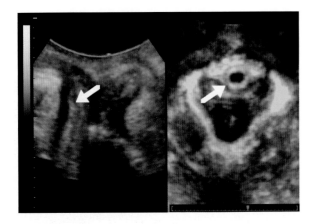

Fig. 38.11 The urethral rhabdosphincter (*arrow*) is much more easily seen in the axial plane (*right*) than in the midsagittal plane (*left*), due to poor tissue discrimination between fibrofatty tissue anterior to the urethra and the rhabdosphincter. In the axial plane the ring structure of the sphincter is surprisingly obvious on this slice of 3 mm thickness obtained by Volume Contrast Imaging™

urethral diverticulum. Prior voiding often fills a collapsed diverticulum, and often a Valsalva maneuver will help in improving visibility, allowing insonation of the structure from varying angles. If spatial relationships remain unclear, transvaginal ultrasound using higher frequencies may be preferred. Standard textbooks suggest that magnetic resonance is the investigation of choice in women suspected of having a urethral diverticulum, but it is difficult to see what advantages magnetic resonance should have over ultrasound for this indication.

Unfortunately, the condition is too uncommon to allow studies of diagnostic efficacy.

38.2.7 Detrusor Wall Thickness

The thickness of the bladder wall (bladder wall thickness, BWT, or detrusor wall thickness, DWT) can easily be determined on translabial ultrasound (Fig. 38.12). As increasing bladder filling reduces BWT due to distension, measurements should only be undertaken at bladder volumes of ≤ 50 mL [29].

While DWT has probably been overrated as a diagnostic tool in the context of detrusor overactivity [30, 31], increased DWT is associated with symptoms of the overactive bladder [31, 32], and may be a predictor of postoperative de novo urge incontinence

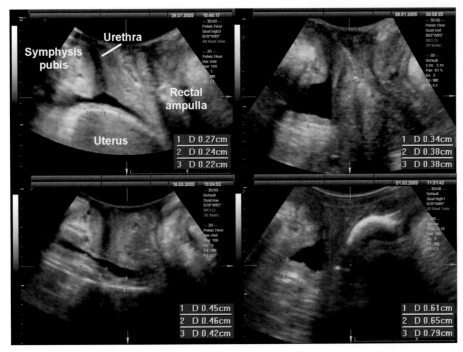

Fig. 38.12 Measurement of bladder wall thickness at the dome in four women with non-neuropathic bladder dysfunction. In all cases residual urine is well below 50 mL. From [31], with permission

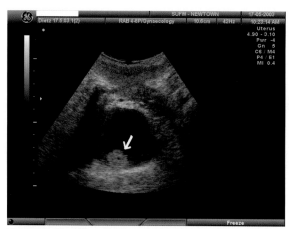

Fig. 38.13 Transitional cell carcinoma of the bladder as seen on parasagittal translabial ultrasound (*arrow*). From [1], with permission

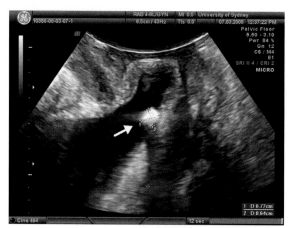

Fig. 38.14 Bladder stone as visualized in the midsagittal plane (*arrow*)

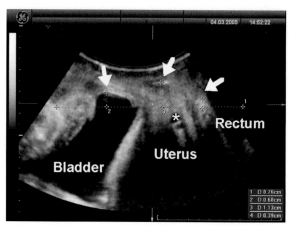

Fig. 38.15 Three-compartment prolapse on translabial ultrasound. The line of reference is placed through the inferior margin of the symphysis pubis. Measurements indicate descent of the bladder to 6.8 mm below the symphysis pubis, of the uterus to 11.3 mm, and of the rectal ampulla to 3.9 mm below the symphysis pubis. *Arrows* indicate the leading edges of those organs. There is a small nabothian follicle in the cervical os, evident as a small cystic structure (*). The clinical examination showed a second-degree uterine prolapse and first-degree anterior and posterior compartment descent. From [39], with permission

and/or detrusor overactivity after anti-incontinence procedures [33].

As opposed to the situation in the male, DWT in women is not predictive of voiding dysfunction [34].

38.2.8 Other Bladder Pathology

Occasionally a foreign body, eroded mesh, or even a bladder tumor (Fig. 38.13) may be picked up on translabial ultrasound [35], and a careful examination using parasagittal planes may show bladder diverticula.

A cystic structure that varies markedly over seconds or minutes and is located 1–3 cm lateral and posterior to the bladder neck is likely to be a uretero-cele, a generally harmless sacculation of the distal ureter due to stenosis of the ureterovesical junction. If the respective upper tract appears normal on renal ultrasound, then no further action is required. A bladder stone is visible as a strongly hyperechogenic structure with distal shadowing (Fig. 38.14).

38.3 The Central Compartment

38.3.1 Uterine Descent

Tranbslabial ultrasound is of relatively limited use in the assessment of central compartment prolapse. Generally, uterine prolapse is obvious clinically, as it is vault descent. An unusually low cervix is isoechoic, its distal margin is evident as a specular line, and it often causes acoustic shadowing. In premenopausal women the cervix often contains Nabothian follicles (Fig. 38.15) that are evident as cystic spaces within the cervix and can occasionally measure several centimeters in diameter.

A Valsalva maneuver will result in relative movement, distinguishing a Nabothian follicle from Gartner duct cysts or urethral diverticula. A low uterus may compress the posterior compartment sufficiently to hide a rectocele or even a recto-enterocele, reducing the diagnostic accuracy of imaging methods and underscoring the fact that clinical and imaging assessments are complementary.

Translabial ultrasound can graphically show the effect of an anteriorized cervix in women with an enlarged, retroverted uterus, explaining symptoms of voiding dysfunction, and supporting surgical intervention in order to improve voiding in a patient with a retroverted fibroid uterus. On the other hand, mild descent of an anteverted uterus may result in compression and inversion of the rectal ampulla, explaining symptoms of obstructed defecation – a situation that is termed a "colpocele" on defecation proctogram. The result is a rectal intussusception, with the intussuscipiens propelled not by small bowel (as usual), but by the cervix.

38.3.2 Vault Prolapse

It is frequently possible to image vault descent in women after hysterectomy, but just as often the thin iso- to hypoechoic structure of the vaginal wall is obscured by a descending rectocele or enterocele.

38.4 The Posterior Compartment

The discrepancy between clinical assessment, i.e. surface anatomy, and imaging is most clearly demonstrated in the posterior compartment. Clinically we diagnose posterior compartment descent as "rectocele",

quite unaware that at least five different conditions can lead to apparent or actual prolapse of the posterior vaginal wall. A second-degree rectocele may be due to a true rectocele, i.e. a defect of the rectovaginal septum (most common, and associated with symptoms of prolapse, incomplete bowel emptying, and straining at stool) [35], due to an abnormally distensible or laterally detached but otherwise intact rectovaginal septum (common and associated only with prolapse symptoms), a combined recto-enterocele (less common), an isolated enterocele (uncommon), or just a deficient perineum giving the impression of a "bulge" [36]. Occasionally, a "rectocele" turns out to be due to rectal intussusception, an early stage of rectal prolapse, where the wall of the rectum is inverted and enters the anal canal on Valsalva maneuver.

38.4.1 Rectocele

An anterior rectocele is evident as a diverticulum of the anterior wall of the rectal ampulla into the vagina, which is generally much more evident on Valsalva than at rest. Posterior rectoceles are uncommon in adult women and may be a form of intussusception rather than an actual rectocele. A rectocele usually contains iso- to hyperechoic feces, and often there is bowel gas as well, resulting in specular echoes and reverberations. Occasionally there is no stool in the ampulla that could be propelled into the rectocele, and as a result it remains smaller and filled only with

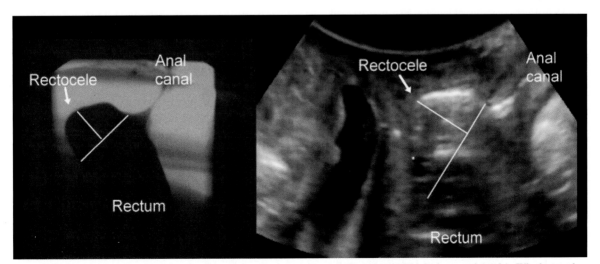

Fig. 38.16 A typical true rectocele as seen on defecation proctogram (*left*) and translabial ultrasound (*right*). Whether such a rectocele is symptomatic may depend on stool quality, and many are asymptomatic. From [38], with permission

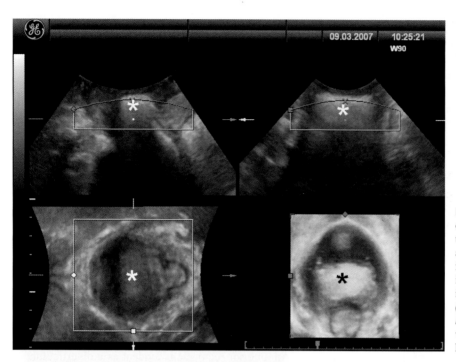

Fig. 38.17 A true rectocele on 3D imaging, showing the spatial extent and symmetry of this typical finding. The rectocele is marked by an *asterisk* in all orthogonal planes (*top left, top right,* and *bottom left*) as well as in a rendered volume (*bottom right*). From [39], with permission

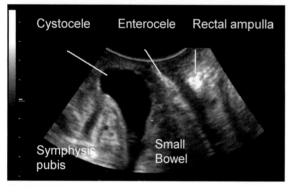

Fig. 38.18 Three-compartment prolapse after hysterectomy. The iso-echoic area between the bladder (*left*) and rectal ampulla (*right*) represents an enterocele. There also is a third-degree cystocele with marked urethral kinking visible on the left, showing an almost inverted bladder neck

rectal mucosa. Since distension of a rectocele will depend on the presence and quality of stool, appearances may vary considerably from one day to the next. The severity of a rectocele can be quantified by measuring maximal descent relative to the inferior symphyseal margin, and by determining the maximal depth of the sacculation as seen in Fig. 38.16 [38], which compares ultrasound and radiological findings in a patient with rectocele. Fig. 38.17 [39] shows a typical symmetrical rectocele in the three orthogonal planes as well as in a rendered volume (*bottom right*).

38.4.2 Enterocele

An enterocele is visualized as downwards displacement of abdominal contents into the vagina, ventral to the anal canal. Small bowel may be identifiable due to its peristalsis, and sometimes intraperitoneal fluid outlines the apex of the enterocele. Distal shadowing is much less common than with rectocele, and often the contents have an irregular isoechoic or ground-glass-like appearance (Fig. 38.18). A sigmoid enterocele tends to show coarser patterns, as seen in Fig. 38.19 in a patient with rectal intussusception.

38.4.3 Rectal Intussusception and Prolapse

An intussusception is seen as splaying of the normally tubular anal canal, with the anterior wall of the rectal ampulla (and occasionally the posterior wall as well) being inverted and propelled into the opening anal canal. Fig. 38.19 shows a comparison of radiological and ultrasound findings in a patient with rectal intussusception.

Usually, a rectal intussusception is due to an enterocele of small bowel that progresses down the anal canal, but other abdominal contents such as sigmoid (as in Fig. 38.19), omentum, and even the uterus can act in a similar way. Ultimately, rectal mucosa and

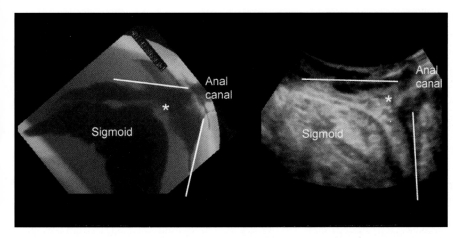

Fig. 38.19 A rectal intussusception (indicated by *) due to a sigmoid enterocele as seen on defecation proctogram (*left*) and translabial ultrasound (*right*). It is generally not possible to distinguish as to what part of the small or large bowel propels the intussuscipiens, although the coarse appearances of the intussuscipiens are suggestive of large rather than small bowel. From [38], with permission

muscularis may protrude from the anus, resulting in rectal prolapse.

When a rectocele or rectal intussusception is identified on translabial imaging, one may want to provide the patient with visual biofeedback. Demonstrating that straining at stool is obviously counterproductive (propelling feces not into the anal canal but into the vagina, or pushing down not feces but small bowel) may help in modifying behavior. Several studies have recently shown that ultrasound is much better tolerated than defecation proctography, and of course it is much cheaper.

As a result it is likely that ultrasound will replace the radiological technique in the initial investigation of women with defecation disorders. If there is a rectocele or a rectal intussusception/prolapse on ultrasound, this condition is very likely to be found on x-ray imaging [38, 40, 41]. In addition, anismus may be evident as an inability to relax the levator ani, which can be diagnosed qualitatively, or by measuring the anorectal angle [42], although it is often not clear whether observations on

diagnostic imaging bear any relation to what happens during defecation.

Assessment of the anal sphincter is covered elsewhere and will not be discussed in any detail here. The anal sphincter is generally imaged by endoanal ultrasound. This method is firmly established as one of the cornerstones of a colorectal diagnostic workup for anal incontinence and is beyond the scope of this chapter. Due to the limited availability of such probes in gynecology, obstetricians and gynecologists often use high-frequency curved array or endovaginal probes placed exoanally, i.e. transperineally, in the coronal rather than the midsagittal plane [43–46]. Lately, 3D pelvic floor imaging has also been used to demonstrate the anal canal [45, 47] and tomographic ultrasound seems to be particularly useful for demonstrating the entire sphincter in one single series of 8 slices.

There are advantages to this approach – not just from the point of view of the patient. Exoanal imaging (Fig. 38.20) [48] reduces distortion of the anal canal

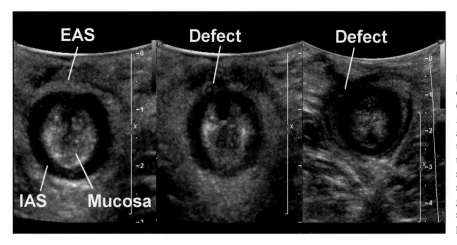

Fig. 38.20 Translabial imaging of the external anal sphincter (*EAS*), coronal plane. All three patients were seen after repair of third-degree tears. As illustrated by this figure, appearances after surgical repair of anal sphincter tears can vary greatly. *IAS*, internal anal sphincter. From [48], with permission

and allows dynamic evaluation of the anal sphincter and mucosa at rest and on sphincter contraction, which seems to enhance the definition of muscular defects. However, resolutions are likely to be inferior [49] to those obtained by endoanal ultrasound, and good comparative studies are still lacking.

38.5 Postoperative Findings

38.5.1 Anterior Colporrhaphy/Vaginal Paravaginal Repair

Anatomical results after traditional anterior repair and vaginal paravaginal repair are highly variable. There are no distinct ultrasonographic features. In the short term, fluid collections are frequently seen and usually do not require any action. Suture material, detritus, and patient discomfort will impair imaging conditions for the first few postoperative weeks. In the medium term, ultrasound imaging sometimes demonstrates no significant change after such surgery. This is true even for patients who consider themselves cured of their prolapse symptoms, raising the possibility that symptom relief may at times be due to vaginal wall denervation rather than altered anatomy. Recurrence is common, easily detected on ultrasound, and associated with levator trauma [50].

38.5.2 Colposuspension

Contrary to the situation with anterior repair, ultrasound findings after colposuspension are quite distinct (Fig. 38.21). Bladder neck mobility is often greatly reduced, and the internal meatus of the urethra anteriorized to a

varying degree, depending on surgical technique. The urethra is straightened and sometimes obviously compressed, and the trigone distorted to a varying degree. Recurrent hypermobility is uncommon – anatomical changes after open Burch colposuspension are usually permanent and result in highly unphysiological sonographic appearances. Occasionally, the bladder neck is pulled up and anteriorized so far that it is difficult to image behind the symphysis pubis. Such appearances are associated with postoperative voiding dysfunction and possibly with symptoms of bladder overactivity [11, 51], although the latter may only be true for markedly overelevated colposuspensions [52].

After laparoscopic colposuspension, similar findings are observed, although overelevation seems very difficult to achieve by the laparoscopic route, and recurrent bladder neck hypermobility may be more common [53]. The typical appearance is most obvious on Valsalva maneuver, in the form of a "colposuspension ridge" underneath the trigone [11, 54–56] as seen in Fig. 38.21.

After Marshall Marchetti urethropexies and laparoscopic urethropexy, there usually is no distinct "colposuspension ridge". While the bladder neck is more (Marshall Marchetti) or less (laparoscopic urethropexy) immobilized, there is no support underneath the trigone, resulting in a sharply sloping trigone on Valsalva and also a low retrovesical angle (80 degrees or less) on Valsalva [57] (Fig. 38.22).

38.5.3 Fascial/Synthetic Traditional Slings

Synthetic or fascial traditional bladder neck slings performed according to the Aldridge technique often result in complete fixation of the bladder neck. There is little

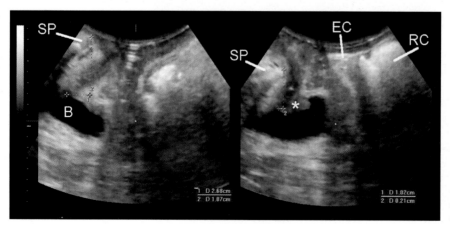

Fig. 38.21 Typical appearances after Burch colposuspension, with the "colposuspension ridge" under the trigone clearly seen on Valsalva maneuver (indicated by *). There also is a recto-enterocele. *B*, bladder; *EC*, enterocele; *RC*, rectocele; *SP*, symphysis pubis

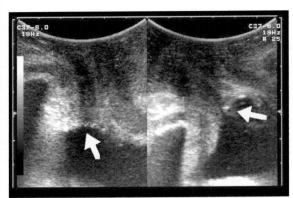

Fig. 38.22 Typical appearances after urethropexy: due to more anterior suture placement, the bladder neck (*arrow*) assumes a particularly unusual appearance, with a retrovesical angle of well below 90 degrees on Valsalva maneuver

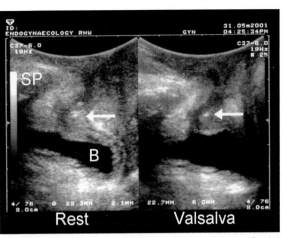

Fig. 38.23 Typical appearances after an Aldridge-type fascial sling. The bladder neck is immobilized, and there is obvious urethral compression. In this case the location of the sling is indicated by a hyperechoic area (*arrow*), but this is not a consistent finding. *B*, bladder; *SP*, symphysis pubis

mobility or change in the retrovesical angle on Valsalva maneuver (Fig. 38.23), and appearances are similar to those after Burch colposuspension. Fascial implants are of varying visibility, but synthetic implants are generally hyperechoic and show distal shadowing. Due to the highly abnormal anatomy, voiding function is often poor, resulting in a chronic residual or retention.

38.5.4 Injectables

The echogenicity of injectables varies considerably. Due to the small market share of those procedures

after the introduction of modern suburethral slings, the literature on sonographic appearances is very scant. Collagen injections do not seem to cause longer- term changes visible on ultrasound, but silicone macroparticles (Macroplastique™) remain visible permanently as a hyperechogenic donut shape surrounding the urethra (Fig. 38.24). Highly peculiar findings are sterile abscesses after Zuidex injection – cystic or polycycstic structures of hypo- to isoechoic appearance that resemble endometriomata.

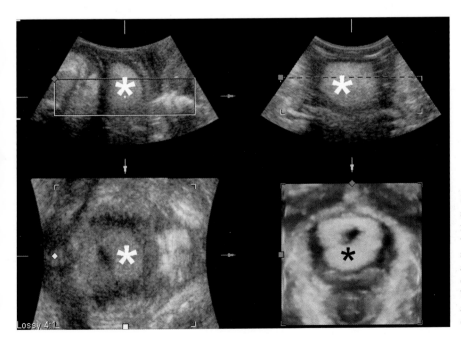

Fig. 38.24 Macroplastique silicone macroparticles used in incontinence surgery are very echogenic and located surrounding the urethra both anteriorly and posteriorly (marked with *) as seen both in sectional planes and rendered volume (*bottom right*)

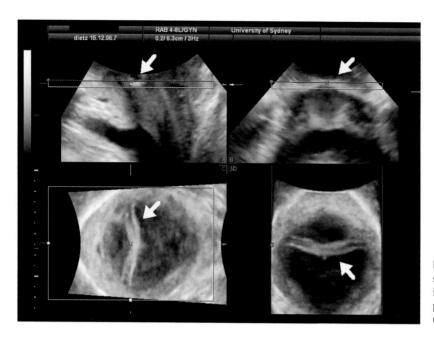

Fig. 38.25 A transobturator suburethral sling (*arrow*) imaged in the three orthogonal planes and in a rendered volume (*bottom right*)

38.5.5 Suburethral Slings

Synthetic suburethral slings such as the tension-free vaginal tape (TVT™), intravaginal sling (IVS™), suprapubic arc sling (SPARC™), TVT obturator (TVT-O™), Monarc™, etc, have replaced colposuspensions as the commonest surgical procedures for the treatment of urodynamic stress incontinence. Ultrasound can confirm the presence of such a sling (see Fig. 38.25 for a 3D representation of a typical transobturator sling), distinguish between transobturator and transretzius implants [58], especially when examining the axial plane (Fig. 38.26), and even allow an educated guess regarding the exact

type and material of the tape [59]. As these implants are highly echogenic, ultrasound is superior to magnetic resonance in identifying such meshes [60] and has helped elucidate their mode of action [61]. A successful sling reduces urethral mobility on Valsalva maneuver, especially mobility of the midurethra [6] and funneling [62], although the latter is often still visible postoperatively and certainly does not imply failure. The location of the tape relative to the urethra does not seem to matter much [63–65], and dislodgment or migration of suburethral wide-weave polypropylene tapes is highly unlikely [66].

Ultrasound is particularly useful in women who present with postoperative complications such as voiding

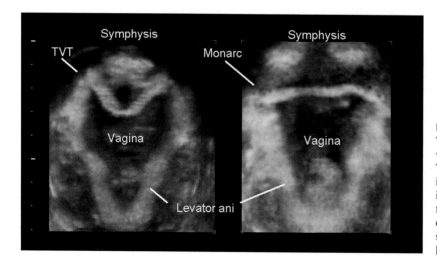

Fig. 38.26 Monarc sling (*right*) vs. TVT sling (*left*) in rendered volumes of the levator hiatus. The difference in placement is obvious: the Monarc sling is inserted through the obturator foramen, the TVT through the space of Retzius. As a result the latter is situated much more medially. From [48], with permission

dysfunction, symptoms of the overactive bladder, recurrent urinary tract infections, and pain [67, 68]. Urethral kinking is sometimes very marked and on its own does not necessarily imply that there is a problem. However, a tape that is curled into a tight "C"-shape at rest, that shows minimal mobility, and that leaves a gap of less than 8 cm between the tape and the symphysis pubis, is more likely to cause voiding dysfunction. Having said this, transobturator tapes somehow seem to follow a different set of rules. A small gap between transobturator tapes and the symphysis pubis on Valsalva maneuver does not usually seem to be a problem, and results in less rather than more urge incontinence [69]. This may be due to the fact that (for reasons of applied physics) transobturator tapes are unlikely to result in clinically relevant voiding dysfunction in women with normal detrusor function [70].

After TVT and other transretzius slings, and occasionally after transobturator slings, persistent voiding dysfunction or de novo symptoms of the overactive bladder sometimes necessitate tape division. Ultrasound may help in locating implants if a tape division is contemplated and confirm tape division if the success of such a procedure is in question.

38.5.6 Mesh Implants in Prolapse Surgery

There is a worldwide trend towards implantation of permanent vaginal wall meshes, especially for recurrent prolapse, and complications such as support failure, chronic pain, and mesh erosion are not uncommon. Polypropylene meshes such as the Perigee™, Prolift™, Avaulta™, and Apogee™ are highly echogenic, and their visibility is limited only by persistent prolapse and transducer distance (Figs. 38.27, 38.28). 3D translabial ultrasound has demonstrated that the implanted mesh is often surprisingly short in the sagittal plane. This is probably most often due to mesh folding on implantation, and to deformation once the mesh comes under tension as soon as the patient coughs or stands up [71, 72]. It is often assumed that implanted mesh may contract or retract, although so far

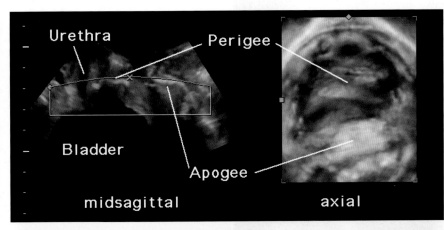

Fig. 38.27 Perigee and Apogee mesh in patient with massive levator ballooning and, despite this, successful prolapse repair. Both implants appear flat and smooth and are clearly functional, blocking a large part of the hiatus on Valsalva maneuver

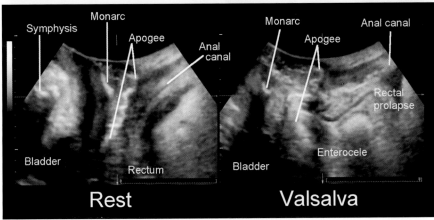

Fig. 38.28 Suburethral sling (*Monarc*) and posterior compartment mesh repair (*Apogee*) in a patient with clinical prolapse cure and symptoms of obstructed defecation 6 months postoperatively. The *right-hand* image shows a rectal intussusception that is due to an enterocele barred from developing into the vagina. From [39], with permission

there is no proof for this [73–74]. Surgical technique seems to play a role in determining appearances, as fixation of mesh to underlying tissues results in a flatter, more even appearance. This may also have an effect on the likelihood of postoperative stress urinary incontinence. The closer the mesh is to the symphysis pubis, and the higher it remains on Valsalva, the lower the prevalence of postoperative stress incontinence [75].

The position, extent, and mobility of vaginal wall mesh can be determined with translabial ultrasound, helping with the assessment of individual technique, and ultrasound may uncover complications such as dislodgment of anchoring arms [71]. Another clinically inapparent form of "failure" is shown in Fig. 38.28. The patient is cured of her symptoms of vaginal prolapse after a clinically successful posterior compartment mesh. However, she now complains of symptoms of obstructed defecation – and the reason is an enterocele that now descends into the anal canal rather than the vagina, causing a rectal in-

tussusception. Clearly, translabial 4D ultrasound will be useful in determining the functional outcome and location of implants, and will help in optimizing both implant design and surgical technique.

38.6 The Levator Hiatus and Muscle

The main current use of 3D translabial ultrasound and axial plane imaging is the assessment of the levator ani muscle, occasionally extending to paraurethral tissues in patients with diverticula or strictures. Translabial ultrasound has confirmed 65-year old clinical data [76] and magnetic resonance imaging studies [77] showing that major morphological abnormalities of levator structure and function are common in vaginally parous women [78]. Clearly such morphological abnormalities are due to vaginal delivery [79] (see Fig. 38.29 for a comparison of antepartum and postpartum findings in

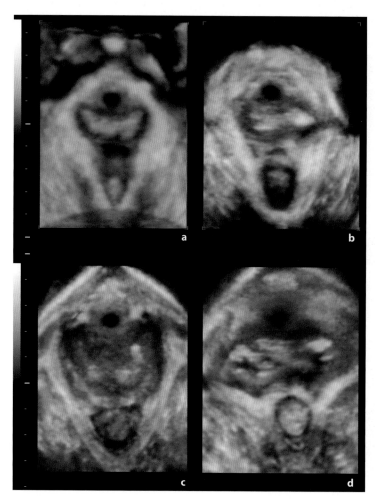

Fig. 38.29 Small left-sided unilateral levator avulsion as evident in rendered volumes. **a** Normal antepartum findings on *left*. **b** Postpartum state on the *right*. **c, d** The same comparison in a patient with a major bilateral levator avulsion as imaged in rendered volumes

patients with unilateral and bilateral avulsion injuries and Fig. 38.30 [80] for clinical findings, ultrasound, and magnetic resonance imaging in a patient with unilateral levator avulsion diagnosed immediately postpartum). The effect on distensibility of the hiatus is evident on Valsalva as shown in Fig. 38.31 [81]. Such trauma can be documented on 2D ultrasound – either with a side-firing endocavitary probe [82] or with a parasagittal probe orientation [83] using abdominal transducers. When using a standard 2D abdominal probe for parasagittal imaging, the probe has to be tilted laterally in order to follow the "V"-shape of the puborectalis muscle between the inferior pubic ramus anteriorly and the anal canal posteriorly (see Figs. 7.7 and 7.8). Fig. 38.32 shows 2D parasagittal findings in women with intact muscle (Fig. 38.32a), and unilateral

(Fig. 38.32b) and bilateral trauma (Fig. 38.32c), as verified by tomographic ultrasound. While levator trauma can be seen on 2D imaging, the most convenient and reproducible approach is by using an abdominal 3D probe. Just as when imaging a fetal face, a rendered volume, with the rendering direction set from distally to proximally, results in evocative, easily understood images that provide the illusion of depth and therefore facilitate interpretation.

Major delivery-related levator trauma, affecting the inferomedial aspects of the puborectalis muscle ("avulsion injury") is clearly part of the missing link between vaginal childbirth and prolapse. While there are other factors, probably including microtrauma or altered biomechanics of otherwise intact muscle, levator trauma seems to enlarge the hiatus [84] and results

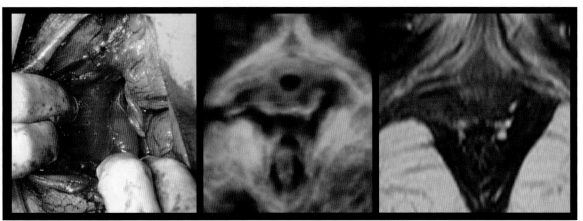

Fig. 38.30 Typical right-sided levator avulsion injury as diagnosed in the delivery suite after a normal vaginal delivery at term (*left*), on 3D ultrasound (*center*) and on magnetic resonance imaging (*right*) three months postpartum. This patient was asymptomatic apart from deep dyspareunia. From [80], with permssion

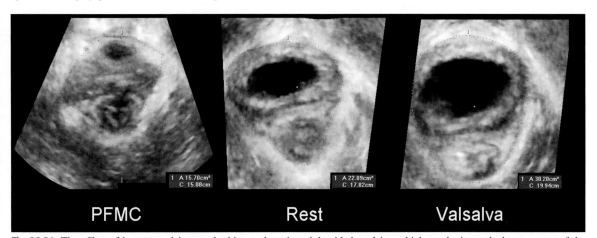

Fig. 38.31 The effect of levator avulsion on the hiatus: there is a right-sided avulsion which results in marked asymmetry of the hiatus as seen in the axial plane on pelvic floor contraction (PFMC, *left*), at rest (*middle*), and on Valsalva (*right*). From [89], with permission

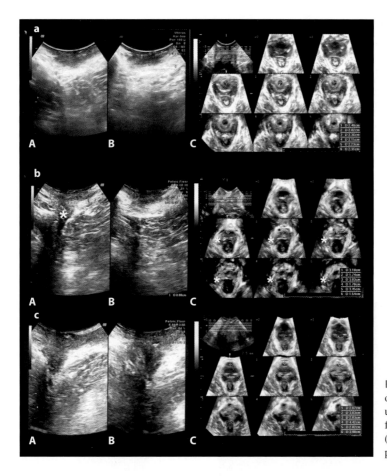

Fig. 38.32 2D parasagittal imaging (*left pairs* of images, *A* and *B*) and tomographic ultrasound (*C*) of a patient with normal findings (**a**), a unilateral right-sided avulsion (**b**) and a bilateral avulsion (**c**), worse on the patient's left. From [89], with permission

in anterior and central compartment prolapse [78]. Patients with avulsion defects are 2.3 times more likely to have a significant cystocele, and four times as likely to have uterine prolapse [85]. Avulsion reduces pelvic floor muscle function by about one-third [86, 87], and has a marked effect on hiatal biometry and distensibility [81] (Fig. 38.31). In the past it was generally assumed that abnormal muscle function was due to neuropathy, but damage to the innervation of the levator ani muscle is likely to play a much smaller role compared to direct trauma [88].

The larger the defect, the higher is the likelihood of prolapse [84], as quantified on multislice or tomographic ultrasound (Fig. 38.32). Levator defects seem to be associated with cystocele recurrence after anterior repair [50, 89] and may well be a risk factor for prolapse development or recurrence after pelvic surgery in general [90].

These defects are palpable (Fig. 38.33) [91], but palpation requires significant teaching [92, 93] and is clearly less repeatable (κ = 0.41) [91] than identifica-

tion by ultrasound (κ = 0.83 on analysis of whole volumes and κ = 0.61 for single slices in own data) [94, 95]. Fig. 38.34 shows a proforma we use for mapping puborectalis muscle defects on palpation. Identification

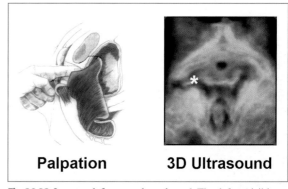

Palpation   **3D Ultrasound**

Fig. 38.33 Levator defects can be palpated. The defect visible on ultrasound (* *right image*) is evident as a widened gap between the urethra and the insertion of the puborectalis muscle on the pelvic sidewall on vaginal examination as illustrated on the left. A full avulsion is defined as a complete absence of muscle fibers on the inferior pubic ramus. From [91], with permission

of an avulsion injury is aided by measurement of the "levator–urethra gap" (Fig. 38.35), the distance from the center of the urethral lumen to the most medial aspect of the puborectalis muscle [96], analogous to the measurement of the levator–symphysis gap (LSG) on magnetic resonance imaging [97].

Avulsion injury does not seem to be associated with stress urinary incontinence and urodynamic stress incontinence, a highly counterintuitive finding in view of the role of pelvic floor muscle exercises in the treatment of this condition [98], nor does it seem to matter much for fecal incontinence [99]. Despite this, there seems to be a high prevalence of levator defects in women with anal sphincter defects, which is not really surprising given the overlap in risk factors [100, 101]. Bilateral defects (see Fig. 38.36 for a comparison of ultrasound and magnetic resonance in a patient with bilateral trauma) are more difficult to detect since there is no normal side to compare with, but they have a particularly severe impact on pelvic floor function and organ support.

Another factor that is only apparent on axial plane imaging is the degree of hiatal distension on Valsalva maneuver. Hiatal dimensions are obtained by determining the plane of minimal hiatal dimensions in the A plane and then locating the same plane in the C plane [102] (see Fig. 7.5) or in a rendered volume [103].

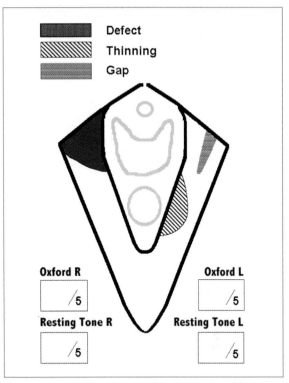

Fig. 38.34 Schematic proforma used for the mapping of the inferior aspects of the levator ani muscle. A typical right-sided avulsion is shown on the left of the image, and the slit-like "gap" shown on the patient's left (*right hand side of the graph*) represents a typical form of partial trauma. From [91], with permission

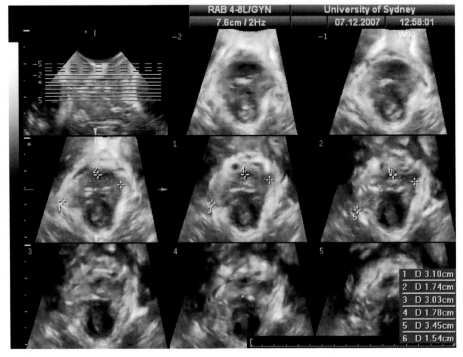

Fig. 38.35 The levator–urethra gap is determined by measuring the minimal distance between the center of the urethra and the puborectalis muscle on the sidewall, and may help in identifying levator trauma in doubtful cases. This tomographic representation of a typical right-sided avulsion demonstrates abnormal gap measurements on the right (3–3.5 cm) versus normal measurements on the left (1.54–1.78 cm)

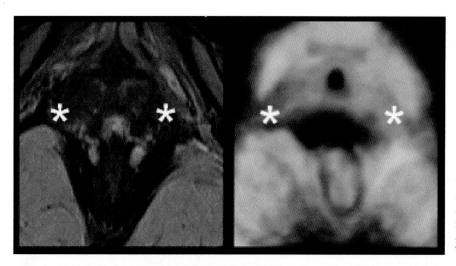

Fig. 38.36 A bilateral avulsion which was identified in the delivery suite and followed up with magnetic resonance (*left*) and 3D ultrasound (*right*). The defects are indicated by *

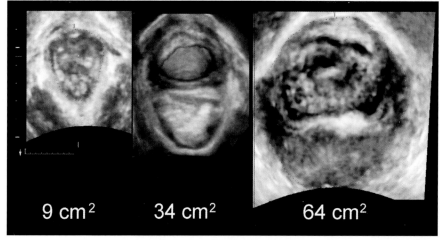

9 cm²   34 cm²   64 cm²

Fig. 38.37 Ballooning of the levator hiatus as measured in the plane of minimal dimensions on maximal Valsalva maneuver. The *left image* illustrates an unusually narrow hiatus in a patient with normal pelvic organ support, the *middle image* shows moderate ballooning, and the *left* demonstrates severe ballooning in a patient with recurrent pelvic organ prolapse and bilateral avulsions

Fig. 38.37 gives an impression of the range of hiatal area measurements in patients attending a pelvic floor clinic. Measures of hiatal dimensions seem highly repeatable [102, 104–107] and correlate well with findings on magnetic resonance imaging [108]. Hiatal enlargement to over 25 cm² on Valsalva maneuver is defined as "ballooning" on the basis of receiver operator characteristics statistics [109] and normative data in young nulliparous women [102, 104]. A simplified method allows determination of hiatal diameters and area in rendered volumes [103], and this may be more reproducible, and possibly even more valid than the original method of using an adjusted C plane, since the true plane of minimal hiatal dimensions is non-Euclidean, i.e. warped rather than flat [110].

Hiatal dimensions are associated with the length of the second stage of labor, and may be a surrogate measure of soft tissue compliance of the birth canal [111, 112], although biometric parameters do not seem to predict trauma [113]. During childbirth the hiatus has to distend to about 68 cm² to allow delivery of a term-sized Caucasian baby, even in the best-case scenario of an occipito-anterior presentation, and data obtained in late pregnancy imply that the required distension in nulliparous women varies enormously, from 61 % to 274 % over the dimensions at rest [114].

The degree of distension observed on Valsalva maneuver is strongly associated with prolapse [115] and symptoms of prolapse [109]. It seems that ballooning is associated with prolapse recurrence after rectocele repair [116], and the same probably holds for other forms of prolapse surgery. However, the role of "ballooning" is likely to be much more complex than the role of avulsion. Clearly, excessive distensibility of the hiatus can be congenital. The author has documented severe ballooning of 52 cm² in a 26-year-old nulliparous

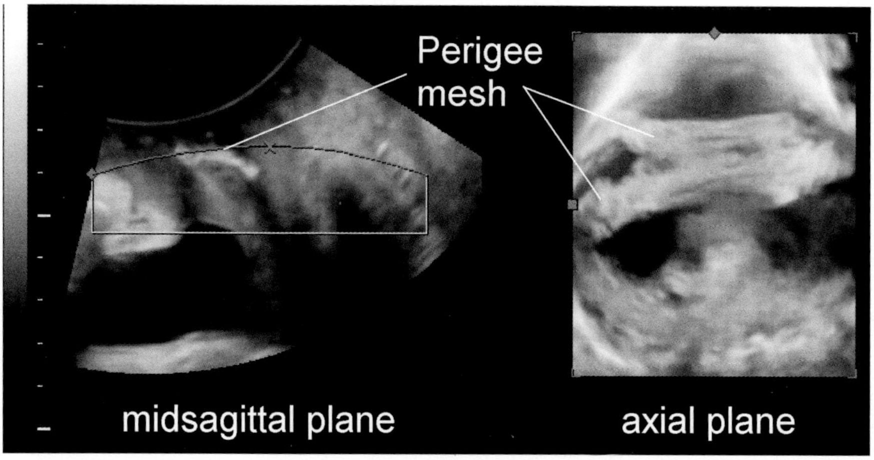

Fig. 38.38 Perigee anterior compartment mesh in a patient with severe bilateral avulsion, shown on maximal Valsalva maneuver. In the axial plane (*right*), the mesh is seen to traverse a hiatus that is enormously enlarged in the coronal plane (*from left to right*) due to the avulsion. Despite the severe trauma, the cystocele is completely reduced, as shown in the midsagittal plane on the left. From [48], with permission

woman. Avulsion increases the hiatal area on Valsalva by about 5–6 cm^2 [81], but there is an additional effect of childbirth that is probably due to traumatic overdistension and that adds on average about 3–4 cm^2 [117]. Finally, it is not at all clear how much of this effect is active, i.e. a cause, rather than passive, i.e. a result of pelvic organ prolapse.

If delivery-related trauma and excessive distensibility of the levator are indeed risk factors for female pelvic organ prolapse and recurrence after reconstructive surgery, then of course we should know about it preoperatively and adjust our surgical approach accordingly. Some forms of prolapse are probably impossible to cure using conventional surgical techniques, unless one uses mesh implants such as the transobturator mesh shown in Fig. 38.38, reducing the effective size of the hiatus by bridging the defects. In future, we should aim to develop surgical methods that reduce the size and distensibility of the hiatus or reconnect the detached muscle in an attempt to prevent recurrence – and this is now a realistic goal that very likely will be reached within a year or two. First attempts to achieve a primary repair immediately after childbirth, however, have proven unsuccessful [80], and secondary repair will probably have to utilize mesh or autologous fascia.

38.7 Outlook

Even before the widespread introduction of 3D/4D imaging, pelvic floor ultrasound was a highly useful diagnostic tool for physicians dealing with pelvic floor disorders. While the uptake of this diagnostic method has varied from one country to another, and from one specialty to another, there now is a substantial body of literature dealing with translabial/perineal/introital ultrasound and its use in women with pelvic floor dysfunction. The near-universal introduction of 4D ultrasound in obstetrics and gynecology, new software options, and increasing availability of training, will lead to more general acceptance of ultrasound as a standard diagnostic option in pelvic floor medicine. The issue of levator trauma, one of the most significant developments in clinical obstetrics since the introduction of fetal monitoring, will take pelvic floor ultrasound from a niche application into the mainstream, and speed the convergence of clinical specialties dealing with pelvic floor disorders. Very likely, ultrasound imaging will help us to resolve some of the many open questions in pelvic floor medicine and lead to improvements in clinical skills and surgical techniques. The crucial factor, as always, is teaching and the provision of up-to-date resources.

For further information see my website (www.med-fac.usyd.edu.au/people/academics/profiles/pdietz.php) and the textbook: Dietz HP, Steensma AB, Hoyte L (eds) Atlas of pelvic floor ultrasound. Springer-Verlag, London, 2007.

References

1. Dietz H. Ultrasound imaging of the pelvic floor: part 1: 2D aspects. Ultrasound Obstet Gynecol 2004;23:80–92.
2. Schaer GN, Siegwart R, Perucchini D, DeLancey JO. Examination of voiding in seated women using a remote-controlled ultrasound probe. Obstet Gynecol 1998;91:297–301.
3. Pirpiris A, Shek K, Dietz HP. Urethral mobility and its relationship with urodynamic diagnosis. Neurourol Urodyn 2009;28:851-852.

4. Dietz HP, Bennett MJ. The effect of childbirth on pelvic organ mobility [comment]. Obstet Gynecol 2003;102:223–228.

5. Shek KL, Dietz HP. The urethral motion profile: a novel method to evaluate urethral support and mobility. Aust N Z J Obstet Gynaecol 2008;48:337–342.

6. Shek KL, Chantarasorn V, Dietz HP. The urethral motion profile before and after Monarc suburethral sling placement. Abstract. Annual Meeting of the International Continence Society, San Francisco, USA, 29 September to 3 October 2009.

7. Haylen BT, Frazer MI, Sutherst JR, West CR. Transvaginal ultrasound in the assessment of bladder volumes in women. Preliminary report. Br J Urol 1989;63:149–151.

8. Schaer GN, Koechli OR, Schuessler B, Haller U. Perineal ultrasound for evaluating the bladder neck in urinary stress incontinence. Obstet Gynecol 1995;85:220–224.

9. Dietz HP, Wilson PD. Anatomical assessment of the bladder outlet and proximal urethra using ultrasound and videocystourethrography. Int Urogynecol J 1998;9:365–369.

10. Dietz HP, Wilson PD. The influence of bladder volume on the position and mobility of the urethrovesical junction. Int Urogynecol J 1999;10:3–6.

11. Martan A, Masata J, Halaska M, Voigt R. Ultrasound imaging of the lower urinary system in women after Burch colposuspension. Ultrasound Obstet Gynecol 2001; 17:58–64.

12. Dietz HP, Eldridge A, Grace M, Clarke B. Pelvic organ descent in young nulligravid women. Am J Obstet Gynecol 2004;191:95–99.

13. Oerno A, Dietz H. Levator co-activation is a significant confounder of pelvic organ descent on Valsalva maneuver. Ultrasound Obstet Gynecol 2007;30:346–350.

14. Reed H, Waterfield A, Freeman RM, Adekanmi OA. Bladder neck mobility in continent nulliparous women: normal references. Int Urogynecol J 2002;13:S4.

15. Brandt FT, Albuquerque CD, Lorenzato FR, Amaral FJ. Perineal assessment of urethrovesical junction mobility in young continent females. Int Urogynecol J 2000;11:18–22.

16. Peschers UM, Fanger G, Schaer GN et al. Bladder neck mobility in continent nulliparous women. BJOG 2001; 108:320–324.

17. Dietz HP, Hansell N, Grace M et al. Bladder neck mobility is a heritable trait. Br J Obstet Gynaecol 2005;112:334–339.

18. Peschers U, Schaer G, Anthuber C et al. Changes in vesical neck mobility following vaginal delivery. Obstet Gynecol 1996;88:1001–1006.

19. Dietz HP, Clarke B, Vancaillie TG. Vaginal childbirth and bladder neck mobility. Aust N Z J Obstet Gynaecol 2002;42:522–525.

20. Huang WC, Yang JM. Bladder neck funneling on ultrasound cystourethrography in primary stress urinary incontinence: a sign associated with urethral hypermobility and intrinsic sphincter deficiency. Urology 2003;61:936–941.

21. Masata J, Martan A, Halaska M et al. Ultrasound imaging of urethral funneling. Int Urogynecol J 1999;10(suppl):S62.

22. Dietz HP, Clarke B. The urethral pressure profile and ultrasound parameters of bladder neck mobility. Int Urogynecol J 1998;17:374–375.

23. Dietz HP, McKnoulty L, Clarke B. Translabial color Doppler for imaging in urogynecology: a preliminary report. Ultrasound Obstet Gynecol 1999;14:144–147.

24. Dietz HP, Clarke B. Translabial color Doppler urodynamics. Int Urogynecol J 2001;12:304–307.

25. Masata J, Martan A, Halaska M et al. Detection of Valsalva leak point pressure with colour Doppler- new method for routine use. Neurourol Urodyn 2001;20:494–496.

26. Dietz HP, Haylen BT, Vancaillie TG. Female pelvic organ prolapse and voiding function. Int Urogynecol J 2002;13:284–288.

27. Eisenberg V, Chantarasorn V, Dietz HP. Avulsion defect and cystocele: is there a link? Ultrasound Obstet Gynecol 2009;3(suppl 1):8.

28. Tsai M, Tsai K, Liu C et al. Perineal ultrasonography in diagnosing anterior vaginal leiomyoma resembling a cystocele. Ultrasound Obstet Gynecol 2007;30:1013–1014.

29. Khullar V, Cardozo L. Imaging in urogynaecology. Br J Obstet Gynaecol 1996;103:1061–1067.

30. Yang JM, Huang WC. Bladder wall thickness on ultrasonographic cystourethrography: affecting factors and their implications. J Ultrasound Med 2003;22:777–782.

31. Lekskulchai O, Dietz H. Detrusor wall thickness as a test for detrusor overactivity in women. Ultrasound Obstet Gynecol 2008;32:535–539.

32. Robinson D, Anders K, Cardozo L et al. Can ultrasound replace ambulatory urodynamics when investigating women with irritative urinary symptoms? BJOG 2002;109:145–148.

33. Robinson D, Khullar V, Cardozo L. Can bladder wall thickness predict postoperative detrusor overactivity? Int Urogynecol J 2005;16:S106.

34. Lekskulchai O, Dietz HP. Is detrusor hypertrophy in women associated with voiding dysfunction? Aust N Z J Obstet Gynaecol 2009;49:653-666.

35. Tunn R, Petri E. Introital and transvaginal ultrasound as the main tool in the assessment of urogenital and pelvic floor dysfunction: an imaging panel and practical approach. Ultrasound Obstet Gynecol 2003;22:205–213.

36. Dietz HP, Korda A. Which bowel symptoms are most strongly associated with a true rectocele? Aust N Z J Obstet Gynaecol 2005;45:505–508.

37. Dietz HP, Steensma AB. Posterior compartment prolapse on two- dimensional and three-dimensional pelvic floor ultrasound: the distinction between true rectocele, perineal hypermobility and enterocele. Ultrasound Obstet Gynecol 2010;202:321–334.

38. Perniola G, Shek K, Chong CC et al. Defecation proctography and translabial ultrasound in the investigation of defecatory disorders. Ultrasound Obstet Gynecol 2007;31:567–571.

39. Dietz HP. Pelvic floor ultrasound: a review. Am J Obstet Gynecol 2010;202:321-334.

40. Steensma AB, Oom DMJ, Burger CW, Schouten WR. Comparison of defecography and 3D/ 4D translabial ultrasound in patients with pelvic organ prolapse and/ or evacuation disorders. Ultrasound Obstet Gynecol 2007;30:447.

41. Konstantinovic ML, Steensma AB, Domali E et al. Correlation between 3D/4D translabial ultrasound and colpocystodefecography in diagnosis of posterior compartment prolapse. Ultrasound Obstet Gynecol 2007;30:448.

42. Grasso R, Piciucchi S, Quattrocchi C et al. Posterior pelvic floor disorders: a prospective comparison using introital ultrasound and colpocystodefecography. Ultrasound Obstet Gynecol 2007;30:86–94.

43. Peschers UM, DeLancey JO, Schaer GN, Schuessler B. Exoanal ultrasound of the anal sphincter: normal anatomy and sphincter defects. Br J Obstet Gynaecol 1997;104:999–1003.

44. Kleinubing H, Jr., Jannini JF, Malafaia O et al. Transperineal ultrasonography: new method to image the anorectal region. Dis Colon Rectum 2000;43:1572–1574.

45. Yagel S, Valsky DV. Three-dimensional transperineal sonography for evaluation of the anal sphincter complex: another dimension in understanding peripartum sphincter trauma. Ultrasound Obstet Gynecol 2006;27:119–123.

46. Hall RJ, Rogers RG, Saiz L, Qualls C. Translabial ultrasound assessment of the anal sphincter complex: normal measurements of the internal and external anal sphincters at the proximal, mid- and distal levels. Int Urogynecol J 2007;18:881–888.

47. Lee J, Pretorius D, Weinstein MM et al. Transperineal three-dimensional ultrasound in evaluating anal sphincter muscles. Ultrasound Obstet Gynecol 2007;30:201–209.

48. Dietz HP. Pelvic floor ultrasound. Australasian Society for Ultrasound Medicine Bulletin 2007;10:17–23.

49. Cornelia L, Stephan B, Michel B et al. Trans-perineal versus endo-anal ultrasound in the detection of anal sphincter tears. Eur J Obstetrics Gynecol Reprod Biol 2002;103:79–82.

50. Dietz HP, Chantarasorn V, Shek KL. Levator avulsion is a risk factor for cystocele recurrence. Ultrasound Obstet Gynecol 2010;accepted 1.12.09.

51. Bombieri L, Freeman RM, Perkins EP et al. Why do women have voiding dysfunction and de novo detrusor instability after colposuspension? Br J Obstet Gynaecol 2002; 109:402–412.

52. Dietz HP, Wilson PD, Clarke B, Haylen BT. Irritative symptoms after colposuspension: are they due to distortion or overelevation of the anterior vaginal wall and trigone? Int Urogynecol J 2001;12:232–235; discussion 235–236.

53. Dietz H, Wilson P. Laparoscopic colposuspension vs. urethropexy: a case control series. Int Urogynecol J 2005;16:15–18; discussion 18.

54. Dietz HP, Wilson PD. Colposuspension success and failure: a long-term objective follow-up study. Int Urogynecol J 2000;11:346–351.

55. Bombieri L, Freeman RM, Perkins EP et al. Objective assessment of bladder neck elevation and urethral compression at colposuspension. BJOG 2002;109:395–401.

56. Viereck V, Pauer HU, Bader W et al. Introital ultrasound of the lower genital tract before and after colposuspension: a 4-year objective follow-up. Ultrasound Obstet Gynecol 2004;23:277–283.

57. Dietz H, Wilson P. Long-term success after open and laparoscopic colposuspension: a case control study. Gyn Endoscopy 2002;11:81–84.

58. Dietz H, Barry C, Lim Y, Rane A. TVT vs Monarc: a comparative study. Int Urogynecol J 2006;17:566–569.

59. Dietz HP, Barry C, Lim YN, Rane A. Two-dimensional and three-dimensional ultrasound imaging of suburethral slings. Ultrasound Obstet Gynecol 2005;26:175–179.

60. Schuettoff S, Beyersdorff D, Gauruder-Burmester A, Tunn R. Visibility of the polypropylene tape after TVT (tension-free vaginal tape) procedure in women with stress urinary incontinence: comparison of introital ultrasound and MRI in vitro and in patients. Ultrasound Obstet Gynecol 2006; 27:687–692.

61. Dietz HP, Wilson PD. The "iris effect": how two-dimensional

and three-dimensional ultrasound can help us understand anti-incontinence procedures. Ultrasound Obstet Gynecol 2004;23:267–271.

62. Masata J, Martan A, Svabik K et al. Ultrasound imaging of the lower urinary tract after successful tension-free vaginal tape (TVT) procedure. Ultrasound Obstet Gynecol 2006; 28:221–228.

63. Dietz HP, Mouritsen L, Ellis G, Wilson PD. How important is TVT location? Acta Obstet Gynecol Scand 2004;83:904–908.

64. de Tayrac R, Deffieux X, Resten A et al. A transvaginal ultrasound study comparing transobturator tape and tension-free vaginal tape after surgical treatment of female stress urinary incontinence. Int Urogynecol J 2006;17:466–471.

65. Ng C, Lee L, Han H. Use of three- dimensional ultrasound scan to assess the importance of midurethral placement of the tension- free vaginal tape (TVT) for treatment of incontinence. Int Urogynecol J 2006;16:220–225.

66. Dietz HP, Mouritsen L, Ellis G, Wilson PD. Does the tension-free vaginal tape stay where you put it? Am J Obstet Gynecol 2003;188:950–953.

67. Harms L, Emons G, Bader W et al. Funneling before and after anti-incontinence surgery – a prognostic indicator? Part 2: tension-free vaginal tape. Int Urogynecol J 2007; 18:189–294.

68. Tunn R, Gauruder-Burmester A, Koelle D. Ultrasound diagnosis of intra-urethral tension-free vaginal tape (TVT) position as a cause of postoperative voiding dysfunction and retropubic pain. Ultrasound Obstet Gynecol 2004;23:298–301.

69. Chantarasorn V, Shek KL, Dietz HP. Sonographic appearance of transobturator slings: implications for function and dysfunction. Abstract. Annual Meeting of the Internation Continence Society, San Francisco, 29 September to 3 October 2009.

70. Jurgens J, Steller J. Theoretisch-mathematische Modelle zur Kräftewirkung bei alloplastischen Bandsystemen in der Inkontinenztherapie. Gynäkol Geburtshilfliche Rundsch 2005; 45:257–261.

71. Shek KL, Dietz HP, Rane A, Balakrishnan S. Transobturator mesh repair for large and recurrent cystocele. Ultrasound Obst Gynecol 2008;32:82–86.

72. Tunn R, Picot A, Marschke J, Gauruder-Burmester A. Sonomorphological evaluation of polypropylene mesh implants after vaginal mesh repair in women with cystocele or rectocele. Ultrasound Obstet Gynecol 2007;29:449–452.

73. Svabik K, Martan A, Masata J, ElHaddad R. Vaginal mesh shrinking-ultrasound assessment and quantification. Int Urogynecol J 2009;20:S166.

74. Erdmann M, Shek K, Dietz H. Mesh contraction: myth or reality? Int Urogynecol J 2010; in print.

75. Shek C, Rane A, Goh JTW, Dietz HP. Stress urinary incontinence after transobturator mesh for cystocele repair. Int Urogynecol J 2009;20:421–425.

76. Gainey HL. Post-partum observation of pelvic tissue damage. Am J Obstet Gynecol 1943;46:457–466.

77. DeLancey JO, Kearney R, Chou Q et al. The appearance of levator ani muscle abnormalities in magnetic resonance images after vaginal delivery. Obstet Gynecol 2003;101:46–53.

78. Dietz H, Steensma A. The prevalence of major abnormalities of the levator ani in urogynaecological patients. Br J Obstet Gynaecol 2006;113:225–230.

79. Dietz H, Lanzarone V. Levator trauma after vaginal delivery. Obstet Gynecol 2005;106:707–712.

80. Dietz H, Gillespie A, Phadke P. Avulsion of the pubovisceral muscle associated with large vaginal tear after normal vaginal delivery at term. Aust N Z J Obstet Gynaecol 2007; 47:341–344.

81. Abdool Z, Shek K, Dietz H. The effect of levator avulsion on hiatal dimensions and function. Am J Obstet Gynecol 2009;201:89.e1–89.e5.

82. Athanasiou S, Chaliha C, Toozs-Hobson P et al. Direct imaging of the pelvic floor muscles using two-dimensional ultrasound: a comparison of women with urogenital prolapse versus controls. BJOG 2007;114:882–888.

83. Dietz HP, Shek KL. Levator trauma can be diagnosed by 2D translabial ultrasound. Int Urogynecol J 2009;20:807–811.

84. Dietz HP. Quantification of major morphological abnormalities of the levator ani. Ultrasound Obstet Gynaecol 2007; 29:329–334.

85. Dietz HP, Simpson J. Levator trauma is associated with pelvic organ prolapse. BJOG 2008;115:979–984.

86. DeLancey J, Morgan D, Fenner D et al. Comparison of levator ani muscle defects and function in women with and without pelvic organ prolapse. Obstet Gynecol 2007; 109:295–302.

87. Dietz HP, Shek C. Levator avulsion and grading of pelvic floor muscle strength. Int Urogynecol J 2008;19:633–636.

88. Sarma S, Hersch M, Siva S et al. Women who cannot contract their pelvic floor muscles: avulsion or denervation? Neurourol Urodyn 2009;28(suppl 1):680–681.

89. Adekanmi OA, Freeman R, Puckett M, Jackson S. Cystocele: does anterior repair fail because we fail to correct the fascial defects? A clinical and radiological study. Int Urogynecol J 2005;16:S73.

90. Model A, Shek KL, Dietz HP. Do levator defects increase the risk of prolapse recurrence after pelvic floor surgery? Neurourol Urodyn 2009;28(suppl 1):888–889.

91. Dietz HP, Shek KL. Validity and reproducibility of the digital detection of levator trauma. Int Urogynecol J 2008;19:1097–1101.

92. Dietz HP, Hyland G, Hay-Smith J. The assessment of levator trauma: a comparison between palpation and 4D pelvic floor ultrasound. Neurourol Urodyn 2006;25:424–427.

93. Kearney R, Miller JM, Delancey JO. Interrater reliability and physical examination of the pubovisceral portion of the levator ani muscle, validity comparisons using MR imaging. Neurourol Urodyn 2006;25:50–54.

94. Dietz H. Quantification of major morphological abnormalities of the levator ani. Ultrasound Obstet Gynecol 2007; 29:329–334.

95. Weinstein MM, Pretorius D, Nager CW, Mittal R. Inter-rater reliability of pelvic floor muscle imaging abnormalities with 3D ultrasound. Ultrasound Obstet Gynecol 2007;30:538.

96. Dietz H, Abbu A, Shek K. The levator urethral gap measurement: an objective means of determining levator avulsion? Ultrasound Obstet Gynecol 2008;32:941-945.

97. Singh K, Jakab M, Reid W et al. Three-dimensional magnetic resonance imaging assessment of levator animorphologic features in different grades of prolapse. Am J Obstet Gynecol 2003;188:910–915.

98. Dietz HP, Kirby A, Shek KL, Bedwell P. Does avulsion of puborectalis muscle affect bladder function? Int Urogynecol J 2009;20:967-972.

99. Chantarasorn V, Shek KL, Dietz HP. Levator avulsion is not associated with fecal incontinence. Int Urogynecol J 2009;20(suppl 2):S169–170.

100. Weinstein MM, Pretorius D, Jung SY et al. Anatomic defects in the puborectalis muscle in women with fecal incontinence. Ultrasound Obstet Gynecol 2007;30:637.

101. Steensma AB, Schweitzer KJ, Burger CW, Schouten WR. Are anal sphincter injuries related to levator abnormalities? Ultrasound Obstet Gynecol 2007;30:448.

102. Dietz H, Shek K, Clarke B. Biometry of the pubovisceral muscle and levator hiatus by three-dimensional pelvic floor ultrasound. Ultrasound Obstet Gynecol 2005;25:580–585.

103. Wong V, Shek KL, Dietz HP. A simplified method for the determination of levator hiatal dimensions. Int Urogynecol J 2009;20(suppl 2):S145–156.

104. Yang J, Yang S, Huang W. Biometry of the pubovisceral muscle and levator hiatus in nulliparous Chinese women. Ultrsound Obstet Gynecol 2006;26:710–716.

105. Hoff Braekken I, Majida M, Ellstrom Engh M et al. Test-retest and intra-observer reliability of two- three- and four-dimensional perineal ultrasound of pelvic floor muscle anatomy and function. Int Urogynecol J 2008;227-235.

106. Guaderrama N, Liu J, Nager C et al. Evidence for the innervation of pelvic floor muscles by the pudendal nerve. Obstet Gynecol 2006;106:774–781.

107. Kruger J, Dietz H, Murphy B. Pelvic floor function in elite nulliparous athletes and controls. Ultrasound Obstet Gynecol 2007;30:81–85.

108. Kruger J, Heap X, Dietz HP. A comparison of MRI and ultrasound in the assessment of the levator hiatus. Ultrasound Obstet Gynecol 2007;30:447.

109. Dietz HP, Shek KL, De Leon J, Steensma A. Ballooning of the levator hiatus. Ultrasound Obstet Gynecol 2008;31:676–680.

110. Kruger J, Heap X, Murphy B, Dietz H. Pelvic floor function in nulliparous women using 3-dimensional ultrasound and magnetic resonance imaging. Obstet Gynecol 2008;111:631–638.

111. Lanzarone V, Dietz H. 3-Dimensional ultrasound imaging of the levator hiatus in late pregnancy and associations with delivery outcomes. Aust N Z J Obstet Gynaecol 2007; 47:176–180.

112. Balmforth J, Toosz-Hobson P, Cardozo L. Ask not what childbirth can do to your pelvic floor but what your pelvic floor can do in childbirth. Neurourol Urodyn 2003;22: 540–542.

113. Shek KL, Chantarasorn V, Dietz HP. Can levator avulsion be predicted antenatally? Accepted, Am J Obstet Gynecol 15.9.09.

114. Svabik K, Shek KL, Dietz HP. How much does the puborectalis muscle have to stretch in childbirth? BJOG 2009; 116:1657-1662.

115. Dietz H, Steensma A. Dimensions of the levator hiatus in symptomatic women. Ultrasound Obstet Gynecol 2005; 26:369–370.

116. Barry C, Dietz H, Lim Y, Rane A. A short-term independent audit of mesh repair for the treatment of rectocele in women, using 3-dimensional volume hiatal ultrasound: a pilot study. Aust N Z Continence J 2006;12:94–99.

117. Shek KL, Dietz HP. The effect of childbirth on hiatal dimensions: a prospective observational study. Obstet Gynecol 2009;113:1272-1278.

Cystography and Defecography

39

Vittorio L. Piloni

Abstract Perineal sonography and fast magnetic resonance imaging (MRI) are currently confronting conventional x-ray studies in the diagnosis of pelvic organ prolapse including cystocele, enterocele, peritoneocele, and rectocele, with no evidence of substantial discrepancies among the three modalities. Contrast-enhanced studies still serve as the standard of reference in specific cases such as genuine stress urinary incontinence, voiding dysfunctions, neurogenic bladder, poor emptying, and obstructed defecation syndrome in the postoperative anorectum. The advent of three-dimensional (3D) ultrasound and the availability of a remote-controlled, mobile vertically oriented MR system are expected to reduce the inaccuracy rate of these modalities in the diagnosis of advanced pelvic organ prolapse, making conventional studies almost obsolete within a few years.

Keywords Contrast-enhanced radiography • Defecography • Double contrast cystourethrography • Dynamic radiology • Fast MR imaging of the pelvis • Pelvic organ prolapse • Perineal sonography

39.1 Introduction

In the past 20 years, innovations in pelvic floor imaging have been numerous, and the ability to generate spatial information with energy sources other than x-ray, such as ultrasound (US) and magnetic resonance imaging (MRI), has drastically changed the role of conventional radiology in this field. As a consequence, it is no wonder that traditional radiologic procedures including retrograde and voiding cystourethrography, defecography, and colpocystoenterodefecography, no longer seem so interesting or clinically pertinent. Currently, there appears to be a general agreement in the literature that new knowledge in pelvic floor imaging will be gained most exclusively with US and MRI

[1–8]. On the other hand, in most hospitals in Italy, traditional radiologic procedures and contrast examinations still comprise between 70% and 80% of all "basic" imaging studies in such patients. Assuming that current trends in the use of US and MRI continue, a realistic prediction is that this decline in conventional radiology will continue until contrast x-ray examinations are considered almost obsolete.

This chapter examines specific indications for conventional studies of the lower urinary and alimentary tracts, to determine in what conditions they have pertinence and enduring value.

39.2 Lower Urinary Tract Conditions

Several techniques for performing dynamic examination of the lower urinary tract have been described,

V.L. Piloni
Diagnostic Imaging Centre "Villa Silvia" Clinic, Senigallia, Italy

G.A. Santoro, A.P. Wieczorek, C.I. Bartram (eds.) *Pelvic Floor Disorders*
© Springer-Verlag Italia 2010

including retrograde and voiding cystourethrography and metallic bead-chain urethrocystography [9–14]. The two conditions for which contrast radiography studies were traditionally considered most helpful are female urinary incontinence associated with excessive vesical neck motion, and voiding obstructive syndromes. An additional interesting field of study is represented by patients with voiding disorders of neurologic origin.

Provided the above-mentioned diagnostic tests are not obtained uncritically, they still seem to have enduring value in specific cases. For the purpose of improving quantification of vesical descent and identifying the associated leakage of urine at rest and under provocative maneuvers such as coughing or straining, in a less invasive way with respect to bead-chain cystography, we have developed a new method called double-contrast cystourethrography (DCCU), which can be performed easily and rapidly in any radiologic department. The following is a description of our protocol and diagnostic criteria.

39.2.1 Imaging Technique

The examination is usually carried out on an all-purpose gastrointestinal tract remote-controlled x-ray apparatus (Opera T30cs, GMM, Senigallia, Italy). Prior to imaging, the patient is asked to void and the residue registered after insertion into the bladder of a 14 French foley. The same catheter is subsequently used for water-soluble radiopaque contrast administration, with the patient in a dorsolithotomy position on the x-ray table. For DCCU, the empty bladder is firstly filled with 10 mL of 37 mg/mL meglumine iodamide (Iopamidolo 370, Bracco Industria Chimica Spa, Milan, Italy) at body temperature, using a syringe; this is followed by instillation by gravity drip at a rate of 15 mL/min of an additional amount of 15 mg/mL contrast (Iomeron 150) until the patient expresses the desire to micturate (mean 300 mL, range 200–480 mL). According to Fotter et al [15], contrast medium is dripped into the bladder from a constant height of 30 cm above the level of the bladder, thus acting as a sort of manometer when observing the speed of the infusion. Any cessation or even reversal of flow in the tubing is noted and, depending on the volume infused, is considered to be evidence of an unhinibited detrusor contraction. Then, after catheter withdrawal, the table

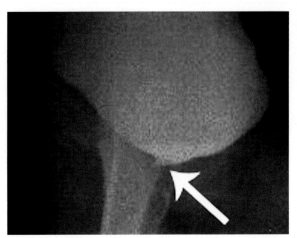

Fig. 39.1 Double contrast cystourethrography (DCCU) in a 38-year-old woman with no evidence of stress incontinence. Lateral upright film on straining. The radiopaque fluid–fluid level visible at the bottom of the bladder depicts the closed bladder neck (*arrow*)

is tilted upright under continuous fluoroscopy and videorecording, while the patient stands up on the foot rest of the radiographic unit. Typically, due to the different iodine concentration, a fluid–fluid level becomes apparent at this moment, the higher-density contrast being seen at the most dependent portion of the bladder (Fig. 39.1). Thereafter, upright lateral and oblique views are taken while the patient is coughing and straining forcefully for evidence of leakage. To prevent embarrassment by the patient, a pad is held between the legs just below the perineal region, to collect any material. In case of urinary loss, the patient is asked to hold back in an attempt to stop the stream (stop test). Seated imaging is also an integral part of the examination for evaluation of the entire voiding performance.

39.2.2 Image Analysis

Evaluation of the overall anatomical situation of the opacified bladder, and the degree of bladder neck mobility are noted. The posterior urethrovesical angle (beta angle) and the angle between the vertical axis and urethral axis (alpha angle) are measured at rest and on straining. The posterior urethrovesical angle is described as the angle between the urethral axis and the floor of the bladder axis one-third closer to the urethra. By using the posterior edge of the symphysis pubis as a reference point, the bladder neck mobility is evaluated at the cephalocaudal plane by measuring the descensus diameter.

In continent subjects the vesical neck and proximal urethra are closed at rest and situated at or above the superior margin of the symphysis pubis; on exertion, the vertical component of urethrovesical junction mobility is no more than 4.0 mm, and failure to demonstrate urinary leakage is a distinctive feature of subjects with normal urine control.

In case of hypermobility and associated loss of urine, the urethrovesical junction makes a rotational movement during stress on both the ventro-dorsal and cephalo-caudal axes, while the higher-density contrast is seen to leak out. Interestingly, in patients with genuine stress incontinence, leakage of contrast is simultaneous with the increase in abdominal pressure, as opposed to evidence of a variable 15–50 s delay between the provocative maneuver and leakage occurring in those with incontinence involving a detrusor-uninhibited contraction.

Additional features of genuine urinary incontinence include a wider posterior urethrovesical angle, which is usually found to differ significantly between incontinent subjects and control groups both at rest and on straining (121.6 ± 17.8 vs. 109.2 ± 7.5 degrees and 166.8 ± 33.3 vs. 123.1 ± 8.9 degrees, P = 0.010 and 0.001, respectively), and the angle between the vertical axis and urethral axis, which differs significantly between the two groups on straining only (51.0 ± 14.0 vs. 31.3 ± 11.7 degrees, P = 0.001). The cephalo-caudal distance (descensus diameter) is also longer in patients with stress urinary incontinence (27.4 ± 7.2 vs. 11.2 ± 4.4 mm, P = 0.001).

According to Blaivas and Olsson [16], a first-degree urinary incontinence is diagnosed if the vesical neck and proximal urethra are closed at rest and are situated at or above the inferior margin of the symphysis pubis. On straining, the vesical neck opens and descends less than 2 cm, and is accompanied by distinctive evidence of radiopaque contrast loss with little or no cystocele. A second-degree urinary incontinence is characterized by the vesical neck being closed at rest which is seen above (2nd a) or below (2nd b) the symphysis pubis. During stress, the vesical neck opens and descends more than 2 cm. Leakage of contrast is most frequently associated with obvious cystourethrocele. A third-degree urinary incontinence is diagnosed when the vesical neck is open at rest and the proximal urethra assumes a funnel shape.

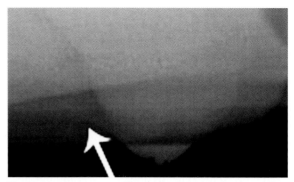

Fig. 39.2 Forty-two-year-old woman with hypermobility of the bladder neck at physical examination and history of recurrent cystitis. Voiding cystouretrography in the sitting position. After repeated voiding attempts assisted by abdominal straining, the higher-density contrast remains entrapped within the most dependent portion of the bladder base and the urethra is seen to describe an arc upward (*arrow*) before reaching the external orifice

In cases of urinary retention, the radiographic documentation taken with the patient sitting sideways while voiding the contrast, allows easy identification of the mechanism involved when the condition is due to a rotational movement and hypermobility of the urethrovesical junction on both the ventro-dorsal and cephalo-caudal axes. The voiding pattern (whether split or continuous), the total voiding time, and the residue are also noted (Fig. 39.2).

Radiologic evaluation of the bladder and urethra in patients with neurologic conditions [17] affecting the brain or any of the neural pathways connecting the brain with the lower urinary tract (spinal cord injuries, tumors, or inflammatory and degenerative diseases), is focused on the size and geometrical configuration of the bladder, the filling sensation, the maximum tolerable volume, the capacity at first leakage, and the characteristics of the voiding pattern. More particularly, based on the reflexivity of the bladder, a detrusor hyperreflexia can be inferred at retrograde cystouretrography, when a small-size, round-shaped bladder is seen with uncontrollable urine loss at low distending volume. This pattern is most frequently observed in patients with damage occurring above the level of the sacral level arc (upper motor neuron). Conversely, a bladder detrusor areflexia often reveals a smooth, thin-walled bladder with increased capacity, extending high into the abdomen in the absence of any characteristic filling sensation. This pattern is seen in cases with lower motor neuron lesions, typically in diabetic patients. Often, these patients are also unable to void spontaneously unless abdominal straining is attempted and the amount of residual urine is high. The voiding phase varies depending on whether the external sphincter at the level of the urogenital diaphragm is seen to contract inappropriately or not.

39.3 Evacuation Conditions

Intermittent fluoroscopy and videorecording during coughing, squeezing, straining, and emptying after opacification of the anorectosigmoid junction combined with opacification of other pelvic viscera (colpocystoenterodefecography) [18, 19] was traditionally considered the imaging technique of choice for investigating pelvic organ prolapse (Fig. 39.3), until the advent of dynamic MRI [20, 21]. The absence of ionizing radiation and the superior reproducibility in measuring the parameters of anorectal configuration by MRI make it preferable when assessing patients with evacuation disorders, despite the less physiological position, i.e. horizontal, assumed by the patient during the examination. Currently, dynamic MR defecography in the cine-loop presentation and the use of a computer ensure better depiction of the entire pelvic floor anatomy and quantification of organ pro-

lapse, together with similar detection rates for the most clinically relevant abnormalities such as rectal intussusception, features of anismus, rectocele, and enterocele, etc. Conversely, radiographic methods for measurements of distances from anatomical landmarks, and organ size and angles are only made possible by incorporating a radiopaque centimeter ruler within the field of view. In addition, identification of the ischial tuberosities as a landmark to measure the position of the anorectal junction can be difficult because of glare in the lower part of the radiographic images. Moreover, on fluoroscopic examination, the pubococcygeal line is often difficult to identify. This problem is caused by lack of clarity of the inferior margin of the symphysis on lateral radiographs, which may affect the anterior point of the pubococcygeal line in some patients.

One unequivocal area in which evacuation proctography, due to its superior spatial resolution, still maintains specific major advantages over MRI, is in the diagnosis of derangements of the anal mucosal pattern, including tears, fissures, strictures, and fold thickening (Fig. 39.4). Occasionally, identification of the internal opening of an ano-perianal fistula is better appreciated on defecographic series, thanks to the penetration of radiopaque contrast within the sinus tract (Fig. 39.5).

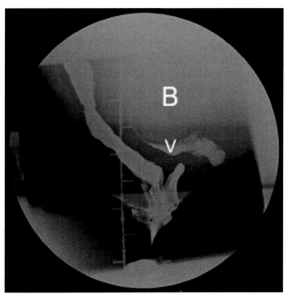

Fig. 39.3 Colpocystodefecography, once considered the main examination to document occult internal intussusception, no longer seems so exclusive for imaging pelvic organ descent. The same evidence can be obtained non-invasively with perineal sonography and, more recently, with MRI. *B*, bladder; *V*, vagina

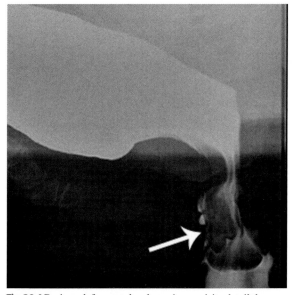

Fig. 39.4 Barium-defecography shows in exquisite detail the prolapsed mucosal folds and hemorrhoids as a filling defect (*arrow*) at the posterior aspect of the distal anal canal. Note also the persistent impression on the rectal wall due to a puborectalis muscle failing to relax during defecation

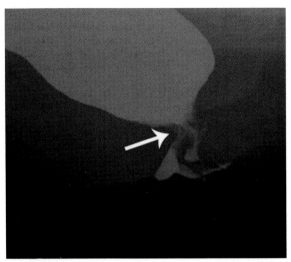

Fig. 39.5 Barium penetration (*arrow*) within the internal opening of a perianal sinus tract was found by chance at defecography in a 28-year-old man with nocturnal episodes of pain of unknown origin and no symptoms of obstructed defecation

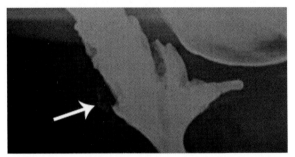

Fig. 39.6 Anastomotic stricture and persistent finger-shaped deformity of the anterior rectal wall, also known as "rectal pocket syndrome" after stapled transanal rectal resection (STARR) procedure for rectocele repair. Note the anastomotic chain (*arrow*)

In addition, the advantage of evacuation proctography over MRI is commonly recognized when evaluating the anorectal configuration of postoperative patients following specific reconstructive procedures such as low resection and anastomosis for rectal cancer, ileo-anal pouch for ulcerative colitis and familial polyposis, and stapled transanal rectal resection (STARR) for rectocele and mucous prolapse. More specifically, x-ray pouchogram is an effective tool to assess early pouch failure due to dehiscence, anastomotic stricture, or fistula, as well as long-term function in patients with poor emptying. With respect to MR defecography, evacuation proctography offers superior information on the dynamic, completeness, and speed of evacuation, and the presence of any deformity of the anorectal configuration (Fig. 39.6). Finally, in patients with impaired control

of stools and gas, a simple diagnostic test such as administering a standard dose of thick barium paste into the rectum and identifying the leakage of contrast outside the anus [22], may add information that can otherwise only be obtained with more sophisticated methods– i.e. anorectal manometry – concerning the factor involved, and whether there is a reduced rectal capacity, an excessive sigmoid propulsion, weakness of the pelvic floor musculature, or sphincteric damage. This, in turn, helps the clinician to plan therapy.

39.4   Conclusions

Imaging in patients with pelvic organ prolapse today can properly be accomplished by a combination of perineal sonography and dynamic fast MRI. Currently, these modalities are well established and are touted as being superior to conventional (radiographic) studies in the diagnosis of cystocele, enterocele, and peritoneocele. The present report represents a backlash, in which the shortcomings of the new techniques and their inferiority to prior modalities in specific conditions are stressed, in order to reach an equilibrium among them when choosing the most cost-effective procedure in individual cases.

More specifically, underestimation of rectocele size and the lower detection rate of external rectal prolapse by US and MRI when compared to x-ray defecography, probably due to a supine straining as opposed to an upright straining position, are well known. In addition, one area in which contrast-enhanced radiologic studies are superior is in the diagnosis of distortion of the mucosal anal infolding, tears, postoperative strictures, depiction of the internal opening of ano-perianal fistula, and involuntary loss of either rectal or bladder contrast. As such, using the equipment currently available in most radiology departments, a modified voiding cystourethrography, i.e. DCCU, can be properly standardized to provide a practical urodynamic evaluation of urinary incontinence, neurogenic bladder dysfunctions, and urinary retention. Similarly, x-ray defecography can still be considered the benchmark test against which to test other newer modalities in cases of fecal incontinence with no objective evidence of sphincteric derangements, and poor emptying syndromes following rectoanal surgery including coloanal anastomosis, ileoanal pouch reconstruction, and STARR.

References

1. Dietz HP, Steensma AB. Posterior compartment prolapse on two-dimensional and three-dimensional pelvic floor ultrasound: the distinction between true rectocele, perineal hypermobility and enterocele. Ultrasound Obstet Gynecol 2005;26:73–77.

2. Kolbl H, Bernaschek G, Wolf G. A comparative study of perineal scan and urethrocystography in patients with genuine stress incontinence. Arch Gynecol Obstet 1988;244:39–45.

3. Schaer GN, Koechli OR, Schuessler B, Haller U. Perineal ultrasound for evaluating the bladder neck in urinary stress incontinence. Obstet Gynecol 1995;85:220–224.

4. Sandridge DA, Thorp JM. Vaginal endosonography in the assessment of the anorectum. Obstet Gynecol 1995;86:1007–1009.

5. Kelvin FM, Maglinte DT, Hale DS, Benson JT. Female pelvic organ prolapse: a comparison of triphasic dynamic MR imaging and triphasic fluoroscopic cystocolpoproctography. AJR Am J Roentgenol 2000;174:81–88.

6. Stoker J, Halligan S, Bartram CI. Pelvic floor imaging. Radiology 2001;218:621–641.

7. Healy JC, Halligan S, Reznek RH et al. Patterns of prolapse in women with symptoms of pelvic floor weakness: assessment with MR imaging. Radiology 1997;203:77–81.

8. Fielding JR. Practical MRI imaging of female pelvic floor weakness. Radiographics 2002;22:295–304.

9. Ala-Ketola L. Roentgen diagnosis of female stress urinary incontinence. Roentgenological and clinical study. Acta Obstet Gynecol Scand Suppl 1973;23:1–59.

10. Pelsang RE, Bonney WW. Voiding cystourethrography in female stress incontinence. AJR Am J Roentgenol 1996;166:561–565.

11. Kuzmarov IW. Urodynamic assessment and chain cystogram in women with stress urinary incontinence: clinical significance of detrusor instability. Urology 1984;24:236–238.

12. Fantl JA, Hurt WG, Beachley MC et al. Bead-chain cystourethrogram: an evaluation. Obstet Gynecol 1981;58:237–240.

13. Henriksson L, Aspelin P, Ulmstein U. Combined urethrocystometry and cinefluorography in continent and incontinent women. Radiology 1979;130:607–611.

14. Westby M, Ulmsten U, Asmussen M. Dynamic urethrocystography in women. Urol Int 1983;38:329–336.

15. Fotter R, Kopp W, Klein E et al. Unstable bladder in children: functional evaluation by modified voiding cystourethrography. Radiology 1986;161:811–813.

16. Blaivas JG, Olsson CA. Stress incontinence: classification and surgical approach. J Urol 1988;139:727–731 .

17. Amis ES, Blaivas JG. Neurogenic bladder simplified. Rad Clin North Am 1991;29:571–580.

18. Kelvin FM, Maglinte DT, Benson JT et al. Dynamic cystoproctography: a technique for assessing disorders of the pelvic floor in women. AJR Am J Roentgenol 1994;163:368–370.

19. Maglinte DDT, Kelvin FM, Fitzgerald K et al. Association of compartment defects in pelvic floor dysfunction. AJR Am J Roentgenol 1997;172:439–444.

20. Lienemann A, Anthuber C, Baron A et al. Dynamic MR colpocystoproctography assessing pelvic floor descent. Eur Radiol 1997;7:1309–1317.

21. Bartram CI. Functional anorectal imaging. Abdom Imaging 2005;30:195–203.

22. Piloni V, Gesuita R, Fioravanti P et al. Diagnosis of fecal incontinence by defecography: receiver operating characteristic (ROC) analysis. Techn Coloproct 1995;2:70–72.

Magnetic Resonance Imaging

40

Dominik Weishaupt and Caecilia S. Reiner

Abstract Pelvic floor dysfunction is a frequent condition that primarily affects women. Dynamic magnetic resonance imaging (MRI) of the pelvic floor is an excellent tool for evaluation of pelvic organ prolapse and patients with outlet obstruction. Findings reported at dynamic MRI of the pelvic floor are valuable for selecting patients who are candidates for surgical treatment and for choosing the appropriate surgery. This chapter reviews MRI imaging findings of pelvic prolapse as well as findings in patients with obstructed defecation.

Keywords Dynamic magnetic resonance imaging • Magnetic resonance imaging • Obstructed defecation • Pelvic floor • Pelvic floor dysfunction • Pelvic organ prolapse

40.1 Introduction

The term "outlet obstruction" (synonym: obstructed defecation syndrome, ODS) encompasses all pelvic floor dysfunctions or abnormalities that are responsible for incomplete evacuation of fecal contents from the rectum (Table 40.1). Outlet obstruction is a functional cause of constipation. Hence, a correct assessment of constipation includes evaluation of the presence of outlet obstruction.

Patients with outlet obstruction often present with generalized pelvic floor relaxation and pelvic organ prolapse. This means that in patients with ODS, concurrent abnormalities of the anterior and middle compartments of the pelvic floor can be observed. In light of this fact, it makes sense to discuss obstructed defecation and pelvic organ prolapse within a common context.

Traditionally, outlet obstruction has been investigated by conventional defecography to assess for rectocele, internal prolapse (intussusception), and enterocele. In early days, imaging was not considered important for evaluation of pelvic floor relaxation and pelvic organ prolapse. Most clinicians use a clinical grading system approved by the International Continence Society, the American Urogynecology Society, and the Society of Gynecologic Surgeons, known as the Pelvic Organ Quantification System [1–3] for grading pelvic floor relaxation and pelvic organ prolapse. Although this grading system is widely accepted, it may underestimate the degree of organ prolapse or the number of failed interventions. In a study by Kelvin et al [4] comparing physical examination with dynamic cystoproctograpahy, physical examination failed to detect 36 of 155 rectoceles (23%), 23 of 47 enteroceles (49%), 8 of 8 sigmoidoceles (100%), and 27 of 159 cystoceles (17%).

As discussed in Section II, magnetic resonance imaging (MRI), and in particular dynamic MRI, is

D. Weishaupt
Institute of Radiology, Triemli Hospital Zurich, Switzerland

G.A. Santoro, A.P. Wieczorek, C.I. Bartram (eds.) *Pelvic Floor Disorders*
© Springer-Verlag Italia 2010

Table 40.1 Causes of outlet obstruction

Functional causes of outlet obstruction	Morphological causes of outlet obstruction
Dyssynergic defecation	Rectocele
Hirschprung's disease	Enterocele
Chagas' disease	Rectal prolapse
Hereditary internal sphincter myopathy	Pelvic floor relaxation
Central nervous lesions	Rectal tumors
	Post-therapeutic stenosis of the ano-rectum

highly useful to assess the pelvic floor and its abnormalities.

In this chapter, we describe MRI features (and in particular dynamic MRI features) of various findings that may be observed in patients with outlet obstruction. In addition, MRI criteria, which are used to grade pelvic floor relaxation and organ prolapse, will be discussed. For classification of the imaging findings we use the three-compartment-model of the pelvic floor: the anterior compartment (bladder and urethra), middle compartment (vagina and uterus), and posterior (anorectal) compartment [5, 6]. Pelvic organ prolapse is defined as any protrusion of a given organ (bladder,

urethra, vagina, uterus, small bowel, or rectum) below the pubococcygeal line (PCL), or below the H line of the HMO system as described in Chapter 11 [7, 8]. Measurements are performed on midsagittal MR images obtained at maximal strain, or during defecation.

40.2 Pelvic Organ Prolapse versus Pelvic Floor Relaxation

Pelvic organ prolapse and pelvic floor relaxation are two related and often coexistent but separate pathologic entities (Fig. 40.1). Pelvic organ prolapse is the

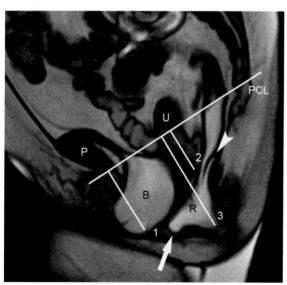

Fig. 40.1 Fifty-nine-year-old female patient with descending perineum syndrom (pelvic floor relaxation). Midsagittal balanced steady-state free precession T2-weighted MR image obtained during maximal straining shows a bulging of the whole pelvic floor with a moderate descent of the anterior compartment (*1*: 5.5 cm) and the middle compartment (*2*: 4 cm), and a large descent of the posterior compartment (*3*: 8 cm). In addition, a small anterior rectocele (*arrow*) and intussusception of the posterior rectal wall (*arrowhead*) are seen. *B*, bladder; *P*, symphysis pubis; *PCL*, pubococcygeal line; *R*, rectum; *U*, uterus

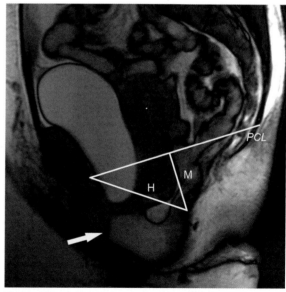

Fig. 40.2 Forty-eight-year-old female patient with symptoms of obstructed defecation syndrome. Midsagittal T2-weighted trueFISP MR image obtained during defecation shows pelvic floor relaxation with pelvic floor descent (M line: 5.3 cm) and hiatal widening (H line: 8.3 cm). According to the HMO system, a small cystocele is evident with prolapse of the bladder below the H line. A large anterior rectocele (*arrow*) and a rectal descent evolve. *H*, H line; *M*, M line; *PCL*, pubococcygeal line

abnormal protrusion of a pelvic organ through its respective hiatus. Organ prolapse can involve any of the following: the bladder (cystocele), vaginal vault or cervix (vaginal vault prolapse), uterus (uterine prolapse, rectum (rectocele), sigmoid colon (sigmoidocele), or small bowel (enterocele).

In pelvic floor relaxation (also termed descending perineum syndrome), the pelvic sling, which includes active and passive pelvic support structures including muscles and connective tissue, becomes widened. There are two components of pelvic floor relaxation: pelvic floor (hiatal) descent, measured with the M line, and hiatal widening, measured with the H line of the HMO system described in Chapter 11. Abnormal pelvic floor relaxation is present when the M line exceeds 2 cm, and when the H line exceeds 5 cm in length [7] (Fig. 40.2).

40.3 Anterior Compartment Abnormalities

40.3.1 Cystocele

Cystoceles are the most common pathology of the anterior compartment of the pelvic floor and occur in postmenopausal women (Fig. 40.3). Cystocele is defined as a bladder base descent below the border of the pubic symphysis, and represents organ prolapse of the anterior pelvic compartment through its respective hiatus. Quantification of a cystocele using dynamic MRI can be made in two different ways, depending on the classification system used. In both systems, measurements are performed on sagittal MR sections through the pelvis. If the cystocele is graded with respect to the position of the bladder base below the PCL, the following three grades can be distinguished: small, if the bladder base extends less than 3 cm below the PCL; moderate, if the extension is between 3 cm and 6 cm; and large, if it is 6 cm or more [5].

In cystoceles, the bladder base occupies part of the width of the levator hiatus, thus displacing the uterus and ano-rectal junction posteriorly and inferiorly. As a consequence, the H and M lines of the HMO system (see Chapter 11) are elongated on MR images, exceeding 5 cm and 2 cm, respectively [7]. Using the HMO system, cystoceles are graded based on the distance of the bladder base relative to the H line as follows: grade 0 (no prolapse), bladder base above the H

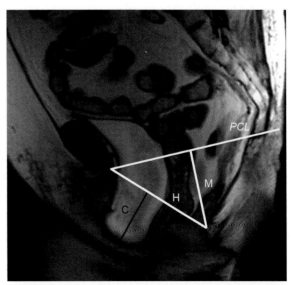

Fig. 40.3 Seventy-nine-year-old female patient with a large cystocele and pelvic floor relaxation. MR image obtained during defecation shows a large cystocele (*C, black line*) with the bladder base > 4 cm below the H line according to the HMO system. In addition, the H (8 cm) and M line (5 cm) are enlarged. *H*, H line; *M*, M line; *PCL*, pubococcygeal line

line; grade 1 (mild or small cystocele), bladder base 0–2 cm below the H line; grade 2 (moderate), bladder base 2–4 cm below the H line, and grade 3 (severe or large cystocele), bladder base 4 cm or more below the H line [5].

40.4 Middle Compartment Abnormalities

Middle compartment abnormalities represent uterine or vaginal vault prolapse. Vaginal prolapse is defined as descent of the vaginal vault below the PCL [5]. The degree of prolapse is graded as mild if the vaginal vault or cervix extends less than 3 cm below the PCL, moderate if it extends between 3 and 6 cm, and severe if it extends 6 cm or more below the PCL. In complete uterine prolapse, the vaginal walls are everted and the uterus is visible as a bulging mass outside the external genitalia (Fig. 40.4).

In cases of uterine prolapse, the H and M lines are elongated on sagittal images. On axial images, the cervix is often at the level of the pubic symphysis and there is loss of the normal H shape of the vagina, often with posterior displacement of the fornix on the affected side. As previously discussed for cystocele,

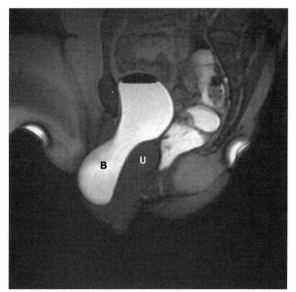

Fig. 40.4 Large cystocele and complete uterine prolapse in a 38-year-old female. *B*, bladder; *U*, uterus

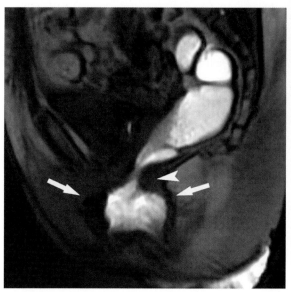

Fig. 40.5 Fifty-eight-year-old female patient with anterior and posterior rectocele. Midsagittal T1-weighted gradient recalled echo MR image obtained during defecation shows bulging of the anterior and posterior rectal wall (*arrows*) evolving during massive straining effort due to paradoxial sphincter contraction (*arrowhead*). In addition, a large rectal descent is evident

grading for uterine prolapse according to the HMO system is based on the distance of the vaginal vault relative to the H line. The same reference values are used for grading uterine prolapse as for grading of cystocele (grade 0, no prolapse; grade 1, 0–2 cm below the H line; grade 2, 2–4 cm below the H line; grade 2, ≥ 4 cm below the H line).

40.5 Posterior Compartment Abnormalities

40.5.1 Rectocele

Rectoceles are defined as an outpouching of the rectal wall. The anterior wall is most commonly affected, but a rectocele may also be located in the posterior rectal wall (Fig. 40.5), where it is also termed posterior perineal hernia because the defect occurs through the levator plate [9]. Most rectoceles become apparent only during defecation.

Rectoceles are common, and some degree of rectocele formation is present in most symptomatic women. Rectoceles are measured as the depth of wall protrusion beyond the expected margin of the normal ano-rectal wall. Based on sagittal MR sections through the mid-pelvis, rectoceles are graded as small if they measure less than 2 cm, moderate if they measure 2–4 cm, and large if they measure 4 cm or more [5]. Small recto-

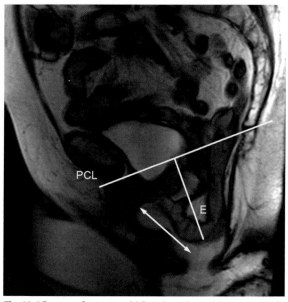

Fig. 40.6 Seventy-four-year-old female patient with an enterocele and anterior rectocele. Midsagittal T2-weighted trueFISP MR image during defecation shows protrusion of a large enterocele (7 cm) (*E*) into the extended perineum, leading to compression of the distal rectum resulting in outlet obstruction. The large anterior rectocele shows retention of contrast medium due to compression by the enterocele. The extension of the anterior rectocele is measured as the maximum wall protrusion beyond the expected margin of the normal anterior rectal wall (*white arrow*). *E*, enterocele; *PCL*, pubococcygeal line

celes are seen in asymptomatic women and most likely represent normal variation [10]. Rectoceles may develop due to weakness of the rectovaginal fascia, promoted by different factors such as chronic constipation, complicated vaginal delivery, hysterectomy, congenital or constitutional weakness of the pelvic floor, or ageing.

A rectocele does not necessarily impede evacuation, but retention of stool within a rectocele may lead to a sense of incomplete evacuation (Fig. 40.6). The clinical relevance may be determined by different criteria, such as the size, retention of contrast medium, need for evacuation assistance, and reproducibility of outlet obstruction.

40.5.2 Enterocele

An enterocele is defined as a herniation of the peritoneal sac, which contains omental fat (peritoneocele), small bowel (enterocele), or sigmoid (sigmoidocele), into the rectovaginal or rectovesical space below the PCL. The prevalence of enteroceles in patients with pelvic floor disorders ranges from 17% to 37% [11, 12]. Women are more frequently affected and often have a history of vaginal or abdominal hysterectomy [13]. Symptoms vary and are largely dependent on the size and location of the enterocele. Patients may present with constipation, a feeling of incomplete evacuation, or a sensation of a heavy feeling in the vagina. Large enteroceles may follow the sacral curve and lead to compression of the ano-rectum, resulting in outlet obstruction (Fig. 40.6). MRI is ideally suited for the evaluation of enteroceles, being superior to conventional cystocolpoproctography [14]. Because of its inherent soft tissue contrast, dynamic pelvic MRI allows for differentiation between peritoneocele, enterocele, and sigmoidocele, without filling the small or large bowel with contrast agent. Enteroceles may result in progressive symptoms and in the need for another operation [12].

Enteroceles are typically seen at the end of defecation as a consequence of increased intra-abdominal pressure, and are often concomitant findings of other pathologies of the pelvic floor. The size of an enterocele is usually measured in relation to the PCL. The largest distance between the PCL and the most inferior point of the enterocele is measured with a perpendicular line. Depending on this distance, small (< 3 cm),

moderate (3–6 cm), and large (> 6 cm) enteroceles are distinguished [5].

40.5.3 Intussusception and Rectal Prolapse

Rectal prolapse is defined as an infolding of the rectal wall. An inner rectal prolapse (intussusception) is distinguished from an external rectal prolapse (corresponding to the widely used clinical term "rectal prolapse") [15].

An intussuception is infolding of the rectal mucosa occurring during defecation. Depending on the location, an intrarectal intussusception (Fig. 40.7), limited to the rectum, is distinguished from an intra-anal intussusception extending into the anal canal. The location of the intussusception may be anterior, posterior, or circumferential. The intussusception either involves only the mucosa or the full thickness of the rectal wall. Patients may present with constipation or a feeling of incomplete evacuation as their main symptom, due to outlet obstruction, or with fecal incontinence. Small intussusceptions may be detected in asymptomatic volunteers [10].

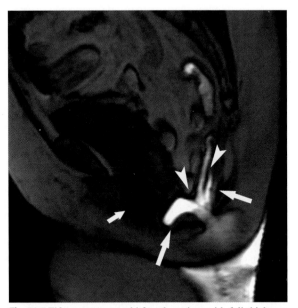

Fig. 40.7 Fifty-seven-year-old female patient with full-thickness intrarectal intussusception. MR image during defecation shows a circumferential mural intussusception, which extends into the rectum (intra-rectal, full-thickness intussusception) (*arrowheads*). Associated anterior and posterior rectoceles are seen (*large arrows*). In addition, a cystocele evolves during defecation (*small arrow*)

Using dynamic pelvic MRI, differentiation between a mucosal intussusception and a full-thickness intussusception is possible. This was shown in a study by Dvorkin et al, where two of ten patients diagnosed with full-thickness intussusception at conventional defecography showed only mucosal intussusception at MR defecography [16]. The differentiation of mucosal and full-thickness intussusception is of clinical relevance, because the two different forms entail different treatment strategies [17, 18]. In up to 30% of patients with intussusception, associated anterior or middle pelvic floor compartment descent has been shown [16]. Thus, dynamic pelvic MRI provides useful additional information, especially if surgery is planned. However, as already mentioned,

MR defecography performed in a supine position may miss intussusception, probably due to the lack of gravity. Therefore, with regard to intussusceptions, we recommend performing conventional defecography in patients with equivocal findings at MR defecography.

External rectal prolapse is defined as an infolding of rectal mucosa that protrudes through the anal canal outwards (Fig. 40.8). The incidence is 4:1000 and is higher in women than in men (women:men = 6:1) [19]. Common symptoms include constipation, a sensation of incomplete evacuation, fecal incontinence, and rectal ulceration with bleeding. External prolapse is a clinical diagnosis, and dynamic pelvic MRI is performed for diagnosing associated pathologies and surgical planning.

40.5.4 Dyssynergic Defecation

Dyssynergic defecation produces functional outlet obstruction during defecation and is one of the causes of chronic constipation. Dyssynergic defecation is a functional disorder characterized by either paradoxical contraction or an inability to relax the anal sphincter and/or puborectalis muscle. In the literature, many other terms such as dyskinetic puborectalis muscle [13], non-relaxing puborectalis syndrome [20], spastic pelvic floor syndrome [21, 22], pelvic floor dyssynergia [23], and anismus [24] have been used. In order to take into account that this dysfunction is not confined to a single muscle, an expert group (Rome III) [25] recently proposed the term "dyssynergic defecation" to appropri-

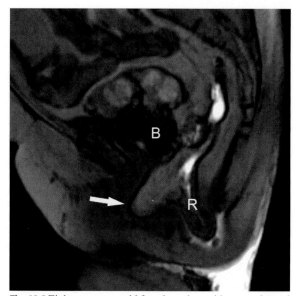

Fig. 40.8 Eighty-two-year-old female patient with external rectal prolapse. MR image obtained during defecation shows an external rectal prolapse and an additional peritoneocele in the rectovesical space (*arrow*). *B*, bladder; *R*, rectum

ately describe the failure of coordination or dyssynergia of the abdominal and pelvic floor muscles involved in defecation.

Patients with dyssynergic defecation present with a variety of symptoms, centering on constipation including rectal evacuation difficulties such as excessive straining, a sensation of blockage, a feeling of incomplete evacuation, a need for manually assisted defecation, and frequent use of enemas or suppositories [26]. The exact cause of dyssynergic defecation is still unclear, but there seems to be an association between dyssynergic defecation and pelvic surgery, previous sexual abuse, anxiety, and psychological stress in some patients [27].

The diagnosis of dyssynergic defecation is notoriously difficult. Most authorities recommend using a combination of clinical history and diagnostic tests, including electromyography, the balloon expulsion test, manometry, and defecography. The individual weight of each of the tests for the final diagnosis of dyssynergic defecation is not exactly defined.

Functional imaging with conventional defecography or dynamic pelvic MRI is considered to be a useful adjunct in establishing the diagnosis of dyssynergic defecation. Different structural imaging findings in conventional defecography have been described in patients with dyssynergic defecation, which can be also

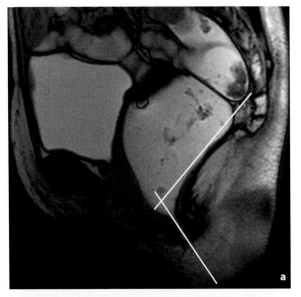

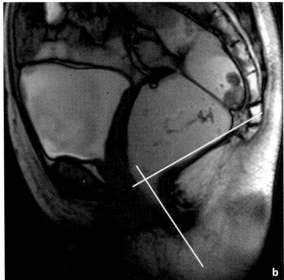

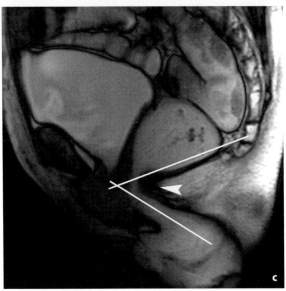

Fig. 40.9 Sixty-six-year-old female patient with clinical suspicion of dyssynergic defecation. On MR images obtained at rest (**a**), the ano-rectal angle measures 115°, whereas the ano-rectal angle during squeezing is 85° (**b**). During evacuation, a pathologic decrease of the anorectal angle (52°) is seen (**c**). Paradoxical sphincter contraction is noted with impression of the dorsal ano-rectal wall during evacuation (*arrowhead* in **c**). The patient was able to evacuate only less than two-thirds of the contrast agent

seen on dynamic pelvic MRI, including a prominent impression of the puborectal sling, narrow anal canal, prolonged evacuation, lack of descent of the pelvic floor, and thus a failure to increase the ano-rectal angle (Fig. 40.9) [22, 28].

However, the usefulness of these findings is controversial [24, 28, 29]. In addition, defecography can be performed to rule out structural rectal abnormalities, and provides an estimate of the degree of rectal emptying.

Delayed initiation of evacuation, and impaired evacuation in particular, as seen on conventional defecography, are present in patients with dyssynergia [24, 30]. Impaired evacuation, which was defined by Halligan et al [30] as an inability to evacuate two-thirds of the contrast enema within 30 s, is especially highly suggestive for the presence of dyssynergic defecation.

References

1. Bump RC, Mattiasson A, Bo K et al. The standardization of terminology of female pelvic organ prolapse and pelvic floor dysfunction. Am J Obstet Gynecol 1996;175:10–17.
2. Kelvin FM, Hale DS, Maglinte DD et al. Female pelvic organ prolapse: diagnostic contribution of dynamic cysto-

proctography and comparison with physical examination. AJR Am J Roentgenol 1999;173:31–37.

3. Weber AM, Richter HE. Pelvic organ prolapse. Obstet Gynecol 2005;106:615–634.

4. Kelvin FM, Maglinte DD, Hale DS, Benson JT. Female pelvic organ prolapse: a comparison of triphasic dynamic MR imaging and triphasic fluoroscopic cystocolpoproctography. AJR Am J Roentgenol 2000;174:81–88.

5. Roos JE, Weishaupt D, Wildermuth S et al. Experience of 4 years with open MR defecography: pictorial review of anorectal anatomy and disease. Radiographics 2002; 22:817–832.

6. Weber AM, Abrams P, Brubaker L et al. The standardization of terminology for researchers in female pelvic floor disorders. Int Urogynecol J Pelvic Floor Dysfunct 2001;12:178–186.

7. Boyadzhyan L, Raman SS, Raz S. Role of static and dynamic MR imaging in surgical pelvic floor dysfunction. Radiographics 2008;28:949–967.

8. Comiter CV, Vasavada SP, Barbaric ZL et al. Grading pelvic prolapse and pelvic floor relaxation using dynamic magnetic resonance imaging. Urology 1999;54:454–457.

9. Mahieu P, Pringot J, Bodart P. Defecography: II. Contribution to the diagnosis of defecation disorders. Gastrointest Radiol 1984;9:253–261.

10. Shorvon PJ, McHugh S, Diamant NE et al. Defecography in normal volunteers: results and implications. Gut 1989; 30:1737–1749.

11. Hock D, Lombard R, Jehaes C et al. Colpocystodefecography. Dis Colon Rectum 1993;36:1015–1021.

12. Kelvin FM, Maglinte DD, Hornback JA, Benson JT. Pelvic prolapse: assessment with evacuation proctography (defecography). Radiology 1992;184:547–551.

13. Karasick S, Karasick D, Karasick SR. Functional disorders of the anus and rectum: findings on defecography. AJR Am J Roentgenol 1993;160:777–782.

14. Lienemann A, Anthuber C, Baron A, Reiser M. Diagnosing enteroceles using dynamic magnetic resonance imaging. Dis Colon Rectum 2000;43:205–212; discussion 12–13.

15. Stoker J, Halligan S, Bartram CI. Pelvic floor imaging. Radiology 2001;218:621–641.

16. Dvorkin LS, Hetzer F, Scott SM et al. Open-magnet MR defaecography compared with evacuation proctography in the diagnosis and management of patients with rectal intussusception. Colorectal Dis 2004;6:45–53.

17. McCue JL, Thomson JP. Rectopexy for internal rectal intussusception. Br J Surg 1990;77:632–634.

18. Tsiaoussis J, Chrysos E, Glynos M et al. Pathophysiology and treatment of anterior rectal mucosal prolapse syndrome. Br J Surg 1998;85:1699–1702.

19. Fengler SA, Pearl RK, Prasad ML et al. Management of recurrent rectal prolapse. Dis Colon Rectum 1997;40:832–834.

20. Jorge JM, Wexner SD, Ger GC et al. Cinedefecography and electromyography in the diagnosis of nonrelaxing puborectalis syndrome. Dis Colon Rectum 1993;36:668–676.

21. Kelvin FM, Maglinte DD, Benson JT. Evacuation proctography (defecography): an aid to the investigation of pelvic floor disorders. Obstet Gynecol 1994;83:307–314.

22. Kuijpers HC, Bleijenberg G. The spastic pelvic floor syndrome. A cause of constipation. Dis Colon Rectum 1985; 28:669–672.

23. Whitehead WE, Wald A, Diamant NE et al. Functional disorders of the anus and rectum. Gut 1999;45(suppl 2):II55–59.

24. Halligan S, Bartram CI, Park HJ, Kamm MA. Proctographic features of anismus. Radiology 1995;197:679–682.

25. Bharucha AE, Wald A, Enck P, Rao S. Functional anorectal disorders. Gastroenterology 2006;130:1510–1518.

26. Rao SS, Mudipalli RS, Stessman M, Zimmerman B. Investigation of the utility of colorectal function tests and Rome II criteria in dyssynergic defecation (anismus). Neurogastroenterol Motil 2004;16:589–596.

27. Bolog N, Weishaupt D. Dynamic MR imaging of outlet obstruction. Rom J Gastroenterol 2005;14:293–302.

28. Karlbom U, Pahlman L, Nilsson S, Graf W. Relationships between defecographic findings, rectal emptying, and colonic transit time in constipated patients. Gut 1995; 36:907–912.

29. Karlbom U, Nilsson S, Pahlman L, Graf W. Defecographic study of rectal evacuation in constipated patients and control subjects. Radiology 1999;210:103–108.

30. Halligan S, Malouf A, Bartram CI et al. Predictive value of impaired evacuation at proctography in diagnosing anismus. AJR Am J Roentgenol 2001;177:633–636.

Invited Commentary

Julia R. Fielding

As the author elegantly discusses in Chapter 36, the pelvic floor is a complex structure with multiple possible defects. Testing should be used to elucidate compartmental damage based on physical examination and patient complaints. In my hospital, we triage patients according to symptomatology.

1. Stress incontinence or detrusor instability
   - Urinary leakage with coughing or laughing is virtually diagnostic of stress incontinence. The patient should be assessed for cystocele using, in most cases, a physical examination. When no significant cystocele is identified, treatment is usually a Burch colposuspension of the bladder neck to the pelvic sidewalls.
   - Detrusor instability is unwanted bladder contractions leading to urinary leakage. It occurs more often in the elderly patient often in association with stress incontinence. When necessary, it is diagnosed using videourodynamics, which can detect detrusor wall contractions. Treatment is medical and usually consists of drying agents.
2. Prolapse of the bladder (cystocele) and vaginal vault
   - This is a common scenario in the perimenopausal patient when ageing aggravates organ descent. Large cystoceles often require a paravaginal fascial repair. Hypermobility of the urethra indicates loss of anterior support at the symphysis and can easily be seen using magnetic resonance imaging (MRI). The repair is usually a sling or tape procedure. A long strip of rectus fascia or tape extends from the parasymphyseal bony region pos-

terior to the rectum and inserts anteriorly on the ilium on the opposite side of the bladder.
3. Prolapse of the colon (enterocele, rectocele, sigmoidocele)
   - Fecal incontinence, often associated with constipation, is often the presenting complaint. Evaluation includes manometry for rectal tone, endoanal ultrasonography to detect sphincter disruption, and defecography to assess for colonic motion and defects. Standard fluoroscopic defecography is a useful test for postmenopausal women presenting with bowel symptoms only and an otherwise intact pelvic floor. For women of menstrual age, radiation is to be avoided when possible, and an MRI is the test of choice.
4. Symptomatic global pelvic floor prolapse or failed surgery
   - Because these cases will often require a team approach consisting of a urologist and gynecologist to reapproximate supporting ligaments, elevate the bowel and bladder and repair muscular defects, MRI in the sagittal and axial plane is the test of choice.

Fluoroscopic cystography, described in Chapter 39, is now rarely performed in the radiology department. Exceptions include assessment for vesicoureteral reflux and bladder rupture in pelvic trauma. Patients with simple stress incontinence, which is associated with a cough or laughing, may be directed towards needle suspension surgery without imaging. Those with an associated cystocele and urethral rotation may undergo voiding cystourethrography to identify loss of anterior urethral supports. These patients may require a sling procedure and paravaginal repair.

J.R. Fielding
Department of Radiology, University of North Carolina
at Chapel Hill, NC, USA

When urge incontinence secondary to detrusor instability is suspected, patients undergo videourodynamics. Pressure-sensitive catheters are placed within the rectum and bladder. Subtraction of the intravesicular pressure from the rectal pressure (a simulation of abdominal pressure) yields the detrusor pressure. As the bladder is filled in a retrograde fashion, fluoroscopic video is reviewed for focal bladder wall contractions. Detrusor pressure is then compared with the fluoroscopic findings. Urge incontinence is associated with bladder wall trabeculation in men and women. In a minority of cases it is caused by surgery to repair stress incontinence.

Fluoroscopic defecography remains a useful tool for postmenopausal women with constipation or fecal incontinence, findings that are isolated to the posterior compartment of the pelvis. The upright positioning best reproduces the symptoms and the patient can perform pelvic floor contractions and release to directly visualize floor motion. The angle of the ano-rectal junction is not useful because of its variability within the healthy population. When the patient evacuates, enteroceles, rectoceles and instussuceptions can be readily identified. Anal ulcer or inflammation and sphincter dyssynergia remain difficult diagnoses. Because of the high radiation dose, women of menstrual age should usually be examined using cine MRI at rest, strain, and usually post-evacuation.

Dynamic MRI of the pelvic floor, as reported in Chapter 40, allows the examiner to view descent of the pelvic organs and evacuation mimicking the physiologic state. In our institution, MRI is performed in the left lateral decubitus position with 60 mL ultrasound gel within the rectum as a positive contrast agent. Using ½ acquisition rapid acquisition relaxation enhanced (RARE) or true fast imaging with steady-state precession (FISP) sequence, multiple images of the pelvis are obtained as the patient defecates. Images are obtained at a rate of one per second. Many patients need to Valsalva several times in order to evacuate; therefore it is prudent to repeat the sequence scan two or three times. In most cases, existing enteroceles and rectoceles are identified. Rectoceles are considered significant when they are > 2 cm beyond the expected location of the rectal wall and when they retain fecal contents following defecation. Enteroceles can give a persistent feeling of rectal fullness, leading to a cycle of straining, which may progress to complete prolapse or involvement of multiple pelvic floor compartments. If the patient has difficulty evacuating in the left lateral decubitus position, she can be sent to the commode and re-imaged to locate any abnormalities. Review of the images in the cine mode allows for detection of association of cystocele and vaginal vault prolapse. Perineal hernias are usually best seen with the patient in the supine position. Sagittal images at rest and at maximal strain usually reveal the hernia, its contents and its depth. Axial images show detached or torn muscles, usually the puborectalis.

In some patients, evacuation is just not possible in the MR suite. For these women, standard defecography is an excellent tool. The patient is in the seated, upright position, which is often more comfortable, and gravity may accentuate descent of the bowel. We have found rectal intussusception and dyssynergia of the anal sphincter to be difficult diagnoses using both fluoroscopic and MR defecography. Intussusception may only be identified in one plane and neither fluoroscopic equipment nor MRI can obtain three planes simultaneously. In the future, as three-dimensional acquisitions become more routine, MRI may become more accurate. Dyssynergia, or spastic pelvic floor, may be functional or neuropathic in origin. We consider imaging is of little use in its diagnosis other than to exclude other pathology.

Invited Commentary

Andrea Maier

Fecal incontinence is often multifactoral. Clinical examination may not detect the cause in at least 25% of patients. The choice of an optimal therapy is determined on the basis of a proper assessment, especially accurate images of the anal sphincter complex. Over the last decade, technical advances in anal imaging have increased the significant impact of imaging on the management of patients with fecal incontinence. As described in the preceding chapters, a number of imaging methods, such as defecography, endoanal ultrasonography, dynamic and three-dimensional (3D)-endoluminal ultrasonography, transperineal and transvaginal ultrasonography, and dynamic magnetic resonance imaging (MRI), are employed for the diagnosis of incontinence.

All the authors have highlighted their described method with advantages and disadvantages. Endoanal ultrasonography has replaced the invasive method of electromyography and is valuable as a screening procedure to detect sphincter tears that are amenable to surgical treatment. Endosonography is the method of choice to show damage to the anal sphincter muscles, either with general thinning as found in degeneration, or from focal discontinuities due to any cause of trauma. In addition, new technical developments such as 3D-endoluminal and 3D-transvaginal ultrasonography improve the application of the method. In particular, 3D-transvaginal ultrasonography provides excellent anatomical details of the anterior, central, and posterior compartment.

Endoanal ultrasonography and MRI are complementary with regard to surgical decision making. The advantages of endosonography are that it is a cheaper,

more widely available, and faster technique than MRI.

However, MRI has also been shown to be accurate in delineating the anatomy of the sphincter complex. It is a powerful tool with which to investigate weakness of the pelvic floor generally and atrophy of the external sphincter, an important predictive factor for the outcome of sphincter repair. Recently, dynamic MRI, with the advantages of a dynamic analysis of the pelvic floor organs and soft tissue, decreased invasiveness, and lack of ionizing radiation, has been introduced for ano-rectal disease. The limitations of MRI are that it requires patients to be in the supine position and it may underestimate rectal abnormalities. Interest in this modality for pelvic floor imaging has been relatively recent, and validation of the accuracy of MRI as well as the optimal technique for the study is still in the process of being determined. When MRI has been compared to evacuation proctography, the results have been variable. Studies in larger numbers will help to clarify the sensitivity and accuracy of MRI compared to proctography, which is the traditional test.

On the other hand, conventional defecography still has an important role for the accurate diagnosis of intussusceptions and rectoceles. Defecography provides both structural and functional information for rectal voiding and prolapse. It may demonstrate pelvic floor and sphincter weakness by abnormal descent at rest and anal leakage.

Furthermore, defecography still remains the standard test in specific postoperative cases.

Nevertheless, 3D-ultrasonography and dynamic MRI will diminish the role of defecography within the next few years.

In these articles, a multiplicity of imaging modalities for the evaluation of pelvic floor disorders, in-

A. Maier
Department of Radiology, Medical University of Wien, Austria

cluding 3D-ultrasonography, 3D-transvaginal ultrasonograpy, dynamic transvaginal ultrasonography, perineal sonography, cystourethrography, defecography, and dynamic MRI imaging, are described. Not all modalities are available in all hospitals or in expert centres. However, the lack of a particular imaging modality can be replaced by the use of existing equipment.

Overall, pelvic floor imaging is an innovative field for finding the best imaging modality for selected patients.

Anorectal Manometry

41

Filippo Pucciani

Abstract It is useful to perform an anorectal manometry in individuals with pelvic organ prolapse who have substantial defecatory symptoms or fecal incontinence. Manometric evaluation can provide functional anorectal data in patients who are affected by posterior prolapse (rectocele, enterocele, sigmoidocele): anal sphincter activity, rectal compliance, and rectal sensation may be tested. Manometric signs of defective anal sphincter function or impaired anal relaxation may be detected, depending on concomitant rectal pathologies.

Keywords Anorectal manometry • Descending perineum syndrome • Enterocele • Fecal incontinence • Obstructed defecation • Pelvic floor dyssynergia • Posterior prolapse • Rectocele • Rehabilitation • Sigmoidocele

Pelvic organ prolapse, also called uterovaginal prolapse, is a downward descent of the pelvic organs that results in a protrusion of the vagina, uterus, or both [1]. It is distinct from rectal prolapse, in which the rectum protrudes beyond the anal canal [2]. Women with pelvic organ prolapse may have symptoms that are related to bowel function. Fecal incontinence and defecatory dysfunction are frequently reported (79.7% of women with posterior vaginal wall prolapse), but there is a weak or no relationship between symptoms and the degree of prolapse [3, 4]. This observation reinforces the notion that bowel symptoms are not related to pelvic organ prolapse and that they seem to be attributed predominantly to abnormal anorectal function [5]. In fact, defecatory disorders appear to be an important factor in the pathogenesis of uterovaginal prolapse [6]. Therefore it would be useful

to perform anorectal manometry, defecography, or both, in the context of a structured program in individuals with pelvic organ prolapse who have substantial defecatory symptoms, and to carry out an anorectal manometry, combined with endoanal ultrasound, when an anal sphincter defect is suspected [1], in patients with fecal incontinence.

Posterior vaginal wall prolapse concerns the rectum (rectocele) but can also include the small (enterocele) or large bowel (sigmoidocele). Anorectal manometry can provide useful data for evaluation of anorectal function in patients affected by posterior prolapse: sphincter activity, rectal compliance, and rectal sensation may be tested (see details in Chapter 27).

Anterior rectoceles represent a herniation of the anterior rectum into the posterior wall of the vagina. Nichols and Ponchak [7] have suggested that there are two types of anterior rectocele: the "distension" rectocele, where the vaginal vault and uterus are in a normal position within the pelvis, and the "displacement" rectocele, which occurs when the posterior

F. Pucciani
Department of Medical and Surgical Critical Care, University of Firenze, Italy

vaginal wall follows the descent of the vaginal vault. Anorectal dysfunction may be noted in both types of rectocele: the distension rectocele is related to a pelvic floor dyssynergia, and a collapse of the pelvic floor connotes the displacement rectocele [8]. Equivalent anorectal manometry provides different reports: paradoxical sphincter response (impaired anal relaxation at straining) is detected as a marker of pelvic floor dyssynergia [9]; low pressures of the anal canal are recorded, at rest and during maximal voluntary contraction, in patients with displacement rectocele [8]. Therefore manometric evaluation, supplemented by other physiologic and morphologic tests, is indispensable for the therapeutic strategy. When there are signs of paradoxical sphincter response, a rehabilitative attempt is essential; on the other hand, surgical repair of the large rectocele may be considered in the absence of dyssynergic defecation, or after failed rehabilitative treatment [10].

Enterocele and sigmoidocele are defecographic findings in patients affected by obstructed defecation. Enterocele is a peritoneal sac containing the small intestine, which in women lies between the posterior vaginal wall and the anterior rectal wall. A deep rectogenital pouch is common in constipated patients, and just over half such pouches fill with viscera forming an enterocele [11]. Pelvic surgery, especially hysterectomy, may be a risk factor for development of an enterocele. The obstructed defecation might be due to mechanical compression of the rectum, but enterocele is often accompanied by other causes of impaired evacuation such as rectal intussusception (55%) and rectal prolapse (38%) [12]. These explain the meaning of aspecific manometric data which may be recorded from time to time. Manometric signs of defective anal sphincter function or impaired anal relaxation may be detected, depending on concomitant rectal pathologies. The same principles may be applied in patients affected by sigmoidocele, where a loop of sigmoid extending caudally is entangled in the deep rectogenital pouch. Several mechanisms may be involved in obstructed defecation, including collapse of the rectum, direct compression by hernia contents, and stasis in the sigmoid [13]. Manometric evaluation can only identify those patients whose outlet obstruction is sustained by concomitant anorectal dysfunction.

Pelvic organ prolapse is related to impairment of the anatomical support of the pelvic viscera provided by the levator ani muscle complex and the connective tissue attachments of the pelvic organs (endopelvic fascia) [1]. Disruption or dysfunction of one or both of these components may also occur in descending perineum syndrome. This complex disorder of the pelvic floor was first outlined by Parks et al [14], who described excessive descent of the perineum during a straining effort. Several defects may coexist, including anterior rectocele, rectoanal intussusception, cystocele, and vaginal or uterine prolapse. A previous study [15] showed that some degree of genital relaxation was present in 92.8% of women with descending perineum, and therefore a relationship between pelvic organ prolapse and descending perineum syndrome may be suspected. Weak pelvic floor is the common denominator for any objective report regarding both disorders, and therefore some doubts might be raised. The question "is it a simple problem of terminology used by coloproctologists and gynecologists?" seems to be justifiable. A useful starting point to providing an answer may be an overall evaluation of defecation disorders, descending perineum, and the degree of pelvic organ support in a general population of women [15].

References

1. Jelovsek JE, Maher C, Barber MD. Pelvic organ prolapse. Lancet 2007;369:1027–1038.
2. Peters WA, Smith RM, Drescher CW. Rectal prolapse in women with other defects of pelvic floor support. Am J Obstet Gynecol 2001;184:1488–1495.
3. Weber AM, Walters MD, Ballard LA et al. Posterior vaginal wall prolapse and bowel function. Am J Obstet Gynecol 1998;179:1446–1450.
4. Ellerkmann RM, Cundiff GW, Melick CE et al. Correlation of symptoms with location and severity of pelvic organ prolapse. Am J Obstet Gynecol 2001;185:1332–1338.
5. Marques da Silva G, Gurland B, Sleemi A et al. Posterior vaginal wall prolapse does not correlate with fecal symptoms or objective measures of anorectal function. Am J Obstet Gynecol 2006;195:1742–1747.
6. Spence-Jones C, Kamm MA, Henry MM et al. Bowel dysfunction: a pathogenic factor in uterovaginal prolapse and urinary stress incontinence. BJOG 2005;101:147–152.
7. Nichols DH, Ponchak S. Anterior and posterior colporraphy. In: Nyhus LM, Baker RJ (eds) Mastery of surgery. Little Brown and Company, Boston, 1992, pp 1532–1549.
8. Pucciani F, Rottoli ML, Bologna A et al. Anterior rectocele and anorectal dysfunction. Int J Colorectal Dis 1996;11:1–9.
9. Siproudhis L, Dautrème S, Ropert A. Dyschezia and rectocele – a marriage of convenience? Physiologic evaluation of the rectocele in a group of 52 women complaining of difficulty in evacuation. Dis Colon Rectum 1993;36:1030–1036.

10. Boccasanta P, Venturi M, Stuso A. et al. Stapled transanal rectal resection for outlet obstruction: a prospective multicenter trial. Dis Colon Rectum 2004;47:1285–1296.

11. Halligan S, Bartram C, Hall C et al. Enterocele revealed by simultaneous evacuation proctography and peritoneography: does "defecation block" exist? AJR Am J Roentgenol 1996;167:461–466.

12. Mellgren A, Johansson C, Dolk A et al. Enterocele demonstrated by defaecography is associated with other pelvic floor disorders. Int J Colorectal Dis 1994;9:121–124.

13. Jorge JMN, Yang YK, Wexner SD. Incidence and clinical significance of sigmoidoceles as determined by a new classification system. Dis Colon Rectum 1994;37:1112–1117.

14. Parks AG, Porter NH, Hardcastle J. The syndrome of descending perineum. Proc R Soc Med 1966;59:477–482.

15. Pucciani F, Boni D, Perna F et al. Descending perineum syndrome: are abdominal hysterectomy and bowel habits linked? Dis Colon Rectum 2005;48:2094–2099.

Invited Commentary

Anton Emmanuel

The critical role of anorectal physiological tests in patients with pelvic organ prolapse is to identify occult gut dysfunction. It is these patients in particular who need to have their management, surgical or conservative, tailored to include consideration of the whole pelvic floor.

The second putative role of anorectal physiology testing is to provide diagnostic information that alters decision making. In particular, those with fecal incontinence in association with pelvic organ prolapse should undergo physiological and imaging assessment of the anal sphincters. But, as discussed in Chapter 27, the place of such testing in fecal incontinence, whether comorbid with pelvic organ prolapse, is already established.

What is clear is that any physiological abnormalities identified in the various publications about anorectal testing cannot differentiate between chicken and egg; in other words, what is causative of pelvic floor weakness and what is a consequence of this? The most frequently observed abnormalities are reduced anal sphincter pressures and reduced rectal distension sensitivity. If anything, these seem to be bystander abnormalities, in that they are equally present in pelvic organ prolapse patients both with and without constipation. Furthermore, studies have failed to show an association between the degree of dysfunction and the degree of pelvic organ prolapse.

One key potential development in pelvic organ prolapse patients with constipation is to determine the value of emerging anorectal investigative tools in this subgroup.

Puborectalis dynamometry as an assessor of levator ani function would be potentially revealing. Correlation with magnetic resonance proctography would be especially interesting.

In summary, the role of anorectal physiology testing in the fecally incontinent patient with pelvic organ prolapse is well established; its value in patients who are constipated or have evacuation difficulty and prolapse is negligible, with currently used clinical testing methods.

A. Emmanuel
GI Physiology Unit, University College Hospital, London, UK

G.A. Santoro, A.P. Wieczorek, C.I. Bartram (eds.) *Pelvic Floor Disorders*
© Springer-Verlag Italia 2010

Management of Pelvic Organ Prolapse: a Unitary or Multidisciplinary Approach?

42

Giuseppe Dodi, Luca Amadio and Erica Stocco

Abstract Until recently urologists, gynecologists, proctologists, and colorectal surgeons had worked independently in their pelvic compartments neglecting the other specialties. In the last two decades, studies of the role of muscles, connective tissue, and innervations of the pelvic floor have radically changed the methods for coping with perineal dysfunctions. The new approach, whether a transdisciplinary or a interdisciplinary one, needs to consider the perineum as a unit. Often pelvic dysfunctions involve more than one compartment, and an organ-specific approach may fail to recognize a more complex problem resulting in a partial or incorrect treatment. In order to improve the study of the perineum, it is mandatory to better understand the interactions between the compartments, to create a common language, and to use randomized controlled studies with long follow-up to evaluate the anatomical and functional results of the new prosthestic surgery. Expert physicians and surgeons are needed in this new specialty, which we call perineology.

Keywords Holistic • Integral theory • Multidisciplinary approach • IPGH (Incontinence, Pelvic floor and Prolapse, General factors, Handicap) • Pelviperineology • TAPE (Three Axis Perineal Evaluation)

42.1 Introduction

The anatomy of the pelvic floor was traditionally considered as divided into three compartments in the domains of urology, gynecology, and coloproctology. From the anatomical and functional points of view, however, the pelvic floor is now seen as a single unit, as in many conditions the three compartments are deeply interrelated.

DeLancey's functional anatomic studies [1–3] and the Integral Theory proposed in 1990 by Petros and

Ulmsten [4] gave a new interpretation of female pelvic floor dysfunction and laid the foundation of new corrective surgical treatment [5–8].

42.2 Why a Multidisciplinary Approach?

The need for a multidisciplinary approach is confirmed by the frequent coexistence of dysfunctions in the three compartments. Many patients treated for functional colorectal diseases also have urogynaecologic symptoms. Epidemiological surveys have shown that, of patients treated for anal incontinence, 53% and 18% respectively complain of urinary incontinence

G. Dodi
Department of Oncological and Surgical Science, 2nd Surgical Clinic, University of Padova, Italy

and genital prolapse. Among all patients operated for rectal prolapse, 65% have urinary incontinence and 34% genital prolapse [9–11]. Genital prolapse (halfway system ≥ 2) is observed in 44% of constipated women, whose risk of posterior colpocele is significantly higher than in the control population [12].

Based on these data, an integrated multidisciplinary approach seems to be mandatory for an adequate diagnosis and for treating pelvic floor dysfunctions. However, this is often not adopted among specialists, who frequently work on a more individual basis. This is confirmed by the data collected at the 12th Annual Cleveland Clinic Colorectal Symposium which revealed that, although 96% of colorectal surgeons inquire about urinary incontinence while evaluating women with fecal incontinence or rectal prolapse, only 50% cooperate with a urologist or urogynaecologist for treating the pelvic defects, and only 44% perform simultaneous operations for urinary, genital, and/or colorectal dysfunctions [13]. Combined urologic, gynecologic and colorectal reconstructive procedures can safely be undertaken during the same surgical session, with no increase of morbidity, and there is a good possibility of an enhanced success rate, and shortened recovery time when all pelvic floor dysfunctions are treated in the same operative session [14]. Between 42% and 77% of women with urinary incontinence also need another procedure for treating genital prolapse [15, 16]. All clinicians who work in this field must remember that surgery alone does not cure pelvic floor dysfunctions in all cases. An attempt to use treatment with rehabilitation is often useful, as it may be effective and the patient may avoid an operation, which always carry some risk.

42.3   The Present and Future

The multidisciplinary approach, rather than a transdisciplinary or interdisciplinary one, limits urologists, gynecologists and colorectal surgeons in their integrated view of the pelvic floor. In order to manage the dysfunctions in this area in the best way, a full evaluation of the urinary, genital, colorectal, sexual, and neuromuscular problems is needed. As stated by Davila [17], however, one clinician alone cannot afford this commitment – a problem that can be overcome by a team of specialists cooperating in the diagnosis and treatment. A good example of this attitude is the Pelvic Floor Team of the Cleveland Clinic in Florida where a urogynecologist, a urologist, a colorectal surgeon, a gastroenterologist, a physiotherapist, a sexual dysfunction therapist, and a mental health specialist cooperate with clinical and research fellows and nursing personnel. Each case is then discussed in a joint meeting on the basis of the history and physical examination, in order to create the most convenient diagnostic and therapeutic program.

The need for a new approach to pelvic floor problems was underlined in 1990 by an editorial that appeared in the Italian Journal of Coloproctology (today Pelviperineology), where the neologism "perineology" indicated that a "super-specialty" was born, willing to evaluate, in a unitary way, the diseases of the anterior, middle, and posterior pelvic floor [18].

In Italy, an interdisciplinary approach was introduced in 1998 by five specialists, a urologist, a gynecologist, a colorectal surgeon, a physiatrist, and a geriatrician: W. Artibani, R. Milani, G. Dodi, P. Di Benedetto, and F. Benvenuti, who founded the Società Interdisciplinare del Pavimento Pelvico. The aims of this society were the study of pelvic floor dysfunctions, the training of pelvic floor specialists, and the use of diagnostic and therapeutic procedures for the treatment of female pelvic diseases conforming to the ICS (International Continence Society) and the ICI (International Consultation on Incontinence). An important step in this field has been the organization of the pelviperineology unit. This is a "transverse" structure aimed at facilitating an integration among urologists, gynaecologists, colorectal surgeons, physiatrists, and physiotherapists. Its purposes are: to favor the correct enrolment of the patients in the different services, coordination of the diagnostic pathway and of the multidisciplinary consultations (urologic, gynaecologic, and colorectal), collaboration among different specialists in the operating theatre, training of a specialist in this field through the specialty schools of the universities, and training of the "pelviperineal coordinating nurse". The pelviperineal coordinating nurse is in charge of connecting the patient with the different specialists and departments. This role is considered to be extremely important during both the diagnostic and therapeutic procedures. He or she must be able to perform manometry, electromyography, urodynamic examinations, etc, to assist the patients with sacral neurostimulation, artificial sphincters, and rehabilitation therapies (for urinary or anal incontinence, pelvic and perineal pain, constipation), and to help in the prevention of pelvic floor damage. The requirements for setting up a pelviperineology unit are: cooperation between the services of urology, gynecology, colorectal surgery, and rehabilitation; experience in the field of functional surgery; and the availability of diagnostic tools with a standardized method of clinical data collection.

42.4 The Need for a Common Language

As indicated by Albo et al [19], the discrepancy in diagnosis and definition is an unresolved question in female pelvic floor medicine. The need for a classification system and common terminology has been brought to various international attempts (ICS, etc) for measuring the severity of the diseases and their impact on patients' quality of life [20]. There is still a lack of an internationally accepted grading system to evaluate the anatomy and function of the three pelvic compartments in a transdisciplinary way. The IPGH system (Incontinence, Pelvic floor and Prolapse, General factors, Handicap) is a standardized method defining the severity of the dysfunctions in each compartment [21]. It is useful for planning treatment, evaluating results, and favoring the exchange of information among specialists. Each acronym defines the severity of the problem in the different domains. This classification system is part of the data collection in the pelvic floor computerized chart that is being used in our institution. In the chart, the scores are applied automatically, making evaluation of individual cases and comparison between the symptoms before and after treatment much easier [22]. In 2002, Beco and Mouchel highlighted that in perineology "everybody has to speak the same language" [23]. To find a solution to this they invented the TAPE (Three Axis Perineal Evaluation) diagram. This tool takes into account six standard perineal disorders (sexual difficulties, dysuria, anal incontinence, prolapse, urinary incontinence, and dyschesia) presented in three axes: gynecological, urological, and coloproctologial.

42.5 Pelviperineology: an Evolving Discipline

Due to the great interest and rapid advancement that pelviperineology has gained in the international scientific world in the last few years, the amount of information and the rapidity of the progress in this discipline requires an adequate cultural background. This must be based on continuous education in theory and practice. The Pelvic Floor Digest (www.pelvicfloordigest.org) is a pool in which a large number of abstracts of scientific articles can be found online, selected from the international literature and divided into ten main chapters: pelvic floor general; functional anatomy; diagnosis; prolapses; retentions; incontinence; pain; fistulae; behaviour, psychology, sexology; and basic science, miscellaneous. In 2005, the Pelvic Floor Digest published 2548 abstracts from 159 international scientific journals.

Basic and clinical research is very important in pelviperineology. The most interesting topics currently are the responsible use of prostheses and the evaluation of minimally invasive surgical procedures. Only well planned and carefully performed clinical randomized studies conforming to the criteria of evidence-based medicine can be valued in these years of great technological progress and strong marketing pressures. Basic research is also needed to find new therapeutic approaches, such as with stem cells or tissue engineering [19].

42.6 The Need for a Holistic Vision

The relationship between mind and body is an ever-present issue in medicine. The pelvic floor is no exception, and this is an important topic of research into the dysfunctions of the posterior compartment. There are conditions, such as severe constipation, in which a precise etiology cannot be found, but the psychological features are becoming increasingly interesting due to the connections between the nervous system and the patient's life experiences. Quite often, digestive dysfunctions without evident organic lesions (at least with the instruments now available) are treated unsuccessfully with drugs or surgery. In these cases modern psychoanalysis allows a holistic view of the human being, considering the possible meaning of the disease. Psychotherapy may then reduce the pain, also improving the so-called functional alterations – bowel dysfunction, for instance. About 50% of women undergoing a consultation for irritable bowel syndrome are thought to have suffered some sort of sexual abuse in their life, including their childhood. The pelvic floor diseases, therefore, are not only due to defects of the pelvic organs from the anatomic point of view, but may also depend on important interactions between cortical and psychic functions [24, 25]. The etiology of the idiopathic forms of incontinence, constipation, retention, and pelviperineal pain can probably be considered, at least in part, as multifactorial, and the "central" aspects may have quite an important role. Sacral neural stimulation in the treatment of these dysfunctions probably acts both locally and, through afferent pathways, in the central nervous system [26–29].

The field of pelvic floor medicine is in rapid evolution and advancement. In the future, more surgeon-scientists will train and research to try to answer the long list of questions in female pelvic floor dysfunctions, using new practice patterns and a high level of scientific achievement.

References

1. Wei JT, DeLancey JOL. Functional anatomy of the pelvic floor and lower urinary tract. Clinic Obstet Gynecol 2004;47:3–17.
2. Ashton-Miller JA, DeLancey JOL. Functional anatomy of the pelvic floor. Ann N Y Acad Sci 2007;1101:266–296.
3. DeLancey JOL. Structural anatomy of the posterior pelvic compartement as it relates to rectocele. Am J Obstet Gynecol 1999;180:815–823.
4. Petros PE, Ulmsten U. An Integral Theory of female urinary incontinence. Acta Obstet Gynecol Scand Suppl 1990;153:1–79.
5. Papa Petros PE. The female pelvic floor. Function, dysfunction and management according to the Integral Theory. 2nd edn. Springer, Heidelberg, 2007.
6. Petros P, Swash M. A Muscolo-Elastic Theory of anorectal function and dysfunction in the female. Pelviperineology 2008;27:86–87.
7. Petros P, Swash M. The Muscolo-Elastic Theory of anorectal function and dysfunction. Pelviperineology 2008;27:89–93.
8. Petros P, Swash M. Experimental Study No. 1: Directional muscle forces activate anorectal continence and defecation in the female. Pelviperineology 2008;27:94–97.
9. Gonzalez-Argente FX, Jain A, Nogueras JJ et al. Prevalence and severity of urinary incontinence and pelvic genital prolapse in females with anal incontinence or rectal prolapse. Dis Colon Rectum 2001;44:920–926.
10. Meschia M, Buonaguidi A, Pifarotti P et al. Prevalence of anal incontinence in women with symptoms of urinary incontinence and genital prolapse. Obstet Gynecol 2002; 100:719–723.
11. Altman D, Zetterstrom J, Schultz I et al. Pelvic organ prolapse and urinary incontinence in women with surgically managed rectal prolapse: a population-based case-control study. Dis Colon Rectum 2005;49:28–35.
12. Soligo M, Salvatore S, Emmanuel AV et al. Patterns of constipation in urogynecology: Clinical importance and pathophysiologic insights. Am J Obstet Gynecol 2006;195:50–55.
13. Kapoor DS, Davila GW, Ghoniem GG. Practice patterns of colorectal surgeons in the management of voiding and sexual dysfunction. Int Urogynecol J 2001;12:S30.
14. Sun JH, Aguirre AO, Davila GW. Team approach to pelvic floor dysfunction benefit the patients. Dis Colon Rectum 1999;42:A15.
15. Christopher NG, Rackley RR, Appell RA. Incidence of concomitant procedures for pelvic organ prolapse and reconstruction in women who undergo surgery for stress urinary incontinence. Urology 2001;57:911–913.
16. Hart SR, Moore RD, Miklos JR et al. Incidence of concomitant surgery for pelvic organ prolapse in patients surgically treated for stress urinary incontinence. J Reprod Med 2006;51:521–524.
17. Davila GW. Concept of the pelvic floor as a unit: the case for multidisciplinary pelvic floor centers. In: Becher HD, Stenzl A, Wallwiener and Zittel TT. Urinary and fecal incontinence. An interdisciplinary approach. Springer-Verlag, Berlin, Heidelberg, 2005, pp 458–464.
18. Dodi G. Perineologia: un neologismo? Riv It Colproct 1990;9:113.
19. Albo M, Brubaker L, Daneshgari F. Open and unresolved clinical questions in female pelvic medicine and reconstructive surgery. BJU Int 2006 98;S1:110–116.
20. Bump RC, Mattiasson A, Bo K et al. The standardization of terminology of female pelvic organ prolapse and pelvic floor dysfunction. Am J Obstet Gynecol 1996;175:10–17.
21. Artibani W, Benvenuti F, Di Benedetto P et al. Staging of female urinary incontinence and pelvic floor disorders. Proposal of IPGH system. Urodinamica, Neurourology, Urodynamics & Continence 1996;6:1–5.
22. Dodi G, Lucio P, Spella M et al. La raccolta dati nel paziente pelvi-perineologico. Pelvi-Perineologia 2006;25:19–27.
23. Beco J, Mouchel J. Understanding the Concept of Perineology. Int Urogynecol J 2002;13:275–277.
24. Pescatori M. Dialogo di un presidente onorario (il passeggere disincantato) e di un giovin chirurgo (il venditore di almanacchi). Pelvi-Perineologia 2006;25:149–152.
25. Miliacca C, Lombardi AM, Bilali S, Pescatori M. Il test del disegno della famiglia nella valutazione dei pazienti con patologia colorettale. Pelvi-Perineologia 2006;25:15–18.
26. Malaguti S. Il ruolo della neurofisiologia del pavimento pelvico: nuove prospettive. Pelvi-Perineologia 2006;25:67–69.
27. Lombardi G, Macchiarella A, Celso M, Del Popolo G. La NMS nei pazienti neurologici: effetti sulla funzione urinaria, colorettale e sessuale. Pelvi-Perineologia 2006;25:86–88.
28. Ratto C. La neuromodulazione sacrale nel trattamento dell'incontinenza fecale: l'esperienza del GINS. Pelvi-Perineologia 2006;25:95–99.
29. Spinelli M. Il futuro della neuromodulazione sacrale: Pelvi-Perineologia 2006;25:106–108.

The Abdominal Approach to Urogenital Prolapse

43

Dennis H. Kim and Gamal M. Ghoniem

Abstract In deciding which surgical approach to use in repairing pelvic organ prolapse (POP), it is essential to have a complete understanding not only of the relevant anatomy, but also of the pathogenesis of POP. A detailed discussion of pelvic floor anatomy and physiology was presented earlier. There is no ideal approach or repair for POP. The choice of operation is made after careful consideration of a series of factors related to the patient's anatomy, medical history, and goals of surgery. To further complicate matters, laparoscopic and robotic surgery are new techniques available to the pelvic reconstructive surgeon. These newer techniques will be discussed in detail in a later Chapter. Finally, the traditional view that hysterectomy is part of POP repair is being challenged.

Keywords Abdominal sacrocolpopexy • Pelvic organ prolapse • Uterine preservation

43.1 Introduction

Generally speaking, the surgical repair of pelvic organ prolapse (POP) can be accomplished through two routes – a vaginal or an abdominal incision. Reconstructive pelvic surgeons need to be proficient with both routes of surgical access. In choosing the optimal surgical approach, several factors need to be considered.

First and foremost is the type of prolapse present. Specific types of prolapse or combinations of prolapse may dictate the optimal route of repair. With more complex prolapse, sometimes a combined vaginal and abdominal approach is needed.

The vaginal approach can be used to repair prolapse through all compartments – anterior, apical, and posterior. Specifically, the vaginal approach can be used to repair central and lateral cystoceles, vaginal vault prolapse, uterine prolapse, enteroceles, and rectoceles, and to reconstruct the perineal body. Additionally, sling procedures to address concomitant stress urinary incontinence can be easily performed.

An abdominal approach, on the other hand, is required if concurrent intra-abdominal pathology exists that needs to be addressed. However, not all prolapse can be repaired through an abdominal approach. This approach can only be used to repair apical prolapse and lateral cystoceles. Central cystoceles, most rectoceles unless very high, and perineal body defects cannot be readily accessed and repaired through the abdominal route alone.

43.2 The Abdominal Approach

When we speak of an abdominal approach, we must first examine what we mean, because not all incisions

G.M. Ghoniem
Department of Urology, Cleveland Clinic Florida, Weston, FL, USA

G.A. Santoro, A.P. Wieczorek, C.I. Bartram (eds.) *Pelvic Floor Disorders*
© Springer-Verlag Italia 2010

through the abdominal wall are the same. The dissection can be either a transperitoneal approach, opening the peritoneal cavity and gaining access to the bowels, or an extraperitoneal retropubic approach, where the peritoneal cavity is not entered.

Some centers still perform retropubic paravaginal cystocele repairs. If these women also have stress urinary incontinence, a Burch colposuspension can also be done via this approach, obviating the need for a separate vaginal incision in order to place a sling. Given the added morbidity of an abdominal incision though, it has become increasingly less common to perform a retropubic paravaginal cystocele repair, especially given all the advantages of doing the same repair transvaginally. Additionally, the ability to accurately classify a cystocele as a result of a central or lateral defect has been questioned [1]. Preoperative exam findings have been shown to not correlate well with actual intraoperative findings. A study of 117 women found that those who were thought to have normal paravaginal support at physical exam tended to have normal support at surgery, but less than two-thirds of women who were identified as have a paravaginal defect at physical exam actually had a paravaginal defect at surgery [2]. This is of particular significance since central-type defects cannot be accessed and repaired abdominally. Finally, with the advent of commercially available kits for the repair of anterior wall prolapse, the distinction between central and lateral defects has become less important, as these kits are all used transvaginally and correct both types of fascial defects.

Likewise, a transperitoneal abdominal enterocele repair is rarely done as an isolated procedure. An enterocele, if it exists, can be repaired through either the vaginal or abdominal route, so it is often repaired in conjunction with other procedures that usually dictate the surgical approach.

From a practical standpoint then, when we speak of the abdominal approach to prolapse repair, we are essentially referring to the repair of the vaginal apex – either vaginal vault prolapse or uterine prolapse; specifically we are speaking of a transperitoneal abdominal approach. Since this remains the main indication for the abdominal approach to prolapse, this will be the focus of the remainder of the chapter.

43.3   The Surgical Approach to the Vaginal Apex

Table 43.1 lists all the surgical options for correcting apical prolapse. There is no one ideal procedure for all patients, and so the surgical approach should be customized to the overall evaluation of each patient's spectrum of prolapse, continence, and goals of surgery. Additionally, each case must consider several important patient-related factors.

Some of the main patient-related factors include age, overall health, medical comorbidities, level of activity, whether the patient is sexually active, and finally the patient's expectations and goals of surgery.

Certain technical and anatomic factors are also important and may influence the surgical approach. A failed prior repair of the apex would favor an abdominal approach as a repeat procedure. A short or relatively scarred non-pliable vagina would also favor an abdominal approach, as the vaginal apex would need to reach the sacrospinous ligament in order to do a sacrospinous fixation. Finally, long vaginal length would also favor the abdominal approach, as a vaginal procedure may result in shortening.

Table 43.1 Surgical options for correcting apical prolapse

Surgical approach		Technique
Abdominal	Reconstructive	Sacrocolpopexy
		Uterosacral suspension
		Laparoscopic
		Robotic
Vaginal	Reconstructive	Sacrospinous fixation
		Uterosacral suspension
		Ileococcygeus suspension
		Posterior intravaginal slingplasty
	Obliterative	LeFort colpocleisis

Table 43.2 Surgical success of sacrospinous fixation and uterosacral suspension

Author	Year	Technique	Success (%)
Benson et al [3]	1996	Sacrospinous fixation	88
Lo and Wang [4]	1998	Sacrospinous fixation	80
Maher et al [5]	2004	Sacrospinous fixation	91
Schull et al [6]	2000	Uterosacral suspension	87
Karram et al [7]	2001	Uterosacral suspension	89
Barber et al [8]	2000	Uterosacral suspension	90

A final consideration is the experience of the surgeon. The vaginal approach to apical prolapse repair may be unfamiliar if a surgeon was not trained on the anatomy and techniques. In this regard the abdominal approach may be preferred as the anatomy is more familiar.

The vaginal route does have several advantages. It is less morbid than an abdominal approach, allowing a faster recovery for the patient. It can be done under regional anesthesia, and the operative time and blood loss is less compared to the abdominal approach. The other main advantage of the vaginal approach is that multiple compartments can be accessed and repaired concurrently.

Comparing the results of apical prolapse repair between the transvaginal and abdominal routes, however, shows the superiority of the abdominal route in terms of anatomic and subjective cure rates. Additionally, there can be a higher incidence of dyspareunia with the vaginal approach [3–5].

So, when it comes to apical prolapse repair, there is a slight trade-off for the less-invasive vaginal route in terms of surgical success rates compared to the abdominal approach.

An abdominal sacrocolpopexy (ASC) would be a better choice in a healthy woman who has failed a prior vault suspension procedure and has no other significant compartment defects, and who wants the most durable results with the least risk of dyspareunia. A younger woman with vault prolapse is a good candidate for ASC since she may inherently have genetically weak supporting structures. An older woman who is less active, has had multiple prior abdominal surgeries, and has multiple compartment defects may be a better candidate for a vaginal sacrospinous fixation procedure. Finally, an elderly woman with significant medical comorbidities and advanced multicompartment prolapse, who no longer has any desire to be sexually active may best be treated with vaginal colpocleisis.

Currently, no studies define who would benefit most from an abdominal sacrocolpopexy.

The vaginal apex can be repaired via the vaginal route, utilizing either a reconstructive approach that attempts to maintain and restore normal vaginal anatomy, or an obliterative approach whereby the prolapse is repaired by inverting the vagina and permanently securing the potential space in the vagina, such that the vaginal lumen is closed and the prolapse will not recur. Consequently, the obliterative approach should never be done on a woman who is or plans to be sexually active.

Of the vaginal reconstructive approaches, sacrospinous fixation and uterosacral suspension are the most commonly performed, with comparable success rates (Table 43.2) [3–8]. No randomized controlled trials comparing vaginal uterosacral suspension to abdominal sacrocolpopexy have been done to date. More recently, commercially available kits utilizing synthetic mesh and biologic grafts have become available, specifically to elevate the vaginal apex. Since these kits are a relatively new development, long-term data are lacking; however, early data show that they are effective in repairing apical prolapse [9].

Debate is currently ongoing as to the safety of these kits. Mesh-related complications have been reported, such as mesh erosions, vaginal scarring, and dyspareunia [9]. As more experience is accrued, the ultimate efficacy and safety of the kits remains to be determined.

Recent refinements in laparoscopic surgery, and the evolution of robotic surgery, have made these techniques more commonplace in performing vaginal vault and uterine prolapse surgery.

Although these minimally invasive techniques will continue to supplant the more traditional open approach to surgery, the open approach can still, today, be considered the gold standard by which all other techniques will be judged.

43.4   Abdominal Sacrocolpopexy

Women with vaginal vault or apical prolapse are very likely to have prolapse through other compartments as well. Prior to proceeding with surgery, a careful assessment should also include evaluation of the anterior and posterior compartments as well as the perineal body, and assessment for any degree of urinary incontinence. Even though a woman may not complain of urinary incontinence, women with high degrees of prolapse should have an assessment for so-called occult urinary incontinence. Following prolapse surgery, as many as 60% of women develop stress incontinence postoperatively [10, 11]. Evaluation for occult incontinence entails reduction of the prolapse with either a vaginal pack or a sponge stick elevating the vaginal apex to its usual anatomic position, and testing to assess for stress incontinence [12]. Often, simple provocative maneuvers such as straining and coughing with the prolapse reduced will reveal the incontinence. Urodynamic testing can also be used to specifically quantify the leak point pressure as well as to to assess overall bladder function. Although to date no studies have specifically validated urodynamics in the prolapse population, their clinical use is still widespread.

Symptoms related to pelvic organ prolapse include feeling a vaginal bulge or pelvic pressure or fullness. Occasionally, women experience low back pain. Other times, symptoms pertaining to voiding or defecation, specifically incontinence or having a sense of incomplete emptying or a need to strain, are present [13]. The degree of prolapse and severity of symptoms do not correlate. Some women with advanced prolapse are relatively asymptomatic. A prior history of stress incontinence with spontaneous resolution suggests kinking of the urethra with advancing prolapse, and one would expect to find occult incontinence with the prolapse reduced [14].

The use of magnetic resonance imaging (MRI) can be useful in selected cases of pelvic organ prolapse, but its application lacks uniform protocols, is not useful in identifying specific fascial defects, and has not been shown to influence or improve surgical outcomes. Thus, a careful physical exam is the cornerstone of the assessment of the type and degree of prolapse present.

The physical exam should be done in a systematic fashion. Standardized staging for pelvic organ prolapse has been described, and currently the International Continence Society (ICS) recommends use of the POP-Q (Pelvic Organ Prolapse Quantification) system [15]. The anterior compartment should be checked for prolapse and urethral hypermobility.

Apical descent, as well as the posterior wall and degree of perineal descent should be assessed, as concomitant procedures via the vaginal route would be needed to address these at the time of vault prolapse surgery.

Since the surgical approach is through the peritoneal cavity, it is helpful if patients are placed on clear liquids and given a mechanical bowel prep the day before surgery to decompress the bowels. Patients are given prophylactic antibiotics and placed in sequential compression devices for prophylaxis of deep vein thrombosis prior to the induction of anesthesia. Patients are positioned in a low lithotomy position with the aid of adjustable leg stirrups. Should there also be a need to perform a vaginal procedure, the stirrups can easily be elevated. The abdomen and vagina are thoroughly prepped in the surgical field and a Foley catheter is placed into the bladder under sterile conditions.

The choice of incision largely depends on surgeon preference. Either an infra-umbilical midline or Pfannenstiel incision can be used. A midline incision may be needed if the patient is obese, or may be preferable if there is a prior midline scar from earlier surgery.

If a paravaginal defect is found or a Burch colposuspension is needed, this can be performed first in the retropubic space, prior to entry of the peritoneal cavity for the sacrocolpopexy.

Entry into the peritoneal cavity is done sharply to avoid thermal injury from the bovie to the underlying bowel. Adhesions, if present, are taken down such that the bowel can be safely packed into the abdominal cavity exposing the sacral promontory. Some type of self-retaining retractor is useful in this regard. Next, the aorta, vena cava, and iliac vessels are noted, as well as the right ureter. The posterior peritoneum is elevated and opened sharply just above the sacral promontory. Care must be made to avoid the great vessels as well as the middle sacral vessels, as severe bleeding will occur if these are injured. Dissection inferiorly into the presacral space is avoided, so as not to disturb the presacral venous plexus, which can also cause troublesome venous bleeding from the sacrum. Some surgeons prefer to carry the peritoneal opening down into the pelvis, taking care of the right ureter to the right and the rectum to the left. Others do not open the peritoneum, and simply create a tunnel underneath extending down to the vaginal apex. We prefer the latter technique.

A sponge stick or Lucite rod or an EEA™ sizer is placed in the vagina to fully expand and identify the vaginal apex. The overlying peritoneum is opened transversely. A combination of sharp and blunt dissection is used to dissect the bladder free off the anterior vaginal wall. Partially filling the bladder with sterile irrigation can partially distend it and help in identifying the correct plane. Care is taken not to create fascial defects in the endopelvic fascia surrounding the vagina.

Next the peritoneum is similarly dissected from the posterior vaginal wall down to the rectovaginal septum. Another EEA sizer can be placed in the rectum to aid in its identification. Defects in the endopelvic fascia are now repaired using delayed absorbable suture.

Macroporous polypropylene mesh is now fashioned in a "Y"-shaped configuration, with one end of the "Y" covering the vagina anteriorly and the other end extending posteriorly (Figs. 43.1, 43.2). Most surgeons make the posterior arm slightly longer as a way to reduce the risk of posterior compartment prolapse following sacrocolpopexy. In fact, high rectoceles, when present, can be repaired at this time with this technique. The arms of the mesh are attached to the vaginal apex, starting with the posterior arm as distally as possible and working proximally up to the apex. Some surgeons deliberately place the suture through the full-thickness vaginal wall; others make an attempt to avoid the vaginal lumen. Most use permanent suture but others use a delayed absorbable suture. Once the posterior wall is attached, the anterior wall is attached in a similar fashion. The mesh is then configured in the pelvis to reach

the sacral promontory. If the posterior peritoneum was not opened, the mesh is now tunneled underneath the peritoneum to reach the sacral promontory. The mesh should lie without any tension along the hollow of the sacrum. Excess length is then trimmed and the proximal end of the mesh is now attached, with permanent suture, to the anterior spinous ligament at the level of the sacral promontory. The use of bone anchors at his point is a variation in technique for fixing the proximal end of the mesh to the sacrum [16]. Bone anchors are purported to lower the risk of bleeding, as there is more precision in their placement [17]. Bone anchors have been known to dislodge or migrate, which could lead to failure of the repair [18, 19]. No randomized trials to date have addressed the superiority of suture over bone anchors in sacrocolpopexy.

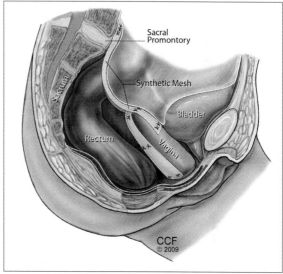

Fig 43.1 The mesh has two layers; the anterior layer extends to the level of bladder base, and the posterior layer can extend all the way to the top of perineal body

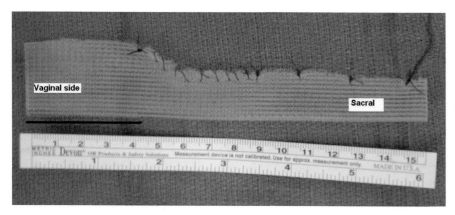

Fig 43.2 Polypropylene mesh can be made cheaply out of hernia mesh. A cut piece (4 × 15 cm) is folded and the vaginal end is opened to form anterior and posterior layers. The edges are sutured together. The length is adjusted intraoperatively

If the posterior peritoneum was opened to place the mesh, it is then closed at this point, to avoid the possibility of small bowel slipping behind the mesh and causing bowel obstruction. The abdominal cavity is now closed, and additional vaginal procedures such as cystocele repair, rectocele repair, placement of a sling, or reconstruction of the perineal body are done at this time.

Typically, patients are kept in hospital for 2–3 days, and discharged home once they are tolerating food, ambulatory, in good pain control on oral analgesics, and without a Foley catheter.

Abdominal sacrocolpopexy has a high success rate. Anatomic success with respect to the vaginal apex ranges from 78% to 100%. When the development of postoperative prolapse through any compartment is considered, the rate drops to 58–100%. In terms of patient satisfaction in relation to resolution of their symptoms, success rates are similarly high at 85–100% [20]. The procedure has also been shown to be durable, with success rates ranging from 74% to 91%, with an average follow-up of 14 years [21, 22]. Table 43.3 [23-31] lists contemporary results from larger series with ASC.

Anatomic failures, when they occur, affect other compartments, most commonly the posterior compartment, with a frequency as high as 57% in one study [32]. This has been true despite attempts to reduce this risk by extending the mesh further inferiorly along the posterior vaginal wall. Failure can also occur, albeit less commonly, in the anterior compartment, with one study reporting a frequency as high as 29% [33]. Beer and Kuhn [34] summarized 2008 patients who underwent colposacropexy and found the site of recurrent prolapse was the apical compartment in 1.9%, the anterior compartment in 2.3%, and the posterior compartment in 4.1% of patients.

This illustrates the point that although sacrocolpopexy is a durable and effective surgical technique for repairing the vaginal apex, additional surgery may be required later for failure in other compartments. Additionally, the fact that concominant prolapse surgery to correct pre-existing anterior or posterior defects is often done at the same time as the original colposacropexy, makes the interpretation of anatomic failure data difficult. It is not possible to know whether the recurrent prolapse through the anterior or posterior compartment is a result of the sacrocolpopexy, or of deficiencies of technique in performing the original anterior or posterior compartment repair.

Complications have been previously reported by an exhaustive review and are presented in Table 43.4. Mesh erosion has been a well-described complication. Its incidence has been found to depend on the type of mesh used. The overall rate is 3.4% and it usually occurs in the first two years after surgery, although late erosions have been described [35]. Autologous or cadaveric fascia has the lowest rate of erosion (0%), whereas the highest rates are noted with microporous polyfilament mesh (5%) [20]. Although autologous or cadaveric fascia has virtually no risk of erosion, the added time and morbidity of harvesting autologous mesh, and the problem with failure due to autolysis or the breakdown of autologous or cadaveric fascia, make this material a poor choice [36, 37]. Culligan et al [38] randomized 100 women undergoing abdominal sacrocolpopexy to receive either cadaveric fascia lata or prolene mesh. At 12 months of follow-up, the anatomic cure rate was 91% in the mesh group and 68% in the fascia group (P = 0.007). We do not recommend the use of biologic mesh for ASC.

At the present time there is no ideal mesh type. Currently, the use of a macroporous polypropylene

Table 43.3 Contemporary results with ASC from larger series

Author	Year	Patients	Follow-up (months)	Success Rate (%)
Snyder and Krantz [23]	1991	147	43	93
Sullivan et al [24]	2001	236	64	100
Culligan et al [25]	2002	245	61.2	85
Brizzolara and Pillai-Allen [26]	2003	124	36	98
Timmons et al [27]	1992	163	33	99
Lecuru et al [28]	1994	203	32.5	86.7
Occelli et al [29]	1999	271	66	97.7
Patsner [30]	1999	175	12	97
Lindeque and Nel [31]	2002	262	16	99

Table 43.4 Complications of ASC [20]

Complication	Incidence (%)
Intraoperative	
Cystotomy	3.1
Enterotomy or rectotomy	1.6
Ureteral injury	1.0
Bleeding or transfusion	4.4
Postoperative	
Urinary tract infection	10.9
Wound infection, hematoma, or dehiscence	4.6
Ileus	3.6
Deep vein thrombosis or pulmonary embolus	3.3
Bowel obstruction	1.1
Incisional hernia	5.0

mesh appears to be the best option. It is easy to use, inexpensive, and has a low rate of erosion 0.5% [20].

To reduce the risk of mesh erosion the vaginal tissue quality should be maximized preoperatively. Atrophic tissue should be treated with estrogen cream. Pessary use should be discontinued to allow for healing and recovery of any erosive vaginal lesions. Biologic grafts can be used to support any thin or attenuated tissue. Mesh should be placed without tension, to avoid ischemic breakdown of the tissue.

If mesh erosion occurs, a trial of conservative treatment with granulation tissue fulguration with silver nitrate and estrogen cream treatment may resolve the erosion. If the erosion is large or persistent, surgical excision of the exposed mesh may be required. There is little risk of prolapse repair failure after local excision of eroded mesh [39].

In those who have a uterus and suffer from uterine prolapse, it is currently controversial whether there is a need to perform hysterectomy at the time of sacrocolpopexy. Originally, it was believed that the uterus was the cause of the prolapse and therefore must be removed. Now the uterus is more viewed as a "passenger along for the ride", in that the prolapse occurs due to defects in support, and as the apex loses support and descends, so does the uterus. This changing view, along with recognition of the increase in complications with hysterectomy performed at the time of sacrocolpopexy, has called into question this once standard component of prolapse repair. The main concern is one of mesh erosion, with reported rates ranging from 0% to 27% if a hysterectomy is done concomitantly [20, 40]. To decrease this risk, some have advocated

a supracervical hysterectomy, closing the vaginal cuff in multiple layers, using biologic graft instead of synthetic mesh to attach the apex to the sacrum, or placing an intervening piece of biologic graft in between the cuff and the mesh. Currently no data exist to support the efficacy of these techniques.

43.5 Results Compared to the Vaginal Approach

To date there are three randomized trials comparing abdominal sacrocolpopexy to vaginal sacrospinous fixation. Benson et al [3] were the first to compare the two procedures, performing abdominal sacrocolpopexy in one group and bilateral sacrospinous fixation in another. In a total of 80 patients with a mean follow-up of 29 months, the surgical success rate, which was defined as no prolapse symptoms and no anatomic defect beyond the hymenal ring, was 58% in the abdominal sacrocolpopexy group and 29% in the vaginal sacrospinous fixation group. When failures occurred, they were noted to take place sooner with the vaginal approach. The reoperation rate for recurrent prolapse was higher in the vaginal group, 33% versus 16% in the abdominal group. Lo and Wang [4] compared abdominal sacrocolpopexy to unilateral sacrospinous fixation in 118 women. At 25 months, the surgical success rate was 94% in the abdominal sacrocolpopexy group and 80% in the sacrospinous fixation group. The most favorable results for the vaginal approach came from Maher et al [5], who randomized 95 women and at two years of follow-up found the anatomic (76% versus 69%) and patient-reported subjective success rates (94% versus 91%) to be similar. The degree of failure, however, was notable, in that the vaginal group had a higher proportion of cystoceles and failures that reached the introitus, when compared with the abdominal group (17% versus 4%).

The relatively high occurrence of anterior compartment prolapse has been noted by several authors, with reported rates ranging between 22% and 92% [41–43]. This may be caused by the retroverted vaginal axis exposing the anterior wall to increased abdominal pressure.

Beer and Kuhn [34] performed a review on surgical techniques for vault prolapse. Of 2390 women who had sacrospinous fixation, they found recurrent prolapse at the apex in 3.6%, the anterior compartment in 4.6%, and the posterior compartment in 1.5%.

A more detailed discussion of the vaginal approach to the repair of pelvic organ prolapse will follow in the next chapter.

43.6 Uterine Sparing

As previously mentioned, the traditional treatment for uterine prolapse included hysterectomy. The rationale in postmenopausal women included removal of a non-functional organ that may harbor uterine or cervical pathology. It was also believed that if the uterus was left behind, this would compromise the prolapse repair. There is a lack of evidence to suggest that leaving the uterus behind negatively affects surgical outcomes [44]. Alternatively, the removal of the uterus may actually increase the risk of later prolapse by disrupting the natural support structures such as the cardinal uterosacral ligaments [45]. Certainly, in a young woman with uterine prolapse who wishes to preserve her fertility, the uterus should be preserved. Uterine preservation is an option only after uterine pathology has been excluded.

Recently there has been great debate as to the degree that hysterectomy can affect a woman's sexual well-being. The traditional view from Masters and Johnson states that removal of the uterus and cervix can lead to sexual and orgasmic dysfunction [46]. One study did report an increase in sexual dysfunction in those who had a total versus supracervical hysterectomy [47]. Randomized trials have shown, however, that there is no difference with respect to sexual function [48, 49]. Other studies have even shown an improvement in sexual function after total hysterectomy, presumably due to resolution of prolapse and correction of the vaginal anatomy itself [50–52].

Like the repair of the prolapsed apex, either the vaginal, abdominal, or laparoscopic approach can be used for preservation of the prolapsed uterus.

For the transvaginal route, the technique of sacrospinous fixation or Lefort colpocleisis is essentially the same. For the abdominal or laparoscopic route, synthetic mesh is attached to the uterus and cervix, and attached to the sacrum in much the same way as ASC is performed.

The debate for hysterectomy at the time of prolapse surgery, as well as the optimal route of prolapse repair,

will continue, reflecting changes in social attitudes towards surgery, as surgical techniques become more refined, and more data become available. Ultimately, individual patients' goals and expectations from surgery need to be balanced with the medical indications, through a personalized discussion between the patient and surgeon.

43.7 Conclusions

There are several approaches to repairing POP – abdominally, transvaginally, and now laparoscopically. There is no one optimal approach for repairing prolapse in all women. Whatever the approach, a thorough understanding of the relevant anatomy is required. Matching the patient's goals and expectations with the surgical approach will help to maximize the success of surgery.

References

1. Whiteside JL, Barber MD, Paraiso MF et al. Clinical evaluation of anterior vaginal wall support defect: interexaminer and intraexaminer reliability. Am J Obstet Gynecol 2004;191:100–104.
2. Barber MD, Cundiff GW, Weidner AC et al. Accuracy of clinical assessment of paravaginal defects in women with anterior vaginal wall prolapse. Am J Obstet Gynecol 1999; 181:87–90.
3. Benson JT, Lucente V, McClellan E. Vaginal versus abdominal reconstructive surgery for the treatment of pelvic support defects: a prospective randomized study with long-term outcome evaluation. Am J Obstet Gynecol 1996; 175:1481–1422.
4. Lo TS, Wang AC. Abdominal colposacropexy and sacrospinous ligament suspension for severe uterovaginal prolapse: a comparison. J Gynecol Surg 1998;14:59–64.
5. Maher CF, Qatawneh AM, Dwyer PL et al. Abdominal sacral colpopexy or vaginal sacrospinous colpopexy for vaginal vault prolapse: a prospective randomized study. Am J Obstet Gynecol 2004;190:20–26.
6. Shull BL, Bachofen C, Coates KW et al. Transvaginal approach to repair of apical and other associated sites of pelvic organ prolapse with uterosacral ligaments. Am J Obstet Gynecol 2000;183:1365–1373.
7. Karram M, Goldwasser S, Kleeman S et al. High uterosacral vaginal vault suspension with fascial reconstruction for vaginal repair of enterocele and vaginal vault prolapse. Am J Obstet Gynecol 2001;185:1339–1342.
8. Barber MD, Visco AG, Weidner AC et al. Bilateral uterosacral ligament vaginal vault suspension with site-specific endopelvic fascia defect repair for treatment of pelvic organ

prolapse. Am J Obstet Gynecol 2000;183:1402–1410.

9. Feiner B, Jelovsek JE, Maher C. Efficacy and safety of transvaginal mesh kits in the treatment of prolapse of the vaginal apex: a systematic review. BJOG 2009;116:15–24.

10. Gallentine ML, Cespedes RD. Occult stress urinary incontinence and the effect of vaginal vault prolapse on abdominal leak point pressures. Urology 2001;57:40–44.

11. Bergman A, Koonings PP, Baddard CA. Predicting postoperative urinary incontinence development in women undergoing operation for genitourinary prolapse. Am J Obstet Gynecol 1988;158:1171–1175.

12. Ghoniem GM, Walters F, Lewis V. The value of the vaginal pack test in large cystoceles. J Urol 1994;152:931–934.

13. American College of Obstetricians and Gynecologists. Pelvic organ prolapse. ACOG Technical Bulletin. American College of Obstetricians and Gynecologists, Washington DC, 1995.

14. Ellerkamann RM, Cundiff GW, Melick CF et al. Correlation of symptoms with location and severity of pelvic organ prolapse. Am J Obstet Gynecol 2001;185:1332–1338.

15. Bump RC, Mattiasson A, Bo K et al. The standardization of terminology of female pelvic organ prolapse and pelvic organ dysfunction. Am J Obstet Gynecol 1996;175:10–17.

16. van der Weiden RM, Withagen MI, Bergkamp AB et al. A new device for bone anchor fixation in laparoscopic sacrocolpopexy: the Franciscan laparoscopic bone anchor inserter. Surg Endosc 2005;19:594–597.

17. Smith MR. Colposacropexy: an alternative technique. Am J Obstet Gynecol 1997;176:1374–1375.

18. Ghoniem GM, Bryan W. Male perineal sling. Tech Urol 2001;7:229–232.

19. Park HB, Keyurapan E, Gill HS et al. Suture anchors and tacks for shoulder surgery, part II: the prevention and treatment of complications. Am J Sports Med 2006;34:136–144.

20. Nygaard IE, McCreery R, Brubaker L et al. Abdominal sacrocolpopexy: a comprehensive review. Obstet Gynecol 2004;104:805–823.

21. Hilger WS, Poulson M, Norton PA. Long-term results of abdominal sacrocolpopexy. Am J Obstet Gynecol 2003; 189:1606–1610.

22. Lefranc JP, Atallah D, Camatte S. Long-term follow-up of posthysterectomy vaginal vault prolapse abdominal repair: a report of 85 cases. J Am Coll Surg 2002;195:352–358.

23. Snyder TE, Krantz KE. Abdominal-retroperitoneal sacral colpopexy for the correction of vaginal prolapse. Obstet Gynecol 1991;77:944–949.

24. Sullivan ES, Longaker CJ, Lee PY. Total pelvic mesh repair: a ten-year experience. Dis Colon Rectum 2001;44:857–863.

25. Culligan PJ, Murphy M, Blackwell L et al. Long-term success of abdominal sacral colpopexy using synthetic mesh. Am J Obstet Gynecol 2002;187:1473–1480.

26. Brizzolara S, Pillai-Allen A. Risk of mesh erosion with sacral colpopexy and concurrent hysterectomy. Obstet Gynecol 2003;102:306–310.

27. Timmons MC, Addison WA, Addison SB et al. Abdominal sacral colpopexy in 163 women with posthysterectomy vaginal vault prolapse and enterocele: evolution of operative techniques. J Reprod Med 1992;37:323–327.

28. Lecuru F, Taurelle R, Clouard C et al. Surgical treatment of genito-urinary prolapses by abdominal approach: results

in a continuous series of 203 operations Ann Chir 1994; 48:1013–1019.

29. Occelli B, Narducci F, Cosson M et al. Abdominal colposacropexy for the treament of vaginal vault prolapse with or without urinary stress incontinence. Ann Chir 1999; 53:367–377.

30. Patsner B. Abdominal sacral colpopexy in patients with gynecologic cancer: report of 25 cases with long-term follow-up and literature review. Gynecol Oncol 1999;75:504–508.

31. Lindeque BG, Nel WS. Sacrocolpopexy- a report on 262 consecutive operations. S Afr Med J 2002;92:982–985.

32. Baessler K, Schuessler B. Abdominal sacrocolpopexy and anatomy and function of the posterior compartment. Obstet Gynecol 200197:678–684.

33. Brubaker L. Sacrocolpopexy and the anterior compartment: support and function. Am J Obstet Gynecol 1995; 173:1690–1696.

34. Beer M, Kuhn A. Surgical techniques for vault prolapse: a review of the literature. Eur J Obstet Gynecol Reprod Biol 2005;119:144–155.

35. Visco AG, Weidner AC, Barber MD et al. Vaginal mesh erosion after abdominal sacral colpopexy. Am J Obstet Gynecol 2001;184:297–302.

36. Fitzgerald MP, Edwards SR, Fenner D. Medium-term follow-up on use of freeze-dried, irradiated donor fascia for sacrocolpopexy and sling procedures. Int Urogynecol J Pelvic Floor Dysfunct 2004;15:238–242.

37. Fitzgerald MP, Mollenhauer J, Bitterman P et al. Functional failure of fascia lata allografts. Am J Obstet Gynecol 1999;181:1339–1344.

38. Culligan PJ, Blackwell L, Goldsmith LJ et al. A randomized controlled trial comparing facia lata and synthetic mesh for sacral colpopexy. Obstet Gynecol 2005;106:29–37.

39. Hurt WG. Abdominal sacral colpopexies complicated by vaginal graft erosion. Obstet Gyencol 2004;103:1033–1034.

40. Cundiff GW, Varner E, Visco AG et al. Risk factors for mesh/suture erosion following sacral colpopexy. Am J Obstet Gynecol 2008;199:688.e1–5.

41. Morley GW, DeLancey JO. Sacrospinous ligament fixation for eversion of the vagina. Am J Obstet Gynecol 1988;158:872–881.

42. Shull BL, Capen CV, Riggs MW et al. Preoperative and postoperative analysis of site-specific support defects in 81 women treated with sacrospinous ligament suspension and pelvic reconstruction. Am J Obstet Gynecol 1992; 166:1764–1768.

43. Holley RL, Varner RE, Gleason BP et al. Recurrent pelvic support defects after sacrospinous ligament fixation for vaginal vault prolapse. J Am Coll Surg 1995;180:444–448.

44. Langer R, Ron-El R, Neuman M et al. The value of simultaneous hysterectomy during Burch colposuspension for urinary stress incontinence. Obstet Gynecol 1988; 72:866–869.

45. Nesbitt RE. Uterine preservation in the surgical management of genuine stress urinary incontinence associated with uterovaginal prolapse. Surg Gyencol Obstet 1989;168:143–147.

46. Masters WH, Johnson VE. Human sexual response. Little Brown, Boston, 1966.

47. Saini J, Kuczynski E, Gretz HF et al. Supracervical hysterectomy versus total abdominal hysterectomy: perceived

effects on sexual function. BMC Womens Health 2002;2:1.

48. Thakar R, Ayers S, Clarkson P et al. Outcomes after total versus subtotal abdominal hysterectomy. N Engl J Med 2002;347:1318–1325.

49. Zobbe V, Gimbel H, Andersen MA et al. Sexuality after total vs. subtotal hysterectomy. Acta Obstet Gynecol Scand 2004;83:191–196.

50. Rhodes JC, Kjerulff KH, Langenberg PW et al. Hysterectomy and sexual functioning. JAMA 1999;282:1934–1941.

51. Roovers JP, van der Bom JG, van Der Vaart CH et al. Hysterectomy and sexual wellbeing: prospective observational study of vaginal hysterectomy, subtotal abdominal hysterectomy, and total abdominal hysterectomy. BMJ 2003;327:774–778.

52. Gutl P, Greimel ER, Roth R et al. Women's sexual behavior, body image and satisfaction with surgical outcomes after hysterectomy: a comparison of vaginal and abdominal surgery. J Psychosom Obstet Gynecol 2002;23:51–59.

Tomasz Rechberger

Abstract The increase in the prevalence of pelvic organ prolapse and urinary incontinence, associated with modern population demographics, is leading to a different set of urogynecological surgical challenges. Nowadays, traditional techniques for pelvic floor repair are being steadily replaced by several new procedures involving the use of different meshes or grafts, with or without introducer kits. The surgical management of multicompartment prolapse is challenging and often requires a combination of techniques in order to achieve a proper anatomical and functional outcome. Since 1996, prosthetic meshes have become increasingly popular for transvaginal surgical cure of genital prolapse. This chapter reports available data and highlights more specifically the consequences of surgery with mesh reinforcement, which is currently an important issue particularly when surgery is performed by a vaginal approach. While evidence is accumulating that using a polypropylene mesh inserted via the vaginal route has a lower rate of prolapse recurrence, the lack of data on the real rate of complications and patient quality of life is still a main limitation of this type of surgery. However, in light of the growing number of proposed techniques and new resorbable and non-resorbable meshes, further widespread use of these techniques is expected in the near future.

Keywords Meshes • Midurethral slings • Reconstructive vaginal surgery • Vaginal surgical kits

44.1 Introduction

During the last 20 years, surgeons involved in the urogynecology field have almost completely changed their attitude to principles of pelvic floor surgery. Classical operations with massive tissue removal, including vaginal hysterectomy in the case of complete prolapse, have been replaced by reconstructive surgery, paying special attention not only to restoring anatomy but also to the functioning of organs located within the pelvis. This approach has not only revolutionized surgeons' work, but has also changed patients' attitude to this kind of surgery. How were such great changes possible in such a short time? In my opinion three fundamental causes have revolutionized the field of urogynecology within the last decade:

1. better understanding of the physiology of the pelvic floor (pioneering work of DeLancey – the hammock theory) and a new approach to reconstructive sur-

T. Rechberger
2nd Department of Gynecology, Medical University of Lublin, Poland

gery based on the Integral Theory of Petros and Ulmsten [1, 2]

2. rapid development of medical technology with the introduction of new prosthetic materials used in reconstructive urogynecologiacal surgery

3. introduction into clinical practice of relatively simple surgical "kits", which enable anatomical correction of prolapse, paying special attention to the functional outcome.

44.2 Theoretical Background of Modern Reconstructive Urogynecological Surgery Based on Integral Theory

Improper functioning of the female pelvic organs could be divided into structural problems, which result in their descent or prolapse (with or without functional disturbances), or intrinsic changes, which are clinically manifested by normal, or almost normal, anatomy but with improper function.

According to the main principles of Integral Theory, there is a close relationship between anatomy and function, and functional disturbances are the result of improper functioning of supportive connective tissue (fascia and ligaments) and muscles of the pelvic floor. These disturbances could be caused genetically or epigenetically, with pregnancy and labor being a leading causative factor for damage. To simplify this, forces generated by the muscles stabilize the pelvic organs in their normal position, according to current requirements, and therefore damage to the ligaments and fascia results in improper opening and closure (urinary and fecal incontinence) or improper function (coital capacity), and these are manifested by a marked decrease in the patient's quality of life. Therefore, in most cases, restoration of normal anatomy should result in the patient regaining normal function. According to this main principle, properly placed synthetic or xenogenic tapes reinforce and restore the function of the pubourethral ligament (PUL), uterosacral ligaments (USL), and arcus tendineus fascia pelvis (ATFP). A special diagnostic algorithm helps the clinician to recognize the site of the defect [3]. Of course several controversies exist in relation to whether the Integral Theory could really scientifically explain all the abnormalities and symptoms related to anatomical disturbances, but there is no doubt that the principles of this theory fully apply to the clinical effectiveness of the midurethral sling, which is currently the gold standard in the surgical treatment of stress urinary incontinence (SUI). All necessary information can be found at www.integraltheory.org.

44.3 Prostheses in Urogynecology

The current trend in modern urogynecological surgery is the use of synthetic and/or xenogenic prostheses in order to achieve a longlasting clinical effect that will not deteriorate with ageing. This is especially true among women who have undergone previous unsuccessful classical operation due to pelvic organ prolapse (POP), since this group usually accepts mesh augmentation in order to increase the probability of success [4]. The practical background in favor of using synthetic prostheses in pelvic reconstructive surgery is the fact that after classical operation utilizing native tissues, the recurrence rate markedly exceeds 30%, which definitely calls for improvement [5, 6]. This is probably caused by the fact that among women with severe prolapse (Pelvic Organ Prolapse Quantification score (POP-Q) III and IV), the composition of connective tissues responsible for the positioning of pelvic organs is defective, and therefore the ligaments and fascias used for reconstruction cannot function normally. Moreover, it should be stressed that in urogynecological surgery, the goal is to restore not only anatomy but also urinary and fecal continence, and also to maintain coital capacity.

Today, several synthetic and xenogenic materials are used in pelvic reconstructive surgery. However, polypropylene (Marlex), which was introduced into the medical market in 1958, is still the most popular and commonly used [7].

Theoretically, the ideal urogynecological prosthesis, which is, of course, not currently available, should have several characteristic features such as:

- biocompatibility
- it should induce only minimal local inflammation
- it should not change its biomechanical characteristic with ageing
- it should be easy to sterilize
- it should be resistant to bacterial infections
- it should be easy to use, e.g. its shape should be compatible to supported or reinforced organs
- and finally, it should be relatively cheap.

Taking into account all the above-mentioned features, one can expect that the biophysical characteristics of the material from which the prosthesis is made are of critical importance. The porosity of synthetic materials was a background for the currently used classification of prostheses proposed by Amid [8]. According to this classification, all prostheses are divided into four types:

- type I: macroporous (e.g. Atrium, Marlex, Prolen) – porosity greater than 75 μm, which allows for penetration of macrophages and fibroblasts, and also for ingrowth of extracellular matrix (ECM) components into the scaffold created by the prosthesis
- type II: microporous (e.g. Goretex) – porosity less than 10 μm, which makes tissue ingrowth practically impossible; currently not in clinical use
- type III: combination of macroporous and microporous materials which is a result of multifilament structure of fibers (e.g. PTFE = Teflon, Dacron = Mersilen or SurgiPro)
- type IV: submicroporous (e.g. Silastic, Cellgard).

Of course, the porosity of the mesh influences not only the possibility of immune cells penetrating but also the biomechanical characteristics of the prosthesis [9, 10]. Currently only meshes and tapes belonging to the type I prosthesis family are commonly used in pelvic reconstructive surgery, since they allow penetration of leukocytes (size 9–15 μm) and macrophages (size 16–20 μm) and this minimizes the possibility of infection. As was mentioned earlier, the ideal prosthesis should evoke only minimal inflammation, which should drive recruitment of fibroblasts in order to create de novo ECM elements on the scaffold created by the prosthesis. The proper incorporation of the prosthesis into host tissues should be characterized by a high rate of fibroblast recruitment, which is a biological indicator of the acceptance of a prosthesis, with the ideal graft showing little inflammatory response with early infiltration of fibroblasts. Fibroblasts are the source of many substances that might influence wound healing and graft incorporation by secreting a number of potentially beneficial molecules for repair, e.g. growth factors, including vascular endothelial growth factor (VEGF), platelet-derived growth factor (PDGF-A), insulin-like growth factor (IGF)-1, granulocyte/macrophage colony-stimulating factor (GM-CSF), interleukin (IL)-8, IL-6, tumor necrosis factor (TNF), transforming growth factor-beta (TGF β), and matrix proteins involved in the wound-healing process [11–14]. Problems relating to the erosion of sling material, through either the vagina or the urethra, have been encountered with almost all kinds of synthetic sling materials. Commonly known risk factors for inappropriate graft incorporation into host tissues include infection, inadequate surgical technique, vaginal atrophy caused by estrogen depletion, and inappropriate choice of suture material. However, some women might have genetic differences that predispose them to mesh erosion after reconstructive pelvic surgery. These differences are reflected in altered production of proinflammatory Th1 cytokines, which alter the ECM repair pathways of wound healing. Moreover, accumulated evidence suggests that T cells produce Th2 cytokines (IL-3, IL-4, IL-5, IL-6, IL-10, IL-13, TGFβ-2,3-related factors, and other related cytokines) or cytotoxic, proinflammatory Th1 cytokines (IL-2, TNF-α, interferon (INF)-γ), and the balance between Th1 and Th2 cytokines is crucial in cell homeostasis during proper wound healing [15].

Reported rates of tape and mesh erosion range from 1% for polypropylene to 6–12% for Goretex, which calls for new, better tolerated material [16]. Several new prosthetic materials are currently being tested in clinical trials (e.g. absorbable, such as Polyglactin 910, or combined absorbable Vypro I and II (50% Polyglactin 919 and 50% polypropylene)).

44.4 The Surgical Perineal Approach

44.4.1 Urogenital Prolapse and Functional Abnormalities

The basic principles of modern vaginal urogynecological reconstructive surgery with the use of synthetic prostheses are as follows:

- replacement or reinforcement of the pelvic ligaments and fascia with prosthetic materials, which serve as a scaffold for newly synthesized ECM elements
- restoration of functional integrity between damaged elements of pelvic supportive structures
- restoration of the continence mechanism by tape reinforcement of the pubourethral ligament
- stabilization (without tension) of the vaginal hammock

in its natural anatomical position, which is feasible due to the anatomical proximity of the foramen obturatorius and ATFP.

44.4.2 Urinary Incontinence

Since its introduction into clinical practice in 1961, Burch colposuspension has been the gold standard in the treatment of SUI [17]. It is still a method with established clinical effectiveness, but it is technically challenging and therefore a long learning curve is required. The retropubic synthetic midurethral sling, which became a clinical reality in 1995, was a revolution in the treatment of SUI [18]. A very simple vaginal technique, short learning curve, and near-total lack of possibility for individual modification by surgeons, meant that, regardless of the center, the method was reproducible and was characterized by very high efficacy compared to Burch colposuspension. The probability of bladder injury was almost reduced to zero when, in 2002, DeLorme introduced his transobturator method of midurethral tape placement [19]. The technical aspects of both methods are presented in Table 44.1.

It should, however, be mentioned that in some cases of type III SUI (intrinsic sphincteric deficiency (ISD)), the classical retropubic sling might be more efficient [20]. The new minimally invasive surgical kits for treatment of female SUI are currently being tested clinically, and their real clinical effectiveness should soon be established [21, 22]. It should be stressed that correct positioning of the tape under the midurethra, accompanied by its proper tensioning, is critical for clinical effectiveness (see Chapter 17).

44.4.3 Urogenital Prolapse

At present, surgery is the only effective treatment for POP and can be performed by an abdominal or vaginal approach. For years the only efficient way to surgically correct uterovaginal prolapse was sacrocolpopexy, either classical (abdominal) or laparoscopic and Richter sacrocolpofixation, but both of these methods are technically difficult and therefore require a long learning curve and good surgical experience, which obviously limits their use in routine clinical practice [23]. The vaginal approach, while less invasive, is less efficient and still demands significant surgical skills as well as local or general anesthesia and – in the majority of cases – hospitalization of at least 1–3 days [24]. Over the last ten years, many new, potentially more effective, treatments have been developed, mainly based on the introduction of artificial polypropylene as well as xenogenic prostheses in order to reinforce connective tissue support of the female pelvic organs [25]. Moreover, this new type of surgery, besides being less invasive, pays much more attention to both the anatomical and functional outcome of the procedure, especially in terms of bladder and bowel functions, as well as vaginal coital capacity. The real step forward in the surgical treatment of advanced uterovaginal prolapse was infracoccygeal sacropexy, described for the first time in 1990 by Petros and coworkers [26, 27]. This is a minimally invasive and a technically simple vaginal operation, which enables the restoration of all three levels that support the vagina in a normal anatomical position; however, it does not properly address the vaginal hammock defect. The technical solution in effective treatment of cystocele with restoration of the ATFP and anterior vaginal wall is the "double TOT (transobturator tape)" operation, which

Table 44.1 Comparison of technical aspects of retropubic and transobturator midurethral slings

	Retropubic sling	Transobturator sling
Surgical treatment of SUI	Yes	Yes
Short general or local anesthesia required	Yes	Yes
Probability of bladder perforation	Yes	Sporadic
Probability of iliac vessels damage	Yes (very low)	No
Probability of bowel damage	Sporadic	No
Probability of retropubic hematoma	Yes	Sporadic
Postoperative de novo overactive bladder syndrome	Yes	Yes
Intraoperative cystoscopy	Yes routinely	No
Mean surgery time	20–30 min	10–15 min
Infection and/or erosion of tape	Yes (< 1–2%)	Yes (< 1–2%)

enables anatomical correction of the vaginal hammock by transobturator placement of four-arm mesh, which restores damaged pubocervical fascia and reattaches it to the AFTP. Nowadays, several surgical kits enable complex restoration of the female pelvic supportive structure, but all of them use (with some minor modifications) the same surgical rules using a transperineal approach:

- correction of vaginal hammock with a prosthesis based on double transobturator mesh placement and, if necessary, also restoration of the pubourethral ligament with a midurethral sling
- reinforcement of the uterosacral ligaments and rectovaginal fascia by the insertion of two-arm mesh through both the ischiorectal fossa (with or without attachment to the ischiosacral ligaments), which is in fact a further development of the original idea of Petros' classical infracoccygeal sacropexy.

After more than ten years of clinical application, suburethral slings, either retropubic or transobturator, are currently considered the gold standards in the treatment of female SUI. However, the gold surgical standard in the treatment of severe uterovaginal prolapse is still to be established, since no currently used methods are free of some complications and recurrences. It should be stressed that in a recently published Cochrane review concerning surgical management of POP, in terms of evidence-based medicine, sacrocolpopexy is still considered the best surgical option for a long-term effect [28]. Based on literature review, the authors agreed that abdominal sacrocolpopexy is associated with a lower rate of recurrent vault prolapse and dyspareunia than the vaginal sacrospinous colpopexy; however, these benefits must be balanced against the longer operating time, longer time to return to activities of daily living, and increased cost of the abdominal approach. A panel of experts stated that the use of mesh or graft inlays at the time of anterior vaginal wall repair may reduce the risk of recurrent cystocele, and the addition of a continence procedure to a prolapse repair operation may reduce the incidence of postoperative urinary incontinence, but this benefit needs to be balanced against possible differences in costs and adverse effects [28]. The best surgical approach to vaginal vault prolapse still remains unknown. Surgeon comfort and preference, as well as proper patient selection remain critical. However, the use of graft materials in pelvic floor reconstruction opens up a new field in surgical strategy in terms of pelvic floor disorders. There is definitely a need for well-powered, controlled, long-term, randomized studies, with patient-generated quality-of-life questionnaires comparing the short- and long-term outcomes of these techniques.

Great progress has been made in the last 20 years, but several pivotal questions still need to be answered in the future.

1. What is the optimal surgical material for vaginal reconstructive surgery: synthetic, xenogenic or allogenic?
2. Should the use of prostheses be limited only to recurrences after classical operations, or can we safely apply this method to all patients regardless of their age and advancement of prolapse? In this strategy, only a few procedures will be performed and on the patients in which the dissection is the most difficult. This involves poor results because few cases on extraordinary patients mean non-standardized procedures and lack of a learning curve in easier patients. On the other hand, if we consider the strategy to only use meshes in patients with risk factors for recurrence, we should clearly define these risk factors. In the literature, recurrence occurs in almost 30% of patients, requiring a second operation, and this percentage is unacceptably high.
3. Can we really safely offer prosthesis reconstruction to young sexually active women without fear that in some cases unpredictable excessive fibrosis could hamper their quality of life? Some surgeons may have concerns about inserting meshes in patients aged under 50 years, wondering about the future of the mesh after 20 or 30 years. They will therefore apply a traditional, vagina-narrowing technique with a high risk of recurrence in a very active patient. This seems to be illogical; a young active woman needs a long-term effective technique that preserves the coital capacity of the vagina. Currently only mesh surgery can provide this.

Almost 50 years ago TeLinde wrote: "Every honest surgeon of extensive and long experience will have to admit that he is not entirely and absolutely satisfied with his long-term results of all his operations for prolapsed and allied conditions", and despite all the new achievements in POP surgery this statement is still valid [29]. Therefore, a lot of clinical questions still need to be answered before we can effectively treat both the anatomical abnormalities and patients' symptoms related to POP.

References

1. DeLancey JOL. Structural supprt of the urethra as it relates to stress urinary incontinence: the hammock hypothesis. Am J Obstet Gynecol 1994;170:1713–1720.
2. Petros PEP, Ulmsten U. An Integral Theory of female urinary incontinence. Experimental and clinical considerations. Acta Obstet Gynecol Scand Suppl 69 1990;153:7–31.
3. Petros PE. Diagnosis of connective tissue damage. In: Petros PE (ed) The female pelvic floor. Function, dysfunction and management according to the Integral Theory. Springer-Verlag, Heidelberg, 2004, pp 48–76.
4. Srikrishna S, Robinson D, Cardozo L, Thiagamoorthy G. The vagina dialogues: Womens expectations of prolapse treatment. Int Urogynecol J 2009;20(suppl 2):S174.
5. Paraiso MF, Ballard LA, Walters MD et al. Pelvic support defects and visceral and sexual function in women with sacrospinous ligament pelvic reconstruction. Am J Obstet Gynecol 1996;175:1423–1431.
6. Olsen AL, Smith VG, Bergstrom JO et al. Epidemiology of surgically managed pelvic organ prolapse and incontinence. Obstet Gynecol 1997;89:501–506.
7. Usher FC, Ochsner J, Tuttle Jr LLD. Use of Marlex mesh in the repair of incisional hernias. Am Surg 1958;24:969.
8. Amid PK. Classification of biomaterials and their related complication in abdominal wall surgery. Hernia 1997;1:15–21.
9. Poureddeyhimi B. Porosity of surgical mesh fabrics: new technology. J Biomed Mater Res 1989;23:145–152.
10. Chu CC, Welch L. Characterisation of morphological and mechanical properties of surgical meshfabrics. J Biomed Res 1985;19:903–916.
11. Mansbridge JN, Liu K, Pinney RE. Growth factors secreted by fibroblasts: role in healing diabetic foot ulcers. Diabetes Obes Metab 1999;1:265–279.
12. Mansbridge J, Liu K, Patch R. Three-dimensional fibroblast culture implant for the treatment of diabetic foot ulcers: metabolic activity and therapeutic range. Tissue Eng 1998;4:403–414.
13. Jimenez PA, Jimenez SE. Tissue and cellular approaches to wound repair. The American Journal of Surgery 2004; 187(suppl May):56S–64S.
14. Gath HJ, Hell B, Zarrinbal R. Regeneration of intraoral defects after tumor resection with a bioengineered human dermal replacement (Dermagraft). Plast Reconstr Surg 2002;109:889–893.
15. Chapel H, Haeney M, Misbah S, Snowden N (eds). Essentials of clinical immunology, 5 edn. Blackwell Publishing Ltd, Boston, MA, 2006.
16. Clemens JQ, DeLancey JO, Faerber GJ et al. Urinary tract erosions after synthetic pubovaginal slings: diagnosis and management strategy. Urology 2000;56:589–595.
17. Burch JC. Urethrovaginal fixation to Coopers ligament for correction of stress incontinence, cystocele and prolapse. Am J Obstet Gynecol 1961;81:281–290.
18. Petros P, Ulmsten U. Intravaginal slingoplasty. An ambulatory surgical procedure for treatment of female urinary stress incontinence. Scand J Urol Nephrol 1995;29:75–82.
19. DeLorme E. La bandelette transoburatrice: un procede mini-invasif pour traiter l'incontinence urinaire de la femme. Prog Urol 2001;11:1306–1313.
20. Miller JJ, Botros SM, Akl MN et al. Is transobturator tape as effective as tension-free vaginal tape in patients with borderline maximum urethral closure pressure? Am J Obstet Gynecol 2006;195:1799–804.
21. Petros PEP, Richardson PA. Tissue fixation system posterior sling for repair of uterine/vault prolapse – a preliminary report. Aust N Z J Obs Gynaecol 2005;45:376–379.
22. Rechberger T, Bogusiewicz M, Jankiewicz K. Tissue fixation system – letter to editor. Aust N Z J Obs Gynaecol 2006; 46:177–178.
23. Richter K. Die operative Behandlung des prolabierten Scheidengrunades nach Uterusextripation Beittarg zur Vaginae fixation Sacrotuberalis nach Amreich. Geburtshilfe Frauenheilked 1967;27:941–947.
24. Davila GW, Guerette N. Current treatment options for female urinary incontinence – a review. Int J Fertil Womens Med 2004;49:102–112.
25. Birch C, Fynes MM. The role of synthetic and biological prostheses in reconstructive pelvic floor surgery. Curr Opin Obstet Gynecol 2002;14:527–535.
26. Petros PE, Ulmsten U, Papadimitriou J. The autogenic neo-ligament procedure: a technique for planned formation of an artificial neo-ligament. Acta Obstet Gynecol Scand 69 (Suppl) 1990;153:43–51.
27. Petros PE. Vault prolapse II. Restoration of dynamic vaginal supports by infracoccygeal sacropexy, an axial day-case vaginal procedure. Int Urogynecol J 2001;12:296–303.
28. Maher C, Baessler K, Glazener CM et al. Surgical management of pelvic organ prolapse in women: a short version Cochrane review. Neurourol Urodyn 2008;27:3–12.
29. TeLinde RW. Prolapse of the uterus and allied conditions. Am J Obstet Gynecol 1966;94:444–463.

The Laparoscopic Approach to Pelvic Floor Surgery

45

Erika Werbrouck, Filip Claerhout, Jasper Verguts, Joan Veldman, Frank Van der Aa, Dirk De Ridder and Jan Deprest

Abstract Laparoscopy offers great exposure and surgical detail, and reduces blood loss and the need for excessive abdominal packing and bowel manipulation, making it an excellent modality for performing pelvic floor surgery. Though laparoscopic colposuspension has been shown to be equally effective as an open procedure at two years' follow-up, it is less practiced since the introduction of transvaginal tape procedures. Laparoscopic repair of level I or apical vaginal defects may be challenging, due to the need for extensive dissection and advanced suturing skills. However, it offers the advantages of abdominal sacrocolpopexy, such as lower recurrence rates and less dyspareunia.

Keywords Colposuspension • Graft-related complications • Laparoscopy • Learning curve • Mesh • Prolapse • Sacrocolpopexy • Urinary Incontinence

45.1 Laparoscopy and Pelvic Floor Surgery

Laparoscopy may yield better exposure and surgical detail, and reduce blood loss and the need for excessive abdominal packing and bowel manipulation, all of which may result in a lower morbidity [1]. Laparoscopy has gradually found its way into the field of urogynecology, but scientific validation of this approach has been poor for a long time. Recently, laparoscopic colposuspension was shown to be equally effective as an open procedure at two years' follow-up [2]. Today, the procedure may be less practiced since the transvaginal tension-free tape (TVT) procedure has been shown to be equally effective as open colposuspension and is even less invasive and less expensive [3–6]. It has there-

fore become the gold standard for treating stress urinary incontinence, leaving laparoscopic colposuspension in our unit as a procedure that is only offered to patients who are simultaneously undergoing other procedures by laparoscopy.

However, other urogynecologic procedures may still benefit from an abdominal approach. Surgical repair of level I or apical vaginal defects, which also preserves vaginal function, can be performed either vaginally or through an abdominal approach [7]. Randomized trials, however, have shown that sacrocolpopexy offers lower recurrence rates and less dyspareunia than sacrospinous fixation, but at the expense of a longer recovery time [8].

Logically, a laparoscopic modification for sacrocolpopexy (LSC) may reduce the morbidity of sacrocolpopexy. However, LSC was embraced later than colposuspension, probably because vault prolapse occurs more rarely and LSC needs extensive dissection and advanced suturing skills, limiting this

J. Deprest
Pelvic Floor Unit, UZ Gasthuisberg, Leuven, Belgium

as a procedure within reach of the general gynecologist or urologist [9].

45.2 Stress Urinary Incontinence: Laparoscopic Colposuspension

45.2.1 Introduction

For many women, urinary incontinence is a common and often debilitating problem. Around one-third of women of child-bearing age have some degree of stress incontinence [10]. Continence is achieved by a combination of anatomical and physiological properties of the bladder and urethra and the sphincteric complex, as well as other pelvic floor muscles and structures, including a normally functioning nervous system. Disruption of any of these components may lead to incontinence.

Stress urinary incontinence is typically referred to as the involuntary loss of urine associated with physical activities that increase intra-abdominal pressure. The International Continence Society (ICS) defines "genuine stress incontinence" (GSI) as the involuntary leakage of urine during increased abdominal pressure in the absence of a detrusor contraction, noted during urodynamic testing, which actually hints at the pathophysiologic mechanism believed to be behind GSI [11].

The most likely causes of genuine stress incontinence are:

- abnormal descent of the bladder neck and proximal urethra, with or without laxity of suburethral support
- a diminished intra-urethral pressure, e.g. as a result of former surgery and radiation.

Non-surgical treatments for stress urinary incontinence include conservative and pharmalogical therapies, which are beyond the scope of this chapter. Surgical therapy for treating GIS aims to elevate and support the urethra-vesical junction and increase bladder outlet resistance, reproducing normal continence mechanisms. Numerous surgical techniques for treating GSI have been described. The first retropubic approach was described by Burch and colleagues [12]. Laparoscopic modification of the typical Burch colposuspension was first described by the Belgian researcher Vancaillie in the early 1990s, who claimed the advantages of avoiding large incisions, shorter hospitalization, and faster return to normal activities [13].

45.2.2 The Technique of Laparoscopic Colposuspension

45.2.2.1 Patient's Preparation and Positioning

The patient is prescribed a soft diet three days prior to the surgery, to reduce intraoperative bowel distension. We use a single shot of cefazolin 2 g administered intravenously 1 h before to the first incision. After general anesthesia, the patient is positioned in a modified lithotomy position. After disinfection and sterile draping, a Foley catheter is introduced to empty the bladder, to enable identification of the bladder neck. A three-way catheter can be used to fill the bladder with dyed sterile water at any time during the operation. This allows easy recognition of an accidental bladder perforation. Four trocars are used: one subumbilical primary port, two lateral 5 mm ports, and one trocar halfway between the symphysis and the umbilicus, allowing needle passage (7 mm or more).

45.2.2.2 Preperitoneal or Transperitoneal Approach

It is uncertain whether an extraperitoneal approach has advantages over a transperitoneal one [14]. The preperitoneal approach is mainly performed when colposuspension is the only procedure to be performed. The transperitoneal approach can be performed primarily, when concomitant intraperitoneal procedures are done, or secondarily, after failure of the preperitoneal approach. First, the anterior peritoneum is incised about 3 cm above the symphysis. Then the urachus is coagulated and an incision from the left to the right obliterated umbilical artery is made.

The dissection in the space of Retzius is first oriented towards the symphysis, hence keeping the midline. Lateral dissection does not contribute and may cause laceration of venous structures. A thin fascial layer must be pierced to reach the posterior aspect of the rectus muscles to avoid entering the dome of the bladder. In cases of previous abdominal surgery, the top of the bladder may be attached to the abdominal wall and peritoneal scar. In such a case, filling the bladder may help to identify the upper margin of the bladder and locate the best place for peritoneal incision.

45.2.2.3 Dissection of the Operative Field

The symphysis pubis is used as a landmark. From there, the dissection extends laterally to the ileopectineal ligaments and downwards along the midline into the retropubic area until the Cooper's ligaments can be identified. The bladder neck and the vaginal vault are the next landmarks. Dissection of the Retzius space is done by blunt dissection. When dissecting the vagina, all fatty tissue is removed to allow perfect visualization and grasping of an appropriate bite of perivaginal tissue. It may also enhance postoperative fibrosis.

45.2.2.4 Suture Suspension Technique, by either Staplers or Meshes

The use of sutures appears more effective than mesh and staples [15]. There is only one study comparing the number of sutures used. When one paravaginal suture was used on each side of the bladder neck and urethra, an objective cure rate of only 58% was observed, whereas with two sutures this was 83%. Subjective cure rates were 65% and 89% respectively [16].

The sutures are placed after dissection and meticulous hemostasis. To facilitate proper placement of the sutures, the anterior vaginal wall is lifted with the aid of two fingers in the vagina. The needle is inserted with the needle holder 2 cm beyond the suture end of the needle. We use Ethibond 0 sutures (Ethicon), which are 90 cm or more in length to allow extracorporeal suturing. Vancaillie et al [13] proposed the use of Weston clinch knots. These allow tightening of the knot at any degree of elevation of the vagina, also without approximation to the ileopectineal ligament. We use at least two single-bite sutures placed approximately 2.0 cm lateral to each side of the urethra and 2.0 cm distal to the bladder neck, as described in the Tanagho modification [17].

45.2.2.5 End of Operation and Postoperative Regimen

After checking haemostasis and the integrity of the bladder, the peritoneum is closed with a running suture. For this purpose we use a monofilament suture with a large needle, such as Monocryl (Ethicon) 0 suture, because this slips easily when tying the knot.

We remove the catheter after 48 h, following which the voided and residual volumes are checked. When the preoperative residual bladder volume was normal, we target for a residual volume < 125 mL. If too large, the catheter is reinserted temporarily, or intermittent self-catheterization is preferred. We have empirically forbidden heavy lifting or sports for 6 weeks postoperatively.

45.2.2.6 Complications

Hemorrhage rarely occurs, and should be addressed appropriately. It rarely leads to discontinuation of the laparoscopic procedure. Lower urinary tract injury is the most common complication of colposuspension, in particular bladder lesions. The majority of these lesions can be easily sutured endoscopically but may cause prolonged catheterization. Ureteral obstruction has been described but it is rare.

Urinary tract infection is a common complication after this surgery. Other infectious complications such as wound infections or retropubic abscesses are rare, but are a source of serious morbidity. Urinary retention, de novo urge, and voiding dysfunctions may occur.

Later development of enterocele is less documented for laparoscopic procedures, but there is no reason to believe this would be less likely than observed earlier for open surgery.

45.2.3 Results

Several studies have demonstrated clinical outcomes that were comparable to those observed following open colposuspension [18–23]. In a randomized controlled trial by Kitchener and colleagues [20], the objective cure rates for open and laparoscopic colposuspension were 70.1% and 79.7% respectively. The subjective cure rates after 24 months in that study were 54.6% and 54.9 %.

Although laparoscopy usually requires a longer operation time, it is associated with less pain, less blood loss during surgery, and a faster return to normal activities [23, 24].

Apart from a trend towards more bladder lesions, the laparoscopic approach seems to result in fewer perioperative complications [20, 24].

In terms of cost-effectiveness, laparoscopic procedures may be cost-effective in the long term. One study demonstrated that laparoscopic surgery has a higher average cost (within 6 months of the operation) compared to open colposuspension, due to high operation room costs, mainly because of the cost of disposable instruments.

However, considering all costs up to 24 months, laparoscopic procedures may be a cost-effective alternative, provided that their failure rates are equal to those achieved by open surgery [25].

45.2.4 Conclusions

There is now level I evidence that the clinical outcomes from laparoscopic colposuspension are comparable to those from its open counterpart [20]. Like other laparoscopic procedures, laparoscopic colposuspension appears to have short-term benefits over open surgery, such as quicker recovery, less pain, and fewer serious perioperative complications. On the other hand, proper training in laparoscopy (especially mastering the suturing skills) is necessary to minimize perioperative complications, reduce operation time, achieve proper results, and make the operation cost-effective. However, the clinical relevance of colposuspension per se has been reduced since the widespread acceptance of sling procedures for GSI.

45.3   Laparoscopy and Uterine and Vault Prolapse

45.3.1 Introduction

Support of the cervix and, in its absence, the apex of the vagina, is provided by vertically orientated fibers that have a broad origin at the sacrum and lateral pelvic wall. These structures are better known as the uterosacral and cardinal ligaments, described by De-Lancey as level I support [7]. When these fail, uterine or vaginal vault prolapse occurs. Loss of apical support is associated with concomitant defects of the anterior or posterior wall in 67–100% of cases [7, 26].

The leading risk factor for development of post-hysterectomy vault prolapse is the prior presence of uterine prolapse at the time of hysterectomy. The prevalence of vault prolapse in women with prior hysterectomy because of prolapse is as high as 11.6%, whereas it is only 1.8% when the hysterectomy was done for another reason (overall incidence 4.4%) [27]. Other risk factors for vaginal vault prolapse include more generic causes, such as chronic pulmonary disease, but not obesity [28, 29]. Adequate prophylactic suspension of the vault by a proper culdoplasty at the time of hysterectomy prevents the occurrence of post-hysterectomy vault prolapse [28–30].

The clinical presentation of apical prolapse can vary from being asymptomatic to having a multitude of symptoms. The common denominator is feeling or seeing a vaginal lump. Frequently, urinary, defaecatory, or sexual symptoms may coexist. The prevalence of symptoms of stress urinary incontinence, overactive bladder, and voiding dysfunction varies and is around 30% for each one [31]. One in three patients has constipation, and around one in five experiences dyspareunia, but their relationship remains difficult to explain.

Vault prolapse can be treated by pessaries, but with limited success. A variety of abdominal and vaginal operations restoring level I support have been described. Vaginal repairs include uterosacral ligament suspension, ileococcygeal suspension, sacrospinous fixation, and infracoccygeal sacropexy. These are of less relevance to this chapter. Suspension at the uterosacral ligaments involves suturing the vaginal vault to the remnants of the uterosacral ligaments as high as possible [32]. Abdominal techniques involve uterosacral ligament suspension [33], sacrospinous fixation [34], and sacrocolpopexy [35]. Historically, these techniques were first described via laparotomy, and laparoscopic modifications were only recently described. In the uterosacral ligament fixation, the apex is suspended by shortening the ligaments with helical sutures. Abdominal sacrocolpopexy involves fixation of the vault to the anterior longitudinal ligament by the interposition of a graft, and historical reports of this procedure go back as far the late 19th century, by Freund in 1889 and Kustner in 1890. Cutaneous flaps were initially used by Huguier and Scali in 1958, and a synthetic graft was first described by Scali in 1974.

A Cochrane systematic review concluded that abdominal sacrocolpopexy is associated with less recurrence at the vaginal vault (risk ratio (RR) 0.23, 95% confidence interval (CI) 0.07–0.77) and less dyspareunia (RR 0.39, 95% CI 0.18–0.86) than vaginal sacrospinous fixation [8]. Conversely, open abdominal sacrocolpopexy was associated with a longer operating time, longer hospital stay, and higher cost than vaginal suspension. Logically, laparoscopic sacrocolpopexy may reduce the morbidity of the procedure.

45.3.2 Technique of Laparoscopic Sacrocolpopexy

45.3.2.1 Patient's Preparation and Positioning

We operate only on symptomatic vault prolapse, minimally presenting as stage II prolapse of the apex or upper posterior wall of the vagina according to the Pelvic

Organ Prolapse-Quantification system (POP-Q) [36]. In cases of associated rectal prolapse, a rectopexy may be performed (Fig. 45.1). Patient preparation is as for laparoscopic colposuspension, but bowel preparation may be even more important. Good exposure of the promontory is easier with adequate bowel preparation (Fig. 45.2). For this procedure we give both cefazolin (2 g) and metronidazole (1500 mg) prophylaxis. After induction of general anesthesia, the patient is positioned in a modified lithotomy position giving access to the vagina and rectum. After disinfection and sterile draping, a three-way Foley catheter is inserted to empty the bladder. The additional channels allow for bladder filling with dyed saline, to exclude bladder lesions or for

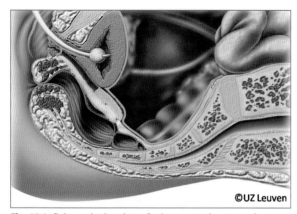

Fig. 45.1 Schematic drawing of a laparoscopic sacrocolpopexy. In this case, the posterior implant is extended over the entire posterior wall and sutured at the level of the sphincteric complex. From [37], with permission

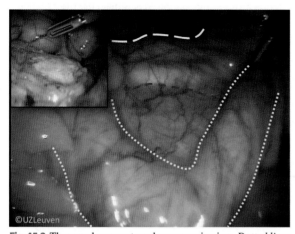

Fig. 45.2 The sacral promontory, laparoscopic view. *Dotted lines* demarcate the major arteries, the red line is the inferior border of the venous bifurcation, and the white line is the inferior border of the promontory. Insert: promontory following dissection. From [37], with permission

identifying the bladder margins. At least four trocars are necessary: one primary subumbilical 10 mm cannula, two lateral 5 mm trocars, and one trocar halfway between the symphysis and the umbilicus. The latter one is used for suturing, and should have leak-proof seals; we use Excel trocars for that purpose (Ethicon, Johnson and Johnson).

45.3.2.2 Retroperitoneal Dissection

After careful identification of L5–S1, the inferior limit of the left common iliac vein, and the right ureter, the dissection of the promontory commences (Fig. 45.2). First the prevertebral parietal peritoneum is incised with 5 mm monopolar scissors vertically. Retroperitoneal fat is dissected to allow exposure of the anterior vertebral ligament. An area as large as required for fixing the mesh needs to be dissected on the promontory just right from the midline. Pitfalls are the median sacral vessels, or, when moving any distance laterally, the ureter, or, to the left, the main vessels. Occasionally, bipolar forceps are used for this purpose.

The peritoneal incision at the promontory is then extended along the rectosigmoid to continue over the deepest part of the cul-de-sac, opening the recto- and vesicovaginal space (Fig. 45.3). Some prefer to create a tunnel under the peritoneum, avoiding later suturing. The lateral incision, as well as the dissection downward towards the perineal body, can be extended as far as required. This will be necessary when there is a large rectocele or when a concomitant rectopexy is required for rectal prolapse.

45.3.2.3 Mesh and Suturing Technique

At this point, we change gloves to prevent contamination of the mesh. Two separate meshes are sutured to the posterior and anterior aspect of the vagina (Fig. 45.3), using a knot pusher, needle holder, and assistant needle holder. As much as possible we try to avoid perforating the vagina while suturing. Because this might not always be avoided, we have also moved away from braided sutures such as Ethibond, and now use PDS sutures which were made for this purpose (Ethicon, 120 cm). Today, double-legged meshes are commercially available, such as Y-mesh (AMS) and Alyte (Bard). If not available, one can easily cut a larger mesh to the appropriate size, e.g. Ultrapro 15×15 cm implants (Ethicon). The posterior mesh can be fixed as laterally

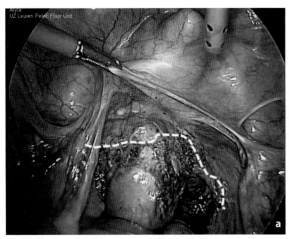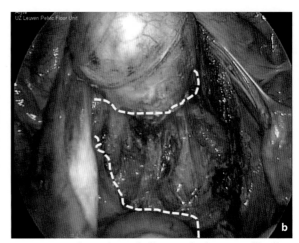

Fig. 45.3 Anterior (**a**) and posterior (**b**) dissection of the peritoneum to expose the vagina and allow mesh placement. The *lines* indicate the peritoneal incisional borders

as the levator muscle. There is no agreement on the size of the meshes that should be used, or on the number of sutures required for this operation, but we usually place between 9 and 16 sutures. It may be necessary to palpate the rectum and vagina to define their borders. Once this is finished, the vault is positioned by the rectal pusher (placed in the vagina) at the level of the ischial spines and then fixed in a tension-free position. We use either staples or tackers to fix the mesh to the promontory; however, sutures can be used as well. At this point, one needs to be alert to avoid hemorrhage from the presacral vessels. We then close the peritoneum with both a running suture and the staples left over from the sacral fixation (Fig. 45.4). This will avoid adhesions to the mesh. At the end of the procedure we pack the vagina.

45.3.2.4 End of Operation and Postoperative Regimen

We remove the vaginal packing and urinary catheter after 48 h. Postoperatively, low molecular weight heparin injections as well as a stool-softener macrogol 3.350, 13.25 g (Movicol, Norgine) are continued for six postoperative weeks to prevent heavy pushing. Also, sexual inactivity is recommended until the 3-month postoperative visit. All these measures were empirically determined.

In patients with uterine prolapse, a laparoscopic supracervical hysterectomy can be performed. This avoids opening of the vagina and might decrease the risk of erosion [38]. In patients where hysterectomy

should be avoided, a hysteropexy is performed instead [39]. A mesh is then placed both anteriorly and posteriorly, but they are connected to each other through the ligamentum latum.

45.3.2.5 Complications

At the promontory, large vessel or venous injury should be avoided. During dissection of the vesicovaginal space, hemorrhage or a bladder lesion can occur. Ureteric lesions are uncommon, but may occur when the dissection is performed too laterally.

Dissection of the rectovaginal space may lead to hemorrhage and rectal injury. Appropriate traction and dissection close to the vagina may reduce the risk. Also, the use of a rectal probe helps in identifying these structures.

Postoperative wound infections are rarely seen. De novo stress incontinence may be the result of excessive correction and traction backwards, opening the urethrovesical angle. De novo urge incontinence may occur, with a relatively unpredictable course.

The use of a mesh, remaining as a foreign body, can lead to graft-related complications. Pain or dyspareunia related to the mesh can occur. Exposure of suture material or mesh erosions (< 6%) may occur and require reintervention. Infections of the mesh, leading to sepsis or spondylodiscitis are rare but feared complications. Intravenous antibiotics are started, and reintervention with removal of the infected mesh may be required. Constipation may be due to extensive dissection or damage to the sacral plexus, but the majority of patients have this condition present before the operation.

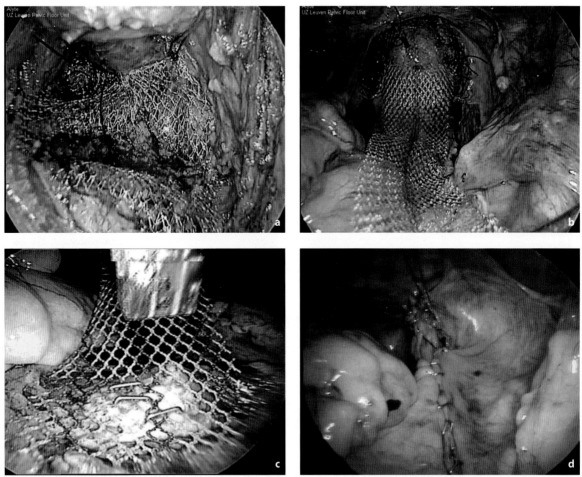

Fig. 45.4 Suturing of the mesh to the posterior (**a**) and anterior (**b**) aspect of the vagina. Tension-free suspension of the mesh by stapling it to the promontory (**c**). The remainder of the staples are used to close the peritoneum, which is finished by a purse string (**d**). From [37], with permission

45.3.3 Results

Data on LSC were initially limited to observational studies of variable size [40–48]. They covered issues such as perioperative parameters, reported short-term results, and were usually retrospective in design. In the largest retrospective study (n = 363), the anatomical cure rate was 96% at a mean follow-up of 14.6 months [44]. Over a longer term, Higgs and coworkers observed 8% recurrence at the level of the vault, but over one in three recurrences in the anterior or posterior compartment [45]. The overall reoperation rate for prolapse was 16% [45].

We recently reported our prospective experience with all consecutive LSCs beyond our learning curve (Tables 45.1, 45.2) [49]. LSC was introduced in our Unit in 1996. Since then, laparoscopy has been used as the primary access route. In order to avoid an effect on outcome of the inherent learning process that such a procedure involves, we used the cumulative sum analysis method to determine the learning curve [50]. Based on a 90% rate of avoiding conversion to laparotomy or occurrence of perioperative complications, our prior learning curve was set at 60 cases. Later cases (> 61) were included in a prospective consecutive series of 132 women.

They all had vaginal vault prolapse, defined as minimally presenting as stage II apical prolapse. They underwent LSC using an Amid type I polypropylene implant over a 5-year-period and were prospectively followed-up by a standardized protocol to determine anatomical cure (≤ POP-Q Stage I), subjective cure, and impact on quality of life, as measured by a standardized interview and a prolapse- specific question-

Table 45.1 Perioperative characteristics and complications in a prospective series of 132 LSCs [49]

Characteristic	Mean or N	SD or %
Operation time (min), mean (SD)	180.5	(46)
Blood loss (mL), mean (SD)	185	(124)
Inpatient days, mean (SD)	5.7	(1.9)
Conversion, n (%)	1	(0.7)
Completely by laparoscopy, n (%)	131	(99)
Perioperative complications, n (%)	0	(0)
Complications in the early postoperative (< 6 weeks) period, n (%)		
Bleeding	1	(0.75)
Nerve lesions	3	(2.3)
Local problems	2	(1.5)
Complications in the late postoperative (6 weeks to 59 months) period, n (%)		
Reintervention related to the mesh	9	(6.8)
Mesh erosion	6	(4.5)
Pain related to mesh	3	(2.3)
Reintervention for genital prolapse, n (%)	0	(0)

Table 45.2 Anatomical findings prior to and 3 months after surgery and at study closure in a prospective series of 132 LSCs [49]

POP-Q	Preoperative	3 months	Study closure
Number of patients at each time point	132	132	99
POP-Q ≥ –1 at any compartment, n (%)	132 (100)	7 (5.3)	22 (22)
POP-Q point Ba ≥ –1, n (%)	72 (54.5)	1 (0.8)	3 (3)
POP-Q point C ≥ –1, n (%)	87 (66)	0 (0)	2 (2)
POP-Q point Bp ≥ –1, n (%)	124 (94)	6 (4.5)	18 (18)

naire (P-QoL) before and after the operation [51, 52]. The standardized interview consists of 28 questions related to prolapse, bladder, bowel, and sexual function. P-QoL assesses the impact of prolapse on different quality-of-life domains, with scores for each domain ranging between 0 and 100. Postoperative assessment was done after 3, 6, and 12 months, and annually thereafter by a single independent assessor. De novo symptoms were defined as symptoms that were not present before surgery but that were present at the 3-months visit.

At study closure, all patients were asked to complete the P-QoL. If patients did not attend their planned follow-up visits, they were phoned to come for clinical assessment, and if that was not possible, a telephone interview was undertaken to document the functional outcome.

Women reporting "never" or "rarely" for the occurrence of prolapse symptoms (questions 1, 2 or 3 of the standardized interview) were classified as subjectively cured.

45.3.4 Choice of the Mesh Material

Different types of mesh have been suggested, either xenografts or synthetics. A comprehensive review reported an overall rate of mesh erosion of 3.4% when synthetic permanent materials are used [53]. The nature of the material used has been identified as a risk factor for the occurrence of graft-related complications. For this reason, surgeons have moved away from type II (microporous – e.g. Expanded PTFE, Gore-Tex) and type III (macroporous with microporous or multifilamentous components – e.g. polyethylene tetraphthalate, Mersilene), because of their increased risk for infection and erosion, and their poor integration into the host. Therefore, type I macroporous polypropylene grafts are used most frequently nowadays and provide excellent long-term anatomical results.

There now is also some evidence that synthetic grafts are superior to xenografts. They do not reduce the number of graft-related complication events, neither are they equally effective in terms of recurrence for this type of prolapse. We conducted a controlled study on a consecutive number of patients implanted with xenografts [54]. Anatomical and subjective outcomes were compared to outcomes from consecutive controls operated with a polypropylene mesh either before the xenograft cohort, or after (to allow an overall comparable follow-up period). After a mean follow-up of 33 months, the anatomical failure rate at the level of the vault was significantly higher (21% versus 3%, P < 0.01. There were also significantly more posterior compartment (36% versus 19%, P < 0.05) prolapses. There was a trend for an increased recurrence at any stage as well. There were also significantly more reoperations for recurrence. Functional outcomes were equal. Though a cross-linked (resistant to collagenase) as well as a non-cross-linked graft was used, the recurrence rates were similar. We concluded that substitution of polypropylene grafts by xenografts did not yield equally good objective outcomes, nor did it reduce the number of graft-related complications. Though functional outcomes are comparable, we have moved away from the routine use of xenografts for this operation and hope a more ideal "biological" mesh will be designed in the near future.

45.3.5 The Learning Process and Robotic Surgery

We studied the feasibility and the learning process of LSC by documenting our entire experience, i.e. from the first laparoscopic case onwards [55]. As outcome measures we used a variety of relevant indicators of surgical performance, including the number of laparotomies, complication rate, operation time, and anatomical failure. We analyzed these by different statistical methods, including "moving average" and "cumulative sum" analysis. We demonstrated that LSC can be implemented without increasing the complication rate. We defined the endpoint for the learning curve as the moment that the surgeon was able to complete the procedure by laparoscopy, without complications and with good anatomical outcome in at least 90% of patients. With this as an endpoint, the surgeon required 60 cases. This is fairly high and can be explained by the high number of laparotomies in our series. The majority of laparotomies were, however, performed as a precaution: only 2 (6%) were converted for complications. It is possible that this would be less today, since we now

have far more background laparoscopy experience than at that time, in 1996.

Operation time can also be used as a sole endpoint. This declined rapidly over the first 30 procedures, declining more slowly thereafter, to reach a steady state after 90 cases (175 min). This rather long learning curve motivated us to get better insight into the limiting factors or challenging steps of the procedure. To investigate this we studied the learning curve of a colleague who was familiar with advanced laparoscopic surgery but not LSC. Instead of only focusing on total operation time and complication rate, we split the operation empirically into five steps: (1) dissection of the promontory; (2) dissection of the right parasigmoidal, pararectal gutter and the vaginal vault; (3) fixation of the implant to the vault, which involves the placement of several sutures; (4) fixation of the implant to the promontory; and (5) reperitonealization. For each step we analyzed the operation time, performance, and complication rate. Taking operation time as the outcome measure, we found an apparent learning curve for all steps of the procedure, except for the dissection of and fixation to the promontory. The most challenging step was the dissection of the vault. It took the trainee 31 procedures to achieve an operation time that was comparable to that of an experienced surgeon. After a skills lab for suturing, the trainee could suture the implant to the vault as quickly as the teacher.

Robotic surgery is increasingly being used in gynecology and urology, and many hospitals have invested into the required hardware. It can also be used to perform LSC [56]. It is possible that, for surgeons who are not

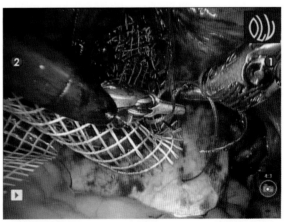

Fig. 45.5 View of a robotic sacrocolpopexy. The mesh is being sewn in with the robotic intstruments. Supplied courtesy of Dr A Mottrie, Onze-Lieve-Vrouw Ziekenhuis, Aalst, Belgium

familiar with endoscopic suturing, robotic surgery reduces their learning time. The cost associated with robotic surgery, however, remains an obstacle for the wider implementation of the operation. The surgical technique involves four to five laparoscopic ports: three to four for the da Vinci robot and two for the assistant. Suturing is intracorporeal (Fig. 45.5). Elliot et al [57] published their experience in 30 patients. In their preliminary report, they docked the robot only for the suturing of the mesh, which helped them overcome problems with endoscopic suturing [58]. On average, the operation took over 3 h (range 2.15–4.75 h). Recurrent grade 3 rectocele developed in one patient, one had recurrent vault prolapse, and two had vaginal extrusion of mesh.

A smaller series from Kramer [59] showed similar operation times, with one recurrence in a series of 21 patients, and over half of the patients had recurrent surgery for prolapse in other compartments. It remains to be seen the advantages of this technique for centers that already have a lot of experience with laparoscopy, and how effective the operation is.

45.3.6 Conclusions

Laparoscopic sacrocolpopexy yields objective and subjective cure rates that are equally as good as those for open surgery. At present there is no randomized controlled trial proving this, but one is under way. Observational data are, however, reassuring. Patients benefit from the low perioperative complications and quick recovery. However, extensive laparoscopic skills are necessary for this type of surgery, and the turnover required to become proficient may be a limiting factor to making this operation a reasonable goal for the average gynecologist or urologist. The place for robotic sacrocolpopexy, which makes suturing more intuitive, remains to be established.

References

1. Garry R, Fountain J, Mason S et al. The eVALuate study: two parallel randomised trials, one comparing laparoscopic with abdominal hysterectomy, the other comparing laparoscopic with vaginal hysterectomy. BMJ 2004;328:129–136.
2. Tan E, Tekkis PP, Cornish J et al. Laparoscopic versus open colposuspension for urodynamic stress incontinence. Neurourol Urodyn 2007;26:158–169.
3. Maher C, Qatawneh A, Baessler K et al. Laparoscopic colposuspension or tension-free vaginal tape for recurrent stress urinary incontinence and/or intrinsic sphincter deficiency- a randomized controlled trial. Neurourol Urodyn 2004; 23:433–434.
4. Paraiso MF, Walters M, Karram M et al. Laparoscopic Burch colposuspension versus the tension-free vaginal tape procedure: a randomised controlled trial. Neurourol Urodyn 2004;22:487–488.
5. Jelovsek JE, Barber MD, Karram MM et al. Randomized trial of laparoscopic Burch colposuspension versus tension-free vaginal tape: long term follow up. BJOG 2008;115:219–225.
6. Dean N, Herbison P, Ellis G et al. Laparoscopic colposuspension and tension-free vaginal tape: a systematic review. BJOG 2006;113:1345–1353.
7. DeLancey JOL. Anatomic aspects of vaginal eversion after hysterectomy. Am J Obstet Gynecol 1992;166:1717–1728.
8. Maher C, Baessler K, Glazener CMA et al. Surgical management of pelvic organ prolapse in women. Cochrane Database Syst Rev 2007;(3):CD004014.
9. Nezhat CH, Nezhat F, Nezhat C. Laparoscopic sacral colpopexy for vaginal vault prolapse. Obstet Gynecol 1994; 84:885–888.
10. Wilson PD, Herbison RM, Herbison GP. Obstetric practice and the prevalence of urinary incontinence three months after delivery. BJOG 1996;103:154–161.
11. Abrams P, Cardozo L, Fall M et al. Lower urinary tract function: standardisaton of terminology. Neurourol Urodyn 2002;21:167–178.
12. Burch JC, Moehrer B, Carey M et al. Cooper's ligament urethrovesical suspension for stress incontinence. Am J Obstet Gynecol 1968;100:764–774.
13. Vancaillie TG, Schuessler W. Laparoscopic bladder neck suspension. J Laparoendosc Surg 1991;1:169–173.
14. Wallwiener D, Grischke EM, Rimbach S et al. Endoscopic retropubic colposuspension: "Retziusscopy" versus laparoscopy – a reasonable enlargement of the operative spectrum in the management of recurrent stress incontinence. Endosc Surg Allied Technol 1995;3:115–118.
15. Ankerdahl M, Milsom I, Stjerndahl JH, Engh ME. A three-armed randomized trial comparing open Burch colposuspension using sutures with laparoscopic colposuspension using sutures and laparoscopic colposuspension using mesh and staples in women with stress urinary incontinence. Acta Obstet Gynecol Scand 2005;84:773–779.
16. Persson J. Stress urinary incontinence among women: aspects of risk factors, evaluation and surgical treatment. PhD thesis. Department of Obstetrics and Gynaecology Lund University, 2001, pp 1–61.
17. Deprest J, Brollman H, De Ridder D et al. Laparoscopic colposuspension. In: Timmerman D, Deprest J, Bourne T (eds) Ultrasound and endoscopic surgery in obstetrics and gynaecology. A combined approach to diagnosis and management: a combined approach to diagnosis and treatment. Springer-Verlag, New York, 2002, pp 122–131.
18. Morris AR, Reilly ETC, Hassab A et al. 5–7 year follow-up of a randomized trial comparing laparoscopic colposuspension and open colposuspension in the treatment of genuine stress incontinence. Int Urogynecol J 2001;13(suppl 3):S6.
19. Carey MP, Goh JT, Rosamilia A et al. Laparoscopic versus open Burch colposuspension: a randomized controlled trial. BJOG 2006;113:999–1006.

20. Kitchener HC, Dunn G, Lawton V et al. Laparoscopic versus open colposuspension-results of prospective randomized controlled trial. BJOG 2006;113:1007–1013.

21. Reid F, Smith A. Laparoscopic versus open colposuspension: which one should we choose? Curr Opin Obstet Gynecol 2007;19:345–349.

22. Tan E, Tekkis PP, Cornish J et al. Laparoscopic versus open colposuspension for urodynamic stress incontinence. Neurourol Urodyn 2007;26:158–169.

23. Dean N, Ellis G, Herbison GP, Wilson D. Laparoscopic colposuspension for urinary incontinence in women. Cochrane Database Syst Rev 2006;19(3):CD002239.

24. Carey MP, Goh JT, Rosamilia A et al. Laparoscopic versus open Burch colposuspension: a randomized controlled trial. BJOG 2006;113:999–1006.

25. Dumville JC, Manca A, Kitchener HC et al. Cost effectiveness analysis of open colposuspension versus laparoscopic colposuspension in the treatment of urodynamic stress incontinence. BJOG 2006;113:1014–1022.

26. Shull BL. Pelvic organ prolapse: anterior, superior and posterior vaginal segment defects. Am J Obstet Gynecol 1999;181:6–11.

27. Marchionni M, Bracco GL, Checcucci V et al. True incidence of vaginal vault prolapse. Thirteen years of experience. J Reprod Med 1999;44:679–684.

28. Dällenbach P, Kaelin-Gambirasio I, Jacob S et al. Incidence rate and risk factors for vaginal vault prolapse repair after hysterectomy. Int Urogynecol J Pelvic Floor Dysfunct 2008;19:1623–1629.

29. Blandon RE, Bharucha AE, Melton LJ 3rd et al. Risk factors for pelvic floor repair after hysterectomy. Obstet Gynecol 2009;113:601–608.

30. Cruikshank SH. Preventing posthysterectomy vaginal vault prolapse and enterocele during vaginal hysterectomy. Am J Obstet Gynecol 1987;156:1433–1440.

31. Maher CF, Qatawneh AM, Dwyer PL et al. Abdominal sacral colpopexy or vaginal sacrospinous colpopexy for vaginal vault prolapse: a prospective randomized study. Am J Obstet Gynecol 2004;190:20–26.

32. Shull BL, Bachofen C, Coates KW, Kuehl TJ. A transvaginal approach to repair of apical and other associated sites of pelvic organ prolapse with uterosacral ligaments. Am J Obstet Gynecol 2000;183:1365–1373; discussion 1373–1374.

33. Karram MM, Sze EH, Walters MD. Surgical treatment of vaginal vault prolapse. In: Walters MD, Karram MM (eds) Urogynecology and reconstructive pelvic surgery, 2 edn. Mosby, St Louis, 1999, pp 235–256.

34. Hale DS, Rogers RM Jr. Abdominal sacrospinous ligament colposuspension. Obstet Gynecol 1999; 94:1039–1041.

35. Addison WA, Livengood CH 3rd, Sutton GP, Parker RT. Abdominal sacral colpopexy with Mersilene mesh in the retroperitoneal position in the management of posthysterectomy vaginal vault prolapse and enterocele. Am J Obstet Gynecol 1985;153:140–146.

36. Bump R, Mattiasson A, Bø K et al. The standardization of terminology of female pelvic organ prolapse and pelvic floor dysfunction. Am J Obstet Gynecol 1996;175:10–17.

37. Claerhout F. The introduction of laparoscopy and novel biomatrices for surgical repair of vaginal vault prolapse by sacral colpopexy. PhD thesis, UZ Leuven. Leuven Academia Press, Leuven, 2010, p 190.

38. Visco AJ, Weidner AC, Barber MD et al. Vaginal mesh erosion after abdominal sacral colpopexy. Am J Obstet Gynecol 2001;184:297–302.

39. Krause HG, Goh JT, Sloane K et al. Laparoscopic sacral suture hysteropexy for uterine prolapse. Int Urogynecol J Pelvic Floor Dysfunct 2006;17:378–381.

40. Cosson M, Rajabally R, Bogaert E et al. Laparoscopic sacrocolpopexy, hysterectomy and Burch colposuspension: feasibility and short-term complications of 77 procedures. J Soc Lap Surg 2002;6:115–119.

41. Elliott DS, Frank I, DiMarco DS, Chow GK. Gynecologic use of robotically assisted laparoscopy: sacrocolpopexy for the treatment of high-grade vaginal vault prolapse. Am J Surg 2004;188:52S–56S.

42. Antiphon P, Elard S, Benyoussef A et al. Laparoscopic promontory sacral colpopexy: Is the posterior recto-vaginal mesh mandatory? Eur Urol 2004;45:655–661.

43. Gadonneix P, Ercoli A, Salet-Lizée D et al. Laparoscopic sacrocolpopexy with two separate meshes along the anterior and posterior vaginal walls for multicompartment pelvic organ prolapse. J Am Assoc Gynecol Laparosc 2004;11:29–35.

44. Rozet F, Mandron E, Arroyo C et al. Laparoscopic sacral colpopexy approach for genito-urinary prolapse: experience with 363 cases. Eur Urology 2005;47:230–236.

45. Higgs PJ, Chua HL, Smith ARB. Long term review of laparoscopic sacrocolpopexy. BJOG 2005;112:1134–1138.

46. Paraiso MF, Walters MD, Rackley RR et al. Laparoscopic and abdominal sacral colpopexies: a comparative cohort study. Am J Obstet Gynecol 2005;192:1752–1758.

47. Rivoire C, Botchorishvili, Canis M et al. Complete laparoscopic treatment of genital prolapse with meshes including vaginal promontofixation and anterior repair: a series of 138 patients. J Minim Invasive Gynecol 2007;14:712–718.

48. Agarwala N, Hasiak N, Shade M. Laparoscopic sacral colpopexy with Gynemesh as graft material – experience and results. J Minim Invasive Gynecol 2007;14:577–583.

49. Claerhout F, De Ridder D, Roovers JP et al. Medium-term anatomic and functional results of laparoscopic sacrocolpopexy beyond the learning curve. Eur Urol 2009;55:1459–1467.

50. Ramsay CR, Wallace SA, Garthwaite PH et al. Assessing the learning curve effect in health technologies. Lessons from the nonclinical literature. Int J Technol Assess Health Care 2002;18:1–10.

51. Digesu GA, Khullar V, Cardozo L et al. P-QOL: a validated questionnaire to assess the symptoms and quality of life of women with urogenital prolapse. Int Urogynecol J 2005;6:176–181.

52. Claerhout F, Moons P, Ghesquiere S et al. Validity, reliability and responsiveness of a Dutch version of the prolapse quality-of-life questionnaire. Int Urogynaecol J Pelvic Floor Dysfunction 2010;21:569-578.

53. Nygaard IE, McCreery R, Brubaker L et al, for the Pelvic Floor Disorders Network. Abdominal sacrocolpopexy: a comprehensive review. Obstet Gynecol 2004;104:805–823.

54. Deprest J, De Ridder D, Roovers JP et al. Medium term outcome of laparoscopic sacrocolpopexy with xenografts compared to synthetic grafts. J Urol 2009;182:2362–2368.

55. Claerhout F, Lewi P, Verguts J et al. Analysis of the learning curve for laparoscopic sacrocolpopexy: identification of challenging steps. Int Urogynecol J 2009;20(suppl 2): S202–S203.

56. Mottrie A, Martens P, Bollens R et al. Laparoscopic colpopromontofixation. Aktuelle Urol 2005;36:157–165.

57. Elliott DS, Krambeck AE, Chow GK. Long-term results of robotic assisted laparoscopic sacrocolpopexy for the treatment of high grade vaginal vault prolapse. J Urol 2006; 176:655–659.

58. Di Marco DS, Chow GK, Gettman MT, Elliott DS. Robotic-assisted laparoscopic sacrocolpopexy for treatment of vaginal vault prolapse. Urology 2004;63:373–376.

59. Kramer BA, Whelan CM, Powell TM, Schwartz BF. Robot-assisted laparoscopic sacrocolpopexy as management for pelvic organ prolapse. J Endourol 2009;23:655–658.

Total Pelvic Floor Reconstruction

46

Peter Papa Petros

Abstract The pelvic organs are suspended by ligaments. Pelvic muscle forces stretch the organs against these ligaments to give them shape, strength, and function, much like a trampoline or suspension bridge. Childbirth stretches the ligaments and fascia laterally to cause fascial damage and ligamentous laxity. One consequence of this damage is organ prolapse. Another is organ dysfunction, because the ligaments also function as insertion points for the muscle forces that open or close the bladder and rectum. The core aims of this chapter are to present the anatomical principles of surgical repair and the importance of tissue tension in the restoration of both structure and function. Existing surgical options for total pelvic floor reconstruction are analyzed. The tissue fixation system (TFS) is presented as the next step in pelvic floor reconstruction. The TFS is a new minimally invasive technique. It uses a different bioengineering support principle, akin to that of a cathedral ceiling, for pelvic organ prolapse. Specific suspensory ligaments are reinforced with tensioned tapes, without vaginal excision. The surgical restoration of the prolapse is anatomically precise, with good restoration of organ function. The TFS allows normal organ movement, and few of the problems associated with major mesh reconstructions, such as mesh shrinkage, dyspareunia, and erosion have been reported.

Keywords Apical prolapse • Cystocele • Fascia • Integral Theory • Ligaments • Mesh • Prolapse • Rectocele • Total pelvic floor reconstruction • TFS • Uterine prolapse • Vaginal repair • Vault prolapse

46.1   Introduction

Cut away from the pelvic bones, the organs, bladder, uterus, vagina and rectum, have no structure and no form (Fig. 46.1).

The organs, bladder, uterus, vagina and rectum, are suspended from the bony pelvis by ligaments, and tensioned by pelvic muscles against these ligaments to give them shape, strength, and function, much like a suspension bridge (Fig. 46.2).

The organs are tightly bound to each other (Fig. 46.3) and to ligaments and muscles with fibromuscular tissue.

These tissues, and the ligaments themselves, are composed of collagen, elastin, smooth muscle, nerves, and blood vessels.

P. Papa Petros
Formerly Department of Gynecology, Royal Perth Hospital,
School of Engineering, University of Western Australia,
Crawley, Australia

G.A. Santoro, A.P. Wieczorek, C.I. Bartram (eds.) *Pelvic Floor Disorders*

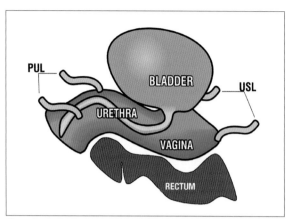

Fig. 46.1 Unsuspended from the pelvis, the organs have no shape, form, or structure. *PUL*, pubourethral ligament; *USL*, uterosacral ligament

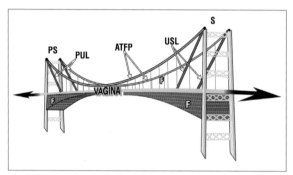

Fig 46.2 The biomechanics of organ structure: the suspension bridge analogy. *F*, fibromuscular attachments; *PS*, pubic symphysis; *PUL*, pubourethral ligament; *S*, sacrum; *USL*, uterosacral ligament

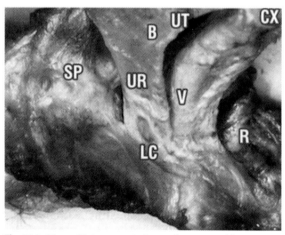

Fig. 46.3 Normal interconnectedness of organs and levator crus by fibromuscular tissue – lateral view, cadaveric specimen. The vagina (*V*), urethra (*UR*), and rectum (*R*) are tightly bound to each other and to the levator crus (*LC*) by connective tissue. *CX*, cervix; *SP*, symphysis pubis; *UT*, uterus. From [1], with permission.

46.2 Pathogenesis

Childbirth stretches the ligaments and fascia laterally. Stretching may cause laxity, organ prolapse, and dysfunction (Figs. 46.4 and 46.5). Therefore, any total prolapse repair must, in some way, recreate the relevant suspensory ligaments, and perineal body, where indicated.

The pathogenesis of rectocoele and enterocoele is described in Fig. 46.6.

46.3 Diagnosis

Fig. 46.7 incorporates a three-zone system which summarizes the anatomical relationships between lax suspensory ligaments, prolapse, and organ dysfunction (symptoms).

46.4 Total Pelvic Floor Reconstruction

"Restore the structure, and you will restore the function" is a fundamental rule of reconstructive surgery.

Therefore, any surgical repair must mimic the normal anatomy as precisely as possible. As regards prolapse causation, the key structures (Fig. 46.7) are the

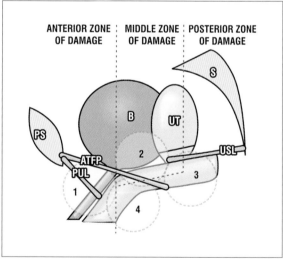

Fig. 46.4 Connective tissue damage at childbirth. Schematic representation of ligament and fascial damage by the fetal head (circles) as it descends through the vagina. 1: *PUL*, pubourethral ligament (stress incontinence); 2: *ATFP*, arcus tendineus fascia pelvis and pubocervical fascia (cystocele); 3: *USL*, uterosacral ligament (uterine prolapse); 4: perineal body/rectovaginal fascia (rectocele). *B*, bladder; *S*, sacrum; *UT*, uterus

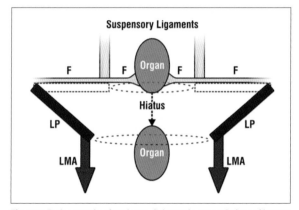

Fig.46.5 Pathogenesis of prolapse. Schematic coronal view of levator hiatus (straining). During straining, the levator plate (*LP*) is angulated downwards by the longitudinal muscle of the anus (*LMA*) vector, opening out the levator hiatus. If the suspensory ligaments and the fibromuscular attachments (*F*) are weak, the organs prolapse through the widened hiatus. As the elastin and collagen weaken with time, the prolapsed position becomes permanent. Therefore, any prolapse repair ideally should approximate and stabilize the laterally displaced tissue (*F*), to prevent outward displacement during straining.

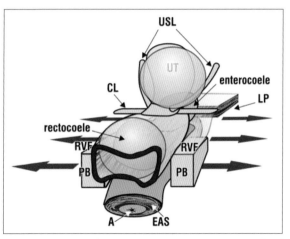

Fig.46.6 Pathogenesis of rectocele and enterocele. The perineal body (*PB*) supports > 50% of the posterior vaginal wall. Separation of perineal body below and uterosacral ligaments (*USL*) above create potential defects for rectocele and enterocele. When these structures are separated laterally, a rectocele/enterocele protrudes. *A*, anus; *CL*, cardinal ligament; *EAS*, external anal sphincter; *L*, levator plate; *RVF*, rectovaginal fascia; *UT*, uterus

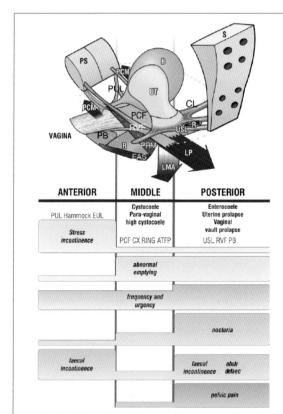

Pelvic Floor Laxities which can be repaired

Pubourethral ligament (*PUL*); hammock; external urethral ligament (*EUL*)

Pubocervical fascia (*PCF*); arcus tendineus fascia pelvis (*ATFP*); cardinal ligament/cervical ring (*CL*)

Uterosacral ligament (*USL*); rectovaginal fascia (*RVF*); perineal body (*PB*)

Fig.46.7 Pictorial diagnostic algorithm summarizing the relationships between structural damage in the three zones and symptoms. The size of the bar gives an approximate indication of the prevalence (probability) of the symptom. The same connective tissue structures in each zone (*red lettering*) may cause prolapse and abnormal symptoms. Anterior zone, external meatus to bladder neck; middle zone, bladder neck to anterior cervical ring; posterior zone, apex to perineal body. *B*, bladder; *EAS*, external anal sphincter; *LMA*, longitudinal muscle of the anus; *LP*, levator plate; *PCM*, pubococcygeus muscle; *PS*, pubic symphysis; *R*, rectum; *S*, sacrum; *UT*, uterus

arcus tendineus fascia pelvis (ATFP) and cardinal ligament (CL) in the middle zone, and the uterosacral ligaments (USL) and perineal body (PB) in the posterior zone. Repair of these structures and their attached fascia is sufficient for even fourth-degree prolapse.

46.5 Surgical Principles for Organ Prolapse Repair

1. Creation of artificial collagenous neoligaments is the key to all major prolapse repairs. Special instruments insert polypropylene tapes in the position of the damaged ligaments. These provoke a collagenous foreign body reaction to reinforce the ligament. Any prolapse repair should ideally approximate and stabilize the laterally displaced tissue ("F", Fig. 46.5), to prevent outward displacement during straining.
2. Vaginal excision and suturing under tension should be avoided. The former shortens the vagina. The latter may provoke pelvic pain.
3. Surgery and mesh application at the bladder neck area of the vagina ("zone of critical elasticity") should be avoided. Scar tissue may cause the posterior vectors, (*arrows*, Fig. 46.7) to overpower the anterior vectors, causing massive urine loss on effort ("tethered vagina syndrome") [2]. At least 1.5 cm of vaginal tissue should be left free at the bladder neck.
4. Conservation of the uterus where possible. The uterus (Fig. 46.7) is like the keystone of an arch, the direct insertion point of the cardinal and uterosacral ligaments, and the pubocervical fascia, and should be conserved where possible. Total hysterectomy predisposes to prolapse and posterior zone symptoms, such as urgency and pelvic pain. Subtotal hysterectomy is a preferable option.

In the next sections, surgical options for total pelvic floor reconstruction are analysed against these principles.

46.6 Traditional Vaginal Repairs

46.6.1 Vaginal Excision and Suturing

This is the worst possible operation and has no place in any type of vaginal surgery. Severe scarring, chronic

pain, vaginal shortening and narrowing may occur, as well as functional problems such a "tethered vagina syndrome [2]. Salvage operations may be difficult.

46.6.2 The Manchester Repair

The Manchester repair shortens and re-attaches the cardinal and uterosacral ligaments. The problem is that damaged tissue is approximated to damaged tissue. Traditionally, a coexisting cystocele and rectocele were repaired by a wedge excision of tissue. The perineal bodies ("levators"), were forcibly approximated. It is best to perform the vaginal repair component without tissue excision. Excision of tissue only weakens it further. Excess tissue is usually vaginal epithelium with a laterally dislocated fibromuscular (or "fascial") layer. Re-attaching the epithelial layer to the laterally displaced fibromuscular "fascial" layer is a far better option, as the tissue tension created by the muscle forces rearranges the "ground substance" with time. Subsequent interventions are not greatly compromised.

46.6.2.1 "Levator Approximation"

"Levator approximation" is performed as part of the Manchester repair. It is actually the laterally displaced perineal bodies which are forcibly approximated. This operation is extremely painful, and the perineal bodies generally return to their laterally displaced position some months after surgery.

46.7 Abdominal or Laparoscopic Repairs for Cystocoele or Apical/Uterine Prolapse

Damaged lateral pubocervical fascia causing cystocele is re-attached to the ATFP. This technique may work with a site-specific lateral fascial defect, but not if there is also a significant central defect. A mesh attached to the apex for apical/uterine prolapse stretches it towards the sacral promontory. This is a major procedure, with significant morbidity [3]. Uterine prolapse is like an intussusception. Therefore, the sidewall fascial and ligamentous supports require reconstruction so as to also address coexisting cystocele, rectocele, or perineal body defect, whether clinical or subclinical. It is difficult to do this laparoscopically. Furthermore, the sacral promontory is at least 6–7 cm cranial to the insertion site of the uterosacral ligaments. Major problems may occur with organ function in patients with short or inelastic vaginas. Complications include erosion, neourgency, and even intestinal obstruction [3].

46.8 Posterior Sling Suspensions: Infracoccygeal Sacropexy for Uterine/Vault Prolapse

The first posterior suspensory operation, the infracoccygeal sacropexy ("posterior IVS" or PIVS), was performed in 1992, as a day-care procedure [4]. Using a transperineal approach, the vaginal apex was attached to the posterior levator muscles just medial to the sacrospinous ligament (SSL), by means of polypropylene tapes. Of critical importance for symptom cure and minimization of erosion was the approximation of laterally displaced fascia to cover the tape, and tension the fascia. A central "bridge repair" in patients was successfully used in patients with large rectoceles. The PIVS is axial, but not quite anatomical, as the pelvic muscles and sacrospinous ligaments are some 3 cm lower than the USL in that position. Erosion rates between 5% and 17%, and, rarely, rectal perforations (usually inconsequential) have been reported. High cure rates have been reported for the vault prolapse, but also symptoms such as urge incontinence [5], nocturia, and urine evacuation problems. A postoperative cystocele rate of 16% has been reported. Dyspareunia was generally only a problem in patients with inflammation due to erosion, as the rectovaginal space was not altered.

46.9 Large Mesh Repairs

These can be suspended via the obturator membrane (Delorme approach) or sacrospinous ligament via a transperineal approach as per the PIVS [4], or simply left free. They work by providing an obstruction. They do not approximate the laterally displaced fascia, and so are far less likely to cure the associated specific symptoms detailed in Fig. 46.7. A greatly decreased symptom cure rate with posterior mesh attached to the tape, compared to a simple infracoccygeal sacropexy, has been reported [6]. Mesh rigidity prevents the musculoelastic stretching of the vaginal membrane required

to balance the organ control mechanisms. All repairs that use large mesh have potential problems with mesh shrinkage, scar tissue adhesions, erosion, and dyspareunia [7].

A major concern of these large mesh insertions is obliteration of the organ spaces. It is important for the organs to be able to move independently of each other for intercourse, and for adequate support of the bladder base stretch receptors for urge control.

46.10 Direct Repair of the Suspensory Ligaments by the Tissue Fixation System: a New Direction for Total Pelvic Floor Repair

The tissue fixation system (TFS) is a universal system for pelvic ligament repair (Fig. 46.8). It comprises a non-stretch monofilament polypropylene tape tensioned via a one-way system at the base of the anchor (Fig. 46.8). It is positioned adjacent to damaged ligaments as described in Fig. 46.7, up to the fourth grade of prolapse [8]. Because the tapes are laterally applied (Figs. 46.9–46.11), there is little possibility of anteroposterior shrinkage, a major problem with large mesh implantation. The operations are minimally invasive, with little postoperative pain and retention. Three-year data [9] for vault prolapse repair indicate longer-term effectiveness.

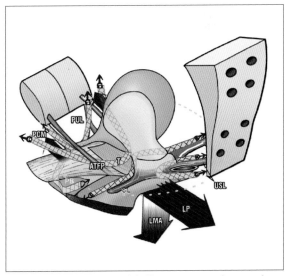

Fig. 46.8 Tensioned TFS mini-sling tapes approximate and tension laterally displaced ligaments and their attached fascia. For abbreviations see Fig. 46.7

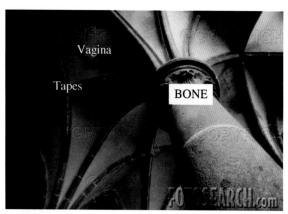

Fig. 46.9 Buttressed cathedral ceiling structure. The pillars (bone) provide the anchoring point for the beams (tapes), which in turn provide sufficient support for the weaker plaster board (vagina). Like a wire suspension bridge, tensioned tapes provide a much stronger support than "tension-free" meshes, which have a tendency to sag

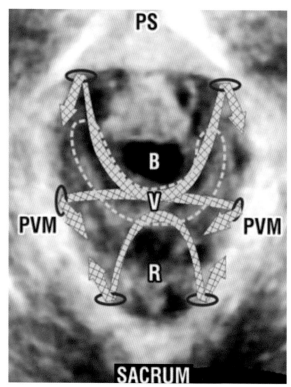

Fig. 46.10 Modus operandi of the "tensioned tape" surgical system, analogous to a buttressed cathedral ceiling. Schematic view. From the top, tissue fixation system (TFS) U-Sling (ATFP), cardinal ligament TFS, posterior (uterosacral ligament) TFS sling. *Arrows* indicate the direction of tensioning through the one-way system (*blue ovoid shapes*), the aim being restoration of normal tissue tension, and prevention of further separation of the levator hiatus (space between the pubovesical muscles "PVM"). Ultrasound kindly supplied by HP Dietz. *B*, bladder; *PS*, pubic symphysis; *R*, rectum; *V*, vagina

46.10.1 Prolapse Applications of the TFS Mini-sling System

- Central and lateral cystocele
- High cystocele (cardinal ligament/cervical ring defect)
- Uterine prolapse (uterosacral ligament defect)
- Apical prolapse and enterocele (uterosacral ligament defect)
- Rectocele (uterosacral ligament and perineal body defect)

Tensioned TFS mini-sling tapes (Fig. 46.8) approximate and tension laterally displaced ligaments and fascia. The laterally positioned tapes do not limit the backward stretching of the muscle forces (*arrows*), and act much like the tensioned beams of a cathedral ceiling (Figs. 46.9, 46.10) to provide support for prolapsed organs.

46.10.2 Large Rectocele Repair

Lateral separation of the upper ligamentous supports (uterosacral ligaments) and also the lower supports (perineal bodies) (Fig. 46.11), allows protrusion of a high, mid, or low rectocele [10]. The TFS approximates the laterally displaced structures, and reduces the rectocele (Fig. 46.11).

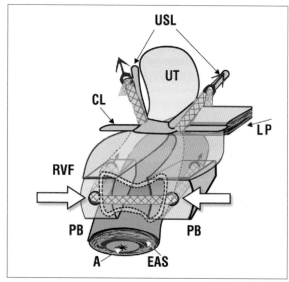

Fig. 46.11 Approximation of the perineal body (*PB*) and uterosacral ligaments (*USL*) by tightening the TFS, effectively blocks entry of the rectocoele into the vagina. *A*, anus; *CL*, cardinal ligament; *EAS*, external anal sphincter; *LP*, levator plate; *RVF*, rectovaginal fascia; *UT*, uterus

46.11 Conclusions

The introduction of site-specific tapes to reinforce otherwise unrepairable suspensory ligaments [11], has created an entirely new direction for pelvic floor reconstruction. Inevitably, some wrong directions are taken, one of which seems to be large mesh applications. Repair of specific ligaments using tensioned tapes such as the TFS seems to avoid many of the major problems associated with large mesh.

However, this system too must be tested widely, before it can be generally accepted as an improvement on existing methods.

References

1. Zacharin RF. Pelvic floor anatomy and cure of pulsion enterocoele. Springer-Verlag, Wien, 1985.
2. Petros PE, Ulmsten U. The free graft procedure for cure of the tethered vagina syndrome. Scand J Urol Nephrol 1993;153(suppl):85–87.
3. Sze EH, Karram MM. Transvaginal repair of vault prolapse: a review. Obstet Gynecol 1997;89:466–475.
4. Petros PE. Vault prolapse II: restoration of dynamic vaginal supports by the infracoccygeal sacropexy: an axial day-care vaginal procedure. Int J Urogynecol Pelvic Floor 2001; 12:296–303.
5. Neuman M, Lavy Y. Posterior intra-vaginal slingplasty for the treatment of vaginal apex prolapse: Medium-term results of 140 operations with a novel procedure. Eur J Obstet Gynecol Reprod Biol 2008;140:230–233.
6. Farnsworth FB, Parodi M. Total vaginal reconstruction with polypropylene mesh. Objective and functional outcomes assessment. Int Urogyn J 2005;16(suppl 2):55.
7. Milani R, Salvatore S, Soligo S et al. Functional and anatomical outcome of anterior and posterior vaginal prolapse repair with prolene mesh BJOG 2005;112:107–111.
8. Petros PEP, Richardson PA, Goeschen K, Abendstein B. The Tissue Fixation System (TFS) provides a new structural method for cystocoele repair – a preliminary report. Aust N Z J Obstet Gynaecol 2006;46:474–478.
9. Petros PE, Richardson PA. A 3 year follow-up review of uterine/vault prolapsed repair using the TFS minisling. Aust N Z J Obstet Gynaecol 2009;49:439–440.
10. Abendstein B, Petros PEP, Richardson PA et al. The surgical anatomy of rectocele and anterior rectal wall intussusception, Int Urogynecol J 2008;19:513–517.
11. Petros PE, Ulmsten U, Papadimitriou J. The autogenic neo-ligament procedure: a technique for planned formation of an artificial neo-ligament. Acta Obst Gynecol Scand Suppl 153 1990;69:43–51.

Invited Commentary

Paul Riss

There is some discrepancy between what gynecologists and what other specialties mean by "perineum". To an obstetrician/gynecologist, the term perineum denotes the area between the vaginal introitus (the posterior fourchette) and the anus. This area is stretched during vaginal childbirth, is cut when an episiotomy is done, and may be torn during vaginal childbirth. For this reason, the term "perineology" has not yet become popular in urogynecology, because gynecologists feel that they always should look at the whole pelvic floor and the organs in the small pelvis.

One can only agree with the authors of Chapter 42 that a combined effort by different specialties is called for when dealing with problems of the pelvic floor. Indeed, one of the major advances in recent years has been the realization that symptoms of the pelvic floor are interconnected, and that the evaluation and treatment of pelvic floor disorders calls for the availability and close collaboration of gynecologists, urologists, and colorectal surgeons. The challenge, of course, is how such an approach by different specialties can be implemented in a hospital or clinic. The support of the hospital is required to provide the necessary infrastructure and instruments, and on a personal level good communication skills are a prerequisite for a successful pelvic floor clinic. The authors are correct in pointing out the need for a "common language" between the different specialties. This can be a classification system (for example the IPGH (Incontinence, Pelvic floor and Prolapse, General factors, Handicap) system), or a special diagram (for example the Three Axis Perineal Evaluation diagram proposed

by Beco). Time will tell which system will find wide acceptance but this is certainly an idea whose time has come. A common language and terminology will be extremely helpful in encouraging and even forcing the different specialties to work together.

In Chapter 43, there is a very balanced discussion of the various aspects of the abdominal approach to surgery for urogenital prolapse. It is obvious that the preferred approach for anterior and posterior compartment repair is the vaginal route. The abdominal route is only considered in cases of post-hysterectomy vault prolapse or massive enterocele.

As the authors are correct in pointing out, there are two main reasons why the abdominal approach is no longer considered by most surgeons for anterior compartment repair. First the concept of paravaginal defect is not used by most surgeons because a so-called paravaginal defect is almost impossible to substantiate during evaluation of a patient or during surgery. As a consequence, even the pioneers of the paravaginal concept no longer propagate the use of this concept when planning surgery. Second, the differentiation between a central and a lateral defect (pulsation and traction cystocele) is not useful or even necessary when employing a prolene mesh or a mesh kit to repair an anterior defect. Whatever the underlying anatomical defect or functional pathology, the placement of a mesh will take care of any defect and provide a very good support of the anterior compartment.

Although randomized controlled trials are now available comparing the abdominal with the vaginal approach for level I defects (vault prolapse), both routes are commonly used. The reason is that the vaginal approach – in particular the vaginal sacrospinous fixation – is a standardized, relatively easy to perform

P. Riss
Department of Obstetrics and Gynecology,
Landesklinikum Thermenregion Moedling, Moedling, Austria

surgery with a very low complication rate and rapid patient recovery. The abdominal approach still requires laparotomy and is technically more challenging, and even more so when the laparoscopic route is chosen.

The authors summarize the current view on hysterectomy in conjunction with repair of a level I defect. There is ample data from well-conceived and executed randomized controlled trials that hysterectomy per se does not cause subsequent pelvic organ prolapse and does not have a negative impact on sexual function. However, when the uterus is prolapsed but the patient is too young to be a candidate for hysterectomy, abdominal sacropexy is an excellent option to repair the prolapse while keeping the uterus and preserving childbearing potential.

Chapter 44 looks at the use of meshes in pelvic reconstructive surgery. The starting point is that the vaginal approach is the best route for pelvic reconstructive surgery. When considering the anatomical defects responsible for pelvic organ prolapse or stress urinary incontinence, one soon realizes that current vaginal methods cannot address all anatomical defects properly, are not standardized, and have a relatively high failure rate depending on the location of the anatomical defect.

Not everyone takes this pessimistic view. Many surgeons point out that vaginal operations can be standardized and are successful when the execution is based on a thorough knowledge of the anatomy and use of appropriate connective tissue. It is very important to identify planes of connective tissue, to isolate them, and to use them for reconstruction. Only then will there be good support of the anterior or posterior vaginal wall.

Still, it is tempting to view prolene meshes as a god-sent addition to the surgical armamentarium. It is easy to see why: instead of meticulous identification and dissection of connective tissue planes, the surgeon only has to open the relevant spaces in order to be able to insert a mesh, usually in a pre-cut form or from a commercial kit.

Whatever the cause of the pelvic organ prolapse, a mesh is thought to provide solid support of the whole compartment.

Not everyone will agree with the statement that traditional vaginal techniques are vagina-narrowing with a high risk of recurrence. On the contrary, many vaginal surgeons feel that vaginal reconstructive surgery has evolved, and offers better and reproducible results. Some techniques have been discarded, and our current understanding of the pelvic floor has helped to put vaginal pelvic floor reconstructive surgery on a new footing.

The author points out the complications related to mesh placement and the factors limiting their widespread use. Not the least important factor is the relatively high cost which precludes the use of commercial kits in developing countries. The challenge remains to identify and practice the best methods in vaginal pelvic floor reconstructive surgery – with or without the use of meshes.

In Chapter 46, Peter Petros presents his unified theory of the pelvic floor. Over the years this theory has been widely publicized and attracted widespread interest. There seems to be a genuine interest in having a theory that explains everything related to the pelvic floor: which ligaments are important, which fascial planes support the abdomen, which spaces connect the different structures, and, above all, how these structures work together to build and maintain the pelvic floor as we know it. The suspension bridge analogy (Fig. 46.2) seems intuitive, but a look at the more complex diagram may leave some clinicians confused. One reason is that clinicians look for explanations of what they see when examining a patient. If the theory behind a well-circumscribed pathology – e.g. prolapse of the anterior vaginal wall – becomes too complicated, clinicians have a tendency to look for a useful description of the pathology and not worry too much whether ligament A or arcus B is involved.

Clinicians are also mistrustful of theories that claim to explain everything. Experience teaches that prolapse is often multifactorial, including the quality of the tissues involved, strength of suspensory mechanisms, involvement of the muscles of the pelvic floor, and various risk factors and lifestyle influences. The theory becomes even more problematic when it is applied directly to surgical principles and specific operations. It is also not helpful when the author makes claims that are not generally accepted or based on evidence. For example, the statement that the uterus should always be conserved in pelvic reconstructive surgery, and that subtotal hysterectomy is the preferred option is not generally accepted, and there are good data showing that the removal of the uterus does not negatively impact on the pelvic floor. On the contrary, after subtotal hysterectomy, the cervix can prolapse in a small minority of patients [1].

When the author's Integral Theory of the pelvic floor is applied to surgical principles, it seems that the posterior sling suspension of the vaginal vault has proved a clearly defined, standardized, and easy-to-perform operation. This operation is very effective as a treatment for post-hysterectomy vault prolapse. It is easier to perform than vaginal sacrospinous fixation or abdominal or laparoscopic sacropexy, and it gives excellent results.

The author certainly is to be congratulated on his innovative approach to the use of tapes or meshes in pelvic reconstructive surgery, in particular in view of the fact that the widespread use of large meshes with or without kits has proven somewhat disappointing. However, the author himself realizes that only time will tell, and states that that his new tissue fixation system must be tested widely before it can be generally accepted as an improvement on existing methods.

References

1. Thakar R, Ayers S, Clarkson P et al. Outcomes after total versus subtotal abdominal hysterectomy. N Engl J Med 2002;347:1318–1325.

The Abdominal Approach to Rectal Prolapse

47

Sthela M. Murad-Regadas, Rodrigo A. Pinto and Steven D. Wexner

Abstract Numerous approaches have been described for the treatment of rectal prolapse. The two basic categories of operation are transabdominal and perineal. The former type tends to be more durable with lower recurrence rates but at the expense of higher morbidity. The latter group tends to be safer but is associated with higher recurrence rates and less functional recovery. More recently, the abdominal approaches have been modified to be laparoscopically accomplished in most cases. The indications for, technical details of, and results following these abdominal operations will be described and discussed.

Keywords Abdominal approach • Constipation • Fecal incontinence • Functional results • Laparoscopy • Mesh rectopexy • Rectal prolapse • Resection rectopexy • Recurrence • Surgical management • Suture rectopexy • Surgical techniques

47.1 Introduction

Full-thickness rectal prolapse is defined as the protrusion of all layers of the rectal wall through the anal sphincters [1]. If the prolapsed rectal wall does not protrude through the anus it is called intussusception or internal rectal prolapse [2, 3]. Mucosal prolapse is the protrusion of only rectal mucosa.

Complete rectal prolapse has been reported since the Egyptian and Greek ancient civilizations [4]. The first written report dates from 1500 BC, by Ebers Papyrus [5]. Over the years, multiple treatments came and went. Mickulicz [6] popularized the perineal amputation in 1888, and Lockhart-Mummery [7], in 1910, performed a perineal procedure for the treatment of rectal prolapse. In 1912, Moschowitz [8] started the abdominal repair.

The estimated incidence of rectal prolapse is 4 per 1000 population, being more common in elderly females after the fifth decade. The female to male ratio ranges from 6:1 to 10:1. Among children, males and females are equally affected, usually by the age of 3 years [9, 10].

47.2 Etiology

The anatomical basis for rectal prolapse is a deficient pelvic floor through which the rectum herniates [3, 11–13]. The exact way that the prolapse takes place is not completely understood, thus it is based on theories.

Rectal prolapse as an intussusception of the rectal wall was first described by Hunter [14] and confirmed by Broden and Snellman [11] with cineradiography. Complete rectal prolapse is thought to be a process that starts within 6–8 cm of the anal verge, continuing through the anal canal, and everting onto the perineum

S.D. Wexner
Division of Colon and Rectal Surgery,
Cleveland Clinic Florida, Weston, FL, USA

G.A. Santoro, A.P. Wieczorek, C.I. Bartram (eds.) *Pelvic Floor Disorders*
© Springer-Verlag Italia 2010

[11, 15, 16]. The lower rest and squeeze pressures found in the anal manometries of these patients compared to normal control subjects support this theory [17]. However, defecographic studies have found that in patients with intussusception, the risk of developing rectal prolapse was small, which contradicts this theory [18, 19].

Parks et al support the theory that repeated stretching of the pelvic floor muscles can injure the pudendal nerves and can be a part of the cause of rectal prolapse [20]. This theory is supported by some surgeons who have detected a frequent association between neurogenic fecal incontinence and rectal prolapse [12, 13]. However, the improvement of fecal incontinence after surgery, and the electromyographic findings of normal innervation in patients with rectal prolapse challenge this theory.

Lax lateral ligaments combined with an atonic condition of the muscles of the pelvic floor and the anal canal could be the main cause of rectal prolapse [11, 12]. In addition, the lack of normal fixation of the rectum, with a mobile mesorectum and a laxity of the lateral ligaments, may predispose to and/or be associated with rectal prolapse [12, 21, 22].

Regardless of which theory is chosen, the following anatomic findings are commonly associated with rectal prolapse: abnormally deep cul-de-sac, loss of posterior fixation of the rectum, laxity of the anal sphincters, and redundant sigmoid colon. All of the procedures described to date attempt to correct some or all these abnormalities.

47.3 Assessment of Patients with Rectal Prolapse and Associated Symptoms

The evaluation of patients with rectal prolapse is based on a complete history and physical examination; a search for particular risk factors should also be considered. The prolapse may be easily visible on anorectal examination. Otherwise, the patient is asked to sit down on a commode, leaning forward, with the examiner standing behind to confirm the diagnosis.

Evaluation of the colon with colonoscopy and barium enema is recommended to exclude coexisting conditions, such as polyps, cancer, and diverticular disease, that may influence the choice of procedure. The colonic transit study is important, especially in patients with associated constipation. Madoff [23] suggested that slow colonic transit time is the primary factor associated with constipation in patients with rectal prolapse. It has also been postulated that an increased sigmoid transit is a significant factor associated with fecal incontinence in patients with rectal prolapse [24]. Symptoms of obstructive defecation usually require the use of cinedefecography for investigation; however, this investigation has limited impact in decision making for the management of rectal prolapse. In addition, the patient may be completely unable to hold the contrast, making for a messy and embarrassing failed evaluation. Thus, we do not employ cinefecography unless there is some very specific reason to conduct this study.

The preoperative physiologic evaluation with anorectal manometry, electromyography, and endoanal ultrasound is important to evaluate the pelvic floor muscles, particularly in patients with preoperative fecal incontinence.

Reducible protrusion that may be associated with mucous discharge is a common sign of initial prolapse. Prolapse may theoretically be due to bowel movements, straining, and increased intra-abdominal pressure. After the diagnosis of prolapse has been made, patients may experience loss of control of stool because of stretching of the sphincter muscles and the pudendal nerves. In addition, bleeding may develop if the rectum remains exposed and therefore becomes traumatized.

Other pelvic floor disorders may be present in 8% to 27% of patients with rectal prolapse [25]. Altman et al [25] observed an incidence of 48% of genital prolapse and 31% of urinary incontinence in patients with rectal prolapse (Fig. 47.1). Gonzalez-Argente et al [26] observed a higher incidence of urinary incontinence (58%)

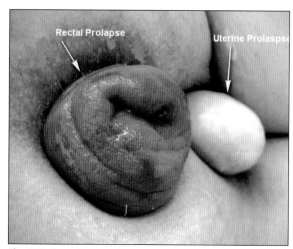

Fig. 47.1 Rectal and uterine prolapse

and genital prolapse (24%) in patients operated for rectal prolapse. Previous pelvic surgery, obstetric trauma, elevated intra-abdominal pressure, increasing age, and chronic constipation are some factors allied with rectal and genital prolapse [25].

Up to 75% patients with rectal prolapse experience fecal incontinence, and 25–50% have significant constipation [23, 24, 27, 28]. Metcalf and Loening-Baucke [28] supposed that an increased external sphincter activity seen by electromyography could be a cause of outlet obstruction and constipation. Although it is not life-threatening, rectal prolapse is a distressing condition that affects patients' quality of life; therefore, surgical treatment should be considered even in high-risk patients.

47.4 Selection of Patients for Abdominal Procedures

Surgical management of full-thickness rectal prolapse aims to eradicate the external prolapse, limit the risk of recurrence, and limit any impairment to bowel function and continence. Additionally, morbidity and mortality rates should be minimal. The lack of any one treatment as a panacea is why multiple surgical approaches are in common use.

Perineal procedures are advocated for elderly patients with significant comorbidity, as they are associated with limited surgical stress and relatively low postoperative morbidity. Nevertheless, recurrence rates up to 58%, and persistent bowel dysfunction, are commonly reported [29–31].

Conversely, the abdominal approaches are associated with lower recurrence rates, which vary from 0% to 20% among different surgeons [32–37]. The reason for this superior durability is not clearly known, but is attributed to the ability to perform a complete rectal mobilization and fixation under direct vision, with no sacrifice to the rectal reservoir. It also offers a more accurate determination of whether to excise or fix any additional redundant bowel that may prolapse [38]. Abdominal procedures are also related to symptomatic improvement and better functional results than perineal operations [30, 33, 39, 40].

The surgical options can be summarized as suture or mesh rectopexy, with or without sigmoid resection. The abdominal approach can be performed with either an open or a laparoscopic aproach. Some authors have reported higher morbidity rates, of 15%, with open techniques [30, 33, 37]. Furthermore, the laparoscopic approach, first introduced by Berman [41] in 1992, tried to integrate the surgical stress reduction associated with the perineal approach with the lower recurrence rates achieved with abdominal repair.

The decision as to whether or not to perform sigmoid resection is based on bowel function and sphincter muscle status. If the patient has normal bowel function, or constipation associated with normal anal tone, a resection is preferred. Whenever diarrhea or sphincter damage are suspected, maintenance of the sigmoid colon seems to be correlated with better functional results.

Choosing the optimal repair for rectal prolapse involves consideration of the patient's health and the pre-existing bowel function as well as any history or physical findings consistent with either constipation or fecal incontinence.

Lastly, the individual surgeon's experience is always an important factor in the decision-making process as to which procedure is most appropriate for the individual patient. This chapter addresses the abdominal approaches for rectal prolapse.

47.5 Abdominal Procedures

Multiple abdominal operations for the treatment of rectal prolapse have been described since the beginning of the past century. The procedures that have persisted, and are mostly commonly reported in the literature at the present time, are discussed below.

47.5.1 Ripstein Procedure (Anterior Sling Rectopexy)

First described by Ripstein [42] in 1952, the procedure consists of insertion of a synthetic mesh or fascia lata to the anterior wall of the mobilized rectum, fixing the mesh to the sacral promontory and promoting an encirclement of the rectum. The technique restores the posterior curve of the rectum and provides a stiff anterior support (Fig. 47.2). The major problem with this procedure is the development of obstruction due to the anterior mesh, which can cause rectal stenosis and erosion of the mesh into the rectal wall, followed by fistula formation. Kuijpers [12] observed a 7% incidence of stenosis in his experience. Aiming to reduce this com-

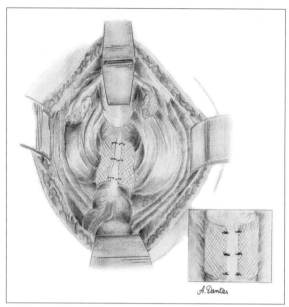

Fig. 47.2 Mesh placement in the Ripstein procedure. Supplied courtesy of Dr Amanda M. Dantas

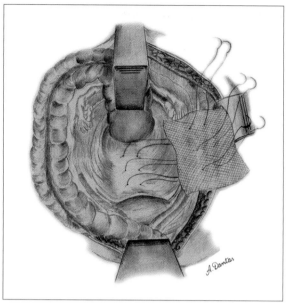

Fig. 47.3 Posterior mesh fixation of the sacral promontory in the Wells procedure. Supplied courtesy of Dr Amanda M. Dantas

plication, Ripstein [42] modified the procedure by including a posterior fixation of the mesh to the sacrum and an intraoperative calibration with a proctoscope to prevent the narrowing. Despite this modification, the complication rate remained high, significantly limiting the use of the technique.

Roberts et al [43] reviewed their experience with the Ripstein procedure in 135 patients and reported a 52% complication rate and an overall recurrence rate of 10%. Furthermore, a review by Madiba et al [44] also showed a high complication rate, with mortality ranging from 0% to 2.8%, and recurrence rates ranging from 0% to 13%.

47.5.2 Posterior Mesh Rectopexy

First described by Wells [45] in 1959, this technique was popular in the UK. The procedure consists of placement of a prosthetic Ivalon® (polyvinyl alcohol) sponge between the rectum and the promontory in either side of the rectum, after mobilization of the posterior rectal wall (Fig. 47.3). The anterior part of the rectum must stay free to prevent stenosis. The parietal peritoneum is closed to isolate the mesh from the peritoneal cavity. The well-built fibrous reaction promoted by the presence of a foreign body restores the anorectal angle.

Novell et al [46], in a prospective randomized trial comparing the Ivalon sponge to sutured rectopexy, showed similar recurrence rates and higher wound infection in the mesh group. They failed to demonstrate any advantage of the Ivalon rectopexy over the simpler sutured rectopexy.

Other non-absorbable and even absorbable meshes have been introduced, and have undergone evaluation with similar results, including mortality ranging from 0% to 1% and recurrence rates ranging from 0% to 6%, using absorbable [47–49] or non-absorbable [22, 24, 47–51] meshes.

The main concern about the presence of a foreign material is the development of infection and sepsis. The reported sepsis occurrence after mesh placement has varied from 2% to 16% [11, 12, 48, 52–57]. The performance of a resection associated with de novo mesh insertion may be associated with an increased risk of infection because of the presence of an anastomosis and a new foreign body; thus the placement of a mesh for rectopexy seems to be reasonable without resection, due to lower mortality and infection rates [48, 54, 58].

The placement of a drain in the presacral space is also recommended while inserting a mesh to prevent infected collections or hematomas [46, 48, 54]. Whenever sepsis occurs it is worthwhile to remove the mesh [48, 49, 53, 55–57].

47.5.3 Suture Rectopexy

First described by Cutait [59] in 1959, the operation involves a mobilization and upward fixation of the rectum to the sacral promontory with tow to three unabsorbable sutures on either side of the rectum (Fig. 47.4). The healing process by fibrosis keeps the rectum fixed in the elevated position, preventing recurrence [1].

Despite the sound theory, the recurrence rates range from 0% to 27% [46, 59–63]; however, the majority of reports have included recurrence rates ranging from 0% to 3%.

The effect of rectopexy on constipation may include exacerbation constipation and sometimes the development of a new onset of constipation [64, 65]. Currently, the lower complication rates and similar long-term outcomes associated with the suture rectopexy compared to mesh placement, have led surgeons to prefer sutures to foreign material.

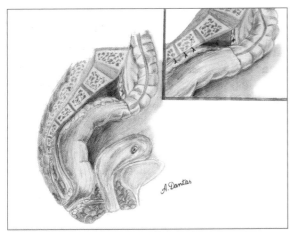

Fig. 47.4 Stitches placed onto the sacral promontory in suture rectopexy. Supplied courtesy of Dr Amanda M. Dantas

47.5.4 Sigmoid Resection Associated with Rectopexy

Originally described by Fryckman [32] in 1955 and championed by Goldberg, commonly known as resection rectopexy or Fryckman-Goldberg procedure, the addition of a sigmoid resection combines the advantages of rectal mobilization and fixation to an excision of the redundant sigmoid. The sutures can be applied before the bowel resection and secured after the anastomosis. Some studies have shown improvement in constipation compared to rectopexy alone [34, 47]. Mckee et al [34] associated rectopexy alone to a higher incidence of constipation, due to a kinking between the redundant sigmoid and the rectum in the rectosigmoid junction. The sigmoidectomy seemed to alleviate this possibility, which could cause delay in the passage of intestinal content. However, there are risks of higher morbidity from anastomotic complications and longer hospital stay, due to the presence of an intraperitoneal anastomosis [66, 67]. Table 47.1 summarizes the postoperative results of rectopexy with and without sigmoid resection.

47.6 Abdominal Surgical Techniques

Patients are placed in a Lloyd-Davis position with split legs, and the prolapse is reduced before starting the procedure. For an open approach, an infra-umbilical midline incision is usually preferred, although some surgeons use a pfanestiel incision to perform the rectopexy.

In the case of laparoscopy, the pneumoperitoneum is established with a Veress needle or opened under

Table 47.1 Results of rectopexy with and without sigmoid resection

Author	Year	Resection	Number	Complication (%)	Mortality (%)	Success (%)	Recurrence (%)
Solla et al [31]	1989	Yes	102	4	0	98.1	1.9
Stevenson et al [68]	1998	Yes	34	13	3	92	7 (MP)
Aitola et al [50]	1999	No	112	15	1	–	6 (FT); 12 (MP)
Heah et al [69]	2000	No	25	12	0	60	0
Lechaux et al [65]	2005	Yes	48	5	0	72	4
Ashari et al [70]	2005	Yes	117	9	< 1	80	2.5 (FT); 18 (MP)
Carpelan Holmström et al [71]	2006	Yes	85	0	0	84 wo; 92 w	2.3
Kariv et al [72]	2006	No	111	–	–	75 LR; 89 OR	9.3 LR; 4.7 OR
Dulucq et al [64]	2007	No	77	0	0	89	1.3

FT, full thickness; *LR*, laparoscopic rectopexy; *MP*, mucosal prolapse; *OR*, open rectopexy; *w*, with resection; *wo*, without resection

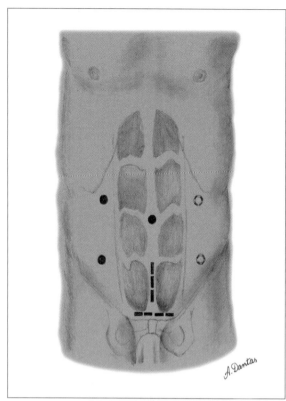

Fig. 47.5 Placement of ports for the laparoscopic approach. Supplied courtesy of Dr Amanda M. Dantas

direct vision using a Hasson trocar. The surgeon and the camera-holder stay on the right side of the patient, while the assistant surgeon stands between the legs, and the monitor is placed in the left side of the patient. Placement of three to five trocars is described by different authors. Usually one 10 mm umbilical port is positioned for the camera, and two 5 mm or 10 mm ports in the right lower quadrant (12 mm if a stapler device is used) and in the right upper quadrant. An additional 10 mm port can be placed in the left lower quadrant to help facilitate the exposure, particularly in obese patients (Fig. 47.5). The patient is positioned in a modified supine position to facilitate the exposure, retracting the small bowel, the omentum, and the redundant sigmoid from the pelvis.

Either the medial to lateral or lateral to medial dissection is acceptable, as are diathermy scissors, harmonic scalpel (Ethicon Endo-Surgery, Cincinnati, OH, USA), or Ligasure (Valleylab, Tyco Healthcare Group Lp, Boulder, CO, USA). The posterior dissection is undertaken anteriorly from the promontory distal to the pouch of Douglas after identifying the ureters, in a

plane surrounding the mesorectum between the parietal and visceral fascial planes of the pelvis. During the dissection, care has to be taken to identify and preserve the pelvic splanchnic nerves (superior hypogastric nerves, the autonomic branches of S2, S3, S4, and the pelvic autonomic nerve plexus). The posterior dissection is carried down to the levator plane. The lateral ligaments of the rectum should preferably be preserved.

The promontory is exposed to visualize the presacral fascia. If the sigmoid is going to be excised, some surgeons prefer a lateral to medial laparoscopic dissection. The superior hemorrhoid artery may be preserved and the rectum can be transected at the rectosigmoid junction, followed by construction of a circular stapled colorectal anastmosis.

The rectopexy can be performed with the placement of a mesh, usually when there is no resection, or by a suture rectopexy. The mesh is placed in the right posterior side of the rectum, usually fixed with sutures or with staples. A simple suture rectopexy can be an option, and two to four stitches are placed in the posterior side of the mesorectum or in the lateral rectal wall, and fixed to the periostium of the sacral promontory, taking care to avoid injury of the middle sacral artery with the needle. At the end of the procedure the peritoneum can be closed with absorbable running sutures. The 10 or 12 mm ports, or the open incision, are then closed, and a drain may be placed into the pelvis. The open dissection is performed similarly in an identical manner, except that most surgeons routinely mobilize from lateral to medial instead of medial to lateral during laparotomy.

Some technical aspects seem to be directly related to patients' postoperative functional outcomes, especially exacerbation of constipation. Some authors consider preservation of the lateral ligaments of the rectum for normal evacuation after surgery to avoid the parasympathetic denervation that may be responsible for rectosigmoid dysmotility [73–77]. Bruch et al [74] reported that preservation of the lateral ligaments leads to a significant improvement in constipation after resection rectopexy and suture rectopexy. Darzi et al [75] observed persistence of constipation in 18% of patients who underwent resection rectopexy with division of the lateral stalk of the rectum. A Cochrane meta-analysis of ten randomized controlled trials comprising 324 patients concluded that division of the lateral ligaments of the colon was associated with less prolapse recurrence, but more postoperative constipation [78].

Other features related to constipation may be functional obstruction caused by kinking of the redundant sigmoid left in place, and fibrosis related to the rectal dissection or the use of a mesh, creating stenosis [34, 79]. Mckee et al [34] suggest that the redundant or kinking sigmoid colon could cause delayed colonic transit, which eventually leads to persistent constipation.

47.7   Minimally Invasive Approach

During the last 20 years, due to the advent of laparoscopy, abdominal rectopexy for the management of rectal prolapse has become one of the earliest procedures. The results are comparable with the open approach, with the advantages associated with a minimally invasive approach. Rectopexy alone can be performed as a completely laparoscopic procedure since there is no specimen to be retrieved.

Recent reports have compared laparoscopic to open procedures and have shown reduced postoperative pain, earlier recovery, and shorter length of hospital stay for laparoscopy [76, 80–83], despite a longer operative time and higher direct costs [80, 82–85]. However, Salkeld et al [84] stated that laparoscopy is associated with an overall cost saving per patient from faster recovery, less use of pain medications, and shorter stay in hospital. Forty-four per cent of the additional operative costs for laparoscopy were attributed to longer operative times.

Carpelan-Holmström et al [71] addressed the abdominal approach for elderly high-risk patients, evaluating 65 patients operated by laparoscopy and 10 patients operated in an open fashion. Half of the patients were American Society of Anesthesiologists (ASA) classification III and IV. The operative time was similar overall, although, the laparoscopic resection rectopexies were more time consuming (150 vs. 80 min; P = 0.07). The hospital stay and intraoperative bleeding were significantly shorter for laparoscopic procedures. Sixty-eight patients were selected for follow-up, after a mean of 1.8 years, and the results were comparable between laparoscopic and open procedures. Full-thickness rectal prolapse recurrence occurred in two patients. There was no difference in constipation after the procedures, and continence was fully restored in 86% of patients who underwent rectopexy and 79% of patients who underwent resection rectopexy.

The authors concluded that laparoscopic procedures can be safely performed and well tolerated by elderly patients.

Solomon et al [85] performed a randomized controlled trial with 39 patients allocated to either open (19) or laparoscopic (20) mesh rectopexies, and analyzed some objective parameters related to stress response to surgery. Acute-phase reactants, such as urinary catecholamines, interleukin-6 (IL-6), serum cortisol and C-reactive protein favored laparoscopy. Respiratory function was comparable between the groups, whereas respiratory morbidity was greater in the open group. The overall and the major morbidity incidence also favored laparoscopy (overall 3% vs. 9% and major 0% vs. 4%, respectively for laparoscopic and open groups). Likewise, Stage et al [86] observed no difference in respiratory function, and decreased pain scores and morphine requirements for laparoscopy. There was also minor stress response represented by IL-6 and C-reactive protein, and shorter hospital stay (5 vs. 8 days for laparoscopy and open, respectively), favoring laparoscopy. In contrast, Milsom et al [87] reported improvement in respiratory function with laparoscopic rectopexy, but similar hospital stay (6 vs. 7 days for laparoscopy and open, respectively).

Regarding constipation after surgery, Kariv et al [72], reviewing the experience of Cleveland Clinic Foundation, noticed that laparoscopic cases were related to better improvement of constipation (74% vs. 54%, respectively in laparoscopy and open procedures) and lower worsening of constipation (3% vs. 17%, respectively in laparoscopy and open procedures) compared to open cases. Postoperative constipation rates also seemed better following laparoscopy (35% vs. 53%, respectively in laparoscopy and open procedures). However, anterior mesh placement in open cases may contribute to higher constipation rates. Within the laparoscopy data, resection and no resection outcomes were comparable in terms of constipation (70% vs. 59% improvement, P = 0.53; respectively in patients without and with resection).

The latest meta-analysis comparing open to laparoscopic abdominal rectopexy included six studies and 195 patients (98 open and 97 laparoscopic cases) [88]. The length of hospital stay was significantly shorter in the laparoscopic group, while the operative time was 60.38 min longer. There was no difference in morbidity or recurrence rates in the studies included in the analysis. Cost was addressed by two studies that favored the laparoscopic group. The long-term functional results

Table 47.2 Follow-up and functional results in open and laparoscopic abdominal approaches

Author	Year	N	Procedure	Follow-up (months)	Constipation (improve %)	Incontinence (improve %)	Recurrence (%)
McKee et al [34]	1992	9	RR	20	50	0	0
Duthie and Bartolo [33]	1992	29	RR	6	Yes	78	n.s.
Madoff [23]	1992	47	RR	65	50	30	FT 6; MP 8
Deen et al [37]	1994	10	RR + PFR	17	Yes	90	FT 0; MP 10
Huber et al [40]	1995	39	RR	54	42	65	FT 0; MP 0
Cirocco et al [89]	1995	41	AR+FRM	72	18	48	Total 7
Benoist et al* [90]	2001	18	LARR	20	82	100	n.s.
Kellokumpu et al* [66]	2000	17	LARR	24	64	80	n.s.
Ashari et al* [70]	2005	117	LARR	62	69	62	FT 2.5; MP 18
Kariv et al* [72]	2006	136	LARR/OR	56 LR; 63 OR	74 LR; 54 OR	48 LR; 35 OR	9.3 LR; 4.7 OR
Madbouly et al* [76]	2003	24	LARR/LWP	18.1	95	80	0
Lechaux et al* [65]	2005	48	LARR	36	3 (23% worse)	31	4.2 FT; 4.2 MP
Dulucq et al* [64]	2007	68	LWP	34	36	89	1.5

*Laparoscopy-assisted procedures. *AR*, anterior resection; *FRM*, full rectal mobilization without fixation; *FT*, full thickness; *LARR*, laparoscopy-assisted resection rectopexy; *LWP*, laparoscopic Wells procedure; *MP*, mucosal prolapse; n.s., not specified; *OR*, open rectopexy; *PFR*, pelvic floor repair; *RR*, resection rectopexy

reported with open and laparoscopic approaches are described in Table 47.2.

New minimally invasive techniques are emerging, such as robotic-assisted and single trocar laparoscopy; however, no benefit has yet been proven; in fact, one recent study found a higher recurrence rate after robotic compared to laparoscopic rectopexy [91]. Heemskerk et al [92] recently reviewed 14 robotic-assisted rectopexies and compared them to 19 laparoscopic cases. The authors found the new approach to be 39 minutes longer than laparoscopy and it was associated with an increased charge of $745 per patient, while the postoperative morbidity was similar. The lack of experience, and hence publications, and the influence of a learning curve process limit further conclusions about these new procedures.

47.8 Incontinence Improvements and Mechanisms

Fecal incontinence in patients with rectal prolapse is attributed to pudendal nerve neuropathy causing sphincter denervation [90], direct sphincter trauma caused by intussuscepting rectum, and chronic rectoanal inhibition and abnormal anorectal sensations [33, 80, 90, 93, 94]. Associated factors that may be present are impaired internal anal sphincter, pelvic floor muscle dysfunction, and abnormal somatic nerve stimulation [20, 32]

The anal sphincters usually start to regain tone approximately 1 month after surgery, and responsive pa-

tients are fully continent in 2 to 3 months [24]. Functional improvement after surgery is seen in 60% to 90% of patients, although the exact mechanism is not well established [47, 48, 66, 89, 90, 94–96]. Some authors have suggested that the restoration of internal anal sphincter function and improved anorectal sensation or rectal compliance after surgery contribute to the patient's regain of continence [33].

Different abdominal procedures have shown similar improvement of anal continence. Benoist et al [90] reported no difference in incontinence improvement among different laparoscopic techniques (suture, mesh, and resection) in a two-year follow-up period, with 75% of the patients having better continence after surgery.

47.9 Management of Recurrent Rectal Prolapse

The mean reported time period for complete rectal prolapse recurrence is between two and three years after surgery. Early surgical failures are generally attributed to technical problems [97, 98]. The reported surgical management of prolapse recurrence is limited. Steele et al [98] reviewed the management of 78 recurrences in 685 patients operated for initial rectal prolapse, and compared the abdominal to the perineal approach. The incidence of re-recurrence was 29% and was significantly higher in the perineal cases (37.3 vs. 14.8%, P = 0.03, respectively for perineal and abdominal approaches). The authors concluded that abdominal re-pair has consistently lower re-recurrence rates for recurrent rectal prolapse, independently of the number of previous repairs, and suggested that whenever possible the abdominal approach for recurrent prolapse should be undertaken, if the patient's risk profile permits.

Whenever performing surgery for recurrent prolapse, it is important to be aware of the previous procedure. If there is any prior resection involved, either perineal rectosigmoidectomy or resection rectopexy, and another resection is planned, the surgeon has to preferably excise the previous anastomosis to avoid desvitalization of the remaining colonic segment.

47.10 Conclusions

Rectal prolapse is a fairly uncommon pathology that mainly affects female adults after the fifth decade. The etiology is poorly understood and most patients present with an abnormally deep cul-de-sac, loss of posterior fixation of the rectum, laxity of the anal sphincters, and a redundant sigmoid colon. The diagnosis is based on anorectal examination, with the patient straining seated in a commode as needed. Complementary exams help to access associated conditions, such as compromise of the sphincter and pelvic floor muscles, constipation, and obstructed defecation; nevertheless, these have limited impact in decision making for the management of rectal prolapse. Surgical treatment should be considered even in high-risk patients, once rectal prolapse has become a distressing condition that affects the patient's quality of life.

Choosing the optimal repair for rectal prolapse involves consideration of the patient's health and the pre-existing bowel function related to a history of constipation or fecal incontinence, and also compromise of the sphincter muscles at the anorectal evaluation. Among the abdominal procedures, suture or mesh rectopexies are the option for patients with normal or increased bowel function or atonic sphincter. Resection rectopexy is preferred for constipated patients or those with normal sphincter tonus. Abdominal approaches are associated with low morbidity rates, even among elderly patients, and lower long-term recurrence rates compared to the perineal approach.

During the last two decades, laparoscopy has augmented the low morbidity rates and reduced the surgical stress related to perineal approaches, maintaining the long-term efficacy of abdominal procedures. Currently, laparoscopy is the preferred approach for the abdominal management of complete rectal prolapse.

References

1. Jacobs LK, Lin YJ, Orkin BA. The best operation for rectal prolapse. Surg Clin North Am 1997;77:49–70.
2. Felt-Bersma RJ, Cuesta MA. Rectal prolapse, rectal intussusception, rectocele and solitary ulcer syndrome. Gastroenterol Clin North Am 2001;30:199–222.
3. Roig JV, Buch E, Alós R et al. Anorectal function in patients with complete rectal prolapse: differences between continent and incontinent individuals. Rev Esp Enferm Dig 1998; 90:794–805.
4. Boutsis C, Ellis H. The Ivalon-sponge-wrap operation for rectal prolapse: an experience with 26 patients. Dis Colon Rectum 1974;17:21–37.
5. Moody RL. Rectal prolapse. In: Morson BC (ed) Diseases of the colon, rectum and anus. Appleton-Century-Crofts, New York, 1969, pp 238–250.
6. Mikulicz J. Zur operativen behandlung dis prolapsus recti et coli invaginati. Arch Klin Chir 1889;38:74–97.
7. Lockhart-Mummery JP. A new operation for prolapse of the rectum. Lancet 1910;1:641.
8. Moschcowitz AV. The pathogenesis, anatomy and cure of prolapse of the rectum. Surg Gynecol Obstet 1912;15:7–21.
9. Flowers LK. Rectal prolapse. In: E-medicine 2002. Available at: http://www.emedicine.com/emerg/topic496.htm (accessed 7 October 2009).
10. Senapati A. Rectal prolapse. In: Phillips RK (ed) Colorectal surgery. WB Saunders, London, 2001, pp 251–271.
11. Broden B, Snellman B. Procidentia of the rectum studied with cineradiography. Dis Colon Rectum 1968;11:330–347.
12. Kuijpers HC. Treatment of complete rectal prolapse: to narrow, to wrap, to suspend, to fix, to encircle, to plicate or to resect? World J Surg 1992;16:826–830.
13. Nicholls RJ. Rectal prolapse and the solitary ulcer syndrome. Ann Ital Chir 1994;65:157–162.
14. Monro A. The morbid anatomy of the human gullet, stomach, and intestines. Archibald Constable & Co, Edinburgh, 1811, p 363.
15. Devadhar DSC. A new concept of mechanism and treatment of rectal procidentia. Dis Colon Rectum 1965;8:75–81.
16. Pantowitz D, Levine E. The mechanism of rectal prolapse. S Afr J Surg 1975;13:53–56.
17. Sun WM, Read NW, Donnelly TC et al. A common pathophysiology for full thickness rectal prolapse, anterior mucosal prolapse and solitary rectal ulcer. Br J Surg 1989;76: 290–295.
18. Mellgren A, Schultz I, Johansson C, Dolk A. Internal rectal intussusception seldom develops into total rectal prolapse. Dis Colon Rectum 1997;40:817–820.
19. Ihre T, Seligson U. Intussusception of the rectum-internal procidentia: treatment and results in 90 patients. Dis Colon Rectum 1975;18:391–396.
20. Parks AG, Swash M, Urich H. Sphincter denervation in ano-

rectal incontinence and rectal prolapse. Gut 1977;18:656–665.

21. Wassef R, Rothenberger DA, Goldberg SM. Rectal prolapse. Curr Probl Surg 1986;23:397–451.

22. Yakut M, Kaymakciioglu N, Simsek A et al. Surgical treatment of rectal prolapse: a retrospective analysis of 94 cases. Int Surg 1998;83:53–55.

23. Madoff RD. Rectal prolapse and intussusception. In: Beck SD, Wexner SD (eds) Fundamentals of anorectal surgery. Mc Graw Hill, New York, 1992, pp 89–103.

24. Keighley MRB, Shouler PJ. Abnormalities of colonic function in patients with rectal prolapse and faecal incontinence. Br J Surg 1984;71:892–895.

25. Altman D, Zetterstrom J, Schultz I et al. Pelvic organ prolapse and urinary incontinence in women with surgically managed rectal prolapse: a population-based case-control study. Dis Colon Rectum 2006;49:28–35.

26. Gonzalez-Argente XF, Jain A, Nogueras JJ et al. Prevalence and severity of urinary incontinence and pelvic genital prolapse in females with anal incontinence or rectal prolapse. Dis Colon Rectum 2001;44:920–926.

27. Madden MV, Kamm MA, Nicholls RJ et al. Abdominal rectopexy for complete rectal prolapse: prospective study evaluating changes in symptoms and anorectal function. Dis Colon Rectum 1995;35:301–307.

28. Metcalf AM, Loening-Baucke V. Anorectal function and defecation dynamics in patients with rectal prolapse. Am J Surg 1988;155:206–210.

29. Johansen OB, Wexner SD, Daniel N et al. Perineal rectosigmoidectomy in the elderly. Dis Colon Rectum 1993;36:767–772.

30. Watts JD, Rothenberger DA, Buls JG et al. The management of procidentia: 30 years experience. Dis Colon Rectum 1985;28:96–102.

31. Solla JA, Rothenberger DA, Goldberg SM. Surgical techniques in prolapse of the rectum. Langenbecks Arch Chir 1989;6:370–6.

32. Frykman HM, Goldberg SM. The surgical treatment of rectal procidentia. Surg Gynecol Obstet 1969;129:1225–30.

33. Duthie GS, Bartolo DC. Abdominal rectopexy for rectal prolapse: a comparison of techniques. Br J Surg 1992; 79:107–113.

34. Mckee RF, Lauder JC, Poon FW et al. A prospective randomized study of abdominal rectopexy with and without sigmoidectomy in rectal prolapse. Surg Gynecol Obstet 1992;174:145–8.

35. Atkinson KG, Tylor DC. Wells procedure for complete rectal prolapse: a 10 year experience. Dis Colon Rectum 1984; 27:96–98.

36. Penfold JCB, Hawley PR. Experience of Ivalon-sponge implant for complete rectal prolapse at St. Mark's Hospital, 1960–1970. Br J Surg 1972;59:846–848.

37. Deen KI, Grant E, Billingham C, Keighley MR. Abdominal resection rectopexy with pelvic floor repair versus perineal rectosigmoidectomy and pelvic floor repair for full thickness rectal prolapse. Br J Surg 1994;81:302–304.

38. Eu K-W, Seow-Choen F. Functional problems in adult rectal prolapse and controversies in surgical treatment [review]. Br J Surg 1997;84:904–911.

39. Bartolo CC. Rectal prolapse. Br J Surg 1996;83:3–5.

40. Huber FT, Stein H, Siewert JR. Functional results after tre-
atment of rectal prolapse with rectopexy and sigmoid resection. World J Surg 1995;19:138–143.

41. Berman IR. Sutureless laparoscopic rectopexy for procidentia: technique and implications. Dis Colon Rectum 1992; 35:689–693.

42. Ripstein CB. Treatment of massive rectal prolapse. Am J Surg 1952;83:68–71.

43. Roberts PL, Schoetz DJ, Coller JA et al. Ripstein procedure: Lahey clinic experience: 1963–1985. Arch Surg 1988; 123:554–557.

44. Madiba TE, Baig MK, Wexner SD. Surgical management of rectal prolapse. Arch Surg 2005;140:63–73.

45. Wells C. New operation for rectal prolapse. Proc R Soc Med 1959;52:602–603.

46. Novell JR, Osborne MJ, Winslet MC, Lewis AAM. Prospective randomized trail of Ivalon sponge versus sutured rectopexy for full thickness rectal prolapse. Br J Surg 1994; 81:904–906.

47. Luukkonen P, Mikkonen U, Järvinen H. Abdominal rectopexy with sigmoidectomy vs. rectopexy alone for rectal prolapse: a prospective, randomised study. Int J Colorectal Dis 1992;7:219–222.

48. Winde G, Reers H, Nottberg H et al. Clinical and functional results of abdominal rectopexy with absorbable mesh-graft for treatment of complete rectal prolapse. Eur J Surg 1993;159:301–305.

49. Galili Y, Rabau M. Comparison of polyglycolic acid and polypropylene mesh for rectopexy in the treatment of rectal prolapse. Eur J Surg 1997;163:445–448.

50. Aitola PT, Hiltunen KM, Matikainen MJ. Functional results of operative treatment of rectal prolapse over an 11-year period: emphasis on transabdominal approach. Dis Colon Rectum 1999;42:655–660.

51. Scaglia M, Fasth S, Hallgren T et al. Abdominal rectopexy for rectal prolapse: influence of surgical technique on functional outcome. Dis Colon Rectum 1994; 37:805–813.

52. Morgan CN, Porter NH, Klugman DJ. Ivalon sponge in the repair of complete rectal prolapse. Br J Surg 1972;59: 841–846.

53. Arndt M, Pircher W. Absorbable mesh in the treatment of rectal prolapse. Int J Colorectal Dis 1988;3:141–143.

54. Athanasiadis S, Weyand G, Heiligers J et al. The risk of infection of three synthetic materials used in rectopexy with or without colonic resection for rectal prolapse. Int J Colorectal Dis 1996;11:42–44.

55. Lake SP, Hancock BD, Lewis AA. Management of pelvic sepsis after Ivalon rectopexy. Dis Colon Rectum 1984; 27:589–590.

56. Ross AH, Thomson JPS. Management of infection after prosthetic abdominal rectopexy (Wells' procedure). Br J Surg 1989;76:610–612.

57. Wedell J, Schlageter M, Meier zu Eissen P et al. Die Problematik der pelvinen Sepsis nach Rectopexie mittels Kunstoff und ihre Behandlung. Chirurg 1987;58:423–427.

58. Speakman CT, Madden MV, Nichols RJ, Kamm MA. Lateral ligament division during rectopexy causes constipation but prevents recurrence: results of a prospective randomized study. Br J Surg 1991;78:1431–1433.

59. Cutait D. Sacro-promontory fixation of the rectum for

complete rectal prolapse. Proc R Soc Med 1959; 52(suppl):105.

60. Briel JW, Schouten WR, Boerma MO. Long-term results of suture rectopexy in patients with fecal incontinence associated with incomplete rectal prolapse. Dis Colon Rectum 1997;40:1228–1232.

61. Carter AE. Rectosacral suture fixation for complete prolapse in the elderly, the frail and the demented. Br J Surg 1983;70:522–523.

62. Graf W, Karlbom U, Påhlman L et al. Functional results after abdominal suture rectopexy for rectal prolapse or intussusception. Eur J Surg 1996;162:905–911.

63. Khanna AK, Misra MK, Kumar K. Simplified sutured sacral rectopexy for complete rectal prolapse in adults. Eur J Surg 1996;162:143–146.

64. Dulucq JL, Wintringer P, Mahajna A. Clinical and functional outcome of laparoscopic posterior rectopexy (Wells) for full-thickness rectal prolapse. A prospective study. Surg Endosc 2007;21:2226–2230.

65. Lechaux D, Trebuchet G, Siproudhis L, Campion JP. Laparoscopic rectopexy for full-thickness rectal prolapse. A single-institution retrospective study evaluating surgical outcome. Surg Endosc 2005;19:514–518.

66. Kellokumpu IH, Vironen J, Scheinin T. Laparoscopic repair of rectal prolapse: a prospective study evaluating surgical outcome and changes in symptoms and bowel function. Surg Endosc 2000;14:634–640.

67. Xynos E, Chrysos J, Tsiaoussis J et al. Resection rectopexy for rectal prolapse: the laparoscopic approach. Surg Endosc 1999;13:862–864.

68. Stevenson AR, Stitz RW, Lumley JW. Laparoscopic assisted resection rectopexy for rectal prolapse: early and medium follow-up. Dis Colon Rectum 1998;41:46–54.

69. Heah SM, Hartley JE, Hurley J et al. Laparoscopic suture rectopexy without resection is effective treatment for full-thickness rectal prolapse. Dis Colon Rectum 2000;43:638–643.

70. Ashari LH, Lumley JW, Stevenson ARL, Stitz RW. Laparoscopic assisted resection rectopexy for rectal prolapse: ten year experience. Dis Colon Rectum 2005;48:982–987.

71. Carpelan-Holmström M, Kruuna O, Scheinin T. Laparoscopic rectal prolapse surgery combined with short hospital stay is safe in elderly and debilitated patients. Surg Endosc 2006;20:1353–1359.

72. Kariv Y, Delaney CP, Casillas S et al. Long term outcomes after laparoscopic and open surgery for rectal prolapse. Surg Endosc 2006;20:35–42.

73. Dolk A, Broden G, Holmstrom B et al. Slow transit of the colon associated with severe constipation after the Ripstien procedure. A clinical and physiologic study. Dis Colon Rectum 1990;33:786–790.

74. Bruch HP, Herold A, Schiedeck T, Schwander O. Laparoscopic surgery for rectal prolapse and outlet obstruction. Dis Colon Rectum 1999;42:1189–1195.

75. Darzi A, Henry MM, Guillou PJ et al. Stapled laparoscopic rectopexy for rectal prolapse. Surg Endosc 1995; 9:301–303.

76. Madbouly KM, Senagore AJ, Delaney CP et al. Clinically based management of rectal prolapse. Surg Endosc 2003;17:99–103.

77. Boulos PB, Strykers SJ, Nicholls RJ. The long-term results of polyvinyl alcohol (Ivalon) sponge for rectal prolapse in young patients. Br J Surg 1984;71:213–214.

78. Brazzilli M, Bachoo P, Grant A. Surgery for complete rectal prolapse in adults. Cochrane Database Sys Rev 2000; (2):CD001758.

79. Allen-Mersh TG, Turner MJ, Mann CV. Effect of abdominal Ivalon rectopexy on bowel habit and rectal wall. Dis Colon Rectum 1990;33:550–553.

80. Baker R, Senagore AJ, Luchtefeld MA. Laparoscopic assisted vs. open resection: rectopexy offers excellent results. Dis Colon Rectum 1995;38:199–201.

81. Senagore AJ. Management of rectal prolapse: the role of laparoscopic approaches. Semin Laparosc Surg 2003;10: 197–202.

82. Boccasanta P, Venturi M, Reitano MC et al. Laparotomic vs laparoscopic rectopexy in complete rectal prolapse. Dig. Surg 1999;16:415–419.

83. Kairaluoma MV, Viljakka MT, Kellokumpu IH. Open vs. laparoscopic surgery for rectal prolapse: a case–controlled study assessing short-term outcome. Dis Colon Rectum 2003;46:353–360.

84. Salkeld G, Bagia M, Solomon M. Economic impact of laparoscopic versus open abdominal rectopexy. Br J Surg 2004;91:1188–1191.

85. Solomon MJ, Young CJ, Eyers AA, Roberts RA. Randomized clinical trial of laparoscopic versus open abdominal rectopexy for rectal prolapse. Br J Surg 2002;89:35–39.

86. Stage JG, Schulze S, Moller P et al. Prospective randomized study of laparoscopy vs. open colonic resection for adenocarcinoma. Br J Surg 1997;84:392–396.

87. Milsom JW, Bohm B, Hammerhofer KA et al. A prospective, randomized trial comparing laparoscopic versus conventional techniques in colorectal cancer surgery: a preliminary report. J Am Coll Surg 1998;187:46–54.

88. Purkayastha S, Tekkis P, Athanasiou T et al. A comparison of open vs. lap abdominal rectopexy for full-thickness rectal prolapse: a meta-analysis. Dis Colon Rectum 2005; 48:1930–1940.

89. Cirocco WC, Brown AC. Anterior resection for the treatment of rectal prolapse: a 20-year experience. Am Surg 1993; 59:265–269.

90. Benoist S, Taffinder N, Gould S et al. Functional results two years after laparoscopic rectopexy. Am J Surg 2001;182: 168–173.

91. de Hoog DHeemskerkJ, Nieman FH et al. Recurrence and functional results after open versus conventional laparoscopic versus robot-assisted laparoscopic rectopexy for rectal prolapse: a case-control study. Int J Colorectal Dis 2009; 24:1201–1206.

92. Heemskerk J, de Hoog DE, van Gemert WG et al. Robot-assisted vs. conventional laparoscopic rectopexy for rectal prolapse: a comparative study on costs and time. Dis Colon Rectum 2007;50:1825–1830.

93. Farouk R, Duthie GS, Bartolo DC, MacGregor AB. Restoration of continence following rectopexy for rectal prolapse and recovery of the internal anal sphincter electromyogram. Br J Surg 1992;79:439–440.

94. Zittel TT, Manncke K, Haug S et al. Functional results after laparoscopic rectopexy for rectal prolapse. J Gastrointest Surg 2000;4:632–641.

95. Hiltunen KM, Matikainen M. Improvement of continence after abdominal rectopexy for rectal prolapse. Int J Colorectal Dis 1992;7:8–10.

96. Tjandra JJ, Fazio VW, Church JM et al. Ripstein procedure is an effective treatment for rectal prolapse without constipation. Dis Colon Rectum 1993;36:501–507.

97. Hool GR, Hull TL, Fazio VW. Surgical treatment of recurrent complete rectal prolapse: a thirty-year experience. Dis Colon Rectum 1997;40:270–272.

98. Steele SR, Goetz LH, Minami S. Management of recurrent rectal prolapse: surgical approach influences outcome. Dis Colon Rectum 2006;49:440–445.

The Perineal Approach to Rectal Prolapse

Mario Trompetto and Silvia Cornaglia

Abstract Surgical treatment of rectal prolapse has unpredictable results, whatever approach the surgeon decides to use. Perineal operations are safer than abdominal ones but carry a higher likelihood of recurrence of the prolapse. Functional results probably depend more on the initial severity of the disorder than on the type of operation.

Keywords Altemeier's operation • Constipation • Delorme's operation • Fecal incontinence • Rectal prolapse

48.1 Introduction

Both external (complete) and internal rectal prolapse are common perianal conditions that occur in conjunction with many functional disorders of defecation, mainly fecal incontinence and constipation. The goal of treating these conditions is to solve or at least greatly improve both the anatomical and functional disorders. Complete rectal prolapse is defined as a full-thickness protrusion of the rectal wall through the anal canal, while different types of internal prolapse have been described, depending on many different features. Among internal prolapses, different degrees of disturbance are considered, from a simple mucosal prolapse to the so-called rectal intussusception.

It is a matter of debate whether these minor prolapses can lead to a complete external procidentia, but there are no studies clearly demonstrating this anatomical evolution.

The so-called internal prolapses are very difficult to define clinically and radiologically and their surgical treatment is quite controversial.

Complete rectal prolapse is more common in older females but can occur in both sexes and at any age. Surgical treatment of the anatomical disorder has been of great interest for colorectal surgeons for a long time. Because the mechanisms by which prolapse occurs remain poorly understood, an optimal surgical approach has not been yet determined, so more than 100 procedures have been reported. Geographic factors and personal opinions have increasingly confused the results of proposed treatments. The goals of surgery are to prevent recurrent prolapse and to improve continence and bowel function. Unfortunately, surgical results are very often considered satisfactory when the anatomical solution is achieved without any real benefit from the functional point of view.

The main procedures can be grouped into perineal and abdominal operations. The choice between the two approaches must also take into consideration elements that are not directly related to the surgical treatment, involving other important factors such as age, general health, comorbidity, social factors, and life expectancy of the patients, as well as their history of

M. Trompetto
Colorectal Eporediensis Centre, "Santa Rita" Clinic, Vercelli,
Policlinic of Monza, Italy

G.A. Santoro, A.P. Wieczorek, C.I. Bartram (eds.) *Pelvic Floor Disorders*
© Springer-Verlag Italia 2010

constipation or different degrees of fecal incontinence.

The functional results and percentage of recurrence are better in abdominal approaches and this has been confirmed by some new studies [1], but a recent Cochrane review failed to identify or refute any clinically important differences between the alternative surgical operations [2].

The most frequently used perineal procedures are the Delorme's and Altemeier's operations.

48.2 Delorme's Operation

This is an operation that was first described by Delorme more than one century ago, then modified and improved by other surgeons in the 1950s.

Its main anatomical indication is a complete rectal prolapse not exceeding more than 10 cm from the anal verge. Its low morbidity and the possibility to perform it also as a day case surgery make it the first choice for old, frail patients as well as in cases where an abdominal approach could result in possible pelvic morbidity such as nerve or ureteral damage.

The operation starts with a circular incision of the mucosal and submucosal layers at 1 cm above the dentate line. A cylinder of mucosubmucosa is then stripped, beginning at this level and continuing up above the prolapsing segment. The length of the removed cylinder must be twice the length of the clinical procidentia. Submucosal infiltration with diluted epinephrine prior to mucosal incision and during mucosal dissection may reduce perioperative bleeding. The rectal muscle is then plicated with concertina-type stitches, and finally the

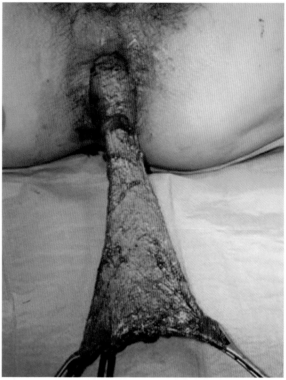

Fig. 48.2 The correct length of submucosal cylinder

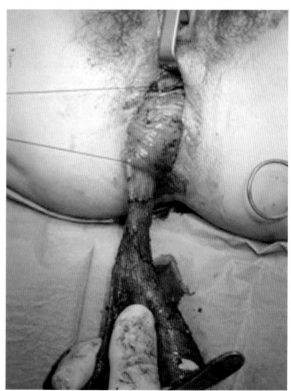

Fig. 48.3 The start of vertical plication

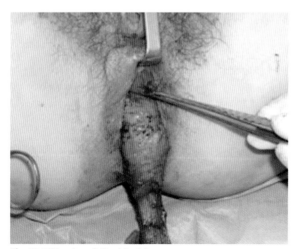

Fig. 48.1 The site of distal incision

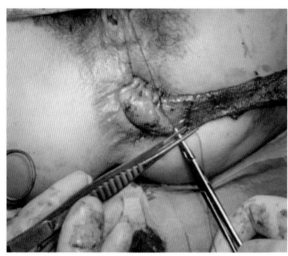

Fig. 48.4 Vertical plication

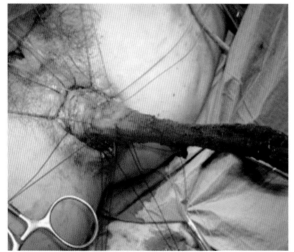

Fig. 48.5 Final step of plication

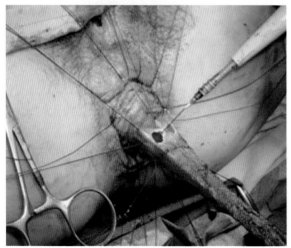

Fig. 48.6 Section of the submucosal cylinder

Box 48.1 Delorme's operation – surgical steps

1. Incision of the mucosa at least 1 cm above the dentate line
2. Dissection of a mucosal cylinder twice the length of the rectal prolapse
3. Muscular vertical plication
4. Mucosal resection
5. Suture of the two mucosal limbs

Table 48.1 Delorme's operation – results

Author	Number of patients	Recurrence %
Oliver et al, 1994 [3]	40	22
Lechaux et al, 1995 [4]	85	13.5
Tsunoda et al, 2003 [5]	31	13
Pascual et al, 2006 [6]	21	9.5
Lieberth et al, 2009 [7]	66	14.5

mucosa is anastomosed to the distal margin of mucosal resection (Figs. 48.1–48.6).

The surgical steps of the operation are described in the Box 48.1. The surgical results reported regarding the percentage of recurrence and improvement in bowel function after Delorme's operation have not dramatically improved in recent years, and some new tools and modifications of the well-known technique have failed to obtain better results (Table 48.1).

48.3 Altemeier's Operation

This operation consists of a rectosigmoid perineal resection with subsequent coloanal anastomosis and it is the only possible option in major rectal prolapse that is not suitable for an abdominal approach (Fig. 48.7).

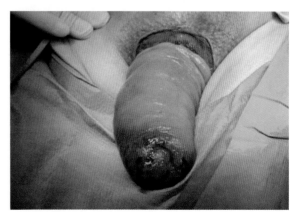

Fig. 48.7 Huge complete rectal prolapse

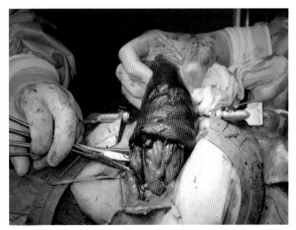

Fig. 48.8 Full-thickness circular incision and opening of the pouch of Douglas

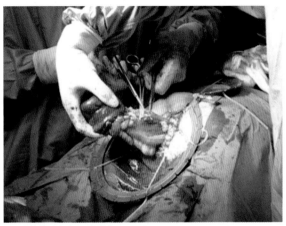

Fig. 48.9 Vascular ligature close to the bowel wall

This procedure was popularized by Altemeier in the 1950s and 1960s [8–10] and is the most used approach for the treatment of complete rectal prolapse in the US, while it is infrequently applied in European countries where the Delorme's operation is considered the operation of choice.

The operation begins with a circular incision of the complete rectal wall, 2 cm above the dentate line. When the pouch of Douglas is opened (Fig. 48.8), dissection of the rectosigmoid junction and then of the sigmoid colon can be easily performed, with careful vascular ligature of the mesorectum and mesosigma (Fig. 48.9). Care must be taken to stay very close to the bowel wall during all the stages of the operation, to avoid dangerous bleeding from major sigmoid vessels. The dissection is carried out gradually, using a continuous gentle traction of the colon, until the required length for the section is reached (Fig. 48.10); this can be done in different ways depending on the type of subsequent anastomosis the surgeon chooses to perform. An end-to-end hand-sewn anastomosis is the technique most frequently used, although some surgeons prefer a mechanical anastomosis according to the method of Knight-Griffen. The anastomosis technique does not seem to influence the long-term results of the operation [11]. A small colonic J-pouch can possibly achieve better functional results in the short term, with the addition of a levatorplasty (Figs. 48.11, 48.12). The final result of the procedure is shown in Fig. 48.13.

A comparison between the two main perineal ap-

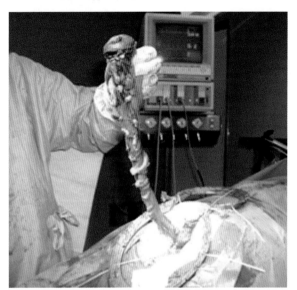

Fig. 48.10 Length of the possible bowel removal

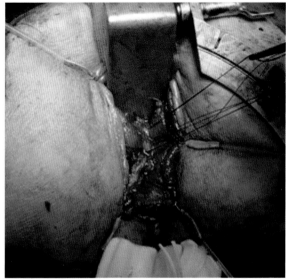

Fig. 48.11 Levatorplasty

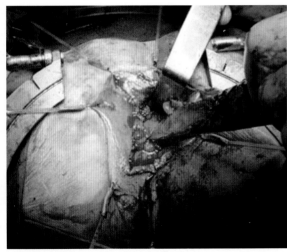

Fig. 48.12 Closure of the levatorplasty

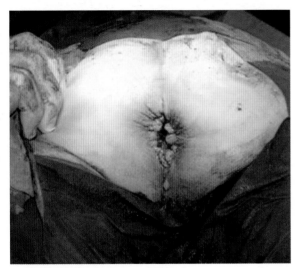

Fig. 48.13 Final view of the anoperineal area

proaches regarding recurrences favors the Altemeier's procedure [12, 13], although the possible complications associated with this approach can result in a worse outcome [14].

48.4   Other Operations

The old rectal encirclement known as Thiersch repair has been completely abandoned. Its unacceptably high morbidity (breakage, infection, erosion) and recurrence rate (20–60%) confine it as a simple historical memory, although some case reports can still be found, albeit rarely, in the literature [15].

Some new techniques, such as the so-called "Ex-

press procedure", and some technical modifications of the old approaches [16, 17] need future evaluation before achieving a significant place in the armamentarium for the treatment of complete rectal prolapse.

A less invasive, alternative management for the treatment of very high-risk patients complaining of rectal prolapse could be the simple use of a specially designed anal plug that can avoid fecal leakage and procidentia. No adverse effects of the approach have been reported, but its poor tolerance by patients is a very important limitation for its routine use [18].

References

1. Hoel AT, Skarstein A, Ovrebo KK. Prolapse of the rectum, long-term results of surgical treatment. Int J Colorectal Dis 2009;24:201–207.
2. Tou S, Brown SR, Malik AI, Nelson RL. Surgery for complete rectal prolapse in adults. Cochrane Database Syst Rev 2008;(8):CD001758.
3. Oliver GC, Vachon D, Eisenstat TE et al. Delorme's procedure for complete rectal prolapse in severely debilitated patients. An analysis of 41 cases. Dis Colon Rectum 1994;37: 461–467.
4. Lechaux JP, Lechaud P, Perez M. Results of Delorme's procedure for rectal prolapse. Advantages of a modified technique. Dis Colon Rectum 1995;38:301–307.
5. Tsunoda A, Yasuda N, Yokoyama N et al. Delorme's procedure for rectal prolapse: clinical and physiological analysis. Dis Colon Rectum 2003;46:1260–1265.
6. Pascual Montero JA, Martinez Puente MC, Pascual I et al. Complete rectal prolapse: clinical and functional outcome with Delorme's procedure. Rev Esp Enferm Dig 2006; 98:837–843.
7. Lieberth M, Kondylis LA, Reilly JC, Kondylis PD. The Delorme repair for full-thickness rectal prolapse: a retrospective review. Am J Surg 2009;197:418–423.
8. Altemeier WA, Giuseffi J, Hoxworth P. Treatment of extensive prolapse of the rectum in aged or debilitated patients. AMA Arch Surg 1952;65:72–80.
9. Altemeier WA, Hoxworth P, Giuseffi J. Further experiences with the treatment of prolapse of the rectum. Surg Clin North Am 1955;Nationwide No:1437–1447.
10. Altemeier WA, Culbertson WR, Alexander JW. One-stage perineal repair of rectal prolapse. Twelve years' experience. Arch Surg 1964;89:6–16.
11. Boccasanta P, Venturi M, Barbieri S, Roviaro G. Impact of new technologies on the clinical and functional outcome of Altemeier's procedure: a randomized, controlled trial. Dis Colon Rectum 2006;49:652–660.
12. Kimmins MH, Evetts BK, Isler J, Billingham R. The Altemeier repair: outpatient treatment of rectal prolapse. Dis Colon Rectum 2001;44:565–570.
13. Glasgow SC, Birnbaum EH, Kodner IJ et al. Recurrence and quality of life following perineal proctectomy for rectal prolapse. J Gastrointest Surg 2008;12:1446–1451.
14. Altomare DF, Binda G, Ganio E et al, Rectal Prolapse Study

Group. Long-term outcome of Altemeier's procedure for rectal prolapse. Dis Colon Rectum 2009;54:698–703 .

15. Shoab SS, Saravanan B, Neminathan S, Grsaa T. Thiersch repair of a spontaneous rupture of rectal prolapse with evisceration of small bowel through anus- a case report. Ann R Coll Surg Engl 2007;89:W6–8.

16. Williams NS, Giordano P, Dvorkin LS et al. External pelvic rectal suspension (the Express procedure) for full tickness rectal prolapse: evolution of a new technique. Dis Colon Rectum 2005;48:307–316.

17. Romano G, Bianco F, Caggiano L. Modified perineal stapled rectal resection with Contour Transtar for full tickness rectal prolapse. Colorectal Dis 2009;11:878–881.

18. Parés D, Vial M, Grande L. An alternative management for high-risk patients with rectal prolapse. Colorectal Dis 2009;11:531–532.

Invited Commentary

Andrew P. Zbar

The chapter by Murad-Regadas, Pinto and Wexner comprehensively centers the place of the common abdominal procedures for the treatment of rectal prolapse, particularly examining the role of more minimally invasive approaches. The emergence of some of these newer technologies has, somewhat paradoxically, made the choice for patients presenting with full-thickness rectal prolapse a little more complicated, since there is scarce prospective trialling of some of these novel techniques with any durable outcomes available. I believe that the authors make the case on available literature for primary laparoscopic use when there are no contraindications. Despite recent meta-analysis showing similarities between laparoscopic and open arms of retrospectively analyzed and non-randomized data for morbidity and mortality, with an advantage of shorter hospital stay in the laparoscopic groups [1], there are still few available prospectively randomized clinical trials comparing the two main techniques. The laparoscopic approach is accompanied by an overall earlier return to bowel function and less postoperative analgesic requirement [2], along with the potential (as discussed by the authors) of overall cost-benefit where reduced hospital stay (and its accompaniments) offset more prolonged operative times and the capital expenditure of laparoscopic disposables. In this respect, Byrne and colleagues from Sydney have shown laparoscopic rectopexy to have durably low recurrence rates with equivalent functional outcomes (in terms of postoperative evacuatory difficulty and incontinence) when compared with open abdominal approaches [3]. This sort of data can be read alongside durable single-center long-term

outcomes selected from prospective laparoscopic databases [4], and even the use of a laparoscopic benefit of day-case rectopexy in small numbers of younger selected cases [5].

But there is much in the sophisticated analysis of this literature that we do not yet know. It is accepted that the choice for laparoscopy may be deliberately made for those with significant underlying comorbidity (particularly cardiac in nature), but it is unknown whether the more difficult resection rectopexy which has so gained favor in open surgery will be transcribed for those more routinely using minimally invasive techniques. The open data, as discussed in this chapter, show sufficient complications with mesh (and its removal) to probably eschew its use, with equivalent (or better) results for simple suture rectopexy. The latter technique, when performed open, is best done in my opinion to the lumbosacral disk, taking care of the middle sacral artery when present rather than performing any sort of presacral fixation with its occasional potential for serious bleeding. In this context, although discussed by the authors, the arguments concerning division of the lateral ligaments improving recurrence rates but leading to a higher incidence of postoperative constipation probably reflect more the technique of the closeness of rectal dissection, given the lack of really definable 'ligaments' as such, where some patients may develop an autonomic neuropathy following such rectal dissection, and others with significant preoperative constipation and disordered sigmoidorectal transit may not have been fully assessed [6].

With the advent of minimally invasive approaches, however, the place for mesh insertion, its type and its design features has become more fluid. This has arisen for several reasons. Firstly, there is an increased use of minimalist approaches with mesh insertions for a range

A.P. Zbar
Division of Colon and Rectal Surgery, Universities
of New England and New Castle, NSW, Australia

G.A. Santoro, A.P. Wieczorek, C.I. Bartram (eds.) *Pelvic Floor Disorders*
© Springer-Verlag Italia 2010

of patients with uterogenital prolapse, the indications and outcomes of which remain to be seen [7]. These are an eclectic group of patients often presenting with complex symptomatology including urinary and anal incontinence, evacuatory and urinary difficulty, and dyspareunia, and a lot of this literature will be difficult to dissect for practising coloproctologists. There will, however, I suspect, be an interest by colorectal surgeons in translating some of this minimally invasive mesh use to the treatment of more isolated rectal prolapse, as is already occurring without clear management guidelines for rectocele and enterocele patients who present with evacuatory difficulty [8, 9]. Secondly, for isolated rectal prolapse, these approaches that dissect and then fixate the rectum adequately are likely to provide durable success, but the morass of developing literature analyzing the right procedure (if that exists) for those presenting with mixed prolapse and preoperative symptoms of obstructed defaecation is currently difficult to interpret. Thirdly, it is more likely in these patients that the mesh design will need to be more complicated, being interposed in the rectogenital septum and providing coincident sacrocolpopexy, rectopexy, obliteration of the peritoneal cul-de-sac, and even vesico-uterine support. Such an approach will need a combined abdomino-perineal technique with two surgeons.

Laparoscopic sigmoid resection will, in this minefield, likely be re-evaluated over time as we come to understand better the associated conditions that contribute to preoperative constipation. As the authors quite rightly state, it is mandatory if resection is contemplated in a recurrent case to excise the old anastomosis of a prior resection (however that has been performed), because of the inherent risks of ischemia.

Further, there are data to show from a single study [4] that recurrence rates are particularly high when laparoscopic resection rectopexy is performed in patients who have undergone a prior perineal procedure for prolapse.

This latter finding has not generally been noted using an open approach after a failed perineal procedure [10], and probably reflects the fact that some reported results of laparoscopy are likely to be technique dependent in their early learning phase. Given that incontinence is likely to be 'cured' in at least two-thirds of patients by efficient prolapse removal, this appears to be less of an issue with the abdominal approach except when it is very severe. Add to this

the role of NOSE (natural orifice specimen extraction) therapy, and we may be re-examining the place of sigmoidectomy [11] as we may use entirely transvaginal surgery for this condition [12].

And what of the robot in this scenario? The answer at this stage is that we simply do not know its place. Superficially, it may seem that robotic advantage in coloproctology (as has been translated from cardiac surgery), might lie in the performance of both repetitive and very precise tasks, and that therefore its role is questionable, but this would be a simplistic view. The lessons learned from stepwise robot-assisted radical prostatectomy could be translated to the formulaic surgical treatment of benign colorectal conditions like rectal prolapse where close and extended rectal dissection, secure rectopexy, and peritoneal cul-de-sac closure all feature as prominent and necessary parts of the procedure. As the authors clearly state, it is feasible, safe and durable, but such an approach will, over time, influence referral practices where there is a substantial learning curve [13] and limited availability of the necessary equipment, where we will need to assess the acquisitional tools of the trade [14] and where there may be market forces pushing for the technology well before the scientific analysis itself is developed [15].

The excellent chapter by Trompetto and Cornaglia describes the most common perineal approaches towards the primary surgical treatment of full-thickness rectal prolapse. We need to separate cases presenting with full-thickness rectal prolapse from those patients presenting with what used to be referred to as occult or concealed rectal prolapse [16]. This is a specific group which is currently designated as internal rectal prolapse and is representative of a constellation of combined pelvic floor and perineal soft-tissue disorders resulting in the clinical "final common pathway" of evacuatory dysfunction [17]. As the authors quite rightly state, the choice of over 130 different surgical options for one condition reflects the fact that no procedure is definitive and that prospective, randomized, controlled trials are unavailable to guide the coloproctologist in the management of patient subgroups. Indeed, the attempts at this through the recent PROSPER (PROlapse Surgery: PErineal or Rectopexy) trial conducted in the UK make some analysis available for the most commonly performed perineal and abdominal procedures where there is broadest experience, although there is no consensus regarding the true incidence of recurrence and postoperative continence (and other functional) disturbance, and this trial reveals bias in the randomization that is somewhat dependent upon surgical preferences and training as well as on preoperative patient comorbidity [18, 19].

Of the two main perineal procedures performed for rectal prolapse (Delorme's mucosectomy and imbrication versus Altemeier's rectosigmoidectomy), it is still unclear which is more suitable and for which patient. It would appear that the perineal rectosigmoidectomy is easier to perform if the prolapse is large, and that either a complete Delorme's procedure or a hemi-Delorme's modification is technically suitable for almost all extents of rectal prolapse, being readily performed under regional blockade in those patients with high perioperative risk. In non-randomized reports we know that these main perineal approaches are associated with a higher overall full-thickness recurrence when compared with abdominal approaches over time [20, 21].

Although there is no clear evidence that partial prolapse inexorably leads to full-thickness prolapse if untreated [22], there is some physiologic data that links the two conditions [23]; however, many of the physiological effects of perineal operations in these patient cohorts, which may adversely affect functional status (particularly in those cases initially presenting with significant fecal incontinence), are unknown [24]. Since the etiology of incontinence is varied, the effects of extensive perineal surgery can be unpredictable, with some patients suffering sphincter damage [25] or pudendal neuropathy [26], while others demonstrate excessive internal anal sphincter relaxation induced by the prolapsed mass [27]. Some patients demonstrate high-pressure prolapse waves [28], some distortion of the recto-anal pressure gradient [29], and still others show reproducible abnormal recovery of the rectoanal inhibitory reflex that is indicative of internal anal sphincter damage [30]. In particular, the effects on neo-rectal physiology following perineal resection are poorly understood or examined [31] but it is this reviewer's opinion that these physiological changes in rectal prolapse (based on no available prospective data), can provide practical clinical insight into the selective preoperative use of both basic anal manometry and endoanal sonography to guide against certain perineal procedures. Correction of the prolapsed mass itself is likely to revert much of this pathophysiology and assist in the restoration of continence postoperatively in those cases that are operatively successful;

however, I would caution against perineal rectal excision in those patients with severe preoperative incontinence where there is no sign of internal anal sphincter function, as occasioned by extremely low resting anal pressure or by an absent rectoanal inhibitory reflex [19, 32]. Equally, I would favour an expectant approach in those presenting with preoperative incontinence, rather than the use of a coincident levatorplasty, although the addition of the latter procedure has, in one study, shown reduced prolapse recurrence rates and a delayed time to recurrence when combined with an Altemeier's procedure alone [33], despite the potential morbidity of requiring a second perineal incision.

We do know, at least, that if an Altemeier's procedure is successfully performed alone and unaccompanied by significant perioperative morbidity, that it is associated with an improved general and constipation-specific quality of life and subjective health status [34], despite some recent concerns regarding its longer-term success [35] but this itself would not be a specific endorsement for the less selective use of this operation when it is deemed safest to perform a perineal procedure. It is likely that any perineal procedure when deemed appropriate will, if successful, improve the patient's quality of life. In adoption of a perineal operation to treat prolapse, we do not yet know the advantage of some new advances, as the authors quite rightly point out. I would caution at this stage about the use of stapled technology for rectal resection as has recently been advocated, until there is more prospective and randomized data [36, 37]. Equally, we do not yet know the long-term outcome or indications for the use of tunneled transperineal Permacol mesh in the enduring control of full-thickness as opposed to internal rectal prolapse [38]. We are also going to have to await the prospective outcome of advantage in elderly patients not deemed normally fit for a conventional open abdominal procedure over perineally performed surgery of laparoscopic ventral (non-resectional) rectopexy in well-selected cases. As yet, these interesting data are non-randomized, but they suggest that the laparoscopic approach is equally valuable and safe with a markedly reduced recurrence rate on medium-term follow-up when compared with our much-loved perineal procedures [39]. Whether these perineal procedures could become almost redundant remains to be seen.

References

1. Sajid M, Siddiqui M, Baig M. Open versus laparoscopic repair of full thickness rectal prolapse: a re-meta-analysis. Colorectal Dis 2009;13 April epub ahead of print.

2. Hong D, Lewis M, Tabet J, Anvari M. Prospective comparison of laparoscopic versus open resection for benign colorectal disease. Surg Laparosc Endosc Percutan Tech 2002;12:238–242.

3. Byrne CM, Smith SR, Solomon MJ et al. Long-term functional outcomes after laparoscopic and open rectopexy for the treatment of rectal prolapse. Dis Colon Rectum 2008;51:1597–1604.

4. Laubert T, Kleemann M, Schorcht A et al. Laparoscopic resection rectopexy for rectal prolapse: a single-center study during 16 years. Surg Endosc 2010;23 February 3pub ahead of print.

5. Vijay V, Halbert J, Zissimopoulos A et al. Day case laparoscopic rectopexy is feasible, safe and cost effective for selected patients. Surg Endosc 2008;22:1237–1240.

6. Livanage CA, Rathnayake G, Deen KI. A new technique for suture rectopexy without resection for rectal prolapse. Tech Coloproctol 2009;13:27–33.

7. Wetta LA, Gerten KA, Wheeler TL 2nd et al. Synthetic graft use in vaginal prolapse surgery: objective and subjective outcomes. Int Urogynecol J Pelvic Floor Dysfunct 2009; 20:1307–1312.

8. Slawik S, Soulsby R, Carter H et al. Laparoscopic ventral rectopexy, posterior colporrhaphy and vaginal sacrocolpopexy for the treatment of recto-genital prolapse and mechanical outlet obstruction. Colorectal Dis 2008;10:138–143.

9. D'Hoore A, Vanbeckevoort D, Penninckx F. Clinical, physiological and radiological assessment of rectovaginal septum reinforcement with mesh for complex rectocele. Br J Surg 2008;95:1264–1272.

10. Pikarsky AJ, Joo JS, Wexner SD et al. Recurrent rectal prolapse: what is the next good option? Dis Colon Rectum 2000;43:1273–1276.

11. Sanchez JE, Rasheid SH, Krieger BR et al. Laparoscopic-assisted transvaginal approach for sigmoidectomy and rectocolpopexy. JSLS 2009;13:217–220.

12. Gurland B, Garrett KA, Firoozi F, Goldman HB. Transvaginal sacrospinous rectopexy: initial clinical experience. Tech Coloproctol 2010;23 March epub ahead of print.

13. Akl MN, Long JB, Giles DL et al. Robotic-assisted sacrocolpopexy: technique and learning curve. Surg Endosc 2009;23:2390–2394.

14. Muffly T, McCormick TC, Dean J et al. An evaluation of knot integrity when tied robotically and conventionally. Am J Obstet Gynecol 2009;200:e18–20.

15. Zbar AP. Innovations in coloproctology. Tech Coloproctol 2009;13:331–332.

16. Cuthbertson AM. Concealed rectal prolapse. Aust N Z J Surg 1980;50:116–117.

17. Pescatori M, Zbar A. Tailored surgery for internal and external rectal prolapse: functional results of 268 patients operated upon by a single surgeon over a 21 year period. Int J Colorectal Dis 2009;11:410–419.

18. Phillips RKS. Rectal prolapse – update on the PROSPER trial. Royal Australian College of Surgeons Annual Scientific Congress, 2004. A N Z J Surg 2004;74(suppl):A37(CR 33).

19. Zbar AP, Nguyen H. Management guidelines for full-thickness rectal prolapse. In: Altomare D, Pucciani F (eds) Rectal prolapse. Springer-Verlag, Milan, 2008: pp 201–206.

20. Raftopoulos Y, Senagore AJ, Di Giuro G, Bergamaschi R; Rectal Prolapse Recurrence Study Group. Recurrence rates after abdominal surgery for complete rectal prolapse: a multicenter pooled analysis of 643 individual patient data. Dis Colon Rectum 2005;48:1200–1206.

21. Rianuswan W, Hull TL, Bast J et al. Comparison of perineal operations with abdominal operations for full-thickness rectal prolapse. World J Surg 2010;34:1116-1122.

22. Wijffels NA, Collinson R, Cunningham C, Lindsey I. What is the natural history of internal rectal prolapse? Colorectal Dis 2009;13 April epub ahead of print.

23. Sun WM, Read NW, Donnelly TC et al. A common pathophysiology for full thickness rectal prolapse, anterior mucosal prolapse and solitary rectal ulcer. Br J Surg 1989;76:290–295.

24. Zbar AP, Takashima S, Hasegawa T, Kitabayashi K. Perineal rectosigmoidectomy (Altemeier's procedure): a review of physiology, technique and outcome. Tech Coloproctol 2002;6:109–116.

25. Williams JG, Wong WD, Jenzen L et al. Incontinence and rectal prolapse: a prospective manometric study. Dis Colon Rectum 1991;34:209–216.

26. Birnbaum EH, Stamm L, Rafferty JF et al. Pudendal nerve terminal motor latency influences surgical outcome in treatment of rectal prolapse. Dis Colon Rectum 1996;39:1215–1221.

27. Sun WM, Read N, Miner PB et al. The role of transient internal anal sphincter relaxation in faecal incontinence. Int J Colorectal Dis 1990;5:31–36.

28. Broden G, Dolk A, Hölmstrom B. Recovery of the internal anal sphincter following rectopexy: a possible explanation for continence improvement. Int J Colorectal Dis 1988;3:23–28.

29. Goes RN, Simons AJ, Beart RW Jr. Level of highest mean pressure segment in the anal canal. A quantitative assessment of anal sphincter function. Dis Colon Rectum 1996;39:289–293.

30. Zbar AP, Aslam M, Gold DM et al. Parameters of the rectoanal inhibitory reflex in patients with idiopathic fecal incontinence and chronic constipation. Dis Colon Rectum 1998;41:200–208.

31. Siproudhis L, Bellissant E, Juguet F et al. Rectal adaptation to distension in patients with overt rectal prolapse. Br J Surg 1998;85:1527–1532.

32. Glasgow SC, Birnbaum EH, Kodner IJ et al. Preoperative anal manometry predicts continence after perineal proctectomy for rectal prolapse. Dis Colon Rectum 2006;49:1052–1058.

33. Chun SW, Pikarsky AJ, You SY et al. Perineal rectosigmoidectomy for rectal prolapse: role of levatorplasty. Tech Coloproctol 2004;8:3–9.

34. Kim M, Reibetanz J, Boenicke L et al. Quality of life after transperineal rectosigmoidectomy. Br J Surg 2010;97:269–272.

35. Altomare DF, Binda G, Ganio E et al; Rectal Prolapse Study Group. Long-term outcome of Altemeier's procedure for rectal prolapsed. Dis Colon Rectum 2009;52:698–703.

36. Boccasanta P, Venturi M, Barbieri S, Roviaro G. Impact of new technologies on the clinical and functional outcome of Altemeier's procedure: a randomized, controlled trial. Dis Colon Rectum 2006;49:652–660.

37. Romano G, Bianco F, Caggiano L. Modified perineal stapled rectal resection with Contour Transtar for full-thickness rectal prolapse. Colorectal Dis 2009;11:878–881.

38. Dench JE, Scott SM, Lunniss PJ et al. Multimedia article. External pelvic rectal suspension (the express procedure) for internal rectal prolapse, with or without concomitant rectocele repair: a video demonstration. Dis Colon Rectum 2006; 49:1922–1926.

39. Wijffels N, Cunningham C, Dixon A et al. Laparoscopic anterior rectopexy for external rectal prolapse is safe and effective in the elderly. Does this make perineal procedures obsolete? Colorectal Dis 2010;20 February epub ahead of print.

The Laparoscopic Approach to Rectal Prolapse

49

Joshua R. Karas and Roberto Bergamaschi,
on behalf of the Rectal Prolapse Recurrence Study Group

Abstract This chapter represents a current opinion on the impact laparoscopy may have on the outcomes of full-thickness rectal prolapse (FTRP) surgery, and presents a concise insight on laparoscopic surgical technique, the authors' personal experience, and an overview of the literature dealing with this specific subject.

Patients with FTRP are a heterogenous group with a variety of symptoms, and a variety of treatment options are available. As part of the preoperative evaluation, it is necessary to perform a detailed risk assessment. Physical examination will detect anal pathology, sphincter tone assessment, and squeeze pressures, which is important to aid the surgeon in choosing the appropriate procedure for each patient. Tests that are useful in evaluating the patient with rectal prolapse include defecography, colorectal transit time, colonoscopy, and anal manometry.

Controversies remain as to which step of the abdominal surgery for FTRP contributes most to containment of recurrence rates. Rectal mobilization with suture rectopexy, performed to control prolapse and prevent impaired evacuation, can be performed via an open or laparoscopic approach. The procedure for laparoscopic suture rectopexy is reviewed, as well as laparoscopic sigmoid resection sparing the superior rectal artery.

The laparoscopic approach for the treatment of rectal prolapse is the standard of care. Recurrence rates are not clearly improved by adding rectopexy, resection, or both to rectal mobilization only. Most importantly, the surgeon must choose the surgical approach according to the needs of each individual patient and consider the type of previous surgery in cases of recurrence.

Keywords Full-thickness rectal prolapse surgery • Laparoscopy • Mobilization • Randomized control trials • Rectum • Recurrence • POSSUM score • Surgery

R. Bergamaschi
Division of Colon and Rectal Surgery, State University of New York, Stony Brook, NY, USA

G.A. Santoro, A.P. Wieczorek, C.I. Bartram (eds.) *Pelvic Floor Disorders*
© Springer-Verlag Italia 2010

49.1 Introduction

More than 150 years have elapsed since the first report on full-thickness rectal prolapse surgery (FTRP) appeared in the literature [1]. There are a number of abdominal procedures available for the treatment of FTRP, which differ technically as to whether rectopexy is added to mobilization of the rectum. A meta-analysis of randomized controlled trials by the Cochrane Library concluded that at present there is not enough evidence to support one form of abdominal surgical procedure over another with regard to recurrence rates [2]. This chapter represents a current opinion on the impact laparoscopy may have on the outcomes of FTRP.

The Chapter does not provide a systematic review of the evidence available in the literature; the objective is to present a concise insight on laparoscopic surgical technique, the authors' personal experience, and an overview of the literature dealing with this specific subject.

49.2 Preoperative Evaluation

49.2.1 Risk Assessment

Patients with FTRP are a heterogeneous group with a variety of additional symptoms. Hence, a single treatment would not be appropriate [3], and treatment options should be selected. The first step of the algorithm is to evaluate the risk of death for a specific individual undergoing surgery. This evaluation should be based on the colorectal Physiologic and Operative Severity Score for the enUmeration of Mortality (POSSUM) score [4], rather than on the American Society of Anesthesiologists (ASA) score. The colorectal POSSUM score can be quickly evaluated online [5], entering four physiological and four operative data points. If the patient is unfit for abdominal surgery under general anesthesia, a perineal procedure under spinal anesthesia can be offered. All patients who are fit for general anesthesia should be offered an abdominal procedure, regardless of chronological age. One exception to this rule is the occasional male patient with true FTRP. The risk of iatrogenic impotence in abdominal surgery should be thoroughly explained to male patients, and the advantages and disadvantages of perineal procedures considered individually. There are four risk areas of autonomic nerve damage during rectal dissection [6].

Damage to the sympathetic nerves may occur when dissecting the inferior mesenteric artery, and during posterior rectal mobilization at the promontory close to the hypogastric nerves. Damage to the parasympathetic nerves may occur during dissection of the lateral stalks of the rectum and anterior rectal mobilization from the seminal vesicles and prostate.

49.2.2 Workup

The patient with rectal prolapse may present with a myriad of different symptoms that range from constipation and straining to fecal incontinence. Therefore, it is of utmost importance that all patients undergo a complete preoperative workup before surgery.

Upon physical examination, inspection may reveal an obvious rectal prolapse, especially during straining. However, FTRP must be differentiated from mucosal prolapse. The mucosal prolapse can be differentiated from the full-thickness presentation because of the radially oriented grooves, while the FTRP has concentric grooves. In order to measure the prolapse adequately, the patient is asked to position themself in a squatting position. The patient is then asked to increase straining and the prolapse enlarges and lengthens. While the patient is straining, the distance from the perianal skin to the top of the prolapse is measured. Digital rectal examination may also add valuable information by detecting anal pathology and assessing sphincter tone and squeeze pressures. This information is important and aids the surgeon choosing the appropriate procedure for each individual patient.

49.2.2.1 Defecography

Although not a standard test ordered for the evaluation of a patient with rectal prolapse, defecography provides the surgeon with valuable anatomic and functional information for pelvic floor abnormalities. In addition, the results may indicate the presence of sigmoidocoele or enterocoele.

49.2.2.2 Colorectal Transit Time

This test provides essential information when confronted with a patient with concomitant constipation. Among the different methods for establishing the colorectal transit time, we recommend the method described by Gore et al [7]. The patient receives six numbered daypacks. The five first packs contain 10 rings and the sixth contains 10 rings and 20 cylinders. Each day, at the same time, a pack is ingested. A plain abdominal radiography is taken on day 7. Rings are counted and the transit time is measured by the hospital's radiology department protocol.

49.2.2.3 Colonoscopy

This procedure must be performed in order to rule out any mucosal abnormality, especially in patients with a prior diagnosis of diverticulitis, inflammatory bowel disease, or cancer.

49.2.2.4 Anal Manometry

Manometry is important in evaluating the patient with a longstanding history of rectal prolapse and incontinence. Patients with pudendal nerve damage, from either obstetric trauma, diabetes, or neoplasms, must also undergo manometric evaluation prior to surgery.

49.3 Treatment Options

49.3.1 Rectopexy versus Mobilization Only

Controversies have not yet been resolved as to which step of the abdominal surgery for FTRP contributes the most to containment of recurrence rates. Although the addition of rectopexy to mobilization of the rectum is thought to decrease recurrences, there is currently no evidence to support this claim [2]. Moreover, the additional rectopexy may have disadvantages such as added operating time, implantation of foreign material, bleeding from the sacral veins, and nerve injury to the presacral plexus. On the other hand, the literature data on rectal mobilization only (without rectopexy) are very limited, if data on resection are not taken into account. A series of 13 patients undergoing rectal mobilization only for FTRP had a 15% recurrence rate during a median follow-up of 1.09 years (range 0.39–1.88 years) [8]. Furthermore, published recurrence rates are often unreliable. In a recent meta-analysis on individual patient data, published recurrence rates differed by as much as 47% from recurrence rates re-estimated by actuarial analysis [9]. Therefore, a recent randomized

controlled trial evaluates whether the addition of rectopexy to mobilization of the rectum significantly decreases recurrence rates [10].

49.3.2 Suture Rectopexy

Suture rectopexy was first described by Cutait in 1959 [11] (personal communication, Rectal Prolapse Recurrence Study Group, 2007). The rationale of using sutures has been to keep the rectum in its new position to allow its eventual fixation to the sacrum by scar tissue [12]. There are a few technical details about the surgical technique of suture rectopexy that need our attention. Most authors would suture the posterior mesorectum to the presacral fascia [12–14]. Some would also include a partial thickness of the posterior rectum [12]. We prefer to suture the right and left peritoneal flaps to the presacral fascia. We agree with some authors [14] that the sutures may be placed on the sacral promontory. The exact location on the promontory is lateral to the hypogastric nerves and medial to the ureter on both sides of the rectum (Fig. 49.1). Alternative sites on the

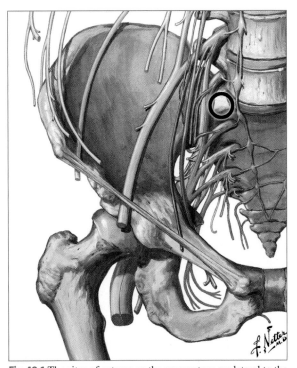

Fig. 49.1 The sites of sutures on the promontory are lateral to the hypogastric nerves and medial to the ureter on both sides of the rectum; right side shown at *black circle*. Reprinted from www.netterimages.com © Elsevier Inc., with permission

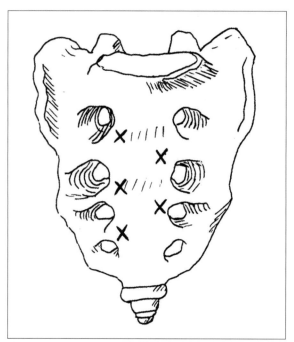

Fig. 49.2 Schematic diagram of the sacrum with the sites of sutures indicated with crosses. Reprinted from [14], with permission

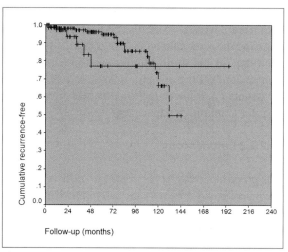

Follow-up (months)

Fig. 49.3 Recurrence-free rates comparing suture rectopexy to mesh rectopexy. Log-rank test, p = 0.2494; *n* = 261 patients; *short line*, suture rectopexy; *dotted line*, mesh rectopexy. Reprinted from [16], with permission

sacrum below the promontory have been suggested (Fig. 49.2). Most authors would agree that two sutures are adequate [12, 14].

49.3.3 Mesh Rectopexy

The authors concur with the literature suggesting that rectopexy is just as effective with sutures as it is with mesh [2, 15, 16]. A multicenter pooled analysis of 643 patients showed no difference in recurrence rates between suture rectopexy and mesh rectopexy [16] (Fig. 49.3). This leads to the question of whether a mesh should be used at all, as it may increase the rates of postoperative constipation, and also carry the potential risk of infection [17].

49.3.4 Sigmoid Resection

Sigmoid resection is suggested only in cases of well-documented constipation and should be strictly avoided in incontinent patients. However, adding resection to rectopexy does not seem to decrease recurrence rates as compared to rectopexy alone [2]. In addition to a significant history of constipation, clustering of rings

in the sigmoid should be documented at the colorectal transit time. If resection is indicated, it should be kept at a minimum without mobilizing the sigmoid colon. The superior rectal artery should be spared [18], since preserving the blood supply to a long rectal stump may in fact minimize the risk of anastomotic leak and its related morbidity. Therefore, by obviating the need to divide the mesorectum at the rectosigmoid junction, this may prove to have a favorable impact on anasto-

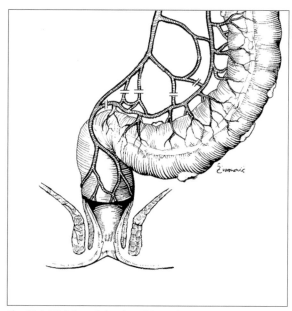

Fig. 49.4 Division of the sigmoid arteries and sparing of the superior rectal artery. Reprinted from [18], with permission

motic leak rates. Moreover, avoiding dissection of the inferior mesenteric artery is particularly relevant in male patients undergoing resection for rectal prolapse due to potential damage to the sympathetic nerves (Fig. 49.4).

49.4 Surgical Technique

Rectal mobilization with suture rectopexy to repair FTRP is an abdominal procedure that can be performed via an open or laparoscopic approach. The procedure involves mobilization of the rectum followed by suture fixation of the rectum to the sacral promontory, restoring the anatomic position of the rectum. The goal of the procedure is to control the prolapse and prevent impaired evacuation.

49.4.1 Preoperative Care

The day before the planned surgical intervention, the patient should be restricted to a clear diet. It is the author's preference to administer a bowel preparation the day before surgery. The patient is instructed to take nothing by mouth as of midnight before surgery and to evacuate the rectum with an enema prior to traveling to the hospital. In the preoperative area, the patient should receive intravenous fluids, as the bowel preparation often contributes to dehydration. Epidural analgesia should also be offered to the patient, especially if the surgery entails a bowel resection. General endotracheal anesthesia is administered by the anesthesiologist, and a Foley catheter and oral-gastric tube are inserted.

The patient is positioned on top of a bean bag in lithotomy, with both arms tucked and padded to the side. It is important that the height of the knee and the torso is maintained, to avoid any impediment while the surgeon is operating. For obese patients, the surgeon may want to consider strapping the patient to the operating table at the chest. Prior to creating a sterile field, the surgeon must verify that the patient is secured to the table.

This is accomplished by maneuvering the remote control of the operating room table and positioning the patient in a steep Trendelenburg position. Antibiotics should be administered intravenously within the hour prior to the planned incision.

49.4.2 Laparoscopic Suture Rectopexy

If the rectum is prolapsed it should be reduced prior to starting the procedure. The abdomen and perineum are then prepped and draped in a sterile fashion. The stirrups securing the patient's legs are also draped. Prior to the incision, the name of the patient, the scheduled procedure, and the operating surgeon are identified. It is the author's preference to achieve the pneumoperitoneum through an open technique as opposed to using a Veress needle. A 10 mm incision is made just below the umbilicus, and the umbilical stalk is dissected and then grasped with a Kocher clamp and pulled in a cephalad direction. The fascia is incised with a knife in a longitudinal fashion under direct visual control. A bladeless Hasson trocar is then inserted into the peritoneal cavity. The trocar is secured in place by two stitches placed on each side of the incision. It is not necessary to go beyond 10 mmHg and achieve high intra-abdominal pressures, since most of the procedure will be done in the bony structure of the pelvis.

Two ports (10 mm and 5 mm) are placed in the right lower quadrant of the patient's abdomen in a triangulating fashion with the umbilical site. The 10 mm port allows the surgeon to insert the curved needle of the suture into the abdominal cavity for the rectopexy. A final 5 mm port is placed in the left lower quadrant, for the assistant's instruments. The patient is placed in the Trendelenburg position, which facilitates removal of the small bowel and omentum out of the pelvis into the upper abdominal cavity.

The assistant proceeds to lift the rectosigmoid colon from the epiploic appendages. The sigmoid colon should not be mobilized. The second step includes close identification of the left ureter. This is facilitated by prior insertion of lighted ureteral stents. Visualization of the iliac bifurcation as well as the gonadal vessels can also facilitate this identification. The peritoneum should be opened into the pelvic sulcus, toward the pouch of Douglas. This will define the extent of the lateral dissection.

Medial dissection is begun above the level of the sacral promontory. The peritoneum is divided at least 2 cm from the rectum in order to create peritoneal "wings" to be used for pexy. The peritoneum of the sigmoid mesentery is opened and connected with the lateral dissection just posterior to the inferior mesenteric pedicle, which is elevated as the rectosigmoid colon is maintained on stretch. The medial peritoneal dissection is extended over the sacral promontory along the sulcus toward the pouch of Douglas, to mirror the lateral dissection. At the level of the sacral promontory, the hypogastric nerves are amenable to injury. To avoid such an injury, the dissection is kept close to the fascia propria of the rectum. The surgeon continues to lift and provide appropriate tension to the rectosigmoid colon. This dissection is often facilitated by the abnormal lack of fixation in this area, which has contributed to the prolapse. The presacral fascia and hypogastric nerves should remain away from the area of dissection.

It is important to be mindful of the presacral vessels as the dissection approaches the pelvic floor. As the levator ani muscles become visible, the rectum will become parallel to the pelvic floor and the angle of dissection should be adjusted to avoid injury to the presacral vessels. Diffuse bleeding may occur if these vessels are inadvertently injured. The posterior dissection is completed to the level of the coccyx. The lateral dissection should spare the lateral stalks (ligaments). The rectum is lifted by the assistant and a point is selected for the rectopexy. The rectum should not be placed on tension, but the prolapse defect should be reduced. Non-absorbable silk sutures are secured to the right and left sacral promontory. The sites of sutures on the promontory are lateral to the hypogastric nerves and medial to the ureter on both sides of the rectum (Fig. 49.1). Attention to the position of the hypogastric nerves and the presacral vessels will guide the suture placement. The surgical assistant will maintain the anatomic position of the rectum while the surgeon secures the two previously placed sutures to the peritoneal "wings".

Once the mobilization and rectopexy are complete, hemostasis should be reaffirmed. The pelvis is irrigated with saline. There should be no reason to place a drain in the pelvis.

The wound is cleaned and dressed, and the patient is extubated and taken to recovery. The Foley catheter should be left in place, but the oral-gastric tube may be discontinued.

49.4.3 Laparoscopic Sigmoid Resection Sparing the Superior Rectal Artery

The previously mentioned technical steps remain the same, yet there are some important points worth describing. While performing the circumferential rectal mobilization, the mesorectum is dissected off the posterior wall of the rectum at approximately 14 cm from the anal verge. This distance is verified by an intraoperative rigid sigmoidoscopy.

The sigmoid colon is then divided by a laparoscopic linear stapler that is positioned perpendicular to the axis of the sigmoid colon. The mesentery of the sigmoid colon is divided close to the bowel, and the mesorectum is not divided, therefore sparing the superior rectal artery (Fig. 49.4). The specimen is retrieved through a pfannestiel incision. We then proceed to perform a double-stapled colorectal anastomosis without the need to re-establish pneumoperitoneum.

49.4.4 Postoperative Care

Postoperatively, the usual considerations are addressed. Early activity and incentive spirometry are encouraged. Pain is initially controlled with an epidural catheter with local anesthetic. Diet is advanced with the return of bowel function, and the pain medication is transitioned to oral formulations. The Foley catheter can be removed on the first postoperative day unless other comorbidities are present.

Upon discharge, the patient is instructed to avoid heavy lifting. Dietary goals should be addressed. Avoidance of constipation or overly loose stool should be discussed. The patient should be seen in the office within 1 to 2 weeks of discharge. Continued follow-up will assist the surgeon in his or her evaluation of the success of the repair.

49.5 Outcomes

In an unpublished retrospective multicenter study conducted by the author, laparoscopic rectopexy for FTRP was evaluated, to determine its impact on recurrence rates. Data from 1992 to 2002 were reviewed. Laparoscopic rectopexy consisted of mobilization of the rectum and suture rectopexy. There were 179 patients with a median age of 62 years (range 15–93 years). There were 154 females and 25 males. One hundred and thirty-eight patients underwent laparoscopic rectopexy, whereas 41 patients had a resection in addition to rectopexy. There were no deaths; 30-day complications occurred in 7 (4%) patients and included pneumonia ($n = 1$), urinary tract infection ($n = 2$), urinary retention ($n = 1$), wound infection ($n = 1$), and left ureter partial injury ($n = 1$). Seven (3.9%) patients were lost to follow-up, 172 (96%) were available at a median follow-up of 15.5 months, and only 10 (5.8%) patients had a recurrence. In comparison, Ashari et al [19] reported a recurrence rate of 2.5% in 117 patients with laparoscopically assisted resection rectopexy. However, their overall morbidity was 9% (10 patients), with one mortality.

49.6 Conclusions

The laparoscopic approach provides the surgeon with a magnified vision deep into the pelvis, with the added benefit of a relatively weak fixation of the rectal fascia to the sacrum. In spite of these benefits, different studies have demonstrated comparable data in terms of recurrence and associated morbidity when comparing laparoscopy to conventional surgery. However, caution must be used when interpreting available data. In a recent meta-analysis study analyzing individual patient data, published recurrence rates differed as much as 47% by actuarial analysis [9]. Moreover, procedures with added steps such as rectopexy, resection, or both do not appear to offer any clear advantage in terms of recurrence rates. On the contrary, rectopexy may have some disadvantages such as: longer operating time, implant of foreign material (mesh, tacks, sutures), possible bleeding from sacral veins, and possible nerve injury of the presacral plexus.

In conclusion, the surgeon must choose his surgical approach according to each individual patient, taking account of gender, comorbidities, the presence of constipation, prior abdominal surgery, and recurrence. If the case is a recurrence, it is of utmost importance to know what surgery was performed previously, to allow the surgeon to plan the procedure adequately with knowledge of the available blood supply.

References

1. Madoff RD, Mellgren A. One hundred years of rectal prolapse surgery. Dis Colon Rectum 1999;42:441–450.
2. Ton S, Brown SR, Malik A, Nelson RL. Surgery for complete rectal prolapse in adults. Cochrane Database Syst Review 2008;(4):CD001758. DOI:101002/14651858. CD001758. pub. 2.
3. Brown AJ, Anderson JH. Strategy for selection of type of operation for rectal prolapse based on clinical criteria. Dis Colon Rectum 2004;47:103–107.
4. Vather R, Zargar-Shoshtari K, Adegbola S, Hill AG. Comparison of the possum, P-POSSUM and Cr-POSSUM scoring systems as predictors of postoperative mortality in patients undergoing major colorectal surgery. ANZ J Surg 2006; 76:812–816.
5. Smith JJ, Tekkis PP. Risk Prediction in Surgery. Colorectal-POSSUM scoring. www.riskprediction.org.uk/index-cr.php (accessed 19 December 2009).
6. Lindsey I, Mortensen NJ. Iatrogenic impotence and rectal dissection. Br J Surg 2002;89:1493–1494.
7. Gore RN, Levine MS, Laufer I (eds). Textbook of gastrointestinal radiology. WB Saunders, Philadelphia (PA), 1994.
8. Nelson R, Spitz J, Pearl RK, Abcarian H. What role does full rectal mobilization alone play in the treatment of rectal prolapse? Tech Coloproctol 2001;5:33–35.
9. DiGiuro G, Ignjatovic D, Brogger J, Bergamaschi R. Rectal Prolapse Recurrence Study Group. How accurate are published recurrence rates after rectal prolapse surgery? A meta-analysis of individual patient data. Am J Surg 2006;191:773–778.
10. Karas JR, Uranues S, Altomare DF, Sökmen S, MD, Krivokapic Z, Hoch J, Bartha I, Bergamaschi R, Rectal Prolapse Recurrence Study Group. No rectopexy versus rectopexy for full-thickness rectal prolapse: a randomized multicenter trial. Presented at the American Society of Colon and Rectal Surgeons (ASCRS) 2010 annual meeting, Minneapolis, MN, May 15-19, 2010, S23.
11. Cutait D. Sacro-promontory fixation of the rectum for complete prolapse. J R Soc Med 1959;52(suppl):105.
12. Khanna AK, Misra MK, Kumar K. Simplified sutured sacral rectopexy for complete rectal prolapse in adults. Eur J Surg 1996;162:143–146.
13. Graf W, Stefansson T, Arvidsson D, Pahlman L. Laparoscopic suture rectopexy. Dis Colon Rectum 1995;38:211–212.
14. Heah SM, Hartley JE, Hurley J et al. Laparoscopic suture rectopexy without resection is effective treatment for full-thickness rectal prolapse. Dis Colon Rectum 2000;43:638–643.
15. Duthie GS, Bartolo DC. Abdominal rectopexy for rectal prolapse: a comparison of techniques. Br J Surg 1992;79:107–113.
16. Raftopoulos Y, Senagore AJ, Di Giuro G, Bergamaschi R. Rectal Prolapse Recurrence Study Group. Recurrence rates after abdominal surgery for complete rectal prolapse: a multicenter pooled analysis of 643 individual patient data. Dis Colon Rectum 2005;48:1200–1206.
17. Sayfan J, Pinho M, Alexander-Williams J, Keighley MR. Sutured posterior abdominal rectopexy with sigmoidectomy compared with Marlex rectopexy for rectal prolapse. Br J Surg 1990;7:143–145.
18. Bergamaschi R, Lovvik K, Marvik R. Preserving the superior rectal artery in laparoscopic sigmoid resection for complete rectal prolapse. Surg Laparosc Endosc Percutan Tech 2003; 13:374–376.
19. Ashari LH, Lumley JW, Stevenson ARL, Stitz RW. Laparoscopically assisted resection rectopexy for rectal prolapse: ten years' experience. Dis Colon Rectum 2005; 48:982–987.

Invited Commentary

Conor P. Delaney

It is a great pleasure to be asked to write a commentary on the paper by Drs Karas and Bergamaschi discussing laparoscopic approaches to rectal prolapse. This is a focused article describing practical approaches to prolapse.

The chapter is particularly important, as evidence-based opinions on rectal prolapse are relatively few, and the opinions of experts like Dr Bergamaschi are of significant importance in trying to steer beteween the varying opinions in the literature.

The authors carefully describe work-up, surgical options, and postoperative care for patients with rectal prolapse. Much as the authors do, we also feel that preoperative consideration of the degree of constipation and levels of incontinence is of primary importance. Based on this, we have reported outcomes using an algorithm for the laparoscopic approach. Briefly, resection is reserved for those with significant symptoms from constipation, or evidence of documented slow transit. Those with diarrhea or incontinence never receive resection. Those without particular symptoms of either diarrhea or incontinence receive a suspensory operation.

As the authors describe, there are various approaches to surgical fixation. I perform an initial posterior mobilization down to the ano-rectal junction, followed by a lateral or anterior mobilization, sufficient to complete reduction of the prolapsed segment on digital examination.

Some patients have a more distal prolapse than others, and require a more distal mobilization. I fix the rectum using a posterior mesh, with a small piece of prolene mesh being tacked to the anterior sacrum below the promontory, and fixed to the mesorectum on each side with two sutures.

Our results with this have been favorable. Short-term outcomes and morbidity and hospital stay have all been excellent, and recurrence rates low. This spares the patient the morbidity of an abdominal wound, and appears to derive the same benefits of low recurrence rates seen with open abdominal surgery. We have even used this laparoscopic approach on patients referred with recurrent prolapse, and with prior resections, preserving the old anastomosis and using a small posterior mesh. Diarrhea and incontinence tend to be improved in most patients, once the regular dilating effect of the prolapse has been removed.

These thoughts are similar to those carefully described in this chapter by Karas and Bergamaschi. This is a useful chapter, which will be of practical interest to surgeons managing patients with diseases of the pelvic floor.

Suggested Reading

1. Delaney CP, Senagore AJ. Rectal prolapse. In: Fazio VW, Church JM, Delaney CP (eds) Current therapy in colon and rectal surgery, 2 edn. Elsevier, Mosby Inc., Philadelphia, PA, 2005, pp 131–134.
2. Madbouly KM, Senagore AJ, Delaney CP et al. Clinically based management of rectal prolapse: comparison of the laparoscopic Wells procedure and laparoscopic resection with rectopexy. Surg Endosc 2003;17:99–103.
3. Kariv Y, Delaney CP, Casillas S et al. Long-term outcome after laparoscopic and open surgery for rectal prolapse. Surg Endosc 2006;20:35–42.
4. Marderstein E, Delaney CP. Management of rectal prolapse. Nature Clin Pract – Gastroenterol Hepatol 2007;4(10):552–561.

C.P. Delaney
Division of Colorectal Surgery, Case Medical Center, Cleveland, OH, USA

Pelvic Floor Muscle Training in Prevention and Treatment of Pelvic Organ Prolapse

Kari Bø and Ingeborg Hoff Brækken

Abstract This chapter describes the four randomized controlled trials (RCTs) published on the effect of pelvic floor muscle training (PFMT) to treat pelvic organ prolapse (POP) and symptoms of prolapse. The results of all four trials show a significant effect of PFMT. However, to date there is only one full-scale RCT using the gold standard Pelvic Organ Prolapse Quantification (POP-Q) system to evaluate stage of prolapse and a validated symptom questionnaire to assess the results. The same research group also used ultrasound to assess the position of the bladder and the rectal ampulla at rest, in addition to assessment of morphological changes of the pelvic floor muscles. There was a significant reduction in stage of prolapse, symptoms, and bother, and increase in pelvic floor muscle strength. Significant hypertrophy of the pelvic floor muscles, shortening of muscle length, and constriction of the levator hiatus were found in the treatment group only. The four RCTs in this area differ in training dosage such as intensity of the contractions, duration of the training period, and therapist contact, factors that are all known to affect outcome. The results of PFMT in treatment of POP are promising. Further studies are needed to understand differences between responders and non-responders and especially the role of PFMT in primary prevention of POP.

Keywords Effect • Evidence • Pelvic floor muscle training • Pelvic organ prolapse • Randomized controlled trials

50.1 Introduction

The prevalence of symptomatic pelvic organ prolapse (POP) is reported to be 3–28% [1–5]. Mechanical symptoms such as vaginal bulging and pelvic pressure are the most specific symptoms of POP [6, 7], and these symptoms may greatly impair quality of life with restriction of participation in, for example, physical activity. POP may occur in the anterior, middle, and/or posterior compartment of the pelvic floor and it is defined as descent of the anterior vaginal wall (bladder, urethra), posterior vaginal wall (bowel), and/or apex of the vagina (cervix, uterus).

Absence of prolapse is defined as stage 0 support; prolapse can be staged from stage I to stage IV (total eversion) [8, 9].

It is estimated that approximately 50% of all women lose some of the supportive mechanisms of the pelvic floor due to childbirth, leading to different degrees of pelvic organ prolapse (POP) [10]. In the UK, POP ac-

K. Bø
Department of Sports Medicine, Norwegian School of Sport Sciences, Oslo, Norway

G.A. Santoro, A.P. Wieczorek, C.I. Bartram (eds.) *Pelvic Floor Disorders*
© Springer-Verlag Italia 2010

counts for 20% of women on waiting lists for major gynecological surgery [11]. Prolapse recurs in up to 58% of women after surgery [12], and about one-third of operated women undergo at least one more surgical procedure for prolapse [13]. The high prevalence and its increase with age highlight the need for prevention measures that could reduce both the incidence and the impact of POP.

However, prolapse may be asymptomatic until the descending organ is through the introitus, and therefore POP may not be recognized until an advanced condition is present [6, 10]. In some women, the prolapse advances rapidly, while others remain stable for many years. Most clinicians have considered that POP does not seem to regress [10]. However, Handa et al [14] found that spontaneous regression is common, especially for minor prolapse.

Treatment of POP can be conservative (lifestyle interventions and/or pelvic floor muscle training (PFMT)), mechanical (use of a pessary), or surgical [16, 17]. While systematic reviews and randomized controlled trials (RCTs) have shown convincing effect of PFMT for stress and mixed urinary incontinence [18, 19], there seems to be a paucity of research for POP and other conditions caused by pelvic floor dysfunction. A survey of UK women's health physiotherapists showed that several women attending physiotherapy practice presented with a mixture of pelvic floor dysfunctions such as stress urinary incontinence and prolapse, and that 92% of the physiotherapists assessed and treated women with POP [20]. The most commonly used treatment was PFMT with and without biofeedback. However, there were no available guidelines to follow for treatment of POP in clinical practice. A Cochrane review on PFMT for POP concluded that the most pressing need was for guidance regarding the effectiveness of PFMT [16].

The aim of the present chapter is to give an up-to-date systematic review of RCTs on PFMT to prevent and treat POP.

50.2 Methods

The basis for this review is a search on the Cochrane database, PubMed and the abstract books from the International Continence Society and International Urogynecology Annual Meetings from 2009, for RCTs on PFMT to prevent or treat POP.

50.3 Results

No RCTs or studies using other designs have been found in evaluating the effect of PFMT on POP in primary prevention (stop prolapse from developing). Table 50.1 [21-26] shows the four RCTs assessing PFMT to treat POP or POP symptoms. The RCTs are all in favor of PFMT demonstrating statistically significant improvement in symptoms [21–23] and/or prolapse stage [21, 23, 24].

The only full-scale RCT showed a 19% improvement in prolapse stage measured by POP-Q, compared to 4% in the control group receiving lifestyle advice only [23].

50.4 Discussion

Based on the four RCTs in this area, the results in relation to the effect of PFMT on POP stages and POP symptoms are promising. All studies are in favor of the PFMT group.

To date, there is only one full-scale RCT evaluating both stage of prolapse and symptoms [23]. This examiner-blinded trial found significant improvement in a group of women with stage I, II, and III POP receiving supervised PFMT compared to a group receiving advice not to strain while defecating, in addition to encouragement to pre-contract the pelvic floor muscles (PFM) before an increase in intra-abdominal pressure. The published studies only reported short-term effects. To maintain the effect, it is expected that PFMT must be continued, although to a lesser degree with a reduced frequency of training, to avoid relapse [27].

There are two main hypotheses for mechanisms as to how PFMT may be effective in prevention and treatment of stress urinary incontinence [28, 29], and the same theories may apply for a possible effect of PFMT to prevent and treat POP.

The two hypotheses are: (1) women learn to consciously contract before and during increases in abdominal pressure (also termed "bracing" or "performing the Knack"), and continue to perform such contractions as a behavior modification to prevent descent of the pelvic floor; and (2) women are taught to perform regular strength training in order to build up "stiffness" and structural support of the pelvic floor over time [28].

50.4.1 Conscious Contraction (Bracing or "Performing the Knack") to Prevent and Treat POP

Research on basic and functional anatomy supports conscious contraction of the PFM as an effective maneuver to stabilize the pelvic floor [30, 31]. However, to date, there are no studies on how much strength or what neuromotor control strategies are necessary to prevent descent during cough and other physical exertions, nor how to prevent gradual descent due to activities of daily living or over time. Brækken et al [23] found that advice to do "the Knack" and not to strain on defecation improved prolapse stage in 4% [23], but no morphological changes of the PFM were found after this training modality [25].

An interesting, but difficult hypothesis to test, is whether women at risk for POP can prevent development of prolapse by performing "the Knack" during a rise in intra-abdominal pressure. Since it is possible to learn to hold a hand over the mouth before and during coughing, one would expect that it is possible to learn to pre-contract the PFM before and during simple and single tasks such as coughing, lifting, and isolated exercises such as performing abdominal exercises. However, multiple task activities and repetitive movements such as running, playing tennis, aerobics, and dance activities cannot be conducted with intentional co-contractions of the PFM.

50.4.2 Strength Training

The theoretical rationale for intensive strength training of the PFM to treat POP is that strength training may build up the structural support of the pelvis by:

- elevating the levator plate to a permanently higher location inside the pelvis
- enhancing hypertrophy and stiffness of the PFM and connective tissue, reducing muscle length
- constricting the levator hiatus.

As described by DeLancey [32] in the "boat in dry dock" theory, the connective tissue support of the pelvic organs fails if the PFM relax or are damaged, and organ descent occurs. This underpins the concept of elevation of the PFM and closure of the urogenital hiatus as important elements in conservative management of POP.

All the RCTs in this area have used strength training principles in the treatment protocols. However, Brækken et al [23] was the only research group measuring PFM strength increase in both randomized arms. They found a significant and huge increase in strength in the PFMT group only. They also found statistically significant increases in muscle volume, shortening of the muscle length, constriction of the levator hiatus, and lifting of the bladder neck and rectal ampulla [25], factors that may be essential in prevention and reversion of POP (Table 50.1).

50.5 Should PFMT be an Adjunct to Prolapse Surgery?

Surgery for POP is common, with a lifetime risk of undergoing a single operation for either prolapse or incontinence by the age of 80 years of 11.1% [13]. However, rates of recurrence of POP after surgery are found to be up to 58% [12]. The accurate recurrence rate is not known, as many women do not re-present for repeat surgery, despite the recurrence of POP. A 29.2% re-operation rate for POP has been found [13].

Jarvis et al [33] studied the effect of PFMT and bladder/bowel training on women undergoing surgery for POP/urinary incontinence, with an RCT of 60 women. Thirty women were randomized to each of the treatment and control groups. The intervention consisted of PFMT, functional bracing of PFM prior to rises in abdominal pressure, bladder/bowel training, and advice to reduce straining during voiding and defecation. Significant improvements in quality of life and symptom-specific scores were found in the treatment group. Subjects in the treatment group also demonstrated an increase in digital palpation score and maximum vaginal squeeze pressure compared with subjects in the control group, who showed a decrease in squeeze pressure.

In an assessor-blinded RCT comparing the effect of POP surgery with and without a structured physiotherapy program, Frawley et al [34] did not find any significant effect of PFMT at one-year follow-up after surgery. The physiotherapy intervention comprised a PFM strength-training protocol, supplemented by bladder and bowel advice.

This was provided over eight sessions: one preoperative and seven postoperative sessions – day 3 postoperatively, weeks 6, 7, 8, 10, and 12, and a final appointment at 9 months postoperatively.

Table 50.1 Randomized controlled trials (RCTs) on pelvic floor muscle training (PFMT) to treat pelvic organ prolapse (POP)

Author, year	Design	Population	Intervention
Piya-Anant et al, 2003 [24]	RCT	654 women > 60 years in Thailand; anterior vaginal wall POP	(1) PFMT: 2 years of 30 contractions/day + eat more fruit and vegetables and drink 2 L water/ day; (2) control: no intervention, same follow-up
Hagen et al, 2004 [21]	Assessor-blinded RCT	47 women, mean age 56 years (SD 9 years) in UK, with symptomatic stages I and II POP UK; all kinds of POP	(1) PFMT for 16 weeks, 5 visits with physiotherapist, 6 sets of 10 maximal contractions/day, use of diary + lifestyle advice sheet; (2) lifestyle advice sheet
Ghroubi et al, 2008 [22]	RCT	47 women mean age 53.4 years (SD 11 years) from Tunis; stages I and II anterior vaginal wall POP	(1) PFMT + advice on healthy living; (2) control: no treatment
Brækken et al, 2009 [25]	Assessor-blinded RCT	109 women, mean age 48.8 years (SD 11.8 years), mean BMI 25.6 kg/m^2 (SD 4.5 kg/m^2), mean parity 2.4 (0.7), with POP-Q stages I, II, and III; all kinds of POP	(1) PFMT: information on not to strain on toilet + "the Knack"; 3 sets of 8–12 contractions/day, diary; weekly visits with physiotherapist for 3 months, then every second week for 3 months; (2) control: instruction not to strain on toilet; "the Knack"

BMI, body mass index; *ICIQ UI-SF*, International Consultation on Incontinence Questionnaire, Urinary Incontinence Short Form; *QOL*, quality of life; *SD*, standard deviation; *VAS*, visual analog scale

Adherence and drop-out	Outcome measures	Results
Adherence: not reported; drop-out: not reported; no report of how many drank water and ate more vegetables	No, mild or severe prolapse assessed by Valsalva maneuver on vaginal examination	PFMT: 27% worsening; control: 72% worsening; P = 0.005; effect only seen in severe prolapse
Drop-out not reported; POP-Q data missing for 27/47; 91% attended at least 3 physiotherapy sessions, 65% attended 5 visits; 61% rated as good/moderate compliers	POP-Q; prolapse sysmptoms; QoL/interference of daily living; self report of change in POP; Oxford grading for PFM strength only in exercise group	PFMT significantly more likely to have improved POP stage (45% vs. 0%, P = 0.04), significant greater decrease in POP symptoms (3.5 vs. 0.1, P = 0.021), significantly more likely to say their POP was better (63% vs. 24%); no difference in urinary, bowel or vaginal symptoms; Oxford grading ($n = 15$): significant improvement in exercise group: mean 0.5 (95% CI: 0.2–0.8)
Drop-out and adherence not known	Clinical examination; "urinary handicap scale" maximal urethral pressure; urodynamic tests; Ditrovie quality of life scale; patient satisfaction (VAS)	PFMT: heaviness – 18.5%; control: heaviness 70%; significantly better report on urinary handicap in PFMT; pelvic heaviness: 18.5% in PFMT and 70% in control after treatment, P < 0.001; uroflowmetry showed significant improvement in maximum flow rate
One drop-out in each group; 79% adhered to ≥ 80% of exercise sessions	POP-Q; ultrasound of bladder and rectal position at rest; symptoms and bother [25]); ICIQ UI-SF; muscle strength	POP-Q stage: 11 (19%) in the PFMT vs. 4 (8%) controls improved one stage (P = 0.04); elevation of the bladder neck: ↑ 2.3 mm vs. ↓0.6 mm; difference: 3.0 mm (95% CI 1.5–4.4), P < 0.001; elevation of the rectal ampulla: ↑4.4 mm vs. ↓1.1 mm, difference: 5.5 mm (95% CI 1.4–7.3), P = 0.02; symptoms: • vaginal bulging/heaviness: ↓ frequency: 32/43 vs. 8/26; P < 0.01 • ↓bother: 29/43 vs. 11/26; P < 0.01; ICIQ-UI-SF: effect size 0.66 in favour of PFMT, difference 2.63 (95% CI 0.95–4.30), P < 0.01; bowel symptoms: no effect on emptying or solid fecal incontinence; flatus frequency: difference 31.2% (95% CI 0.7–55) P < 0.01; bother: difference 25.3% (95% CI 1.5–49.1) P < 0.01; loose fecal incontinence, frequency: difference 68.6% (95% CI 40.2–97.0) P < 0.01; bother: difference 64.3% (95% CI 39.2–89.4) P < 0.01; strength (P < 0.01): • PFMT: ↑13.1 cmH_2O (95% CI: 10.6–15.5) • control: ↑1.1 cm H_2O (95% CI 0.4–2.7), effect size 1.21 ; endurance (P < 0.01): • PFMT: ↑107 cmH_2O sec (95% CI 77.0–136.4) • control: ↑8 cmH_2O sec (95% CI –7.4–24.1), effect size 0.96

50.6   Conclusions

To date there are only four RCTs in the area of PFMT and treatment of POP, and only one of these is a full-scale study using POP and ultrasound to assess POP stage and bladder and bowel position. The study showed that significantly more women in the PFMT group improved one POP stage compared to the control group. In addition, the study demonstrated significant reduction of POP symptoms (heaviness and bulging) and bladder and bowel sysmptoms. The overall results are supported by the three other RCTs of lower methodological quality. Further studies are needed to address which women respond to training and if POP can be prevented. A suggested primary prevention strategy for the general female population would be to avoid straining, to learn to contract the PFM during an increase in intra-abdominal pressure, and to conduct regular strength training of the PFM.

References

1. Hunskaar S, Burigo K, Clark A et al. Epidemiology of POP. In: Abrams P, Cardozo L, Khoury S, Wein A (eds) Incontinence. Health Publication Ltd, Plymouth, 2005, pp 290–298.
2. Nygaard I, Barber MD, Burgio KL et al. Prevalence of symptomatic pelvic floor disorders in US women. JAMA 2008;300:1311–1316.
3. Tegerstedt G, Maehle-Schmidt M, Nyren O, Hammarstrom M. Prevalence of symptomatic pelvic organ prolapse in a Swedish population. Int Urogynecol J Pelvic Floor Dysfunct 2005;16:497–503.
4. Slieker-Ten Hove MC, Pool-Goudzwaard AL, Eijkemans MJ et al. Symptomatic pelvic organ prolapse and possible risk factors in a general population. Am J Obstet Gynecol 2009;200:184–187.
5. Lawrence JM, Lukacz ES, Nager CW et al. Prevalence and co-occurrence of pelvic floor disorders in community-dwelling women. Obstet Gynecol 2008;111:678–685.
6. Mouritsen L. Classification and evaluation of prolapse. Best Pract Res Clin Obstet Gynaecol 2005;19:895–911.
7. Srikrishna S, Robinson D, Cardozo L. Validation of the patient global impression of improvement for urogenital prolapse. Int Urogynecol J 2009;20(suppl 2):S95.
8. Abrams P, Cardozo L, Fall M et al. The standardisation of terminology of lower urinary tract function: report from the Standardisation Sub-committee of the International Continence Society. Neurourol Urodyn 2002;21:167–178.
9. Weber AM, Abrams P, Brubaker L et al. The standardization of terminology for researchers in female pelvic floor disorders. Int Urogynecol J Pelvic Floor Dysfunct 2001;12: 178–186.
10. Brubaker L, Bump RC, Jacquetin B et al. Pelvic organ prolapse. In: Abrams P, Cardozo L, Khoury S, Wein A (eds) Incontinence: 2nd International Consultation on Incontinence, 2 edn. Health Publication Ltd, Plymouth, 2002, pp 243–266.
11. Thakar R, Stanton S. Management of genital prolapse. BMJ 2002;324:1258–1262.
12. Whiteside JL, Weber AM, Meyn LA, Walters MD. Risk factors for prolapse recurrence after vaginal repair. Am J Obstet Gynecol 2004;191:1533–1538.
13. Olsen AL, Smith VJ, Bergstrom JO et al. Epidemiology of surgically managed pelvic organ prolapse and urinary incontinence. Obstet Gynecol 1997;89:501–506.
14. Handa VL, Garrett E, Hendrix S et al. Progression and remission of pelvic organ prolapse: a longitudinal study of menopausal women. Am J Obstet Gynecol 2004;190:27–32.
15. Hahn I, Myrhage R. Bekkenbotten. Bygnad, funktion och traning. AnaKomp AB, Goethenburg, 1999, p 39.
16. Maher C, Baessler K, Glazener CM et al. Surgical management of pelvic organ prolapse in women. Cochrane Database Syst Rev 2007;(3):CD004014.
17. Hagen S, Stark D, Maher C, Adams E. Conservative management of pelvic organ prolapse in women. Cochrane Database Syst Rev 2006;(4):CD003882.
18. Dumoulin C, Hay-Smith J. Pelvic floor muscle training versus no treatment for urinary incontinence in women. A Cochrane systematic review. Eur J Phys Rehabil Med 2008; 44:47–63.
19. Hay Smith J, Berghmans B, Burgio K et al. Adult conservative management. In: Abrams P, Cardozo L, Khoury S, Wein A (eds) Incontinence: 4th International Consultation on Incontinence, 4th edn. Health Publication Ltd, Plymouth, 2009, pp 1025–1108.
20. Hagen S, Stark D, Cattermole D. A United Kingdom-wide survey of physiotherapy practice in the treatment of pelvic organ prolapse. Physiotherapy 2004;90:19–26.
21. Hagen S, Stark D, Glazener C et al. A randomized controlled trial of pelvic floor muscle training for stages I and II pelvic organ prolapse. Int Urogynecol J Pelvic Floor Dysfunct 2009;20:45–51.
22. Ghroubi S, Kharrat O, Chaari M. Effect of conservative treatment in the management of low-degree urogenital prolapse. Ann Readapt Med Phys 2008;51:96–102.
23. Brækken IH, Majida M, Ellstrom-Engh M, Bø K. Pelvic floor muscle training in treatment of pelvic organ prolapse - A single blind randomised controlled trial. Neurourol Urodyn 2009;28:663–664.
24. Piya-Anant M, Therasakvichya S, Leelaphatanadit C, Techatrisak K. Integrated health research program for the Thai elderly: prevalence of genital prolapse and effectiveness of pelvic floor exercise to prevent worsening of genital prolapse in elderly women. J Med Assos Thail 2003;86:509–515.
25. Brækken IH, Majida M, Ellstrom-Engh M, Bø K. Morphological changes after pelvic floor muscle training measured by 3-dimensional ultrasound: a randomized controlled trial. Obstet Gynecol 2010; 115, Part I: 317-324.
26. Mouritsen, L, Larsen JP. Symptoms, bother and POPQ in women referred with pelvic organ prolapse. Int Urogynecol J 2003;4:122–127.
27. Bø K, Aschehoug A. Pelvic floor and exercise science -

strength training. In: Bo K, Berghmans B, Morkved S, Kampen MV (eds) Evidence-based physical therapy for the pelvic floor. Elsevier, Edinburgh, 2007, pp 119–132.

28. Bø K. Pelvic floor muscle training is effective in treatment of female stress urinary incontinence, but how does it work? Int Urogynecol J Pelvic Floor Dysfunct 2004;15:76–84.

29. Bø K. Pelvic floor muscle training for stress urinary incontinence. In: Bo K, Berghmans B, Morkved S, Kampen MV (eds) Evidence-based physical therapy for the pelvic floor. Elsevier, Edinburgh, 2007, pp 171–187.

30. Miller JM, Perucchini D, Carchidi LT et al. Pelvic floor muscle contraction during a cough and decreased vesical neck mobility. Obstet Gynecol 2001;97:255–260.

31. Peschers UM, Fanger G, Schaer GN et al. Bladder neck mobility in continent nulliparous women. BJOG 2001;108:320–324.

32. DeLancey JO. Anatomy and biomechanics of genital prolapse. Clin Obstet Gynecol 1993;36:897–909.

33. Jarvis SK, Hallam TK, Dietz HP, Vancaille TG. Pre and postoperative physiotherapy intervention for gynaecological surgery: a single blind randomized controlled trial (abstract 65). J Am Assoc Gynecol Laparosc 2004;11(3 suppl):S23.

34. Frawley HC, Phillips BA, Bø K, Galea MP. Physiotherapy as an adjunct to prolapse surgery: An assessor-blinded randomized controlled trial. Neurourol Urodyn 2009; 8 Oct epub ahead of print.

Medical Treatment of Irritable Bowel Syndrome, Constipation, and Obstructed Defecation

51

Pier Francesco Almerigi, Mauro Menarini and Gabriele Bazzocchi

Abstract The treatment of bowel dysfunction is a common medical challenge, due to the high prevalence and complexity of constipation among the populations of western countries. The aim of this chapter is to point out the main elements of the medical treatment of the bowel functional disorders that may afflict the pelvic floor. Irritable bowel syndrome (IBS) may feature constipation (IBS-C) or diarrhea (IBS-D) as predominant dysfunction, or even alternating symptoms (IBS-A). IBS can be treated with traditional therapies (antidiarrheals, dietary modifications, fiber supplementation, bulking agents, osmotic laxatives, tricyclic antidepressants, and antispasmodics). Currently, evaluation of new agents (agonists and antagonists of serotonin receptors, adrenergic modulators, chloride channel activators, probiotics, and others) is in progress. The treatment of slow transit constipation (STC) may feature therapy of the comorbidities that may result in constipation – dietary suggestions, lifestyle changes, correction of bowel habits, and laxatives, but new agents are also taken in consideration. Obstructed defecation (OD) can be treated by aiming to decrease the consistency of the stool and facilitate rectal evacuation. Many patients affected by OD and correctly treated with conservative therapies can obtain relief from their symptoms and avoid surgical treatment.

Keywords Bulking agents • Chloride channel activators • Irritable bowel syndrome • Laxatives • Lubiprostone • Medical treatment • Obstructed defecation • Probiotics • Serotonin receptors • Slow transit constipation

51.1 Introduction

The treatment of bowel dysfunction is a common medical challenge, due to the broad range of different forms of constipation and their high prevalence among the populations of western countries (from 2% to 27%, with a female predominance) [1]. The aim of this chapter is to point out the main elements of the extremely complex medical treatment of this range of functional disorders that may primarily or secondarily afflict the pelvic floor.

51.2 Medical Treatment of Irritable Bowel Syndrome

Irritable bowel syndrome (IBS) is a gastrointestinal disorder characterized by abdominal pain and discomfort in association with altered bowel habits. IBS can

G. Bazzocchi
Unit of Visceral Disorders and Anatomic Dysfunction,
Montecatone Rehabilitation Institute, University of Bologna,
Imola, Italy

G.A. Santoro, A.P. Wieczorek, C.I. Bartram (eds.) *Pelvic Floor Disorders*
© Springer-Verlag Italia 2010

feature constipation as the predominant dysfunction (IBS-C) or diarrhea (IBS-D), or even alternating symptoms of constipation and diarrhea (IBS-A) [2]. The pathophysiology of IBS is considered to be multifactorial, involving disturbances of the brain–gut axis: IBS has been associated with abnormal gastrointestinal motor functions, visceral hypersensitivity, psychosocial factors, autonomic dysfunction, and mucosal inflammation [3].

The general goal of treatment is to alleviate the symptoms of abdominal pain, altered bowel transit (diarrhea or constipation), and any associated symptoms such as bloating and fecal incontinence [2].

In all cases, it is of great importance to educate the patient about the nature of his syndrome and the origin of symptoms. The patient should be aware that his condition is a real medical disorder and that a single drug is not likely to eradicate all symptoms, but also has to know that IBS is a benign process associated with a normal life expectancy [4].

51.2.1 Traditional Therapies

The traditional IBS therapies are directed mainly at the relief of symptoms. They include antidiarrheals (diphenoxylate, loperamide, etc), dietary modifications, fiber supplementation, bulking agents, osmotic laxatives (magnesium salt, lactulose, polyethylene glycol, etc), tricyclic antidepressants (desipramine, amitriptyline, etc), and antispasmodics. These treatments are not always completely successful and have been subject of much discussion.

Loperamide is probably the most widely used drug for IBS-D, but although it decreases stool frequency and improves stool consistency, it does not affect abdominal pain in IBS-D, and should be considered only in painless diarrhea.

The use of bulking agents and fiber is also commonly considered for the treatment of IBS-D, but it remains a controversial issue due to methodological limitations in clinical trials. Bulking agents can result in abnormal bacterial fermentation and may cause bloating and abdominal pain, worsening the clinical outcome of IBS patients. The American College of Gastroenterology Functional Gastrointestinal Disorders Task Force (ACG-CCTF) currently recommends the use of fiber in constipation but not in IBS [5].

For some of these agents (antidepressants and antispasmodics), a poor study design and methodological flaws in clinical trials make it difficult to judge their real therapeutic value [3].

The development of knowledge on the pathophysiology of IBS is leading to the introduction of many new therapeutics approaches, although most need further large trials before reaching a proven efficacy [3].

51.2.2 New Agents – Serotonin Axis

Serotonin (5-hydroxytryptamine, 5-HT) is the most important neurotrasmitter in the pathogenesis of IBS. While its exact role in this disorder is not yet fully understood, pharmacotherapy directed at modulating its activity has proved to be an effective way of treating many IBS symptoms [2]. Antagonists of the 5-HT3 receptor (alosetron, ramosetron) are effective in decreasing small bowel and colonic transit time, increasing stool firmness, and reducing intestinal secretion and visceral pain. These agents are indicated in the treatment of IBS-D [6, 7].

Piboserod, a 5-HT4 antagonist, tends to delay colonic transit time in patients affected by IBS-D, but further studies are needed to confirm these results [8].

Agonists of the 5-HT4 receptor (tegaserod, prucalopride) stimulate intestinal secretion of water and chloride, and decrease the nociceptive response to rectal distension. The use of these agents seems to be effective in women with IBS-C but does not result in improvement of bowel symptoms in men [9, 10].

Mixed 5-HT4 agonist/5-HT3 antagonists (renzapride and mosapride) have shown promise for patients with IBS-C and IBS-A, and further studies are under way [11, 12].

ATI-7505 is a potent agonist of the 5-HT4 receptor, and preliminary data seem to show good effectiveness in IBS-C [13].

51.2.3 New Agents – Adrenergic Modulators

Clonidine, an $\alpha 2$ agonist originally developed as antihypertensive agent, has been shown to increase colonic compliance, delay small bowel transit, and reduce colonic tone and sensitivity to distension. It may play a role in the treatment of IBS-D but few data are currently available [14].

51.2.4 New Agents – Future Research

Many other different agents are currently under development for clinical use in IBS. The main areas of research are investigating the use of octreotide, opioid agents, corticotropin-releasing hormone receptor antagonists, chloride channel activators (lubiprostone), cholecystokinin antagonists, neurokinin antagonists, benzodiazepines, and antibiotics [2].

51.2.5 The Use of Probiotics in the Treatment of IBS

The utility of probiotics in the treatment of IBS has been suggested by many authors. The rationale for this kind of therapy is based on the presence of low-grade inflammation and immune activation in some patients with IBS, which suggests that alterations in indigenous gut flora may play a role in this disorder. Probiotics may work by qualitative and quantitative restoration of intestinal flora. Unfortunately, a large number of studies with poor methodological and statistical design have been published [15]. The most rigorous studies have shown good efficacy of Bifidobacterium infantis [16, 17], the probiotic cocktail VSL#3 [18], and Lactobacillus plantarum alone [19] or in combination with Bifidobacterium breve or L. acidophilus [20].

Although the evidence is still limited, the absence of dangerous side-effects suggests consideration of probiotics in the treatment of IBS [21].

51.3 Medical Treatment of Slow-transit Constipation

Slow-transit constipation (STC) is a bowel dysfunction characterized by prolongation of transit time through the colon [22]. Causes of STC are often multifactorial: endocrine or metabolic disorders, neurologic disorders (Parkinson's disease, multiple sclerosis, spinal lesions, autonomic neuropathy, etc), psychiatric disorders (depression and eating disorders), pharmacologic agents (opiates, anticholinergics and antidepressants), and lifestyle factors (dietary, repressed urge to defecate, physical inactivity).

The medical treatment of this kind of bowel dysfunction must be integrated with therapy of the comorbidities that may result in constipation. It must begin with advice to increase the intake of fluids (1.5–2 L/day), fiber (20–25 g/day of bran, psyllium, methylcellulose, or polycarbophil), and probiotics, a minimal physical activity and correction of bowel habits, responding to the urge to defecate without excessive delay or prolonged sitting and straining.

Despite its widespread use, fiber supplementation is sufficiently effective in only a subset of patients [23]. Two recent systematic reviews [24, 25] have shown a lack of high-quality data demonstrating the efficacy of the most commonly used kind of fiber. The ACG-CCTF recommends the use of psyllium in chronic constipation as the only bulking agent of proven efficacy in increasing stool frequency. Rankumar and Rao, following the parameters established by the US Providence Services Task Force found evidence of the efficacy of psyllium, calcium polycarbophil, methylcellulose, and bran [25].

A second level is based on the use of laxatives: osmotic laxatives are effective but not always well tolerated because of poor efficacy on abdominal cramping, bloating, and flatulence [23]; magnesium or sodium phosphate are also effective but can only be used for limited periods due to adverse effects; lactulose is very effective but may exacerbate bloating because of its metabolism along the colon; stimulant laxatives (senna, bisacodyl, etc) may be considered after failure of the previous agents, but data supporting their long-term use are inadequate [22, 23].

The newest agents used for the treatment of chronic idiopathic constipation, which have shown proven efficacy, are the neurotransmitter serotonin receptor agonists. Among these, tegaserod is the one that has shown the best clinical results and long-term safety and efficacy [23].

Lubiprostone (a selective chloride channel activator), inducing intestinal water secretion, is effective in the treatment of chronic constipation as demonstrated in several trials [26–28], but its clinical applicability is still to be determined.

It has been suggested that probiotics should be considered for treatment of STC. As for IBS, the real efficacy is still not completely clear because of a lack of high-quality large trials. The most reliable data showing good results are those obtained with Bifidobacterium infantis [16, 17], the probiotic cocktail VSL#3 [18], and Lactobacillus plantarum alone [19] or in combination with Bifidobacterium breve or

L. acidophilus [20]. Absolute changes in defecation and other symptoms are always very rare in these studies, making the clinical use of probiotics a treatment that still has uncertain results.

In particular situations, such as spinal cord injuries, it has been shown that transanal irrigation can result in a better improvement of constipation and quality of life compared to conservative bowel management [29].

51.4   Medical Treatment of Obstructed Defecation

Obstructed defecation (OD) is the inability to evacuate contents from the rectum and may be the symptomatic expression of many underlying pathological conditions. This disorder is commonly known by numerous terms such as anismus, outlet obstruction, pelvic floor dyssynergia, paradoxical puborectalis syndrome, and others. Most commonly, these terms are not completely exact or are insufficient to define this disorder because they usually seem to focus on a certain dysfunction of the muscular motility of the pelvic floor during defecation straining, while this is very often only a part of the problem. OD may feature rectoanal intussusception, pelvic organ prolapse, rectocele, sigmoidocele, enterocele, solitary rectal ulcer syndrome, and a descending perineum. In the majority of cases, these anatomical abnormalities can be detected, as well as a real lack of coordination of the pelvic floor muscles (dyssynergia), which may lead to missed sphincter and puborectalis relaxation during defecation or even to a paradoxical contraction [1]. A muscular dyssynergia may lead to anatomical consequences but the opposite is also possible. Pathological behaviors or chronic slow colon transit constipation or an association of these features may lead to repeated prolonged and unsuccessful straining attempts that may result in pelvic organ prolapse and then to dyssynergia.

In any case of OD, the initial therapy is always conservative. The aim is to decrease the consistency of the stool and facilitate rectal evacuation. This treatment includes adequate hydration (1.5–2 L/day), a high fiber intake (20–30 g/day), the use of probiotics, regular physical activity, enemas, and laxatives. It has been shown that polyethylene glycol (PEG) improves the symptoms of OD in a large proportion of patients with "organic" ano-rectal disease in which

surgical treatment was taken into consideration [30].

Biofeedback training may be added to the first-line therapy, particularly in cases of dyssynergia [1].

References

1. Khaikin M, Wexner SD. Treatment strategies in obstructed defecation and fecal incontinence. World J Gastroenterol 2006;12:3168–3173.
2. Hammerle CW, Surawicz CM. Updates on treatment of irritable bowel syndrome. World J Gastroenterol 2008;14:2639–2649.
3. Pohl D, Tutuian R, Fried M. Pharmacologic treatment of constipation: what is new? Curr Opin Pharmacol 2008; 8:724–728.
4. Owens DM, Nelson DK, Talley NJ. The irritable bowel syndrome: long term prognosis and the physician-patient interaction. Ann Intern Med 1995;122:107–112.
5. Brandt LJ, Bjorkman D, Fennerty MB et al. Systematic review on the management of irritable bowel syndrome in North America. Am J Gastroenterol 2002;97:S7–S26.
6. Camilleri M, Mayer EA, Drossman DA et al. Improvement in pain and bowel function in female irritable bowel patients with alosetron, a 5-HT3 receptor antagonist. Aliment Pharmacol Ther 1999;13:1149–1159.
7. Hirata T, Keto Y, Funatsu T et al. Evaluation of the pharmacological profile of ramosetron, a novel therapeutic agent for irritable bowel syndrome. J Pharmacol Sci 2007;104:263–273.
8. Bharucha AE, Camilleri M, Haydock S et al. Effects of a serotonin 5-HT(4) receptor antagonist SB-207266 on gastrointestinal motor and sensory function in humans. Gut 2000;47:667–674.
9. Prather CM, Camilleri M, Zinsmeister AR et al. Tegaserod accelerates orocecal transit in patients with constipation-predominant irritable bowel syndrome. Gastroenterology 2000;118:463–468.
10. Coremans G, Kerstens R, De Pauw M et al. Prucalopride is effective in patients with severe chronic constipation in whom laxatives fail to provide adequate relief. Results of a double-blind, placebo-controlled clinical trial. Digestion 2003; 67:82–89.
11. Camilleri M, McKinzie S, Fox J et al. Effect of renzapride on transit in constipation-predominant irritable bowel syndrome. Clin Gastroenterol Hepatol 2004;2:895–904.
12. Liu Z, Sabakibara R, Odaka T et al. Mosapride citrate, a novel 5-HT4 agonist and partial 5-HT3 antagonist, ameliorates constipation in parkinsonian patients. Mov Disord 2005;20:680–686.
13. Foxx-Orenstein AE, Camilleri M, Szarka LA et al. Does coadministration of a non-selective opiate antagonist enhance acceleration of transit by a 5-HT4 agonist in constipation-predominant irritable bowel syndrome? A randomised controlled trial. Neurogastroenterol Motil 2007;19:821–830.
14. Camilleri M, Kim DY, McKinzie S et al. A randomised, controlled exploratory study of clonidine in diarrhea-predominant irritable bowel syndrome. Clin Gastroenterol Hepatol 2003;1:111–121.
15. Brenner DM, Moeller MJ, Chey WD et al. The utility of probiotics in the treatment of irritable bowel syndrome: a systematic review. Am J Gastroenterol 2009;104:1033–1049.

16. O'Mahony L, McCarthy J, Kelly P et al. Lactobacillus and bifidobacterium in irritable bowel syndrome: symptom responses and relationship to cytokine profiles. Gastroenterology 2005;128:541–51.

17. Whorwell PJ, Altringer, L, Morel J et al. Efficacy of an encapsulated probiotic Bifidobacterium infantis 35624 in women with irritable bowel syndrome. Am J Gastroenterol 2006;101:1581–1590.

18. Kim HJ, Camilleri M, McKinzie S et al. A randomized controlled trial of a probiotic, VSL#3, on gut transit and symptoms in diarrhea-predominant irritable bowel syndrome. Aliment Pharmacol Ther 2003;17:895–904.

19. Nidzielin K, Kordecki H, Birkenfeld B. A controlled, doubleblind, randomized study on the efficacy of lactobacillus plantarum 299V in patients with irritable bowel syndrome. Eur J Gastroenterol Hepatol 2001;13:1143–1147.

20. Saggioro A. Probiotics in the treatment of irritable bowel syndrome. J Clin Gastroenterol 2004;38(6 suppl):S104–S106.

21. Andresen V, Camilleri M. Irritable bowel syndrome. Recent and novel therapeutic approaches. Drugs 2006;66:1073–1088.

22. Wong SW, Lubowski DZ. Slow-transit constipation: evaluation and treatment. A N Z J Surg 2007;77:320–328.

23. Johanson JF. Review of the treatment options for chronic constipation. MedGenMed 2007;9:25.

24. Brandt LJ, Schoenfeld P, Prather CM et al. Evidenced-based position statement on the management of chronic constipation in North America. Am J Gastroenterol 2005; 100(suppl):S1–S21.

25. Ramkumar D, Rao SSC. Efficacy and safety of traditional medical therapies for chronic constipation: systematic review. Am J Gastroenterol 2005;100:936–971.

26. Johanson JF, Gargano MA, Holland PC et al. Phase III study of lubiprostone, a chloride channel 2 (CIC-2) activator for the treatment of constipation: safety and primary efficacy. Am J Gastroenterol 2005;100(suppl):S328–S329.

27. Johanson JF, Gargano MA, Holland PC et al. Initial and sustained effects of lubiprostone, a chloride channel-2 (CIC-2) activator for the treatment of constipation: data from a 4-weeks phase III study. Am J Gastroenterol 2005;100(suppl): S324–S325.

28. Johanson JF, Gargano MA, Holland PC. Phase III efficacy and safety of RU-0211, a novel chloride channel activator, for the treatment of constipation Gastroenterology 2003;124:A104.

29. Christensen P, Bazzocchi G, Coggrave M et al. A randomised, controlled trial of transanal irrigation versus conservative bowel management in spinal cord-injured patients Gastroenterology 2006;131:738–747.

30. Bazzocchi G. Polyethylene glycol solution in subgroups of chronic constipation patients: experience in obstructed defaecation. Ital J Gasroenterol Hepatol 1999;31(suppl 3): S257–S259.

The concept of the "boat in dry dock" pioneered by John DeLancey has come to be recognized as central to our understanding of the biomechanics of the female pelvic floor. Failure, or more rarely rupture, of the connective tissue "ropes" allows the pelvic organs to descend through the urogenital hiatus. Additionally, collapse of the anterior vaginal wall allows formation of a cystocele, and if this affects the posterior vaginal wall a rectocele results. Frequently, but not invariably, these anatomical deficits result in symptoms – bladder or bowel evacuation and continence difficulties, and sexual dysfunction, as well as symptoms related to the physical presence of the prolapse. Quality of life is almost inevitably impaired, and over 10% of women from developed countries (in a society of increasing age) have undergone corrective pelvic floor surgery by the age of 80 years. The importance of conservative therapies for this condition is, therefore, of vital importance.

Pelvic floor retraining is inevitably directed at muscle function, and cannot directly target connective tissue. However, surgical correction of connective tissues is often fraught, not least as many individuals are known to have benign joint hypermobility. The role of muscle retraining as an adjuvant to pelvic floor surgery has not been formally studied, and such trials would inevitably be very difficult to undertake with sufficient clinical rigor. In considering pelvic floor muscle retraining for prolapse, there is an inherent problem. More severe prolapse occurs in patients with more severe pelvic floor weakness, who are able to exercise less well. Equally, the downward prolapse of the organs onto the pelvic musculature will further compromise the function of these muscles by causing passive lengthening of the muscle fibers.

The randomized controlled trials of this intervention to date have been well summarized in Kari Bø's chapter (Chapter 50). Benefit is seen in terms of reducing both the severity of the prolapse, and, more easily, the severity of symptoms associated with prolapse. The shortcomings of randomized studies in this field are also well described in the chapter. One additional factor is that women with prolapse are often co-treated with vaginal pessaries. As such, an ideal trial would also account and stratify for those women with such mechanical support devices. One other critical factor that has been little addressed in outcome measures of these studies is the issue of bowel function. It is well described that women with pelvic organ prolapse often have fecal incontinence, and as many as one-third have bowel-evacuation difficulties. The studies to date have generally failed to address this important comorbidity. A final factor relates to the need for a large – probably multicenter – study to assess the role of pelvic floor muscle retraining in prevention of prolapse and prolapse symptoms. This would need to be a study not only of a large number of patients, but also over a long period to meet clinically meaningful endpoints.

Several whole textbooks have been devoted to the medical management of each of the three conditions irritable bowel syndrome (IBS), anismus, and constipation, so summarizing a topic into one chapter is an impossible challenge. This commentary will inevitably suffer from the same fault of omission, and will inevitably just reflect personal viewpoints.

The various options for medical therapy of IBS have been outlined in Chapter 51. The critical question relates to the sequence of treatments, especially in view of the fact that most treatments benefit only a minority. As such it is often pragmatic to prescribe the safest and most inexpensive options. A clinical trial investigating the efficacy of initiating such an algorithmic ap-

A. Emmanuel
GI Physiology Unit, University College Hospital, London, UK

proach would be beneficial. In most IBS subjects, reducing dietary fiber, especially insoluble cereal fiber, can be beneficial. Tricyclic agents are frequently used, and with a "number needed to treat" of 4, they represent a cost-effective and efficacious option. Hypnotherapy has a particular place in medical management, as although not widely available, it is of proven efficacy in the majority of patients. It offers long-lasting symptom improvements and is especially effective in patients without psychiatric comorbidity. Apart from these medical interventions aimed at definitive relief of IBS, the general approach is to focus on the predominant symptom: anti-diarrheals for IBS with diarrhea, laxatives for IBS with constipation, and anti-spasmodics where pain is predominant. Bloating represents a frequently encountered and difficult to treat comorbidity. Newer serotonin-receptor agents and probiotics are aimed at specific subgroups of IBS patients, but are often aimed at addressing more general pathophysiological disturbances associated with the diagnosis of IBS.

The issues surrounding newer agents being developed for IBS, and prokinetics for slow-transit constipation relate to two key questions. First is the issue of the safety of the proposed agents – this is vitally important given that the disorders they are treating are benign ones. The ischemic colitis and cardiac toxicity of drugs such as alosetron and tegaserod have seen these agents withdrawn from the market shortly after release, and underlie the importance of this issue. The second key question relates to the duration of treatment. These are chronic conditions with long-term symptom persistence. As such the efficacy of drugs needs to be considered in longer terms than the standard 12 weeks of clinical studies. The cost of these drugs must also be taken into account when considering long-term use, even with agents such as probiotics.

The management of evacuation difficulties revolves around identifying whether there is a substantial anatomical defect that needs addressing. In situations where this is not the case, biofeedback and pelvic floor muscle training is central to management. Suppositories and enemas offer long-term options for managing symptoms in patients who are refractory to biofeedback or where it is not available. Transanal irrigation for nonneurogenic bowel dysfunction is a controversial option given the rare, but serious, complication of bowel perforation. Again, for benign conditions, albeit with significant impact on quality of life, the use of interventions with significant adverse effects must be especially carefully considered.

Section VII
Pelvic Pain

Pelvic Pain: Introduction

Ewa Kuligowska

Chronic pelvic pain is a common, disabling problem among women. Although chronic pelvic pain can be produced by many conditions, some causes are frequently overlooked and under-diagnosed, resulting in inappropriate referral and inadequate treatment.

Patients with chronic pelvic pain can present both diagnostic and therapeutic challenges for the clinician. Chronic pelvic pain is a common and disabling condition that is defined as non-menstrual pain of at least 6 months' duration [1, 2]. The sources of pelvic pain are multifactorial, and their causes are difficult to determine.

The prevalence of chronic pelvic pain is 15% in women between the ages of 18 and 50 years [2]. Chronic pelvic pain accounts for 10–40% of all gynecological outpatient visits [2]. In the United States, 35% of diagnostic laparoscopies and 15% of all hysterectomies are performed because of chronic pelvic pain [1]. Interestingly, black women have a lower risk of developing this condition (0.73; confidence interval, 0.55–0.99) [1]. Women over 35 years of age also have lower odds of developing this problem (0.72; confidence interval, 0.60–0.85) [1].

The economic impact of chronic pelvic pain is substantial: 15% of women with chronic pelvic pain miss an average 12.8 hours of work per month in the United States, which accounts for $14 billion of lost productivity per year [1, 3]. The total cost of potentially unnecessary medical, surgical, and psychiatric care or hospitalization amounts to $128 million per year. It is estimated that the total cost of care for women with chronic pelvic pain constitutes $38 billion per year [1, 3].

Many conditions produce chronic pelvic pain in women. These conditions range from problems in the gastrointestinal track to gynecological disorders and urologic abnormalities. Some of these conditions are easily diagnosed, but the other causes of chronic pelvic pain are extremely difficult to recognize. These conditions have often been overlooked and under-diagnosed in the past.

There are a number of diagnostic radiologic modalities that can be used for evaluation of patients presenting with pelvic pain, including ultrasonography, computed tomography (CT), and magnetic resonance imaging (MRI). Recent advances in radiologic imaging and therapeutic procedures make it possible to diagnose accurately the conditions producing chronic pain in most women, and to guide effective treatment.

Radiologists familiar with the clinical, pathologic, and radiologic characteristics of the underlying causes of chronic pelvic pain will be able to make an accurate diagnosis in most cases and facilitate referral for appropriate therapy.

References

1. Association of Professors of Gynecology and Obstetrics (APGO) Educational Series on Women's Health Issues. Chronic pelvic pain: an integrated approach. APGO, Crofton, MD, 2000.
2. Harris RD, Holtzman SR, Poppe AM. Clinical outcome in female patients with pelvic pain and normal pelvic US findings. Radiology 2000;216:440–443.
3. Wenof M, Perry C. Chronic pelvic pain: a patient education booklet. International Pelvic Pain Society, Birmingham, AL, 1999.
4. Kuligowska E, Deeds L, Lu K. Pelvic pain: over-looked and under diagnosed gynecological conditions. RadioGraphics 2005;25:3–20.

E. Kuligowska
Department of Radiology, Boston Medical Center, Boston University School of Medicine, Boston, MA, USA

Painful Bladder Syndrome

52

Mauro Cervigni, Franca Natale, Albert Mako
and Loredana Nasta

Abstract Painful bladder syndrome/interstitial cystitis (PBS/IC), also known as bladder pain syndrome (BPS/IC), is primarily based on symptoms of urgency, frequency, and pain in the bladder and/or pelvis. Its etiology is not known and clinical characteristics vary among patients. Early recognition of BPS/IC is very important because the symptoms are quite disabling, affecting quality of life and resulting in patients being visited by a variety of specialists. Several and controversial etiologic theories have been proposed but one aspect has been emphasised: the multifactorial etiology of the disease. Physical evaluation is a critical component of diagnosing BPS/IC. Questionnaires can be helpful in screening. The most commonly used screening tools are the Pelvic Pain, Urgency, Frequency patient questionnaire (PUF) and O'Leary–Sant Symptom and Problem Index. Local cystoscopy is not mandatory but is a good preliminary investigation to rule out other conditions. Cystoscopy with hydrodistension under anesthesia is now considered too restrictive, however it remains the most common procedure performed in patients with BPS/IC especially in Europe. There are currently no specific blood or urine markers available for diagnosis. The therapeutic strategy is to reduce or eliminate the symptoms of BPS/IC, so improving quality of life and interfering with the potential disease mechanism. Therapies include conservative, medical (oral, subcutaneous, and intravesical), or interventional procedures. A multimodal approach seems to be more effective. A surgical approach should be the ultimate option for refractory BPS/IC patients.

Keywords Allodynia • Bladder hypersensitivity (BH) • Bladder pain syndrome (BPS) • Chronic prostatitis (CP) • Chronic pelvic pain (CPP) • Chronic pelvic pain syndrome (CPPS) • Dyspareunia • Interstitial cystitis (IC) • Painful bladder syndrome (PBS) • Vulvodynia

52.1 Introduction

Painful bladder syndrome/interstitial cystitis (PBS/IC), also known as bladder pain syndrome (BPS/IC), is a syndrome primarily based on symptoms of urgency, frequency, and pain in the bladder and/or pelvis. These collective terms describe debilitating, chronic bladder disorders of unknown causes with an exclusion of confusable diseases. Current data show that the condition is much more prevalent than previously thought. BPS/IC is also a disorder of the pelvic floor occurring

M. Cervigni
Division of Urogynecology, San Carlo-IDI Hospital, Roma, Italy

G.A. Santoro, A.P. Wieczorek, C.I. Bartram (eds.) *Pelvic Floor Disorders*
© Springer-Verlag Italia 2010

mostly (> 90%) in women) [1, 2]. A number of studies have identified the bladder as one of major causes of chronic pelvic pain (CPP) [3–7].

Misdiagnosis and ineffective treatments are common, leaving patients with persistent pain and the potential for neuropathic upregulation and allodynia. Currently BPS/IC is considered a diagnosis of exclusion because its etiology is not known and clinical characteristics vary among patients. Voiding often relieves the typical symptoms of pain, pressure, or discomfort involving the lower pelvic area including gastrointestinal organs. The symptoms have to be present for no less than 6 months, obviously in the absence of urinary tract infection (UTI) [1]. Early recognition of BPS/IC is very important because symptoms are quite disabling, affecting quality of life and leading to patients being seen by a variety of specialists (usually between five and seven times in a period of 3–5 years). The syndrome is also exacerbated by the high incidence of other comorbid diseases including: allergies, asthma, atopic dermatitis, inflammatory bowel syndrome (IBS), systemic lupus erythematosus (SLE), Sjögren's syndrome, chronic fatigue syndrome, and fibromyalgia [8–11]. Vulvodynia may also be present in 20% of cases [4], as well as endometriosis in 45–65% of women with pelvic pain of bladder origin [5]. BPS/IC may also be present in men (2.2% of the population using the National Institutes of Health Chronic Prostatitis Symptom Index (NIH-CPSI)) with less frequent urgency and frequency of urination (type 3 prostatitis, non-bacterial prostatitis, or chronic prostatitis) [12].

52.2 Definition

The National Institute of Diabetes and Digestive Kidney Diseases (NIDDK) established a set of consensus criteria, which were developed to ensure the comparability of patients enrolled in clinical studies [13]. These included:

- Hunner's ulcers
- any two of:
  - pain on bladder filling, relieved by emptying
  - suprapubic, pelvic, urethral, vaginal, or perineal pain for 9 months
  - glomerulations on endoscopy or upon hydrodistension under spinal or general anesthesia.

However, over 60% of patients with possible BPS/IC

appear to fail these criteria expanding the definition [14].

The International Continence Society (ICS) in 2002 defined the term painful bladder syndrome as "The complaint of suprapubic pain related to bladder filling, accompanied by other symptoms such as frequency and nocturia in the absence of proven pathologies" [15].

Most recently, the European Society for the Study of Interstitial Cystitis (ESSIC) named this disease bladder pain syndrome [16] according to the definition by the International Association for the Study of Pain (IASP) [17].

Sometimes a significant proportion of BPS/IC patients do not complain of pain but relate their feelings to pressure and discomfort [18]. In this situation, patients not complaining of pain would remain undiagnosed for IC if only pain syndromes are applicable to a diagnosis of BPS/IC; therefore in May 2009, the Asian Society published clinical guidelines for IC, proposing a new definition of the syndrome as "hypersensitive bladder syndrome" (HBS) – bladder hypersensitivity, usually associated with urinary frequency, with or without bladder pain [19].

52.3 Epidemiology

The prevalence of BPS/IC was estimated in the past at 18.1/100,000 women [20]. Subsequent studies in 2002 indicated it was 450 per 100,000 (0.45%), and more recently it was 680 per 100,000 (0.68%) for a probable IC and 300 per 100,000 (0.3%) for a definite diagnosis of IC [21, 22].

A recent study of 981 urban females in Vienna showed an overall prevalence of 306 per 100,000 (0.3%), with the highest number in the 40–59 years age group [23]. BPS/IC has also been reported in children and adolescents [24–26]. In Japan the prevalence reported from a questionnaire survey of 300 major hospitals was only 2 per 100,000 patients [27]. The patients were older (52.9 years on average) than those in Europe and the United States [28]. This may indicate that patients have had symptoms for a long time before diagnosis. However, a recent epidemiological investigation in Japan found that 1.0% of the general population experienced bladder pain every day [29]. There is some evidence of genetic predisposition; the prevalence of BPS/IC in first-degree relatives has been shown to be 17 times higher than in the general population [30].

52.4 Etiology and Pathogenesis

Several etiologic theories have been proposed in recent years, although they remain somewhat speculative and controversial, and the precise causes of BPS/IC are still unknown. One aspect has been emphasised: the multifactorial etiology of the disease. Interaction between nervous, immune, and endocrine factors creates a vicious cycle, provoking and maintaining the inflammatory effect in the bladder.

52.4.1 Infection

To date, no infectious etiology has been identified using reverse transcriptase polymerase chain reaction (RT-PCR) for *Chlamydia trachomatis*, adenovirus, cytomegalovirus, herpes simplex virus, papillomavirus, or *Gardnerella vaginalis* [31, 32]. It is well known that antibiotic treatment is ineffective for BPS/IC. Flare-up of symptoms can occasionally be elicited by an infection, as an associated factor that initiates or exacerbates IC [33].

52.4.2 Mastocytosis

An increased number of activated bladder mast cells has been reported repeatedly in BPS/IC [34]. There are twice as many mast cells in the urothelium of BPS/IC patients and ten times more in the detrusor as compared to controls [35]. In addition, more than 70% of bladder mast cells were activated in BPS/IC as compared to less than 10% in controls [34]. In fact the mast cells play a pivotal role in the inflammatory process: they release potent inflammatory mediators such as histamine, leukotriene, and serotonin, and also interact with immunoglobulin E (IgE) antibodies, other inflammatory cells, and the nervous system [35, 36].

52.4.3 Dysfunctional Bladder Epithelium

The protective inner layer of the bladder is made up of glycosaminoglycans (GAGs), chondroitin sulphate (CS), and sodium hyaluronate (SH). This GAG component is hydrophilic and binds a layer of water molecules that is thought to protect the urothelium from potentially harmful agents, including bacteria, proteins, and ions. Proponents of the leaky endothelium theory suggest that the GAG layer may be damaged in BPS/IC [37, 38]; this deficiency allows irritants in the urine to leak through the urothelium and causes inflammation, irritation, and numerous, other reactions [39].

Increased urinary levels of CS and SH have been reported in some BPS/IC patients [40, 41], with concomitant decrease of mucosal glycoprotein GP1 [42].

The etiology of the defect in the GAG layer is currently unknown. Antiproliferative factors (APFs), detected in the urine of IC patients, downregulate expression of genes that stimulate proliferation of bladder epithelial cells, and upregulate genes that inhibit proliferation, leading to urothelial undermaturation and dysfunction [43, 44].

52.4.4 Neurogenic Inflammation

BPS/IC is not an end-organ condition; it should be considered a condition of the peripheral and central nervous systems as they relate to acute or chronic pain. The initiating event is a noxious stimulus such as trauma, infection, or inflammation. Acute pain is associated with nociception, which results in pain perception modulated in the peripheral and central nervous systems. Conversion of acute to chronic pain begins with activation of visceral silent unmyelinated C-fibers by prolonged noxious stimulation and inflammation. The neurotransmitter glutamate is released, which activates N-methyl-d-aspartate receptors. A chronic pain cycle begins as dorsal horn neurons are activated (wind-up), which causes exaggerated responses to less noxious stimuli (hyperalgesia), or a painful response to normally innocuous stimuli (allodynia), as small volumes of urine in the bladder are perceived as a full bladder. The neurotransmitter substance P stimulates the release of histamine and nitric oxide, which causes neurogenic inflammation. Once the dorsal horn becomes hypersensitive, the pain syndrome becomes a chronic pain syndrome. Prolonged noxious stimuli can cause dorsal horn cells to transmit efferent signals to peripheral nerve terminals (antidromic transmission). Thus a self-perpetuating signal is established as a visceral CPPS, causing expression of genes such as c-Fos in the spinal cord and loss of inhibitory neurons, resulting in a decreased threshold for activation.

52.4.5 Reduced Vascularization

A decrease in the microvascular density has been observed in the suburothelium in patients with BPS/IC [45]. Bladder vascular perfusion is reduced by bladder filling in BPS/IC, while it is slightly increased in controls [46].

A recent paper showed that hyperbaric therapy seems to relieve the symptoms of BPS/IC [47], confirming indirectly that a reduced blood supply may cause a decrease in epithelial function as well as epithelial thinning and denudation [48]. It is reasonable that the impaired blood circulation in the bladder is related to BPS/IC and the apoptotic activity of microvascular endothelial cells is increased [49].

52.4.6 Pelvic Floor Dysfunction

Women with BPS/IC have often a history of hysterectomy, cesarean section, miscarriage, stillbirth, or abortion [50, 51]. Pelvic surgery can be the trigger for symptom development. The symptoms are likely to be affected by the menstrual cycle [50]. Another frequent association of BPS/IC is with irritable bowel syndrome (IBS); both are improved by treating small-intestinal bacterial overgrowth, which probably potentiates visceral hypersensitivity [52]. On the other hand, vulvodynia, dyspareunia, scrotal and perineal pain are one of the expressions of the exaggerated muscle tone activity, contributing to the maintenance of the noxious stimuli.

52.4.7 Autoimmunity

Many of the clinical features of BPS/IC reflect an autoimmune component of the disease process. Investigators have also reported concomitant association of BPS/IC and other autoimmune diseases, such as SLE, rheumatoid arthritis, and Sjögren's syndrome [53–55].

52.5   Diagnosis

It is important to keep in mind that BPS/IC patients may present with only one of the symptoms, particularly early in the course of the disease. Up to 30% with BPS/IC present without pelvic pain [56], and ap-

proximately 15% present with pain as the only symptom [57].

The diagnosis of BPS/IC is symptom driven by exclusion, but should not necessarily be organ oriented, considering the large number of confusable diseases (Table 52.1). A comprehensive medical history should include suprapubic pain, pressure, and discomfort related to bladder filling, as well as frequency and urgency in the absence of UTI or other pathology [58]. Table 52.1 shows which disease could be confused with BPS/IC.

A retrospective analysis from the IC Database (ICDB) pointed out the most common baseline pain site was lower abdominal (80%), urethral (74%), and low back (65%), with the majority of patients describing their pain as intermittent [59].

Questionnaires can be helpful in screening for BPS/IC. The most commonly used screening tools are the Pelvic Pain, Urgency, Frequency symptom scale (PUF) and O'Leary–Sant Symptom and Problem Index [60, 61]. Both surveys include questions regarding pain, urgency, frequency, and nocturia and how these symptoms impact on quality of life.

Physical evaluation is a critical component of diagnosing BPS/IC. Since the bladder is a pain generator, tenderness with single-digit examination of the trigonal area can help establish a diagnosis of BPS/IC [62] as

Table 52.1 Confusable diseases in BPS/IC

Disease type	Confusable diseases
Bladder diseases	Overactive bladder
	Neurogenic bladder
	Radiation cystitis
	Bladder calculus
	Bladder cancer
Prostate and urethral diseases	Benign prostatic hypertrophy
	Prostate cancer
	Urethral stenosis
	Urethral diverticulum
Genitourinary infections	Bacterial cystitis
	Urethritis
	Prostatitis
Gynecologic diseases	Endometriosis
	Uterine myoma
	Vaginitis
	Postmenopausal syndrome
Other conditions	Polyuria
	Hypertonic pelvic floor

pelvic floor tenderness at the trigger point in the levator muscles [63]. Physical examination should also address high tone of the pelvic floor muscles, and hypersensitivity of the perineal area using the Kaufman Qtip touch sensitivity test that might screen for the presence of vulvarvestibulodynia (VVS) [64]. Urine analysis can rule out hematuria, and urine culture is required to identify bladder infection as cytology can help rule out bladder cancer. Several optional diagnostic tests are also used but diagnostic evaluation varies among urologists/urogynecologists, in different centers [65–67] and between the US, Europe, and Asia [19, 68].

Urodynamic studies can highlight detrusor overactivity or reduced bladder capacity without detrusor overactivity (bladder hypersensitivity) suggestive of BPS/IC [69–71]. A mild impaired voiding phase with detrusor-sphincter discoordination is probably related to the dysfunctional pelvic floor behavior.

Local cystoscopy is not mandatory but is a good preliminary investigation to rule out other conditions (e.g. bladder stone, hematuria, or cancer). Cystoscopy is also needed to identify Hunner's ulcer [72], the positive specific finding of BPS/IC. Typically, an ulcer is recognized as a well-demarcated reddish mucosal lesion lacking the normal capillary structure. In addition, some scars or fissures with a rich hypervascularization or a pale mucosal aspect may be found, and are an indirect index of hypovascularization.

Cystoscopy with hydrodistension under anesthesia is proposed by the NIDDK research criteria, but is now considered too restrictive [67]; however, it remains the most common procedure performed in patients with BPS/IC especially in Europe [73]. Hydrodistension is also done using different methodologies, making comparison between studies difficult [64, 74, 75]. It may be necessary to exclude other pathologies and to identify the presence of "classic" BPS/IC with "Hunner's ulcers", and document urothelial bleeding (glomerulations), even though these have also been noted in the bladders of normal women undergoing tubal ligation [76].

Bladder biopsy has to be performed after hydrodistension to avoid the risk of bladder rupture, to prove the presence of mast cell infiltration, and to orientate toward a more specific therapy. Biopsy with histopathology may be necessary to exclude neoplasm and eosinophilic or tuberculosis cystitis. A count of tryptase-positive bladder mast cells is recommended by the European Society, with > 28 mast cells/mm constituting detrusor mastocytosis, which is considered diagnostic

for BPS/IC [67, 77, 74]. An increased number of mast cells was also recently proposed as a diagnostic criterion for vulvar vestibulitis [78].

There are no specific blood or urine markers available for diagnosis. An APF, recently identified as a frizzled-8 surface sialoglycopeptide [79], was increased in BPS/IC urine as determined by its ability to decrease in vitro proliferation of bladder epithelial cells, and could distinguish BPS/IC from other urologic disorders [80]. Urine APF levels also apparently distinguished BPS/IC from CPPS in men [81].

However, APF still needs to be validated and independently reproduced. Classic BPS/IC might be differentiated from nonulcer disease by elevated urine nitric oxide (NO) [82].

Other urinary markers include heparin-binding epidermal growth factor-like growth factor (HB-EGF), histamine, methylhistamine, and interleukin-6 (IL-6) [83, 84]. Four proteins that differed significantly between IC and controls have been identified, with uromodulin and two kininogens found to be higher for controls and inter-alphatrypsin inhibitor heavy chain H4 higher for IC [85]. Urinary concentration of neutrophile elastase is increased in patients with pain and small bladder capacity [86]. These markers are not necessarily precise predictors of ulcer and/or symptom severity [87].

Intravesical administration of 40 mL of a solution of 40 mEq of potassium chloride in 100 mL of water (potassium sensitivity test – PST), with pain and urgency scored by the patient as compared to administration of sterile water has been proposed for BPS/IC diagnosis [60]. However, this test's sensitivity and specificity is only about 75% and the participants at the International IC Consultation in Rome recommended that it should not be used for diagnostic purposes because of its low prognostic value [88].

52.6 Treatment

There is no curative therapy for BPS/IC [89–92]. This is consistent with the fact that the causes of BPS/IC are yet not understood and the pathophysiology remains uncertain.

Therefore, the therapeutic strategy is to reduce or eliminate the symptoms of BPS/IC, thereby interfering with the potential disease mechanism and improving quality of life.

Because IC is a chronic disease, patients should

be counselled regarding realistic expectation of treatment. Remission may be attained but should not be expected, and even when it is attainable, months of medical treatment may be required [93].

Exacerbations during periods of remission are common and patients need to be encouraged that therapy is not failing.

52.6.1 Conservative Therapy

Behavioral modification may have modest benefit for IC patients (grade of recommendation B). Barbalias et al looked at a type of bladder training as an adjunct to treatment with intravesical oxybutynin in patients with IC; there was a modest improvement in O'Leary–Sant questionnaire at 6 months [94]. Chaiken et al reported similar results with diary-timed voiding and pelvic floor muscle training [95]. There are no randomized controlled trials (RCTs) attesting the efficacy of pelvic floor physical therapy. Biofeedback and soft tissue massage may aid in muscle relaxation of the pelvic floor [96].

Manual physical therapy (grade of recommendation C) to the pelvic floor myofascial trigger points twice per week for 8–12 weeks also resulted in moderate to marked improvement in 7/10 BPS/IC patients [97].

Modified Thiele intravaginal massage of high-tone pelvic floor muscle trigger points twice per week for 5 weeks, has been shown to improve the O'Leary–Sant Index [98].

Common-sense dietary changes, especially avoidance of potential bladder irritancy as identified by individual patients may be beneficial (grade of recommendation B).

A majority of BPS/IC patients seem to have symptom exacerbation related to the intake of specific foods and beverages: coffee, spicy foods, and alcoholic beverages [99].

However, different patients seem to be affected to different degrees by specific foods and beverages and patients should avoid only those foods and beverages that they find worsen their symptoms.

52.6.2 Medical Therapy

Medical therapies for BPS/IC include oral, subcutaneous, and intravesical agents. These drugs are categorized according to their intended point of action within the disease process.

52.6.2.1 Protection of the Mucosal Surface

One of the theories in the pathogenesis of IC is that deficiency of the GAG layer causes symptoms related to the increased permeability of the urothelium. Therefore, a number of agents have been used to improve the integrity of the mucosal surface.

- Pentosan polysulfate (PPS), a branched polysaccharide presumably acting to "replenish" the GAG layer, is the only oral drug approved in the US for BPS/IC (grade of recommendation B, level of evidence 2). One study of PPS (300 mg/day) used for 3 years showed it was twice as potent as placebo (18%) in reducing pain but the placebo response was unusually low [1, 90]. A randomized double-blind multicenter study, with a range of doses (300, 600 or 900 mg per day) for 32 months, of 380 BPS/IC patients with > 6 months' symptoms and positive cystoscopic examination but no placebo control, reported that 45–50% of all patients were classified as responders (50% or greater improvement on the Patients' Overall Rating of Symptoms Index – PORIS), irrespective of the dose [100]. In a recent prospective study, 41 patients with BPS/IC were divided into three groups according to their response to PPS (major, intermediate, minor); they were administered 3 × 5000 IU subcutaneous heparin per day for 2 days, followed by 2 × 5000 IU per day for 12 days plus 300 mg PPS per day, compared to 17 nonmatched patients taking PPS alone; 32% of the patients in the minor response group reported a significant improvement in "overall well-being" over that of PPS alone [101].
- Hydroxyzine is a histamine1 receptor antagonist, with additional anxiolytic, sedative, anticholinergic, and mast cell inhibitory properties (grade of recommendation D, level of evidence 1). It has been shown to reduce neurogenic bladder inflammation [102]. Hydroxyzine has shown mixed results in treating BPS/IC symptoms. One open label study showed a 55% reduction in symptoms, particularly in patients who suffered from allergies [103].
- Cimetidine is a histamine-2 receptor antagonist (grade of recommendation D, level of evidence 4). It was reported to decrease the median symptom score in 34 BPS/IC patients studied, but with no apparent histological changes in the bladder mucosa [104].
- l-Arginine is a natural substrate of nitric oxide

synthase (NOS) (grade of recommendation D). It may re-activate NOS activity, which is suppressed in IC, and relieve symptoms [105]. No significant effect was observed in double-blind studies [106, 107]. More detailed results of the use of oral drugs in BPS/IC patients are reported in Table 52.2.

52.6.2.2 Intravesical Instillation or Bladder Wall Injection

Intravesical and subcutaneous heparin has been used for the treatment of IC since early 1960. It is either instilled or administered subcutaneously. When instilled, heparin does not have systemic anticoagulant effects. In one study, 48 patients with IC self-administered intravesical heparin (10,000 IU in 10 mL sterile water 3 times weekly for 3 months). Fifty-six per cent of the patients attained clinical remission after 3 months [108]. Subcutaneous heparin has been demonstrated to produce rapid relief of symptoms in eight patients, who reported long-term benefit over 1 year [109].

- Intravesical dimethylsulfoxide (DMSO) remains the basis of intravesical therapy for IC (grade of recommendation B, level of evidence 2). It has been shown to reduce symptoms for up to 3 months [110]. Its multiple effects include an anti-inflammatory and analgesic effect, muscle relaxation, mast cell inhibition, and collagen dissolution [111]. Patients treated with DMSO have experienced a 50–70 % reduction of symptoms, although the relapse rate is 35–40%. Administration in combination with various other agents including hydrocortisone, heparin,

and sodium bicarbonate has been recommended to improve the response to DMSO [1].

- Intravesical hyaluronic acid (grade of recommendation C, level of evidence 4), has been used with a long-lasting moderate efficacy with no side-effects, but a recent multicenter study found no significant efficacy (Interstitial Cystitis Association – Physician perspectives, unpublished data).
- Chondroitin sulfate (grade of recommendation C, level of evidence 3) demonstrated a 33% response rate [112]. Combined instillation of hyaluronic acid and chondroitin sulfate in refractory interstitial cystitis resulted in significant symptomatic improvement [113].
- Botulinum toxin (grade of recommendation C, level of evidence 4) inhibits the release of calcitonin gene-related peptide and substance P from afferent nerves, and weakens pain [114, 115]. Small studies of intravesical Botox into the bladder wall indicated symptom relief in IC patients, without significant adverse events [116]. Table 52.3 shows the results of drugs administered intravesically for the treatment of BPS/IC.

52.6.2.3 Pain Modulation

Tricyclic antidepressants (TCAs), especially amitriptyline, are known to have pain-reducing effects (grade of recommendation B, level of evidence 2). One recent RCT of amitriptyline evaluated 50 patients with IC. Improvement in overall symptom scores was significantly greater in the treatment group, as well reduction in pain and urgency ($P < 0.001$) [117].

Table 52.2 Oral medications for treatment of BPS/IC: results[a]

Drug	RCT	Success (%)
Amitriptyline; tricyclic antidepressant	Yes	42
Antibiotics	Yes	48
Cimetidine	Yes	65
Hydrocortisone	No	80
Ciclosporin	No	90
Hydroxyzine	Yes	31
l-Arginine	Yes	Not effective
Nifedipine	No	87
Quercetin	No	92
Sodium pentosanpolysulfate	Yes	33
Suplatast tosilate	No	86

[a]Adapted from [58]

Table 52.3 Intravesical medications for treatment of BPS/ic: results[a]

Drug	RCT	Success (%)
DMSO	Yes	70
BCG	Yes	Conflicting RCT data as to efficacy
Resiniferatoxin	Yes	No proven efficacy
Hyaluronic acid	Yes	No proven efficacy
Heparin	No	60
Chondroitin Sulfate	No	33
Lidocaine	No	65
PPS	Yes	Suggestion of possible efficacy 40

[a]Adapted from [58]

52.6.2.4 Immunologic Modulation

Immune stimulants and suppressants have been used in BPS/IC.

- Intravesical Bacillus Calmette–Guérin (BCG) (grade of recommendation D, level of evidence – no efficacy) was initially reported to have some benefit in BPS/IC [118]; however, a subsequent randomized placebocontrolled trial of BPS/IC patients, who met the NIDDK research criteria, showed that there was no statistical difference at 34 weeks [119].
- Ciclosporin is an immunosuppressant used in organ transplantation (grade of recommendation C, level of evidence 2). It was tested in a small, open-label study of 11 patients. The results were largely positive and bladder pain decreased or stopped completely in 10 patients [120].
- Suplataste tosilate (IPD-1151T) is a new immunoregulator that selectively suppresses IgE, IL-4 and IL-5 (grade of recommendation C, level of evidence 4). Treatment for one year in 14 women resulted in a significantly increased bladder capacity and decreased urgency, frequency, and pain [121].

52.6.2.5 Multimodal Medical Therapy

To manage the multiple pathological features of IC, a multimodal approach, combining agents from different classes, is suggested to improve the therapeutic response by attacking the disease at several points. One common multimodal approach is:

1. to restore epithelial funtion with heparinoid
2. to treat neural activation and pain with TCA
3. to control allergies with an anthistamine.

In advanced form, intravesical treatment may be required. Combination intravesical therapy is also indicated for patients who experience significant flare of symptoms after remission.

52.6.3 Procedural Intervention

BPS/IC is a chronic and debilitating disease with an impairment of quality of life due to disabling symptoms. Surgical options should be considered only when all conservative treatment has failed.

Laser resection, augmentation cystoplasty, cystolysis, cystectomy, and urinary diversion may be the ultimate option for refractory BPS/IC patients [93]. Continent diversion may have better cosmetic and lifestyle outcome, but recurrence is a real possibility.

Posterior tibial nerve stimulation somewhat improved less than half of patients [122].

Sacral nerve neuromodulation as a treatment for BPS/IC in initial stadies seems to relieve the symptoms of IC. Further stadies are needed [123].

52.7 Conclusions

BPS/IC is a chronic, multifactorial disorder with symptoms of urinary frequency, urgency, and pelvic pain, often associated with other painful diseases, which profoundly affects patients' quality of life due to its disabling aspects. Pelvic pain in BPS/IC is a visceral pain syndrome with multiple pain generators, which can make the diagnosis difficult. Patients with a history of recurrent UTIs that are culture negative, those with endometriosis and significant bladder symptoms, with overactive bladder syndrome who have responded poorly to therapy, or with vulvodynia or chronic pelvic pain are all likely to have untreated BPS/IC. The primary providers of care for women with pelvic pain must consider the bladder as a very important source of pain. The earlier the diagnosis is made and therapy begun, the sooner patients with BPS/IC will experience improvement of their symptoms.

References

1. Hanno P. Interstitial cystitis and related disorders. In: Walsh PC (ed) Campbell's urology. Elsevier, Philadelphia PA, 2002, pp 631–668.
2. Sant GR. Etiology, pathogenesis and diagnosis of interstitial cystitis. Rev Urol 2002;4(suppl 1):S9–S15.
3. Paulson JD, Delgado M. Chronic pelvic pain: the occurrence of interstitial cystitis in a gynecological population. J Soc Laparosc Surg 2005;9:426–430.
4. Stanford EJ, Koziol J, Fang A. The prevalence of interstitial cystitis, endometriosis, adhesions and vulvar pain in women with chronic pelvic pain. J Minim Invasive Gynecol 2005; 12:43–49.
5. Chung MK, Chung RP, Gordon D. Interstitial cystitis and endometriosis in patients with chronic pelvic pain: the "evil twins" syndrome. J Soc Laparosc Surg 2005;9:25–29.
6. Sand PK. Chronic pain syndromes of gynecologic origin. J Reprod Med 2004;49:230–234.
7. Parsons CL, Dell J, Stanford EJ et al. The prevalence of interstitial cystitis in gynecological patients with pelvic pain, as detected by intravesical potassium sensitivity. Am J Obstet Gynecol 2002;187:1395–1400.
8. Yamada T. Significance of complications of allergic diseases in young patients with interstitial cystitis. Int J Urol 2003;10(suppl):S56–S58.
9. Peeker R, Atansiu L, Logadottir Y. Intercurrent autoimmune conditions in classic and non-ulcer interstitial cystitis. Scand J Urol Nephrol 2003;137:60–63.
10. Novi JM, Jeronis S, Srinivas S et al. Risk of irritable bowel syndrome and depression in women with interstitial cystitis: a case control study. J Urol 2005:174:937–940.
11. Alagiri M, Chottiner S, Ratner V et al. Interstitial cystitis: unexplained associations with other chronic disease and pain syndrome. Urology 1997;49:52–57.
12. Schaeffer AJ. Clinical practice. Chronic prostatitis and the chronic pelvic pain syndrome. N Engl J Med 2006; 355:1690–1698.
13. Hanno PM, Landis JR, Matthews-Cook Y et al. The diagnosis of interstitial cystitis revisited: lessons learned from the National Institutes of Health Interstitial Cystitis Database Study. J Urol 1999;161:553–557.
14. Sant GR, Hanno PM. Interstitial cystitis: current issues and controversies in diagnosis. Urology 2001;57:82–88.
15. Abrams P, Cardozo L, Fall M et al. The standardisation of terminology of lower urinary tract function: report from the Standardisation Sub-committee of the International Continence Society. Neurourol Urodyn 2002;21:167–178.
16. van de Merwe JP, Nordling J, Bouchelouche P et al. Diagnostic criteria, classification, and nomenclature for painful bladder syndrome/interstitial cystitis: an ESSIC proposal. Eur Urol 2008;53:60–67.
17. Merskey H, Bogduk N (eds) International Association for the Study of Pain Part III: pain terms: a current list with definitions and notes on usage. In: Classification of Chronic Pain, 2 edn. IASP Task Force on Taxonomy, IASP Press, Seattle, 1994, pp 209–214.
18. Warren JW, Meyer WA, Greenberg P et al. Using the International Continence Society's definition of painful bladder syndrome. Urology 2006;67:1138–1142 ; discussion 1142–1143.
19. Homma Y, Ueda T, Tomoe H et al. Clinical guidelines for interstitial cystitis and hypersensitive bladder syndrome. Int J Urol 2009;16:597–615.
20. Oravisto KJ. Epidemiology of interstitial cystitis. Ann Chir Gynaecol Fenn 1975;64:75–77.
21. Leppilahti M, Tammela TL, Huhtala H, Auvinen A. Prevalence of symptoms related to interstitial cystitis in women: a population based study in Finland. J Urol 2002;168:139–143.
22. Leppilahti M, Sairanen J, Tammela TL et al. Prevalence of clinically confirmed interstitial cystitis in women: a population based study in Finland. J Urol 2005;174:581–583.
23. Temml C, Wehrberger C, Riedl C et al. Prevalence and correlates for interstitial cystitis symptoms in women participating in a health screening project. Eur Urol 2007;51:803–808; discussion 809.
24. Close CE, Carr MC, Burns MW et al. Interstitial cystitis in children. J Urol 1996;156:860–862.
25. Farkas A, Waisman J, Goodwin WE. Interstitial cystitis in adolescent girls. J Urol 1977;118:837–838.
26. Mattoks TF. Interstitial cystitis in adolescents and children: a review. J Pediatr Adolesc Gynecol 2004;17:7–11.
27. Ito T, Miki M, Yamada T. Interstitial cystitis in Japan. BJU Int 2000;86:634–637.
28. Ito T, Ueda T, Homma Y, Takei M. Recent trends in patient characteristics and therapeutic choices for interstitial cystitis: analysis of 282 Japanese patients. Int J Urol 2007;14:1068–1070.
29. Homma Y, Yamaguchi O, Hayashi K. Epidemiologic survey of lower urinary tract symptoms in Japan. Urology 2006;68:560–564.
30. Warren JW, Jackson TL, Langenberg P et al. Prevalence of interstitial cystitis in first-degree relatives of patients with interstitial cystitis. Urology 2004;63:17–21.
31. AlHadithi HN, Williams H, Hart CA et al. Absence of bacterial and viral DNA in bladder biopsies from patients with interstitial cystitis/chronic pelvic pain syndrome. J Urol 2005;174:151–154.
32. Agarwal M, Dixon RA. A study to detect Gardnerella vaginalis DNA in interstitial cystitis. BJU Int 2001;88:868–870.
33. Warren JW, Brown V, Jacobs S et al. Urinary tract infection

and inflammation at onset of interstitial cystitis/painful bladder syndrome. Urology 2008;71:1085–1090.

34. Theoharides TC, Kempuraj D, Sant GR. Mast cell involvement in interstitial cystitis: a review of human and experimental evidence. Urology 2001;57(6 suppl 1):47–55.

35. Peeker R, Enerbäck L, Fall M, Aldenborg F. Recruitment, distribution and phenotypes of mast cells in interstitial cystitis. Urology 2000;163:1009–1015.

36. Hofmeister MA, He F, Ratliff TL et al. Mast cells and nerve fibers in interstitial cystitis (IC): an algorithm for histologic diagnosis via quantitative image analysis and morphometry (QIAM). Urology 1997;49:41–47.

37. Parsons CL, Stauffer C, Schmidt JD. Bladdersurface glycosaminoglycans: an efficient mechanism of environmental adaptation. Science 1980;208:605–607.

38. Parsons CL, Lilly JD, Stein P. Epithelial dysfunction in nonbacterial cystitis (interstitial cystitis). J Urol 1991; 145:732–735.

39. Metts JF. Interstitial cystitis: urgency and frequency syndrome. Am Fam Physician 2001;64:1199–1206.

40. Wel DC, Politano VA, Seizer MG, Lokeshwar VB. The association of elevated urinary total to sulfated glycosaminoglycan ratio and high molecular mass hyaluronic acid with interstitial cystitis. J Urol 2000;163:1577–1583.

41. Erickson DR, Sheykhnazan M, Ordille S, Bhavanandan VP. Increased urinary hyaluronic acid and interstitial cystitis. J Urol 1998;160:1282–1284.

42. Moskowitz MO, Byrne DS, Callahan HJ et al. Decreased expression of a glycoprotein component of bladder surface mucin (GPI) in interestitial cystitis. J Urol 1994; 151:343–345.

43. Keay S, Kleinberg M, Zhang CO et al. Bladder epithelial cells from patients with interstitial cystitis produce an inhibitor of heparin-binding epidermal growth factor-like growth factor production. J Urol 2000;164:2112–2118.

44. Keay S, Seillier-Moiseiwitsch F, Zhang CO et al. Changes in human bladder epithelial cell gene expression associated with interstitial cystitis or antiproliferative factor treatment. Physiol Genomics 2003;14:107–115.

45. Rosamilia A, Cann L, Scurry J et al. Bladder microvasculature and the effects of hydrodistention in interstitial cystitis. Urology 2001;57:132.

46. Pontari MA, Hanno PM, Ruggieri MR. Comparison of bladder blood flow in patients with and without interstitial cystitis. J Urol 1999;162:330–334.

47. van Ophoven A, Rossbach G, Pajonk F, Hertle L. Safety and efficacy of hyperbaric oxygen therapy for the treatment of interstitial cystitis: a randomized, sham controlled, double-blind trial. J Urol 2006;176:1442–1446.

48. Cervigni M, Zoppetti G, Nasta L et al. Reduced vascularization in the bladder mucosa of bladder pain syndrome/interstitial cystitis patients. In: Proceedings of the ESSIC Annual Meeting, Göteborg, Sweden, 4–6 June 2009.

49. Yamada T, Nishimura M, Mita H. Increased number of apoptotic endothelial cells in bladder of interstitial cystitis patients. World J Urol 2007;25:407–413.

50. Peters KM, Carrico DJ, Diokno AC. Characterization of a clinical cohort of 87 women with interstitial cystitis/painful bladder syndrome. Urology 2008;71:634–640.

51. Hall SA, Link CL, Pulliam SJ et al. The relationship of common medical conditions and medication use with symptoms of painful bladder syndrome: results from the Boston area community health survey. J Urol 2008;180:593–598.

52. Weinstock LB, Klutke CG, Lin HC. Small intestinal bacterial overgrowth in patients with interstitial cystitis and gastrointestinal symptoms. Dig Dis Sci 2008;53:1246–1251.

53. Fister GM. Similarity of interstitial cystitis (Hunner's ulcer) to lupus erythematosus. J Urol 1938;40:37–51.

54. Silk MR. Bladder antibodies in interstitial cystitis. J Urol 1970;103:307–309.

55. Leppilahti M, Tammela TL, Huhtala H et al. Interstitial cystitis-like urinary symptoms among patients with Sjogren's syndrome: a population-based study in Finland. Am J Med 2003;115:62–65.

56. Parsons CL. Interstitial cystitis: epidemiology and clinical presentation. Clin Obstet Gynecol 2002;45:242–249.

57. Parsons CL, Bullen M, Kahn BS et al. Gynecologic presentation of interstitial cystitis as detected by intravesical potassium sensitivity. Obstet Gynecol 2001;98:127–132.

58. Hanno P, Baranowski A, Fall M et al. Painful bladder syndrome (including interstitial cystitis). In: Abrams P, Cardozo L, Khoury S, Wein A (eds) Incontinence. Health Publication Ltd, Plymouth, 2005, pp 1457–1520.

59. Fitzgerald MP, Brensinger C, Brubaker L et al. What is the pain of interstitial cystitis like? Int Urogynecol J Pelvic Floor Dysfunct 2005;17:69–72.

60. Parsons CL, Del J, Stanford AJ et al. Increased prevalence of interstitial cystitis: previously un-recognized urologic and gynecologic cases identified using a new symptoms questionnaire and intravesical potassium sensitivity. Urology 2002;60:573–578.

61. O'Leary MP, Sant GR, Fowler FJ Jr et al. The interstitial cystitis symptom index and problem index. Urology 1997;49(suppl 5A):58–63.

62. Howard FM. Physical examination. In: Howard FM, Perry CP, Carter JA et al (eds) Pelvic pain: diagnosis and management. Lippincott Williams and Wilkins, Philadelphia PA, 2000, pp 26–42.

63. Howard FM. Chronic pelvic pain. Obstet Gynecol 2003;101:594–611.

64. Kaufman RH, Friedrich EG, Gardner HL. Nonneoplastic epithelial disorders of the vulvar skin and mucosa; miscellaneous vulvar disorders. In: Kaufman RH, Friedrich EG, Gardner HL (eds) Benign diseases of the vulva and vagina. Chicago Yearbook, Chicago, IL, 1989, pp 299–360.

65. Hanno PM, Levin RM, Monson FC et al. Diagnosis of interstitial cystitis. J Urol 1990;143:278–281.

66. Turner KJ, Stewart LH. How do you stretch a bladder? A survey of UK practice, a literature review, and a recommendation of a standard approach. Neurourol Urodyn 2005;24:74–76.

67. Erickson DR, Tornaszewski JE, Kunselman AR et al. Do the National Institute of Diabetes and Digestive and Kidney Diseases cystoscopic criteria associate with other clinical and objective features of interstitial cystitis? J Urol 2005;173:93–97.

68. Nordling J, Anjum FH, Bade JJ et al. Primary evaluation of

patients suspected of having interstitial cystitis (IC). Eur Urol 2004;45:662–669.

69. Frazer MI, Haylen BT, Sissons M. Do women with idiopathic sensory urgency have early interstitial cystitis? Br J Urol 1990;66:274–278.

70. Awad SA, MacDiarmid S, Gajewski JB, Gupta R. Idiopathic reduced bladder storage versus interstitial cystitis. J Urol 1992;148:1409–1412.

71. Al-Hadithi H, Tincello DG, Vince GS et al. Leukocyte populations in interstitial cystitis and idiopathic reduced bladder storage. Urology 2002;59:851–855.

72. Braunstein R, Shapiro E, Kaye J, Moldwin R. The role of cystoscopy in the diagnosis of Hunner's ulcer disease. J Urol 2008;180:1383–1386.

73. Moldwin R. How to define the interstitial cystitis patients. Int Urogynecol J Pelvic Floor Dysfunct 2005;16(suppl 1):S8–S9.

74. Nordling J, Anjum FH, Bade JJ et al. Primary evaluation of patients suspected of having interstitial cystitis (IC). Eur Urol 2004;45:662–669.

75. Payne CK, Terai A, Komatsu K. Research criteria versus clinical criteria for interstitial cystitis. Int J Urol 2003; 10(suppl):S7–S10.

76. Waxman JA, Sulak PJ, Kuehl TJ. Cystoscopic findings consistent with interstitial cystitis in normal women undergoing tubal ligation. J Urol 1998;160:1663–1667.

77. Bouchelouche K. Mast cells in PBS/IC. International Symposium: Frontiers in Painful Bladder Syndrome and Interstitial Cystitis. 26–27 October 2006, Bethesda, MD.

78. Bomstein J, Gotdschmid N, Sabo E. Hyperinnervation and mast cell activation may be used as histopathologic diagnostic criteria for vulvar vestibulitis. Gynecol Obstet Invest 2004;58:171–178.

79. Keay SK, Szekely Z, Conrads TP et al. An antiproliferative factor from interstitial cystitis patients is a frizzled 8 proteinrelated sialoglycopeptide. Proc Natl Acad Sci U S A 2004;101:11803–11808.

80. Keay SK, Zhang CO, Shoenfelt J et al. Sensitivity and specificity of antiproliferative factor, heparinbinding epidermal growth factorlike growth factor, and epidermal growth factor as urine markers for interstitial cystitis. Urology 2001; 57:9–14.

81. Keay S, Zhang CO, Chai T et al. Antiproliferative factor, heparinbinding epidermal growth factorlike growth factor, and epidermal growth factor in men with interstitial cystitis versus chronic pelvic pain syndrome. Urology 2004; 63:22–26.

82. Logadottir YR, Ehren I, Fall M et al. Intravesical nitric oxide production discriminates between classic and nonulcer interstitial cystitis. J Urol 2004;171:1148–1150.

83. Hosseini A, Ehren I, Wiklund NP. Nitric oxide as an objective marker for evaluation of treatment response in patients with classic interstitial cystitis. J Urol 2004;172:2261–2265.

84. Lamale LM, Lutgendorf SK, Zimmerman MB, Kreder KJ. Interleukin-6, histamine, and methylhistamine as diagnostic markers for interstitial cystitis. Urology 2006;68:702–706.

85. Canter MP, Graham CA, Heit MH et al. Proteomic techniques identify urine proteins that differentiate patients with interstitial cystitis from asymptomatic control subjects. Am J Obstet Gynecol 2008;198:553 e1–6.

86. Kuromitsu S, Yokota H, Hiramoto M et al. Increased concentration of neutrophil elastase in urine from patients with interstitial cystitis. Scand J Urol Nephrol 2008;42:455–461.

87. Erickson DR, Tomaszewski JE, Kunselman AR et al. Urine markers do not predict biopsy findings or presence of bladder ulcers in interstitial cystitis/painful bladder syndrome. J Urol 2008;179:1850–1856.

88. Hanno P. International Consultation on IC Rome, September 2004/Forging an International Consensus: progress in painful bladder syndrome/interstitial cystitis. Int Urogynecol J Pelvic Floor Dysfunct 2005;16(suppl 1):S2–S5.

89. Lukban JC, Whitmore KE, Sant GR. Current management of interstitial cystitis. Urol Clin North Am 2002; 29:649–660.

90. Phatak S, Foster HE Jr. The management of interstitial cystitis: an update. Nat Clin Pract Urol 2006;3:45–53.

91. Theoharides TC, Sant GR. New agents for the medical treatment of interstitial cystitis. Expert Opin Investig Drugs 2001;10:521–546.

92. Theoharides TC, Sant GR. Immunomodulators for the treatment of interstitial cystitis. Urology 2005;65:633–638.

93. Moldwin RM, Sant GR. Interstitial cystitis: a pathophysiology and treatment update. Clin Obstet Gynecol 2002;45:259–272.

94. Barbalias GA, Liatsikos EN, Athanasopoulos A, Nikiforidis G. Interstitial cystitis: bladder training with intravesical oxibutinin. J Urol 2000;163:1818–1822.

95. Chaiken DC, Blaivas JG, Blaivas ST. Behavioral therapy for the treatment of refractory interstitial cystitis. J Urol 1993;149:1445–1448.

96. Mendelowitz F, Moldwin R. Complementary approaches in the management of interstitial cystitis. In: Sant GR (ed) Interstitial cystitis. Lippincott-Raven, Philadelphia PA, 1997, pp 235–239.

97. Weiss JM. Pelvic floor myofascial trigger points: manual therapy for interstitial cystitis and the urgency-frequency syndrome. J Urol 2001;166:2226–2231.

98. Oyama IA, Rejba A, Lukban JC et al. Modified Thiele massage as therapeutic intervention for female patients with interstitial cystitis and hightone pelvic floor dysfunction. Urology 2004;64:862–865.

99. Koziol JA. Epidemiology of interstitial cystitis. Urol Clin North Am 1994;21:7–20.

100. Nickel JC, Barkin J, Forrest J et al. Randomized, doubleblind, dose-ranging study of pentosan polysulfate sodium for interstitial cystitis. Urology 2005;65:654–668.

101. van Ophoven A, Heinecke A, Hertle L. Safety and efficacy of concurrent application of oral pentosan polysulfate and subcutaneous lowdose heparin for patients with interstitial cystitis. Urology 2005;66:707–711.

102. Minogiannis P, ElMansoury M, Betances JA et al. Hydroxyzine inhibits neurogenic bladder mast cell activation. Int J lmmunopharmacol 1998;20:553–563.

103. Theoharides TC. Hydroxyzine for interstitial cystitis. J Allergy Clin Immunol 1993;91:686–687.

104. Thilagarajah R, Witherow RO, Walker MM. Oral cimetidine gives effective symptom relief in painful bladder disease: a prospective, randomized, doubleblind placebocontrolled trial. BJU Int 2001;87:207–212.

105. Smith SD, Wheeler MA, Foster HE Jr, Weiss RM. Effect of

long-term oral l-arginine on the nitric oxide synthase pathway in the urine from patients with interstitial cystitis. J Urol 1997;158:2045–2050.

106. Korting GE, Smith SD, Wheeler MA et al. A randomized double-blind trial of oral l-arginine for treatment of interstitial cystitis. J Urol 1999;161:558–565.

107. Cartledge JJ, Davies AM, Eardley I. A randomized double-blind placebo-controlled crossover trial of the efficacy of L-arginine in the treatment of interstitial cystitis. BJU Int 2000;85:421–426.

108. Parson CL, Housley T, Schmidt JD et al. Treatment of interstitial cystitis with intravesical heparin. Br J Urol 1994;73.504–507.

109. Loose G, Jespersen J, Frandsen B et al. Subcutaneous heparin in the treatment of interstitial cystitis. Scand J Urol Nephrol 1985;19:27–29.

110. Ghoniem GM, McBride D, Sood OR, Lewis V. Clinical experience with multiagent intravesical therapy in interstitial cystitis patients unresponsive to singleagent therapy. World J Urol 1993;11:178–182.

111. Sant GR, Larock DR. Standard intravesical therapies for interstitial cystitis. Urol Clin North Am 1994;21:73–83.

112. Steinhoff G, Ittah B, Rowan S. The efficacy of condroitin-sulfate 0.2% in treating interstitial cystitis. Can J Urol 2002;9:1454–1458.

113. Cervigni M, Natale F, Nasta L et al. A combined intravesical therapy with hyaluronic acid and chondroitin for refractory painful bladder syndrome/interstitial cystitis. Int Urogynecol J Pelvic Floor Dysfunct 2008;19:943–947.

114. Chuang YC, Yoshimura N, Huang CC et al. Intravesical botulinum toxin a administration produces analgesia against acetic acid induced bladder pain responses in rats. J Urol 2004;172:1529–1532.

115. Lucioni A, Bales GT, Lotan TL et al. Botulinum toxin type A inhibits sensory neuropeptide release in rat bladder models of acute injury and chronic inflammation. BJU Int 2008;101:366–370.

116. Smith CP, Radziszewski P, Chancellor MB et al. Botulinum toxin a has antinociceptive effects in treating interstitial cystitis. Urology 2004;64:871–875; discussion 875.

117. van Ophoven A, Pokupic S, Heineke A et al. A prospective randomized placebo controlled, double blind study of amytriptiline for the treatment of interstitial cystitis. J Urol 2004;172:533–536.

118. Peeker R, Haghsheno MA, Holmang S, Fall M. Intravesical bacillus CalmetteGuerin and dimethyl sulfoxide for treatment of classic and nonulcer interstitial cystitis: a prospective, randomized doubleblind study. J Urol 2000;164:1912–1916.

119. Mayer R, Propert KJ, Peters KM et al. A randomized controlled trial of intravesical bacillus CalmetteGuerin for treatment refractory interstitial cystitis. J Urol 2005;173:1186–1191.

120. Sairanen J, Forsell T, Ruutu M. Long-term outcome of patients with interstitial cystitis treated with low dose cyclosporine A. J Urol 2004;171:2138–2141.

121. Ueda T, Tamaki M, Ogawa O et al. Improvement of interstitial cystitis symptoms and problems that developed during treatment with oral IPD-1151T. J Urol 2000;164:1917–1920.

122. Zhao J, Bai J, Zhou Y et al. Posterior tibial nerve stimulation twice a week in patients with interstitial cystitis. Urology 2008;71:1080–1084.

123. Peters KM, Feber KM, Bennett RC. A prospective, single-blind, randomized crossover trial of sacral vs pudendal nerve stimulation for interstitial cystitis. BJU Int 2007; 100:835–839.

Pelvic Pain Associated with a Gynecologic Etiology

53

Sondra L. Summers and Elizabeth R. Mueller

Abstract Healthcare practitioners often treat women with coexistent gynecological pelvic pain which may be attributed, by the patient, to a pelvic floor disorder. This chapter presents an algorithm for categorizing pelvic pain disorders into acute and chronic, based on the duration of the symptoms. Further categorization is based on the location of the pain.

Keywords Chronic pelvic pain • Endometriosis • Pelvic floor disorders • Pelvic pain

53.1 Introduction

Understanding pelvic pain, and all of its manifestations, is an essential part of clinical practice for healthcare providers treating women. Pelvic pain (PP) is formally defined as *discomfort localized to the pelvic compartment, abdominal wall, or perineum, which causes a woman to seek medical attention or affects her ability to function*. For most clinicians in non-gynecologic specialties, and even the seasoned gynecologist, the workup and management of a woman who presents with pelvic pain can be daunting. A thought process that we have found helpful is to first categorize the pelvic pain as acute or chronic. We triage the acute pain into emergent and non-emergent, and differentiate the chronic pain complaints into a cyclic or non-cyclic pattern (Fig. 53.1). In this chapter we will provide the framework for the evaluation and management of women who present with pelvic pain not associated with bladder or rectal pain, as these topics are covered in the previous and subsequent chapters.

E.R. Mueller
Female Pelvic Medicine and Reconstructive Surgery,
Departments of Urology, Obstetrics and Gynecology, Loyola
University Stritch School of Medicine, Chicago, IL, USA

53.2 Etiology of Pelvic Pain

53.2.1 Acute Pelvic Pain

As demonstrated in Fig. 53.1, patients who present with new-onset pelvic pain and the findings of acute abdomen (elevated white blood cell count and peritoneal signs) warrant evaluation in an emergency room situation. They usually have a source for their peritoneal irritation, such as pelvic inflammatory disease, intra-abdominal bleeding, ovarian cyst rupture, or ovarian torsion. Although an ectopic pregnancy can present without evidence of acute abdomen, it is important to rule out this diagnosis in reproductive-aged women due to the potential for serious consequences if left untreated.

When it has been determined that the PP is acute but not emergent, the clinician can pursue the identification of the cause in the outpatient setting. Patients presenting with complaints of acute pain of the vulva and perineum should be evaluated for causes of acute irritation such as infection or allergic dermatitis. Evaluation and treatments of common pelvic infections are listed in Table 53.1. Herpes simplex virus (HSV) infection presents with extremely painful vesicles and ulcers on the vulva; the first infection is usually ac-

G.A. Santoro, A.P. Wieczorek, C.I. Bartram (eds.) *Pelvic Floor Disorders*
© Springer-Verlag Italia 2010

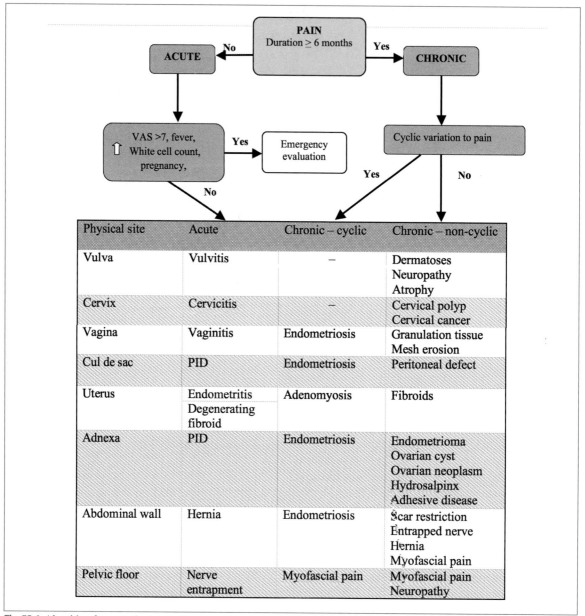

Fig. 53.1 Algorithm for outpatient evaluation of pain

companied by fever, myalgias, and enlarged inguinal lymph nodes. Recurrent outbreaks of HSV are usually less severe and are characterized by similar lesions distributed in a dermatome pattern. Candidal vulvovaginitis is most frequently caused by C. albicans and presents with an erythematous appearance, with swollen and small excoriations on the perineum, which can cause external dysuria. Treatment with topical antifungals such as the azoles, although effective in 80% of such patients, may be painful due to local irritation; oral ter-

conazole may be preferred if there are no contraindications to this medication [1]. Allergic dermatitis will also present as a non-specific erythematous rash on the perineum and may be difficult to distinguish from a candidal infection.

Other pelvic infections that can cause acute onset of mild pelvic pain are infections of the lower urinary tract and pelvic structures. Infections can be minor, such as vaginitis or urethritis, which nonetheless cause inflammation resulting in pelvic pain. A malodorous

Table 53.1 Evaluation and treatment of common pelvic infections

	Type	Method and diagnosis	Treatment
Vulvitis	Candida	Exam: erythema; satellite lesions	Fluconazole 150 mg po × 1
		Test: fungal culture	Topical azole (multiple regimens)
	Herpes simplex	Exam: ulcers or blisters	Aciclovir 400 mg po bd × 5 days
		Test: Herpes culture	Famciclovir 250 mg po bd × 5 days
		Valaciclovir 1 g po orally qd × 5	
Vaginitis	Candida	Exam: thick white discharge	Fluconazole 150 mg po × 1
		Microscopy with KOH: hyphae	Topical azole multiple regimens
		pH > 5.0	
		Test: fungal culture	
	Trichomonas	Exam: thick white discharge	Metronidazole 2 g po × 1
		Microscopy: Trichomonas	Metronidazole 500 mg po bd for 7 days
		pH < 4.5	
	Bacterial vaginosis	Exam: fish odor, yellow brown discharge	Metronidazole 500 mg po bd × 7 days gel, 0.75%, qds × 5 days (5 g) intravaginally
		Microscopy: clue cells, no lactobacilli	Clindamycin cream, 2% (5 g), intravaginally every night × 7 days
		pH < 4.5	Metrogel (various regimens)
Cervicitis, urethritis	Chlamydia	Test: nucleic acid amplification (NAAT)	Azithromycin 1 g po × 1 Doxycycline 100 mg po bd × 7–10 days
	Gonorrhea	Test: NAAT	Ceftriaxone 125 mg IM × 1 Cefixime 400 mg po × 1
Urinary tract infection	Bacterial	Test: urine culture	(Dependent upon sensitivities of culture)
Pelvic inflammatory disease	Multibacterial	Exam: purulent cervical discharge, cervical motion tenderness	Treat empirically for gonorrhea/Chlamydia
		Test: NAAT for Chlamydia/gonorrhea	Consult CDC guideline (www.cdc.gov)

vaginal discharge is usually bacterial in origin, such as Trichomonas or bacterial vaginosis. The diagnosis is made by inspection of the vaginal vault with a speculum and collection of vaginal discharge for examination with microscopy and pH testing. Cervicitis is characterized by a friable, inflamed cervix with purulent discharge. Pelvic pain, as differentiated from vulvar pain from vaginal candidiasis, is unusual.

Pelvic inflammatory disease (PID) is a multibacterial infection of the internal pelvic organs usually initiated by a sexually transmitted infection such as chlamydia or gonorrhea. Symptoms can be mild discomfort initially with urethritis or dysuria symptoms and occasionally a vaginal discharge. Acute PID can present with more severe pain and a purulent discharge with tenderness localized to the lower uterine segment/cervix

and adnexal regions. If an acute episode of PID results in peritubal adhesions, hydrosalpinx or tubo-ovarian abscess formation, the patient can experience chronic pelvic pain (CPP).

53.2.2 Chronic Pelvic Pain

53.2.2.1 Cyclic Chronic Pelvic Pain

Once it is determined that the patient's pain is chronic (≥ 6 months), we categorize the pain based on whether or not it is cyclic. Pain associated with the menstrual cycle is often assumed to be caused by endometriosis, which is the presence of endometrial glands and stroma located outside of the endometrial cavity. One hypothesis is that endometriosis is due to retrograde flow of menstrual effluent through the fallopian tubes into the peritoneal cavity, although many theories take into account a possible genetic and immunological association [2]. The pelvic pain occurs when these implants of the endometrial tissue, which grow and invade into pelvic tissues, are stimulated during menses.

Chronic pelvic pain affects one out of seven women in the US, is as prevalent as migraine, back pain, and asthma in the UK, and accounts for as much as 25% of gynecologic office visits [3]. The prevalence of endometriosis is believed to be 1–7% [4], although one study of 50 asymptomatic women undergoing a laparoscopic tubal ligation demonstrated a 15% incidence of endometrial implants at the time of surgery [5]. That said, most experts agree that endometriosis is associated predominantly with cyclic, menstrual pain. The high prevalence of CPP, along with the not-infrequent finding of endometriosis during diagnostic laparoscopy, has resulted in the symptom of CPP being associated with the physical finding of endometriosis, and the clinician is cautioned to proceed carefully before assuming a cause and effect relationship between these two entities.

Hurd proposes that the following three criteria be met prior to associating the pain to endometriosis: the pain should be cyclic, endometriosis should be diagnosed surgically, and appropriate treatment of the endometriosis should result in prolonged pain relief (for example, medical therapy has been shown to provide relief for 10 months after cessation of therapy) [6]. This definition only allows for the diagnosis of endometriosis after laparoscopy and successful treatment, and may not be as helpful in clinical practice as it is in research protocols.

Ectopic implants of endometriosis can also be found in locations other than the peritoneal cavity. A condition related to endometriosis known as adenomyosis involves endometriotic implants within the muscular wall of the uterus itself and not only causes pain during menses but can also be associated with increased menstrual flow and a tender uterus during examination. Endometriosis has been found in abdominal incisions, most commonly after a cesarean section with the theorized etiology from direct implantation of the tissue at the time of surgery [7].

Some women may complain of cyclic recurrent PP which occurs mid-cycle. This pattern is known as "mittelschmerz" and is thought to be related to ovulation.

The pain is usually short-lived, lasting about 24 hours, and usually responds to analgesics [8].

Other causes of cyclic variations in pain may be due to interactions between somatic structures (muscle/skin) or between somatic and visceral structures (somatovisceral) [9]. These interactions are believed to provide a mechanism by which pathology in one organ influences the function of another organ (viscerovisceral). Researchers have demonstrated that acute inflammation of the rat colon or prostate, as well as chronic abdominal pathology (surgically induced endometriosis), produces inflammation in an otherwise healthy bladder [10–13]. This finding may help explain why patients with pelvic pain often have coexisting visceral pain syndromes such as painful bladder or irritable bowel.

In fact, every structure in the abdomen and pelvis could have a role in the etiology of CPP. Therefore, it is essential to think beyond the organs of the reproductive, genitourinary, and gastrointestinal tracts and also consider contributions from the peripheral and central nervous system, the blood vessels, and the muscles and fascia of the abdominal and pelvic floor. Although the assessment of pain in the pelvic musculoskeletal system currently lacks standardization or even objective measurements, most experts agree that it can be a primary or secondary cause of CPP [14].

When discussing the possible eitiologies of cyclic pelvic pain, it is important to remember that many pain syndromes (including non-pelvic pain syndromes such as migraines) appear to have a cyclic nature associated with an increase in estriol levels. Studies have also demonstrated that the somatovisceral and viscerovisceral effects that have been seen in rats are at least partially centrally mediated [9]. Such effects could be contributing to the occurrence and cyclicity of pelvic floor disorders in women.

53.2.2.2 Non-Cyclic Chronic Pelvic Pain

Chronic pelvic pain that presents without an association to the menstrual cycle and is non-cyclic has a variety of causes. We have organized these sources of pain by pelvic structure listed in Fig. 53.1, starting with the external genitalia.

Chronic vulvar pain can be part of a pain syndrome known as vulvodynia, which is defined by the International Society for the Study of Vulvovaginal Disease

(ISSVD) as: "vulvar discomfort, most often described as burning pain, occurring in the absence of relevant visible findings or a specific, clinically identifiable, neurologic disorder". Typically this complex can be divided into four categories by etiology: (1) periorificial dermatitis (etiology is cyclic vulvovaginitis, rebound dermatitis after use of topical steroids or lichen sclerosus); (2) vulvar vestibulitis/vaginismus (etiology most likely neuropathic); (3) pudendal neuralgia (etiology is metabolic, traumatic or idiopathic); and (4) vulvar neuroma formation (etiology is traumatic or iatrogenic transaction of peripheral nerve fibers) [15]. The key points are first to determine whether there are any vulvar skin changes. If so, then the etiology is most likely recurrent candidiasis or a skin disorder such as steroid rebound, lichen sclerosus, or irritant/contact allergy. In clinical studies that have looked at biopsies performed on all patients with vulvodynia, 70% of these women were found to have a dermatological cause for their symptoms, with lichen sclerosus being the most common finding, followed by dermatitis [16].

Without skin changes, the etiology is most likely neuropathic and the diagnosis is best helped by history and physical exam findings. Vulvar vestibulitis is typically associated with penetration dyspareunia, while vaginismus is associated with an involuntary spasm of the pelvic floor musculature. Pudendal neuralgias are associated with chronic burning pain in the dermatome of this sensory nerve and are usually not associated with dyspareunia. Vulvar neuromas can often be palpated as a tiny nodule at an area of point tenderness identified by the patient.

Causes for CPP originating from the cervix include inflammatory conditions such as cervicitis, cervical cancer, or postoperative tissue changes such as granulation tissue formation after a cone biopsy. Cervical and endometrial polyps are typically benign and are not a cause of CPP unless the patient has had previous surgery. Cervical and endometrial polyps tend to be asymptomatic, and when symptomatic they present with intermenstrual or post-coital bleeding.

Uterine fibroids are benign tumors of the uterine smooth muscle and are the most common tumors of the female pelvis, occurring in one of every four or five women [17]. Most uterine fibroids are asymptomatic; however, 10–40% produce abnormal uterine bleeding, infertility, or pain. Pain associated with myomas is most often characterized as pelvic pressure or associated with the menses. Although fibroids can undergo a degeneration process which can cause acute pain and fever, this is usually a self-limited process and it is atypical for a patient with a fibroid to have CPP as the presenting symptom. A patient presenting with CPP and uterine fibroids should have an evaluation to rule out other causes of her pain. The clinician must also be aware that the differential diagnosis of pelvic masses thought to be fibroids includes pregnancy, ovarian masses, and colorectal neoplasia.

Ovarian causes for CPP include ovarian remnant and retention syndromes, ovarian neoplasms, and torsion of the ovarian vasculature. The ovarian remnant syndrome is defined as the persistence of functional ovarian tissue after intended extirpation of both ovaries with or without hysterectomy. The ovarian retention syndrome is defined as the presence of ovarian tissue after intended conservation of one or both ovaries at the time of hysterectomy [18]. The etiology of pain in the ovarian retention syndromes is felt to be entrapment of the ovary by adhesions, although this is somewhat controversial. In a combined retrospective analysis representing 487 women in 10 studies, El-Minawi and Howard found that 68% of women with ovarian retention syndrome presented with pelvic pain, 20% with dyspareunia, 21% with asymptomatic mass, 31% with pain and mass, and 4% had other symptoms. The pelvic pain was typically referred to the side of the retained ovary and often radiated to the lower back and down into the legs. The most important physical exam finding was a tender pelvic mass at the vaginal vault.

Ovarian remnant syndrome is also felt to be an under-recognized cause of pelvic pain in women. A combined retrospective analysis of 117 women from seven studies diagnosed with ovarian remnant syndrome demonstrated that 93% of the women presented with pelvic pain, 79% with pelvic mass, 65% with dyspareunia, 30% with pain on defecation, 19% with dysuria, and 33% with other symptoms [18]. The pain was felt to be chronic and non-cyclic in most cases, with the location most often ipsilateral to the retained ovary. The absence of hot flashes in women not receiving hormonal replacement following a bilateral oophorectomy is found in the majority of the women with ovarian remnant syndrome.

Enlargement of the ovarian capsule, in and of itself, is not thought to be a cause for CPP, as evidenced by the common observation that large ovarian neoplasms and carcinomas present without pain. However, a mass effect of an enlarged ovary, especially one fixed in the pelvis by adhesive disease, can cause CPP. The most likely etiology of CPP associated with an enlarged ovary is intermittent torsion of the ovarian vasculature. An enlarged or tortuous fallopian tube can also be a cause for CPP.

Pelvic congestion syndrome is defined as retrograde flow in an incompetent ovarian vein and is felt by some to be a cause of CPP. It has been hypothesized that the effect of this process can cause venous stasis, and flow reversal, and can act much as a varicose vein in pain causation. The diagnosis has historically only been made with venography or laparoscopy though now these dilated ovarian veins can be imaged with ultrasonography (US), computed tomography (CT) and magnetic resonance imaging (MRI) [19]. Expert opinion and case series are the primary evidence supporting the existence of pelvic congestion syndromes.

Adhesions are defined as a fibrous tissue by which anatomic structures abnormally adhere to each other. The role of adhesions in any pain syndrome, including CPP, is controversial. In a combined series of 1,318 patients with CPP and 1,103 patients without, the incidence of adhesions at the time of laparoscopy was found to be 25% versus 17%, respectively [20], suggesting an association between adhesions and CPP. A prospective trial of 48 women diagnosed with adhesive disease by laparoscopy and then randomized to either laparoscopic adhesiolysis or observation failed to show any benefit to adhesiolysis. After one year of follow-up, there was improvement in both groups, with no difference in any pain measurements between the groups. The authors concluded that there is no benefit to adhesiolysis for the alleviation of CPP in women.

53.3 Initial Assessment

Evaluation of the patient with CPP is best done in a multidisciplinary clinic with protocols developed from evidence-based approaches [21, 22]. Flor and Turk [23] evaluated this model for the management of low back pain in a meta-analysis, and found that patients with chronic low back pain treated in a multidisciplinary clinic had reduced pain severity, shorter time off of work, and decreased use of healthcare facilities. More recently, Kapoor and associates [21] evaluated this approach for complex pelvic floor disorders and found that patients experienced improvement in their symptoms for a longer period of time, which resulted in

overall higher quality-of-life parameters [11]. This model has been evaluated specifically for CPP by Peters et al with a prospective randomized trial that found similar results [24].

Patients who come for a clinical consultation are often keenly aware that there is no simple treatment for their pain. At our center, women are asked to list their "personal goals for treatment" and then to rank them in the order of priority. We reported on the patient-selected goals process in new patients presenting to a urogynecological clinic with pelvic floor disorders [25]. During the 5-month study, 305 new patients listed 635 goals for treatment. The majority of the goals could be categorized as symptom related (67%), followed by information seeking (12%), lifestyle (11%), or emotional goals (4%). Women seeking a non-surgical treatment were more likely to list "information seeking" as a primary goal than those who choose surgery. We believe that by having a discussion focused on the patient goals, clinicians can gain valuable insight about the patient expectations for care and can build trust in a process that often seems tiresome.

53.4 Evaluation of Pelvic Pain of Gynecologic Origin

53.4.1 History

The evaluation of PP involves the typical components of a history and physical exam, and at a minimum should include a visual analogue scale (VAS) for the assessment of pain. A complete history of the pain should also include the components of the pain: location, characterization, exacerbating and alleviating activities, and radiation pattern. We will discuss the components of this evaluation and how this can be an essential part of the evaluation of the patient with PP.

Many clinicians utilize a patient questionnaire which includes an anatomical diagram to identify the location of the CPP. It is helpful to ask patients to point out the location of the pain during the interview and examination. For instance, chronic unilateral pelvic pain can be caused by enlargement of an adnexal structure with intermittent torsion or a degenerating uterine leiomyoma located on that side of the uterus. Chronic right-sided pelvic pain can be caused by gastrointestinal conditions such as diverticulosis or chronic appendicitis. Pain localized at the site of previous abdominal surgical incisions can be caused by an incisional hernia or endometrioma of the abdominal wall, neuroma, or entrapped nerve. It is also possible for musculoskeletal strain or myofascial disorder (MFD) involving a specific muscle or muscle group to present as pain localized to the anatomical location of the muscle, its tendons, and site of insertion.

It is just as important that the patient identifies the site of tenderness on the vulva or perineum as with the abdominal exam. A diffuse pattern of CPP on the perineum suggests either a chronic irritant such as dermatoses, or a neuropathic cause found with a MFD such as levator ani syndrome [14]. Pain localized to one area of the vulva may be caused by a specific neuropathy such as pudendal neuralgia. Chronic recurrent painful ulcerative lesions can be found with Behçet's syndrome, HSV, or excoriations found with the "scratch–itch" syndrome of a non-specific irritation.

The patient's description of the location of radiation of her pain can also be helpful in assessing the cause of the pain. Pelvic structures in the posterior portion of the pelvis can cause pain to radiate into the back; for instance, a posterior uterine fibroid can present with a dull backache. Pain which radiates into the lower extremities, specifically the anterior/medial aspect, can be originating from a disease process located along the pelvic sidewall, such as endometriosis [26].

The patient's description of exacerbating events is an important piece of the clinical puzzle. As mentioned above, movement can elicit pain for many patients and may suggest either musculoskeletal origin or adhesive disease. A common exacerbating event for pelvic pain is intercourse, a complaint known as "dyspareunia". The pain can occur during the sex act or minutes, or even hours, later. Introital pain with initial penetration is indicative of a vulvar source of the pain, and extensive evaluation of these causes should be done. Pain which begins during or after penetration suggests a condition that is irritated with contact, such as cervicitis or other infections, endometriosis, or peritoneal defect of the cul de sac, or adenomyosis. Examination of the patient in these cases can find a cause for this irritation and if the examiner can recreate the pain, this can be very helpful. When the onset of pain is hours after intercourse, the cause is more difficult to discern during examination. Many of these women suffer from MFD of the pelvic floor and the pain after intercourse that lingers for an additional day or two is actually the pain from muscle straining.

Alleviating factors are an important component of the history but may not be especially helpful in creating a differential diagnosis. The use of analgesics, narcotics, rest, and heat can be non-specific therapies which help with many types of pain. It is imperative to document any pain medications the patient has used in the past, as well as current medications with dosing schedule and strength.

The patient's qualitative description of the pain can also be helpful. It is thought that the neurophysiological mechanism of pain caused by injury to an anatomic structure can determine the type of pain experienced by the patient. For instance, pain originating from somatic structures such as musculoskeletal injury is described as dull or aching, due to transmission along sensory fibers. Visceral organs transmit pain sensation via sympathetic fibers of the autonomic nervous system, which is perceived as diffuse and crampy. Patients many times use the descriptive term "burning", "tingling", or another term associated with a dysthesia, when their pain is caused by neuropathy [27].

53.4.2 Physical Exam

The clinician should initiate the physical exam of a CPP patient after establishing a rapport during the interview process. The exam may elicit significant pain for the patient, so effective communication and trust need to be developed. It is also important to note that patients will respond to a painful examination with guarding, which may thus render the remainder of the exam difficult to interpret. We prefer a systematic, gentle approach with maneuvers that are thought to cause pain performed last. Physical examination of the patient is critical to directing further evaluation and formulating a treatment plan, and thus is a crucial part of the patient evaluation.

The exam typically starts with the patient seated on the exam table. The back is carefully inspected for sacral defects, tenderness over the spine or sacroiliac joint, and normal spinal alignment. Gentle but firm palpation at the costavertebral angle is performed to elicit tenderness. An exam of the lower extremities can then be performed and is indicated in patients who present with a potential neurological cause to their symptoms.

The abdominal exam is performed after the patient has been assisted into the supine position and appropriately draped. Relaxation during this part of the exam is paramount, as guarding in response to and in anticipation of pain can cause spurious findings. The examination of the abdomen begins with visual inspection: note abdominal scars and any superficial masses or skin retraction. The next step will isolate the anterior abdominal wall and is initiated by asking the patient to engage her abdominal wall muscles by lifting her head or legs off the exam table. This maneuver will allow the examiner to evaluate the anterior abdominal wall for causes of pain such as trigger points in the rectus muscles, abdominal wall endometriomas, neuromas, or entrapped nerves near incisions. The Valsalva effect will also elicit a bulge if there is a hernia present. If there is significant tenderness with this portion of the exam, allow the patient to relax prior to any deep palpation.

Deep palpation should begin at the point furthest away from the site of pain. The examiner should look for an abdominal or pelvic mass, evidence for distention caused by constipated stool in the colon, ascites, and a full bladder as he or she is isolating the location of the tenderness. Percussion of the lower abdomen can also help identify the bladder edge. Deep palpation can also elicit a referred pattern of pain which can be helpful.

Inspection of the female genitourinary structures is performed in the dorsal lithotomy position with the physician seated. The external genitalia, specifically the vulva and the perineum, should be inspected for any visible lesion or skin breakdown. If the pain is localized, the patient may be asked to point out the site of symptoms. Any suspicious skin lesion should be biopsied or referred for consultation to rule out malignancy. A Q-tip test is used to faintly stroke the vulva and hymenal opening in order to note any dys-esthesia found with many vulvodynia syndromes. Visual examination of the urethra may demonstrate a small rim of urethral mucosa posteriorly, which is called a urethral caruncle. If the mucosa appears circumferentially around the urethra, it is referred to as urethral prolapse. Both of these findings are benign and often require no treatment. Patients may attribute their symptoms to this finding, especially if they have been performing self-examination, but usually some reassurance is necessary. The neurourologic exam should include assessment of sensation of the genitalia and inner thighs. The bulbocavernosus reflex is elicited by squeezing the clitoris and looking for an anal wink. While the presence of the bulbocavernosus reflex assures that the reflex arc is intact, it is common to find a negative reflex in patients who are neurologically normal.

The post-void residual urine volume should be measured to rule out urinary retention which can be a cause of diffuse suprapubic pain. This can be done by straight catheterization or bladder ultrasound within ten minutes of voiding. Any urine specimen obtained should be tested for the microscopic presence of red and white blood cells and the presence of bacteria, since urinary tract infections and bladder tumors can present with urinary symptoms and pelvic pain.

A double-bladed speculum exam is indicated for women who present for evaluation of pelvic pain. Visualization of the vaginal walls will allow you to see erosion or extrusion of synthetic materials used during prolapse or incontinence procedures. The vagina and cervix will be visualized in order to take samples for microscopy, cultures, and cytology.

Following the speculum exam, the physician should perform a systematic examination of the urethra, perineal muscles, and pelvic floor with a single digit inserted into the vagina. Tell the patient that you are going to push on some muscles in her vagina to check for tenderness. Demonstrate the amount of pressure you will use by firmly pushing on her thigh muscles. Ask her to rate her tenderness on a scale of 0–10, where 0 is no pain and 10 is the worst pain imaginable. Use a single digit to firmly palpate the muscles of the posterior, lateral, and anterior pelvic walls, looking for trigger points or myofascial tenderness. Sweep anteriorly to evaluate the urethra, and anterior vaginal and abdominal wall for similar findings. The digital exam concludes with isolation of the posterior cul de sac and cervix, with attempts to evaluate these deep structures without eliciting pain in the pelvic floor. A simple touching of the cervix with movement can evaluate for PID; nodularity and tenderness in the cul de sac can raise suspicion for endometriosis, and a retroverted uterus can be best palpated in this manner. Palpation of a circumferential mass in the anterior vaginal wall may indicate periurethral leiomyoma, vaginal wall cyst, urethral diverticulum, or urethral carcinoma. The anterior vaginal cavity can also be palpated for the presence of a foreign body such as an extruded mesh.

To complete the evaluation of the internal pelvic structures and to localize pain, place two fingers of the dominant hand beneath the cervix and elevate the vaginal apex. By gently placing the non-dominant hand suprapubically, one can elicit uterine tenderness and evaluate uterine size. By sweeping these digits anterolaterally, one can evaluate for tenderness or mass in the adnexal region, again using the abdominal hand gently to guide these structures for palpation. In women with obesity, guarding, and menopause, it may not be realistic to expect to palpate ovaries; the transvaginal ultrasound will allow effective and diagnostic visualization and many clinicians make this part of their protocol for women presenting with CPP.

53.4.3 Office Testing

After obtaining a thorough history and performing a directed physical exam, office testing can be initiated, depending upon clinical suspicion. Pregnancy tests are an imperative first step and will rule out pregnancy prior to any prescribing or imaging. In many instances, the pain may be difficult to localize and protocols will call for urinalysis, cultures, and other sexually transmitted infection testing to assure complete evaluation. Table 53.1 lists the types of pelvic infections, findings and diagnostic testing with appropriate treatment regimens.

Complete evaluation of perineal and vulvar pain should include biopsies which may be directed by colposcopy [16]. Vulvar ulcers should be tested for herpes and can be biopsied if other etiologies are a possibility. When a vaginal discharge is noted that is suspicious for infection, a sample should be sent for culture and, if a microscope is available, evaluated by microscopy and pH testing. Cervical cytology should be sent routinely if the patient is not up to date on her cervical cancer screening, or to evaluate any cervical lesions; likewise a cervical biopsy could be considered. Testing for *Chlamydia* and gonorrhea is performed with a swab at the cervical os and a nucleic acid amplification test (please note that urine can also be tested in a patient for whom a pelvic exam is not appropriate).

53.4.4 Imaging

Pelvic ultrasonography with transvaginal imaging is one of the most useful tools in the assessment of the woman with PP, and is the optimal method of visualizing pelvic structures to identify a structural cause of pain. The positive predictive value (PPV) of ultrasonography for determining the cause of pelvic pain has been evaluated in patients prior to undergoing laparoscopy

for definitive diagnosis. One series of 316 women with CPP who were enrolled in the study found that the PPV of ultrasonography was 82% and the negative predictive value was 46.9% [28]. Another series which looked at "soft signs" noted at the time of pelvic ultrasonography done prior to laparoscopy in 87 patients found the PPV of ultrasound to be only 25% until factors such as site-specific pelvic tenderness, free fluid in the pelvis, and immobile ovaries were taken into account; the PPV then rose to 78% [29].

CT scan of the pelvic structures is not as specific or sensitive for structural disorders of the pelvis but can be used to diagnose other causes of pain such as diverticulosis, hernia, or an abdominal wall mass such as endometrioma. The use of a pelvic MRI scan can be helpful in identifying the exact nature of an adnexal mass such as hydrosalpinx (which can have the appearance of complex mass on pelvic ultrasound), ovarian mass as with an endometrioma, uterine mass such as adenomyosis or fibroid, or, less frequently, retroperitoneal neoplasms not imaged with ultrasono-graphy [28, 30].

53.4.5 Surgical Evaluation

Laparoscopy is indicated in the evaluation and potential treatment of many women suffering from CPP. Laparoscopy can detect many causes of CPP when all other testing has been negative, including adhesive disease, PID, and, most importantly, the findings of endometriosis including blue, clear, or red endometriotic implants or peritoneal defects [20]. Although laparoscopy accounts for almost half of all gynecologic laparoscopic procedures, there are many instances when the findings are normal or inconclusive [28]. Laparoscopy is considered the optimal method to diagnose endometriotic implants, as these will not show up on any imaging technology, but as a diagnostic test it lacks sensitivity and specificity. Even when visual findings of endometriosis are made, the biopsies are not always confirmatory [31], and 15 to 40% of asymptomatic women have been found to have signs of endometriosis at the time of laparoscopy done for sterilization [5, 29]. Despite these findings, many women experience resolution of their CPP after a normal diagnostic laparoscopy, with theorized etiologies ranging from pelvic relaxation, anesthetic, or placebo effect [6].

53.5 Treatment of Chronic Pelvic Pain of Gynecologic Origin

Many of the causes of CPP cannot be readily identified through conventional methods of history and physical exam, radiological imaging techniques, or lab work. Therefore, it is reassuring to the patient to communicate that a "normal" test result does not indicate that there is no etiology for the pain, and although the "cure" may be elusive, you will continue to provide care with the intent to minimize her symptoms. The use of empirical therapies and protocols can be an effective method that allows for potential alleviation of symptoms while concurrently completing the evaluation.

53.5.1 Infections

The link between acute pelvic pain, chronic non-cyclic pain, and gynecological infections would seem to be self-evident. It is imperative that this diagnosis is made in a timely fashion, given the potential for relief with appropriate care and for significant morbidity if undiagnosed [32].

Vulvovaginal infections are usually easy to diagnose and treat with appropriate medication. Chronic or recurrent vulvovaginal infections require prolonged treatment and further investigation. Candidal infections of the vulva can be especially symptomatic, and application of topical azoles can cause pain to the infected vulva; we recommend oral fluconazole 150 mg unless the patient has contraindications to this medication. A chronic or complicated candidal infection will require prolonged use of antifungal therapies. *Herpes simplex* infections, especially in the primary outbreak, are best treated with antiviral oral medication with analgesics, with some patients requiring narcotics for severe pain and post-herpetic neuropathic pain [32].

For a patient presenting with acute pain consistent with PID, it is sometimes prudent to treat empirically for *Chlamydia* and gonorrhea, especially in the outpatient setting. The nucleic acid amplification testing can take a few days for results, and waiting for the result may miss the window of opportunity to treat an uncomplicated infection. *Chlamydia* is treated with azithromycin 1 g orally for the patient, and for the partner when appropriate; alternatively doxycycline 100 mg bd can be used for 7–10 days, but compliance with the regimen is a concern. Gonorrhea has historically

been treated with ceftriaxone 125 mg IM; it is prudent to check with guidelines in your geographic area for optimal therapy due to many resistant drug strains (www.cdc.gov) [33].

53.5.2 Vulvar Pain

When the targeted evaluation of a patient with acute vulvar pain is suggestive of infection, the guidelines described above and in Table 53.1 should be followed. When a patient fails to respond to an antifungal, or the clinical history is suggestive of an allergic dermatitis, a topical low-potency steroid cream such as betamethasone valerate 0.1% or hydrocortisone 1–2% may alleviate these symptoms. Vulvar pathology such as lichen sclerosus is treated with a high-potency steroid such as clobetasole 0.05% nightly for 1–3 months, with a tapering period depending upon the severity and duration of the symptoms.

Vulvovaginal atrophy can be treated with either systemic estrogen replacement or topical estrogen such as provided by intravaginal creams, ring, or tablets. Most of these local agents have minimal systemic effects due to their limited absorption into the vasculature.

Vulvodynia is a syndrome with no clear etiology, and is best served with a multidisciplinary approach which includes treatment of MFD of the pelvic floor incorporating physical therapy, and neuromodulators such as gabapentin, amitryptiline, or lyrica. Box 53.1 lists the most commonly used neuromodulators and their dosing schedules. For optimal treatment, the patient may require injections of local anesthetic or corticosteroids into trigger points. Levator ani syndrome with tenderness isolated in the levator muscle complex is a good example of a myofascial condition which presents as vulvar pain, and is best treated in this manner [32]. Likewise, pudendal neuropathy presents with vulvar pain which is located along this sensory nerve innervation and may require a transvaginal or transperineal pudendal nerve block. A prospective trial of 27 women reporting vulvar vestibulitis symptoms responded with a significantly decreased sensation of pain after five sessions of these injections [32, 34]. Topical xylocaine or nitroglycerin can also alleviate vulvar pain, although it may not alter the natural history of the symptoms [35].

Many of the patients with chronic pelvic pain have a component of MFD and will require intense physical therapy and/or trigger point or nerve injections. Dis-

Box 53.1 Commonly used medications for pelvic pain

Analgesics
- Ibuprofen 200–800 mg q 6–8 h with max 3200 mg/24 h
- Naproxen 250, 375, 500 mg bd
- Diclofenac 50–75 mg bd
- Mefenamic acid 250 mg every 4–6 h
- Celecoxib 100–200 mg per day

Narcotics[a]
- Hydrocodone 5–10 mg in combination with acetaminofen qds
- Tramadol 50–100 mg every 4–6 h
- Propoxyphene napsylate 100 mg every 4 h

Tricyclics[b]
- Amitriptyline 10 mg at night, may increase up to 150 mg/24 h tds dosing
- Nortriptyline 10 mg HS, may increase to 150 mg/24 h tds dosing

Other
- Gabapentin 300 mg HS, may increase up to 300 mg tds
- Pregabalin 25 mg HS, may increase up to 75 mg bd with max 600 mg/24 h

[a] Narcotics contracts should be signed by patient prior to initiating prescribing or only given by pain clinic which can closely monitor use
[b] Sedative side-effects of tricyclics warrant slow increase over first few days and weeks of use

cussion of this treatment regimen will be addressed in another chapter.

There are many effective medications for treating the symptoms of dysmenorrhea and other pain manifestations presumed secondary to endometriosis. Box 53.1 lists commonly used analgesics for the alleviation of CPP and dysmenorrhea. Optimally, endometriosis would be a diagnosis based upon a biopsy which shows ectopic implants of endometrial tissue identified at the time of laparoscopy [20]. There are, however, many clinical situations where empiric therapy has been shown to be effective [36]. While first-line therapy should be directed toward analgesics such as nonsteroidal agents, narcotics have also been shown to be effective [37, 38].

Hormonal modalities for treatment for presumed or proven endometriosis have been directed towards reducing the stimulation of the estrogen-dependant endometrial implants. Oral contraceptive medications with a low dosage of estrogen, i.e. 20–35 µg of norinyl acetate, have been shown to be effective in the relief of menstrual pain [38].

Other hormonal agents which have an anti-estrogenic effect on implants include progestational agents such as medroxyprogesterone and danazol, which is an androgenic medication [39].

Gonadotropin-releasing hormone (GnRH) agonists act to suppress the pulsatile release of gonadotropins, which inhibits ovulation to induce a hypoestrogenic state. Double-blind placebo-controlled studies have illustrated significant reduction in pain with the use of lupron [37]. As expected, there are short- and long-term effects of this induced state of menopause, including loss of bone density, and multiple studies have shown that addition of oral contraceptive or progestational agents, known as "add-back" therapy, can help alleviate these side-effects without sacrificing efficacy [37].

It is our recommendation that analgesics be offered as first-line therapy for patients with dysmenorrhea; oral contraceptives can be a useful adjunct in the patient who has no contraindications to their use. Patients who fail to respond to these therapies may benefit from a long-acting progestational agent such as offered by the intramuscular or subdermal implant or via a progesterone-coated intrauterine device. If the patient continues to have pain which is suggestive of endometriosis, a discussion should be initiated as to her options for continued empiric treatment with lupron, with or without add-back therapy, versus a diagnostic procedure such as laparoscopy.

53.5.3 Surgical Treatments

53.5.3.1 Laparoscopic Approach

The use of laparoscopic procedures in the treatment of chronic pelvic pain has been the subject of much discussion and investigation. Surgical treatment of endometriosis is indicated if medical therapy, either provided empirically or after biopsy-proven diagnosis, is not effective, or if the patient desires a diagnosis. Treatment of peritoneal implants with fulguration or surgical excision has been shown to be effective, though temporary, in the relief of symptoms [40]. The beneficial effect of laparoscopic adhesiolysis is controversial, with evidence to suggest that significant relief of pain occurs with lysis of severe adhesive disease involving the bowel [41]. Other laparoscopic procedures such as incidental appendectomy, presacral neurectomy (PSN), and laparoscopic uterosacral nerve ablation (LUNA) have been shown to be effective in some surgical outcomes studies [42, 44]. We feel that the laparoscopic procedures involving adhesiolysis, LUNA, and PSN and incidental appendectomy should not be routinely performed for CPP, as they have not been shown definitively to help with CPP and require an expert level of surgical expertise with a potential for significant morbidity.

53.5.3.2 Hysterectomy

The therapeutic benefit of hysterectomy for the relief of pelvic pain with or without bilateral salpingo-oophorectomy appears substantiated in a number of prospective cohort studies, regardless of the etiology of the pain [45, 46]. Hysterectomy alone appears to offer relief from pelvic pain for the majority of women studied and for a prolonged time period [47]. Obviously, hysterectomy should be considered the treatment of last resort for most women suffering from CPP who have completed their child bearing. If there is a component of MFD as an etiology for the pelvic pain, this source of CPP may not be alleviated with a hysterectomy, especially immediately postoperatively. It is important to identify the women with MFD and counsel them preoperatively that they may require continued treatment after surgery.

53.5.3.3 Uterine Leiomyomas

There are many benign pelvic neoplasms that can cause a patient discomfort but that do not require surgery. Uterine fibroids can be treated symptomatically with oral contraceptives, progestational agents such as IM depoprovera, or GnRH agonists, or procedurally with uterine artery embolization, in order to decrease pain. Degeneration of the solid leiomyoma, a process which is characterized by pain, tenderness of the fibroid, fever, and leukocytosis, can have symptoms that require intervention. In many cases, these patients respond to analgesics, anti-inflammatory agents, and antibiotics, and do not require surgical intervention. If it is determined that a uterine fibroid requires surgical excision, a discussion with the patient can determine whether myomectomy or hysterectomy is warranted, given her desire for future childbearing or other concerns. Interventional radiologic procedures such as uterine artery

embolization can also help reduce the size of uterine fibroids and thus decrease the symptoms associated with the fibroids, including pain [48].

53.5.3.4 Ovarian Neoplasms

Ovarian cysts are usually functional, originating in the ovulation cycle, and will disappear over time with expectant therapy. Even solid benign ovarian masses such mature teratomas or endometriomas can be small and followed expectantly for an indeterminate time [49]. Of course, acute exacerbation of the pain can indicate torsion or twisting of the infundibulopelvic ligament and warrant urgent surgical intervention. Rupture of an ovarian cyst with spillage of serous or hemorrhagic material can also cause acute severe abdominopelvic pain and must be differentiated from the former, as ovarian cyst rupture rarely requires surgical intervention; expectant management with analgesics usually suffices.

The ovarian remnant syndrome can be challenging to diagnose, as even the most sensitive imaging techniques may not identify the small remnant of ovarian tissue, and the location of the remnant tissue may not be in the ovarian fossa [50, 51]. Surgical removal of this ovarian remnant tissue is difficult due to adhesive disease and inability to identify the ovarian tissue. Ovarian suppression with hormonal agents may sometimes offer symptomatic relief. Distention of the fallopian tube or hydrosalpinx or its involvement in adhesive complex is an example of a benign, chronic cause of pelvic pain which has no treatment other than surgery but which can easily be followed expectantly without removal.

53.5.3.5 Conditions Caused From Previous Surgery

Conditions that arise from previous surgery such as incisional hernia neuroma, or entrapped nerve or abdominal wall endometrioma will not improve until they are surgically corrected or removed [7]. Similarly, pain from vaginal mesh erosion after surgery for incontinence will require surgical removal for pain relief. Vaginal cuff granulation tissue, which can form after a hysterectomy, can cause significant pelvic pain and is easily treated in the office with a fulgurative procedure, or can be removed in the operating room. It is important to properly identify these causes of pelvic pain in order to choose the appropriate ameliorative procedure. Adhesive disease that arises from previous surgery is not usually an indication for surgical therapy as it has not been shown to offer pain relief.

53.5.4 Psychological Treatments

It has been well established that there is an association between a history of abuse, depression, anxiety, and pelvic pain [52, 53]. Due to this psychological component of CPP, it is imperative that the patient's psychological needs are addressed in any treatment protocol. The patient should be concurrently receiving therapy from a mental healthcare provider.

53.5.5 Alternative Medicine Treatments

There are some non-traditional treatments that have been shown to be effective in relieving pelvic pain. Acupuncture, biofeedback, physical therapy, and relaxation techniques have been used with some success [54]. Herbal and dietary therapies have been discussed, but a Cochrane review of this topic found only that magnesium supplementation may be helpful reducing symptoms of dysmenorrhea [55].

53.6 Summary

The syndrome of CPP is a difficult clinical dilemma and requires the services of a multidisciplinary approach and team. A thorough history that includes a patient intake questionnaire, review of records, and interview by a trained clinician are important first steps. A detailed physical exam which incorporates techniques of pain mapping done in a non-threatening, reassuring manner is also key to developing a protocol that will assist each patient with individualized therapy. An office pregnancy test is an important test to order at the patient's first evaluation and at each visit when appropriate. There is a role for vulvar biopsy if the patient's presentation does not provide immediate diagnosis. Cultures or other testing for infections is paramount, so that treatable sources of pain are not overlooked. Likewise, cytology and biopsies of the cervix can be important in a patient with a friable cervix. Empiric treatment with antibiotics, analgesics, or suppression of the hormonal cycle with oral contraceptives, progestational agents, or GnRH agonists can be an effective first line of therapy and can be initiated during completion of the workup.

Many patients suffering from CPP have a component of MFD. Many of these women will respond to analgesics, physical therapy, and/or neuromodulators. It is imperative that the clinician keeps in close contact with these patients and their physical therapists to assess whether they are responding appropriately to this line of therapy; pain from MFD can be secondary to another primary cause and thus may not be helped with physical therapy alone. Failure to respond to first-line treatments should be followed up with a discussion regarding other parallel protocols such as a change in medication or more invasive therapies such as trigger point injections or surgical evaluation and treatment. Psychotherapists assist our patients in dealing with the stress and possible concomitant depression that can accompany chronic pain syndromes.

Patients with CPP who have a "normal" evaluation or lack of response to empiric therapy can be counselled regarding the role of surgery for their presumed diagnosis. Laparoscopy, and less commonly cystoscopy, can offer a diagnosis and therapeutic benefit. Many women suffering from CPP have tried multiple therapies and may desire laparoscopy in order to identify the cause of their suffering. Similarly, many patients may request hysterectomy in the erroneous belief that all pelvic pain can be cured with removal of the uterus. Intense counseling of the patient is of utmost importance in these situations to ensure she has realistic expectations regarding the outcome and relief of her pain in these surgical situations. As stated before, the relationship between a woman with CPP and her healthcare provider is crucial, especially in those scenarios where the treatment modalities are not improving the quality of life with pain relief; these women will require more therapy and care even if the ultimate outcome does not result in complete pain relief.

References

1. Centers for Disease Control and Prevention. Sexually transmitted diseases treatment guidelines 2006. Diseases characterized by vaginal discharge. Management of patients who have vaginal infections. www.cdc.gov/std/treatment/2006/vaginal-discharge.htm (accessed 28 October 2009).

2. Dmowski WP, Braun DP. Immunology of endometriosis. Best Pract Res Clin Obstet Gyencol 2004;18:245–263.

3. Howard F. The role of laparoscopy in the evaluation of chronic pelvic pain: pitfalls with a negative laparoscopy. J Am Assoc Gynecol Laparosc 1996;4:85–94.

4. Barbieri R. Etiology and epidemiology of endometriosis. Am J Obstet Gynecol 1990;162:565–567.

5. Kresch AJ, Seifer DB, Sachs LB et al. Laparoscopy in 100 women with chronic pelvic pain. Am J Obstet Gynecol 1984;64:672–674.

6. Hurd W. Criteria that indicate endometriosis is the cause of chronic pelvic pain [see comment]. Obstet Gynecol 1998; 92:1029–1032.

7. Kocakusak A, Arpinar E, Arikan S et al. Abdominal wall endometriosis: a diagnostic dilemma for surgeons. Med Princ Pract 2005;14:434–437.

8. Muse K. Cyclic pelvic pain. Obstet Gynecol Clin North Am 1990;17:427–440.

9. Winnard KP, Dmitrieva N, Berkley KJ. Cross-organ interactions between reproductive, gastrointestinal, and urinary tracts: modulation by estrous stage and involvement of the hypogastric nerve. Am J Physiol Regul Integr Comp Physiol 2006;291:R1592–1601.

10. Lamb K, Zhang F, Gebhart GF, Bielefeldt K. Experimental colitis in mice and sensitization of converging visceral and somatic afferent pathways. Am J Phisiol Gastroenteric Liver Physiol 2006;290:6451–6457.

11. Letourneau R, Pang X, Sant GR, Theoharides TC. Intragranular activation of bladder mast cells and their association with nerve processes in interstitial cystitis. Br J Urol 1996;77:41–54.

12. Malykina AD, Qin C, Greenwood-Van Meerveld G et al. Hyperexcitability of convergent colon and bladder dorsal root ganglion neurons after colonic inflammation: mechanism for pelvic organ cross-talk. Neurogastroenterol Motil 2006;68:938–948.

13. Cason AM, Samuelson CL, Berkley KJ. Estrons changes in vaginal nociception in a rat model of endometriosis. Horn Behav 2003;44:123–131.

14. Tu FF, As-Sanie S, Steege JF. Musculoskeletal causes of chronic pelvic pain: a systematic review of diagnosis: part I. Obstet Gynecol Surv 2005;60:379–385.

15. Perry CP. Vulvodynia. In: Howard FM (ed) Pelvic pain diagnosis and management. Lippincott Williams & Williams, Philadelphia PA, 2000, pp 204–210.

16. Bowen AR, Vester A, Marsden L et al. The role of vulvar skin biopsy in the evaluation of chronic vulvar pain. Am J Obstet Gynecol 2008;199:467:e1–e6.

17. Buttram VC Jr, Reiter RC. Uterine leiomyomata: etiology, symptomatology, and management. Fertil Steril 1981; 36:433–445.

18. El-Minawi A, Howard FM. Ovarian retention syndrome. Pelvic pain diagnosis and management. In: Howard FM (ed) Pelvic pain diagnosis and management. Lippincott Williams & Williams, Philadelphia PA, 2000, pp 162–170.

19. Ganeshan A, Upponi S, Hon LQ et al. Chronic pelvic pain due to pelvic congestion syndrome: the role of diagnostic and interventional radiology. Cardiovasc Intervent Radiol 2007;30:1105–1111.

20. Howard F. The role of laparoscopy in chronic pelvic pain: promise and pitfalls. Obstet Gynecol Surv 1993;48:357–387.

21. Kapoor DS, Sultan AH, Thakar R et al. Management of complex pelvic floor disorders in a multidisciplinary pelvic floor clinic. Colorectal Dis 2008;10:118–123.

22. Milburn A, Reiter RC, Rhomberg AT. Multidisciplinary approach to chronic pelvic pain. Obstet Gynecol Clin North Am 1993;20:643–661.

23. Flor H, Fydrich T, Turk DC. Efficacy of multidisciplinary pain treatment centers: a meta-analytic review. Pain 1992; 49:221–230.

24. Peters AA, van Dorst E, Jellis B et al. A randomized clinical trial to compare two different approaches in women with chronic pelvic pain. Obstet Gynecol 1991;77:740–744.

25. Lowenstein L, Fitzgerald MP, Kenton K et al. Patient-selected goals: the fourth dimension in assessment of pelvic floor disorders. Int Urogynecol J 2008;19:81–84.

26. Vilos GA, Vilos AW, Haebe JJ, Laparoscopic findings, management, histopathology, and outcomes in 25 women with cyclic leg pain. J Am Assoc Gynecol Laparosc 2002;9:145–151.

27. Gunter J. Chronic pelvic pain: an integrated approach to diagnosis and treatment. Obstet Gynecol Surv 2003; 58:615–623.

28. Gjelsteen AC, Chimg BH, Meyermann MW et al. CT, MRI, PET, PET/CT, and ultrasound in the evaluation of obstetric and gynecologic patients. Surg Clin North Am 2008; 88:361–390.

29. Zubor P, Szunyogh N, Galo S et al. Laparoscopy in chronic pelvic pain–a prospective clinical study. Ceska Gynekologie 2005;70:225–231.

30. Potter A, Chandrasekhar CA. Abdominal emergencies: US and CT evaluation of acute pelvic pain of gynecologic origin in nonpregnant premenopausal patients. Radiographics 2008;28:1645–1659.

31. Martin D. Endometriosis: correlation between histologic and visual findings at laparoscopy. Am J Obstet Gynecol 2001;184:1407–11; discussion 1411–1413.

32. Faro S, Maccato M. Pelvic pain and infections. Obstet Gynecol Clin North Am 1990;17:441–455.

33. Drugs for sexually transmitted infections. Treat Guidel Med Lett 2004;2(26):67–74.

34. Rapkin AJ, McDonald M, Morgan M. Multilevel local anesthetic nerve blockade for the treatment of vulvar vestibulitis syndrome. Am J Obstet Gynecol 2008;198:41.e1–e5.

35. Walsh KE, Berman JR, Berman LA, Vierregger K. Safety and efficacy of topical nitroglycerin for treatment of vulvar pain in women with vulvodynia: a pilot study. J Gend Specif Med 2002;5:21–27.

36. Stone RW, Mountfield J. Interventions for treating chronic pelvic pain in women. Cochrane Database Syst Rev 2000; (4):CD000387.

37. Howard F. An evidence-based medicine approach to the treatment of endometriosis-associated chronic pelvic pain: placebo-controlled studies. J Am Assoc Gynecol Laparosc 2000;7:477–488.

38. Davis L, Kennedy SS. Modern combined oral contraceptives for pain associated with endometriosis. Cochrane Database Syst Rev 2007;(3):CD001019.

39. Selak V, Farquhar C, Prentice A, Singla A. Danazol for pelvic pain associated with endometriosis. Cochrane Database Syst Rev 2007;(4):CD000068.

40. Hart RJ, Hickey M, Maouris P, Buckett W. Excisional surgery versus ablative surgery for ovarian endometriomata [update of Cochrane Database Syst Rev 2005; (3):CD004992]. Cochrane Database Syst Rev 2008; (2):CD004992.

41. Parazzini F, Mais V, Cipriani S. Adhesions and pain in women with first diagnosis of endometriosis: results from a cross-sectional study. J Minim Invasive Gynecol 2006; 13:49–54.

42. Chandler B, Beegle M, Elfrink RJ, Smith WJ. To leave or not to leave? A retrospective review of appendectomy during diagnostic laparoscopy for chronic pelvic pain. Missouri Medicine 2002;99:502–504.

43. Johnson NP, Farquhar CF, Crossley S et al. A double-blind randomised controlled trial of laparoscopic uterine nerve ablation for women with chronic pelvic pain. BJOG 2004;111:950–959.

44. Zullo F, Palomba S, Zupi E et al. Effectiveness of presacral neurectomy in women with severe dysmenorrhea caused by endometriosis who were treated with laparoscopic conservative surgery: a 1-year prospective randomized double-blind controlled trial. Am J Obstet Gynecol 2003; 189:5–10.

45. Gambone JC, Reiter RC. Hysterectomy: improving the patient's decision-making process. Clin Obstet Gynecol 1997;40:868–877.

46. Reiter R. Evidence-based management of chronic pelvic pain. Clin Obstet Gynecol 1998;41:422–435.

47. Stones RW, Mountfield J. Interventions for treating chronic pelvic pain in women.[update of Cochrane Database Syst Rev 2000;(2):CD000387]. Cochrane Database Syst Rev 2000;(4):CD000387.

48. Goodwin SC, Spies JB, Worthington-Kirsch R et al. Uterine artery embolization for treatment of leiomyomata: long-term outcomes from the FIBROID Registry. Obstet Gynecol 2008; 111:22–33.

49. Shwayder J. Pelvic pain, adnexal masses, and ultrasound. Semin Reprod Med 2008;26:252–265.

50. Kho RM, Magrina JF, Magtibay PM. Pathologic findings and outcomes of a minimally invasive approach to ovarian remnant syndrome. Fertil Steril 2007;87:1005–1009.

51. Magtibay PM, Magrina JF. Ovarian remnant syndrome. Clin Obstet Gynecol 2006;49:526–534.

52. Poleshuck EL, Dworkin R, Howard FM et al. Contributions of physical and sexual abuse to women's experiences with chronic pelvic pain. J Reprod Med 2005; 50:91–100.

53. Collett BJ, Cordle C, Stewart CR, Jagger C. A comparative study of women with chronic pelvic pain, chronic nonpelvic pain and those with no history of pain attending general practitioners. Br J Obstet Gynaecol 1998;105:87–92.

54. Proctor ML, Lathe PM, Farquhar CM, Stones RW, Transcutaneous electrical nerve stimulation and acupuncture for primary dysmenorrhoea. Cochrane Database Syst Rev 2003;(4):CD002123.

55. Proctor ML, Murphy PA. Herbal and dietary therapies for primary and secondary dysmenorrhoea. Cochrane Database Syst Rev 2001;(3):CD002124.

Aldo Infantino and Andrea Lauretta

Abstract Pelvic pain is the most common form of pain experienced by people and
one of the most frequent reasons inducing patients to seek medical attention. Many
conditions are related to anorectal pain: inflammatory disease; functional disease;
pelvic tumors; post operative complications. In inflammatory bowel disease (IBD)
patients experience visceral pain secondary to hyperalgesia and allodynia. Hyperalgesia
is a peculiarity of patients with active ulcerative colitis (UC), while hypoalgesia is
typical of patients with quiescent or mild UC and Crohn's disease (CD). Inflammatory
pelvic diseases such as prostatitis or interstitial cystitis can cause recto-anal pain,
also. "Functional" disorders such as levator ani syndrome, proctalgia fugax, coccygodynia and Alcock's canal syndrome evoke severe anal pain and affect the quality
of life of patients. Irritable bowel syndrome (IBS) patients complain of pelvic pain,
although there are no structural lesions underlying this symptom. The central nervous
system plays a major role in the pathophysiology of IBS, also. Anorectal tumours
commonly cause pain. Radiotherapy has been demonstrated to be an useful mean to
improve pelvic pain significantly. Sexually transmitted infections can cause proctitis.
The most common symptom of infectious proctitis is anorectal pain. Gonorrhoea,
chlamydia, herpes simplex virus and syphilis are the commonest causative infectious
agents. Specific therapy is ideal but not always feasible. Bowel endometriosis causes
a wide variety of symptoms, which range from rectal bleeding to pelvic pain on defecation. Haemorrhoids, anal fissures and anal absceses are the most common proctological diseases associated with anal pain. Chronic proctalgia has been also described
after many surgical procedures such as PPH and STARR.
In summary, pelvic pain involves many visceral organs. Accuracy in collecting medical
informations and in phyisical examination is fundamental. Pelvic pain should be approached by a multidisciplinary team in order to reach the best results in diagnosis
and treatments.

Keywords Pelvic Pain • Visceral Pain • IBD • Functional Ano-rectal Disorder • IBS •
Tumor • Infectious Ano-rectal Disease • Endometriosis

A. Infantino
Department of Surgery, "S. Maria dei Battuti" Hospital,
S. Vito al Tagliamento, Italy

G.A. Santoro, A.P. Wieczorek, C.I. Bartram (eds.) *Pelvic Floor Disorders*
© Springer-Verlag Italia 2010

54.1　Introduction

Pelvic pain is a very common symptom, and most people experience it at least once during their life. It can be caused by many conditions, often not serious, such as hemorrhoids, fissures, or abscesses; sometimes it may be one of the symptoms of ano-rectal neoplasia, or their local relapse expression. It can also be associated with infective and non-infective inflammation disorders, such as occur post-radiotherapy or after surgical procedures. Ano-rectal pain may arise from a functional disorder such as levator ani syndrome, proctalgia fugax, coccygodynia, or pudendal canal syndrome (Alcock's canal syndrome). The causes of pelvic pain are listed in Table 54.1.

It is estimated that, in the US, over nine million women suffer from pelvic pain, resulting in a significant social cost and severe impairment of quality of life [1]. In Europe, important results of a survey aiming to understand pelvic pain were presented at the University of Oxford: women between 18 and 49 years old were subdivided into four groups: (1) chronic pelvic pain only; (2) chronic pelvic pain and irritable bowel syndrome (IBS); (3) chronic pelvic pain and genitourinary symptoms; and (4) chronic pelvic pain,

Table 54.1 Causes of pelvic pain

Inflammatory
- Inflammatory bowel disease (IBD)
- Proctitis (infectious; non-infectious)
- Abscess (perirectal; pelvic)
- Hemorrhoids
- Fissure
- Irritable bowel syndrome (IBS)
- Prostatitis
- Endometriosis
- Post-radiotherapy

Neoplastic
- Rectal
- Anal
- Prostatic
- Ovarian

Mechanical
- Rectal prolapse

Postoperative
- Proctological
- Urological
- Gynecological

genitourinary symptoms, and IBS. When chronic pelvic pain was present it was associated with genitourinary symptoms or IBS, or both, in half of the women. Genital pain was higher among women with chronic pelvic pain in comparison to women without pelvic pain: dysmenorrhea 81% vs. 58% and dyspareunia 41% vs. 14%. These women were diagnosed with IBS and stress in the majority of cases, but 50% of them were not diagnosed [2].

Interest has developed in the urogynecological field and in IBS, where the border with chronic pelvic pain is not always clear. The latter, often separately approached by urogynecologists, gastroenterologists, and surgeons, leads to a workup overload that is often useless and expensive, inefficient treatments, and frustration in patients and doctors [3]. The approach should be multidisciplinary, and it should be acknowledged that patients might suffer from a chronic visceral pain syndrome; the treatment often has to face the difficult management of chronic pelvic pain [4] .

In some cases, pelvic pain is the cause of urgent hospital admission. Due to the different sources of pain, roughly divided into gynecologic and non-gynecologic, and because the afferent nervous pathways are common for the different and complex organ of the pelvis, ultrasonography is the procedure of choice, as it leads to a diagnosis in most cases. Computed tomography (CT) is advised when the information from ultrasonography is not clear or does not correspond to the clinical data [5,6].

54.2　Inflammatory Bowel Disease

Inflammatory bowel disease (IBD) is idiopathic and commonly refers to ulcerative colitis (UC) and Crohn's disease (CD). The cardinal symptom of UC is bloody diarrhea. Associated symptoms of colicky abdominal pain, urgency, or tenesmus may be present. The clinical course of UC is marked by exacerbation and remission.

Symptoms of CD are more heterogeneous, but typically include abdominal pain, diarrhea, and weight loss. Systemic symptoms of malaise, anorexia, or fever are more common with CD than UC. CD may cause intestinal obstruction due to strictures, fistulae (often perianal), or abscesses. Both ulcerative and Crohn's colitis are associated with an increased risk of colonic carcinoma [7].

54.2.1 Visceral Pain and Mechanical Properties of IBS Patient's Colon-rectal Wall

The authors have focused their attention on pain and its mechanism in patients with IBD. It is a kind of pain evoked from the viscera. Visceral pain is the most common form of pain produced by disease and one of the most frequent reasons that induce patients to seek medical attention. We seldom have any sensory experience from our internal organs other than pain and discomfort, and even when other sensations occur, such as bladder or stomach fullness, these can easily evolve towards pain if the stimulus persists. Pain at rest and pain at defecation are prevalent symptoms in patients with ulcerative colitis (UC) [8]. Drewers et al describe two different factors underlying symptoms of active UC [9]: (1) changed mechanical properties of the rectum; and (2) the inflammation per se. During acute exacerbations in UC, the edema and chronic fibrotic changes relating to repeated inflammations may result in changes in the viscoelastic properties of the mucosa and deeper layers of the gut. Increased stiffness of the rectal wall has been observed in patients with both active and inactive disease. This could explain the symptoms, because stiffness of the gut will lead to increased resistance to the normal passage of feces and air in the affected segment, proximal dilatation, and hence pain and urgency [10, 11]. Inflammatory changes can also result in pain because the cascade of cellular and nervous mechanisms may activate the nociceptive system independently of any mechanical changes [12]. This has been confirmed in animal studies [13] which have shown that an induced acute transient inflammation of the colon results in long-lasting changes in mechanosensory function, and these changes persist after histological healing of lesions. These results support the hypothesis of long-term effects of a transient colitis and their key role in the development of visceral hyperalgesia which is a modification of pain-modulation systems. Pain could be a consequence of peripheral sensitization and hyperexcitability of the central nervous system manifested as hyperalgesia and allodynia (painful response to physiological stimuli that are not normally painful) [14, 15]. The increases in excitability of the central nervous system induced by repetitive stimulation will result in increased pain. On the other hand, Drewers et al [9] demonstrated reduced pain rating during experimental tonic distension of the rectum in patients with active UC. They concluded, against the "central hypothesis", that inflammation of the rectum does not lead to increased integration and hyperexcitability of the central nervous system. According to this study, the hyperalgesia in UC is probably related to peripheral factors such as inflammation and/or changes in rectal wall properties caused by the smooth muscle contraction. Hyperalgesia, previously discussed in patients with active UC, was not found in patients with quiescent disease [10, 16], and Chang et al [17] found hypoalgesia to distension in patients with quiescent or mild UC, instead: they concluded that chronic mild inflammation of the gut in humans does not result in pathological perception of visceral distension. Previously we reported different studies which provided evidence to suggest the presence of rectal hypersensitivity in UC patients with active disease [10, 16]. According to these studies, pain and discomfort experienced by UC patients during disease exacerbation are partially related to the greater degree of inflammation present during flares, resulting in transient sensitization of afferent pathways. In contrast, the relative paucity of pain in patients with mild disease activity may be explained by activation of counter-regulatory antinociceptive systems which produce endogenous analgesia.

In summary, acute tissue damage results in transient upregulation of pain sensitivity, while persistence of the peripheral irritation is associated with activation of counter-regulatory mechanisms [17]. These mechanisms include peripheral opioid-mediated mechanisms, decreasing the excitability of nociceptors [18], descending bulbospinal pain inhibitory systems, decreasing the excitability of dorsal horn neurons [19], corticopontine pain-inhibition systems (the right lateral frontal cortex and periaqueductal gray) [20] and modulating the sensory experience by ascending attentional systems [21]. The fact that abdominal pain is not a prominent clinical feature in the majority of UC patients with mild disease, and that most patients become asymptomatic once an acute flare subsides, is consistent with such counter-regulatory systems which work as an adaptive response of the central nervous system to the presence of chronic visceral injury [17]. We can conclude that hyperalgesia is a peculiarity of patients with active UC, while hypoalgesia is typical of patients with quiescent or mild UC. Hypoalgesia was also demonstrated in patients with long-lasting pain resulting from CD. Evaluating visceral sensitivity in patients with CD, Bernstein et al [22] presented evidence for reduced pain sensitivity, possibly related to activation of antinociceptive mechanisms (counter-regulatory mechanisms) in response to persistent intestinal inflammation. Cook et al [23] also reported an increased somatic pain threshold in patients with CD. Chronic abdominal pain is not a frequent symptom of patients with uncomplicated CD, similarly to patients with chronic inflammation of the stomach (peptic ulcer without inflammation), which is associated with hypoalgesia as well [24]. An explanation for these findings is the activation of antinociceptive mechanisms such as the descending bulbospinal inhibition of sacral dorsal horn neurons in response to chronic gut irritation. Alterations in counter-regulatory mechanisms may explain abdominal pain and discomfort in patients with CD who are known to be in remission [22].

54.2.2 Conclusion

In summary, abdominal pain is a common symptom of patients with IBD, sometimes with disabling effects, especially during exacerbation of the disease. More studies are needed to understand and evaluate the mechanisms underlying visceral pain, its causes, transmission, and perception. The findings of research could provide definitive answers and more effective approaches to this difficult clinical issue, changing clinical thought and practice.

54.3   Inflammatory Diseases

Inflammatory diseases of the pelvis such as prostatitis or interstitial cystitis can be the cause of rectal and/or anal pain. Antibiotics are the most frequently used treatment.

Unfortunately, the evaluated workup including culture, and leukocyte and antibody status of prostate-specific specimens does not predict antibiotic response in patients with chronic prostatitis/chronic pelvic pain syndrome: antibiotic therapy response is not related to laboratory work-up [25]. Moreover, leukocytes and bacterial counts do not correlate with the severity of symptoms. Factors other than leukocytes and bacteria also contribute to symptoms associated with chronic pelvic pain syndrome [26].

54.4   "Functional" Anorectal and Pelvic Pain

"Functional" anorectal and pelvic pain has been included in various groups of disorders. These disorders affect the quality of life and represent a challenge to medical knowledge. In the field of non-gynecologic causes we find: levator ani syndrome, proctalgia fugax, coccygodynia [27], and Alcock's canal syndrome.

Levator ani syndrome is characterized by pain without any demonstrable cause; in particular proctalgia fugax is a mainly nocturnal, severe pain, which occurs in few seconds and disappears spontaneously within a few minutes. Usually, patients experienced that digital massage, sitz baths, or attempts to defecate are useful to improve pain; muscle relaxants, electro-galvanic stimulation, and biofeedback are the treatment modalities most frequently described in the literature [28]. In a retrospective study of consecutively treated patients, intravaginal electrical stimulation has been found useful in women complaining of levator ani syndrome, with no difference for age, race, education, or parity [29].

Coccygodynia is pain in the region of the coccyx; in the majority of patients the cause is unknown. Abnormal mobility is demonstrated by dynamic standing and seating radiographs but we are not sure this is the cause of pain; neither CT scans nor magnetic resonance add useful information for the correct diagnosis or for treatment [30]. When pain is intense, local anesthetic and corticosteroid injections should be made into the painful area; manipulation of the coccyx and massage of the levator ani can also be of some help. The application of infrared thermography in 53 patients before and after massage of the levator ani, followed by Maigne's manipulative technique and external physiotherapy (short-wave diathermy) 3 times a week for 8 weeks in an evaluation of conservative treatment, demonstrated a reduction of surface temperatures; these correlated with variations of the intensity of pain, and in particular with improvement of pain (r = 0.67, P < 0.01) [31]. Partial coccygectomy is a good therapeutic option only for post-traumatic coccygodynia; improvement was recorded in the first 15 weeks, with no further improvement after 6 months [32].

Pudendal nerve entrapment in Alcock's canal (Alcock's canal syndrome) has also been suggested when chronic perianal pain occurs unilaterally and pudendal nerve terminal motor latency is prolonged only on that side [33]. Pudendal neuralgia shows continuous spontaneous pain in the perineal area supplied by the pudendal nerve, and is usually associated with paresthesias as well as occasional electric shocks; it is provoked in the sitting position and worse with bicycle riding [34]. A burning sensation often accompanies the pain, which can be felt in any of the organs supplied by the pudendal nerves: the testicle in males, the labia in females, pain in the anus, and a foreign body sensation in both sexes. All these symptoms are usually unilateral and can be an expression of isolated damage of one of the nerve branches. Pressure on the ischial spine releases violent pain, which can spread and reproduce the same pain from which the patient suffers, while in a rectal or vaginal examination, pain can be evoked with pressure in the region of the ischial spine [35]. Cortisonic or anesthetic infiltration of Alcock's canal under CT or radioscopic control, or surgical decompression of the pudendal nerve can achieve pain relief [35, 36]. Fall et al reported that surgical decompression of the nerve rarely relieves the symptoms, instead [37].

54.5 Irritable Bowel Syndrome (IBS)

Patients with irritable bowel syndrome usually complain of pain, although there are no structural lesions underlying these symptoms. There are clinical findings suggesting an increased incidence of IBS after an acute gastrointestinal infection [38, 39]. In fact some patients with IBS identify the onset of their symptoms just after an acute episode of gastroenteritis. This subset of IBS patients (post-infectious IBS) has an enhanced visceral sensitivity following a transient bowel inflammation and this has been identified as a causative mechanism [39]. Transient inflammation alters visceral sensory function, and the duration and severity of the initial inflammatory stimulus appear to be risk factors for post-infectious IBS [39]. This has been confirmed by several studies; Chang et al [17] showed that repetitive noxious sigmoid distension induced rectal hyperalgesia in IBS patients, therefore demonstrating an enhanced rectal sensitivity; Bernstein et al [22], evaluating the response to rectum distension in patients with IBS, found hypersensitivity to phasic distension.

Another field of research in chronic pain in IBS investigates the complex disordered interaction between the digestive and nervous systems. The results of many studies support the hypothesis that the central nervous system plays one of the major roles in the pathophysiology of IBS. Using positron emission tomography (PET) and functional magnetic resonance imaging (fMRI) in a predominantly female population of IBS patients, Bonaz [40] did not evidence any neuronal activation in locations activated in healthy volunteers, while a significant deactivation was observed in the limbic structure, which is involved in emotional activity, such as experience related to anxiety and fear. The connections and the cerebral area of the central nervous system have been studied to understand where and how rectal pain actually activates the human brain. Using a new technique related to functional magnetic resonance imaging – diffusion tensor imaging – in healthy humans, distension of the rectum revealed a network involving the insula, thalamus, somatosensory cortices, anterior cingulate cortex, and prefrontal cortex [41]. It has been demonstrated that a top-down activation of pain-facilitating neurons stemming from the brain, suggests a possible neural circuit for stress-induced hyperalgesia [42]. These results could give an explanation of lower pain threshold after rectal distension in patients with IBS; in an interesting experimental design, rectal pain threshold reduced after repetitive rectal painful distension in patients with IBS but not in normal volunteers or in a group with abdominal pain syndrome. The authors believe this phenomenon may be induced by a comorbid psychological state, and conclude that the rectal hypersensitivity induced by repetitive rectal painful distension may be a reliable marker for IBS [43].

Many attempts have been made to treat functional anorectal pain. Rectal painful distension is at the basis of a study comparing the spasmolytic agents, hyoscine butylbromide and drotaverin, in IBS patients and normal volunteers. Hyoscine butylbromide, oral tablets or suppositories, leads to a significant reduction in pain scores only in IBS patients with predominant diarrhoea (IBS-D), without modifications of rectal and sigmoid motility; both drugs were significantly active in improving the rectal pain threshold but only in IBS-D. These results support the hypothesis that the improvement after the use of these agents is related more to the effects on visceral sensation than on motility [44]. It has been demonstrated that butyrate has a wide spectrum of effects on the large bowel: inhibition of inflammation has been underlined as one of the main way of lowering visceral sensation [45]. After one week of daily self-administration in normal volunteers, butyrate enemas have the effect of a dose-dependent reduction of pain, urge, and discomfort for all the different pressure used [46].

54.6 Tumors

Carcinomas of the anal canal account for 1–2% of colorectal tumors and for 2–12% of anorectal neoplasia. Eighty-five per cent of anal cancers are epidermoid tumors and account for 3% of gastrointestinal carcinomas [47]. Tumors of the anus and the perineum have variable clinical presentation: acute sepsis is one of the most common, with symptoms such as painful mass, fever, and fistulization [48]. Symptoms are sometimes chronic as in cases of neuroendocrine tumors arising from the presacral region that can be associated with tailgut cyst or sacrococcygeal teratoma that sometimes involve the sacrum [49]. Epidermoid carcinomas rarely appear with urgent symptoms: in fact, even at an advanced stage the symptoms are not distinct from chronic benign disorders such as hemorrhoids and fissures; sepsis is usually due to a neglected disease. However, some cases occurring with abscesses and fistulas have been described [50]. Recto-anal pain is the most frequent acute symptom of rare anoperineal cancer, often a cause of incorrect or late diagnosis [51].

For locally advanced cancer, results are poor, with high rates of locoregional recurrence and poor overall survival data; up to now it is not clear which of the proposed treatments, i.e. chemoradiation or thermoradiation or chemoradiation plus hyperthermia, is more effective in controlling local diseases [52].

Pelvic pain from locally advanced cancer may be improved significantly by radiotherapy. In the case of prostatic cancer, 69% of patients affected improved for at least 4 months after radiotherapy, and 75% had a complete remission or significantly improved pelvic symptoms [53]. Radiotherapy of the pelvic organs is a useful and very common treatment for perineal and pelvic cancers, but tenesmus, mucorrhea, bleeding, and radiodermatitis are frequent and temporary complications in the ano-rectal region during or after treatment. Many drugs have been used to cure or at least improve chronic radiation proctitis. Recently, rebamipide, an amino acid derivative of 2(1H)-quinolinone, used for mucosal healing in peptic ulcers and gastritis, has been demostrated to be effective for radiation proctitis. It works by enhancing mucosal defense, scavenging free radicals, and temporarily activating genes encoding cyclooxygenase-2: enemas containing 150 mg rebamipide per dosing were administered after a morning bowel movement, and prior to bedtime, twice daily for 4 weeks. Improvement of the mean bleeding point, teleangectasia, and friable mucosa scores were all statistically significant. The authors conclude that rebamipide should be a first-line treatment or used when other drugs have failed [54].

A different issue is the cancer relapse. The incidence of local rectal cancer relapse has been reduced after total mesorectal excision, introduced by Heald and Ryall [55], and after neoadjuvant radiotherapy-chemotherapy in patients undergoing curative surgery [56], but it has been still reported to range from 9% to 35% [57, 58]. In cases of relapse of rectal cancer in a phase II study, retreatment with radiotherapy has been demonstrated to be useful in controlling the disease, and the association of regional hyperthermy has been found to be useful in overall 1-year and 3-year survival rates: 87% and 30%, respectively; reduction in pain, the main symptom in the majority of the patients, was achieved in 12/17 patients (70%) [59].

Many of the gastroenterological symptoms and ano-rectal pain are often not distinguishable from those of neoplasias, or from relapses, or new diseases; starting treatment without knowing the cause of the symptom is commonly ineffective [60]. For bleeding, the treatment of choice is considered the application of formalin to the rectal mucosa, but, even with the limitations of a retrospective study, it has been suggested that argon plasma coagulation is more effective and safe than topical formalin [61].

54.7 Infectious Diseases

Sexually trasmitted infections (STIs) are increasing in western countries, and pain, as well as bleeding and inflammation, is one of the main symptoms. Infections may involve several anatomic areas. The area from the anal verge up to the anorectal (dentate) line has an extensive supply of sensory nerve endings, and infection is commonly very painful and sometimes results in constipation and tenesmus associated with spasm of the anal sphincter muscle. Infections that involve the rectum but spare the anus are relatively painless, because the rectum itself has few sensory nerve endings. Symptoms may vary depending on the specific infection or pathological process, but can be indistinguishable from those of inflammatory bowel diseases. The most common symptom of proctitis includes anorectal pain or discomfort, anal discharge, which may be purulent, mucoid, or bloodstained, tenesmus, rectal bleeding, and constipation. Davis and Goldstone [62] reported bleeding and pain as the most common symptoms (73% and 62% respectively), and discharge and blood as the most common findings (58% and 54% respectively). Proctitis and proctocolitis have several infectious and non-infectious causes, the infectious pathogens typically being sexually acquired. Infectious proctitis is more common than non-infectious [62]. Specific pathogens have been associated with these diseases (Table 54.2): gonorrhoea, chlamydia, herpes simplex virus and syphilis are the commonest [63]. Specific pathogens most frequently infect specific sites and have different ways of transmission. *Chlamydia trachomatis* and *Neisseria gonorrhoeae* infect columnar epithelium and infect the ano-rectal mucosa via oral–genital and rectal intercourse. These infections are usually asymptomatic (up to 85%) [64]. *Herpes simplex virus* (HSV), *human papilloma virus*, and *Treponema pallidum* infect stratified squamous epithelium and can be transmitted similarly to the ano-rectal region.

These infections occur between the anal verge and the ano-rectal (dentate) line and tend to be extremely painful owing to the abundance of sensory nerve endings in this area. It has been well established that unprotected anal intercourse is the highest-risk activity and the most efficient mode of infections transmission [63]. Factors associated with an increased risk of acquiring any STI also include oro-anal sex (mostly implicated in the transmission of HSV and enteric bacteria), multiple partners, and anonymous partners. In recent years, there have been numerous reports of increasing risk-taking sexual behavior, particularly of unprotected anal intercourse in men who have sex with men (MSM), heterosexual adolescents, illicit drug users, and heterosexual adults [64–67]. These data have been linked to a resurgence of the rates of STI [68]. Klausner et al [69], in a retrospective review of clinical proctitis among 101 MSM, have found that the commonest infectious agent was gonorrhea (30%), followed by chlamydia (19%), herpes (16%), and syphilis (2%). Polymicrobial infection occurred in 18% of cases.

54.7.1 Gonorrhea, Chlamydia

Infectious proctitis secondary to gonorrhea and chlamydia are typically asymptomatic. Non-lymphogranuloma venereum (non-LGV) serovars of Chlamydia trachomatis can cause mild proctitis, with symptoms of rectal discharge, tenesmus, and anorectal pain. The clinical course of LGV can be divided into three stages. The primary lesion is a painless pustule or ulcer at the site of inoculation (most commonly the coronal sulcus of the penis or the penile shaft). The secondary stage occurs 3–6 months after exposure and manifests either as an inguinal syndrome or as an anogenitorectal syndrome. In heterosexuals, the secondary stage is usually characterized by inguinal or femoral lymphadenopathy (bubo). In homosexual men, anorectal symptoms of proctitis and proctocolitis occur, and excruciating pain helps to distinguish it from many other forms of proctitis. Symptoms may include anal discharge, which may be mucous, purulent, or bloody. The tertiary stage occurs in chronic untreated patients and is associated with ano-rectal strictures, perirectal abscess and fistula formation, mimicking Crohn's disease.

Table 54.2 Different infective agents may be involved in case of proctitis and proctocolitis

Variable	Proctitis	Proctocolitis
Symptoms	Rectal pain, discharge, tenesmus	Proctitis symptoms, pain, diarrhea
Pathogens	*Neisseria gonorrheae*	*Entameba hystolitica*
	Chlamydia trachomatis	*Campylobacter jejuni*
	Treponema pallidum	*Shigella flexneri*
	Herpes simplex virus	*C. trachomatis* (LVG)
Anoscopic finding	Rectal exudate ± friability	Rectal exudate, friability that involves the sigmoid colon

54.7.2 Herpes Simplex Virus

HSV infection typically occurs with small vesicular lesions, which evolve to ulceration and then resolve within a few days.

Lesions are usually multiple, but a solitary ulcer may also be the only sign. Clinical symptoms include severe pain, constipation, tenesmus, rectal discharge, and viremic symptoms, such as fever, chills, malaise, and inguinal lymphadenopathy.

54.7.3 Syphilis

Syphilis is the less common cause of clinical proctitis among MSM [62]. Primary syphilis typically presents 9–90 days after exposure, as an ano-rectal chancre. The classic chancre is painless, with well-demarcated edges and clean base.

It may go unnoticed by the patient because it is asymptomatic, or may be associated with itching, bleeding, pain or discomfort, rectal discharge, and tenesmus [70].

54.7.4 Diagnosis and Treatment

Finally, STIs are a common cause of proctitis, and appropriate testing is imperative. Symptoms and physical findings of proctitis are non-specific and are common in different disorders such as hemorrhoids, anal fissure, and IBD. Physicians must be aware both of the possibility of proctitis and the possibility of specific infections, since infectious proctitis is more common than non-infectious. Recently, several studies have shown an increasing incidence of infectious proctitis concurrent with a re-emergence of STI and HIV transmission, especially amongst MSM. Thus, sexually transmitted proctitis should be considered in MSM with rectal symptoms and, although less prevalent in women, it should be considered as well if there is a history of anal sex. Clinicians evaluating patients for ano-rectal complaints must obtain a detailed sexual history, including sexual preference and practices. Complete microbiological evaluation should include the four more common sexually transmitted pathogens: *N. gonorrhea*, *C. trachomatis*, HSV and *T. pallidum*. Specific therapy is ideal but not always immediate since identification of specific pathogens takes time (Table 54.3). Treatment can be started empirically while awaiting microbiological results, thus reducing inflammation and the duration of infection. Furthermore, empiric therapy reduces the chance of spread. Counselling is an important component of STI treatment. Safe sex practices, risk reduction, and partner notification should be discussed with patients, and when properly performed can reduce recurrence and transmission.

54.8 Endometriosis

Endometriosis is the presence and proliferation of endometrial glands or stroma outside the uterine cavity.

Table 54.3 Diagnostic methods and treatments for the more common pathogens

Pathogens	Investigation	Recommended treatment
Neisseria gonorrheae	Culture	Ceftriaxone 250 mg IM, or cefixime 400 mg oral, or spectinomycin 2 g IM
Chlamydia trachomatis, non-LGV serovars	Nucleic acid amplification test (NAAT); if positive refer for genotyping LGV	Azithromycin 1g oral, or doxycycline 100 mg oral bd for 7 days
Chlamydia trachomatis, LGV serovars		Doxycycline 100 mg oral bd for 21 days
Herpes simplex virus	Culture or PCR	Aciclovir 200 mg five times daily for 5 days
Treponema pallidum	Dark ground microscopy; serological test: (1) non-specific cardiolipin antigen tests: VDRL/RPR; (2) specific treponemal antigen tests: EIA/TPPA/TPHA	Procaine penicillin 600.000 U IM daily for 10–14 days, or benzathine penicillin 2.4 million units IM, or doxycycline bd orally for 14 days

EIA: enzyme immunoassay; LGV: Lymphogranuloma Venereum; PCR: Polymerase Chain Reaction; VDRL: Venereal Disease Research Laboratory; RPR: Rapid plasma reagin; TPPA: *Treponema pallidum* Particle Agglutination; TPHA: *Treponema Pallidum* Hemagglutination Test

It affects women during their reproductive years and is estimated to occur in up to 10% of the female population [71]. This disease has also been identified in postmenopausal women and adolescents [72]. Parazzini et al [73] reported a prevalence of endometriosis varying from 12% to 45% in 3684 premenopausal women undergoing laparoscopy or laparotomy in a gynecological service, depending on the indication of surgery.

This disorder has been described as either superficial or deep. Deep endometriosis can involve the bowel, usually the rectum and sigmoid colon, rectovaginal septum, pelvic sidewalls, and bladder. The bowel is involved in 5–37% of patients with endometriosis [74, 75].

The most common site of bowel involvement is the rectum (79–91%), followed by the sigmoid colon (31–47%), appendix (9–17%), small bowel (5–13%), and different colonic sites (2%) [76]. Involvement of the rectum in endometriosis causes a wide variety of symptoms, which range from rectal bleeding, urgency, pelvic pain on defecation, and alteration in bowel habit to obstruction of the colon. Women with deep endometriosis have reported shooting rectal pain and a sense of their insides being pulled down; moreover, individual pain areas were unrelated to the surgical diagnosis, and the area of pain was unrelated to the area of endometriosis [77].

Symptoms may be non-cyclical [78] and frequently overlap with symptoms of interstitial cystitis, and these two conditions may even coexist in the same patient. Therefore, in cases of unresolved endometriosis and persistent pelvic pain, interstitial cystitis should be investigated [79]. The diagnostic tools of the so-called posterior cul-de-sac endometriosis, confirmed by histology, have been retrospectively evaluated on 25 patients.

Two had rectal blood loss and eight had a palpable mass in the posterior cul de sac; all the patients were evaluated by transvaginal ultrasound, which demonstrated some abnormality: lesions appeared round or ovoid, solid and non-compressible, with high vascularity, localized on the serosal surface of the recto-sigmoid with sparing of the mucosa and submucosa, and in 19/25 a spiculated or tethering contour was demonstrated; furthermore, abdominal ultrasound detected thick-walled adnexal cysts in 11 patients, hydronephrosis in eight, and involvement of the ileocecal region in five [80].

54.9 Common Proctological Diseases

In the introduction we mentioned some common "minor" disorders such as hemorrhoids, anal fissure, and abscess, as possible cause of anal pain; although this chapter considers conditions at the border of pelvic pain, we believe it is important to give a short description in order to present an exhaustive landscape for differential diagnosis in the field of pelvic pain.

Hemorrhoids is one the most common proctological diseases of adults in western countries: according to a recent review of the literature, the incidence of anorectal bleeding in the general population is approximately 20% per year, while the number of people seen by a general practitioner (GP) for this reason is 6/1000 per year, and 7/10,000 per year are seen by a specialist. In the literature, hemorrhoids have extremely high ranges of prevalence, 4.4% to 36% [1, 2], which are influenced by the method of the survey, whether by GPs or specialists [81, 82].

It is still an open question whether prolapse is the etio-pathogenetic basis of hemorrhoidal disease or if prolapse itself is secondary to a vascular stasis which can be treated by a reduction of the arterial inflow. Pain is not related to the degree of the prolapse and is sometimes secondary to a complication such as hemorrhoidal thrombosis, or to the contemporary presence of other local diseases such as fissures, proctitis, crypts inflammation, or solitary rectal ulcer. The haemorrhoidal disease score in four degrees by Goligher [83] is practical but insufficient in case of prospective studies; Gaj et al have introduced a more definite classification system that can be the solution to avoid one of the bias of the published papers: the poor homogeneity of the severity of the disease in each Goligher grade [84].

Anal fissures are a cut or a tear, usually located in the anal posterior or anterior commissures; the appearance is drop shaped, with the apex in the proximity of an anal crypt or at the dentate line; signs of chronicity are the presence of a tag of skin, called a sentinel pile, and of a fibromatous polyp at the apex. The main symptom is pain, usually during the passage of stool, followed by a short pause and again by pain that lasts from minutes to hours, and sometimes with a very disabling intensity [85]. Anal spasm due to a contraction of the internal sphincter, an involuntary muscle, may be the cause of the fissure but it is also the consequence, as a reaction to the pain, thereby creating a vicious circle. There is a large spectrum of diseases that can be presented by an anal fissure: anal cancer, leukemia, tuberculosis, viral infection – herpes or cytomegalovirus – and many others sexually transmitted infections such as gonorrhea, chlamydia, and HIV; an anal fissure is the first acute manifestation in about 4% of patients with CD. Many topical treatments have been proposed, such as botulinus toxin injected into the external or internal anal sphincters [86, 87], or glycerin trinitrate ointment [88, 89], or calcium antagonists [90], but long-term results do not seem encouraging. Anal autodilatations using commercial cones are commonly used [91], but there is no scientific evidence in the literature on the efficacy of this method. Internal sphincteromy is still considered the gold standard when conservative treatments fail [92].

Anal abscess is a collection of pus in the anal structures; usually it is cryptoglandular, so called because it originates in the intersphincteric infected glands. The symptoms are pain, perianal lump, and sometimes fever. Pain improves or disappears when pus flows in the skin or in the anal canal, spontaneously or after surgical incision. Less frequent abscess of the rectal wall or of the pelvi-rectal fossa may be difficult to diagnose if digital rectal exploration is not accurate. The workup is useful to demonstrate the correct topography of the abscess with relation to the anal sphincters and the internal orifice. Endoanal ultrasonography has been demonstrated to be accurate and a cost-effective way of planning the best incision and drainage [93, 94].

54.10 Post-surgical Pain

Many surgical procedures have been proposed to reduce postoperative pain. Rubber band ligation for symptomatic internal hemorrhoids is a well-known and effective method, even in long-term follow-up. Forlini and colleagues, after ligation of two or three piles for second- or third-degree hemorrhoids in a single session, reported that 46% of the patients had moderate anal pain for 24 h post procedure and only two patients had severe pain (1%); at 1 year follow-up, no residual symptoms were reported by 90% of the patients with second-degree piles and 75% of patients with third-degree piles; long-term telephone follow-up at 10 and 17 years collected the history of 138 patients: 69% were asymptomatic [95]. The use of warm sitz baths is thought to help relaxation of the anal

sphincter and post-operative anal pain [96], although Gupta demonstrated that they had no effect on the healing process in the treatment of anal fissure, but only on patient's comfort [97]. A meta-analysis evaluation of 36 published papers was not able to demonstrate whether this time-consuming recommendation is beneficial to patients [98]. More recently, a randomized study on the comparison of clinical effects between warm water spray and sitz bath after hemorrhoidectomy demonstrated no significant difference in healing time or in scores for postoperative pain (P = 0.23), irritation (P = 0.48), or hygiene (P = 0.725) between groups; however, the water spray group reported significantly greater convenience (P < 0.05) and higher overall satisfaction (P < 0.05) compared with the sitz bath group [99]. New technologies have been presented for the treatment of hemorrhoids and for rectal intussusception when it is the cause of obstructed defecation: Procedure for Prolapse Haemorroids (PPH), Stapled Transanal Rectal Resection (STARR), and Transanal Rectal Resection with Contour device (TransSTARR) in selected patients and used by experienced dedicated surgeons have been demonstrated to be effective for avoiding severe postoperative pain. Stapled hemorrhoidopexy has been used widely with great patient satisfaction [100–102], despite the fact that the price is frequent bleeding (3.3%), unexplained pain for over a month, external hemorrhoidal thrombosis, anal fissure, anal fistula, rectal stenosis, anal incontinence [101], and a relapse rate that is higher than hemorrhoidectomy [103]. After a review of the literature, chronic proctalgia has been described as difficult to manage after PPH and STARR [104]. Rectal pain after PPH and STARR has been described and is often secondary to retained staples [104], and recently a case has been described where it was due to a portion of rectal wall being sutured in the perirectal adipose tissue [105].

54.11 Additional Notes on Treatments

Many attempts have been made to cure or alleviate chronic pelvic pain. In the treatment of chronic anorectal pain, electrogalvanic therapy associated with biofeedback is insufficiently effective, but linearly polarized near-infrared irradiation has been used with good response on the strongly tender point or few centimeters apart from the skin for ten minutes in 35 patients complaining of vague and deep pain in the anorectum. The patients had history of lower abdominal surgery, and 18 patients had disordered defecation; the authors found excellent or good results in 32 patients, with recurrences in four, and concluded that this technique can be recommended for primary therapy [106]. Neurostimulation methods have recently gained popularity; three methods are currently used in clinical practice: spinal cord stimulation, peripheral nerve stimulation (PNS), and deep brain stimulation. PNS has, according to a large body of literature, the better pain control after other treatment techniques have been used [107]. In particular in the case of non-inflamed pelvic chronic pain syndrome, benefits have been found after high-frequency urethro-anal afferent electrostimulation; the mean pain score significantly decreased and the quality of life profile improved. The technique and the device is simple and it can be self-administered [108]. Recently, the Italian Group for Sacral Neuromodulation (GINS) presented results in 12 patients (10 women and 2 men; mean age, 61.0 ± 10.3 years; range, 48–82 years) implanted with a permanent device for sacral nerve stimulation (SNS) for chronic anal or perianal pain; pharmacological and rehabilitative therapy had yielded poor results; after a mean follow-up of 15 months (range 3–80 months), visual analogue pain scores had significantly improved (from 8.2 ± 1.7 to 2.2 ± 1.3, P < 0.001). SF-36 physical component scores increased from 26.27 ± 5.65 to 38.95 ± 9.08 (P < 0.02). Scores on the mental component showed improvement, although this was not significant. PNS may help a selected population of patients with anal pain [109]. In a minority of patients, "tolerance" to neurostimulation develops after long-term use.

54.12 Conclusions

Pelvic pain involves many visceral organs and cannot be considered separately from primary or secondary nervous or psychological aspects. Accuracy in collecting medical information and in physical examination is mandatory. The workup should be focused to demonstrate or to exclude a disease in each individual patient, although in a small group of patients, failure to reach the correct diagnosis and cure can be frustrating for both the patient and the coloproctologist. These difficulties should be approached together with the gynecologist or urogynecologist in order to reach the best results in diagnosis and treatment.

References

1. Mathias SD, Kuppermann M, Liberman RF et al. Chronic pelvic pain: prevalence, health-related quality of life, and economic correlates. Obstet Gynecol 1996;87:321Y7.
2. Zondervan KT, Yudkin PL, Vessey MP et al. Chronic pelvic pain in the community. Symptoms, investigations, and diagnoses. Am J Obstet Gynecol 2001;184:1149–1155.
3. Kamm MA. Chronic pelvic pain in women--gastroenterological, gynaecological or psychological? Int J Colorectal Dis 1997;12:57–62.
4. Wesselmann U, Czakanski PP. Pelvic pain: a chronic visceral pain syndrome. Curr Pain Headache Rep 2001;5:13–19.
5. Kalish GM, Patel MD, Gunn ML, Dubinsky TJ. Computed tomographic and magnetic resonance features of gynecologic abnormalities in women presenting with acute or chronic abdominal pain. Ultrasound Q 2007;23:167–175.
6. Potter AW, Chandrasekhar CA. US and CT evaluation of acute pelvic pain of gynecologic origin in nonpregnant premenopausal patients. Radiographics 2008;28:1645–1659.
7. Munkholm P, Langholz E, Davidsen M et al. Intestinal cancer risk and mortality in patients with Crohn's disease. Gastroenterology 1993;105:1716–1723.
8. Jewell PD. Ulcerative colitis. In: Feldman M, Friedman LS, Sleisenger MH (eds) Sleisenger & Fordtran's gastrointestinal and liver diseases. WB Saunders, Philadelphia (PA), 2002, pp 2039–2067.
9. Drewers AM, Frøkjer JB, Larsen E et al. Pain and mechanical properties of rectum in patients with active ulcerative colitis. Inflamm Bowel Dis 2006;12:294–302.
10. Loening-Baucke V. Anorectal manometry in active and quiescent ulcerative colitis. Am J Gastroenterol 1989;8:892–897.
11. Denis P, Colin R, Galmiche JP. Elastic properties of the rectal wall in normal adults and in patients with ulcerativecolitis. Gastroenterology 1979;77:45–48.
12. Byers MR, Bonica JJ. Peripheral pain mechanisms and nociceptor plasticity. In: Loeser JD, Butler SH, Chapman CR et al (eds) Bonica's management of pain. Lippincott Williams & Wilkins, Philadelphia (PA), 2001, pp 26–72.
13. Gschossmann JM, Liebregts T, Adam B et al. Long-term effects of transient chemically induced colitis on the visceromotor response to mechanical colorectal distension. Dig Dis Sci 2004;49:96–101.
14. Cervero F, Laird JMA. Visceral Pain. Lancet 1999;353:2145–2148.
15. Cervero F. Sensory Innervation of the viscera: peripheral basis of visceral pain. Physiol Rev 1994;74:95–138.
16. Farthing MJG, Lennard-Jones JE. Sensibility of rectum to distension and anorectal distension reflex in ulcerative-colitis. Gut 1978;19:64–69.
17. Chang L, Munakata J, Mayer EA et al. Perceptual responses in patients with inflammatory and functional bowel disease. Gut 2000;47:497–505.
18. Stein C. The control of pain in peripheral tissue by opioids. N Engl J Med 1995;332:1685–1690.
19. Mayer EA, Gebhart GF. Basic and clinical aspects of visceral hyperalgesia. Gastroenterology 1994;107:271–293.
20. Mayer EA, Berman S, Suyenobu B et al. Differences in brain responses to visceral pain between patients with irri-

table bowel syndrome and ulcerative colitis. Pain 2005; 115:398–409.

21. Dixon NF. Preconscious processing. John Wiley and Sons, New York, 1987.

22. Bernstein CN, Niazi N, Robert M et al. Rectal afferent function in patients with inflammatory and functional intestinal disorders. Pain 1996;66:151–161.

23. Cook IJ, Van Eeden A, Collins SM. Patients with irritable bowel syndrome have greater pain tolerance than normal subjects. Gastroenterology 1987;93:727–733.

24. Mertz H, Fullerton S, Naliboff B et al. Symptoms and visceral perception in severe functional and organic dyspepsia. Gut 1998;42:814–822.

25. Nickel JC, Downey J, Johnston B et al; The Canadian Prostatitis Research Group. Predictors of patient response to antibiotic therapy for the chronic prostatitis/chronic pelvic pain syndrome: a prospective multicenter clinical trial. J Urol 2001;165:1539–1544.

26. Schaeffer AJ, Knauss JS, Landis JR et al; Chronic Prostatitis Collaborative Research Network Study Group. Leukocyte and bacterial counts do not correlate with severity of symptoms in men with chronic prostatitis: the National Institutes of Health Chronic Prostatitis Cohort Study. J Urol 2002;168:1048–1053.

27. Wald A. Functional anorectal and pelvic pain. Gastroenterol Clin North Am 2001;30:243–251.

28. Ng CL. Levator ani syndrome – a case study and literature review. Aust Fam Physician 2007;36:449–452.

29. Fitzwater JB, Kuehl TJ, Schrier JJ. Electrical stimulation in the treatment of pelvic pain due to levator ani spasm. J Reprod Med 2003;48:573–577.

30. Fogel GR, Cunningham PY 3rd, Esses SI. Coccygodynia: evaluation and management. J Am Acad Orthop Surg 2004;12:49–54.

31. Wu CL, Yu KL, Chuang HY et al. The application of infrared thermography in the assessment of patients with coccygodynia before and after manual therapy combined with diathermy. J Manipulative Physiol Ther 2009;32:287–293.

32. Mouhsine E, Garofalo R, Chevalley F et al. Posttraumatic coccygeal instability. Spine J 2006;6:544–549.

33. Pisani R, Stubinski R, Datti R. Entrapment neuropathy of the internal pudendal nerve. Report of two cases. Scand J Urol Nephrol 1997;31:407–410.

34. Amarenco G, Lanoe Y, Ghnassia RT et al. Syndrome du canal d'Alcock et névralgie périnéale. Rev Neurol Paris 1988;144:523–526.

35. Roche B, Robert-Yap J, Skala K, Zufferey G. Pudendal nerve compression syndrome. www.siccr.org 2009;20:172–179.

36. Kovacs P, Gruber H, Piegger J, Bodner G. New, simple, ultrasound-guided infiltration of the pudendal nerve: ultrasonographic technique. Dis Colon Rectum 2001;44:1381–1385.

37. Fall M, Baranowski AP, Elneil S et al. EAU Guidelines on chronic pelvic pain. Eur Urol 2010;57:31–48.

38. McKendrick MW, Read NW. Irritable bowel syndrome-post salmonella infection. J Infect 1994;29:1–3.

39. Gwee KA, Graham JC, McKendrick MW et al. Psychometric scores and persistence of irritable bowel after infectious diarrhoea. Lancet 1996;347:150–153.

40. Bonaz B. Visceral sensitivity perturbation integration in the brain-gut axis in functional digestive disorders. J Physiol Pharmacol 2003;54(suppl 4):27–42.

41. Moisset X, Bouhassira D, Denis D et al. Anatomical connections between brain areas activated during rectal distension in healthy volunteers: a visceral pain network. Eur J Pain 2010;14:142–148.

42. Martenson ME, Cetas JS, Heinricher MM. A possible neural basis for stress-induced hyperalgesia. Pain 2009; 142:236–244.

43. Nozu T, Kudaira M, Kitamori S, Uehara A. Repetitive rectal painful distention induces rectal hypersensitivity in patients with irritable bowel syndrome. J Gastroenterol 2006; 41:217–222.

44. Khalif IL, Quigley EM, Makarchuk PA et al. Interactions between symptoms and motor and visceral sensory responses of irritable bowel syndrome patients to spasmolytics (antispasmodics). J Gastrointestin Liver Dis 2009; 18:17–22.

45. Hamer HM, Jonkers D, Venema K et al. Review article: the role of butyrate on colonic function. Aliment Pharmacol Ther 2008;15;27:104–119.

46. Vanhoutvin SA, Troost FJ, Kilkens TO et al. The effects of butyrate enemas on visceral perception in healthy volunteers. Neurogastroenterol Motil 2009;21:952-e76.

47. Boman BM, Moertel CG. Carcinoma of the anal canal. A clinical and pathologic study of 188 cases. Cancer 1984;54:114–125..

48. Bracey EE, Mathur P, Dooldeniya M et al. Unusual perianal tumours masquerading as abscesses. Int J Clin Pract 2003;57:343–346

49. Dujardin F, Beaussart P, de Muret A et al. Primary neuroendocrine tumor of the sacrum: case report and review of the literature. Skeletal Radiol 2009;38:819–823.

50. Nelson RL, Prasad ML, Abcarian H. Anal carcinoma presenting as a perirectal abscess or fistola. Arch Surg 1985;120:632–635.

51. Infantino A, Pisegna Cerone L. Rare neoplasias of the anus and the perineum: acute manifestations. www.siccr.org 2006;16:135–145.

52. De Haas-Kock DF, Buijsen J, Pijls-Johannesma M et al. Concomitant hyperthermia and radiation therapy for treating locally advanced rectal cancer. Cochrane Database Syst Rev 2009;(3):CD006269.

53. Din OS, Thanvi N, Ferguson CJ, Kirkbride P. Palliative prostate radiotherapy for symptomatic advanced prostate cancer. Radiother Oncol 2009;93:192–196.

54. Kim TO, Song GA, Lee SM et al. Rebampide enema therapy as a treatment for patients with chronic radiation proctitis: initial treatment or when other methods of conservative management have failed. Int J Colorectal Dis 2008; 23:629–633.

55. Heald RJ, Ryall RD. Recurrence and survival after total mesorectal excision for rectal cancer. Lancet 1986; 28:1479–1482.

56. Ceelen W, Fierens K, Van Nieuwenhove Y, Pattyn P. Preoperative chemoradiation versus radiation alone for stage II and III resectable rectal cancer: a systematic review and meta-analysis. Int J Cancer 2009;15;124:2966–2972.

57. Law WL, Chu KW. Anterior resection for rectal cancer

with mesorectal excision: a prospective evaluation of 622 patients. Ann Surg 2004;240:260–268.

58. Hohenberger W, Merkel S, Matzel K et al. The influence of abdomino-peranal (intersphincteric) resection of lower third rectal carcinoma on the rates of sphincter preservation and locoregional recurrence. Colorectal Dis 2006;8:23–33.

59. Milani V, Pazos M, Buecklein V et al. Radiochemotherapy in combination with regional hyperthermia in preirradiated patients with recurrent rectal cancer. Strahlenther Onkol 2008;184:163–168.

60. Andreyev J. Gastrointestinal symptoms pelvic radiotherapy: a new understanding to improve management of symptomatic patients. Lancet Oncol 2007;8:1007–1017.

61. Alfadhli AA, Alazmi WM, Ponich T et al. Efficacy of argon plasma coagulation compared to topical formalin application for chronic radiation proctopathy. Can J Gastroenterol 2008;22:129–132.

62. Davis TW, Goldstone SE. Sexually transmitted infections as a cause of proctitis in men who have sex with men. Dis Colon Rectum 2009;52:507–512.

63. Hamlyn E, Taylor C. Sexually transmitted proctitis. Postgrad Med J 2006;82:733–736.

64. Kent C, Chaw JK, Wong W et al. Prevalence of rectal, urethral, and pharyngeal chlamydia and gonorrhea detected in 2 clinical settings among men who have sex with men: San Francisco, California, 2003. Clin Infect Dis 2005; 41:67–74.

64. Elford J, Bolding G, Davis M et al. Trends in sexual behaviour among London homosexual men 1998–2003: implications for HIV prevention and sexual health promotion. Sex Transm Infect 2004;80:451–454.

65. Moscicki AB, Millstein SG, Broering J, Irwin CE. Risks of human immunodeficiency virus infection among adolescents attending three diverse clinics. J Pediatrics 1993;122:813–820.

66. Kang SY, Magura S, Shapiro JL. Correlates of cocaine/crack use among innercity incarcerated adolescents. Am J Drug Alcohol Abuse 1994;20:413–429.

67. Melnick SL, Jeffery RW, Burke GL et al. Changes in sexual behavior by young urban heterosexual adults in response to the AIDS epidemic. Public Health Reports 1993; 108:582–588.

68. Macdonald N, Dougan S, McGarrigle CA et al. Recent trends in diagnoses of HIV and other sexually transmitted infections in England and Wales among men who have sex with men. Sex Transm Infect 2004;80:492–497.

69. Klausner JD, Kohn R, Kent C. Etiology of clinical proctitis among men who have sex with men. Clin Infect Dis 2004;38:300Y2.

70. Mindel A, Tovey SJ, Timmins DJ, Williams P. Primary and secondary syphilis, 20 years' experience. 2. Clinical features. Genitourin Med 1989;65:1–3.

71. Eskenazi B, Warner ML. Epidemiology of endometriosis. Obstet Gynecol Clin North Am 1997;24:235–258.

72. Valle RF, Sciarra JJ. Endometriosis: treatment strategies. Ann N Y Acad Sci 2003;997:229–239.

73. Parazzini F, Luchini L, Vezzoli F et al. Prevalence and anatomical distribution of endometriosis in women with selected gynaecological conditions: result from a multicentric Italian study. Hum Reprod 1994;6:1158–1162.

74. Azzena A, Litta P, Ferrara A et al. Rectosigmoid endometriosis: diagnosis and surgical management. Clin Exp Obstet Gynecol 1998;25: 94–96.

75. Prystowsky JB, Stryker SJ, Ujiki GT, Poticha SM. Gastrointestinal endometriosis. Incidence and indication for resection. Arch Surg 1988;123:855–858.

76. Urbach DR, Reedijk M, Richard CS et al. Bowel Resection for intestinal endometriosis. Dis Colon Rectum 1998; 41:1158–1164.

77. Ballard K, Lane H, Hudelist G et al. Can specific pain symptoms help in the diagnosis of endometriosis? A cohort study of women with chronic pelvic pain. Fertil Steril 2009;31 March epub ahead of print.

78. Hensen JH, Puylaert JB. Endometriosis of the posterior cul-de-sac: clinical presentation and findings at transvaginal ultrasound. AJR Am J Roentgenol 2009;192:1618–1624.

79. Butrick CW. Patients with chronic pelvic pain: endometriosis or interstitial cystitis/painful bladder syndrome? JSLS 2007;11:182–189.

80. Hudelist G, Oberwinkler KH, Singer CF et al. Combination of transvaginal sonography and clinical examination for preoperative diagnosis of pelvic endometriosis. Hum Reprod 2009;24:1018–1024.

81. Fijten GH, Blijham GH, Knottnerus JA. Occurrence and clinical significance of overt blood loss per rectum in the general population and in medical practice. Br J Gen Pract 1994;44:320–325.

82. Johanson JF, Sonnemberg A. The prevalence of hemorrhoids and chronic costipation. An epidemiological study. Gastroenterology 1990;98:380–386.

83. Goligher JC. Surgery of the anus, rectum and colon, 4th edn. Balliere Tindall, London, 1980, pp 93–135.

84. Gaj F, Trecca A. PATE 2000 Sorrento: a modern, effective instrument for defining haemorrhoids. A multicentre observational study conducted in 930 symptomatic patients. Chir Ital 2004;56:509–515.

85. Giffin N, Acheson AG, Tung P et al. Quality of life in patients with chronic anal fissure. Colorect Dis 2004; 6:39–44.

86. Jost WH. One hundred cases of anal fissure treated with botulinum toxin. Early and long-term results. Dis Colon Rectum 1997;40:1029–1032.

87. Brisinda G, Maria G, Bentivoglio AR et al. A comparison of injection of botulinum toxin and topical nitroglycerine ointment for the treatment of chronic anal fissure. N Eng J Med 1999;341:65–69.

88. Altomare DF, Rinaldi M, Milito G et al. Glyceryl trinitrate for chronic anal fissure-healing or headache? Results of a multicenter, randomized, placebo-controlled, double-blind trial. Dis Colon Rectum 2000;43:174–179.

89. Orsay C, Rakinic J, Perry WB et al. Prepared by The Standard Practice Task Force The American Society of Colon Rectal Surgeons; Practice parameters for the management of anal fissure (revised). Dis Colon Rectum 2004;47:2003–2004.

90. Perrotti P, Bove A, Antropoli C et al. Topical nifedipine with lidocaine ointment vs. active control for treatment of chronic anal fissure: results of a prospective, randomized, double-blind study. Dis Colon Rectum 200245:1468–1475.

91. Gaj F, Trecca A. Evaluation of the efficacy of a new gra-

duated anal dilator in the treatment of acute anal fissures. Chir Ital 2007;59:545–550.

92. Nelson RL. Operative procedures for fissure in ano. Cochrane Database Syst Rev 2005;(2):CD002199.

93. Santoro GA, Di Falco G. Atlas of endoanal and endorectal ultrasonography. Staging and Treatment Options for Anorectal Cancer Springer-Verlag Italia, Milan, 2003, pp 44–45.

94. Dal Corso HM, D'Elia A, De Nardi P et al. Anal endosonography: a survey of equipment, technique and diagnostic criteria adopted in nine Italian centers. Tech Coloproctol 2007;11:26–33.

95. Forlini A, Manzelli A, Quaresima S, Forlini M. Long-term result after rubber band ligation for haemorrhoids. Int J Colorectal Dis 2009;24:1007-1010.

96. Dodi G, Bogoni F, Infantino A et al. Hot or cold in anal pain? A study of the changes in internal anal sphincter pressure profiles. Dis Colon Rectum 1986;29:248–251.

97. Gupta P. Randomized, controlled study comparing sitzbath and no-sitz-bath treatments in patients with acute anal fissures. Aust N Z J Surg 2006;76:718–721.

98. Tejirian T, Abbas MA. Sitz bath: where is the evidence? Scientific basis of a common practice. Dis Colon Rectum 2005;48:2336–2340.

99. Hsu KF, Chia JS, Jao SW et al. Comparison of clinical effects between warm water spray and sitz bath in post-hemorrhoidectomy period. J Gastrointest Surg 2009;13:1274–1278.

100. Tjandra JJ, Chan MK. Systematic review on the procedure for prolapse and hemorrhoids (stapled hemorrhoidopexy). Dis Colon Rectum 2007;50:878–892.

101. Sultan S, Rabahi N, Etienney I, Atienza P. Stapled hae-morrhoidopexy: Six years' experience of a referral centre. Colorectal Dis 2009;13 April epub ahead of print.

102. Isbert C, Reibetanz J, Jayne DG et al. Comparative study of Contour Transtar and STARR procedure for the treatment of obstructed defecation syndrome (ODS) – feasibility, morbidity and early functional results. Colorectal Dis 2009;29 April epub ahead of print.

103. Jayaraman S, Colquhoun PH, Malthaner RA. Stapled hemorrhoidopexy is associated with a higher long-term recurrence rate of internal hemorrhoids compared with conventional excisional hemorrhoid surgery. Dis Colon Rectum 2007;50:1297–1305.

104. Pescatori M, Gagliardi G. Postoperative complications after procedure for prolapsed hemorrhoids (PPH) and stapled transanal rectal resection (STARR) procedures. Tech Coloproctol 2008;12:7–19.

105. De Nardi P, Corsetti M, Staudacher C. Rectal wall exclusion: a new complication after STARR procedure. Colorectal Dis 2009;10 June epub ahead of print.

106. Mibu R, Hotokezaka M, Mihara S, Tanaka M. Results of linearly polarized near-infrared irradiation therapy in patients with intractable anorectal pain. Dis Colon Rectum 2003;46:S50–3.

107. Stojanovic MP. Stimulation methods for neuropathic pain control. Curr Pain Headache Rep 2001;5:130–137.

108. John H, Rüedi C, Kötting S et al. A new high frequency electrostimulation device to treat chronic prostatitis. J Urol 2003;170:1275–1277.

109. Falletto E, Masin A, Lolli P et al; GINS (Italian Group for Sacral Neuromodulation). Is sacral nerve stimulation an effective treatment for chronic idiopathic anal pain? Dis Colon Rectum 2009;52:456–462.

Marek Jantos

Abstract The anatomical and functional complexity of pelvic floor muscles increases the risk of pelvic floor disorders. Chronic pain disorders in the form of idiopathic bladder, vulvar and rectal pain represent three common pain syndromes that affect the anterior, middle, and posterior pelvic compartments respectively. Evidence suggests that these pain disorders are of somatic and muscular origin and are associated with hypertonic pelvic muscle states. Two potential mechanisms by which muscle overactivation gives rise to sensitization and pain include ischemia and myofascial trigger points found in muscle tissue, ligaments and fascia. Clinical modalities essential to the management of these pain disorders include surface electromyography and myofascial therapy. Surface electromyography provides an objective means of evaluating and normalizing pelvic muscle function, while myofascial therapy provides the means of resolving trigger point related pain. This chapter reviews current research in relation to the three pain syndromes, identifies the physiological characteristics of dysfunctional muscle states for each disorder and provides guidelines for normalizing their function in the management of chronic pain.

Keywords Bladder pain syndrome • Levator ani syndrome • Myofascial therapy • Surface electromyography • Vulvodynia

55.1 Introduction

Pelvic floor muscles (PFM) form one of the most complex muscle units in the body [1]. The high level of anatomical and functional complexity significantly increases the risk of pelvic floor disorders. These disorders constitute a cluster of pain, incontinence, and sexual disorders that arise predominantly from structural changes and dysfunctional muscle states, rather than a malfunction of the pelvic organs. Where the integrity of the structural anatomy has not been compromised, pelvic muscles provide support to the abdominal and pelvic organs, maintain continence, enable sexual intercourse, facilitate parturition, provide postural support, and assist with movement [2–4]. Yet, even in the absence of structural defects and with normal laparoscopy findings, chronic pelvic pain syndromes arise. Understanding the mechanisms of causation can lead to more effective treatment strategies and better therapeutic outcomes.

Initial screening needs to distinguish between acute pain symptoms of organic origin and those arising from dysfunctional muscle states and associated with chronic pain. Management of acute pain needs to a

M. Jantos
Behavioural Medicine Institute of Australia,
Adelaide, Australia

G.A. Santoro, A.P. Wieczorek, C.I. Bartram (eds.) *Pelvic Floor Disorders*
© Springer-Verlag Italia 2010

follow established medical practice protocols; however, chronic pain is a more complex phenomenon. Chronic pain is defined by the International Association for the Study of Pain as an "unpleasant sensory and emotional experience" [5], and thus requires a psychophy-siological approach. Characteristic of this approach is the recognition of the impact of mind–body modulators on the experience of pain. Even though the role of emotions in the experience of chronic pain will not be the focus of the discussion, their influence needs to be acknowledged [6, 7].

This chapter will discuss three pelvic pain conditions related to functional changes in PFM and will specifically consider the role of surface electromyography and myofascial therapy in their management. The three conditions include:

- vulvar pain, classified as vulvodynia, subcategories vestibulodynia and clitorodynia
- bladder pain, referred to as interstitial cystitis and bladder pain syndrome
- rectal pain, labeled as levator ani syndrome, proctalgia, or coccygodynia.

These pain syndromes affect three separate pelvic compartments. Bladder and urethral pain affects the anterior pelvic compartment, vulvovaginal pain affects the middle compartment, and anorectal pain affects the posterior compartment. Although each compartment is associated with a specific function (the bladder with elimination of fluid wastes, the vulva and vagina with reproduction and sexual pleasure, the anus and rectum with elimination of solid wastes), what these three compartments share in common are layers of soft tissue, consisting of muscles, fascia, and ligaments. The PFM make up the bulk of the soft tissue contained within the bony pelvis. Functionally, these muscles support abdominal and pelvic organs, maintain continence, and create the orgasmic platform for sexual function.

Surface electromyography (SEMG) provides an objective means of evaluating the functional state of PFM and is an important modality in the re-education and rehabilitation of pelvic muscles. Where dysfunctional muscle states give rise to chronic pain, myofascial therapy (MT) forms an essential component of pain management. MT focuses on the elimination of trigger points in muscles, fascia, and ligaments, while SEMG assists with correcting dysfunctional

states contributing to pain. Both SEMG and MT assist in normalizing PFM function and elimination of pain.

55.2 Sources of Pain

The prevailing question in the mind of the clinician and patient relates to the source of pain. Generally, three common origins of pain are recognized:

- somatic origin – arising from skin, muscles, and bone tissue; patients describe this type of pain as a throbbing, stabbing, or burning
- visceral origin – coming from internal organs; this type of pain tends to be diffuse and more generalized, with patients frequently describing it in more emotive terms as being a tiring or exhausting pain
- neuropathic origin – arising from damaged nerve fibers; the pain is described as numbness, pins and needles, and as producing electric current-like sensation [8].

Of the three sources of pain, the most common is somatic pain. This arises predominantly from muscle tissue and is a sympathetically maintained pain [9].

In the case of chronic pelvic pain syndromes, muscle overactivation has been shown to be a characteristic of vulvodynia, painful bladder syndrome, and rectal pain, and may be the leading cause of pain [10–16]. Muscle overactivation can arise in response to a range of noxious triggers, including inflammation, chemical irritation, deep somatic or visceral disease, and iatrogenic causes [8, 9, 17]. Triggers of chronic pain may initially be acute in nature (e.g. infection or inflammation), but lead to chronic muscle overactivation via spinally mediated reflexes [8–10]. Such overactivation gives rise to progressive neuromuscular tension by which muscle tissue not only responds to acute nociceptive triggers, but progressively becomes the primary "initiator of nociception" and the site of chronic pain [18, 19]. It is estimated that 85% of chronic pain syndromes may be of muscular origin [20].

55.3 Mechanisms of Pain

To place the problem of chronic pelvic pain in the context of muscle dysfunction, it is necessary to view pelvic muscle states as representing a continuum

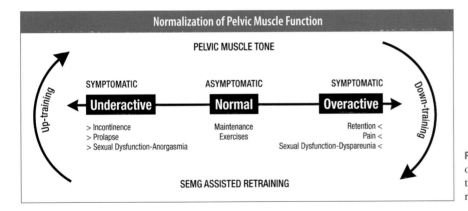

Fig. 55.1 Normalization of pelvic muscle function through SEMG-assisted retraining

(Fig. 55.1). If the midpoint of the continuum represents normal muscle tone and an asymptomatic state, then hypotonic (underactive) and hypertonic (overactive) muscle states form two opposite extremes of that continuum. Hypotonic muscle states are more likely to lead to pelvic disorders associated with muscle weakness, including urinary and fecal incontinence and sexual dysfunctions such as sexual arousal disorder and anorgasmia. Hypertonic muscle states are more likely to be associated with chronic pain disorders in the form of localized pain syndromes affecting the bladder, vulva, and rectum, as well as tension myalgias affecting the abdominal, lower back, groin, and leg areas.

Changes in pelvic muscle tone can be subtle and involuntary. Weakness can occur on account of denervation, overstretching, or atrophy, while overactivation can occur in response to iatrogenic triggers, disease, chemical irritants, or emotional stressors [6–10]. Most of these changes take place without the patient's conscious awareness, and give rise to muscle incompetence, fatigue, instability, irritability, and pain [14].

Two pain mechanisms arise in association with muscular overactivation (hypertonic muscle states). The first of these is ischemia (reduced blood flow), which also leads to hypoxia (reduced oxygen supply) during increased physiological demand (periods of muscle contraction or overactivation). Ischemia leads to deep tissue pain of moderate to high intensity [8, 17, 21, 22]. Ischemic pain is most often described as a "stabbing" and "burning" pain, and results in lower pain thresholds. With lower pain thresholds, patients experience an increased sensitivity to touch consistent with peripheral sensitisation, commonly referred to as hyperalgesia [21, 23]. If a muscle is contracted under ischemic conditions, severe pain can develop within a

minute [8]. Hyperalgesia arising from ischemia can be reversed through conservative therapy based on the deactivation and down-training of muscles (discussed in a later section).

A second mechanism of pain that arises from muscle overactivation is mediated by myofascial trigger points (TrPs), which give rise to myofascial pain syndrome [10, 11, 24]. A TrP is a hyper-irritable nodule usually found within muscle spindles and characterized by electrically active loci and a dysfunctional motor endplate. This nodule is a contraction knot within a taut band of muscle tissue. It is a few millimeters in diameter and can be found at multiple sites in a muscle and muscle fascia. A TrP produces a consistent pattern of referred pain and referred tenderness and can cause motor dysfunction and autonomic phenomena [8, 10, 11]. Pain from TrPs can be felt not only at the site of its origin but in remote areas distant from the source. Since the pain originating from a given muscle tends to exhibit a relatively consistent pattern of pain referral, it is often possible to identify the muscle(s) from which the pain originates if the pattern of pain is clearly delineated by the patient. TrPs are characterized by the following:

- they can arise in response to acute and chronic overload, following physical trauma or result from sympathetically mediated tension (anxiety-related bracing and guarding/splinting)
- they contribute to motor dysfunction by causing increased muscle tension, spasm of neighboring muscles, loss of coordination in affected muscles, substitution patterns in recruitment of muscles, and a weakening of affected muscles
- they cause weakness and limited range of motion; in most cases, the patient is only aware of the

pain but not of the other dysfunctional aspects of muscles

- the intensity and extent of the pain depends on the degree of irritability of the TrPs and not on the size or location of the muscle
- they can disturb the proprioceptive, nociceptive, and autonomic functions of the affected anatomical region.

Pain from TrPs can go unrecognized unless the clinician is prepared to identify them by palpating muscles that harbor these tender points. Palpation of TrPs evokes discomfort and assists the patient to identify "their" pain. This simple and reliable means of identifying the source of pain confirms in the patient's mind that the pain is of muscular origin and not due to other causes. Pelvic musculature is structurally and functionally predisposed to developing myofascial TrPs, due to its workload supporting abdominal and pelvic viscera, maintaining posture, and facilitating movement.

The presence of TrPs in pelvic muscles has been well documented [8, 10, 11]. TrPs in the anterior half of the pelvic floor refer pain to the vagina, bladder, and clitoris. TrPs in muscles of the posterior half of the pelvic floor cause poorly defined pain in the perineal region, and discomfort in the anus, rectum, coccyx, and sacrum [10, 16, 25]. Active TrPs in these muscles can interfere with the function of voiding, movement, and sexual intercourse [10, 16, 25, 26].

55.4 Vulvodynia

Vulvodynia is the most common form of chronic urogenital pain [27]. The condition is defined as unexplained vulvar discomfort, most often described as burning pain for which there is no known physical or neurological explanation [28]. It is a diagnosis of exclusion. The pain is localized in the vulvar area and is most often provoked by pressure application, be it from tight clothing, tampon use, or attempted sexual intercourse. Vulvodynia significantly undermines the quality of life of women and couples [29].

The lifetime prevalence is generally estimated to be in the order of 4–19%, affecting women of all ages but most prevalent among young women [27, 30–32]. In an Australian study of 744 vulvodynia patients, the mean age of women was 30.7 years, and 75% were under the age of 34 years [30]. The prevalence peaked at 24 years

of age and the average age of symptoms onset was 22.8 years, ranging from 5.5 to 45.2 years. Based on these data, it is evident that chronic vulvar pain is not related to parity or commencement of sexual activity, as over 30% of patients in this study reported the onset of symptoms prior to commencement of sexual activity.

For the diagnosis of vulvodynia, two physical criteria show good reliability and validity: the presence of pain on vaginal penetration, and tenderness on pressure application to the vulvar vestibule [33]. Both of these criteria resulted in 90% of cases being correctly classified. A lack of proportionality between the pathology and severity of pain has led some to suggest that vulvodynia may be a somatoform disorder or a sexual dysfunction [34, 35]. There is no evidence to support such hypotheses. Instead, evidence from current research suggests that vulvodynia should be classified as a chronic pain syndrome [36].

55.4.1 SEMG Studies

SEMG studies consistently highlight an association between pelvic muscle dysfunction and symptoms of vulvar pain. SEMG readings show the overactivation of the levator ani muscle to be characteristic, and of diagnostic value [14, 15]. Chronic overactivation of muscles progressively leads to painful decompensation and peripheral sensitization [18, 19]. The mechanisms by which overactivation gives rise to hypersensitivity have been discussed extensively in literature [18, 19].

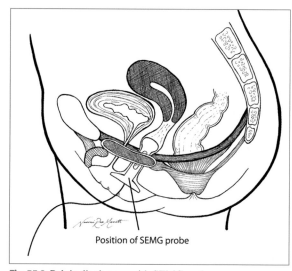

Position of SEMG probe

Fig. 55.2 Pelvic diaphragm with SEMG probe

PFM assessments involving chronic pain syndromes have traditionally used intravaginal probes, as shown in Fig. 55.2.

SEMG functional assessment of pelvic muscles differentiated between vulvodynia patients and controls in the following muscle characteristics:

- elevated resting baselines in 71% of patients, with readings over 2.0 µV
- poor contractile potential in 63% of patients, with readings under 17 µV
- elevated resting standard deviation greater than 0.2 µV in 93% of patients
- poor recruitment and recovery times of over 0.2 s in 86% of patients
- spectral frequency of less than 115 Hz in 69% of patients [14].

Among vulvodynia patients, 88% showed at least three of the above criteria, thus providing objective confirmation for the diagnosis of vulvodynia. Subsequent studies also confirmed that SEMG can differentiate symptomatic patients from asymptomatic controls [37]. Vulvodynia patients showed:

- 32% more amplitude during pretest rest
- 49% more muscle instability during pretest rest
- 46% less amplitude during 3 s phasic contractions
- 49% less amplitude during 12 s tonic contractions.

It is evident from the SEMG studies that the common functional features of PFM in vulvodynia included chronic overactivation, irritability, instability, and fatigue. The SEMG findings were validated by manual assessments of trained physical therapists [38]. Symptomatic women presented with superficial and deeper pelvic floor muscle hypertonicity, reduced muscle strength, and inability to relax, and demonstrated restrictions in the degree of vaginal stretch. The study reported that 90% of the women experiencing pain with intercourse demonstrated pelvic floor pathology. Other comorbidities seen in vulvodynia patients included evacuation difficulties and anal fissures, all symptoms associated with hyper-tonic PFM.

The loss of muscle extensibility that is evident in limited vaginal stretch can be the direct result of chronic overactivation of pelvic muscle tissue. Chronic overactivation gives rise to a shortening of muscle tissue and the development of a muscle contracture. Muscle contracture has been described as consisting of an electrically silent, involuntary state of maintained muscle shortness and decreased extensibility (i.e. loss of elasticity and increased rigidity) of the passive elastic properties of the connective tissue [19]. In the case of vulvodynia, a contracture in the levator ani muscle narrows the urogenital hiatus by compressing the vagina against the pubic bone, closing the lumen of the vagina in a manner similar to that of the other pelvic floor sphincters, thus limiting its extensibility [3, 39].

55.4.2 Management of Vulvodynia

A survey of tertiary specialists working with vulvodynia patients found that 85% expressed concern about the lack of training and information on the management of this pain condition. In relation to treatment, therapeutic drugs were found to be the frontline modality. The most common drugs used were tricyclic antidepressants (89%) and the anticonvulsant, gabapentin (68%). Both of these non-specific pharmaceutical agents were used on the assumption that vulvodynia was caused by a form of neuropathy [40]. The paucity of positive outcomes when using such protocols may be reflected in reports showing that over 64% of the time the interventions tried made the patients' symptoms no better or worse, and no single treatment or combination of treatments was found to improve symptoms [41].

Management of vulvodynia pain needs to incorporate SEMG-assisted normalization of pelvic muscle function using the guidelines discussed in the last section of this chapter. Several studies have shown this to be the most effective approach to the management of the disorder [14–16, 36]. SEMG-assisted normalization of pelvic muscle function resulted in an 83% reduction in symptoms [15]. In a more recent study of 529 vulvodynia patients, SEMG-assisted therapy, in conjunction with release of a functional muscle contracture, enabled 80–90% of patients to resume sexual activity upon conclusion of therapy [36]. Normalization of pelvic muscle function was evident in:

- a decrease in muscle resting baseline
- a decrease in muscle instability
- an increase in phasic contraction amplitude
- an increase in tonic contraction amplitude.

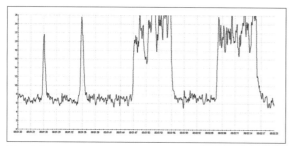

Fig. 55.3 Female, nulliparous, age 31 years, with a three-year history of symptoms. The pretreatment SEMG assessment shows two phasic and two tonic contractions, illustrating a very elevated resting baseline and irritability. Scale range 0–26 μV. For all the SEMG assessments shown in this and subsequent figures, patients rested in a semi-supine position and readings were taken using a single-user vaginal sensor (T6065) connected to a Myo-Trac 3/MyoTrac Infiniti encoder and analysed by computerized software manufactured by Thought Technology Ltd, Montreal, Canada

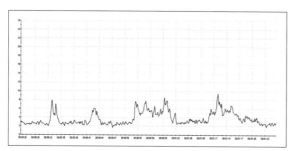

Fig. 55.4 Female, nulliparous, age 24 years, with an early onset of symptoms prior to commencement of sexual activity (primary vulvodynia). The pretreatment SEMG assessment shows two phasic contractions and two tonic contractions, illustrating elevated rest (equivalent to more than 50% of maximum voluntary contraction), poor recruitment and coordination of muscles fibers, low contractile amplitude, and slow recovery indicative of muscle irritability. Scale range 0–26 μV

Figs. 55.3 and 55.4 illustrate typical pretreatment overactivation of PFM. Fig. 55.3 shows overactivation in a patient with a strong pelvic muscles, while Fig. 55.4 identifies overactivation, instability, and fatigue in a patient with inherent muscle weakness.

The post-treatment SEMG readings in Fig. 55.5 illustrate improved resting baseline, good recruitment and coordination of muscle fiber, increased amplitude of phasic and tonic contraction, low irritability, and good recovery post contraction.

Using SEMG retraining of PFM, patients follow a regular home-training protocol of twice-daily exercises using a home-training unit. As readings improve, muscles become more responsive to voluntary control [39]. To restore muscle resilience and elasticity, therapy needs to

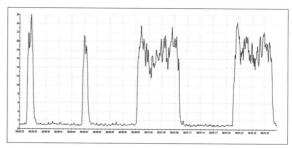

Fig. 55.5 Post-treatment SEMG assessment of same client as in Fig. 55.4, following muscle retraining showing normalization of muscle function and associated with pain-free state. Scale range 0–26 μV

incorporate elements of muscle lengthening and myofascial release [25, 26, 38, 39]. Lengthening can be facilitated through physical therapy exercises or dilator-assisted stretches. In addition to the physiological benefits derived from dilator-assisted lengthening of muscles, dilators have a desensitizing effect and can be used both by the patient alone or with the help of their sexual partner [39, 40, 42]. The clinician needs to review the patient's progress every 2–4 weeks. Significant improvements in SEMG readings are often noted within 3–6 weeks of commencement of therapy. Long-term follow-up studies have shown that SEMG-assisted PFM rehabilitation can lead to long-term normalization of muscle function and resolution of vulvodynia symptoms [43].

55.5 Bladder Pain Syndrome

Bladder pain syndrome, also known as interstitial cystitis and urethral syndrome, is a chronic and debilitating condition. It is characterized by urinary frequency, urgency, nocturia, and suprapubic pressure [44]. Pain occurs in the absence of bacterial infections and urological abnormalities [45, 46]. The diagnosis of bladder pain syndrome is made by excluding all other potential causes of pain. The prevalence of this disorder was found to be 8% in gynecology settings [47]. It is estimated that almost 90% of cases are among women and 30% of these are among women under the age of 30 years [48, 49]. As with vulvodynia, bladder pain has a negative impact on quality of life, with 90% of women reporting impairment in daily activities, 88% suffering sleep disturbances, 79% experiencing work impairment, and 70% confirming problems in relationships and with sexuality [50, 51].

Hypotheses to explain bladder pain have focused

on neurogenic, inflammatory, autoimmune, and psychosomatic causes, but no definitive evidence exists to support any of these hypotheses [52]. However, there is growing evidence showing that dysfunctional muscles contribute significantly to bladder pain [12, 16, 52–54]. Since the early 1980s, evidence has pointed to an association between bladder pain and PFM dysfunctions [54]. In recent studies, examination of pelvic floor muscles was found to reproduce bladder pain symptoms [52–55]. In 87% of cases, pressure applied to the levator ani muscles reproduced referred pain to the suprapubic, bladder, urethra, vulvar, and rectal areas and reproduced urgency and frequency, and in 71% of patients it reproduced symptoms of dyspareunia [52]. Most patients showed lack of control over PFM and poor ability to relax them. The studies concluded that pelvic floor myofascial trigger points may underlie the pathophysiology of bladder symptoms. Muscle overactivation and myofascial changes were seen as not only a source of symptoms, but a trigger for neurogenic inflammation [52, 55]. Most of the patients presenting with bladder pain syndrome also reported an early history of urethral and anal symptoms suggestive of early onset of pelvic floor pathology [16].

55.5.1 SEMG studies

There are very few structured SEMG studies profiling patients with bladder pain. It is an area that requires considerably more research. However, published studies reporting SEMG assessments [16] and physical exams found muscle overactivation, inadequate voluntary control, muscle shortening, and trigger point referred pain, not only as symptoms but possibly also causing bladder pain [25, 26, 52].

Fig. 55.6 illustrates the level of PFM overactivation, instability, irritability, and fatiguing, seen in a SEMG assessment of a patient with an early-onset history of bladder pain with symptoms of urgency and frequency. The pain became so disabling that it disrupted most of her daily activities. The patient was consistently misdiagnosed as suffering from urinary tract infection, and prescribed antibiotics, before undergoing urethral diathermy, urethral scraping, and multiple courses of anti-inflammatory and painkiller medications. The treatments were ineffective in resolving symptoms and resulted in significant scarring

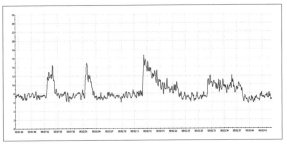

Fig. 55.6 Female, nulliparous, 22 years of age, adolescent onset of bladder pain symptoms. Pretreatment SEMG assessment of two phasic contractions and two tonic contractions. Scale range 0–26 μV

and increased pain.

Following a period of SEMG-assisted muscle retraining and myofascial therapy, the patient no longer complained of urgency and frequency, was able to resume her apprenticeship and was successful with pain-free intercourse.

Chronic pelvic muscle overactivation is characterized by a continuous state of mild contraction. The general mechanisms by which muscle overactivation gives rise to hypersensitivity have been discussed in the literature and in relation to bladder pain [19, 52]. Irrespective of whether muscle tension is due to noxious stimuli, ischemia, visceral–muscular reflexes, build up of neurogenic metabolites and sensitizing agents, inflammation, erythema and edema formation, or emotional tension, each of these agents can act as a trigger that can lead to progressive sensitization and pain [19, 22].

An overactive muscle gives rise to painful trigger points which compromise pelvic muscle function and produce referred pain [16]. These findings have been validated by physical examination carried out by trained nurse practitioners who identified myofascial TrP pain and reproduced the patients' symptoms, noting levator muscle tenderness and palpable taut muscle bands that elicited pain in the bladder, vagina, vulva, or perineum [55].

Another finding that is important to note is the frequency of shared comorbidities among patients with bladder, vulvar, and rectal pain. A significant number of the bladder pain patients also meet the diagnostic criteria for vulvodynia. In one study, medical examinations of the urogenital area carried out by urologists showed that almost 60% of cases reported vulvar pain upon q-tip swab testing in the 5-o'clock and 7-o'clock positions, confirming the presence of vulvodynia [55]. During vaginal examination of the PFM, 94.2% of patients experienced levator pain, 77% reported sexual dysfunction and deep pain with sexual intercourse, 69% described burning pain with or after sexual activity, and 71% reported that the pain could last for hours or days. Another study of 47 bladder pain patients and 47 controls found an even higher prevalence of vulvar pain, with 85.1% of the patients meeting the diagnostic criteria for vulvodynia, whereas only 23.4% reported bladder pain and 51.1% reported urgency and frequency [56]. Again, many of these patients reported childhood histories of voiding difficulties, suggestive of an early onset of pelvic floor dysfunction.

Anatomically and histologically, the bladder and vagina share many common characteristics which may lend support to the concept of a common pain pathway [55, 56]. The bladder, urethra, and vagina derive from the same embryonic urogenital sinus, share the same smooth muscles, collagen, and elastin fibers, and the fibers of the medial portion of the levator muscle interdigitate between the proximal urethra and the vagina.

However, the common embryonic origin of the bladder and vulvovaginal tissue does not explain the common occurrence of rectal pain, as intestinal tissue is not of the same origin. It is more likely that the common denominator in these three pelvic pain conditions is hypertonic pelvic muscles. Because of the lack of awareness of the link between PFM dysfunction and bladder pain, the symptoms are frequently mistaken for gynecologic pain. Based on current research, it has been suggested that bladder pain and vulvar pain may be the same entities mediated by hypertonicity of PFM [55, 56].

55.5.2 Management of Painful Bladder

There are no controlled studies comparing different interventions. Traditional therapies overlooked the muscular component and instead focused on medications, hydrodistention, physical and behavioral therapies, and neuromodulation [57–59]. All of these therapies have been found to be suboptimal in alleviating symptoms, in part because of their failure to address the muscular cause of symptoms [55]. Hydrodistension was shown to significantly reduce symptoms of pain,

but the benefits appeared to be short lived [57, 58]. Medication helped only half of the patients, and heat application and relaxation strategies provided only temporary relief in 34.6% and 25.6% of cases, respectively [55].

Surgery is used as an absolutely last measure [59]. In a study of 52 patients, the reported frequency of ineffective treatments included antibiotics in 55%, urethral dilation in 50%, anticholinergics in 30%, diazepam in 22%, tricyclic antidepressants in 15%, α-blockers in 12.5%, phenazopyridine hydrochloride in 10%, surgery in 5%, and acupuncture in 10% [16]. There are no data showing the frequency with which these treatments were prescribed.

The efficacy of therapies based on pelvic floor muscle normalization using SEMG and myofascial therapy has been documented in several reports [16, 25, 55]. In studies focusing on SEMG retraining, there was a 65% reduction in SEMG resting tone between pre- and post-treatment readings. On average, the pre-treatment resting tone was reduced from 9.73 μV to 3.61 μV post treatment [16]. The retraining of pelvic muscles and elimination of TrPs was associated with a marked reduction in bladder pain, urgency, and frequency symptoms in 70–83% of cases. To date, these are the best reported outcomes, with long-term benefits evident if patients maintained a home program of stress reduction and pelvic floor exercises. In summing up reports on the treatment of bladder pain, one of the primary authors concluded that "it is our experience that the 'taut muscle bands' palpated on exam and trigger points that reproduce the patient's pain are not normal variants. These abnormal areas will often resolve and pain will improve using myofascial release, biofeedback, relaxation techniques, neuromodulation . . . ", and further added that "PFD [pelvic floor dysfunction] and neural upregulation may relate more appropriately to the etiology of the symptoms than an altered glycosaminoglycan layer" [55]. It appears that the bladder may be an "innocent bystander" in a more diffuse process involving pelvic muscle dysfunction [60]. Decreasing PFM tension and eliminating TrP activity appears to effectively ameliorate the symptoms of bladder pain, urgency, and frequency [16, 55]. On the basis of this evidence, SEMG management and myofascial therapy should focus on pelvic floor normalization, using down-training protocols, discussed later in this chapter, and on myofascial TrP release.

55.6 Rectal Pain

The two most common forms of functional anorectal pain include levator ani syndrome (LAS) and proctalgia fugax. Anorectal pain is a poorly understood and managed chronic pelvic pain condition. Based on surveys in the United States, the prevalence of idiopathic rectal pain is estimated at 6% [61], but approximately 90% of affected individuals are female [62]. Pain occurs in the absence of organic disorders, and the pathophysiology is uncertain. The diagnosis of LAS is one of exclusion [63]. In current nomenclature, conditions such as proctalgia fugax (a fleeting rectal pain thought to be caused by spasm of the anal sphincter muscle), LAS (characterized by pain in the rectum and thought to be caused by spasm of levator ani muscles), and coccygodynia (a coccygeal pain most often attributed to skeletal trauma), are seen as distinct pain disorders, yet all three have much in common and present with considerable overlap of symptoms [64]. A number of researchers have consolidated the various syndromes under the one umbrella of tension myalgia of the pelvic floor [65]. The discussion that follows will focus on the most common form of pain, LAS.

LAS is generally accepted as a functional disorder with recurrent pain in the region of the rectum, sacrum, coccyx, and pelvic diaphragm, and possible pain in the gluteal and thigh areas [10]. In a study of 31 patients diagnosed with LAS, the pain was located in the sacrum in 100% of patients, in the pelvic diaphragm in 90%, in the anal region in 68%, and in the gluteal region in 13% [62]. Of all the women presenting with rectal pain, 43% reported pain with sexual intercourse.

An international committee clarified the diagnostic criteria for LAS (Rome II criteria) [66]. LAS was defined as pain of at least 12 weeks' duration (need not be consecutive), occurring in the last 12 months, consisting of chronic or recurrent rectal pain or aching with unexplained pain episodes lasting 20 minutes or longer.

The pain can be exacerbated by extended periods of stress, sitting, constipation (most LAS patients complain of constipation problems), or bowel motions – although patients generally reported alleviation of symptoms following defecation. Diagnosis is suggested primarily by the patient's clinical history and physical examination by a specialist. The proposed mechanisms mediating pain are consistently attributed to levator ani muscle spasm [62, 67–69]. During physical examination the common findings were tenderness and an overly contracted levator ani muscle. The tight levator ani muscle is felt as a tight band, and pain is bilateral in 55% of cases [62], although other reports refer to an asymmetrical distribution in which pain is more commonly reported on the left side [70]. It is a matter of concern that only 29% of individuals suffering from anorectal pain conditions seek assistance and consult a physician [65].

55.6.1 SEMG Findings

Very few SEMG studies have been reported on LAS patients, but those published have confirmed the presence of muscle spasm, increased resting tone, and poor phasic contractions, typically a sign of muscle fatigue due to chronic overactivation [71]. These findings are consistent with SEMG profiles of the other two pelvic pain disorders, vulvodynia and painful bladder [14–16]. Rectal pain is associated with functional changes in PFM, characterized by elevated resting baselines (hypertonicity), higher standard deviation scores at rest (instability), and poor contractile amplitude during phasic and tonic contractions (weakness), and poor recruitment recovery (instability), as shown in Fig. 55.7.

Patients presenting with symptoms of pelvic pain are most often not aware of muscle tension holding, and demonstrate an inability to relax their pelvic muscles [38].

55.6.2 Management of Rectal Pain

Management of LAS has focused on therapies aimed at reducing muscle tension. Traditionally, the most

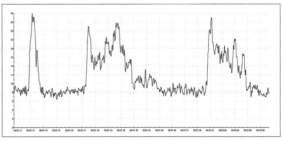

Fig. 55.7 Female, multiparous and menopausal, 48 years of age, presenting with a three-year history of LAS. Tracings show a SEMG assessment with one phasic contraction and two tonic contractions. The SEMG tracing is similar and consistent with those of other pelvic pain syndromes. Scale range 0–26 µV

common therapies include sitz baths, digital massage of the levator muscle, and electrogalvanic stimulation of the levator ani. Massage therapies showed a 68% to 74% improvement if implemented frequently (massage once or twice a week was found to be ineffective) [67]. Electrogalvanic stimulation of the levator muscle (intended to reduce spasm by inducing muscle fatigue) produced mixed outcomes, with reported improvement of 19% to 60% but varying rates of remission [71]. In a comparative study of the effectiveness of triamcinolone and lidocaine injections into tender areas, and of electrogalvanic stimulation therapy, patients receiving the localized injections showed better results in pain scores at the 1 month, 3 month and 6 month follow-up, but there were no statistically significant differences between the two groups at 12 months' follow-up [72].

Ultrasound therapy was also shown to be effective, with 75% of 24 patients reporting being symptomless or experiencing only mild continuing symptoms [62]. Biofeedback using manometric balloon techniques and SEMG was found to be 87% effective in reducing pain, and produced no undesirable side-effects [73]. Studies of SEMG biofeedback reported alleviation of symptoms with no side-effects, but noted that the degree of success depended on the patient's motivation to engage in therapy [74, 75].

55.7 General Guidelines for SEMG Pelvic Floor Protocols

The goal of SEMG-assisted therapy is to restore normal muscle function. To this end, SEMG training focuses on a combination of three primary strategies, namely down-training of overactive muscles (relaxation), up-training of weak muscles (strengthening), and coordination training to improve the relative timing of the recruitment of different muscle groups and fiber types [76]. However, to speak of normalizing muscle function implies working to well-defined criteria that provide a reliable reference point by which the degree of muscle dysfunction can be determined and to which muscles should be restored. In the case of pelvic disorders, this is somewhat difficult due to lack of normative data which would enable comparisons of individuals and categories of pelvic disorders, while still recognizing the significant intra-individual differences.

Individual differences in relation to pelvic muscle function can arise on account of many factors, such as inherited variations in the anatomical location of the pelvic floor, position of muscle attachment, connective tissue composition, cross-sectional area of the pelvic floor muscles, muscle resting length, distribution of slow and fast twitch muscle fibers, medical history, and age [77]. While some normative data for pelvic muscle function exist, they are based on small patient samples. Until more advanced data pools are available, clinicians may need to reconcile themselves to using non-normalized data, while recognizing the limitations of small data pools.

55.7.1 Functional Features of Muscles

The important functional features of muscles include:

- resting baseline tone – refers to the level of muscular energy being expended by the muscle prior to activation; baseline amplitude can be a reliable marker of dysfunction; elevations of resting baselines can be due to histological or emotional factors or a combination of both
- velocity of muscle recruitment – refers to the speed of contraction and depends on the composition and nature of fiber types, innervation ratios, and muscle length; the critical ratio is the ratio of fast-twitch fibers which fire at a rate of 30–50 twitches per second (30–50 Hz), to slow-twitch muscle fibers which fire at a rate of 10–20 twitches per second (10–20 Hz)
- contractile amplitude – is a measure based on the summation of muscle recruitment and is proportional to muscle bulk, innervation ratio, total number of motor units, and resilience to fatigue
- fatigue – refers to the slowing down of conduction velocities of the action potentials along muscle fibers, and is reflected in the muscle twitching less frequently; this can be associated with inadequate perfusion of tissue, the depletion of energy and build-up of metabolites; when a muscle is contracted at 10–50% of maximal voluntary contraction (MVC), the pressure increase is sufficient to compress the small arterioles and deprive the muscle of oxygen and energy
- recovery to baseline – refers to the length of time it takes for muscle activity to return to within 5%

of its pre-baseline levels following activation. In a healthy muscle, a rapid return to the pre-contraction resting level in less than two milliseconds constitutes the expected norm. Failure to return to a relaxed state impacts on the microcirculation and biochemistry of the muscle, potentially leading to sensitization and ischemic pain. When a muscle fails to recover to baseline levels following activation, it reflects post-activation neuromuscular irritability. When muscle tone remains elevated at 10% of maximum voluntary contraction, proprioception can be impaired and muscle fatigue becomes evident, as reflected in slower frequency of muscle twitch in the spectral analysis of SEMG tracing [22, 76].

Overactivation, irritability, and muscle fatigue are common features in pain disorders. In SEMG functional assessments, resting baselines, and muscle stability appear to be more reliable than comparisons of amplitudes.

55.7.2 Important Steps in SEMG Muscle Retraining

The following steps have been adapted from general SEMG muscle assessment and applied to the assessment and re-education of pelvic muscles [22, 76].

1. Isolating muscles – set the screen sensitivity to an appropriate level to assist the patient to detect recruitment of pelvic muscle. Use additional channels to monitor ancillary muscle groups, which may include the abdominal, gluteal, or adductor muscles.
2. Specificity training – while viewing the SEMG signal on the screen, ask the patient to activate the pelvic muscles while limiting the involvement of other muscles. Have the patient perform several repetitions until they become proficient in isolating the correct muscles. The focus of this exercise should be on correct recruitment of pelvic muscle, not on producing MVC. The emphasis needs to be placed on quality rather than quantity of recruitment, with patients being asked not to try too hard, but to focus on the proprioceptive feedback associated with the SEMG signal appearing on the screen.

3. Differentiation between muscles – have the patient deliberately contract other muscle groups, e.g. gluteal, abdominal, and adductor muscles, one group at a time, to assist in learning to differentiate between muscle groups, contrasting inappropriate recruitment with the desired recruitment of pelvic muscles. These exercises will also highlight the impact of tension holding and co-contraction of other muscles on pelvic floor resting tone.
4. Differentiating muscle fiber types – after allowing for a 1–2 min baseline period, ask the patient to produce a series of three to five short, phasic contractions, with each contraction interspersed by at least a 10–30 s rest period. Follow the short contractions with a set of three to five 5–10 s tonic contractions, each interspersed with a rest period. Record average values for the resting baseline, phasic, and tonic contractions and standard deviation measures for baselines pre- and post-contraction. Then explain to the patients the meaning of these measures and encourage correct recruitment of fast-twitch muscle fibers in the onset of contractions, and slow-twitch muscle fibers in the maintenance of tonic contractions.
5. Normalization training – explain the normal amplitude range for resting baselines, expected velocity of muscle recruitment for phasic and tonic contractions, desired contractile amplitudes, significance of fatiguing, post-contraction recovery, and latency of return to baseline.

55.7.3 Relaxation and Deactivation Training (Down-training)

Chronic pelvic pain disorders are often characterized by overactive muscles. Functionally, a muscle is considered to be overactive (or in a hypertonic state) when SEMG reveals excessive muscle effort that is outside the patient's conscious awareness. Chronically overactive muscles show an inability to relax, reduced muscle strength, and a high level of muscle irritability. Overactivity is reflected in low-grade activity of lesser amplitude than seen in muscle spasm or cramp. Because it is chronic and low grade, it cannot be detected during a physical exam but is objectively identified through SEMG assessments. Both chronically overactive muscles and muscle spasm reflect an involuntary increase in motor activity. The main difference between the two dysfunctional states is that a muscle spasm cannot be voluntarily released, whereas a hyperactive muscle can be down-trained. If SEMG assessment is conducted in conjunction with a physical assessment and tension is evident and the muscle is electrically active, then the muscle is clearly overactive. If the muscle is tense and shows no sign of increased electrical activity and is electrically silent, the muscle has become physiologically shortened and may have developed a functional contracture which needs to be released through MT.

SEMG down-training of muscles begins with the patient learning to identify and isolate the correct muscle groups without co-activating ancillary muscles. Several different down-training approaches have been proposed. These include relaxation-based and threshold-based down-training, tension discrimination training, or deactivation training. In-depth discussion of each individual approach is beyond the scope of this chapter but is well covered in SEMG reference literature [22, 76]. Each of the approaches has its merits but two of these techniques have been adapted for down-training of hypertonic pelvic disorders, deactivation training and relaxation-based training.

Deactivation training is focused on teaching patients how to "turn off" their overactive muscles. Chronic pain patients unconsciously maintain muscles in a hypertonic state without allowing for any rest even when there is no need for muscle activity. Patients may for the first time become aware of the hypertonic state of pelvic muscles during the initial SEMG assessment. Deactivation training has two main objectives: a complete reduction in SEMG activity post pelvic contraction, and an immediate return to baseline. The patient is instructed to practice a series of 5–10 s contractions, interspersed with 10–30 s rest periods when cued by the therapist or the computerized protocol. During muscle activation, the patient is instructed to initially practice with low-intensity contractions (30% of MVC) then, upon cue, release so that the SEMG signal drops to the lowest possible level. The patient will gradually progress to moderate- (50% of MVC) and then high-intensity (80–100% MVC) tonic contractions. The duration of exercises begins with 3–5 min per session twice daily, progressively increasing to 10–20 min twice daily by the end of the first 7–10 days. Deactivation training is introduced during in-office consultations and assigned as homework to be carried out with a home-training de-

vice. Home-training devices often have built-in controls for setting thresholds and for presetting activation–rest schedules. The patient continues with the exercises until they demonstrate proficiency in being able to consistently reduce the SEMG activity to a low resting baseline at < 2µV. The exercise protocol produces a well-toned muscle with a low resting amplitude, increased strength, improved endurance, and recruitment and recovery times of < 2 ms [14].

Relaxation-based SEMG training is used to assist patients to become aware of generalized tension holding in the body, and in the pelvic muscle in particular. SEMG activity from the hyperactive pelvic muscles is displayed while the patient is trained in specific relaxation techniques. Techniques like progressive muscle relaxation exercises can be introduced to assist the patient observe progressive reduction in SEMG activity, as body muscles are systematically tightened and relaxed. A technique used by the author utilizes breathing training as a means of relaxing the body and, in particular, the PFM. Patients are instructed in diaphragmatic breathing, learning to effortlessly extend the abdominal muscles during the breath-in phase, and allowing the muscle to return to its resting position with the breath-out phase. While maintaining a slow rhythm of breath, the patient is asked to focus on the gentle descent of the PFM. If the patient has no proprioceptive sense of breath-related pelvic relaxation, they can be asked to perform a Valsalva maneuver. During Valsalva, the downward intra-abdominal pressure enables the levator ani muscle to relax and descend, providing for more proprioceptive awareness. Once the patient becomes aware of the pelvic relaxation sensation, they can focus on more effective release of pelvic tension with each breath. When the pelvic muscle fully relaxes, as reflected in the SEMG signal, it is not uncommon to see breath and pulse artifact in the SEMG tracings. Regular practice of these exercises helps to maintain a relaxed pelvic muscle, and the relaxation technique can be easily generalized to daily activities.

In conclusion, therapists need to note that in chronic pain conditions SEMG biofeedback plays a critical role in muscle re-education and rehabilitation. It is often assumed that it is sufficient to train the patient in the correct recruitment of pelvic muscles and prescribe regular pelvic floor exercises. Such assumptions are often detrimental to the success of therapy. Patients not only recruit the wrong muscles and develop bad exercise practices, but fail to learn to relax their pelvic

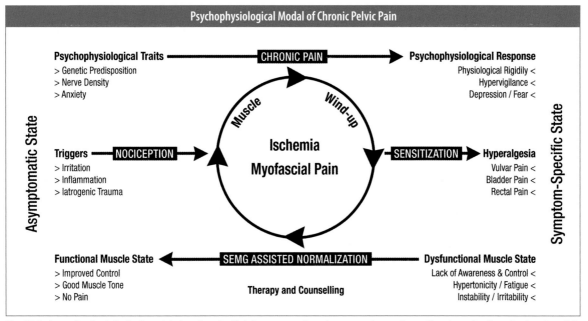

Fig. 55.8 A psychophysiological model showing the link between traits, triggers, and muscle mediated mechanisms in chronic pelvic pain syndromes

muscles and instead produce higher resting amplitudes, which result in exacerbation of pain. These shortcomings are frequently seen among patients where there is no attempt to objectively verify the functional characteristics of pelvic muscles at the commencement of therapy and to monitor progress throughout. SEMG is ideally suited to this purpose as it eliminates much of the guess work, by verifying muscle tone and enabling the patient to accurately discriminate resting amplitude levels that lie outside the sensory capabilities of physical palpation. In chronic pain, precision is essential and can differentiate between success and failure. Due to limitations of space the discussion has focused primarily on the role of SEMG in chronic pain management but a detailed account of myofascial therapy techniques can be found in several recommended specialist reference manuals [8, 10, 11].

55.8 Conclusions

The PFM are anatomically and functionally one of the most complex muscle units in the body. In their dysfunctional overactive state, PFM appear to mediate vulvar, bladder, and rectal pain. Even though these pain syndromes affect three different pelvic compartments and produce varying symptoms, they share common pain mechanisms and common comorbidities. The etiology of chronic pelvic pain may be multifactorial; infections, inflammatory states, trauma, and stress may lead to PFM overactivation (a form of low-level chronic contraction), ischemia, sensitization, and myofascial pain. Though the physiological mechanisms of pain are not fully understood, based on current understanding of these three pain conditions, Fig. 55.8 provides a summary of potential triggers and pain mechanisms and outlines strategies for the management of chronic pelvic pain. SEMG provides an objective means for conducting a functional assessment of PFM and enables a more effective approach to normalizing pelvic muscle function. MT addresses the problem of referred pain and assists in the elimination of TrPs, which are a common source of referred pain. These two modalities provide the two most effective management strategies currently available to clinicians working with idiopathic chronic pelvic pain.

References

1. Dickinson RL. Studies of the levator ani muscle. Am J Dis Wom 1889;22:897–917.
2. DeLancey J. Functional anatomy of the pelvic floor and urinary continence mechanisms. In: Schussler B, Laycock J,

Norton P, Laycock J (eds) Pelvic floor re-education: principles and practice. Springer-Verlag, London, 1994, pp 9–27.

3. Ashton-Miller JA, DeLancey JOL. Functional anatomy of the female pelvic floor. Ann N Y Acad Sci 2007; 1101:266–296.

4. DeLancey JO. Structural anatomy of the posterior pelvic compartment as it relates to rectocele. Am J Obstet Gynecol 1999;180:815–823.

5. Merskey H, Bogduck N. Classification of chronic pain. 2nd edn. IASP Press, Washington DC, 1994.

6. Hoehn-Saric R, McLeod DR. Anxiety and arousal: physiological changes and their perception. J Affect Dis 2000;61:217–224.

7. Keefe FJ, Rumble ME, Scipio CD et al. Psychological aspects of persistent pain: current state of the science. J Pain 2004;5:195–211.

8. Menses S, Simmons DG. Muscle pain: understanding its nature, diagnosis, and treatment. Lippincott, Williams and Wilkins, Baltimore, MD, 2001.

9. Schattschneider J, Binder A, Siebert D et al. Complex regional pain syndromes: the influence of cutaneus and deep somatic sympathetic innervations on pain. Clin J Pain 2006;22:240–244.

10. Travell JG, Simons DG. Myofascial pain and dysfunction: the trigger point manual: the lower extremities. Lippincott, Williams and Wilkins, Baltimore, MD, 1992.

11. Simons DG, Travell TG, Simons LS. The trigger point manual: upper half of body. 2 edn. Lippincott, Williams and Wilkins, Baltimore, MD, 1999.

12. Bernstein AM, Philips HC, Linden W et al. A psychophysiological evaluation of female urethral syndrome: evidence for a muscular abnormality. J Behav Med 1992;15:299–312.

13. Voorham-van der Zalm PJ, Lycklama A, Nijeholt GA et al. Diagnostic investigation of the pelvic floor: a helpful tool in the approach in patients with complaints of micturition, defecation, and/or sexual dysfunction. J Sex Med 2008; 5:864–871.

14. White G, Jantos M, Glazer HI. Establishing the diagnosis of vulvar vestibulitis. J Reprod Med 1997;45:157–160.

15. Glazer HI, Rodke G, Swencionis C et al. Treatment of vulvar vestibulitis syndrome with electromyographic biofeedback of pelvic floor musculature. J Reprod Med 1995;40:283–290.

16. Weiss JM. Pelvic floor myofascial trigger points: manual therapy for interstitial cystitis and the urgency-frequency syndrome. J Urol 2001;166:2226–2231.

17. Graven-Nielsen T, Jansson Y, Segerdahl M et al. Experimental pain by ischemic contractions compared with pain by muscular infusion of adenosine and hypertonic saline. Eur J Pain 2002;7:93–102.

18. Burton RJ, Musculoskeletal pain. In: Raj PP (ed) Pain medicine: a comprehensive review. Mosby, St Louis, MO, 1996, pp 418–429.

19. Calliet R. Soft tissue pain and disability. 3rd edn. FA Davies, Philadelphia, PA, 1996.

20. Slomski AJ. How groups successfully manage pain patients. Med Econ 1996;15:114–127.

21. Coderre TJ, Xanthos DN, Francis L et al. Chronic post ischemic pain (CPOP): a novel model of complex regional pain syndrome-Type 1 (CRPS-1; reflex sympathetic dystrophy) produced by prolonged hindpaw ischemia and reperfusion in the rat. Pain 2004;112:94–105.

22. Cram JR, Kasman GS, Holtz J. Introduction to surface electromyography. Aspen Publishers, Gaithersburg, 1998.

23. Seo H, Kim H, Ro D et al. A new rat model for thrombus induced ischemia pain (TIIP); development of bilateral mechanical allodynia. Pain 2008;139:520–532.

24. Ge H, Zhang Y, Bourdreau S et al. Induction of muscle cramps by nociceptive stimulation of latent trigger points. Exp Brain Res 2008;187:623–629.

25. Fitzgerald MP, Kotarinos R. Rehabilitation of the short pelvic floor I: background and patient evaluation. Int Urogynecol J 2003;14:261–268.

26. Fitzgerald MP, Katarinos R. Rehabilitation of the short pelvic floor II: treatment of the patient with the short pelvic floor. Int Urogynecol J Pelvic Floor Dysfunct 2003;14:269–275.

27. Harlow BL, Stewart EG. A population-based assessment off chronic unexplained vulvar pain: Have we underestimated the prevalence of vulvodynia? J Am Med Womens Assoc 2003;58:82–88.

28. Moyal-Barracco M, Lynch PJ. 2003 ISSVD Terminology and classification of vulvodynia: a historical perspective. J Reprod Med 2004;49:772–777.

29. Dosrosiers M, Bergeron S, Meana M et al. Psychosexula characteristics of vestibulodynia couples: partner solicitousness and hostility associated with pain. J Sex Med 2008;5:418–427.

30. Jantos M, Burns NR. Vulvodynia. Development of a psychosexual profile. J Reprod Med 2007;52:63–71.

31. Bachmann GA, Rosen R, Arnold LD et al. Chronic vulvar and other gynecologic pain: Prevalence and characteristics in a self-reported survey. J Reprod Med 2006;51:3–9 .

32. Goetsch, MF. Vulvar vestibulitis: prevalence and historic features in a general gynecologic practice population. Am J Obstet Gynecol 1991;164:1609–1616.

33. Bergeron S, Binik YM, Khalife S et al. Vulvar vestibulitis syndrome: reliability of diagnosis and evaluation of current diagnostic criteria. Obstet Gynecol 2001;98:54–51.

34. Lynch PJ. Vulvodynia as a somatoform disorder. J Reprod Med 2008;53:390–396.

35. Binik YM, Meana M, Berkley K et al. The sexual pain disorders: Is the pain sexual or is the sex painful. Annu Rev Sex Res 1999;10:210–235.

36. Jantos M. A psychophysiological perspective on vulvodynia. PhD thesis. University of Adelaide, Adelaide, SA, 2009.

37. Glazer HI, Jantos M, Hartman EH et al. Electromyographic comparisons of the pelvic floor in women with dysesthetic vulvodynia and asymptomatic women. J Reprod Med 1998;43:959–962.

38. Reissinger ED, Brown C, Lord MJ et al. Pelvic muscle functioning in women with vulvar vestibulitis syndrome. J Psychosom Obstet Gynecol 2005;26:107–113.

39. Jantos M. Vulvodynia. A psychophysiological profile based on electromyographic assessment. Appl Psychophysiol Biofeedback 2008;33:29–38.

40. Updike GM, Wiesenfield HC. Insight into the treatment of vulvar pain: a survey of clinicians. Am J Obstet Gynecol 2005;193:1404–1409.

41. Sandownik LA. Clinical profile of vulvodynia patients: a prospective study of 300 patients. J Reprod Med 2000; 45:679–684.

42. Murina F, Bernorio R, Palmiotto R. The use of amielle vaginal trainers as adjuvant in the treatment of vestibulodynia:

an observational multicentric study. Medscape J Med 2008; 10:23.

43. Glazer HI. Dysesthetic vulvodynia: long terms follow-up after treatment with surface electromyography-assisted pelvic floor muscle rehabilitation. J Reprod Med 2000;45:798–802.

44. van de Merwe JP, Nordling J, Bouchelouche P et al. Diagnostic criteria, classification, and nomenclature for painful bladder syndrome/interstitial cystitis: an ESSIG proposal. Eur Urol 2008;53:60–57.

45. Nordling J, Anjum FH, Bade JJ et al. Primary evaluation of patients suspected of having interstitial cystitis (IC). Eur Urol 2004;45:662–669 .

46. Daha LK, Riedl CR, Lazar D et al. Do cystometric findings predict the results of the intravesical hyaluronic acid in women with interstitial cystitis? Eur Urol 2005;47:393–397.

47. Stanford EJ, Dell JR, Parsons CL. The emerging presence of interstitial cystitis in gynecologic patients with chronic pelvic pain. Urology 2007;69:53–59.

48. Temml C, Wehrberger C, Reidl C et al. Prevalence and correlates for interstitial cystitis symptoms in women participating in a health screening project. Eur Urol 2007; 51:803–809.

49. Peters-Gee JM. Bladder and urethral syndrome. In: Steege JF, Metzger DA, Levy B (eds) Chronic pelvic pain: an integrated approach. WB Saunders, Philadelphia, PA, 1998, pp 197–204.

50. Koziol JA. Epidemiology of interstitial cystitis. Urol Clin North Am 1994;21:7–20.

51. Michael YL, Kawachi I, Stampfer MJ et al. Quality of life among women with interstitial cystitis. J Urol 2000; 164:423–427.

52. Peters KM, Carrico DJ, Kalinowski SE et al. Prevalence of pelvic floor dysfunction in patients with interstitial cystitis. Urology 2007;70:16–18.

53. Schmidt RA, Vapnek JM. Pelvic floor behaviour and interstitial cystitis. Semin Urol 1991;9:154–159.

54. Schmidt RA, Tanagho EA. Urethral syndrome or urinary tract infection? Urology 1981;18:424–427.

55. Peters KM, Carrico DJ, Ibrahim IA et al. Characterization of a clinical cohort of 87 women with interstitial cystitis/painful bladder syndrome. Urology 2008;71:634–640.

56. Gardella B, Porru D, Ferdeghini F et al. Insight into urogynecologic features of women with interstitial cystitis/painful bladder syndrome. Eur Urol 2008;54:1145–1151.

57. Hsieh CH, Chang CH, Chang ST et al. Treatment of interstitial cystitis with hydrodistension and bladder training. Int Urogynecol J 2008;19:1379–1384.

58. Yamada T, Murayama T, Andoh M. Adjuvent hydrodistension under epidural anaesthesia for interstitial cystitis. Int J Urol 2003;10:463–468.

59. Parsons M, Toozs-Hobson P. The investigation and management of interstitial cystitis. J Br Menopause Soc 2005; 11:132–139.

60. Peters K. Reply to the Letter-to-the-Editor: Prevalence of pelvic floor dysfunction in patients with interstitial cystitis. Urology 2008;71:1232.

61. Drossman DA, Li Z, Andruzzi E et al. US householder survey of functional gastrointestinal disorders: prevalence, sociodemography and health impact. Dig Dis Sci 1993;38:1569–1580.

62. Lilius HG, Valtonen EJ. The lavator ani spasm syndrome: a clinical analysis of 31 cases. Ann Chir Gynaecol Fenn 1973;62:93–97.

63. Wald A. Functional anorectal and pelvic pain. Gastroenterol Clin North Am 2001;30:243–252.

64. Barucha AE, Trabuco E. Functional and chronic anorectal and pelvic pain disorders. Gastroenterol Clin North Am 2008;37:685–696.

65. Sinaki M, Merritt JL, Stillwell GK. Tension myalgias of the pelvic floor. Mayo Clin Proc 1997;52:717–722.

66. Whitehead WE, Wald A, Diament NE et al. Functional disorders of the anus and rectum. Gut 1999;45s:55–59.

67. Thiele GH. Tonic spasm of the levator ani, coccygeus and piriformis muscle: Relationship to coccygodynia and pain in the region of the hip and down the leg. Trans Am Proc Soc 1936;37:145.

68. Thiele GH. Coccygodynia: cause and treatment. Dis Colon Rectum 1963;6:422.

69. Salvati EP. The levator syndrome and its variant. Gastroenterol Clin North Am 1987;16:71.

70. Grant SR, Salvati EP, Rubin RJ. Levator syndrome: an analysis of 316 cases. Dis Colon Rectum 1975;18:161–163.

71. Hull TL, Milson JW, Church J et al. Electrogalvanic stimulation for levator syndrome: How effective is it in the longer term? Dis Colon Rectum 1993;36:731–737.

72. Park DH, Yoon SG, Kim Ku et al. Comparison study between electrogalvanic stimulation and local injection therapy in levator ani syndrome. Int J Colorectal Dis 2005;20:272–276.

73. West L, Abell TL, Cutts T. Anorectal manometry and EMG in the diagnosis of the levator ani syndrome. Gastroenterology 1990;98:A401.

74. Heah SM, Ho YH, Tan M et al. Biofeedback is effective treatment for levator ani syndrome. Dis Colon Rectum 1997;40:187–189.

75. Gilliland R, Heyman JS, Altomare DF et al. Biofeedback for intractable rectal pain: outcome and predictors of success. Dis Colon Rectum 1997;40:190–196.

76. Kassman GS, Cram JR, Wolf SL. Clinical applications in surface electromyography: chronic musculoskeletal pain. Aspen Publishers, Gaithersburg, 1998.

77. Bo K. Pelvic floor muscle training is effective in treatment of female stress urinary incontinence, but how does it work? Int Urogynecol J 2004;15:76–84.

Chronic Pelvic Pain: A Different Perspective

Peter Papa Petros

Abstract A different perspective of chronic lower abdominal pelvic pain, collision dyspareunia, and vulvodynia related to laxity in the uterosacral ligaments is presented. The syndrome presented is quite characteristic: low abdominal 'dragging' pain, usually unilateral, often right-sided, low sacral pain, deep dyspareunia, and post-coital ache, tiredness, and irritability. The pain has been demonstrated to be a referred pain. Injection of local anesthesia in the posterior vaginal fornix causes the pain to disappear temporarily. An initial cure rate of up to 80% has been reported following tensioning and reinforcement of the uterosacral ligaments, most recently with the tissue fixation system (TFS).

Keywords Chronic pelvic pain • Low abdominal pain • Low sacral backache • Tissue fixation system (TFS) • Uterosacral ligaments • Vulvodynia

56.1 Introduction

It is unfortunate how so many painful or distressing conditions of the human organism have been attributed to "psychological stress". In 1998, writing about Helicobacter, HM Spiro [1] commented in the Lancet how stress-related concepts for peptic ulcer causation had led to a half century of wrong management. These comments may well apply equally to chronic pelvic pain in women. The concept of psychological cause [2] has gained such widespread acceptance that many such patients are referred for psychiatric assessment when no gross pathology is found on laparoscopy. And yet it is equally logical for the psychological disturbance to be caused by the pain itself. Chronic pelvic pain is not easy to endure, or to prove objectively. There is no Helicobacter to isolate and present as evidence.

This chapter concerns the role of lax uterosacral ligaments (USLs) in the causation of some types of unexplained chronic pelvic pain.

56.2 Types of Chronic Pelvic Pain

There are essentially two types of pelvic pain:

- explained – endometriosis, pelvic inflammatory disease etc
- unexplained – no obvious cause.

The perspective presented here is of the unexplained type, a summation of a 25-year practical experience in researching and managing hundreds of such cases.

P. Papa Petros
Formerly Department of Gynecology, Royal Perth Hospital,
School of Engineering, University of Western Australia,
Crawley, Australia

G.A. Santoro, A.P. Wieczorek, C.I. Bartram (eds.) *Pelvic Floor Disorders*
© Springer-Verlag Italia 2010

56.3 Types of Unexplained Pelvic Pain

- Low abdominal "dragging" pain and collision dysparuenia
- pain at introitus "vulvodynia" (vulvovestibulitis)
- painful bladder syndrome.

Although many patients may suffer simultaneously with two or more such types of pain, this chapter concerns only the first two. The author's experience with painful bladder syndrome is too limited to discuss it meaningfully.

56.4 Incidence

Unexplained chronic pelvic pain (CPP) comprises up to 10% of outpatient gynecology referrals, and may be an indication for laparoscopy in up to 35% of laparoscopies and 10% of hysterectomies [3]. Up to 30% of women with CPP are found to have a normal pelvis at laparoscopy.

Hysterectomy is commonly prescribed as a treatment for this condition.

56.5 Low Abdominal "Dragging" Pain and Collision Dyspareunia

56.5.1 Perspective

This can be a very severe pain, and it can fluctuate in its severity. It is often found in nulliparas. In a 1996 study [4], six patients were admitted as emergencies, and two out of six were nulliparas.

One patient's description (1996), after cure by uterosacral ligament approximation (see 56.5.7.2) was as follows:

I was almost suicidal after interminable attacks of pain on my right side. It has now been a week since the operation, and I feel like a rabbit that has been released from a trap. My mind keeps scanning up and down my body searching for the pain which so long has been my centre and focus.

This patient's pain had been diagnosed in a London Clinic [2] as psychogenic, and had been treated (unsuccessfully) according to the psychological protocols of that clinic [2].

56.5.2 Characteristics

- low abdominal 'dragging' pain, usually unilateral, often right sided
- low sacral pain
- deep dyspareunia and post-coital ache
- tiredness
- irritability.

The pain worsens during the day, and is relieved by lying down. It is reproduced on palpation of the cervix/posterior fornix. Though the pain is chronic in nature, it varies considerably from time to time. In some patients, the pain is sufficiently severe to require emergency hospital admission. Dyspareunia may occur with deep penetration, or in specific positions. Frequently, the patient complains of a constant lower abdominal pain the day after intercourse. Frequency, nocturia, urgency, and abnormal emptying symptoms are associated symptoms [5], consistent with the Integral Theory's concept of lax USLs as a causative factor.

56.5.3 Relation to Periods

These symptoms are worse during a period. This is explained by depolymerization and 'softening' of the cervical collagen to allow egress of menstrual blood. This 'softening' also causes laxity in the insertions of the uterosacral ligaments. Many patients' symptoms date from the menarche. Laparoscopic findings are invariably negative. Temporary relief of pain in such young women has been reported following division of the USLs, but the pain invariably returns within 12 months, no doubt as a result of nerve regeneration.

56.5.4 Pathogenesis

It is hypothesized that lax USLs cannot support unmyelinated nerve endings. Gravity (G) (Fig. 56.1) pulls on nerves to cause "dragging" pain, so this pain is relieved by lying down.

56.5.5 Diagnosis

Diagnosis is made only by considering other posterior zone symptoms such as urgency, and abnormal emptying

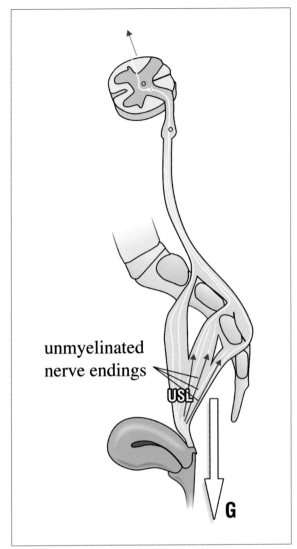

Fig. 56.1 Schematic view of the uterosacral ligament (*USL*) complex. *Red arrows* indicate the unmyelinated nerves. *G* indicates the force of gravity acting on the uterosacral ligaments. A lax ligament will 'droop'

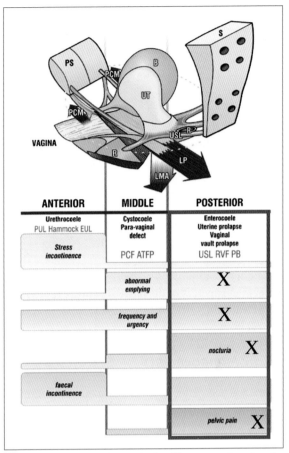

Fig. 56.2 The pictorial diagnostic algorithm summarizes the relationships between structural damage (prolapse) in the three zones and function (symptoms). The size of the bar gives an approximate indication of the prevalence (probability) of the symptom. Laxities (*red lettering*) which can be repaired: pubourethral ligament (*PUL*); external urethral ligament (*EUL*); pubocervical fascia (*PCF*); arcus tendineus fascia pelvis (*ATFP*); uterosacral ligament (*USL*); rectovaginal fascia (*RVF*); perineal body (*PB*). *B*, bladder; *LMA*, longitudinal muscle of the anus; *PCM*, pubococcygeus muscle; *PS*, pubic symphysis; *R*, rectum; *S*, sacrum; *UT*, uterus

(Fig. 56.2) [5]. This type of pain rarely occurs without at least one other posterior zone symptom (Fig. 56.2). Severe pain and other posterior zone symptoms (Fig. 56.2) may occur with even minor degrees of prolapse.

56.5.6 Examination

On examination, one finds lax separated USLs, with an enterocele "bulge" of vaginal tissue on straining; a mobile uterus; and reproduction of the patient's lower abdominal pain by palpating the cervix.

The prolapse is generally not gross, i.e. one would not normally contemplate surgery for the prolapse alone.

It is invariably associated with a lack of gross laparoscopic findings (endometriosis, evidence of pelvic inflammatory disease, etc), although varicosities are frequently seen in the region of the USLs, and also the broad ligament.

This clinical picture applies equally in patients who have undergone hysterectomy. The occurrence of this condition in some nulliparas indicates that such laxity may occur congenitally.

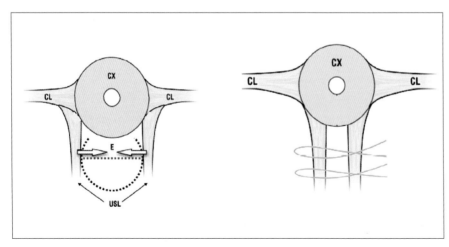

Fig. 56.3 Simple repair of lax uterosacral ligaments. A 3 cm transverse incision (*red broken line*) is made in the posterior vaginal fornix. Using a large no 1 needle, the uterosacral ligaments (*USL*) and attached tissues are grasped laterally on each side and approximated in the midline. This operation is easily performed under local anesthesia as an outpatient procedure. *CL*, cardinal ligament; *CX*, cervix; *E*, enterocele

Findings on examination are:

- uterine/vault prolapse, often first degree only
- gentle palpation of the posterior fornix reproduces pelvic pain.

56.5.7 Management

There are two major problems associated with management:

- physicians do not look for it
- it is diagnosed as "psychological", if laparoscopy is negative.

56.5.7.1 Non-surgical Management

Using a combination of electrical stimulation with a probe in the posterior vaginal fornix, squatting exercises, and sitting on a "fitball" instead of a chair produced a significant improvement in more than 50% of patients with this problem [6]. This regime is especially effective in young nulliparas.

56.5.7.2 Surgery

The important principle is to increase the tension of the USLs. USL approximation achieved an 85% cure at 3 months, decreasing to a 70% cure at 12 months [4], probably due to relaxation of the tissues. This prompted the use of polypropylene tapes to reinforce the USLs. Simple repair of lax USLs is shown in Fig. 56.3.

A posterior intravaginal sling (IVS) achieved an 80% cure of pelvic pain [7].

56.5.7.2.1 Posterior Tissue Fixation System Sling

The tissue fixation system (TFS) comprises a one-way adjustable sling which reinforces the USLs, and simultaneously tightens the fascia, thereby better supporting the unmyelinated nerve fibers (Fig. 56.4).

Results of TFS [8] are summarized in Table 56.1. Of 69 patients operated for uterine/vault prolapse, 46 (64%) had unexplained pelvic pain, 18/46 (39%) had first-degree prolapse only [8].

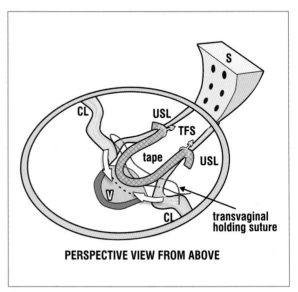

PERSPECTIVE VIEW FROM ABOVE

Fig. 56.4 Posterior TFS sling, perspective view from above. A transverse incision (*broken line*) is made in the posterior vaginal fornix (*V*). The uterosacral ligaments (*USL*) are identified. A channel is made lateral to the USL. The TFS anchor is placed adjacent to the USL, and the tape is tightened to restore tissue tension and to close any enterocele. *CL*, cardinal ligaments; *S*, sacrum

56.6 Vulvodynia ("Vulvar Vestibulitis")

The incidence:of vulvodynia in the general population can be up to 10% of women aged 18–64 years [9].

56.6.1 Definition

Intolerable sensitivity at the vaginal introitus and periurethral area

56.6.2 Experiment 1

In 2005, it was hypothesized that vulvodynia was a referred pain from lax USLs. Five patients were prospectively treated with an infracoccygeal sacropexy operation ("posterior IVS"). All were cured of their vulvodynia and their chronic pelvic pain [10]. Associated symptoms such as nocturia, urgency, abnormal emptying, and frequency were cured or substantially improved.

56.6.3 Experiment 2

The hypothesis was tested more definitively as follows [11]: 2 mL of 2% xylocaine were injected into each of the USLs, at the posterior fornix of the vagina of 10 consecutive patients diagnosed with chronic vulvodynia, diagnosed according to the Friedrich's criteria. The 10 patients were retested after five minutes. Eight patients reported complete disappearance of introital sensitivity, by two separate examiners. In the other two patients, direct testing confirmed that the allodynia (exaggerated sensitivity) had disappeared on one side, but remained on the other side. Retesting the patients showed that the blocking effects disappeared after 30 minutes. We believe that the short-term disappearance of introital pain especially on one side is an important step in further substantiating our hypothesis that vulvodynia may be a referred pain originating from the inability of weakened USLs to support the nerves running along these ligaments.

56.7 Conclusions

- Pelvic pain is rarely psychological.
- It can be cured or improved both surgically and non-surgically.

References

1. Spiro HM. Peptic Ulcer: Moynihan's or Marshall's disease. Lancet 1988;352:645–646.
2. Beard R, Reginald P, Wadsworth J. Clinical features of women with chronic lower abdominal pain and pelvic congestion. Br J Obstet Gynaecol 1988;95:153–161.
3. Reiter RC. A profile of women with chronic pelvic pain. Clin Obstet Gynecol 1990;33:130–136.
4. Petros PE. Severe chronic pelvic pain in women may be caused by ligamentous laxity in the posterior fornix of the vagina. Aust N Z J Obstet Gynaecol 1996;36:351–354.
5. Petros PE, Ulmsten U. The posterior fornix syndrome: a multiple symptom complex of pelvic pain and abnormal urinary symptoms deriving from laxity in the posterior fornix of vagina. Scand J Urol Nephrol 1993;27(suppl 15):89–93.
6. Skilling PM, Petros PE. Synergistic non-surgical management of pelvic floor dysfunction: second report. Int J Urogynecol 2004;15:106–110.
7. Farnsworth BN. Posterior Intravaginal slingplasty (infracoccygeal sacropexy) for severeposthysterectomy vaginal vault prolapse – a preliminary report. Int J Urogynecol 2002;13:4–8.
8. Petros PE. Use of a posterior sling for vaginal vault prolapse. In: Raz S, Rodriguez L (eds) Female urology. WB Saunders, Elsevier, Philadelphia, PA, 2008, pp 689–697.
9. Munday P, Buchan A. Vulvar vestibulitis is a common and poorly recognized cause of dyspareunia. Editorial. BMJ 2004;328:1214–1215.
10. Petros PE, Bornstein J. Vulvar vestibulitis may be a referred pain arising from laxity in the uterosacral ligaments- a hypothesis based on 3 prospective case reports. Aust N Z J Obstet Gynaecol 2004;44:483–486.
11. Bornstein J, Zarfati, D, Petros PEP. Causation of vulvar vestibulitis laxity in the uterosacral ligaments- a hypothesis based on 3 prospective case reports. Aust N Z J Obstet Gynaecol 2005;45:538–541.

Invited Commentary

G. Willy Davila

Pelvic pain, especially when it becomes chronic and a patient has already seen multiple doctors, can be one of the most difficult and frustrating conditions facing a pelvic floor specialist clinician. The fact that multiple chapters in this textbook are dedicated to this complex topic emphasizes the importance of sharing information on current perspectives regarding pathophysiology and treatment options with the clinicians reading the book. It also emphasizes the multifactorial and multisystem nature of this set of conditions.

Painful bladder syndrome (also known as bladder pain syndrome or interstitial cystitis) has been the focus of clinical research and public interest for many years now. It is clearly recognized to be a condition that is frequently associated with pain in other pelvic organs and structures. Evolution of our understanding of this condition has led to a great degree of scientific (and even political) debate and scrutiny of past treatments, but no real novel treatment approaches. Unfortunately, no diagnostic test has been developed to identify those patients with primary "pain of bladder origin". Although various tests are used clinically, including bladder biopsy, potassium chloride infusion into the bladder, and cystoscopy with hydrodilation, none has achieved a scientific or even clinical consensus as a true diagnostic test. Is this because there is such a wide spectrum of disease when it comes to painful bladder syndrome/bladder pain syndrome/interstitital cystitis? Or, is the condition in reality various diseases states with similar and overlapping presenting symptoms? In Chapter 52, Cervigni, Natale, Mako and Nasta present an excellent review of the current state of the art in

painful bladder syndrome, with an extensive reference list for those interested in further reading.

The common embryologic origin of various urogenital structures has led many clinicians to theorize that since a common embryologic origin leads to a common innervation, muscular support, and tissue sensitivity, there must be a commonality to all pain syndromes affecting those urogenital structures. This concept is at least partially confirmed by the common coexistence of vulvar vestibular, urethral, and trigonal sensitivity to urinary irritants and pain. In Chapter 53, Summers and Mueller provide a comprehensive review of urogenital pain which may be most useful for the non-gynecologist treating pelvic floor patients. It covers the various pain syndromes from a urogynecologist's point of view. This chapter does not cover surgery-related pain.

Perhaps even more poorly understood than pain of urogenital origin, ano-rectal pain can have more vertical than horizontal associations. What does this mean? Why is urogenital pain limited to the area anterior to the rectovaginal septum, while ano-rectal pain can be associated with inflammatory bowel disease (IBD) and other gastrointestinal (GI) pain syndromes? In Chapter 54, Infantino and Lauretta use IBD patients as clinical examples of GI and ano-rectal pain syndromes and provide an excellent review for the non-GI specialist. IBD is at least better understood than pelvic floor pain syndromes. Thus, focusing attention on pain and its mechanism in patients with IBD is a rational approach. GI pain is primarily visceral in nature, with unique perception and transmission properties. GI pain can also be caused by other neuromuscular and "functional" conditions that affect the anterior and middle pelvic compartments. These are covered well in this chapter, with particular focus on some extremely frustrating, and thankfully less common, conditions such as coccygeal pain.

G.W. Davila
Department of Gynecology, Urology and Reconstructive Pelvic Surgery, Cleveland Clinic Florida, Weston, FL, USA

G.A. Santoro, A.P. Wieczorek, C.I. Bartram (eds.) *Pelvic Floor Disorders*
© Springer-Verlag Italia 2010

Why is there no general commonality in presentation of "pain of pelvic floor origin"? Clinically, few patients are seen with pain in all compartments concomitantly. Perhaps pain related to the pelvic floor musculature – the levator muscle complex – represents a common condition seen by all pelvic floor specialists. It presents primarily as pain, either focal as found in trigger points, or more generalized myalgias, but the most common feature tends to be resultant disorders of evacuation of urine and/or stool. This myopathic focus is well described and covered in Chapter 55 by Jantos. Whether the increased levator muscle tone that underlies most pain syndromes is the chicken or the egg (primary or secondary) in the patient's presentation will remain a topic of discussion among specialists. However, it is clear that a rehabilitative approach that includes biofeedback is typically beneficial to the majority of patients. Most patients will have some focal areas of identifiable and reproducible pain – designated as trigger points. Addressing these points specifically – either by directed massage and/or injection with local anesthetics or steroids – can be of critical importance in resolving a patient's symptoms. Unfortunately, few physiotherapists and clinicians are adept at identifying and treating focal levator pain. A very gentle and methodical examination is of key importance in identifying trigger points – as once pain is triggered, it promptly becomes more generalized and the examination suboptimal.

A lack of consensus and scientific data regarding the etiology of a chronic and debilitating condition naturally leads to different and diverse concepts and theories regarding the condition's nature. A recent theory designed to explain the pathophysiology of genital prolapse, urinary incontinence, and other pelvic floor problems is the Integral Theory proposed by Petros. Laxity of the uterosacral ligaments and other supporting structures, as argued by Petros in Chapter 56, can lead to pelvic pain syndromes. Restoration of ligamentous support is presented as an option for addressing pelvic pain, including vulvodynia. This, of course, represents a surgical approach to a largely functional set of disorders. Although this approach may be beneficial for patients with overt anatomic alterations, it may be largely dependent on the accurate identification of those patients with pain that is reproducible upon traction of the prolapsing structures. Since prolapse is typically not associated with pain primarily, patients should be counseled as to the possibility of persistence of pain despite surgical anatomic correction.

What about situations where pelvic floor pain and dysfunction can be a secondary manifestation of other systemic diseases or psychological states? Of the conditions that readily come to mind, fibromyalgia – another poorly understood condition – is associated with visceral pain in various body sites, including the pelvic floor. A pelvic floor clinician is likely not qualified to deal with these systemic conditions alone – a team of clinicians including rheumatologists, immunologists, and physiotherapists is required to address these complex patients.

Pelvic pain can also have a somatization factor associated with its etiology and/or exacerbation. This is particularly true of patients who have suffered from any of the various forms of sexual abuse. The pelvic floor structures can thus be extremely sensitive to any even minimally noxious stimuli, and underlying levator hypertonicity can lead to generalized pelvic floor dysfunctions, especially evacuatory and sexual disorders. Here, participation of a mental health specialist may be of crucial importance.

These chapters do not provide a comprehensive "cookbook" approach to the patient presenting with pelvic pain. The future likely holds what may end up being an obvious common etiology that we are currently overlooking (although it may be staring us in the face), or it may confirm that these conditions are indeed extremely heterogeneous and have multiple causative factors. In all likelihood, we are in the infancy of a better understanding of the factors associated with the development of pelvic pain syndromes.

Suggested Reading

1. Butrick CW, Sanford D, Hou Q et al. Chronic pelvic pain syndromes: clinical, urodynamic, and urothelial observations. Int Urogynecol J 2009;20:1047–1053.
2. Butrick CW. Interstitial Cystitis and chronic pelvic pain: new insights in neuropathology, diagnosis, and treatment. Clin Obstet Gynecol 2003;46:811–823.

Invited Commentary

Gian Gaetano Delaini

Pelvic pain is an entity that is difficult to chatacterize and resolve, because it presents numerous issues. Firstly it is complicated for patients to describe all the symptoms involved in a direct way – because of embarrassment in speaking about this kind of problem, and difficulty in localizing the site, type, and frequency of the pain. Patients with pelvic pain who come to our attention are demoralized and confused by their illness because they have already been subjected to many examinations and diagnostic tests; they have already received different diagnoses and treatments that have not solved their basic problems.

As a first step, the correct approach to these patients and to their condition is to help them feel at ease and to listen carefully to what they have to say, without embarrassment. The second step is to take a careful medical history, in order to determinate a set of data, which should ascertain the cause of pelvic pain, including enviromental factors (type of work and posture that the patient takes during the day) and comorbidities.

As noted in Chapter 54 by Infantino and Lauretta, there are different types of intestinal disorders associated with pelvic pain, including ulcerative colitis and Crohn's disease (in which active inflammation causes hyperalgesia and quiescent inflammation determines hypoalgesia), neoplasms (cancer of the rectum, anus, perineum), and previous surgery (procedure for rectal prolapse).

Cervigni, Natale, Mako, and Nasta, in Chapter 52, describe painful bladder syndrome as a major cause of chronic pelvic pain. This syndrome, which has a multifactorial mechanism (nervous, immune, and endocrine), is associated with an increased frequency and urgency of urination and major pelvic pain.

As reported by Summers and Mueller in Chapter 53, there are different gynecological causes of chronic pelvic pain, such as endometriosis, vulvodynia, cervicitis, cervical cancer, and uterine tumors.

A further cause for pelvic pain is to be found in a malfunction of the pelvic floor muscles (PFM). In Chapter 55 Jantos emphasizes that incorrect support of the pelvic organs by the PFM can cause vulvar pain, bladder pain, and rectal pain in the absence of organic changes in these organs.

We must also remember the sexually transmitted infections such as gonorrhea, chlamydia, herpes simplex virus, and syphilis. These can cause ano-rectal pain and tenesmus and are increasing in western countries.

Thus, the importance of a multidisciplinary approach to the study of this condition is evident. By splitting the pelvic area into an anterior, middle, and rear compartment, it is easy to understand the need to involve other professionals such as urologists, gynecologists, and surgeons.

To complete the team, radiologists are also required. Using imaging (ultrasound scan, computerized tomography (CT) scan, magnetic resonance imaging (MRI), entero-MRI, transvaginal scan), they help their colleagues to determine the pathogen responsible for pelvic pain. Three additional professionals should also be present: the endoscopist, who helps in the study of colorectal disorders, the physiotherapist, and finally the psychologist. The psychologist is crucial for determining the psychological component of the disease, which is sometimes relevant in the etiopathogenesis of these disorders, and also for giving psychological support to patients who often have an increased level of anxiety and major depression.

G.G. Delaini
Department of Surgery and Gastroenterology,
University of Verona, Verona, Italy

G.A. Santoro, A.P. Wieczorek, C.I. Bartram (eds.) *Pelvic Floor Disorders*
© Springer-Verlag Italia 2010

Through this multidisciplinary approach, and taking advantage of the numerous investigations, there is the potential to come to an etiological diagnosis of pelvic pain, in order to establish a targeted therapy. However, this is not always possible and in these cases we are forced to start symptomatic therapy with poor results.

As already described, there is a lack of specialists in diseases of the perineum, who would complement the specialist team.

Their task would be to coordinate all other specialists and put into practice a diagnostic and therapeutic algorithm for this difficult disorder.

Section VIII
Fistula

Fistula: Introduction

Tomasz Rechberger

The female genital and urinary tracts share a common embryological origin and therefore the potential for intraoperative and postoperative injury should always be taken into consideration when operating on either one. It has been estimated that urinary tract injuries complicate approximately 1% of all gynecologic procedures and cesarean sections [1]. These injuries are usually divided into two categories:

1. acute intraoperative complications such as a bladder, ureter and/or urethra perforation or laceration that are usually identified immediately during the primary surgery
2. late postoperative (chronic) complications such as various kinds of urinary tract fistulae or stenosis, which can occur later on after the operation or even several years after radiotherapy.

Primary lesions (bladder, ureter, and urethra lacerations) are identified during operation by means of a methylene blue injection and a cystoscope, whereas chronic complications are usually identified through clinical symptoms (constant urine leakage) and finally confirmed by radiological studies [2].

Epidemiology

The real prevalence rate of various types of urogenital fistulae worldwide is unknown because no reliable data are available, especially from third world countries. The prevalence rate of vesicovaginal fistulae (VVFs)

in Africa is over 2 million women, with an annual incidence between 50,000 and 100,000 new cases, and this is mostly the result of poor obstetric care in undeveloped countries [3]. Contrary to that, in developed countries the leading cause of a VVF is a history of pelvic surgery (including cesarean section) or radiotherapy due to pelvic malignancy [4].

When analyzing causes of VVFs among 207 women, hysterectomy was the most common operation (91% of all cases) associated with this pathology. It should be stressed that this complication was much more frequently associated with abdominal (83%) than vaginal hysterectomy (8%). The third causative factor was radiotherapy (4% of all cases), whereas other causes (5% of all cases) including trauma, foreign bodies (neglected pessaries), infection, anti-incontinence procedures, and malignancy were much less common [5].

In a series of 8,824 major gynecological operations analyzed by Bai et al [6], the overall incidence of urinary tract injury was 0.33%. When stratified against the type of surgery, the incidence of urinary tract injury in radical hysterectomy was higher than that for total abdominal hysterectomy (0.76 vs. 0.26%). Of all the cases with urinary tract injury, the most common type of operation was total abdominal hysterectomy ($n = 45$, 67.2%), and the most common indication was uterine myoma ($n = 25$, 36.9%). The most common type of urinary tract injury was bladder injury, including bladder laceration and vesicovaginal fistula ($n = 57$, 76.1%). It should be stressed that in 48.4% of analyzed cases, coexisting pelvic adhesion, distortion of normal pelvic configuration, previous irradiation history, and previous operation history were identified as possible predisposing factors for urinary tract injuries [6].

Recently published personal data by J. Kelly, analyzing 3,072 cases of fistulae (cases of ureterovaginal

T. Rechberger
2nd Department of Gynecology, Medical
University of Lublin, Poland

G.A. Santoro, A.P. Wieczorek, C.I. Bartram (eds.) *Pelvic Floor Disorders*
© Springer-Verlag Italia 2010

fistulae were excluded), revealed that the most common location of the lesion was VVF (2,202 cases – 71.7%) followed by combined vesicovaginal and rectovaginal fistula (756 cases – 24.6%) and finally rectovaginal fistula (114 cases – 3.7%) [7]. When the authors stratified their material against causes of the lesion, the leading cause in developing countries was protracted labor (2,624 cases – 92.4%) when compared to only 12 cases (5.2%) in developed countries with proper medical services. Surgery was the causative factor for the lesion in 84 (3%) patients in developing countries but it accounted for 167 (72%) cases in developed countries. When the clinical material was stratified against malignancy as the causative factor for the lesion, in developing countries 52 (1.8%) cases were found, as compared to 32 (13.8%) patients in developed countries.

Diagnosis

Among all the morbid conditions that can affect women following labor, an obstetric fistula is considered the most debilitating and devastating [8]. This is especially true in developing countries since, as stated by Browning and Patel [9], "At the world's current capacity to repair fistula, it would take at least 400 years to clear the backlog of patients, provided that there are no more new cases"; and by this estimate, the unmet need for surgical treatment could be as high as 99%. This clearly indicates that the majority of women affected by obstetric fistula in developing countries will never have a chance to be operated and finally cured. In developed countries the situation is completely different. Obstetrical fistulae rarely occur but the most common complication, in terms of urinary tract laceration, is the urinary tract–vaginal fistula, detected after pelvic surgery. This is manifested by uncontrolled urine leakage from the vagina and is sometimes accompanied by other general symptoms such as fever, flank pain, and chilling sensations [10]. The common reasons for flank pain or fever are ureter stenosis or deterioration of the ipsilateral renal function. Usually urine leakage from the vagina appears within 1 month after the operation, with variations from 3 to 33 days [11]. Physical examination using a vaginal speculum is an essential aspect of the evaluation if vaginal fistula is suspected. The instillation of methylene blue into the bladder through a Foley catheter is very helpful. The classic finding on speculum examination is pooling of blue urine in the posterior vagina. At that point it is important to recognize the location and size of the fistula, paying special attention to the quality of surrounding tissues and vaginal mucosa. Typically, post-hysterectomy fistulae are located along the anterior vaginal wall and interureteric ridge, whereas postradiation fistulae can be seen distal to the trigone [12]. Cystoscopy is an essential part of the physical examination, helping to determine fistula size, location, and tissue quality. If the fistula is located close to a ureteral orifice, further evaluation is mandatory with intravenous pyelography (IVP) or a retrograde pyelogram. This is of critical importance, since before attempting to close the defect, one should exclude/eliminate the presence of ureterovaginal fistula and also assess a potential need for ureteral reimplant at time of primary correction [13]. Evaluation of the upper tracts by IVP is necessary, since up to 12% of patients have concomitant ureteral injuries or ureterovaginal fistulae [14]. It should be mentioned that the most common site of ureter injury during hysterectomy is its crossing with the uterine artery, when ligation of the uterine artery is performed [15].

Finally, during physical examination special attention should also be paid to the local circumstances, such as the size of the vaginal orifice and length and mobility of the vaginal cuff, since these will be crucial for a decision concerning the route of repair.

Fistula Classifications

In the past, several classification systems were proposed, and nearly all of them were based on descriptions of two factors, namely the size and anatomic location of the defect. However, it should be stressed that such classification systems, while useful in communicating the appearance of a given fistula, do not necessarily give exact information on the difficulty of reconstructive surgery and, what is of critical importance, the prognosis for a successful outcome. The first classification system was proposed by Marion Sims in 19th century and was based purely on the location of injury [16]. Marion Sims classified urogenital tract injuries into four categories:

- urethrovaginal
- fistulae situated at the bladder neck or root of the bladder, destroying the trigone

- fistulae of the body and floor of the bladder
- uterovesical.

This very simple anatomical classification system was later modified by several authors but all these newer systems simply substituted different descriptors of the site or size of the fistula defect [17–20].

In other words, each of these systems preserves the concept of providing information describing the anatomic location and extent of the defect. In 1969, a novel classification system introduced by Hamlin added new information describing the potential difficulty of repair, including terms such as "simple VVFs" and "difficult urinary fistulae" [21]. In that way, this novel classification went beyond an anatomical approach in order to predict how difficult an individual repair would be to perform. Several factors such as "total urethral destruction", "sloughing of the bladder neck and trigone", and "extensive scarring" were taken into account as additional factors that would render an individual approach to predict the difficulty of surgical repair of the defect. Recently also, additional conditions that describe the etiology of damage have been used ("obstetrical", "postsurgical", "postradiative", "malignant", and "infectious"), in order to further facilitate the prognosis for cure. In 2007, Arrowsmith described a novel scoring system based on the degree of scarring (mild – 1; moderate – 2; severe – 3) and the status of the urethra (intact – 0; partial damage – 2; complete loss – 3) as important predictors of the outcome.

When this simple score was stratified against clinical outcome of reparative surgery in 229 Nigerian patients, a striking "break" occurred. Patients with a score less that 3 showed an 83.5% rate of dryness at discharge, compared to a rate of only 40% for those with a score of 3 or higher [22]. These data are of great clinical importance, since the introduction of only two simple physical parameters enables clinicians to predict the success rate in 80% of properly selected cases, whereas patients with score > 3 should be honestly informed that the probability of success is much lower than 50%.

The most precise classification system for vesicovaginal and rectovaginal fistulae was introduced into clinical practice by Goh in 2004 [23]. In this system, not only fistula location and the size of the fistula but also local factors that could compromise clinical outcome are taken into consideration.

Vesicovaginal Fistulae

Type 1   distal edge > 3.5 cm from the external urinary meatus

Type 2   distal edge 2.5–3.5 cm from the external urinary meatus

Type 3   distal edge 1.5 to < 2.5 cm from the external urinary meatus

Type 4   distal edge < 1.5 cm from the external urinary meatus
  a. size < 1.5 cm in the largest diameter
  b. size, 1.5 to 3 cm in the largest diameter
  c. size > 3 cm in the largest diameter
    i.   none or only mild fibrosis (around the fistula and/or vagina), and/or vaginal length > 6 cm with normal capacity
    ii. moderate or severe fibrosis (around the fistula and/or vagina), and/or reduced vaginal length and/or capacity
    iii. special consideration, e.g. postradiation, ureteric involvement, circumferential fistula, or previous repair.

Rectovaginal Fistulae

Type 1   distal edge of fistula > 3.5 cm from the hymen

Type 2   distal edge of fistula 2.5 to 3.5 cm from the hymen

Type 3   distal edge of fistula 1.5 to < 2.5 cm from the hymen

Type 4   distal edge of fistula < 3.5 cm from the hymen
  a. size < 1.5 cm in the largest diameter
  b. size 1.5–3 cm in the largest diameter
  c. size > 3 cm in the largest diameter
    i.   no or mild fibrosis around the fistula and/or vagina
    ii. moderate or severe fibrosis
    iii. special consideration, e.g. postradiation, inflammatory disease, malignancy, or previous repair.

Treatment

The best treatment strategy is certainly prophylaxis. In obstetrics the best strategy is obviously 24-hour access to a properly equipped delivery unit with well-trained medical staff.

This is a reality in the developed world but still a dream in several developing countries in Africa and Asia. Currently, fistulae of the genitourinary tract, either obstetric or surgical, are still a challenge for many surgeons and therefore an optimal treatment strategy is of critical importance.

The Cochrane database published a protocol for the systematic review of surgical management of vesicovaginal and/or urethrovaginal fistulae [24]. It should, however, be stressed that there are no properly designed trials relating to techniques used to repair fistulae. Because of the reasonably high success rates, in good centers [25], the numbers required to show a difference between techniques will be large and therefore difficult to achieve. Approval must be given for case mix, operator expertise, and, often forgotten, the quality of preoperative and postoperative care, including the nutritional status of operated individuals. Obviously rehabilitation, physiotherapy, counseling, and skill building must be also an integral part of the treatment strategy [26].

Surgical procedures performed in order to repair fistulae of different location are either vaginal or abdominal. However, some controversies still exist concerning the type and timing of the procedures, the use or not of a local infiltration containing an analgesic and/or a vasoconstrictor which facilitate tissue preparation, and the need for local flaps for additional support of the repair [27, 28].

There is no doubt that all damage to the bladder, ureters, and urethra recognized during the primary surgery should be repaired immediately. According to current knowledge, all injuries recognized before 72 hours from primary surgery (usually immediately after bladder catheter removal) should also be repaired immediately [29]. However, in most cases diagnosis is made several days or even weeks after surgery, and therefore it is reasonable to wait for the initial acute inflammation to resolve before proceeding with repair [30]. The traditional recommendation is that a 3-month waiting period, which allows the fistula tract to mature, is mandatory in order to achieve success rates from 84% to 100% [31, 32]. This classical concept has recently been challenged by a study comparing the clinical outcome of the closure of vesicovaginal obstetrical fistulae early (before 12 weeks) or late (after 12 weeks), and showing 87.8% success rates for early repair versus 87.2% success rates for late repair [33]. The authors of this report proved that early repair ben-

efited patients both medically and socially, with no detriment to procedure success since there was no significant difference in success rates between patients with early or delayed repair. In the light of these findings, a waiting period longer than 3 months is currently not recommended. Of course if the fistula is small, the closure could be achieved by catheter drainage concomitant with antibiotic treatment [30]. Also with small fistula size, some clinical success is possible after electrocoagulation of the fistula tract cystoscopically [34]. With the advances of new technologies, using placement of cyanoacrylic or fibrin glues might also be of some value in selected cases of VVF [35, 36]. A detailed description of the currently used surgical techniques for optimizing the clinical outcome of patients operated due to urogenital fistulae has recently been published by Cohen and Gousse [37]. According to these authors, the basic principles that warrant successful closure of urogenital fistula are as follows:

- adequate exposure of the operative field (depending on the route of operation – either vaginal or abdominal)
- wide dissection of surrounding tissues with proper separation of the bladder wall from the vagina
- avoidance of overlapping suture lines
- maintenance of the fistula tract, which prevents widening of the fistula
- watertight closure with absorbable suture material with low tissue reactivity (consider tissue interposition when necessary)
- maintenance of watertight closure by using a urethral and/or suprapubic catheter
- proper postoperative care with obligatory bladder drainage, and catheter removal after a cystogram demonstrating no extravasation.

To summarize, when the vaginal approach is considered for fistula repair, a circumscribing incision is made around the fistula, which is exposed on Foley catheter, and the vaginal mucosa is separated from the bladder wall. The fistula tract within the bladder wall is not excised but is closed with interrupted sutures. The second layer of sutures is placed on the perivesical fascia, followed by the third layer which finally closes the vaginal wall.

The bladder Foley catheter is removed 2 weeks later, following a negative postoperative cystogram. For transabdominal fistula closure, the O'Conor technique is generally considered as the gold standard [38]. A recently performed clinical trial comparing the surgical outcome at discharge and at 6 months' follow-up in patients who underwent repair of obstetric fistulae with postoperative bladder catheterization for 10, 12, or 14 days revealed that in less complicated cases bladder catheterization for 10 days is sufficient for proper bladder healing [39].

The most challenging clinical situation for both a surgeon and patient is the repair of combined vesicovaginal and rectovaginal fistulae, which are present in 6–24% of patients with obstetric fistulae [25]. A classical approach involves at least three surgical sessions, all associated with morbidity, and often a colostomy procedure as well. However, this classical approach has recently been challenged by the group of Ojengbede et al who, after a proper preoperative preparation (described below) of the patients, successfully performed one-stage repair of both types of fistulae in a group of 20 women, with 100% success and no temporary colostomy in any case [40]. Prior to surgery, all women were encouraged to drink plenty of water (4–6 L per day). Three to five days before the surgery, bowel preparation was initiated with a low-fiber diet (pap or "fura"), an antimicrobial bowel treatment with 1 g of neomycin every 12 hours, and a laxative every evening. An enema saponis was performed on the night preceding the surgery, and another as a rectal washout on the morning of the surgery. All patients had their repairs performed vaginally in the lithotomy position, using subarachnoid block anesthesia (spinal anesthesia). The authors concluded that in experienced hands such one-step surgery is possible with a very high success rate.

Vesicovaginal fistulae, while still common in developing countries due to lack of professional obstetric care in the developed world, are uncommon but potentially devastating complications of pelvic surgery and radiotherapy.

A conservative treatment by means of bladder catheterization rarely allows resolution to be achieved, and therefore strict adherence to the basic principles of surgical fistula repair is paramount for a successful outcome. Newer techniques involving laparoscopy and robotic-assisted laparoscopy are still at the level of learning curve, and therefore vaginal or transabdominal repairs are the methods of choice when treating this complication.

References

1. Gilmour DT, Dwyer PL, Carey MP. Lower urinary tract injury during gynecologic surgery and its detection by intraoperative cystoscopy. Obstet Gynecol 1999;94:883–889.
2. Michael P, Aronson MD, Teresa M, Bose MD. Urinary tract injury in pelvic surgery. Clin Obstet Gynecol 2002; 45:428–438.
3. Second Meeting of the Working Group for the Prevention and Treatment of Obstetrical Fistula, Addis Ababa, Africa; 30 October 2002. New York: United Nations Population Fund, 2003.
4. Evans DH, Madjar S, Politano VA et al. Interposition flaps in transabdominal fistula repairs: are they really necessary? Urology 2001;57:670–674
5. Eilber KS, Kavaler E, Rodriguez LV et al. Ten-year experience with transvaginal vesicovaginal fistula repair using tissue interposition. J Urol 2003;169:1033–1036.
6. Bai SW, Huh EH, Jung DJ et al. Urinary tract injuries during pelvic surgery: incidence rates and predisposing factors. Int Urogynecol J 2006;17:360–364.
7. Kelly J, Winter HR. Reflections on the knowledge base for obstetric fistula. Int J Gynecol Obstet 2007;99:S21–S24
8. Angioli R, Gomez-Marin O, Cantuaria G, O'Sullivan MJ. Severe perineal lacerations during vaginal delivery: the University of Miami experience. Am J Obstet Gynecol 2000;182:1083–1085.
9. Browning A, Patel TL. FIGO initiative for the prevention and treatment of vaginal fistula. Int J Gynecol Obstet 2004;86:317–322.
10. Lee RA, Symonds RE, Williams TJ. Current status of genitourinary fistula. Obstet Gynecol 1988;72:313–319.
11. Oh BR, Kwon DD, Park KS et al. Late presentation of ureteral injury after laparoscopic surgery. Obstet Gynecol 2000;95:337–339.
12. Boronow RC. Repair of the radiation-induced vaginal fistula utilizing the Martius technique. World J Surg 1986;10: 237–248.
13. Blandy JP, Badenoch DF, Fowler CG et al. Early repair of iatrogenic injury to the ureter or bladder after gynecological surgery. J Urol 1991;146:761–765.
14. Goodwin WE, Scardino PT. Vesicovaginal and ureterovaginal fistulas: a summary of 25 years of experience. J Urol 1980;123:370–374.
15. Liapis A, Bakas P, Giannopoulos V, Creatsas G. Ureteral injuries during gynecological surgery. Int Urogynecol J Pelvic Floor Dysfunct 2001;12:391–394.
16. Sims JM. On the treatment of vesicovaginal fistula. Am J Med Sci 1852;23:59–82.
17. Mahfouz Bey N. Urinary fistulae in women. J Obstet Gynaecol Br Emp 1930;45:405–424.
18. Krishnan RG. A review of a series of 100 cases of vesicovaginal fistulae. J Obstet Gynaecol Br Emp 1949;56:22–27.
19. McConnachie EL. Fistulae of the urinary tract in the female. S Afr Med J 1958;32:524–527.
20. Bird GC (1967) Obstetric vesico-vaginal and allied fistulae: a report on 70 cases. J Obstet Gynaecol Br Commonw 1967;74:749–752.
21. Hamlin RH. Reconstruction of the urethra totally destroyed in labour. BMJ 1969;2:147–150.

22. Arrowsmith SD. The classification of obstetric vesico-vaginal fistulas. A call for an evidence-based approach. Int J Gynecol Obstet 2007;99:S25–S27.

23. Goh JT. A new classification for female genital tract fistula. Aust N Z J Obstet Gynecol 2004;44:502–504.

24. Lapitan MC, Rienhardt G. Surgical management of vesico-vaginal and/or urethrovaginal fistulae (protocol for a Cochrane Review). Cochrane Database Syst Rev 2009(4): CD003307.

25. Wall LL, Karshima JA, Kirschner C, Arrowsmith S. The obstetric vesico-vaginal fistula: characteristics of 899 patients from Jos, Nigeria. Am J Obstet Gynecol 2004;90:1011–1623.

26. Miller S, Lester F, Webster M, Cowan B. Obstetric fistula: a preventable tragedy. J Midwifery Women's Health 2005; 50:286–294.

27. Eilber KS, Kavaler E, Rodriguez LV et al. Ten-year experience with transvaginal vesicovaginal fistula repair using tissue interposition. J Urol 2003;69:1033–1036.

28. Rovner ES. Vesicovaginal and urethrovaginal fistulas. AUA Update Series 2006;25:45–56.

29. Cohen BL, Gousse AE. Current techniques for vesicovaginal fistula repair: surgical pearls to optimize cure rate. Curr Urol Rep 2007;8:413–418.

30. Blaivas JG, Heritz DM, Romanzi LJ. Early versus late repair of vesicovaginal fistulas: vaginal and abdominal approaches. J Urol 1995;153:1110–1112.

31. Raz S, Bregg KJ, Nitti VW, Sussman E. Transvaginal repair of vesicovaginal fistula using a peritoneal flap. J Urol 1993;150:56–59.

32. O'Conor VJ. Transperitoneal transvesical repair of vesico-vaginal fistula with omental interposition. AUA Update Series 1991;10:lesson 13.

33. Melah GS, El-Nafaty AU, Bukar M. Early versus late closure of vesicovaginal fistulas. Int J Gynecol Obstet 2006;93:252–253.

34. Stovsky MD, Ignatoff JM, Blum MD et al. Use of electro-coagulation in the treatment of vesicovaginal fistulas. J Urol 1994;152:1443–1444.

35. Muto G, D'Urso L, Castelli E et al. Cyanoacrylic glue: a minimally invasive nonsurgical first line approach for the treatment of some urinary fistulas. J Urol 2005174:2239–2243.

36. Sharma SK, Perry KT, Turk TMT. Endoscopic injection of fibrin glue for the treatment of urinary-tract pathology. J Endourol 2005;19:419–423.

37. Cohen BL, Gousse AE. Current techniques for vesicovaginal fistula repair: surgical pearls to optimize cure rate. Curr Urol Rep 2007;8:413–418.

38. O'Conor VJ. Review of experience with vesicovaginal fistula repair. J Urol 1980;123:367–369.

39. Nardos R, Browning E, Member B. Duration of bladder catheterization after surgery for obstetric fistula. Int J Gyn Obstet 2000;103:30–32.

40. Ojengbede OA, Morhason-Bello IO, Shittu O. One-stage repair for combined fistulas: myth or reality? Int J Gynecol Obstet 2007;99:S90–S93.

Urogenital Fistulae

57

Dmitry Pushkar, Gevorg Kasyan and Natalia Sumerova

Abstract Urogenital fistulae are a rare condition in western countries. Due to the wide variety and individuality of the clinical manifestations of these injuries, it is practically impossible to find and create common guidelines for treatment. Prevention of urogenital fistulae can be achieved through both improvements in obstetric care and profound training in vaginal surgery. The success of any surgical treatment depends on careful patient selection, and assumes knowledge of all possible treatment options. Potential work needs to be directed towards the application of the newest molecular technologies.

Keywords Latzko colpocleisis • Martius flap • Radiation-induced fistulae • Urethral surgery • Urethrovaginal fistulae • Urinary incontinence • Urogenital fistulae • Vaginal surgery • Vesicovaginal fistulae

57.1 Introduction

Urogenital fistulae (UGFs) remain one of the most challenging problems in modern female urology. Although it is not a life-threatening problem, UGF nonetheless significantly decreases a woman's quality of life. Fortunately, it has become a rare problem in western countries due to improvements in obstetric standards. Childbirth and obstetric traumas were the causes of a majority of genital defects in past centuries [1]. At present, this condition also commonly results from prior surgeries such as anterior colporrhaphy, urethral diverticulectomy, paraurethral cyst removal, anti-incontinence surgery, and so on [2, 3]. Other causes of UGFs include urethral trauma, pelvic surgery, lower urinary tract instrumentation [4] (prolonged catheterization), and radiation. Prolonged

obstructive labor, however, remains a major cause of urethral injury in developing nations [1]. Urogenital fistulae include any coaptation between the urinary tract and genital organs. Vesicovaginal and urethrovaginal fistulae are more common in current practice. Other types of UGF that develop due to damage of the uterus or ureters are much rarer conditions.

57.2 Vesicovaginal Fistulae

The problem of vesicovaginal fistulae resulting from obstetric trauma has almost been eradicated from developed countries, but it remains a major problem in the developing world. In a report from the USA [5], only 5% of genitourinary fistulae were of obstetric origin, while studies from Nigeria [6], India [7], and Pakistan [8] indicate obstetric causes are responsible for 92%, 81%, and 68% of such fistulae respectively [9–11]. The United Nations Population Fund estimates

D. Pushkar
Department of Urology, MSMSU, Moscow, Russia

G.A. Santoro, A.P. Wieczorek, C.I. Bartram (eds.) *Pelvic Floor Disorders*
© Springer-Verlag Italia 2010

that there are more than 2 million women currently living with fistulae in the sub-Saharan belt of Africa, and that another 50,000 to 100,000 join their ranks each year [12].

Vesicovaginal fistula (VVF) has become a rare problem in western countries, due to improvements in obstetric standards. While pelvic radiation used for the treatment of malignant diseases is the primary cause of delayed VVF, radiation-induced VVFs (RVVFs) have recently become more apparent, despite the fact that radiation therapy of the pelvic organs is now less aggressive and more precise. The modern use of ionizing radiation in gynecology is limited to the treatment of malignant diseases. Pelvic radiation is the primary cause of delayed VVF [13]. When radiation is terminated, fibrosis occurs in the bladder lamina propria. Due to these changes, hyalinization of the connective tissues develops. Histologic examinations show the presence of large bizarre fibroblasts, which are described as radiation fibroblasts [14]. Vascular damage of bladder tissue leads to atrophy or necrosis of the bladder epithelium, which causes ulceration, or the formation of fissures. The majority of fistulae become apparent 1.5–2 years after termination of radiotherapy. Some fistulae may not appear for many years after treatment [15].

57.3   Urethrovaginal Fistulae

In adults, the majority of urethrovaginal fistulae are a result of iatrogenic injuries [16–18]. It is a conceptual mistake to consider urethrovaginal fistulae synonymous with VVFs. Urethrovaginal fistulae are a different entity requiring special attention and treatment. The medical literature on this particular subject is sparse, and limited to either clinical cases, or a small series of patients. Due to the wide variety and individuality of the clinical manifestations of these injuries, it is practically impossible to find and create common guidelines for treatment.

In the developing world the vast majority of urethrovaginal fistulae result from obstructed labor [19–22]. Roenneburg describes the traumatic absence of the proximal urethra (TAPU) occurring within this context of a broad-field labor injury in Africa [13]. In the developed world, the more common causes of urethral injury include trauma, iatrogenic injury at urethral diverticulectomy, bladder neck suspension,

endoscopic surgery, and gynecologic surgery, such as vaginal hysterectomy or anterior vaginal repair. Urethral erosion can result from synthetic materials used in these procedures or from anti-incontinence surgery, or it may be due to long-term indwelling catheters in neurologically impaired or comatose patients [23–28]. Urethral damage is also a potential sequela of radiotherapy for pelvic malignancy and related procedures. [29]. The incidence of urethral injury with pelvic fractures ranges from 0% to 6%, and is predominantly caused by high-speed motor vehicle accidents. The reader should be aware that here we are covering only urethrovaginal fistulae, as opposed to acute urethral damage, which, when treated, requires a different, specific approach.

57.4   Vesicovaginal Fistula Repair

Since every fistula is unique and requires an individualized approach, it is difficult to describe a standard fistula repair, but some useful tips and general principles can be summarized. The surgery starts with the patient in the dorsal lithotomic position. The Trendelenburg position can improve visualization of the VVF. A 16 F or 18 F Foley catheter is placed into the bladder. Vaginal examination aims to eliminate the risk of missing any additional small fistulae not found during routine vaginal exams without anesthesia, and to evaluate the condition of the surrounding tissues. As a result of severe pain, proper vaginal examination with a vaginal speculum is only possible under anesthesia. This fact shifts decision making about the volume of surgical interventions and prediction of outcomes to the perioperative period as far as vaginal exams done under anesthesia are concerned. Therefore, it is extremely important to discuss possible treatment options and consequences with the patient prior to surgery.

The principles of VVF surgical repair can be summarized in three points: (1) excision of all scar tissues; (2) splitting of the vaginal and bladder layers; and (3) closure of the fistula without overlapping of the suture lines. These principles are not fully applicable for radiation-induced fistulae management: the area of the vaginal and bladder walls surrounding the fistula is always scarred due to radiation and excision of the fibrotic tissues, and would result in large defects on the area of fistula. When this is the case, Latzko colpocleisis should be applied. Another justification for the Latzko technique is the risk of damaging the ureters during preparation of the scarred bladder wall during manipulations on the bladder wall in the first stage of fistula repair.

A circumferential incision is made around the fistula to separate and mobilize the bladder and vaginal walls. Extensive excision of the fistula tissue in these patients should be avoided, as this may lead to lack of tissue. We do not advise catheterization of the ureters prior to or during surgery as a routine procedure. However, whenever a large mobilization of the bladder wall is required for repair of fistulae, it might be safer to insert ureteral catheters during the operation and to remove them as soon as possible afterwards. In some cases, when the ureteral orifices are localized on the edges of a fistula, and there is a risk of ureteral obstruction through postoperative edema of the surrounding tissues, JJ ureteral stents are applicable. Once the bladder wall is mobilized, sutures are placed on it, preferably in a transverse fashion. Once the first line of sutures is completed, evaluation of the bladder wall with a metallic female catheter allows the surgeon to see the small defects, if any, in the suture line, which must be closed properly in a watertight manner. A second suture line is placed using perivesical tissue. The second layer must cover the first layer as completely as possible. In fact, this is not always possible due to surrounding fibrotic changes. Interpositional tissue should be considered whenever the closure lines or vaginal tissues are of questionable quality.

Fig. 57.1 shows a urethrovaginal fistula before (a) and after (b) management.

57.4.1 Flap Techniques

Different flap techniques are used for genitourinary fistula closure. Flisser and Blaivas advocate single-stage vaginal flap reconstruction with a Martius flap and concomitant pubovaginal sling [30]. Fall describes vaginal wall flap repair in 30 patients who often underwent multiple procedures, including 91% who ultimately achieved successful repair, and 70% who were continent [31]. Candiani et al describe a case of recurrent fistula closed by using a bulbocavernous musculocutaneous flap [32]. Patil and colleagues reported satisfactory surgical results by interposition of viable gracilis muscle and labial fibrofatty tissue at the repair site. The authors used a modified Ingelman–Sundberg procedure [33]. However, this random number of case reports does not allow for systematic review or discussion of the technique. The same is true for the rectus abdominis muscle flap procedure [34]. This technique has been described for refractory fistulae after failed repair with the Martius flap procedure.

Park et al have shown promising results using buccal mucosa grafts for reconstructing difficult urethral female problems. Potentially, buccal mucosa may be successfully used for the closure of extensive urethral damage. These data need to be confirmed in a larger sample group.

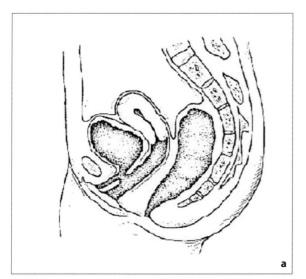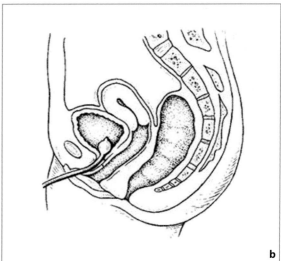

Fig. 57.1 Principles of fistula repair: **a** before and **b** after surgery

The surgeon needs to remember that this area of reconstructive surgery is not only anatomical, but also functional [35].

57.4.1.1 Martius Flap Technique

The surgical technique of labial flap harvesting was described by Martius in 1928 [36]. The procedure starts with a lateral incision on the labia majora pudenda (Fig. 57.2a). The side from which the flap is taken depends on the fistula location. When choosing the side, the shortest distance to the covering area has to be considered because of less tension, a better blood supply for the flap, and better recovery with less recurrence. When a longitudinal incision on the labia majora is done, well-vascularized labial fat is exposed (Fig. 57.2b). Mobilization of the graft should be done taking into consideration the pudendal or epigastric blood supply. From its ventral aspect, the

fat graft is supplied by epigastric vessels, and, if the base of the flap is dorsal, the circulation is furnished by the pudendal basin [37]. These features make the Martius flap a flexible tool for fistula management. After mobilization, the flap is tunneled by a curve clamp under the vaginal wall, from the labia to the vaginal incision (Fig. 57.2c). We use absorbable sutures for fixing the flap over the fistula repair site. Normally the labial flap has excellent mobility and significant bulk effect.

This bulk effect is often quite necessary, but should be considered before flap harvesting. Excessive bulking may provoke problems with the anterior vaginal wall closure. This is why the vaginal wall should be mobilized enough in order to cover the flap without tension. The incision over the labia majora pudenda is sutured (Fig. 57.2d). The final step of the procedure is vaginal wall closure. Any absorbable 3.0 synthetic suture may be used. A Foley

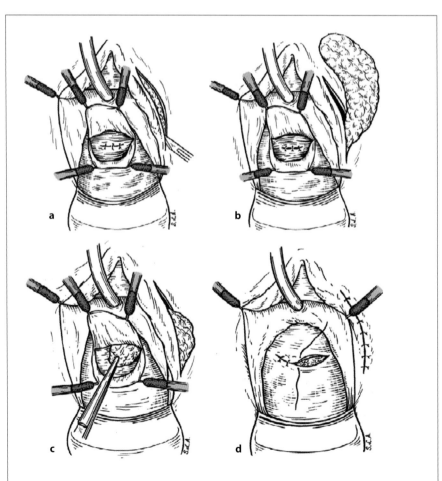

Fig. 57.2 Martius flap technique. **a** A longitudinal incision is made on the labia majora pudenda. **b** Vascularized labial fatty flap is mobilized. **c** The flap is tunneled under the vaginal wall from the labia to the vaginal incision. **d** The vaginal wall is closed over the flap

catheter stays in place for an average of two weeks. All patients receive broad-spectrum antibiotics for one week. They may be discharged from hospital on the second day postoperatively.

57.4.1.2 Latzko Colpocleisis

The Laztko technique, described in 1942 [38], is the treatment of choice for the patient suffering from small radiation-induced VVF with significant trophic disturbances of the vaginal and bladder wall, which do not allow the surgeon to perform traditional splitting repair. Excision of the vaginal epithelium around the fistula site in an oval manner is the first step of the surgery (Fig. 57.3a). It should be emphasized that only vaginal mucosa is excised without going deeper to the bladder wall. This maneuver allows the prevention of any ureteral or bladder trigone injuries during the operation. In some cases, additional incisions on the lateral parts of the oval wound are needed for making the reattached surfaces of the vaginal wall larger. The second stage of the procedure includes closure of the fistula with several layers of absorbable sutures (Vicril 3.0).

The sutures pass through the anterior and posterior vaginal walls, obliterating the upper vagina (Fig. 57.3b and c). Due to the fact that the bladder is not involved in the surgery, ureteral reimplantation should not be required, even if the ureteral orifices are localized on the edges of the fistula while no damage to the upper urinary tract is present.

The Latzko procedure may be classified as upper colpocleisis; therefore, vaginal depth and sexual functions are not significantly compromised by the procedure [39]. In the case of a large fistula, or if there has been significant injury to adjacent areas, additional tissue flaps may be necessary to achieve a proper repair.

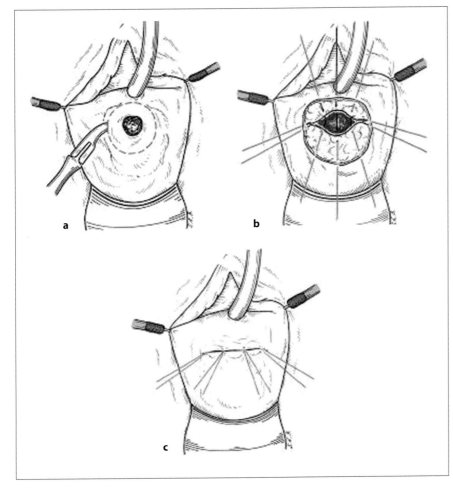

Fig. 57.3 Latzko procedure. **a** Excision of the vaginal epithelium around the fistula is made. **b** Sutures pass through the anterior and posterior vaginal walls. **c** The fistula is closed by upper colpocleisis

57.5 Principles of Urethrovaginal Fistula Repair

Before describing specific surgical treatment methods, we would like to note that treatment procedures are constantly evolving. Therefore we will place special emphasis on the latest technical modifications.

Direct primary anatomical repair may be advised for the patient with minimal anatomical disruption. Flisser and Blaivas have successfully closed 15 urethrovaginal fistulae using this technique [30]. The technique calls for careful vaginal examination immediately prior to the procedure, when the patient is already anesthetized, in order to exclude multiple fistulae. Flisser and Blaivas emphasize the crucial importance of wide mobilization of the urethral wall in order to provide tension-free closure, preferably with two layers of absorbable sutures. Some authors have recently recommended minimizing scar formation postoperatively and facilitating subsequent sling placement if necessary by creating a full-thickness flap from the proximal urethra, or even the bladder, and bringing it in to avoid any tissue tension [7]. During suture placement, the urethral mucosa should be avoided. Non-interrupted sutures with fine monofilament absorbable may be used. Once the first line of sutures is completed, evaluation of the urethra with a metallic urethral sound in place allows the surgeon to see small defects in the suture line, which must also be closed. A second suture line with the same suture material must then be placed using periurethral and perivaginal tissues to provide watertight closure. It should be emphasized that one suture layer is not enough to secure the urethral wall properly; two layers are required to avoid fistula recurrence. The second layer can be either continuous or interrupted sutures, but must cover the first layer as completely as possible. Before final vaginal mucosa closure, careful examination of the suture line with a fine urethral probe should be attempted to detect unsutured places [17, 40–44].

After such a repair, about 50% of patients develop stress urinary incontinence symptoms requiring anti-incontinence procedures. If the full-thickness urethral wall has been used with no tissue tension for fistula closure, tension-free synthetic tape may be considered as an anti-stress procedure for selected patients [17].

Recently, many efforts have been made in the direction of reconstructive urology. Primarily this has affected issues such as tissue engineering, organ regeneration, and graft fabrics. Atala started elegant work on tissue engineering with a cell culture in order to create a urethral tube [45]. Unfortunately, it is too early to fully assess the clinical data. Preliminary findings on fabrication of a urethral graft using reinforced collagen-sponge tubes shows that urethral tissue regeneration depends not only on the biomaterial composition, but also on the fabrication technique [46]. Guan et al state that human vascular endothelial growth factor may be a suitable approach to increase the blood supply in tissue engineering for treatment of urethral damage [47]. Only a limited number of papers on uterovaginal fistula repair are available. The vaginal approach is used in almost all cases [21]. We consider that the use of flaps has a limited role in most cases of uterovaginal fistula. Development of tissue engineering leads to application of the achievements of science in current practice. In our opinion, allograft or autograft cell insertion may be possible in the future for small and narrow fistulae, whereas larger ones might be managed surgically. The role of buccal mucosa autografts is limited to urethral reconstruction, and the possibility of using that in uterovaginal fistula management is not yet evident [35]. In our series, the success rate of fistula repair was 90.14% after one operation and 98.59% after recurrent fistula repair [48].

References

1. Zacharin R. Obstetric fistula. Springer-Verlag, Wien, 1988.
2. Hilton P. Fistulae. In: Shaw R, Souter W, Stanton S (eds) Gynecology, 2 edn. Livingstone, London, 1997, pp 779–801.
3. Lee R, Symmonds R, Williams T. Current status of genitourinary fistula. Obstet Gynecol 1988;71:313–319.
4. Zimmern PE, Handley HR, Leach GE et al. Transvaginal closure of the bladder neck and placement of suprapubic catheter for destroid urethra after long-term indwelling catheter. J Urol 1985;134:554.
5. Atan A, Tuncel A, Aslan Y. Treatment of refractory urethrovaginal fistula using rectus abdominis muscle flap in a six-year-old girl. Urology 2007;69:e11–e384.
6. Liu B, Huang X, Lu J et al. Vaginal calculi secondary to urethrovaginal fistula with vaginal stenosis in a 14-year-old girl. Urol Res 2008;36:73–75.
7. Hoshiyama F, Fujimoto K, Matsushita C et al. Operative position suitable for transvaginal excision of urethral diverticulum or closure of urethrovaginal fistula. Nippon Hinyokika Gakkai Zasshi 2006;97:757–760.
8. Radopoulos DK, Dimitriadis GP, Vakalopoulos IK et al. Our experience with salvage genitourinary fistulae repair: technique and outcomes. Int Urol Nephrol 2009;40:57–63.

9. Rafique M. Genitourinary fistulae of obstetric origin. Int Urol Nephrol 2002;34:489–493.

10. Akman RY, Sargin S, Oezdemir G et al. Vesicovaginal and ureterovaginal fistulas: a review of 39 cases. Int Urol Nephrol 1999;31:321–326.

11. De Ridder D. Vesicovaginal fistula: a major healthcare problem. Curr Opin Urol 2009;19:358–361.

12. Hilton P. Vesico-vaginal fistulas in developing countries. Int J Gynaecol Obstet 2003;82:285–295.

13. Roenneburg ML, Wheeless CR Jr. Traumatic absence of the proximal urethra. Am J Obstet Gynecol 2005; 193:2169–2172.

14. Lawrentschuk N, Koulouris G, Bolton DM. Delineating the anatomy of oncologic postradiation vesico-vaginal fistulae with reconstructed computed tomography. Int Urogynecol J Pelvic Floor Dysfunct 2007;18:955–957.

15. Pushkar D, Dyakov V, Kasyan G. Management of radiation induced vesicovaginal fistula. Eur Urol 2008; 30 April epub ahead of print.

16. Leach GE. Urethrovaginal fistula repair with Martius labial fat pad graft. Urol Clin North Am 1991;18:409–413.

17. Pushkar DY, Dyakov VV, Kosko JW, Kasyan GR. Management of urethrovaginal fistulae. Eur Urol 2006; 50:1000–1005.

18. Biswas A, Bal R, Alauddin M. Genital fistula – our experience. J Indian Med Assoc 2007;105:123–126.

19. Roenneburg ML, Genadry R, Wheeless CR Jr. Repair and outcome of the patient with multiple lower urinary tract fistulae. Annual Meeting of International Continence Society; 28 August to 2 September 2005, Montreal. Abstract 7.

20. Flisser AJ, Blaivas JG. Outcome of urethral reconstructive surgery in a series of 74 women. J Urol 2003; 169:2246–2249.

21. Ahmad S, Nishtar A, Hafeez GA, Khan Z. Management of vesico-vaginal fistulae in women. Int J Gynecol Obstetr 2005;88:71–75.

22. Arrowsmith SD. Genitourinary reconstruction in obstetric fistulae. J Urol 1994;152:403–406.

23. Reisenauer C, Wallwiener D, Stenzl A et al. Urethrovaginal fistula: a rare complication after the placement of a suburethral sling (IVS). Int Urogynecol J 2007; 18:343–346.

24. Kobashi KC, Dmochowski R, Mee SL et al. Erosion of woven polyester pubovaginal sling. J Urol 1999; 162:2070–2072.

25. Glavind K, Larsen EH. Results and complications of tension-free vaginal tape (TVT) for surgical treatment of female stress urinary incontinence. Int Urogynecol J 2001;12:370–372.

26. Golomb J, Leibovitch I, Mor Y et al. Fascial path technique for repair of complicated urethrovaginal fistula. Urology 2006;68:1115–1118.

27. Lowman J, Moore RD, Miklos JR. Tension-free vaginal tape sling with a porcine interposition graft in an irradiated patient with a past history of a urethrovaginal fistula and urethral mesh erosion: a case report. J Reprod Med 2007;52:560–562.

28. Chassagne S, Zimmern P. Transvaginal closure of the bladder neck in women with a neurogenic bladder and destroyed urethra. Prog Urol 1997;7:286–292.

29. Pantaleo-Gandais M, Osorio D. Reconstruction of the urinary tract after radiation fistulae. Prog Clin Biol Res 1991;370:151–155.

30. Flisser AJ, Blaivas JG. Outcome of urethral reconstructive surgery in a series of 74 women. J Urol 2003; 169:2246–2249.

31. Fall M. Vaginal wall bipedicled flap and other techniques in complicated urethral diverticulum and urethrovaginal fistula. J Am Coll Surg 1995;180:150–156.

32. Candiani P, Austoni E, Campiglio GL et al. Repair of a recurrent urethrovaginal fistula with an island bulbocavernous musculocutaneous flap. Plast Reconstr Surg 1993;92:1393–1396.

33. Patil U, Waterhouse K, Laungani G. Management of 18 difficult vesicovaginal and urethrovaginal fistulas with modified Ingelman-Sundberg and Martius operations. J Urol 1980;123:653–656.

34. Bruce RG, El-Galley RE, Galloway NT. Use of rectus abdominis muscle flap for the treatment of complex and refractory urethrovaginal fistulas. J Urol 2000; 163:1212–1215.

35. Park JM, Hendren WH. Construction of female urethra using buccal mucosa graft. J Urol 2001;166:640–643.

36. Martius H. Die operative Wiederherstellung der volkommen fehlenden Harnrehre und des Schiessmuskels derselben. Zentralbl Gynakol 1928;52:480.

37. Hoskins WJ, Park RC, Long R et al. Repair of urinary fistulas with bulbocavernosus myocutaneous flaps. Obstet Gynecol 1984;63:588–91.

38. Latzko W. Postoperative vesicovaginal fistulas: genesis and therapy. Am J Surg 1942;58:211–28.

39. Raz S, Little NA, Juma S. Female urology. In: Walsh PC, Retik AB, Stamey TA (eds) Campbell's urology, 6th edn. WB Saunders, Philadelphia, PA, 1992, pp 2782–2828.

40. Gerber GS, Schoenberg HW. Female urinary tract fistulae. J Urol 1993;149:229–236.

41. Tancer ML. A report of thirty-four instances of urethrovaginal and bladder neck fistulas. Surg Gynecol Obstet 1993;177:77–80.

42. Demirel A, PolatO, Bayraktar Y et al. Transvesical and transvaginal reparation in urinary vaginal fistulas. Int Urol Nephrol 1993;25:439–444.

43. Leng WW, Amundsen CL, McGuire EJ. Management of female genitourinary fistulas: transvesical or transvaginal approach? J Urol 1999;160:1995–1999.

44. Polat O, Gül O, Aksoy Y et al. Iatrogenic injuries to ureter, bladder and urethra during abdominal and pelvic operations. Int Urol Nephrol 1997;29:13–18.

45. Atala A. Tissue engineering, stem cells, and cloning for the regeneration of urologic organs. Clin Plast Surg 2003;30:649–667.

46. Kanatani I, Kanematsu A, Inatsugu Y et al. Fabrication of an optimal urethral graft using collagen-sponge tubes reinforced with copoly (L-lactide/epsiloncaprolactone) fabric. Tissue Eng 2007;13:2933–2940.

47. Guan Y, Ou L, HuG et al. Tissue engineering of urethra using human vascular endothelial growth factor gene-modified bladder urothelial cells. Artif Organs 2008;32:91–99.

48. Pushkar D, Sumerova N, Kasyan G. Management of urethrovaginal fistulae. Curr Opin Urol 2008; 18:389–394.

Rectovaginal Fistulae

58

A. Muti Abulafi and Abdul H. Sultan

Abstract Rectovaginal fistula is a rare condition but with often debilitating symptoms. Surgery is invariably the mainstay treatment with a large number of techniques described. Choice of surgery depends on several factors including the size, location and underlying etiology of the fistula as well as surgeons experience. Multidisciplinary management involving colorectal surgeons, gynecologists and where appropriate gastroenterologists, oncologists and plastic surgeons is key to success.

Keywords Advancement flap • Anovaginal fistula • Rectovaginal fistula • Sphincteroplasty • Vesicovaginal fistula

58.1 Definition

Rectovaginal fistulae (RVF) are abnormal communications between the rectum and vagina. They must be distinguished from ano-vaginal fistulae which are more distal communications between the anal canal and vagina and are considered as a rare type of anorectal fistulae. Fistulae can be either congenital or acquired and this chapter will focus on the management options but also outline the etiology, presentation, diagnosis, and classification of acquired recto- and ano-vaginal fistulae.

58.2 Etiology

Rectovaginal fistulae are rare and account for less than 5% of all ano-rectal fistulae [1, 2]. The causes of recto- and ano-vaginal fistulae are listed in Table 58.1 [1].

A.M. Abulafi
Department of Colorectal Surgery, Mayday University Hospital, Croydon, Surrey, UK

The most common cause of RVF is obstetric trauma, which represents between 50% and 90% of RVF presenting clinically, and occurs in 0.1% of all vaginal deliveries [2]. However, the incidence of RVF in women who sustain a fourth-degree tear is higher and ranges between 0.4% and 3% [3]. In the developing world, it is most frequently related to prolonged obstructive labor due to feto-maternal disproportion and failure of timely intervention. Consequently, tissue ischemia and necrosis lead to the development of a fistula. In case series of patients presenting with vesicovaginal fistulae, between 6% and 24% had concurrent RVF [3, 4]. Other obstetric causes relate to an unidentified fourth-degree obstetric tear at delivery, inadvertent insertion of a rectovaginal suture during repair of perineal trauma, and severe perineal infection, particularly following a repair of a third- or fourth-degree perineal tear. The problem may manifest immediately after delivery due to failed recognition of a fourth-degree tear or inappropriate repair, or more commonly after 7–14 days due to secondary infection of the wound.

The second commonest cause of RVF is Crohn's disease, occurring in up to 23% of patients [5], a figure

Table 58.1 Etiology of rectovaginal fistula, adapted from [1]

Category	Condition	Mechanism
1. Traumatic		
- Obstetric	Obstructed labor	Pressure necrosis of rectovaginal septum
	Midline episiotomy	Extension directed into rectum
	Third/fourth-degree lacerations	Unrecognized RVF or breakdown of repair
- Foreign body	Vaginal pessaries	Pressure necrosis
	Violent coitus	Mechanical perforation
	Sexual abuse	Mechanical perforation
- Iatrogenic	Hysterectomy	Injury to anterior rectal wall
	Stapled colorectal anastomosis	Staple line includes vagina
	Transanal excision of anterior rectal tumor	Deep margin of resection into vagina
	Enemas	Mechanical perforation
	Ano-rectal surgery such as incision and drainage of intramural abscesses	Mechanical perforation
2. Inflammatory	Crohn's disease	Transmural inflammation-perforation
	Pelvic radiation	Early-tumor necrosis
	Pelvic abscess	Late transmural inflammation
	Perirectal abscess	
	Bartholin's abscess	
3. Neoplastic	Rectal tumor	Local tumor growth into neighboring structure
	Cervical tumor	
	Uterine tumor	
	Vaginal tumor	
	Primary or recurrent tumors	
4. Miscellaneous	Fecal impaction	Pressure necrosis/erosion into vagina

that varies depending on the referral pattern of the institution. The problem seems to occur more frequently with large bowel involvement, especially the rectum [6]. Ulcerative colitis is a mucosal disease that rarely causes fistulation unless as a complication of surgery rather than the disease itself, or if it is complicated by tumor. Recurrent RVF following surgery should raise the possibility of underlying occult Crohn's disease, which must be excluded in this situation.

Trauma to the rectum, perineum, or vagina may cause RVF. The commonest form of trauma is during or following surgery, although blunt or penetrating trauma to the perineum or use of a foreign body in the vagina or rectum, are well-recognized causes [7–9]. The use of surgical stapling devices during construction of ileo-anal pouches [10–11], low anterior resections [12], stapled hemorrhoidectomy and stapled transanal rectal resections (STARR) [13] have been implicated. In addition, vaginal or transanal rectocele repair (particularly with the use of mesh) [14, 15],

transanal excision of rectal tumours [16], and vaginal hysterectomy [17] can potentially cause RVF.

Tumours of the perineum, vagina, and ano-rectum may infiltrate and erode the nearby organs and cause fistula formation. In addition, perianal cryptoglandular infection, particularly abscesses and fistulae situated anteriorly, may erode into the vagina to cause an ano-vaginal fistula. Similarly, Bartholin's abscess [18], particularly those extending posteriorly on the perineum or rectovaginal septum, can cause a fistula. The use of bevacizumab (Avastin®) has also been implicated [19].

Finally, one of the most challenging fistulae to treat is radiation-induced fistulae, which usually occur a few years after completing the treatment [20–24]. Thankfully, the incidence has reduced recently with advances in radiotherapy delivery. Radiation therapy of tumors of the cervix, anus, and rectum, particularly those that are locally advanced, have all been implicated. In these situations, one of the first priorities in management is to rule out recurrent disease.

Table 58.2 Classification of rectovaginal fistulae, modified from [27]

Simple rectovaginal fistula	Complex rectovaginal fistula
Low or mid vagina (check rectum) ≤ 2.5cm	High vagina > 2.5cm
Traumatic or infectious cause	Inflammatory bowel disease, irradiation, neoplastic causes, prolonged obstructed labor Failed prior repair

58.3 Classification

There are several classifications reported in the literature, which reflects a lack of unanimity about how best to describe the condition. The two most commonly used classifications are based on the etiology and location of the fistula.

RVF classified according to location is as follows:

- anovaginal – the anal opening of the fistula is situated at or below the dentate line and the fistula tract opens at the posterior fourchette or lower third of the vagina
- rectovaginal – this is further divided into two types, a low and a high fistula. A low RVF is located between the lower third of the rectum and the lower half of the vagina. A high fistula is located between the middle or upper third of the rectum and the posterior vaginal fornix.

RVF classified according to their cause is as follows:

- type I – RVF with or without anal sphincter disruption
- type II – RVF due to inflammatory bowel disease
- type III – RVF due to radiation injury
- type IV – RVF due to postoperative injury.

Obstetric trauma is the most common cause for RVF type I, with an incidence of up to 74% [25]. The incidence of RVF type 4 following previous surgical procedures is reported at 7% of all fistulae [25].

Both classifications are of relevance when planning treatment, and some authors argue for use of one over the other [26]. We would advise that both etiology and location are used when planning treatment; the etiology takes into account the status of the local and adjoining tissues, while the type of surgical approach will depend on the location of the fistula. A convenient classification which takes account of both was proposed by Rothenberger and Goldberg [27] (Table 58.2). They grouped RVF into two categories: simple and complex. Simple fistulae include those that are in a low or mid zone location, are of traumatic or infective nature, and are of < 2.5 cm in diameter. Complex fistulae are high fistulae due to Crohn's disease, pelvic irradiation, or tumours, and are > 2.5 cm in diameter.

58.4 Presentation

Typically, the presenting symptoms of RVF are those of constant passage of liquid stool, foul-smelling brown discharge, or flatus per vagina. This is in contrast with ano-vaginal fistulae when the above symptoms occur only during or shortly after defecation. In addition, patients may complain of discomfort in the pelvis/perineum and during sexual intercourse. Other modes of presentation include recurrent attacks of urinary tract infection, thrush, perineal and vulval irritation, and difficulty keeping the area clean. In addition, patients may also present with other symptoms relating to the underlying etiology of the fistula. For instance, patients with Crohn's disease may present with abdominal pain, diarrhea, and rectal bleeding. Patients with ano-rectal cancers may present with rectal bleeding and change in bowel habit. Radiation proctitis patients may present with rectal bleeding, diarrhea, and pelvic pain.

58.5 Assessment and Investigations

The aim of assessment is to determine the location and etiology of RVF, classify them into simple or complex, and hence determine the mode of surgical intervention. In our opinion this should be undertaken jointly by both a colorectal and gynecological specialist, as is the case in our practice [28]. Clinical assessment starts by taking a careful history, noting the severity of symptoms, previous operations on the ano-rectum and vagina, mode of vaginal delivery, and whether the patient has had pelvic irradiation or is known to have had inflammatory bowel disease. Assessment should also take note of the degree of continence to both urine [29] and stools [30], and take account of any associated comorbidities that could influence management. The degree of symptom interference with daily life is best determined by quality-of-life questionnaires [31]. For instance, patients may have significant comorbidities but minor symptoms that are not interfering with their lifestyle, as is the case with some ano-vaginal fistulae, and therefore the consequences of surgical intervention need to be weighed against potential risks. It is also important to include assessment of prior sexual function, especially dyspareunia, and remember to counsel women who are considering surgery about risks of de novo dyspareunia.

Clinical examination includes careful inspection of the perineum and perianal area for skin rash/excoriation due to constant soiling of liquid stools. Scars from previous ano-rectal surgery, episiotomy, or perineal tears should be noted. Perianal dimpling and/or a "dovetail sign", which consists of perianal folds posterior to the anal opening with smooth mucosa anteriorly, may indicate a disrupted anal sphincter as well as the presence of a fistula [3]. An external opening of the fistula may be seen at the vaginal introitus/fourchette. The anus should be examined to determine the status of anal sphincter function by checking the resting and squeeze pressures. When an ano-vaginal fistula is present, a defect within the anal canal may be felt at this point, whereas in low RVF a defect or thinning may be felt in the lower rectum. Bimanual palpation of the perineum and anal sphincter anteriorly may indicate disruption to the anal sphincter and/or perineal body. In addition, any induration, stenosis, or strictures within the anal canal, rectum, or vagina should be noted. These are usually confirmed on rigid proctosigmoidoscopy or flexible sigmoidoscopy and vaginal speculum examination. Often, examination in the clinic is uncomfortable, making adequate assessment impossible, and in these situations an examination under anesthetic is extremely useful. On rare occasions, the fistula is very fine (pinhole), and therefore may not be easily detected even during examination under anesthetic. Various techniques have been devised to delineate it, including instillation of diluted hydrogen peroxide or mildly soapy water into the rectum and observing bubbles on the vaginal side.

The methylene blue pad test involves injecting dye into the rectum via a Foley catheter and inserting a tampon in the vagina, which is usually stained within 30 minutes if a fistula is present.

Complex RVF invariably require further investigations, not only to confirm the diagnosis but also to help determine the underlying pathology. Contrast studies of either the rectum or vagina [32] are useful in high RVF: computed tomography (CT) with rectal contrast, endoanal ultrasound scan with or without contrast enhancement with hydrogen peroxide [33, 34], or MRI scan with or without endocoil [35].

We would strongly advocate the routine use of endoanal ultrasound scan in these patients not only to delineate the fistula if possible but, more importantly, to identify any associated anal sphincter defects that would influence management. If the diagnosis remains unclear, or if there is discrepancy between imaging and clinical findings, an endoanal/endovaginal/perineal scan can be performed during the examination under anesthesia. Ultrasonographic imaging techniques have already been described in Sections II and VI.

58.6   Treatment

In a few situations, where symptoms are mild and not interfering with lifestyle (as is the case in small ano-vaginal fistulae), conservative treatment should be considered, particularly if there are significant associated comorbidities. In fistulae associated with active Crohn's disease, initial management involves medical treatment aimed at stabilizing the inflammation [36]. The vast majority of patients with RVF have significant and disabling symptoms, and therefore surgical repair is the mainstay treatment. The success of surgical treatment depends on adhering to the known and accepted principles of good surgery, namely accurate diagnosis, choice of appropriate operation, and meticulous surgical technique. The later includes excision of diseased and fibrous tissue, avoiding tension on the suture line, achieving good hemostasis, and ensuring adequate blood supply, if necessary by interposing vascularized tissues.

58.6.1 Surgical Techniques

There are a large number of operations described, reflecting the many combinations of RVF presentations, which depend on the location and diameter of the fistula and the underlying disease process. The operations can be grouped into three main categories, depending on the surgical approach, as shown in Table 58.3.

The patient must be counseled about the benefits, potential risks, and success rates of the proposed surgery. Functional outcomes including sexual function should also be discussed. In abdominal operations, the potential need for a stoma needs to be discussed and agreed.

In general, there has been a recent move away from using mechanical bowel preparation prior to bowel surgery, except where an ultra-low colorectal anastomosis is contemplated. Instead, the rectum is prepared with suppositories or enemas a few hours prior to the surgery, to help exposure and ensure an uncontaminated operative field. Antibiotic prophylaxis is given at induction of anesthesia and continued for 48 h. Deep vein thrombosis (DVT) prophylaxis with low molecular weight heparin is continued until discharge from hospital. The patient is placed either in modified lithotomy, Lloyd Davis or prone jack-knife position, depending on the type of surgery. The abdomen is prepared with alcohol- or water-based antiseptic solution, while the rectal and vaginal lumen are cleansed with water-based antiseptic solution. A Foley catheter is inserted in abdominal operations. For local repair, the area is infiltrated with 1:300,000 adrenalin solution, which will not only reduce the amount of bleeding but facilitate dissection in natural planes.

A stoma is raised either as the first step in treating the fistula or during definitive surgical treatment to cover the surgical repair/anastomosis. The indications for either will be discussed below for each surgical technique.

On discharge, the patients are prescribed bulking agents and fecal softeners to reduce the impact of stool trauma on the repair. Patients should refrain from strenuous physical exercise but continue with gentle exercises. Sexual intercourse and use of tampons should be avoided for 6 weeks after repair.

58.6.1.1 Endorectal Advancement Flap

This technique is most suited for a simple low fistula with the opening above the dentate line. The patient is placed in the prone jack-knife position and the anal canal exposed by opening the anus with an Eisenhammer or Parks' retractor. The fistula is identified by passing a fistula probe through the vaginal opening into the rectum. An adrenalin solution of 1:300,000 is infiltrated into the submucosa around the fistula and cephalad. A U-shaped incision is made around the fistula, with the

Table 58.3 Surgical approaches for rectovaginal fistulae

1. Local	2. Abdominal	3. Tissue interposition
a. Rectal route	a. Simple closure with interposition of omentum	a. Sphincteroplasty
• transrectal advancement flap		b. Labial pad of fat (Martius graft)
• layered closure		c. Gracilis
• rectal sleeve	b. Anterior resection with colorectal/colo-anal anastomosis	d. Sartorius
• Surgisis™ mesh repair		e. Gluteus maximus
• transanal endoscopic microsurgery		f. Rectus
	c. Proctectomy/abdominoperineal excision of rectum and anus	g. Omentum
b. Vaginal route		h. Colon
• transvaginal advancement flap		i. Bricker's onlay colonic patch
• layered closure	d. Diversion colostomy/ileostomy	
• Surgisis™ mesh repair		
	e. Laparoscopic vs. open	
c. Perineal route		
• perineo-proctotomy		
• sphincteroplasty		
• tissue transposition		

base a few centimeters cephalad of the fistula and at least twice the width of the apex to ensure adequate blood supply. The flap is raised by deepening the incision through the mucosa, submucosa, and superficial layers of the circular muscle. Usually, raising the flap is easy and should start laterally, moving medially towards the fistula where dissection and identification of the tissue planes become difficult due to scar tissue around the fistula opening (Fig. 58.1) [37]. Once the flap is raised, the attenuated rectovaginal septum (site of fistula) is exposed. The lateral edges of the rectal mucosa are dissected off the submucosa and internal sphincter muscle, so that these structures are approximated to the midline, with Vicryl sutures closing the fistula defect without any tension. The flap is then advanced over the repaired area and sutured in place after excising the excess flap distally including the site of fistula. The vaginal mucosa is left open for drainage.

The reports in the literature (Table 58.4) [38–55] show mixed results, with healing rates of 41–100%. It is difficult to know conclusively why such variation in results exists but it is possible that it is related to inclusion of complex, Crohn's, and recurrent fistulae.

MacRae et al [38] reported success rates of 85% after first repair, which fell to 55% after a third failed repair. Jones [39] reported healing rates of 77% for fistulae without Crohn's disease, which fell to 60% for fistulae with Crohn's disease. Moreover, Gagliardi and Pescatori [40] reported that in their hands the incorporation of a sphincteroplasty in the repair routinely resulted in 100% success rates compared to 73% for repairs without sphincteroplasty. However, other authors do not recommend the routine use of sphincteroplasty in the repair unless there is evidence of sphincter disruption, so as not to compromise continence [38, 41].

58.6.1.2 Transvaginal Flap

Transvaginal repairs are performed in the lithotomy position. The principles are as follows (Fig. 58.2).

- Invagination of fistula tract: after infiltration of a dilute solution of adrenalin (epinephrine) in saline (1:300,000), an elliptical incision is performed around the fistula orifice. The vaginal epithelium is elevated circumferentially around the opening and is then mobilized from the underlying recto-

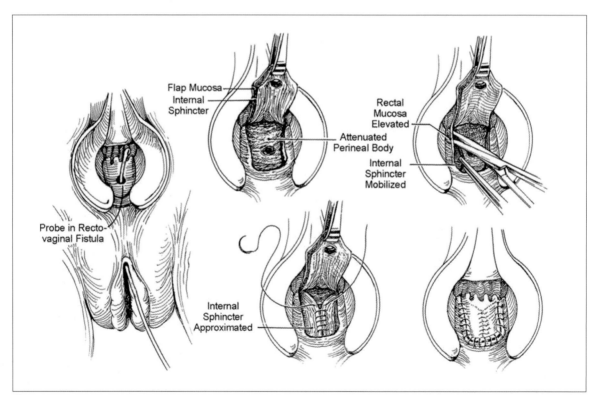

Fig. 58.1 Endorectal advancement flap. Reproduced from [37], with permission

Table 58.4 Summary of surgical outcomes of endorectal advancement flaps in the treatment of RVF

Author	Year	Number of cases	Success rate (%)	Comments
Greenwald and Hoexter [42]	1978	20	100	
Rothenberger et al [41]	1982	35	91	10 with concomitant sphincteroplasty
Hoexter et al [43]	1985	15	100	
Jones et al [39]	1987	23	70	10 patients had Crohn's disease
Lowry et al [25]	1988	81	83	25 with concomitant sphincteroplasty
Wise et al [44]	1991	40	85	15 with concomitant sphincteroplasty
Kodner et al [45]	1993	71	93	
Khanduja et al [46]	1994	16	100	
MacRae et al [38]	1995	28	29	Repair for recurrent fistulae
Mazier et al [47]	1995	19	95	
Watson and Phillips [48]	1995	12	58	
Tsang et al [49]	1998	27	41	
Hyman [50]	1999	12	91	
Joo et al [51]	1998	20	75	Repair for Crohn's fistulae
Baig [52]	2000	19	74	7 concomitant sphincteroplasty
Mizrahi et al [53]	2002	32	56	
Sonoda et al [54]	2002	37	43	
Zimmerman et al [55]	2002	21	48	7 concomitant sphincteroplasty and 12 labial fat
Gagliardi and Pescatori [40]	2007	35	76	10 layered closure and 12 sphincteroplasty

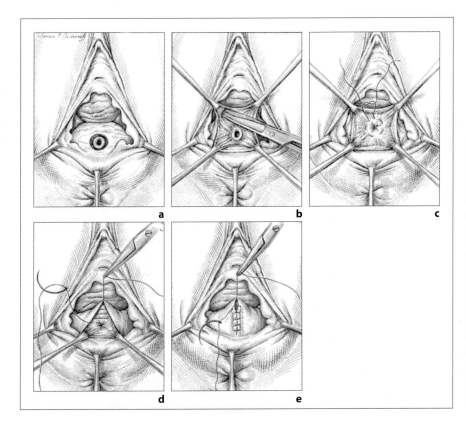

Fig. 58.2 Transvaginal repair of a small rectovaginal fistula. **a** A circular incision is made through the vaginal mucosa around the fistula orifice. **b** The vaginal mucosa is dissected free circumferentially for approximately 2 cm from the margin of the fistula orifice. **c** A pursestring suture is placed around the fistula orifice and tied. **d** The muscularis tissues are approximated with sutures. **e** The vaginal mucosa is closed with a continuous suture. Reproduced from [56], with permission

vaginal fascia for at least 2 cm from the margins of the fistula opening. The opening in the recto-vaginal fascia is then closed by placing a series of purse string sutures (Vicryl 3-0), such that it becomes invaginated into the rectum. A second purse string suture inverts the first. The vaginal epithelium is then closed with a continuous or interrupted sutures. A modification of this technique (the Latzko procedure) is performed for high RVF. Essentially, this technique incorporates both anterior and posterior vaginal walls in the inversion of the fistula into the rectum and closes a portion of the proximal vagina. This technique may therefore not be suitable for a woman who is sexually active.

- Excision of fistula tract: a modification to the above technique is to completely core out the fistula tract and repair the rectal mucosa, the rectovaginal fascia, and vaginal skin in separate layers.
- Vaginal flap: following infiltration with adrenalin solution, a curvilinear U-shaped incision is performed below the fistula opening. The rectovaginal fascial layer is then undermined and mobilized. The margins of the rectal opening are freshened and closed with 3-0 Vicryl sutures. The rectovaginal fascia is then closed as an intervening layer between the rectal and vaginal epithelium. Some surgeons prefer to approximate the levator ani muscles instead, but this can lead to dyspareunia. The fistula is then excised from the vaginal skin flap which is then sutured with interrupted sutures.

58.6.1.3 Excision of Fistula and Layered Closure

A fistula located at or within 1 cm of the dentate line is treated by a modification of the above flap technique as described by Hoexter et al [43], to avoid the potential

of drawing the secreting rectal mucosa into the anal canal and causing the so-called "wet anus". In this situation, the steps are exactly as described above, but a transverse elliptical incision is made around the fistula instead of the U-shaped incision (Fig. 58.3). The fistula tract and a button of vaginal mucosa are excised. The resulting defect is closed with Vicryl in two layers after freeing the lateral edges of the mucosa, as described above, to reduce tension. The rectal mucosal flap is now advanced over the septal repair and sutured. The vaginal mucosa is left open to drain.

58.6.1.4 Rectal Sleeve Advancement Flap

This is a complex operation and should be considered in patients with complex and multiple fistulae, particularly those associated with Crohn's disease. The technique was first described by Berman in 1991 [57] and modified slightly by Marchesa in 1998 [58]. It involves circumferential mobilization of the distal rectum with excision of the diseased rectal mucosa. The patient is positioned in the prone jack-knife position and the anal canal exposed. A circumferential incision is made in normal mucosa, usually below the dentate line, after infiltrating the area with an adrenalin solution of 1:300,000. A full-thickness sleeve flap made of the mucosa and submucosa is then raised to expose the underlying internal sphincter (Fig. 58.4). Invariably, a few fibers of the internal sphincter are included in the raised flap due to associated inflammation from the fistula and Crohn's disease. The submucosal plane is entered and then developed in a cephalad direction circumferentially, passing the ano-rectal ring and levator ani muscle. Further dissection in this plane at the supralevator space, will allow the full thickness of rectum to be mobilized. This is continued if necessary to

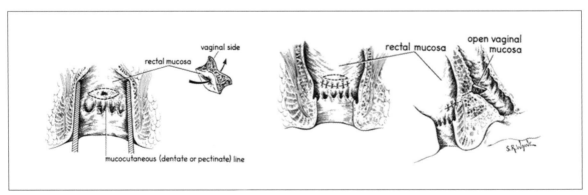

Fig. 58.3 Excision of fistula with layered closure. Schematic drawing of repair. Reproduced from [43], with permission

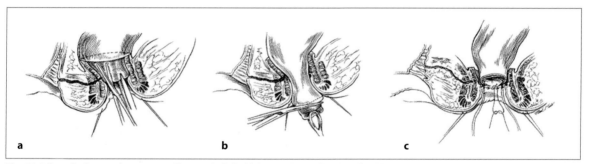

Fig. 58.4 Rectal sleeve advancement flap. **a.** A full-thickness sleeve flap is raised in a cephalad direction resulting in exposed denuded fibers of internal sphincter; dissection is carried into the supralevator space until sufficient mobility is obtained. **b.** After the internal opening of the fistula tract has been cored out and closed, the distal cylinder of diseased tissue is trimmed form the flap. The edge of the flap can then be sutured to the neodentate line. **c.** The distal edge of the flap is sutured to the ridge of the new dentate line using interrupted 3/0 polyglactin sutures. A reinforcing layer of continuous 3/0 polyglactin suture is then add (not shown in this figure). Reproduced from [58] with permission

the level of the peritoneal reflection until healthy rectal tissue can be pulled downward to reach the dentate line without tension. The diseased rectal mucosa is excised, and before suturing the normal rectal mucosa to the dentate line with Vicryl sutures, the underlying fistula tract is excised/cored out and the anal opening is closed (as described earlier for the endorectal advancement flap), leaving the vaginal end open for drainage. It may be necessary to cover the repair with a stoma, especially in patients with Crohn's disease. Reports in the literature describe healing rates of 54–87%, with follow-up longer than two years in one study [51].

58.6.1.5 Episio/perineoproctotomy

This technique is ideally suited for fistulae with associated sphincter disruption, absent perineal body (cloacal defects), or recurrent or failed local (transanal or transvaginal) repair. The principle of the operation consists of identifying the fistula and laying it fully open, followed by layered closure of the divided tissues. The patient is positioned in the lithotomy position, which offers good exposure of both the anus and vagina. The fistula is identified by inserting a fistula probe via the anal canal opening and into the vagina. The tissues superficial to this are then divided fully, thus, in effect, creating a wound similar to that encountered by obstetricians in a fourth-degree perineal tear (Fig. 58.5). The edges of the primary tract are excised and any associated secondary tracts, if present, are identified and excised. The rectal and vaginal mucosa are then freed from the underlying tissues. The edges of the internal and external anal sphincter as

well as the perineal muscles are all identified and mobilized laterally.

The operation is concluded by approximating the rectal mucosa with Vicryl sutures, followed by approximating the internal sphincter to create a high-pressure zone within the anal canal. The external sphincter is then repaired using the overlap technique. Next, the perineum is reconstituted by approximating the perineal muscles and the vaginal mucosa. The final step is to close the perineal skin from the vagina down to the anus.

Reported success rates are good, ranging from 68% to 100% [38, 47, 59]. Exposure is generally excellent with this approach, and it should be considered the first-line approach for those fistulae with associated sphincter/cloacal defects. It should also be considered in patients who have undergone previous failed repairs where exposure via the transanal route may be limited.

58.6.1.6 Tissue Interposition

The principle of this repair is to excise the fistula and interpose healthy vascularized tissue in the space between the rectum and vagina. The surgical approach is performed either through the perineum or the abdomen.

Approaching the fistula via the perineum, the patient is usually in the jack-knife prone position and the perineum is infiltrated with 1:300,000 adrenalin solution. A transverse incision is made on the perineum close to the fourchette. The incision is deepened, and dissection is carried out in the plane between the rectum and vagina, taking particular care to avoid making a button hole in either structure. The fistula is gently separated, and dissection is carried out in this plane cephalad. The rectal and vaginal openings of the fistula are then closed with Vicryl sutures. The chosen tissue is then interposed between the sutured vaginal and rectal defects. The skin is then closed. The most common tissue interposed is an overlapping sphincteroplasty [25, 40, 41, 44, 52, 55], similar to that described above and in Chapter 28. This technique is utilized particularly when there is associated sphincter disruption. In the presence of an intact anal sphincter, this technique of dividing and then performing an overlapping sphincteroplasty should be avoided due to the effect on continence. Other tissues that have been interposed include the gracilis [60], sartorius [61], and rectus abdominis [62] muscles, and labial pad of fat (Martius graft) [63, 64]. If Martius graft is used the patient is positioned in the modified lithotomy position (Fig. 58.6) [65].

Approaching the fistula via the abdomen (see also below), the healthy colon is interposed by undertaking an anterior resection with removal of the diseased rectum beyond the fistula. The vaginal opening is closed and the healthy colon is brought down and anastomosed with the healthy lower rectum directly (an end-to-end or end-to-side colorectal anastomosis or via

construction of a colonic J pouch), or with the anal canal if the whole rectum is removed (coloanal anastomosis or via a colonic J pouch or via the Parks' coloanal anastomosis [38, 66, 67]. The omentum is another structure usually interposed in the space between the rectum and vagina. Bricker reported a technique where the sigmoid colon and rectum is mobilized fully with division of the fistula. The sigmoid is then transected at the midpoint and the distal end folded on itself, and anastomosed to the debrided rectal opening of the fistula.

The proximal end of the transected sigmoid is brought out as a colostomy. Once healing is confirmed by a contrast study, the colostomy end is attached to the folded sigmoid loop as an end-to-side anastomosis [68, 69].

58.6.1.7 Use of Biomaterials

Surgisis™ Mesh Repair
This is a novel technique reported initially by Pye and colleagues in 2004 [70] and more recently modified by Schwandner et al [71]. The technique involves exploring the fistula via a combined transvaginal and transrectal approach. With the patient in lithotomy position, the posterior vaginal wall is opened and the fistula tract identified with a fistula probe. The vagina

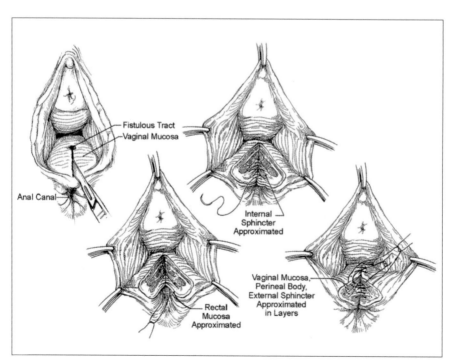

Fig. 58.5 Perineoproctectomy (see text). Reproduced from [37], with permission

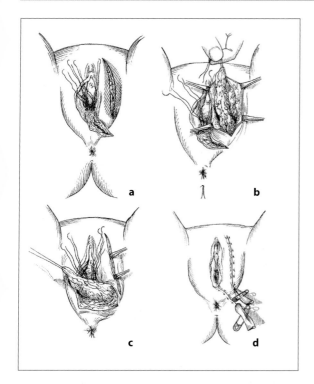

Fig. 58.6 Martius graft. **a** Rectal wall full-thickness closure of the fistula. A skin incision is made over the labia majora and skin flaps developed (hatched area) to expose labial pad of fat. **b** The labial pad of fat is mobilised and developed. **c** The flap is pulled through a subcutaneous tunnel into the fistula wound and placed over the sutured rectal defect. **d** The vaginal, vulvar and episiotomy defects are approximated and drained. Reproduced from [65], with permission

is then dissected off the rectum within the rectovaginal space, approximately 1 cm proximal and distal to the fistula tract. The fistula tract is then completely excised via a combined transvaginal and transrectal approach including a complete "coring-out" of the fistula tissue. The rectal component of the operation consists of an advancement flap repair using PDS 2-0 (muscle layer) and Vicryl 3-0 (rectal mucosa and submucosa) sutures. After completion of the transrectal advancement flap repair, the rectovaginal space is irrigated with antiseptic solution and then a 2 × 2 cm Surgisis™ mesh is placed in the rectovaginal space and fixed with Vicryl 3-0 at each corner. Finally, the posterior vaginal mucosa is closed over the mesh with interrupted Vicryl 3-0 sutures. In the study by Schwandner and colleagues [71], 19 out 21 patients with RVF, most of whom had recurrent fistulae, remained healed at a median period of 12 months; four of those patients healed after a second operation. In another study by Ellis [72], 22 out of 27 patients, half of whom had recurrent fistulae, remained healed at a median period of 12 months (range 6–26 months).

Surgisis™ Fistula Plug

Ellis [72] analyzed seven patients treated with this technique, with a median follow-up of 6 months (range 3–12 months). Six out of seven healed (86%). O'Connor

et al [73] used the fistula plug in two patients with low rectovaginal fistula, although the authors do not elaborate on the outcome in this group specifically. In any case, a large clinical trial with longer follow-up is required before this procedure can be recommended as a standard approach.

58.6.1.8 Abdominal Operations

These operations are indicated for high fistulae and in the case of post-irradiation fistulae, even if the fistula is of the low type, since healthy tissues should be employed to achieve a successful repair.

Direct Closure with Interposed Omental Graft

This operation is undertaken in the case of a simple high fistula due to benign and traumatic causes, particularly those occurring following surgery. The operation involves full mobilization of the rectum posteriorly and anteriorly. In the anterior plane, the rectovaginal plane is entered and the vagina separated from the rectum. At this point, the fistula is encountered, entered, and then divided. The fistula edges are refreshed and then both the rectal and vaginal defects are closed primarily with interrupted Vicryl sutures. The repair is supported by interposing omentum in the intervening space, thus separating the suture lines.

In this operation, the rectum is healthy and is not excised.

Rectal Excision (Anterior Resection) with Colorectal/Colo-anal Anastomosis

This operation is performed in complex high fistulae where the rectal tissue is involved by a pathological process such as cancer, Crohn's disease, or radiation-induced fibrosis. When performing the anterior resection, the dissection is carried out beyond the pathology and fistula until healthy tissues are exposed. This may require removal of only the upper and middle third of the rectum but may also require removal of the whole of the rectum (low anterior resection). Reconstruction is achieved by performing an anastomosis, either stapled or sutured between the descending colon, which is mobilized and brought down into the pelvis without tension and with good blood supply, and the lower rectum or the anus. The defect in the vagina is closed and omentum is interposed in the space between the vagina and rectum.

The Parks' colo-anal sleeve anastomosis [67] is another technique which, in addition to excision of the rectum, involves performing a mucosectomy via the transanal route, then the healthy colon is pulled down the muscular tube of the rectum past the fistula, and a handsewn anastomosis with the anus at the level of the dentate line is performed.

Proctectomy

This involves removal of both the rectum and anus and has been recommended by Goligher [74] as the gold standard to treat inflammatory rectovaginal fistula. However, with advances in surgical techniques, this operation has been used with decreasing frequency but is mentioned here as a last-resort option when all else has failed, particularly if symptoms are troublesome and debilitating and patients' quality of life is poor. The technique involves excising the rectum, as described above, via the abdominal route. The anus is excised via the perineal route using the intersphincteric approach [75], which involves dissection of the intersphincteric plane and removal of the anus with the internal sphincter while leaving the external sphincter behind. Next, the vaginal defect is excised and closed with interrupted Vicryl sutures. The perineal wound is then closed in layers by approximating the levator ani and external anal sphincter muscle. In the presence of sepsis, all tracks should be opened and the perineum left open, to close by secondary intention or by tissue grafting.

Diversion Ileostomy/Colostomy

This is an option that was employed in the past as a primary treatment of a fistula but is now recognized as an option to cover surgical repair whether undertaken via the perineal or abdominal routes. It should be considered in complex and/or repeat repairs.

58.6.1.9 Other Techniques

There are several interesting techniques that have been reported in the literature as a small case series or case reports, and the common theme is the use of minimally invasive surgery to repair the fistula. The use of fibrin sealant was reported but the results are conflicting [76, 77]. The transanal endoscopic microsurgery (TEM) technique was used successfully in a patient with a high fistula and previous history of radiotherapy [78].

Laparoscopic surgery [79] has been employed as an alternative surgical technique to open abdominal operations in the treatment of high RVF. The introduction of robotic surgery may well have a role in the future. Once again, these are case reports, which, if anything, proves that the treatment is technically feasible but long-term outcomes are lacking. As such, these treatments are worth considering as a last resort or in the unfit patient but are not recommended for routine use except in the context of a trial.

58.6.2 Choice of Surgery

There are no comparative studies or randomized trials comparing different operations, and therefore the choice of treatment depends largely on the experience of the surgeon and, as alluded to above, the etiology and location of the fistula, and status of the anal sphincter and ano-rectum.

58.6.2.1 Peripartum Rectovaginal Fistula

RVF secondary to obstructed labor develops after "sloughing" of vaginal tissue that has become necrotic from pressure of the fetal head. Typically, the sloughing follows a week after the delivery of the fetus, after a prolonged labor lasting more than two days. A fistula "field injury" including rectovaginal and/or vesicovaginal fistula, global pelvic floor dysfunction, and foot drop has been described and is indicative of widespread pelvic tissue and neurological damage [3]. A fistula also results following inappropriate/incomplete repair of perineal tears/episiotomy.

As described earlier, it is essential to assess the anatomy and function of the anal sphincter with appropriately directed questions, anal manometry, and endoanal ultrasound scan.

Debridement of the infected wound, removal of residual suture material, and antibiotic therapy should be commenced prior to attempting repair of these fistulae. There is some evidence to suggest that small anovaginal and rectovaginal fistulae may close spontaneously. Rahman et al [80] reported that in their series of 42 women with RVF, 11% healed spontaneously but all these women had a RVF of less than 5 mm.

Although the traditional practice of waiting at least 3–6 months before attempting repair was widely followed, there has been recent evidence to the contrary. Waaldijk [81] reported on 1716 Nigerian women with a vesicovaginal fistula or genital fistula, of whom 211 had a concomitant RVF, presenting between 3 and 75 days after delivery. Successful primary closure was achieved in at least 90%.

Invariably, a fistula associated with obstetric trauma is a simple low fistula and the commonest operation employed is the advancement flap – either endorectal or transvaginal. Most evidence supports approaching the repair via the rectum as this is the site of high pressure. A large number of patients will have an associated sphincter disruption [33, 46, 49], and in these instances a concomitant repair of the sphincter using the overlapping sphincteroplasty technique is advised. Chew and Reiger [82] reported one recurrence out of six operations with a mean follow-up of 24 (range, 11–35) months. Five patients whose Wexner incontinence score was assessed improved from a preoperative mean of 13.4 to 5.6 postoperatively. MacRae et al [38] used this approach for recurrent fistulae, and six out of seven healed completely.

An alternative to this is the use of the perineoproctotomy technique which allows excellent exposure of the structures and meticulous layered repair. Hull et al [59] reported an overall success rate of 74% (100% for those with a cloacal defect and 68% for those with anterior sphincter defect). However, this approach should not be considered if the sphincter is intact or significant anterior muscle is to be divided.

58.6.2.2 Crohn's Disease

In Crohn's disease, RVF are usually a local manifestation of a systemic disease process and this should be taken into consideration during management. There is a wealth of reports in the literature addressing the subject (Table 58.5) [83–94].

Thus, the initial focus of the treatment should be directed at controlling the active disease and any local infective process associated with the fistula, such as abscesses or secondary tracts. In this respect, it is essential to obtain a detailed medical and physical history. The entire gastrointestinal tract, sphincter, and ano-rectal disease status must be assessed prior to consideration of treatment options. A stepwise approach to management as recommended by Hannaway and Hull [36] should start with conservative medical therapies, ideally with involvement of medical gastroenterologists with interest in the disease, and then progress to surgical intervention as needed or when local conditions allow. An exception to this rule is when severe sepsis such as an abscess is present at the initial presentation. In this situation, the abscess should be treated with antibiotics and immediate surgical drainage and, if appropriate, a loose seton should be inserted for drainage.

Specific medical therapy for Crohn's disease includes treatment with steroids and immunomodulators (Table 58.6) [95–104]. This will not only result in controlling the systemic disease but may also result in complete healing of the fistula, or at least may optimize and decrease inflammation in perineal tissues in preparation for surgery. Once sepsis is under control and the active disease is in remission, the type of surgery will depend on the location of the fistula and the presence or absence of sphincter defects, as well as the presence and extent of active disease in the anorectum. In the absence of any sphincter defect and active disease, a fistula in the lower rectum should be closed primarily using the endorectal advancement flap. If a sphincter defect is present but no active disease, an overlapping sphincteroplasty or perineoproctotomy should be considered.

There are no direct comparative studies of these two operations, and therefore the choice of operation depends on the surgeon's own preference and expertise. If mild active disease exists in the rectum, then an advancement sleeve operation should be considered. In a high fistula with or without active disease, an anterior resection with a defunctioning stoma should be considered. If the ano-rectum is severely diseased with active disease/strictures, or in recurrent fistulae, consideration should be given to either an abdomino-perineal excision of the anus and rectum, proctectomy with preservation of the anus if it is not involved with a view to restoring intestinal continuity later on, or even a diverting colostomy/ileostomy.

Although there is no strong evidence to support the use of anal fistula plugs in the treatment of Crohn's RVF, Hannaway and Hull suggested that this could be considered in a simple low fistula with minimal active disease [36].

Table 58.5 Published articles specific to or including the treatment of Crohn's-related RVF, adapted from [36]

Author	Study period	Total n	Crohn's n^a	RVF n^a	Study type
Surgical Treatment					
Morrison et al [83]	1973–1986	12	12	12	Retrospective
O'Leary et al [84]	1991–1996	10	10	10	Retrospective
Penninckx et al [85]	1993–1999	32	32	32	Retrospective
Marchesa et al [58]	1991–1995	13	13	11	Retrospective
Joo et al [51]	1991–1995	26	26	20	Retrospective
Garcia-Olmo et al [86]	2003	1	1	1	Case report
Scott et al [6]	1971–1991	67	67	29	Prospective database review
Simmang et al [87]	1997	2	2	2	Case report
Loungnarath et al [85]^b	1999–2002	39	13	3	Retrospective
Zmora et al [88]^b	1997–2000	37	7	4	Retrospective
Ellis [72]^b	2003–2006	78	7	78	Retrospective review of prospective cohort
Medical Treatment					
Sands et al [90]	2000–2001	25	25	27^c	*Post hoc* analysis of randomized, double-blind, placebo-controlled trial
Korelitz et al [91]	2 years^d	34	34	6	Retrospective review of cohort from randomized, double-blind study
O'Brien et al [92]	1980–1989	35	35	6	Retrospective
Parsi et al [93]	1998–2001	60	60	22	Retrospective
Rusche et al [94]	^{d}	6	6	6	Retrospective

^{a}Numbers reflect those of all subjects and not only those with both Crohn's disease *and* RVF; ^{b}fibrin glue or plug therapy; ^{c}number of fistulae treated; ^{d}dates not stated

Table 58.6 Results of medical treatment of rectovaginal fistula caused by Crohn's disease, adapted from [95]

Study	Agent	Number of patients	Closure	Improvement	Recurrence
Korelitz et al, 1985 [91]	6-Mercaptopurine	6	2	1	
Hanauer and Smith, 1993 [96]	Ciclosporin	5	4	1	2
Present and Lichtiger, 1994 [97]	Ciclosporin	2	1		
Ricart et al, 2001 [98]	Infliximab	15	5	1	
van Bodegraven et al, 2002 [99]	Infliximab	4	0	1	
Ochsenkuhn et al, 2002 [100]	Infliximab	1			
Bell et al, 2003 [101]	Infliximab	2	1		
Topstad et al, 2003 [102]	Infliximab	8	1	5	2
Rasul et al, 2004 [103]	Infliximab	8		6	
Parsi et al, 2004 [93]	Infliximab	14	2	9	
Ardizzone et al, 2004 [104]	Infliximab	7	2		

58.6.2.3 RVF Due to Radiation

Radiation-induced fistulae are a challenging entity to manage. The fistula usually develops several years after radiotherapy and often patients are middle-aged or elderly with considerable comorbidity. Consequently, they may not be suitable for a major operation and therefore require careful preoperative assessment. In addition, since radiation would have been delivered to treat cancer, it is essential to rule out recurrent disease by taking a biopsy of the fistula and surrounding tissue. Once the diagnosis is made, initial treatment starts by raising a defunctioning colostomy which not only will help the patient cope with the debilitating symptom of fecal incontinence but also help resolve any inflammatory process associated with the fistula and surrounding tissues. Often, a colostomy is all that is needed and hence it is important to manage patients' expectations from the beginning. In younger and fitter patients who wish to have definitive treatment, the surgical options, as in Crohn's disease, depend on the location of the fistula and extent of the radiation damage in the rectum. More importantly, any repair should involve interposing well-vascularized tissue, as the blood supply to the surrounding tissues is usually compromised by the radiotherapy. Low fistulae with no or mild radiation damage in the rectum are usually approached via the perineum, with interposition of the anal sphincter muscle (if a defect exists) or a labial fat pad (Martius graft) or the gracilis/sartorius muscle. In a high fistula with no or mild damage, repair is approached via the abdomen with interposition of omentum or colon (Bricker's graft). Bricker reported that 19 out of 26 patients with radiation-induced fistula were healed [69]. If the rectum is severely damaged by radiotherapy (for example the presence of stricture and fibrosis), then an anterior resection/proctectomy should be performed with or without restoration of intestinal continuity, and with interposition of the omentum.

58.6.2.4 RVF Due to Malignancy

Management of RVF associated with malignancy is directed at treating the cancer, which is otherwise a progressive condition. The cancers that may cause RVF are locally advanced tumors arising from the rectum, anus, or cervix. They may be associated with metastases, and therefore patients must be fully staged with magnetic resonance imaging (MRI) of the pelvis and CT scan of the chest, abdomen, and pelvis, and a management plan discussed and agreed in a multidisciplinary setting involving surgeons, oncologists, radiologists, and histopathologists. The initial treatment would involve a defunctioning ileostomy or colostomy with benefits as alluded to above. This is followed by neoadjuvant downstaging chemoradiotherapy along the accepted regimens of the tumor being treated. If the tumor is in the upper or mid-rectum, an anterior resection is undertaken using the techniques described earlier. If the tumor is in the lower rectum, an abdomino-perineal excision of the rectum and anus is the treatment of choice. If the tumor is a squamous cell cancer of the anus and it resolves fully on treatment but the fistula is still present, then a consideration is made for a local repair along the lines discussed for radiotherapy-induced fistula earlier. Ultimately, it may be necessary to undertake a salvage abdomino-perineal excision of the anus and rectum with the use of muscle graft by plastic surgeons to fill the defect in the perineum. In the case of cervical cancer, an anterior resection with en-bloc radical hysterectomy would be required.

58.6.2.5 Postoperative (Iatrogenic) RVF

The commonest causes of postoperative RVF are incorporating the posterior vaginal wall with either sutures or a stapling device during hemorrhoidectomy [13], treatment of obstructed defecation by STARR [13], and reconstruction of the intestinal continuity following low anterior resection or an ileo-anal pouch construction [11, 12]. A leaking anastomosis may result in pelvic sepsis and, rarely, this can lead to fistula formation especially in the irradiated pelvis. Fistulae can also occur following vaginal hysterectomy. In the vast majority of patients, the problem becomes apparent a week or two after initial injury, by which time local sepsis will have set in. In these situations, the treatment starts by raising a defunctioning stoma if one is not already raised to help control the sepsis. Rarely, small fistulae may close spontaneously, but if the fistula persists, a low one is treated by an endorectal or transvaginal advancement flap and a high one by a repeat anterior resection and anastomosis with interposition of omentum. In a low fistula with sphincter disruption, an overlapping sphincteroplasty is used to separate the two suture lines, but interposition of other tissues may be required particularly in recurrent/failed repairs. In the rare situations where the

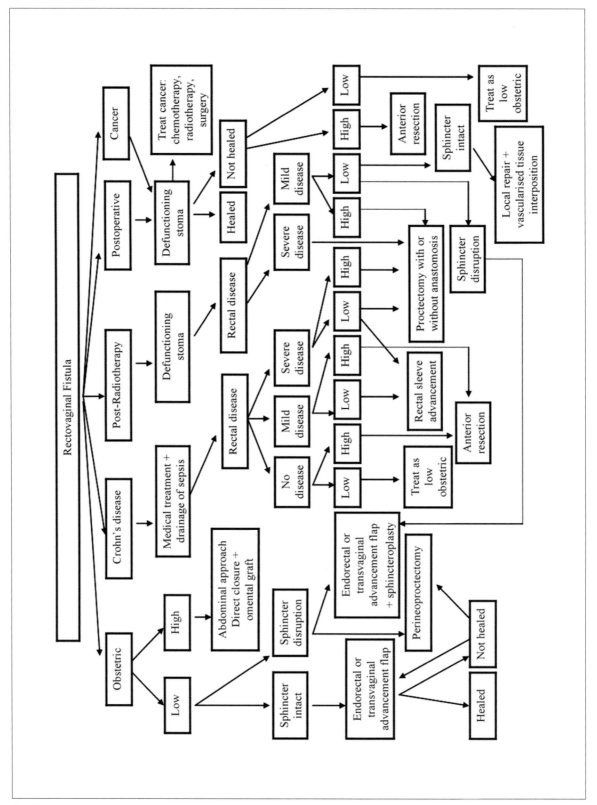

Fig. 58.7 Suggested algorithm to the management of rectovaginal fistula

injury/fistula is recognized at the time of surgery, as may happen during STARR surgery or stapled hemorrhoidectomy, then repair of the fistula should be attempted immediately by undertaking layered closure with repair of the vaginal fascia.

58.6.2.6 Recurrent RVF

The principles of management are similar to of those employed in the management of complex fistulae as discussed earlier. However, the initial choice of treatment should take into account the type of previous failed repair and the surgeon's experience, in addition to other factors such as the location and etiology of the fistula. The two reports in the literature dedicated to this subject employ a variety of techniques via both the local and abdominal routes, with success rates of up to 72% in simple fistulae and 40% in complex ones [38, 77]. It is suggested that repair of fistulae should not be attempted soon after the recurrence develops, but delayed for a few months to allow any inflammatory process to resolve, infection to be treated, and the current status of the fistula to be evaluated. Advancement flaps should not be considered if a previous flap repair has failed and in complex fistulae, because of low success rates of approximately 40%. However, some suggest that this can be considered if only one, or perhaps two, flap repairs have failed.

The success rate of 85% after first failed repair fell to 55% after the third failed repair [25]. Perineoproctotomy, rectal sleeve advancement, and tissue interposition operations should be considered as the initial choice in low fistulae, and rectal resection with or without reconstruction and with and without tissue interposition in high fistulae.

58.6.3 Suggested Algorithm

Figure 58.7 shows a suggested algorithm to the management of rectovaginal fistula. Although rather complex, it provides a quick but concise overview of diagnosis and treatment of the condition.

58.7 Conclusions

RVF can be a potentially difficult problem to manage. Although it is clear that treatment of all fistulae, particularly the complex ones, is best undertaken in specialized units with experience in the condition, we cannot overemphasise the importance of a multidisciplinary approach to management by both gynecologists and colorectal surgeons and, where appropriate, gastroenterologists, clinical oncologists, and plastic surgeons. Unfortunately, there are no comparative studies on the efficacy of various treatment modalities, and therefore treatment should be tailored according to the location, etiology, and status of the sphincter and surrounding tissues, as well as the number of previous repairs. The aim should be to make the first procedure the most appropriate one, as it provides the best chance of success and minimizes the risk of recurrence. Counseling patients regarding outcome and complications is of utmost importance. Although there are no randomized studies, general recommendations are that women who have undergone previous successful continence or vaginal prolapse/fistula surgery should be offered a cesarean section in any subsequent pregnancy [105].

References

1. Stenchever MA, Benson JT (eds) Atlas of clinical gynaecology. McGraw-Hill, New York, 2000.
2. Venkatesh KS, Ramanujam P, Larson DM, Haywood MA. Anorectal complications of vaginal delivery. Dis Colon Rectum 1989;32:1039–1041.
3. Rogers RG, Fenner DE. Rectovaginal fistulas. In: Sultan AH, Thakar R, Fenner D (eds) Perineal and anal sphincter trauma. Springer-Verlag, London, 2007, pp 166–177.
4. De Ridder D, Badlani GH, Browning A. Fistulas in the developing world. In: Abrams P, Cardozo L, Khoury, Wein A (eds) Incontinence, 4 edn. Health Publication Ltd, Plymouth, 2009, pp 1149–1460 .
5. Radcliffe AG, Ritchie JK, Hawley PR et al. Anovaginal and rectovaginal fistulae in Crohn's disease. Dis Colon Rectum 1988;31:94–99.
6. Scott NA, Nair A, Hughes LE. Anovaginal and rectovaginal fistula in patients with Crohn's disease. Br J Surg 1992;79:1379–1380.
7. Singhal SR, Nanda S, Singhal SK. Sexual intercourse: an unusual cause of rectovaginal fistula. Eur J Obstet Gynecol Reprod Biol 2007;131:243–244.
8. Hanavadi S, Durham-Hall A, Oke T, Aston N. Forgotten vaginal pessary eroding into rectum. Ann R Coll Surg Engl 2004;86:W18–19.
9. Purwar B, Panda SN, Odogwu SO, Joseph AT. Recto-vaginal sex leading to colostomy and recto-vaginal repair. Int J STD AIDS 2008;19:57–58.
10. Tsujinaka S, Ruiz D, Wexner SD et al. Surgical management of pouch-vaginal fistula after restorative proctocolectomy. J Am Coll Surg 2006;202:912–918.

11. Heriot AG, Tekkis PP, Smith JJ et al. Management and outcome of pouch-vaginal fistulas following restorative proctocolectomy. Dis Colon Rectum 2005;48:451–458.

12. Tsutsumi N, Yoshida Y, Maehara Y, Kohnoe S. Rectovaginal fistula following double-stapling anastomosis in low anterior resection for rectal cancer. Hepatogastroenterology 2007;54:1682–1683.

13. Pescatori M, Gagliardi G. Postoperative complications after procedure for prolapsed hemorrhoids (PPH) and stapled transanal rectal resection (STARR) procedures. Tech Coloproctol 2008;12:7–19.

14. Hilger WS, Cornella JL. Rectovaginal fistula after posterior intravaginal slingplasty and polypropylene mesh augmented rectocele repair. Int Urogynecol J Pelvic Floor Dysfunct 2006;17:89–92.

15. Huffaker RK, Shull BL, Thomas JS. A serious complication following placement of posterior Prolift. Int Urogynecol J Pelvic Floor Dysfunct 2009;20:1383–1385.

16. Lezoche E, Guerrieri M, Paganini AM, Feliciotti F. Transanal endoscopic microsurgical excision of irradiated and nonirradiated rectal cancer. A 5-year experience. Surg Laparosc Endosc 1998;8:249–256.

17. Perez CA, Grigsby PW, Camel HM et al. Irradiation alone or combined with surgery in stage IB, IIA, and IIB carcinoma of uterine cervix: update of a nonrandomized comparison. Int J Radiat Oncol Biol Phys 1995;31:703–716.

18. Thiele H, Wesch G, Nüsser CJ. Surgical therapy of enterovaginal fistulae following gynecologic primary procedures. Langenbecks Arch Chir 1982;357:35–40.

19. Ley EJ, Vukasin P, Kaiser AM et al. Delayed rectovaginal fistula: a potential complication of bevacizumab (Avastin). Dis Colon Rectum 2007;50:930.

20. Allen-Mersh TG, Wilson EJ, Hope-Stone HF, Mann CV. The management of late radiation-induced rectal injury after treatment of carcinoma of the uterus. Surg Gynecol Obstet 1987;164:521–524.

21. Allal AS, Bieri S, Bründler MA et al. Preoperative hyperfractionated radiotherapy for locally advanced rectal cancers: a phase I-II trial. Int J Radiat Oncol Biol Phys 2002;54:1076–1081.

22. Perez CA, Grigsby PW, Chao C et al. Irradiation in carcinoma of the vulva: factors affecting outcome. Int J Radiat Oncol Biol Phys 1998;42:335–344.

23. Mischinger HJ, Hauser H, Cerwenka H et al. Endocavitary Ir-192 radiation and laser treatment for palliation of obstructive rectal cancer. Eur J Surg Oncol 1997; 23:428–431.

24. Szynglarewicz B, Matkowski R, Gisterek I et al. The impact of pre- or postoperative radiochemotherapy on complication following anterior resection with en bloc excision of female genitalia for T4 rectal cancer. Colorectal Dis 2009;11:377–381.

25. Lowry AC, Thorson AG, Rothenberger DA, Goldberg SM. Repair of simple rectovaginal fistula. Influence of previous repairs. Dis Colon Rectum 1988;31:676–678.

26. Saclarides TJ. Rectovaginal fistula. Surg Clin North Am 2002;82:1261–1272.

27. Rothenberger DA, Goldberg SM The management of rectovaginal fistula. Surg Clin North Am 1983;63:61–79.

28. Kapoor D, Sultan AH, Thakar R et al. Management of complex pelvic floor disorders in a multidisciplinary pelvic floor Clinic. Colorectal Dis 2008;10:118–123.

29. Avery K, Donovan J, Peters TJ et al. ICIQ: a brief and robust measure for evaluating the symptoms and impact of urinary incontinence. Neurourol Urodyn 2004; 3:322–330.

30. Jorge JM, Wexner SD. Etiology and management of fecal incontinence. Dis Colon Rectum 1993;36:77–97.

31. Rockwood TH, Church JM, Fleshman JW et al. Fecal incontinence quality of scale: quality of life instrument for patients with fecal incontinence. Dis Colon Rectum 2000;43:9–17.

32. Giordano P, Drew PJ, Taylor D et al. Vaginography- investigation of choice for clinically suspected vaginal fistulas. Dis Colon Rectum 1996;39:568–572.

33. Yee LF, Birnbaum EH, Read TE et al. Use of endoanal ultrasound in patients with rectovaginal fistulas. Dis Colon Rectum 1999;42:1057–1064.

34. Sudoł-Szopińska I, Jakubowski W, Szczepkowski M. Contrast-enhanced endosonography for the diagnosis of anal and anovaginal fistulas. J Clin Ultrasound 2002;30:145–150.

35. Stoker J, Rociu E, Schouten WR, Laméris JS. Anovaginal and rectovaginal fistulas: endoluminal sonography versus endoluminal MR imaging. AJR Am J Roentgenol. 2002; 178:737–741.

36. Hannaway CD, Hull TL. Current considerations in the management of rectovaginal fistula from Crohn's disease. Colorectal Dis 2008;10:747–755.

37. Lowry AC, Hoexter B. Benign anorectal rectovaginal fistulas. In: Wolff BG, Fleshman JW, Beck DE (eds) The ASCRS textbook of colon and rectal surgery. Springer-Verlag, Berlin 2007, pp 215–227.

38. MacRae HM, McLeod RS, Cohen Z et al. Treatment of rectovaginal fistulas that has failed previous repair attempts. Dis Colon Rectum 1995;38:921–925.

39. Jones IT, Fazio VW, Jagelman DG. The use of transanal rectal advancement flap in the management of fistulas involving the anorectum. Dis Colon Rectum 1987;30:919 – 923.

40. Gagliardi G, Pescatori M. Clinical and functional results after tailored surgery for rectovaginal fistula. Pelviperineology 2007;26:78–81.

41. Rothenberger DA, Christenson CE, Balcos EG et al. Endorectal advancement flap for treatment of simple rectovaginal fistula. Dis Colon Rectum 1982;25:297–300.

42. Greenwald JC, Hoexter B. Repair of rectovaginal fistulas. Surg Gynecol Obstet 1978;146:443–445.

43. Hoexter B, Labow SB, Moseson MD. Transanal rectovaginal fistula repair. Dis Colon Rectum 1985;28:572–575.

44. Wise WE Jr, Aguilar PS, Padmanabhan A et al. Surgical treatment of low rectovaginal fistulas. Dis Colon Rectum 1991;34:271–274.

45. Kodner IJ, Mazor A, Shemesh EI et al. Endorectal advancement flap repair of rectovaginal and other complicated anorectal fistulae. Surgery 1993;114:682–689.

46. Khanduja KS, Yamashita HJ, Wise WE Jr et al. Delayed repair of obstetric injuries of the anorectum and vagina. A stratified surgical approach. Dis Colon Rectum 1994; 37:344–349.

47. Mazier WP, Senagore AJ, Schiesel EC. Operative repair of anovaginal and rectovaginal fistulas. Dis Colon Rectum 1995;38:4–6.

48. Watson SJ, Phillips RK. Non-inflammatory rectovaginal fistula. Br J Surg 1995;82:1641–1643.

49. Tsang CBS, Madoff RD, Wong WD et al. Anal sphincter integrity and function influences outcome in rectovaginal repair. Dis Colon Rectum 1998;41:1141–1146.

50. Hyman N. Endoanal advancement flap repair for complex anorectal fistulas. Am J Surg 1999;178:337–340.

51. Joo JS, Weiss EG, Nogueras JJ, Wexner SD. Endorectal advancement flap in perianal Crohn's disease. Am Surg 1998;64:147–150.

52. Baig MK, Zhao RH, Yuen CH et al. Simple rectovaginal fistulas. Int J Colorectal Dis 2000;15:323–327.

53. Mizrahi N, Wexner SD, Zmora O et al. Endorectal advancement flap: are there predictors of failure? Dis Colon Rectum 2002;45:1616–1621.

54. Sonoda T, Hull T, Piedmonte MR, Fazio VW. Outcomes of primary repair of anorectal and rectovaginal fistulas using the endorectal advancement flap. Dis Colon Rectum 2002;45:1622–1628.

55. Zimmerman DD, Gosselink MP, Briel JW, Schouten WR. The outcome of transanal advancement flap repair is not improved by an additional labial fat flap transposition. Tech Coloproctol 2002;6:37–42.

56. Wiskind AR, Thompson JD. Fecal incontinence and rectovaginal fistulas. In: Rock JA, Thompson JD (eds) Te Linde's Operative Gynaecology, 8th edn. Lippincott-Raven, Philadelphia, PA, 1997, pp 1207-1236.

57. Berman IR. Sleeve advancement anorectoplasty for complicated anorectal/vaginal fistula. Dis Colon Rectum 1991;34:1032–1037.

58. Marchesa P, Hull TL, Fazio VW. Advancement sleeve flaps for treatment of severe perianal Crohn's disease. Br J Surg 1998;85:1695–1698.

59. Hull T, Bartus C, Bast J et al. Success of episioproctotomy for cloaca and rectovaginal fistula. Dis Colon Rectum 2007;50:97–101.

60. Wexner SD, Ruiz DE, Genua J et al. Gracilis muscle interposition for the treatment of rectourethral, rectovaginal, and pouch-vaginal fistulas: results in 53 patients. Ann Surg 2008;248:39–43.

61. Byron RL Jr, Ostergard DR. Sartorius muscle interposition for the treatment of the radiation-induced vaginal fistula. Am J Obstet Gynecol 1969;104:104–107.

62. Tran KT, Kuijpers HC, van Nieuwenhoven EJ et al. Transposition of the rectus abdominis muscle for complicated pouch and rectal fistulas. Dis Colon Rectum1999;42:486–489.

63. Elkins TE, DeLancey JO, McGuire EJ. The use of modified Martius graft as an adjunctive technique in vesicovaginal and rectovaginal fistula repair. Obstet Gynecol 1990;75:727–733.

64. McNevin MS, Lee PY, Bax TW. Martius flap: an adjunct for repair of complex, low rectovaginal fistula. Am J Surg 2007;193:597–599.

65. Boronow RC. Repair of the radiation-induced vaginal fistula utilizing the Martius technique. World J Surg 1986;10:237-248.

66. Kusunoki M, Shoji Y, Yanagi H et al. Colonic J pouch-anal reconstruction with gluteus maximus transposition for a post-irradiation rectovaginal fistula. Hepatogastroenterology 1996;43:1339–1342.

67. Nowacki MP. Ten years of experience with Parks' coloanal sleeve anastomosis for the treatment of post-irradiation rectovaginal fistula. Eur J Surg Oncol 1991;17:563–536.

68. Bricker EM, JohnstonWD. Repair of postirradiation rectovaginal fistula and stricture. Surg Gynecol Obstet 1979;148:499–506.

69. Bricker EM, Kraybill WG, Lopez MJ. Functional results after postirradiation rectal reconstruction. World J Surg1986;10:249–258.

70. Pye PK, Dada T, Duthie G, Phillips K. Surgisistrade mark mesh: a novel approach to repair of a recurrent rectovaginal fistula. Dis Colon Rectum 2004;47:1554–1556.

71. Schwandner O, Fuerst A, Kunstreich K, Scherer R. Innovative technique for the closure of rectovaginal fistula using Surgisis mesh. Tech Coloproctol 2009;13:135–140.

72. Ellis CN. Outcomes after repair of rectovaginal fistulas using bioprosthetics. Dis Colon Rectum 2008; 51:1084–1088.

73. O'Connor L, Champagne BJ, Ferguson MA et al. Efficacy of anal fistula plug in closure of Crohn's anorectal fistulas. Dis Colon Rectum 2006;49:1569–1573.

74. Goligher JC. Rectovaginal fistula and irradiation proctitis and enteritis. In: Goligher JC, Dothie BL, Nixon HH (eds) Surgery of the anus, colon, and rectum. Charles C Thomas, Springfield, IL, 1975, pp 205–255.

75. Lyttle JA, Parks AG. Intersphincteric excision of rectum. Br J Surg 1977;64:413–416.

76. Abel ME, Chiu YS, Russell TR, Volpe PA. Autologous fibrin glue in the treatment of rectovaginal and complex fistulas. Dis Colon Rectum 1993;36:447–449.

77. Halverson AL, Hull TL, Fazio VW et al. Repair of recurrent rectovaginal fistulas. Surgery 2001;130:753–757.

78. Darwood RJ, Borley NR. TEMS: an alternative method for the repair of benign recto-vaginal fistulae. Colorectal Disease 2008;10:619–620.

79. Schwenk W, Böhm B, Gründel K, Müller J. Laparoscopic resection of high rectovaginal fistula with intracorporeal colorectal anastomosis and omentoplasty. Surg Endosc 1997;11:147–149.

80. Rahman MS, Al-Suleiman SA, El-Yahia AR, Rahman J. Surgical treatment of rectovaginal fistula of obstetric origin: a review of 15 years experience in a teaching hospital. J Obstet Gynecol 2003;23:607–610.

81. Waaldijk K. The immediate management of fresh obstetric fistulas. Am J Obstet Gynecol 2004;191:795–799.

82. Chew SS, Reiger NA. Transperineal repair of obstetric-related anovaginal fistula. Aust NZJ Obstet Gynaecol 2004;44:68–71.

83. Morrison JG, Gathright JB Jr, Ray JE et al. Results of operation for rectovaginal fistula in Crohn's disease. Dis Colon Rectum 1989;32:497–499.

84. O'Leary DP, Milroy CE, Durdey P. Definitive repair of anovaginal fistula in Crohn's disease. Ann R Coll Surg Engl 1998;80:250–252.

85. Penninckx F, Moneghini D, D'Hoore A et al. Success and failure after repair of rectovaginal fistula in Crohn's disease: analysis of prognostic factors. Colorectal Dis 2001;3:406-411.

86. Garcia-Olmo D, Garcia-Arranz M, Garcia LG et al. Autologous stem cell transplantation for treatment of rectovaginal fistula in perianal Crohn's disease: a new cell-based therapy.

Int J Colorectal Dis 2003;18:451–454.

87. Simmang CL, Lacey SW, Huber PJ. Rectal sleeve advancement: repair of rectovaginal fistula associated with anorectal stricture in Crohn's disease. Dis Colon Rectum 1998; 41:787–789.

88. Loungnarath R, Dietz DW, Mutch MG et al. Fibrin glue treatment of complex anal fistulae has low success rate. Dis Colon Rectum 2004;47:432–436.

89. Zmora O, Mizrahi N, Rotholtz N et al. Fibrin glue sealing in the treatment of perineal fistulae. Dis Colon Rectum 2003;46:584–589.

90. Sands BE, Blank MA, Patel K, van Deventer SJ. Long-term treatment of rectovaginal fistulae in Crohn's disease: response to infliximab in the ACCENT II Study. Clin Gastroenterol Hepatol 2004;2:912–920.

91. Korelitz B, Present D. Favorable effect of 6-mercaptopurine on fistulae of Crohn's Disease. Dig Dis Sci 1985;30:58–64.

92. O'Brien JJ, Bayless TM, Bayless JA. Use of azathioprine or 6-mercaptopurine in the treatment of Crohn's disease. Gastroenterology 1991;101:39–46.

93. Parsi M, Lashner B, Achkar JP et al. Type of fistula determines response to infliximab in patients with fistulous Crohn's Disease. Am J Gastroenterol 2004;99:445–449.

94. Rusche M, O'Brien JJ. Infliximab in the management of RVF Crohn's disease. Am J Gastroenterol 2001;96(suppl. 9):S306–S307.

95. Andreani SM, Dang HH, Grondona P et al. Rectovaginal fistula in Crohn's disease. Dis Colon Rectum 2007;50: 2215–2222.

96. Hanauer SB, Smith MB. Rapid closure of Crohn's disease fistulas with continuous intravenous cyclosporine A. Am J Gatroenterol 1993;88:646–649.

97. Present DH, Lichtiger S. Efficacy of cyclosporine in treatment of fistula of Crohn's disease. Dig Dis Sci 1994;39:374–380.

98. Ricart E, Panaccione R, Loftus EV. Infliximab for Crohn's disease in clinical practice at the Mayo Clinic: the first 100 patients. Am J Gastroenterol 2001;96:722–729.

99. Van Bodegraven AA, Sloots CE, Felt-Bersma RJ, Meuwissen SG. Endosonographic evidence of persistence of Crohn's disease associated fistulas after inflixmab treatment, irrespective of clinical response. Dis Colon Rectum 2002; 45:39–45.

100. Ochsenkuhn T, Goke B, Sackmann M. Combining infliximab with 6-mercaptopurine/azathioprine for fistula therapy in Crohn's disease. Am J Gastroenterol 2002; 97:2022–2025.

101. Bell SJ, Halligan S, Windsor AC et al. Response of fistulating Crohn's disease to infliximab treatment assessed by MRI. Aliment Pharmacol Ther 2003;17:387–393.

102. Topstad D, Panaccione R, Heine JA et al. Combined seton placement, infliximab infusion and maintenance immunosuppressives improve healing rate in fistulizing anorectal Crohn's disease. A single-center experience. Dis Colon Rectum 2003;46:577–583.

103. Rasul I, Wilson SR, MacRae H et al. Clinical and radiological responses after infliximab treatment for perianal fistulizing Crohn's disease. Am J Gastroenterol 2004;99:89-90.

104. Ardizzone S, Maconi G, Colombo E et al. Perianal fistula following infliximab treatment: clinical and endosonographic outcome. Inflamm Bowel Dis 2004;10:91–96.

105. Sultan AH, Stanton SL. Preserving the pelvic floor and pe-

Anorectal Fistulae

59

Giulio Aniello Santoro, Giuseppe Gizzi, Andrea Rusconi,
Claudio Pastore and Luciano Pellegrini

Abstract The configuration of perianal sepsis and the relationship of abscesses or fistulae with internal and external sphincters are the most important factors influencing the results of surgical management. Preoperative identification of all loculate purulent areas, and definition of the anatomy of the primary fistulous tract, secondary extensions, and the internal opening play an important role in adequate planning of the operative approach, in order to ensure complete drainage of abscesses, prevent early recurrence after surgical treatment, and minimize iatrogenic damage of sphincters and the risk of minor or major degrees of incontinence.

In this chapter, the accuracy and reliability of endoanal ultrasonography and magnetic resonance imaging in the evaluation of perianal abscesses and fistulae will be discussed. The indications for and results of different forms of treatment (fistulotomy, fistulectomy, anal flap, seton positioning, fibrin glue injection, fistula plug) will also be presented and discussed.

Keywords Anal fistulae • Anal flap • Endoanal ultrasonography • Fibrin glue • Fistula plug • Fistulectomy • Fistulotomy • Perianal abscess • Seton positioning

59.1 Introduction

The pathogenesis of anorectal abscesses and fistulae is generally attributed to an infection of the anal glands, usually located in the subepithelial position, the intersphincteric space, or the external sphincter, with ducts that enter at the base of the anal crypts of Morgagni at the dentate line level [1]. Infection of the glands can result in an abscess which can spread in a number of directions, usually along the path of least resistance, and can lead to the subsequent development of anal fistula.

Five presentations of anorectal abscess have been described (Fig. 59.1) [1]:

a. Perianal abscess, which is the most common type of anorectal abscess, occurring in 40–45% of cases and is identified as a superficial, tender mass outside the anal verge. Physical examination reveals an area of erythema, induration, or fluctuance, and anoscopic examination can demonstrate pus exuding at the base of a crypt (Fig. 59.2).

b. Submucosal abscess, which arises from an infected crypt in the anal canal and is located under the mucosa. Rectal examination may reveal a tender submucosal mass, which may not be readily apparent by anoscopy.

c. Intersphincteric abscess, which represents between

G.A. Santoro
Pelvic Floor Unit and Colorectal Service, 1st Department
of General Surgery, Regional Hospital, Treviso, Italy

G.A. Santoro, A.P. Wieczorek, C.I. Bartram (eds.) *Pelvic Floor Disorders*
© Springer-Verlag Italia 2010

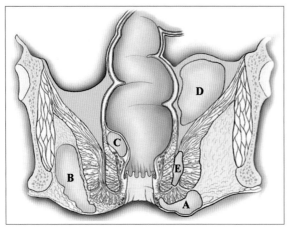

Fig. 59.1 Types of anorectal abscesses: *A,* perianal; *B,* ischioanal; *C,* submucosal; *D,* supralevator; *E,* intersphincteric

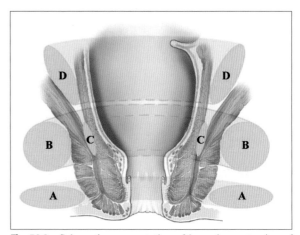

Fig. 59.3 Schematic representation of horseshoe extension of anal sepsis in the different perianal space: *A,* perianal; *B,* ischioanal; *C,* intersphincteric; *D,* supralevator

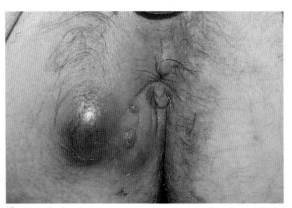

Fig. 59.2 Perianal abscess appears as an area of erythema, induration, or fluctuance

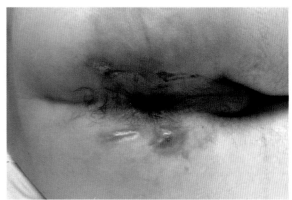

Fig. 59.4 Complex perianal fistula with a number of external orifices

2% and 5% of anorectal abscesses. In this condition, the infection dissects in the intersphincteric plane and can spread cephalad (high type) or caudal (low type).

d. Ischioanal abscess, which is seen in 20–25% of patients and may present as a large, erythematous, indurated, tender mass of the buttock or may be virtually inapparent, the patient complaining only of severe pain or fever.

e. Supralevator and pelvirectal abscesses, which are relatively rare, comprising less than 2.5% of anorectal abscesses. They may occur as a cephalad extension of an intersphincteric or trans-sphincteric abscess, or may be associated with a pelvic inflammatory condition (Crohn's disease, diverticulitis, salpingitis) or pelvic surgery.

Sepsis can spread through the different perianal spaces and become a horseshoe infection (Fig. 59.3).

Anorectal fistula represents a communication between two epithelial surfaces: the perianal skin and the anal canal or rectal mucosa [1]. Any fistula is characterized by an internal opening, a primary tract, and an external or perineal opening (Fig. 59.4). Occasionally the primary tract can present a secondary extension, or a fistula is without a perineal opening. Parks et al [1] classified the main tract of the fistula in relation to the sphincters into four types:

a. Intersphincteric tract (incidence between 55% and 70%). An intersphincteric fistula passes through the internal sphincter and through the intersphincteric plane to the skin (Fig. 59.5a). Only the most superficial portions of the tract pass through the subcutaneous external sphincter. Secondary exten-

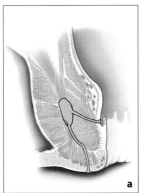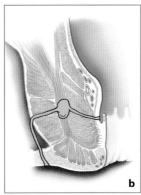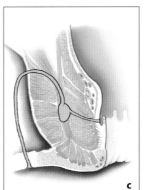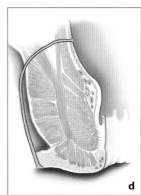

Fig. 59.5 Schematic drawings of differet types of anorectal fistulae. **a** Intersphincteric fistula, **b** trans-sphincteric fistula, **c** suprasphincteric fistula, **d** extrasphincteric fistula

sion may be observed to proceed cephalad in the intersphincteric plane (high blind tract).

b. Trans-sphincteric tract (incidence between 55% and 70%). A trans-sphincteric fistula passes through both the internal and external sphincters, into the ischioanal fossa and to the skin (Fig. 59.5b). The level of the tract determines three types of trans-sphincteric fistula: high (traversing the upper two-thirds of the external sphincter), mid or low. The height of the internal opening, however, does not always reflect the level at which a trans-sphincteric fistula crosses the external anal sphincter [2].

c. Suprasphincteric tract (incidence between 1% and 3%). A suprasphincteric fistula courses above the puborectalis muscle and below the levator after initially passing cephalad as an interphincteric fistula. It then transverses downward through the ischioanal fossa to the skin (Fig. 59.5c).

d. Extrasphincteric tract (incidence between 2% and 3%). An extrasphincteric fistula is described by a direct communication between the perineum and rectum with no anal canal involvement (Fig. 59.5d).

Submucosal fistulae are those in which the tract is subsphincteric and does not involve or pass the sphincter complex. Anovaginal fistulae have an extension toward the vaginal introitus. Secondary tracks may develop in any part of the anal canal or may extend circumferentially in the intersphincteric, ischioanal, or supralevator spaces (horseshoe extensions). The term "complex" fistula is a modification of the Parks' classification, which describes fistulae whose treatment poses a higher risk for impairment of continence.

According to the American Society of Colon and Rectal Surgeons (ASCRS) classification [3], an anal fistula may be termed "complex" when the tract crosses more than 30–50% of the external sphincter (high transsphincteric, suprasphincteric, and extrasphincteric), is anterior in a female, has multiple tracts, is recurrent, or the patient has pre-existing incontinence, local irradiation, or Crohn's disease.

59.2 Assessement of Anorectal Fistulae

The configuration of perianal sepsis and the relationship of abscesses or fistulae with internal and external sphincters are the most important factors influencing the results of surgical management [3]. Preoperative identification of all loculate purulent areas and definition of the anatomy of the primary fistulous tract, secondary extensions, and internal opening plays an important role in adequately planning the operative approach in order to ensure complete drainage of abscesses, to prevent early recurrence after surgical treatment, and to minimize iatrogenic damage of sphincters and the risk of minor or major degrees of incontinence.

59.2.1 Physical Examination

Useful information can be obtained by clinical assessment including digital examination [3]. Physical examination may reveal the fistulous tract proceeding into the anal canal, and anoscopic examination may demonstrate purulent material exuding from the base of the crypt. Intersphincteric tracts usually open externally

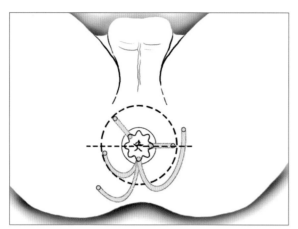

Fig. 59.6 Schematic representation of typical courses of fistula tracts according to Goodsall's rule

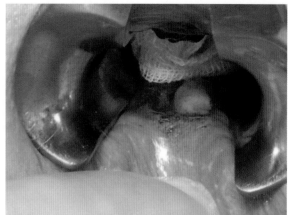

Fig. 59.7 Hydrogen peroxide injection through the external orifice helps to identify the internal orifice

very close to the anal verge, and trans-sphincteric and other more complicated tracts will open further away as they will have to traverse the external anal sphincter first. According to Goodsall's rule [4], when the external opening lies anterior to the transverse plane, the internal opening tends to be located radially and in the same position as the external opening. Conversely, when the external opening lies posterior to this plane, the internal opening is usually located in the posterior midline, irrespective of the site of the external opening (Fig. 59.6). The use of Goodsall's rule alone in decision making before surgical intervention is, however, not recommended because the positive predictive value is 59% for primary fistulae (anterior fistulae: 72%, posterior fistulae: 41%) and 41% for recurrent fistulae (anterior fistulae: 67%, posterior fistulae: 12.5%) [5]. Passage of a probe from both the external and the internal openings may confirm the course of the tract; however, a stenotic or sharply angulated tract may preclude complete passage from either end. Furthermore, this method is potentially dangerous, because a false tract can be made. Methylene blue or hydrogen peroxide injection (Fig. 59.7) through the external opening may confirm the patency of the tract and its communication with an internal opening. The problem with methylene blue is that the material stains the entire mucosa. Staining of the tissue does not occur with hydrogen peroxide, and bubbles may be seen through the internal opening.

Physical examination reaches a very good accuracy in identifying superficial (100%) and trans-sphincteric (100%) tracts, but it appears inadequate for both supralevator (63.6%) and intersphincteric (33.3%) tracts. Deen et al [6] were able to identified only 50% of the internal

openings and 27.3% of the horseshoe tracts by physical examination, and Poen et al [7] reported a correct diagnosis of primary tracts in 38% of patients, with 62% of patients unclassified. Ratto et al [8] also confirmed a low overall accuracy (65.4%) of physical examination for preoperative identification of primary fistulous tracts, and no suprasphincteric or extrasphincteric extensions were correctly described. Moreover, physical examination was unable to identify any of the ischioanal, pelvirectal, and horseshoeing secondary tracts and most of the internal openings.

59.2.2 Fistulography

Fistulography has a very limited role in the assessment of cryptogenic anorectal sepsis and it is little used in clinical practice [3]. It can be helpful in a chronic fistula with an external opening distant from the anus; however, it can offer only indirect and not very reliable information on the involvement of anal sphincters. While the primary track is demonstrated by fistulography, secondary extensions may not fill and the complexity of the fistula may be underestimated. Furthermore, it is not possible on fistulography to determine the relationship between the track and the anorectal junction. Thus, it is not possible to distinguish between sepsis above or below the levator plate. Kuijpers and Schulpen [9] found that fistulograms were correct in only 16% of anal fistulae, with a false-positive rate of 10% and the internal orifice identified in only 24% of patients. They considered fistulography an inaccurate and unreliable procedure and did not recommend it in the diagnosis of fistula-in-ano. In certain patients, however, especially those with either inflammatory bowel disease or an extrasphincteric fistula, fistulography may be helpful as it can show direct communication with the intestine above the levator.

59.2.3 Endoanal Ultrasonography

Endoanal ultrasonography (EAUS) has been demonstrated to be a very helpful diagnostic tool in accurately assessing all fistula or abscess characteristics [3, 5-8, 10, 11]. It can be easily repeated while following patients with perianal sepsis to choose the optimal timing and modality of surgical treatment, to evaluate the integrity of or damage to sphincters after operation, and to identify recurrence of fistula. It also gives information about the state of the anal sphincters, which is valuable in performing successful fistula surgery. A fistula tract affecting minimal muscle can be safely excised, but where the bulk of external sphincter muscle is affected, it is best treated by seton drainage or mucosal advancement flap.

The ultrasound examination is generally started using 10–13 MHz, changing to 7 or 5 MHz to optimize visualization of the deeper structures external to the anal sphincters. The puborectalis muscle, and external, longitudinal, and internal sphincters should always be

identified and used as reference structures for the spatial orientation of the fistula or abscess [11]. An anal abscess appears as a hypoechoic dyshomogeneous area, sometimes with hyperechoic spots within it, possibly in connection with a fistulous tract directed through the anal canal lumen. Abscesses are classified as superficial (Fig. 59.8), intersphincteric (Fig. 59.9), ischioanal (Fig. 59.10), supralevator (Fig. 59.11), pelvirectal (Fig. 59.12), and horseshoe (Fig. 59.13).

An anal fistula appears as a hypoechoic tract, which is followed along its crossing of the subepithelium, internal or external sphincters, and through the perianal spaces. With regard to the anal sphincters, according to Parks' classification [1], the fistulous primary tract can be classified into four types.

a. Intersphincteric tract, which is presented as a band of poor reflectivity within the longitudinal layer, causing widening and distortion of an otherwise narrow intersphincteric plane (Fig. 59.14). The tract goes through the intersphincteric space without traversing the external sphincter fibers

b. Trans-sphincteric tract, appearing as a poorly reflective tract running out through the external sphincter and disrupting its normal architecture (Fig. 59.15). The point at which the main tract of the fistula traverses the sphincters defines the fistula level. The trans-sphincteric fistulae are divided into high,

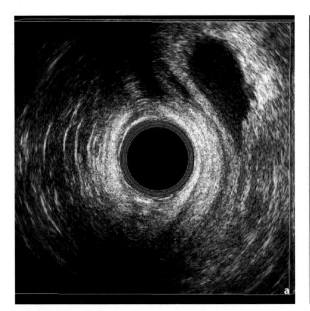
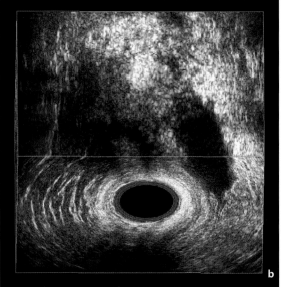

Fig. 59.8 Three-dimensional endoanal ultrasound with rotating probe. Acute abscess in the left anterior perianal space presenting as an area of low reflectivity. **a** Axial plane. **b** Coronal plane

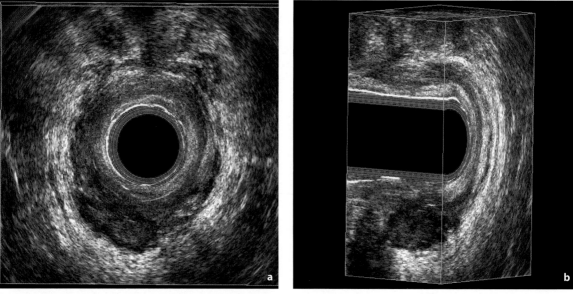

Fig. 59.9 Three-dimensional endoanal ultrasound with rotating probe. Acute intersphincteric abscess presenting as an area of low reflectivity in the posterior intersphincteric space, deep to the hyperechoic ring of the external anal sphincter. **a** Axial plane. **b** Longitudinal plane

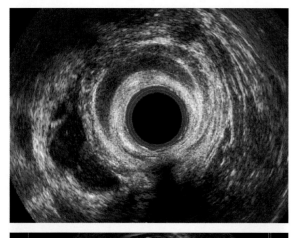

Fig. 59.10 Three-dimensional endoanal ultrasound with rotating probe. Acute abscess in the right ischioanal space in conjunction with a hypoechoic posterior trans-sphincteric tract

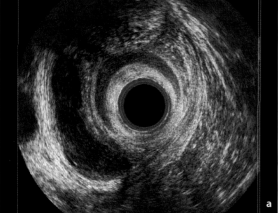

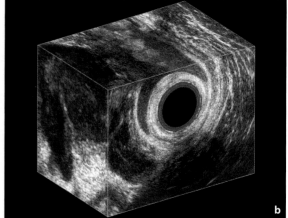

Fig. 59.11 Three-dimensional endoanal ultrasound with rotating probe. Acute supralevator abscess presenting as an area of low reflectivity in the right side of the anal canal, deep to the puborectalis muscle (**a**). The extension of the collection is more easily appreciated in the longitudinal plane (**b**)

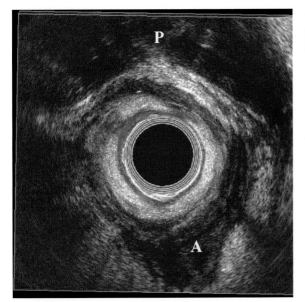

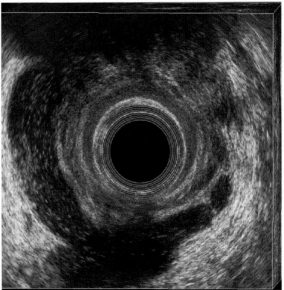

Fig. 59.12 Three-dimensional endoanal ultrasound with rotating probe. Acute left perirectal abscess (*A*). *P*, prostate gland

Fig. 59.13 Three-dimensional endoanal ultrasound with rotating probe. Horseshoe collection in the supralevator space

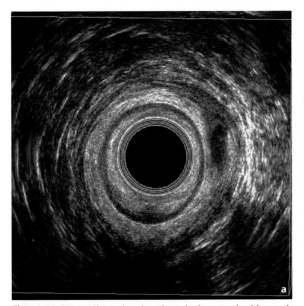

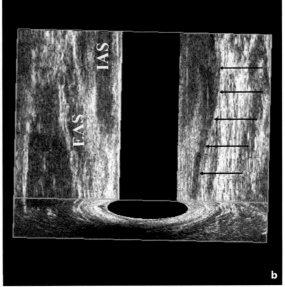

Fig. 59.14 Three-dimensional endoanal ultrasound with rotating probe. A hypoechoic area is present in the left intersphincteric space (3 o'clock) (**a**). Reconstruction in the coronal plane confirms an intersphincteric tract, appearing as a band of poor reflectivity (*arrows*). The tract extends through the intersphincteric space without traversing the external anal sphincter (*EAS*) (**b**). *IAS*, internal anal sphincter

medium or low, corresponding to the ultrasound level of the anal canal. The low trans-sphincteric tract traverses only the distal external sphincter third at the lower portion of the medium anal canal. Medium trans-sphincteric tract traverses both sphincters, external and internal, in the middle part of the medium anal canal (Fig. 59.16). High trans-sphincteric tract traverses both sphincters in the higher part of the medium anal canal, in the space below the puborectalis.

c. Suprasphincteric tract, which goes above or through the puborectalis level (Fig. 59.17). It can be very difficult to determine a suprasphincteric extension because EAUS is not able to visualize

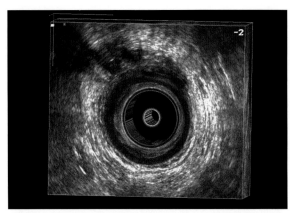

Fig. 59.15 Three-dimensional endoanal ultrasound with rotating probe. An anterior trans-sphincteric tract extending through the external sphincter in the right side of the anal canal

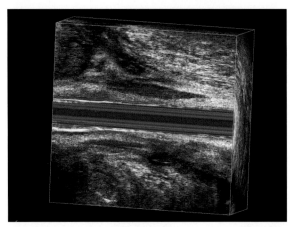

Fig. 59.16 Three-dimensional endoanal ultrasound with rotating probe. Longitudinal reconstruction of the anal canal allows identification of where the tract traverses the external sphincter. In this case, a posterior, medium trans-sphincteric fistula is displayed

the precise position of the levator plate that lies in the same plane as the ultrasound beam.

d. Extrasphincteric tract, which may be seen close to but more laterally placed around the external sphincter (Fig. 59.18).

Differentiation between granulated tracts and scars is sometimes difficult. Straight tracts are easily identified, but smaller and oblique tracts are more difficult to image. Secondary tracts, when present, are related to the main one and are classified as intersphincteric, trans-sphincteric, suprasphincteric, or extrasphincteric (Fig. 59.19). Similarly, horseshoe tracts, when identified, are categorized as intersphincteric, suprasphincteric, or extrasphincteric.

The exact location (radial site and anal canal level)

of the internal opening can be difficult to define, as the dentate line cannot be identified as a discrete anatomical entity on EAUS. It is assumed to lie at approximately mid-anal canal level, which is midway between the superior border of the puborectalis muscle and the most caudal extent of the subcutaneous external sphincter. According to this, the site of the internal opening is categorized as being above, at, or below the dentate line, or in the rectal ampulla. In addition, the site can also be characterized by the clock position, being classified from 1 o'clock to 12 o'clock. The internal opening can be identified as hypoechoic (when acute inflammation is present) or hyperechoic area (when chronically inflamed).

Initial experiences with EAUS [10] reported a good accuracy for the selective identification of fistula (91.7%) and abscess (75%) configurations. However, a significant number of the internal openings (33.3%) were not detected. Worse results in the identification of the internal opening were reported by Poen et al [7] (5.3% accuracy), and Deen et al [6] (11% accuracy). The most probable reason for the poor results in the identification of internal openings by EAUS is the ultrasonographic criteria used. Seow-Choen et al [5] described revised ultrasonographic criteria for identifying an internal opening, which included one or more of the following features: a hypoechoic breach of the subepithelial layer of the anorectum, a defect in the circular muscles of the internal anal sphincter, and a hypoechoic lesion of the normally hyperechoic longitudinal muscle abutting on the normally hypoechoic circular smooth muscle. In spite of the improvement in accuracy (73%) in identifying the internal openings, they found no significant difference between EAUS and digital examination. Cho [12] proposed the following endosonographic criteria to define the site of the internal opening: Criteria 1. an appearance of a root-like budding formed by the intersphincteric tract, which contacts the internal sphincter; Criteria 2. an appearance of a root-like budding with an internal sphincter defect; Criteria 3. a subepithelial breach connected to the intersphincteric tract through an internal sphincter defect. Using a combination of these three criteria, the author reported 94% sensitivity, 87% specificity, and 81% and 96% positive and negative predictive values.

The majority of problems while investigating primary tracts with EAUS occur because of the structural alterations of the anal canal and perianal muscles and tissues, which can overstage the fistula, or poor defi-

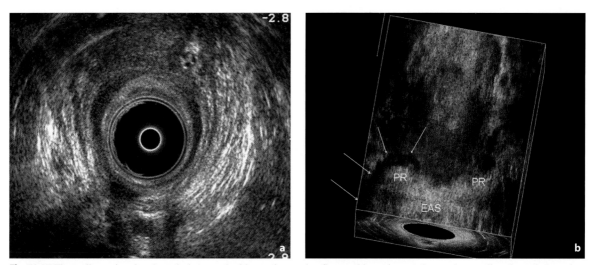

Fig. 59.17 Three-dimensional endoanal ultrasound with rotating probe. Suprasphincteric tract (*arrows*) extending through the pubo-rectalis muscle (*PR*). **a** Axial plane. **b** Coronal plane. *EAS*, external anal sphincter

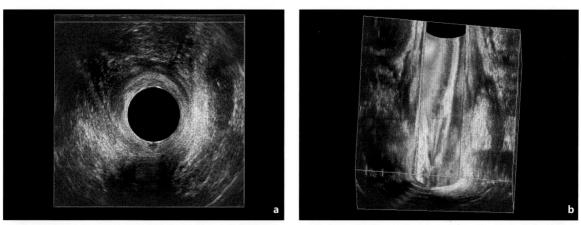

Fig. 59.18 Three-dimensional endoanal ultrasound with rotating probe. A left lateral extrasphincteric fistula, appearing as a hypoechoic area not involving the anal canal (**a**). The longitudinal extension of the tract and the direct communication between the perineum and rectum is identified in the coronal plane (**b**)

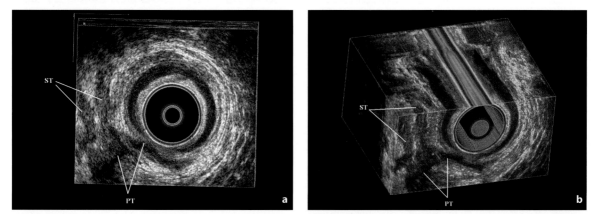

Fig. 59.19 Three-dimensional endoanal ultrasound with rotating probe. Posterior trans-sphincteric fistula (*PT*, primary tract) with two secondary trans-sphincteric tracts (*ST*, secondary tracts) extending through the ischioanal space (**a**). Reconstruction with volume rendering (**b**)

nition of the tract when filled with inflammatory tissue, which can downstage the fistula. The disappointing results of EAUS in diagnosing the extrasphincteric fistulae could be due to the echogenicity of the fistulae, especially those with a narrow lumen, which is practically identical to the fat tissue in the ischioanal fossa, and to the short focal length of the transducer, which prevents imaging of fistulae that are located at large distance from the anal canal. For this reason, performing ultrasonography after injecting 1.0–2.0 mL of 3% hydrogen peroxide (HPUS) through the external opening of the fistula appears to be particularly useful. This technique allows identification of tracts whose presence has not been definitively established, or distinction of an active fistulous tract from postsurgical or post-trauma scar tissue [8]. Gas is a strong ultrasound reflector, and after injection, fistula tracts become hy-

perechoic and the internal opening is identified as an echogenic breach at the submucosa (Fig. 59.20). Because the injected hydrogen peroxide often results in bubbling into the anal canal, which then acts as a barrier to the ultrasound wave, injection should be performed in two phases: an initial injection of a small amount of hydrogen peroxide, and a further injection at a greater pressure [11]. A disadvantage inherent to hydrogen peroxide injection is the very strong reflection that occurs at a gas/tissue interface, which blanks out any detail deep to this interface. The bubbles produced by hydrogen peroxide induce acoustic shadowing deep to the tract, so all information deep to the inner surface of the tract is lost. The reported diagnostic accuracy of HPUS ranges from 71% to 95% for primary tracts and from 63% to 96.1% for secondary tracts, while that of standard EAUS ranges from 50% to 91.7%

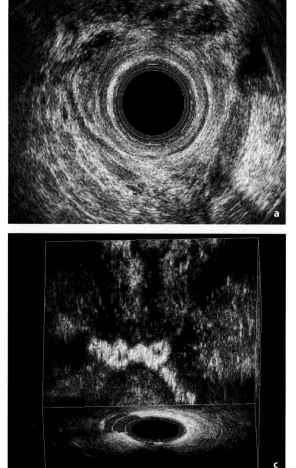

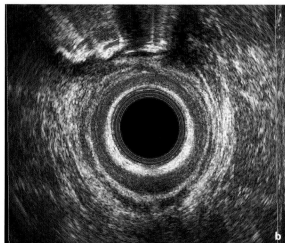

Fig. 59.20 Three-dimensional endoanal ultrasound with rotating probe. The fistulous tract is not clearly visible in this axial image (**a**). After hydrogen peroxide injection through an external orifice, an anterior trans-sphincteric fistula becomes evident as a hyperechoic tract extending through the external sphincter (**b**). Reconstruction in the coronal plane (**c**)

for the primary tract and from 60% to 68% for secondary tracts [7, 8, 13, 14]. The highest concordance is usually reported for primary trans-sphincteric fistulae, while the major diagnostic difficulty is still the adequate identification of primary supra- and extrasphincteric fistulae. Injection can also contribute to a more accurate identification of the internal opening (HPUS accuracy ranging from 48% to 96.6% vs. EAUS accuracy ranging from 5.3% to 93.5%) [13–15].

The availability of a three-dimensional (3D) imaging system has further improved the accuracy of EAUS. With this technique, the operator can follow the pathway of the fistulous tract along all the desired planes (axial, coronal, sagittal, oblique) (Figs. 59.15, 59.17, and 59.19). In addition, volume render mode can facilitate depiction of a tortuous fistula tract after hydrogen peroxide injection, due to the transparency and depth information (Fig. 59.21) [16]. Buchanan et al [17] reported a good accuracy of 3D-EAUS in detecting primary tracts (81%), secondary tracts (68%), and internal openings (90%) in 19 patients with recurrent or complex fistulae. The addition of hydrogen peroxide (3D-HPUS) did not improve these features (accuracies of 71%, 63% and 86%, respectively). Using 3D imaging, Ratto et al [14] reported an accuracy of 98.5% for primary tracts, 98.5% for secondary tracts, and 96.4% for internal openings, compared with 89.4%, 83.3%, and 87.9%, respectively, when the 2D system was used. Our experience [15, 16] on

57 patients with perianal fistulae confirmed that 3D reconstructions improved the accuracy of EAUS in the identification of internal opening compared to 2D-EAUS (89.5% vs. 66.7%; P = 0.0033). Primary tracts, secondary tracts, and abscesses were similarly evaluated by both procedures.

59.2.4 Magnetic Resonance Imaging

In recent years, magnetic resonance imaging (MRI) has emerged as a highly accurate technique in diagnosing perianal fistulae [13, 17]. Active tracts are filled with pus and granulation tissue and thus appear as hyperintense longitudinal structures on T2-weighted or STIR sequences.

Lunniss et al [18] found MRI to be accurate (88% of cases) for determining the presence and course of anal fistulae. Buchanan et al [17] showed that surgery guided by MRI can reduce further recurrence by about 75% in recurrent anal fistulae. They also found that preoperative MRI changed the scheduled surgical approach in 10% of patients presenting with primary fistulae [19].

Differences in detecting the fistulous tract have been described in relation to the technique used (Figs. 59.22, 59.23) [20, 21]. The best spatial resolution is achieved by using dedicated endoluminal anal coils. Their availability remains relatively restricted. Endoluminal coils

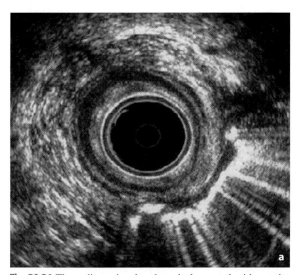
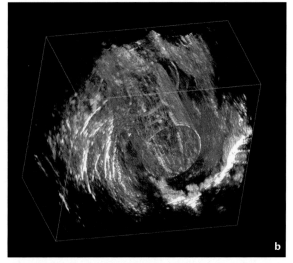

Fig. 59.21 Three-dimensional endoanal ultrasound with rotating probe. After hydrogen peroxide injection into a trans-sphincteric tract, reflections from gas bubbles produce an acoustic shadowing deep to the tract (**a**). To reduce this potential pitfall, rendering of 3D-imaging can facilitate following a tortuous fistula tract due to the transparency and depth information (**b**)

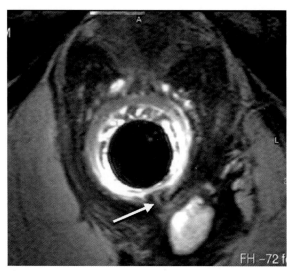

Fig. 59.22 Magnetic resonance with endoanal coil. A trans-sphincteric fistula is visualized in the left posterior aspect of the ischioanal fossa. The internal opening is demonstrated (*arrow*)

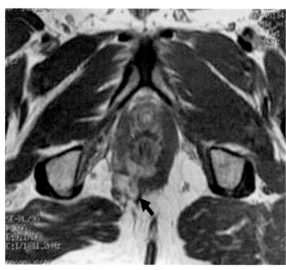

Fig. 59.23 Magnetic resonance with surface coil. A suprasphincteric fistula is diagnosed as a tract extending through the puborectalis (*arrow*)

are susceptible to motion artifact, but this can be reduced by careful patient preparation. A limitation of endoanal coil is the limited field of view (2–3 cm from the coil) [21], so fistulous extensions beyond this range can be missed. When extensive sepsis or supralevator sepsis is suspected, a pelvic phased array coil is more accurate.

De Souza et al [20] compared endoluminal and external phased array coils and found that while the endoluminal coil was superior for classification of the primary tract, extensions were better imaged using the superior field of view of the external coil. These results suggest clearly that a large field of view is necessary whenever extensions are suspected, for example in patients with recurrent fistula or Crohn's disease.

The high spatial resolution of endoluminal coils makes them ideal for demonstrating precisely the location and height of the internal opening, rather like EAUS, and they may have a special role for demonstrating anovaginal or rectovaginal fistulae, which are notoriously difficult to image. Where circumstances allow, it is likely that optimal examination will be achieved using a combination of both external and endoluminal coils.

The most valuable use of MRI is in the assessment of recurrent sepsis not visualized on EAUS [18–21]. A variety of investigators have directly compared EAUS with MRI, both with and without an endoanal

coil, and these comparisons have found EAUS variously superior [22], equivalent [23], or inferior [17]. West et al [13] reported that 3D-HPUS and endoanal MRI were equally adequate for the evaluation of perianal fistulae. The methods agreed in 88% of cases for the primary fistula tract, in 90% for the location of the internal opening, in 78% for secondary tracts, and in 88% for fluid collections. In most studies comparing EAUS and MRI, surgical findings have been used as the gold standard. This, however, may be discussed and questioned, especially for those patients who did not heal after surgery. The difficulty of defining a true reference standard for fistula-in-ano is related to the following potential source of bias: the operators who perform the assessments can have differing levels of experience with EAUS or with MRI and, similarly, the surgeons who perform the operations have different levels of experience. Buchanan et al [17] classified 108 primary tracks using clinical examination, EAUS, and MRI, and compared the findings to a reference standard that was based on ultimate clinical outcome. Digital evaluation correctly classified 61% of primary tracts in comparison to 81% for EAUS and 90% for MRI. While MRI was superior in every comparison made by the authors, EAUS was particularly adapt at correctly predicting the site of the internal opening, achieving this in 91% compared to 97% for MRI. Barker et al [24] showed that 9% of all fistulae do not heal, because fistulous tracts that were identified by endoanal MRI were not recognized during surgery. Therefore, using clinical outcome as the final arbiter can minimize potential biases. Because it is well established that the most common cause of fistula recurrence is infection that has been missed at surgical examination, patients should be followed-up to determine clinical outcome and to identify any patients who require further unplanned surgery because of a failure to heal or further recurrence. Fistula healing is, otherwise, the only definitive assurance that all infection has been identified and treated. Thus, if there is disagreement between findings at EAUS, MRI, and surgical examination, the findings associated to fistula healing should be assumed to be correct. This is defined as the outcome-derived reference standard [17]. Chapple et al [25] found that MRI classification of fistulae into simple and complex enhanced the chance of recurrence being predicted much more accurately than by EAUS alone (positive predictive value 73% vs. 57%). Successful surgery for perianal fistula is contingent upon accurate preoperative classification of the primary tract and its extensions. Sahni et al [26], using an "evidence-based medicine" method, assessed the optimal technique for fistula classification. MRI was found to be more sensitive (0.97) than clinical examination (0.75) but comparable to EAUS (0.92) for discriminating complex from simple fistula. The authors concluded that MRI is the optimal technique for discriminating complex from simple perianal fistula, although EAUS is superior to clinical examination, and may be used if MRI availability is restricted.

Anal endosonography has some clear advantages related to the fact that it is relatively cheap and simple to perform, it is rapid and well tolerated by patients and, unlike MRI, can be performed easily in the outpatient clinic or even on the ward since the machines are easily portable. It is vastly superior to digital examination and is therefore well worth performing. The major advantage of MRI over EAUS is the facility with which it can image extensions that would otherwise be missed since they can travel several centimeters from the primary tract. It is especially important to search for supralevator extensions, since these are not only difficult to detect but pose specific difficulties with treatment. Complex extensions are especially common in patients with recurrent fistulae or those who have Crohn's disease. It should also be borne in mind that MRI and EAUS provide complementary and additive information, and there are no disadvan-

tages to performing both procedures in the same patient where local circumstances, availability, and economics allow this.

59.3 Surgical Treatment of Anorectal Fistulae

The most appropriate management of anorectal sepsis is to eradicate the tract and drain the sepsis while preserving fecal continence. This aim must always be considered when planning treatment. It is fundamental to be cautious and fully inform patients regarding the risk of postoperative anal incontinence as well as recurrence. Success is influenced by the etiology of the fistula (cryptoglandular or related to Crohn's disease), the course of the tract (intersphincteric, trans-sphincteric, suprasphincteric, extrasphincteric), and the initial sphincter status (previous anal surgery, vaginal deliveries, radiation therapy). Multiple techniques have been used, including fistulotomy and fistulectomy, various types of flaps, instillation of fibrin sealant or stem cells, and plug positioning. This high number of available methods attests to the lack of universal success of any single treatment or any combination of treatments. The surgeon should be flexible at all times, given the multiple approaches, and therapy must be tailored to the individual circumstance.

59.3.1 Drainage

Anorectal abscess with evidence of induration, pain, cellulites, or other septic features requires immediate intervention with drainage [3]. Drainage is usually accomplished by making an incision over the area of maximum fluctuance, while also trying to stay close to the ring of external sphincter, while avoiding injury. This allows for the shortest fistula tract if one remains after drainage. The most common drainage methods are insertion of a mushroom-headed catheter into the abscess cavity or performing a wide cruciate incision on the skin over the cavity. Both will allow for complete drainage and prevent premature closure of the skin edges. Onaca et al [27] found in their series of 48 perirectal abscesses that the most common specific causes of early reoperation were inadequate drainage (48%), missed loculation (32%), and missed abscess (8%). This confirms the importance of preoperative imaging to evaluate the anorectal sepsis. Additionally, EAUS can also be performed in the operative suite.

59.3.2 Fistulotomy/Fistulectomy

Fistulotomy has been used for many hundreds of years. It is performed by dividing any muscle enveloped in the tract and laying it open from the internal to the external openings, without excision (Fig. 59.24). Fistule-ctomy is performed by excising the whole tract, without dividing the sphincter muscles (Fig. 59.25). Identification of the internal orifice of the fistula is essential for successful treatment with a fistulotomy/fistulectomy, as the most likely cause of recurrence is failure to identify and adequately deal with the internal opening. If the operative examination fails to demonstrate a drainage of pus from an anal gland, injection of hydrogen peroxide in the external orifice may be useful.

There is great variation in the reported results of fistulotomy/fistulectomy regarding recurrence (0–21%) and incontinence (0–82%) [28]. Chang and Lin [29] considered change in anal incontinence after fistulotomy performed for intersphincteric anal fistula. They studied 45 patients and found a significant decrease in maximal resting anal pressure 6 months after surgery. Division of the external sphincter should always be undertaken with caution, taking account of the sex of the patient, the position of the fistula, previous surgery, and associated diseases. The more proximally the track crosses the sphincter, the greater will be the resulting impairment of continence. Division of more than 30–50% of the external sphincter probably results in a significant functional deficit [3]. Preoperative imaging by MRI has shown that 50% of trans-sphinteric tracts pass obliquely upwards from the internal opening [2]. to the ischioanal fossa, indicating in these cases that more sphincter will be divided by fistulotomy than is suggested by the level of the internal opening [2]. Therefore, fistulotomy is appropriate treatment for intersphincteric fistula and low trans-sphincteric fistula.

Comparing fistulotomy with fistulectomy, the findings are that fistulectomy results in longer healing times and higher rates of impaired continence than fistulotomy (level I of evidence), and it has been recommended (grade A) that the fistula tract should be laid open rather than excised. Regarding fistulotomy in complex fistulae, there may be a limited role for fistulotomy with immediate sphincter reconstruction in the management of this type of fistula and there are no clear guidelines available. Perez et al [30] reported a prospective series of 35 patients who underwent fistulotomy with primary sphincter reconstruction for complex anal fistula (86% high trans-sphincteric; 14% supra- or extrasphincteric). Preoperatively, incontinence was present in 31.4%, and most patients had had previous surgery. Recurrence occurred in 6% and continence was improved after operation. Anal canal pressures improved postoperatively in the incontinent patients and no patient who was continent preoperatively was worse after surgery.

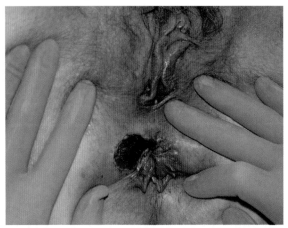

Fig. 59.24 Fistulotomy of a low trans-sphincteric fistula, performed by dividing sphincter muscles enveloped in the tract and laying it open from the internal to the external openings

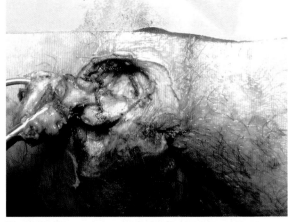

Fig. 59.25 Fistulectomy of a high trans-sphincteric fistula, performed by excising the whole tract, without dividing sphincter muscles

59.3.3 Fistulotomy in Acute Anorectal Sepsis

Treatment of the fistula (fistulotomy or seton positioning) at the time of primary abscess drainage is controversial. Immediate fistulotomy is associated with a lower recurrence rate than simple incision and drainage, and it has been recommended only in patients in whom the internal opening can be found, and the fistula is "simple" (superficial intersphincteric or low trans-sphincteric fistulae). Drainage alone is recommended for high trans-sphincteric or suprasphincteric fistulae [3].

Three studies, comparing initial treatment of drainage and fistulotomy with drainage alone, reported promising results [31–33]. Recurrence was higher with drainage only (Oliver et al [31], 29% vs. 0%; Ho et al [32], 25% vs. 0%; Cox et al [33], 44% vs. 31%), and fecal incontinence rates (Oliver et al [31], 0% vs. 2.8%; Ho et al [32] 0% vs. 0%; Cox et al [33], 21% vs. 21%) were comparable. These results were confirmed by Quah et al [34] in a meta-analysis of five randomized, controlled trials comparing drainage alone with drainage plus fistulotomy (when a fistula was identifiable). Immediate fistulotomy was associated with a significant reduction of recurrent fistula (83%; relative risk 0.17; P < 0.001) but not with significant difference in the risk of incontinence (relative risk 2.46; P = 0.140). While there was no conclusive evidence as to whether either treatment is better in the treatment of anorectal abscess/fistula, a reduction in recurrence of 83% seems more than adequate justification for immediate fistulotomy at the time of abscess drainage in certain situations.

The argument against immediate fistulotomy is based not only on the increased risk of impaired continence, but also on the fact that some individuals would have unnecessary surgery. In a retrospective study of 117 patients with an anorectal abscess treated by drainage alone, there was an overall recurrence rate of 47% (37% fistula formation; 10% recurrent abscess), showing that fistulotomy, if undertaken, would have resulted in unnecessary surgery in over 50% of patients [35]. In another series of 80 patients with ischiorectal abscess, 47.5% were treated by drainage and immediate fistulotomy, with persisting sepsis in 21% compared with 44% after drainage alone [33]. The available data from the literature indicate that immediate fistulotomy at the time of drainage

should be advised in patients in whom the internal opening can be found and where the fistula is submucosal or intersphincteric. Abscesses associated with a more complicated fistula should be simply drained, and subsequent surgery reserved for patients who develop continuing or further sepsis or fistula.

59.3.4 Setons

An inert seton can be inserted through the tract and tied loosely for continued sepsis drainage, or gradually tightened as a cutting seton as definitive treatment (Fig. 59.26). Loose setons, which are later removed, are particularly useful to effectively treat sepsis and to preserve the anus in patients who already complain of incontinence symptoms, in cases of recurrent or Crohn's-related fistulae, or in females with anterior fistula and a history of vaginal deliveries. However, Buchanan et al [36] reported that, at long term follow-up, 80% of patients had recurrent or persistent sepsis after removing a loose seton. Results were similar for cryptoglandular and Crohn's-related causes. Therefore, the aims of a loose seton are to achieve long-term drainage of the fistula to prevent acute septic exacerbations and to allow any secondary tract(s) to heal around the seton lying along the primary tract, before definitive surgery is subsequently undertaken. As part of a staged fistulotomy, in which the sphincter is divided in stages, the seton is used to allow healing of the divided sphincter segment before further division [37]. Garcia-Aguilar et al [38] reported the outcome of 47 patients with high trans-sphincteric (39), suprasphincteric (3), or

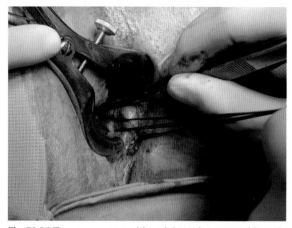

Fig. 59.26 Two setons are positioned through a trans-sphincteric fistula with an external opening and two internal openings

extrasphincteric (5) fistulae treated by two-stage fistulotomy, a loose seton being left in place for at least 6 weeks before the second stage of laying open the tract. There were four recurrences, but 31 patients had imperfect control postoperatively, and 12 patients were incontinent to stool. The frequency and degree of incontinence were, however, no different from those observed in a smaller cohort of 12 patients with similar fistulae treated by the cutting seton method. Williams et al [39] reviewed the experience of seton usage at the University of Minnesota over a 6-year period. Of 24 patients with a cryptoglandular high fistula treated by the two-stage seton technique, there were two recurrences, one with major incontinence. Minor incontinence was reported by 54% of patients.

The loose seton can be also used as a therapeutic strategy in its own right. It is evident from the work of Parks and Stitz [40] that some patients with a high fistula can be treated successfully without recourse to further sphincter division, if effective eradication of intersphincteric space sepsis is achieved and if wounds around the seton heal leaving only the primary track. Kennedy and Zegarra [41] used the same strategy in 32 patients with a high trans- or suprasphincteric fistula, and achieved healing in 25 (78%) without any division of the external sphincter. They observed slower healing rates for posterior than for anterior fistulae. Only 38% of patients were successfully treated and reported no change in continence postoperatively, although none was incontinent to formed stool.

Controversial results are reported in the literature regarding the occurrence of incontinence symptoms using a cutting seton to treat trans-sphincteric fistula. As with all seton techniques, the cutting seton has been mainly used when the risk to continence of a one-stage fistulotomy is felt to be high. Recurrence or persistence rates of 0–18%, using a variety of seton materials and different methods and frequency of seton tightening, have been reported. Disturbance of fine control is common, and in seven studies major incontinence in over 10% of patients was described [37]. Treating 32 patients with cryptoglandular fistula (81% trans-sphincteric) with a cutting seton, Hasegawa et al [42] found that 29% of fistulae recurred and continence disturbances occurred in 54% of patients. Women who had had previous vaginal deliveries complained of major incontinence. The authors concluded that the use of a cutting seton should be avoided in women with an anterior fistula and a history of a vaginal delivery. Isbister and Sanea [43] reported that the use of a cutting seton as treatment of trans-sphincteric fistula was associated with new onset of gas incontinence. Considering patients who were fully continent before surgery, 9.5% were significantly incontinent to gas and 21.4% were occasionally incontinent to gas after the procedure. Mentes et al [44] used a cutting seton for trans-sphincteric fistula involving more than 50% of the sphincter complex. Although only one fistula recurred (5%), 20% of patients reported worsening of anal continence.

59.3.5 Advancement Flaps

High trans-sphincteric or suprasphincteric fistulae or anterior fistula in women may predispose to fecal incontinence if a fistulotomy is performed. To treat these fistulae, advancement flaps should be used. There are multiple variations on the technique. The "advancement rectal flap" involves mobilization of the mucosal and submucosal layers of the rectal wall. The base of the flap must be wide enough (usually twice the width of the apex) to ensure adequate blood supply to the tip of the flap. The flap is raised and the fistula tract cored out. The fistula is then closed on the rectal side with absorbable sutures. The tip of the flap is trimmed to eliminate the area where the fistula had gone through the mobilized tissue of the flap. The flap is advanced down, while avoiding any tension, and sewn to the neodentate line with absorbable sutures. The external opening is left open and may need to be enlarged to ensure adequate drainage. Relative contraindications to the transanal rectal flap include the presence of proctitis, especially in patients with Crohn's disease, undrained sepsis and/or persisting secondary tracts, rectovaginal fistula with a diameter > 3 cm, malignant or radiation-related fistula, fistula of < 4 weeks' duration, stricture of the anorectum, severe sphincter defect, and severe perianal scarring because of previous fistula surgery [45-47].

Zimmerman et al [45] reported that 69% of trans-sphincteric fistulae healed at a median follow-up of 14 months. Ortiz and Marzo [46] reported a recurrence rate of 7% after performing endorectal advancement flaps for high trans-sphincteric or suprasphincteric fistulae. When examining factors affecting success, the level of the fistula did not affect outcome. Continence disturbance was observed in 8% of cases after the surgery. Worse results were reported by Schouten et al [47], who found a recurrence rate of 25% with a disturbance in continence of 35%. A factor associated with success of the endorectal advancement flap was prior drainage with seton.

The creation of the advancement flap may comprise the rectal mucosa only or involve full transection of the rectal wall. A comparison between full-thickness flaps and mucosal flaps was made by Dubsky et al [48], to analyze the defining elements of successful fistula treatment: recurrence rates and anal continence. A retrospective review of 54 consecutive patients with high anal fistula of cryptoglandular origin showed that 24% of all patients suffered from a recurrence. Patients with four or more previous anal surgeries were at highest risk for failure. Recurrence occurred in 5% of the full-thickness vs. 35.3% of the mucosal flap group. The full-thickness endorectal advancement flaps gave an improvement of recurrence rates without higher incontinence rates. To ensure the healing of anal fistulae with a mucosal advancement flap, van der Hagen et al [49] used, in addition, autologous platelet-rich plasma and reported a 90% rate of success at 26 months' follow-up.

The Association of Coloproctology of Great Britain and Ireland (ACPGBI) recommends transanal advancement flap for the treatment of an anal fistula when simple fistulotomy is thought likely to result in impaired continence [37]. At present, rectal advancement is the gold standard for the surgical treatment of high trans-sphincteric perianal fistulae.

Another technique is to perform an "anocutaneous advancement flap" (Fig. 59.27). This procedure has a similar success rate and should be considered an alternative to rectal advancement flap for a high fistula. Using this type of repair in 23 patients with a trans-sphincteric fistula, Zimmerman et al [45] reported successful closure in 46% and deterioration of continence in 30% of cases. Success was inversely correlated with the number of prior attempts at treatment. Better results were reported by Hossack et al [50] (94% success with additionally postoperative continence scores improved in 70% of patients), and Sungurtekin et al [51] (91% success rate with no changes of continence and minimal complications).

59.3.6 Fibrin Sealant

In the treatment algorithm of complex anal fistulae, the use of fibrin glue injection as an alternative to cutting

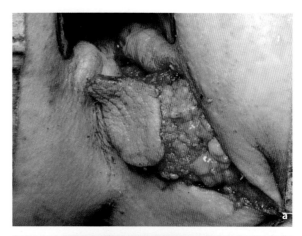
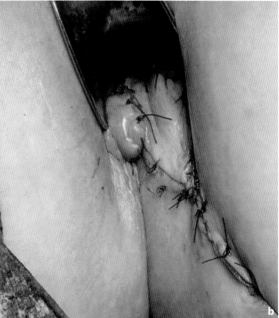

Fig. 59.27 Anocutaneous advancement flap (**a**, **b**)

setons and advancement flaps should be considered (Fig. 59.28). It is simple and carries a low risk of morbidity and can be repeated [37]. However, the success rates reported in the literature are not high at long-term follow-up. At one year, Cintron et al [52] reported that 64% of patients healed after injection of commercial fibrin sealant. Most recurrences occurred by three months, but some continued to recur up to 11 months after treatment. Sentovich [53] observed that 60% of 48 fistulae were closed at a median follow-up of 22 months. Retreatment with fibrin glue increased the closure rate to 69%. Loungnarath et al [54] found that durable healing was achieved only in 31% of cases. Initial healing was

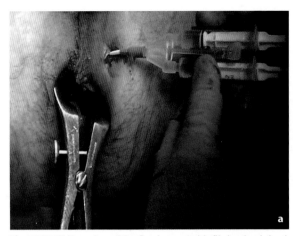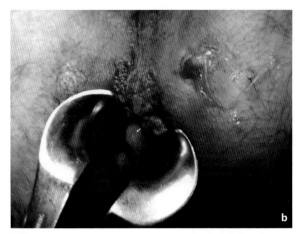

Fig. 59.28 Obliteration of the fistula tract with fibrin glue injection (**a, b**)

common but recurrence was frequent, with most occurring within 3 months. The success rate did not change if patients had failed previous treatment. van Koperen et al [55] conducted a retrospective study to assess the additional value of fibrin glue in combination with transanal advancement flap, compared to advancement flap alone, for the treatment of high trans-sphincteric fistulae of cryptoglandular origin. The overall recurrence rate was 26%. Recurrence rates for advancement flap alone vs. the combination with glue were 13% vs. 56% (P = 0.014) in the group without previous fistula surgery, and 23% vs. 41% (P = 0.216) in the group with previous fistula surgery. The authors concluded that the obliteration of the fistula tract with fibrin glue was associated with worse outcome after rectal advancement flap. Singer et al [56] randomized patients to three groups prospectively: group one received injection of antibiotic plus the sealant, group two had surgical closure of the internal opening, and group three had both. At a mean follow-up of 27 months, initial healing was 21%, 40%, and 31% respectively (P = 0.38). Therefore, neither of these two changes in the technique improved the success rate.

Jain et al [57] reported good results using cyanoacrylate glue to treat complex fistulae. Seventeen out of 20 patients healed with primary injection, two patients required one more injection without signs of discharge thereafter, and one patient with two external openings continued to discharge from one opening even after two injections. Barillari et al [58] reported 71.4% cumulative healing with only one treatment and 90.2% overall healing after more than one session, without any sign of recurrence after 18 months of follow-up.

59.3.7 Anal Plug

Fistula track obliteration with anal plug (AFP) represents a novel approach for complex fistulae. Surgisis® (Cook Surgical, Inc., Bloomington, IN, USA) is a bioabsorbable xenograft made of lyophilized porcine intestinal submucosa: it has a good resistance to infection, produces no foreign body or giant cell reaction, provides a biological scaffold for native cell tissue repair rather than obliteration, and is completely resorbed leaving behind native, site-specific tissue after a period of three months.

To minimize the risk of recurrence, a seton should be positioned for some weeks until there is no evidence of acute inflammation, purulence, or excessive drainage. The debridement, curettage, or brushing of the tract should be carefully performed to facilitate insertion of the plug. The longer the tract is, the lower the risk of plug displacement. A suture is tied around the tail of the AFP for pulling it from the internal opening through the tract to the external opening (Fig. 59.29). Any excess plug should be trimmed at the level of the internal opening (the wide end) and sutured incorporating the underlying internal anal sphincter. The excess external plug should be trimmed flush with the skin without fixation. The external opening is left open to allow continued drainage of the fistula tract. Complete obstruction of the external opening may result in accumulation of fluid, infection, or abscess.

The use of AFP was first reported by Johnson et al [59] in a comparative study between fibrin glue and plug. In this early experience, the conical plug was manually fashioned. Use of the plug was successful in 87%

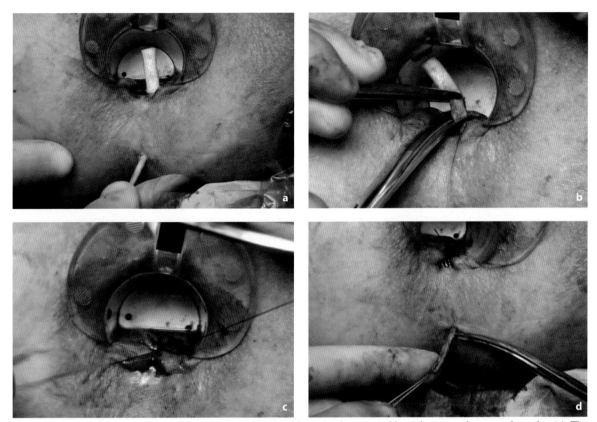

Fig. 59.29 An anal plug is pulled from the internal opening through a posterior trans-sphincteric tract to the external opening (**a**). The head of the plug is cut (**b**) and covered, passing a suture through the mucosa, submucosa, and underlying deep tissue layers (**c**). The narrow end of the plug is cut so that no material protrudes from the secondary opening. The external opening of the tract is left unobstructed to allow continued drainage (**d**)

of patients compared with 40% of the fibrin glue group. Connor et al [60] reported 80% and 83% healing in Crohn's and cryptoglandular anorectal fistulae, respectively, with a higher closure rate in patients with single tract than complex fistulae with multiple primary openings. Most failures occurred during the first 30 days and resulted from dislodgement of the plug due to excessive activity of the patient or inadequate suturing technique. Short tracks may be a critical indication for the AFP procedure: in particular, female patients with straight short anterior anal or anovaginal fistulae and hypermobile perineum may not be optimal candidates because of the higher risk of plug expulsion. In cases of multiple fistulae, each track should be treated independently with a plug, even in the case of fistulae sharing a common internal orifice. Schwandner et al [61] evaluated the efficacy of AFP for the closure of cryptoglandular and Crohn's disease-associated trans-sphincteric anorectal fistulae. The overall success rate was 61% at 9 months

postoperatively, 45.5% in cryptoglandular fistulae, and 85.7% in trans-sphincteric fistulae associated with Crohn's disease. In our experience [62], 60% of patients and 70% of tracts may be treated rapidly, effectively, and cosmetically with the AFP procedure, at the first attempt. The patients' chance of cure may rise to 72%, considering that the procedure may be repeated easily without major tissue manipulation and that in some recurrent cases the plug acts anyway as a support to partial healing, thus leading to fistulotomy without continence impairment. These results are comparable with the experiences of other centers [63, 64]. Thekkinkattil et al [63] examined plug efficacy in a wide spectrum of patients with anorectal, rectovaginal, and pouch vaginal fistulae. The complex nature of the fistula was the main reason for a low success rate (44% of complete healing). Chung at al [64] compared the outcomes of AFP, fibrin glue, advancement flap, and seton drain insertion. Healing rates were 59.3%, 39.1%, 60.4%, and 32.6%, respectively (P < 0.0001), with AFP and anal flap having similar results. Adamina et al [65] conducted a cost-effectiveness analysis showing a fistula healing rate of 50% with AFP vs. 33% with endoanal flap, and demonstrated that AFP is a cost-saving procedure for complex anal fistulae. Reports from various centers, however, do not give consistent results and some authors show negative experiences comparing AFP with advancement flap. Wang et al [66] reported 34% of fistula closure for plugs and 62% for flaps (P = 0.045) and similar results were reported by Christoforidis et al [67], with 32% of fistula closure for plugs and 63% for flaps (P = 0.008). A consensus conference concluded that AFP is a reasonable alternative for the treatment of anal fistula, but should not preclude proceeding to further management options [68]. To achieve the highest possibility of success, accurate patient selection, absence of local infection, and meticulous technique are required. It was recognized, however, that despite apparent healing the rate of subsequent recurrence is unknown.

59.3.8 Other Treatments

Autologous stem cell transplantation for fistula has been reported by Garcia-Olmo et al [69]. These authors conducted a phase II multicenter, randomized controlled trial to investigate the effectiveness and safety of stem cells, obtained from liposuction of abdominal fat, in the treatment of complex perianal cryptoglandular and Crohn's-associated fistulae. Patients were treated by fibrin glue or fibrin glue plus 20 million stem cells. Fistula healing was 71% in the group who received stem cells in addition to fibrin glue, compared with 16% of patients who received fibrin glue alone (P < 0.001). Stem cells were also more effective than fibrin glue alone in patients with a suprasphincteric fistulous tract (P = 0.001). The recurrence rate at one-year follow-up was 17.6 %.

Crohn's-related anal fistulae present a special challenge. Fistulotomy can be performed for superficial fistula in patients with quiescent anal and rectal disease; however, a loose seton is a better choice if continence may be compromised. Advancement flap can be done if the tissue has minimal to no evidence of active Crohn's disease in the anus and rectum (success rate in about 50% of cases). The use of new agents such as infliximab, to reduce the inflammation and active disease, may be successful [70]. Guidi et al

[71] evaluated the efficacy of combined treatment with infliximab and setons for complex perianal fistulae in Crohn's disease. Perianal sepsis was eradicated when necessary and setons were placed before infliximab therapy and removed after ultrasonographic evidence of healing of fistulous tracts. Patients received a mean of 10 ± 2.3 infliximab infusions. At week 6, all patients showed a reduction in mean Crohn's disease activity index (P < 0.005) and perianal disease activity index (P < 0.0001). Complete fistula response was achieved in eight of nine patients. Clinical and EAUS responses persisted at 19.4 ± 8.8 months (range 3–28 months) in five of these patients.

The use of a stoma when doing a complicated repair should also be considered. However, a stoma does not guarantee success and no study has definitely found it offers an advantage.

References

1. Parks AG, Gordon PH, Hardcastle JD. A classification of fistula-in-ano. Br J Surg 1976;63:61–12.
2. Buchanan GN, Williams AB, Bartram CI et al. Potential clinical implications of direction of a trans-sphincteric anal fistula track. Br J Surg 2003;90:1250–1255.
3. Whiteford MH, Kilkenny III J, Hyman N et al. The standards practice task force, the American Society of Colon and Rectal Surgeons. Practice parameters for the treatment of perianal abscess and fistula-in-ano (Revised). Dis Colon Rectum 2005;48:1337–1342.
4. Goodsall DH. Anorectal fistula. In: Goodsall DH, Miles WE (eds) Diseases of the anus and rectum, part I. Longmans, Green & Co, London, 1900, p 92.
5. Seow-Choen F, Burnett S, Bartram CI, Nicholls RJ. Comparison between anal endosonography and digital examination in the evaluation of anal fistulae. Br J Surg 1991;78:445–447.
6. Deen KI, Williams JG, Hutchinson R et al. Fistulas in ano: endoanal ultrasonographic assessment assists decision making for surgery. Gut 1994; 35:391–394.
7. Poen AC, Felt-Bersma RJF, Eijsbouts QA et al. Hydrogen peroxide-enhanced transanal ultrasound in the assessment of fistula-in-ano. Dis Colon Rectum 1998;41:1147–1152.
8. Ratto C, Gentile E, Merico M et al. How can the assessment of fistula-in-ano be improved? Dis Colon Rectum 2000;43:1375–1382.
9. Kuijpers HC, Schulpen T. Fistulography for fistula-in-ano: is it useful? Dis Colon Rectum 1985;28:103–104.
10. Law PJ, Talbot RW, Bartram CI, Northover JMA. Anal endosonography in the evaluation of perianal sepsis and fistula in ano. Br J Surg 1989;76:752–755.
11. Santoro GA, Ratto C. Accuracy and reliability of endoanal ultrasonography in the evaluation of perianal abscesses and fistula-in-ano. In: Santoro GA, Di Falco G. Benign anorectal diseases. Sprinter-Verlag Italia, Milan, 2006, pp 141–157.

12. Cho DY. Endosonographic criteria for an internal opening of fistula-in-ano. Dis Colon Rectum 1999;42:515–518.

13. West RL, Dwarkasing S, Felt-Bersma RJF et al. Hydrogen peroxide-enhanced three-dimensional endoanal ultrasonography and endoanal magnetic resonance imaging in evaluating perianal fistulas: agreement and patient preference. Eur J Gastroenterol Hepat 2004;16:1319–1324.

14. Ratto C, Grillo E, Parello A et al. Endoanal ultrasound-guided surgery for anal fistula. Endoscopy 2005;37:1–7.

15. Santoro GA, Ratto C, Di Falco G. Three-dimensional reconstructions improve the accuracy of endoanal ultrasonography in the identification of internal openings of anal fistulas. Colorectal Dis 2004;6(suppl 2):P214.

16. Santoro GA, Fortling B. The advantages of volume rendering in three-dimensional endosonography of the anorectum. Dis Colon Rectum 2007;50:359–368.

17. Buchanan GN, Halligan S, Bartram CI et al. Clinical examination, endosonography and MR imaging in preoperative assessment of fistula in ano: comparison with outcome-based reference standard. Radiology 2004;233:674–681.

18. Lunniss PJ, Barker PG, Sultan AH et al. Magnetic resonance imaging of fistula-in-ano. Dis Colon Rectum 1994;37:708–718.

19. Buchanan G, Halligan S, Williams A et al. Effect of MRI on clinical outcome of recurrent fistula-in-ano. Lancet 2002;360:1661–1662.

20. deSouza NM, Gilderdale DJ, Coutts GA et al. MRI of fistula-in-ano: a comparison of endoanal coil with external phased array coil techniques. J Comput Assist Tomogr 1998;22:357–363.

21. Halligan S, Bartram CI. MR imaging of fistula in ano: are endoanal coils the gold standard? AJR 1998;171:407–412.

22. Orsoni P, Barthet M, Portier F et al. Prospective comparison of endosonography, magnetic resonance imaging and surgical findings in anorectal fistula and abscess complicating Crohn's disease. Br J Surg 1999;86:360–364.

23. Schwartz DA, Wiersema MJ, Dudiak KM et al. A comparison of endoscopic ultrasound, magnetic resonance imaging, and exam under anesthesia for evaluation of Crohn's perianal fistulas. Gastroenterology 2001;121:1064–1072.

24. Barker PG, Lunniss PJ, Armstrong P et al. Magnetic resonance imaging of fistula in ano: technique, interpretation and accuracy. Clin Radiol 1994;49:7–13.

25. Chapple KS, Spencer JA, Windsor AC et al. Prognostic value of magnetic resonance imaging in the management of fistula-in-ano. Dis Colon Rectum 2000;43:511–516.

26. Sahni VA, Ahmad R, Burling D. Which method is best for imaging of perianal fistula? Abdom Imaging 2008;33:26–30.

27. Onaca N, Hirshberg A, Adar R. Early reoperation for perirectal abscess: a preventable complication. Dis Colon Rectum 2001;45:710–711.

28. Westerterp M, Volkers NA, Poolman RW et al. Anal fistulotomy between Skylla and Charybdis. Colorectal Dis 2003;5:549–551.

29. Chang SC, Lin JK. Change in anal continence after surgery for intersphincteral anal fistula: a functional and manometric study. Int J Colorectal Dis 2003;18:111–115.

30. Perez F, Arroyo A, Serrano P et al. Fistulotomy with primary sphincter reconstruction in the management of complex fistula-in-ano: prospective study of clinical and manometric results. J Am Coll Surg 2005;200:897–903.

31. Oliver I, Lacueva FJ, Vicente FP et al. Randomized clinical trial comparing simple drainage of anorectal abscess with and without fistula track treatment. Int J Colorectal Dis 2003;18:107–110.

32. Ho YH, Tan M, Chui CH et al. Randomized controlled trial of primary fistulotomy with drainage alone for perianal abscesses. Dis Colon Rectum 1997;40:1435–1438.

33. Cox SW, Senagore AJ, Luchtefeld MA, Mazier WP. Outcome after incision and drainage with fistulotomy for ischiorectal abscess. Am J Surg 1997;63:686–689.

34. Quah HM, Tang CL, Eu KW et al. Meta-analysis of randomized clinical trials comparing drainage alone vs. primary sphincter-cutting procedures for anorectal abscess and fistula. Int J Colorectal Dis 2005;30:1–8.

35. Vasilevsky CA, Gordon PH. The incidence of recurrent abscesses or fistula-in-ano following anorectal suppuration. Dis Colon Rectum 1984;27:126–130.

36. Buchanan GN, Owen HA, Torkington J et al. Long-term outcome following loose-seton technique for external sphincter preservation in complex anal fistula. Br J Surg 2004;91:476–480.

37. Williams JG, Farrands PA, Williams AB et al. The treatment of anal fistula: ACPGBI position statement. Colorectal Dis 2007;9(suppl. 4):18–50.

38. Garcia-Aguilar J, Belmonte C, Wong DW et al. Cutting seton versus two-stage seton fistulotomy in the surgical management of high anal fistula. Br J Surg 1998;85:243–245.

39. Williams JG, MacLeod CA, Rothenberger DA et al. Seton treatment of high anal fistulae. Br J Surg 1991;78: 1159–1161.

40. Parks AG, Stitz RW. The treatment of high fistula-in-ano. Dis Colon Rectum 1976;19:487–499.

41. Kennedy HL, Zegarra JP. Fistulotomy without external sphincter division for high anal fistulae. Br J Surg 1990;77: 898–901.

42. Hasegawa H, Radley S, Keighley MR. Long-term results of cutting seton fistulotomy. Acta Chir Iugoslavica 2000; 47:19–21.

43. Isbister WH, Sanea N. The cutting seton: an experience at King Faisal Specialist Hospital. Dis Colon Rectum 2001;44:722–727.

44. Mentes BB, Oktemer S, Tezcaner T et al. Elastic one-stage cutting seton for the treatment of high anal fistulas: preliminary results. Tech Coloproctol 2004;8:159–162.

45. Zimmerman DD, Briel JW, Gosselink MP, Schouten WR. Anocutaneous advancement flap repair of transsphincteric fistulas. Dis Colon Rectum 2001;44:1474–1480.

46. Ortiz H, Marzo J. Endorectal flap advancement repair and fistulectomy for high trans-sphincteric and suprasphincteric fistulas. Br J Surg 2000;87:1680–1683.

47. Schouten WR, Zimmerman DD, Briel JW. Transanal advancement flap repair of transsphincteric fistulas. Dis Colon Rectum 1999;42:1419–1423.

48. Dubsky PC, Stift A, Friedl J et al. Endorectal advancement flaps in the treatment of high anal fistula of cryptoglandular origin: full-thickness vs. mucosal-rectum flaps. Dis Colon Rectum 2008;51:852–857.

49. van der Hagen SJ, Baeten CG, Soeters PB, van Gemert WG. Autologous platelet derived grow factors (platelet rich plasma) as an adjunct to mucosal advancement flap in high cryptoglandular peri-anal fistulae: a pilot study. Colorectal Dis 2009;3 July epub ahead of print.

50. Hossack T, Solomon MJ, Young JM. Ano-cutaneous flap repair for complex and recurrent supra-sphincteric anal fistula. Colorectal Dis 2005;7:187–192.

51. Sungurtekin U, Sungurtekin H, Kabay B et al. Anocutaneous V-Y advancement flap for the treatment of complex perianal fistula. Dis Colon Rectum 2004;47:2178–2183.

52. Cintron JR, Park JJ, Orsay CP et al. Repair of fistulas-in-ano using fibrin adhesive: long-term follow-up. Dis Colon Rectum 2000;43:944–949.

53. Sentovich SM. Fibrin glue for anal fistulas: long-term results. Dis Colon Rectum 2003;46:498–502.

54. Loungnarath R, Dietz DW, Mutch MG et al. Fibrin glue treatment of complex anal fistulas has low success rate. Dis Colon Rectum 2004;47:432–436.

55. van Koperen PJ, Wind J, Bemelman WA, Slors JF. Fibrin glue and transanal rectal advancement flap for high transsphincteric perianal fistulas; is there any advantage? Int J Colorectal Dis 2008;23:697–701.

56. Singer M, Cintron J, Nelson R et al. Treatment of fistulas-in-ano with fibrin sealant in combination with intra-adhesive antibiotics and/or surgical closure of the internal fistula opening. Dis Colon Rectum 2005;48:799–808.

57. Jain SK, Kaza RC, Pahwa M, Bansal S. Role of cyanoacrylate in the management of low fistula in ano: a prospective study. Int J Colorectal Dis 2008;23:355–358 .

58. Barillari P, Basso L, Larcinese A et al. Cyanoacrylate glue in the treatment of ano-rectal fistulas. Int J Colorectal Dis 2006;21:791–794.

59. Johnson EK, Gaw JU, Armstrong DN. Efficacy of anal fistula plug vs. fibrin glue in closure of anorectal fistulas. Dis Colon Rectum 2006;49:371–376.

60. Connor LO, Champagne BJ, Ferguson MA et al. Efficacy of anal fistula plug in closure of Crohn's anorectal fistulas. Dis Colon Rectum 2006;49:1–5.

61. Schwandner O, Stadler F, Dietl O et al. Initial experience on efficacy in closure of cryptoglandular and Crohn's transsphincteric fistulas by the use of the anal fistula plug. Int J Colorectal Dis 2008;23:319–324.

62. Lenisa L, Rusconi A, Mascheroni L et al. Obliterative treatment for cryptoglandular fistula with anal plug. Does it work in Europe? Colorectal Dis 2007;9(suppl 3):54.

63. Thekkinkattil DK, Botterill I, Ambrose NS et al. Efficacy of the anal fistula plug in complex anorectal fistulae. Colorectal Dis 2009;11:584–587.

64. Chung W, Kazemi P, Ko D et al. Anal fistula plug and fibrin glue versus conventional treatment in repair of complex anal fistulas. Am J Surg 2009;197:604–608.

65. Adamina M, Hoch JS, Burnstein MJ. To plug or not to plug: A cost-effectiveness analysis for complex anal fistula. Surgery 2010;147:72-78.

66. Wang JY, Garcia-Aguilar J, Sternberg JA et al. Treatment of transsphincteric anal fistulas: are fistula plugs an acceptable alternative? Dis Colon Rectum 2009;52:692–697.

67. Christoforidis D, Pieh MC, Madoff RD, Mellgren AF. Treatment of transsphincteric anal fistulas by endorectal advancement flap or collagen fistula plug: a comparative study. Dis Colon Rectum 2009;52:18–22.

68. Abcarian H, Bailey HR, Birnbaum EH et al. The surgisis AFPTM anal fistula plug: report of a consensus conference. Colorectal Dis 2007;10:17–20.

69. Garcia-Olmo D, Herreros D, Pascual I et al. Expanded adipose-derived stem cells for the treatment of complex perianal fistula: a phase II clinical trial. Dis Colon Rectum 2009;52:79–86.

70. Present DH, Rutgeers P, Targan S et al. Infliximab for the treatment of fistulas in patients with Crohn's disease. N Engl J Med 1999;340:1398–1405.

71. Guidi L, Ratto C, Semeraro S et al. Combined therapy with infliximab and seton drainage for perianal fistulizing Crohn's disease with anal endosonographic monitoring: a single-centre experience. Tech Coloproctol 2008;12:111–117.

Invited Commentary

Mauro Cervigni

There is nothing more physically and psychologically disabling than the aura of incontinence of urine, gas, and fecal matter. There still remains controversy as to the best primary surgical corrective technique but an even more challenging decision is the approach to the patient who has failed corrective surgery. Before any decision, a precise evaluation is mandatory to: establish the underlying etiology, define the presence and site of the fistula, and identify a concomitant sphincter deficit. The correct timing of a repair is controversial but the decision can be simplified by determining two essential factors. The first is a determination of the overall nutritional health of the patient (especially in the third world population), the second relates to the health of the local tissue, which must be soft, pliable, non-edematous, and uninvolved with active inflammatory bowel disease. Those criteria may be useful to determine if a repair should be immmediate or require a delay of several months. Repairs can be performed through a rectal (mucosal advancement flap, layered closure), vaginal (layered closure, inversion of fistula), perineal (sphincteroplasty, muscle gracilis/ bulbocavernosus interposition), or transabdominal approach. Simple fistulae rarely require a defunctioning stoma or a muscle interposition graft. The selection of the best primary repair may depend upon the indi-

vidual surgeon's experience and preference, but there are potential advantages of each of the techniques. Complex fistulae are best managed according to the specific etiology; decision analysis should incorporate answers to the following questions:

a) should the same type of repair be repeated?
b) does the patient need a stoma?
c) should a muscle interposition be added to the repair?

Firstly, a local repair with a mucosal advancement flap should be considered. But in the case of subsequent unsuccessful repairs, a loop ileostomy should be deferred unless these further attempts fail.

Any subsequent attempt should include a defunctioning stoma, which may be combined with a further local repair, gracilis muscle interposition, or alternatively a transabdominal approach with colo-anal anastomosis.

The myriad of techniques available for repair of a rectovaginal fistula is testimony to the difficult problem that it presents to surgeons. The authors have presented a comprehensive overview of this difficult matter, clearly emphasising that a knowledgeable, rational, and current diagnostic approach, combined with meticolous surgical technique, will minimize failure and provide relief for the disabling symptoms of these complex patients.

Mauro Cervigni
Division of Urogynecology, S. Carlo-IDI Hospital
Roma, Italy

G.A. Santoro, A.P. Wieczorek, C.I. Bartram (eds.) *Pelvic Floor Disorders*
© Springer-Verlag Italia 2010

Invited Commentary

Thang Nguyen and Frank A. Frizelle

The management of fistula is a common and usually a straight forward part of a surgeons practice, however at times can be the most difficult and exasperating part for both patients and surgeons. Different approaches are required depending on the type of fistula, and the patient's status and the surgeon's resources and skill.

Urogenital Fistulae

Urogenital fistulae (UGFs) are uncommon in western societies, where they are usually associated with pelvic surgery, while in developing nations they are more of an issue due to problems with obstetric care (see Chapter 57). Conservative management centers around perineal care, often involving sitz baths, and although bladder catheterization may help with controlling the urinary leak it invariably does not help with closing of the UGF. About 5% of iatrogenic fistulae will close spontaneously, but if the fistula has not closed by three weeks then closure is unlikely to occur without surgical intervention. Estrogen supplements taken orally or as a pessary may help in softening the vagina and improving the vascular supply, particularly in the postmenopausal patient, in preparation for subsequent surgery.

There are essentially four aspects that need to be considered when approaching treatment of a UGF:

1. Timing of the operation.
2. Use of oestrogens/antibiotics.
3. Operative approach – transvaginal, transabdominal, or both.
4. Use of free or pedicled flaps.

The timing of surgery is important as there is trade off between optimizing outcome and psychological distress, particularly in patients with large fistulae. If UGFs are recognized early, which is not often, they can be repaired during the same admission if the patient's health allows it. Early operations are, however, not appropriate in those with significant comorbidities or when the pathology is related to underlying tissue ischemia as occurs in obstructed labor. Most UGFs are detected late and, since the fibrotic process is established, reoperation during the 2nd to 10th week is hazardous, and so delay for at least 3 months is often necessary in order to optimize the outcome. There are also other situations where surgery should be delayed, particularly in those with associated enteric fistulae or pelvic sepsis and those with previous multiple attempts at repair of the UGF.

Preliminary examination and investigation of the patient with a UGF is important. Cystoscopy and vaginoscopy may be aided by filling the bladder with methylene blue to identify the leakage from the vagina. This should be performed under anesthesia, as a biopsy is usually recommended. A retrograde pyelogram, cystogram, and voiding cystourethrogram preoperatively are recommended, as a second fistula (ureterovaginal and vesicovaginal fistula) has been noted in up to 10% of patients. Also, demonstration of vesicoureteric reflux, bladder prolapse, and stress incontinence may warrant consideration of other procedures, which may need to be carried out at the same time as the fistula repair.

Whether the transvaginal or transabdominal approach is used depends on the surgeon's preference but often

F.A. Frizelle
Division of Colorectal Surgery, Department of Academic Surgery, University of Otago, Christchurch, New Zealand

G.A. Santoro, A.P. Wieczorek, C.I. Bartram (eds.) *Pelvic Floor Disorders*
© Springer-Verlag Italia 2010

supratrigonal fistulae (above the interureteric ridge) are dealt with via a transabdominal approach and infratrigonal fistulae via a transvaginal approach. If the UGF tract is not to be excised, then the supratrigonal UGF type may also be approached transvaginally. The transabdominal approach is also appropriate when there is other intra-abdominal pathology that needs to be dealt with, particularly when a contracted urinary bladder, secondary to radiation cystitis, requires a cystoplasty. In our institution, the transvaginal approach is carried out in the prone jack-knife position with a slight Trendelenberg, as not only is access to the anterior vagina, where most fistulae will be located, much easier, but this method also allows maximal use of an assistant, which may be limited if the patient is in the lithotomy position.

Whether the fistulous tract is excised or not during the surgery depends on the surgeon's experience but there is good evidence to suggest that leaving the fistulous tract alone is appropriate. Some would recommend this as they believe that excising the fistula merely creates a larger defect that will bleed a lot. The use of diathermy to control these bleeding sites might compromise the blood supply to the surrounding, residual tissue. With the Martius flap, patients have to be comfortable with the resultant vulval deformity. In addition, there is a compromise between tension and flap vascularity. Another flap worth considering is the gracilis pedicled flap, which involves more thigh dissection. For large bladder defects, there is a potential risk of causing ureteric stenosis, which may involve reimplantation at the time of the UGF repair. Cystoscopy after injection of indigo carmine plus ureteric catherization should be performed if the surgeon has any suspicion of ureteric stenosis. The Latzko technique is preferred by many gynecologists for repair of uncomplicated post-hysterectomy vescicovaginal fistulae, as it is successful in most cases and has a low associated morbidity and an early return to normal activity. Fibrin glue injections have been used by some to treat UGF with limited success. Postoperatively, drains are inserted and removed when drainage is minimal. A urinary catheter, continuously draining, is left in situ until day 10 to 14, when a cystogram is performed demonstrating no leakage of urine. If there is a leak, then the catheter is left in situ and the procedure is repeated 2 weeks later. Anticholinergic drugs are sometimes required to treat bladder spasms and detrusor instability, which may lead to urinary reflux or even dehiscence of the repair. It is recommended that there is no sexual intercourse for at least 6 weeks following the procedure.

The overall success of surgical treatment for UGF tends to be above 90% but is poorer for fistulae arising from radiation-induced injury which may require repeat operations. These operations should always be delayed for some months, at least until the radionecrosis becomes non-progressive. In these cases, biopsies should be performed to rule out any recurrent malignancy or new malignancy secondary to the radiation, particularly if there is a delayed presentation. In the operation, anastomosis of the irradiated tissues to each other should be avoided and so vascularized flaps should be utilized liberally.

Rectovaginal Fistulae

As reported by Abulafi and Sultan in Chapter 58, rectovaginal fistulae are often extremely debilitating. If the opening between the rectum and vagina is wide, it will allow both flatulence and feces to escape through the vagina, leading to gross fecal incontinence with recurrent urinary and vaginal infections. In third world countries, where this is most frequently seen, obstetric fistulae are commonly associated with huge social costs. An obstetric fistula occurring as a result of pressure necrosis of the rectovaginal septum due to a protracted labor is the more common type in third world countries, in contrast to the low rectovaginal fistula that develops as a result of direct tearing during delivery which is more common in developed societies. In western countries there is a greater range of causes for this problem, including Crohn's disease and an increasing number of iatrogenic fistulae following pelvic surgery and radiotherapy. The increasing number of reconstructive procedures for inflammatory bowel disease has led to an increasing incidence of enteric-vaginal fistulae in patients with inflammatory bowel disease. After ileo-anal pouch anastomosis, pouch-vaginal fistula occurs in 6.3% (range, 3.3–15.8%) of female patients [1].

Sepsis and technical factors are the most common contributors and it is the cause of considerable morbidity. Management depends on the level of the fistula, the amount of pelvic scar tissue, and previous treatments [1]. The increased use of radiotherapy for rectal cancers and other pelvic malignancies has similarly led to a growth in these fistulae in what is often a difficult to manage subgroup [2].

As outlined in Chapter 58, in order to optimize the outcome, there is a need for a multidisciplinary approach by a colorectal and gynecological team. Endorectal ultrasonogaphy or magnetic resonance imaging (MRI) and anal manometry are helpful in the workup of these patients, to quantify the strength of the anal musculature and to document sphincter defects that may require repair. Nearly half of patients with rectovaginal fistulae have fecal incontinence [3]. Before embarking on an operation, it is of value to prescribe estrogen cream, particularly to the postmenopausal patient, in order to improve vaginal tissue and vascularity. The timing of the operation depends on the size of the fistula, the general condition of the patient, the underlying cause of the fistula, the health of the surrounding tissue, and the presence or absence of underlying sepsis. The use of fibrin glue and fibrin plugs in the treatment of rectovaginal fistulae often leads to failure, but since they are not associated with much adverse effect it may be considered appropriate to trial them in some patients.

Rectovaginal fistulae can be accessed through the vagina, perineum, and abdomen, or via the ano-rectal canal. The surgeon should pay close attention to tissue handling, hemostasis, and wide mobilization of healthy tissue, as well as closure of the layers with minimum or no tension. If there is associated incontinence and sphincter defect, it is advisable to perform a sphincteroplasty, plus anterior levatorplasty if required. This is best approached through the perineal route. Incontinence usually improves, with less risk of recurrence. The Martius graft, which is a pedicled labial fat graft, not only involves vulval deformity but is often poorly vascularized and under some tension when mobilized to fill the rectovaginal defect. Bleeding is also often a problem when mobilizing such a flap, although this can be controlled with bipolar coagulation or fine sutures. For these reasons, few centers use this approach. The gracilis pedicled flap is more reliable but involves several thigh incisions and other potential risks.

Whether a diverting stoma is required still remains debatable, although there is a trend towards no stoma. Temporary stomas, however, may still have a role in those with recurrent fistulae requiring repair, or in fistulae complicating ano-rectal surgery, particularly those associated with underlying sepsis. In elderly or frail patients, as well as patients who have radiation-inducted fistula, a stoma may well be the definitive management. For a temporary stoma, a laparoscopic diverting loop ileostomy rather than loop colostomy is preferred at our institution, while a sigmoid end colostomy is preferred for a definitive stoma. Before reversal of the stoma, either direct examination or a gastrograffin enema should be performed to ensure that the fistula has healed. Specific postoperative complications include hematoma, which will only require drainage if infected or expanding, and infection, which will require broad-spectrum antibiotics or, if associated with an abscess, drainage. Finally, wound dehiscence is often not the disaster many fear but is usually associated with underlying infection which needs treatment. Repeat surgery is indicated in most recurrent rectovaginal fistulae. Sometimes several attempts may be required in order to achieve success. Conducting more than two procedures, however, is associated with a high failure rate. To maximize success, repeat operations need to incorporate a sphincter repair or interposition graft. Recurrent simple fistulae tend to do better. Before embarking on a repeat repair, the clinician must be mindful of possible underlying predispositions to the recurrence of the rectovaginal fistula, such as Crohn's disease.

Rectovaginal fistulae in Crohn's patients are, at times, difficult to treat and the patient must accept that with any sort of treatment there is a high risk of failure and recurrence. If treated with infliximab or other new biological therapy, the underlying proctitis may subside and will occasionally allow the fistula to heal [4]. There is a growing body of evidence suggesting longer courses of therapy or even maintenance therapy for some. In many, infliximab provides a complete clinical response for the patient without the rectovaginal fistula actually healing [5]. Before biological agents are instituted, however, underlying sepsis must be treated, with or without the use of setons, to optimize the outcome and minimize deterioration of the underlying sepsis while on this medication. To promote healing of the rectovaginal fistula while on infliximab, the seton should be removed when the sepsis has subsided, and before the treatment regime is completed. Repair of the fistula should not be performed with active underlying proctitis, as this will invariably lead to failure. If the symptoms are not unbearable for the patient, rectovaginal fistula in Crohn's patients should left alone. The endovaginal flap has been favored by some in the setting of Crohn's disease, as it firstly does not involve anal dilatation and secondly does not involve dissection around diseased rectal tissue. On the rare occasion when it is associated with severe refractory proctitis and perineal sepsis, a proctectomy is recommended. While many obstetric fistulae are relatively easily fixed with surgery, the increasing complexity of reconstructive surgery in patients with inflammatory bowel disease, and the multidisciplinary management of patients with pelvic tumors, mean that there is an increasing number of patients presenting with complex iatrogenic fistulae that need a considered and individualized approach to a repair.

Perianal Fistulae

What patients want from treatment of their anal fistula is resolution of the perianal sepsis and good fecal continence, as outlined in Chapter 59 by Santoro et al. The management of fistula is a balance of these dual, and at times conflicting, goals. The key to achieving this is good preoperative anatomical knowledge when the fistula is complex, and a range of methods that can be adapted depending on the patient's preoperative function and fistula anatomy.

A fistula usually presents as an acute abscess and is one of the most common acute presentations to hospitals. Males are three times more likely to present with fistula than females and most commonly in their third or fourth decade. While the diagnosis is usually not difficult where there is a history of anal discharge, swelling, or pain, and initial management is simply drainage of sepsis, there are situations where this is difficult. In some patients with an ischiorectal fossa abscess, the diagnosis can be difficult, but suspicion should be roused when a patient has signs of sepsis (fever, tachycardia, raised C-reactive protein (CRP) and/or white cell count), and tender buttock or anal pain; however, imaging (computed tomography (CT)/MRI) may be required to confirm a diagnosis where there is no cutaneous evidence of sepsis. In neutropenic patients there is often no associated pus and hence no discharge or swelling, which makes the diagnosis very difficult.

Ano-rectal fistulae arising from perianal skin infections are more likely to harbor a growth of gram-positive cocci, or staphylococci, as opposed to gut-specific organisms, which are usually not in communication with the dentate line [6, 7]. These infections are therefore less likely to result in fistula formation. In cases without underlying fistula identified, culture of the pus is recommended. Perianal infection and fistulization may occur in any of the following infections and conditions: tuberculosis, actinomycosis, syphilis, gonorrhea, amebiasis, schistosomiasis, Crohn's disease, and malignancy of the ano-rectum. There are other conditions that may mimic perianal fistulous disease, including pilonidal disease, hydradenitis suppurativa of the perineum, perirectal dermoid cyst, and infection of the Bartholin's gland in females. Necrotizing fasciitis is an uncommon complication of perianal sepsis, which should be recognized early so that prompt debridement and fecal diversion can be instituted. A free-floating perineum may also develop when there is extensive horseshoe abscess and tissue loss. The identification of Crohn's disease in patients with perianal sepsis/fistula is important, as unless the Crohn's disease receives some systemic treatment, attempts at resolution of the perianal fistula are often futile, and at times devastating [8]. A good clinical history and examination, clinical suspicion, and pattern recognition, are important in avoiding this pitfall.

The anal glands are usually situated in the intersphincteric space, with a main duct communicating with the anal valves as well as branching ducts spreading to the internal muscle, intersphincteric space, and, rarely, the external sphincter muscle [9, 10]. The conjoined longitudinal muscle fibers usually prevent lateral extension of the infection in the intersphincteric plane. Breach of this results in an ischiorectal abscess. Ischiorectal abscess, however, may also develop from extension from a supralevator source or via caudal extension of the intersphincteric infection under the external sphincter to access the ischiorectal space. Suprasphincteric abscesses are rare and most often arise from a pelvic source. External drainage of ano-rectal abscess does not always result in fistula formation, as obstruction by debris or fibrosis of the internal opening or duct close to this site may have already occurred [11].

While Eisenhammer was able to demonstrate an internal opening of a fistula in 90% of his cases [12], most other studies have shown that fistulae are only demonstrated in between 16% and 44%, with half of these demonstrated at the second anesthetic some days later [13–16]. Fistulae are most readily identified in those with underlying intersphincteric or supralevator abscess [11].

When fistulae are complex, then preoperative knowledge of anatomy is important. This comes down to endoanal ultrasonography (EAUS) and MRI. EAUS is useful for identification of intersphinteric abscess and internal opening, but the restricted focal length prevents its use for identifying pathology beyond the external sphincter. Hence identification and characterization of perianal, ischiorectal, and supralevator abscesses is difficult. Also, in the setting of underlying abscess, the procedure may not be well tolerated. We believe that, when available and interpreted correctly, MRI is a superior investigative modality.

When examining a patient with an ano-rectal fistula, the most effective patient position is the prone jack-knife position. In the acute situation, identification of the internal opening is important but not essential. Aggressive probing may lead to false passages as well leading to significant bleeding at times, because of injury to the inferior rectal artery, especially when there is inflamed and friable tissue around the septic focus.

Using antibiotics alone to treat an abscess, whether large or small, is not recommended. An abscess needs to be drained, and, when associated with cellulitis or systemic sepsis, may benefit from concomitant use of oral or intravenous antibiotics. All that is required is a small cut with elliptical excision of the skin to facilitate drainage, and the wound is left open. A larger incision is occasionally warranted, particularly if the abscess is horseshoe in nature. Fistulotomies in the presence of an acute abscess are generally not recommended, and are performed only if the fistula is very low lying and only in experienced hands, as differentiating a high and low fistula with concurrent sepsis is often difficult, though in simple fistulae it has been shown to be safe and with less risk of abscess recurrence [17, 18]. If there is any doubt about the level of the fistula and any potential risk of incontinence, seton insertion is always a safe option. A second-stage procedure when the local sepsis has subsided is recommended for definitive management of the fistulous tract. For intersphincteric abscess, a strip of internal sphincter muscle is excised and a second examination under anesthesia is required in order to prevent recurrence of the collection.

At our institution we do not often perform fistulectomies. Fistulotomy is considered the gold standard if possible. Certainly, the more extensive the division of the external anal sphincter is made, the greater risk there is of anal incontinence, especially in females with a short sphincter complex which is particularly thin in the anterior portion. Rates of anal incontinence are, however, unlikely to be as high as the 44% reported for fistulotomies involving low internal openings. We also do not often perform primary sphincter repair with a fistulotomy; rather we try to avoid doing fistulotomies on those with significant sphincter involvement that requires such an undertaking, in order to prevent incontinence. Loose setons are safe, effective in preventing recurrence of abscesses, and afford the surgeon time to allow the underlying sepsis to resolve before more definitive procedures are undertaken. Although cutting setons are utilized in selected cases, other modalities (flaps and plugs) are preferred to deal with high fistulae and are associated with lower risk of incontinence. Rectal advancement flaps are discussed in Chapter 59. The flap that is raised should contain mucosa, submucosa, and some underlying internal anal sphincter, and, higher up, only the innermost circular layer of rectal muscle. Alternatively, fibrin glue and, more recently, anal fistula plugs have been used to allow sphincter-sparing eradication of fistulous tracts. The rate of long-term success is now becoming evident, with fibrin glues only demonstrating success in around 10% of cases, while fibrin plugs have increasingly disappointing long-term results after initially favorable short-term results [19–21]. However, as there are few associated complications, some may argue that they are worth trying and even repeating in some instances, if indicated, before the more definitive rectal advancement is performed. More recently, the anal ligation of the intersphincteric fistula tract (LIFT) procedure has been described to treat perianal fistulae, with very impressive results coming out of a handful of institutions [22, 23], although long-term data are not yet available. The procedure involves dissection in the anal intersphincteric plane via the perineal approach to skeletonize the fistulous tract. The tract at this level is then suture ligated. The intervening tract between the ties is then excised and the wound closed. One randomized control trial (RCT) from Thailand has indicated a long-term success rate of above 90% with no long-term incontinence. There is currently a multi-institutional RCT being undertaken in the United States comparing the LIFT procedure with the fibrin plug.

Infliximab and other biological agents have been

important adjuncts in the treatment of Crohn's-related fistulae, with some promising results and without the concomitant risk of incontinence. Setons are often used to ensure drainage of collections and resolution of sepsis. Once the sepsis subsides, the setons are removed to allow the fistula to heal while still being biologically treated.

In patients with complex perianal fistula, incontinence is usually a result of aggressive surgery, not uncontrolled sepsis, so it is important to be conservative with surgery and remember the dual goals of the surgery: control of sepsis but an incontinent patient is not success.

Finally, other modalities including those involving stem cells are in progress and may hopefully one day allow a more straightforward solution without risk of incontinence for patients afflicted with this troubling ailment. It is hoped that these methods will allow both control of sepsis and maintenance of continence to be more easily achieved in what can be a difficult and challenging problem.

References

1. Lolohea S, Lynch AC, Robertson GB et al. Ileal pouch-anal anastomosis-vaginal fistula: a review. Dis Colon Rectum 2005;48:1802–1810.
2. Johnston MJ, Robertson GM, Frizelle FA. Management of late complications of pelvic radiation in the rectum and anus: a review. Dis Colon Rectum 2003;46:247–259.
3. Tsang CB, Madoff RD, Wong WD et al. Anal sphincter integrity and function influences outcome in rectovaginal fistula repair. Dis Colon Rectum 1998;41:1141–1146.
4. Taxonera C, Schwartz DA, García-Olmo D. Emerging treatments for complex perianal fistula in Crohn's disease. World J Gastroenterol 2009;15:4263–4272.
5. Ng SC, Plamondon S, Gupta A et al. Prospective evaluation of anti-tumor necrosis factor therapy guided by magnetic resonance imaging for Crohn's perineal fistulas. Am J Gastroenterol 2009;104:2973–2986.
6. Eykyn SJ, Grace RH. The relevance of microbiology in the management of anorectal sepsis. Ann R Coll Surg Engl 1986;68:237–239.
7. Whitehead SM, Leach RD, Eykyn SJ et al. The aetiology of perirectal sepsis. Br J Surg 1982;69:166–168.
8. Frizelle FA, Santoro GA, Pemberton JH. The management of perianal Crohn's disease. Int J Colorectal Dis 1996;11:227–237.
9. Kratzer Gl. The anal ducts and their clinical significance. Am J Surg 1950;79:32–39.
10. Granet E. Is anal fistula a necessary sequel to perianal abscess? N Y State J Med 1948;48:63–66.
11. Ramanujam PS, Prasad ML, Abcarian H, Tan AB. Perianal abscesses and fistulas. A study of 1023 patients. Dis Colon Rectum 1984;27:593–597.
12. Eisenhammer S. The final evaluation and classification of the surgical treatment of the primary anorectal cryptoglandular intermuscular (intersphincteric) fistulous abscess and fistula. Dis Colon Rectum 1978;21:237–254.
13. Goligher JC, Ellis M, Pissidis AG. A critique of anal glandular infection in the aetiology and treatment of idiopathic anorectal abscesses and fistulas. Br J Surg 1967;54:977–983.
14. Parks AG. Pathogenesis and treatment of fistula-in-ano. Br Med J 1961;18:463–469.
15. Abcarian H. Acute suppurations of the anorectum. Surg Annu 1976;8:305–333.
16. McElwain JW, MacLean MD, Alexander RM et al. Anorectal problems: experience with primary fistulectomy for anorectal abscess, a report of 1000 cases. Dis Colon Rectum 1975;18:646–649.
17. Tang CL, Chew SP, Seow-Choen F. Prospective randomized trial of drainage alone vs. drainage and fistulotomy for acute perianal abscesses with proven internal opening. Dis Colon Rectum 1996;39:1415–1417.
18. Ho YH, Tan M, Chui CH et al. Randomized controlled trial of primary fistulotomy with drainage alone for perianal abscesses. Dis Colon Rectum 1997;40:1435–1438.
19. Thekkinkattil DK, Botterill I, Ambrose NS et al. Efficacy of the anal fistula plug in complex anorectal fistulae. Colorectal Dis 2009;11:584–587.
20. Wang JY, Garcia-Aguilar J, Sternberg JA et al. Treatment of transsphincteric anal fistulas: are fistula plugs an acceptable alternative? Dis Colon Rectum 2009;52:692–697.
21. Schwandner T, Roblick MH, Kierer W et al. Surgical treatment of complex anal fistulas with the anal fistula plug: a prospective, multicenter study. Dis Colon Rectum 2009;52:1578–1583.
22. Rojanasakul A. LIFT procedure: a simplified technique for fistula-in-ano. Tech Colproctol 2009;13:237–240.
23. Shanwani A, Nor AM, Amri N. Ligation of the intersphincteric fistula tract (LIFT): a sphincter-saving technique for fistula-in-ano. Dis Colon Rectum 2010;53:39–42.

Section IX
Failure or Recurrence after Surgical Treatment: What to Do When it All Goes Wrong

Failure or Recurrence after Surgical Treatment: Introduction

Tomasz Rechberger and Andrzej Paweł Wieczorek

Modern urogynecological reconstructive surgery over the last ten years has been dominated by prosthesetic augmentation of destroyed fascias and ligaments, in order to decrease the percentage of recurrences, which, after classical methods, was unacceptably high. According to epidemiological studies, the percentage of failures after primary classical repair of pelvic organ prolapse (POP) markedly exceeds 30%, which makes the development of new and more reliable methods imperative [1–4].

Moreover, it has been estimated that in the near future the need for prolapse surgery may increase by as much as 45%, as a result of demographic trends, and, therefore, more efficient techniques should be introduced into clinical practice in order to decrease the failure rate after primary repair [5]. Additionally, it has been shown that even if the majority of women accept a short-term pelvic floor muscle training (PFMT) and pessaries in order to cure POP, these remain unpopular in the long term, mainly due to lack of lasting clinical efficacy [6]. It is obvious that the percentage of failures and complications will increase with every subsequent surgery. Commonly known risk factors responsible for surgical failure after primary repair of POP include:

- improper patient selection
- bad surgical technique and improper selection of surgical materials, accompanied by lack of experience in pelvic reconstructive surgery
- persistence after surgery of risk factors for POP occurrence, such as obesity, constipation, or chronic coughing

- intrinsic (congenital) defects in extracellular matrix (ECM) components that influence the function of fascias and ligaments
- diminished levator ani contraction strength and a widened genital hiatus > 5 cm [7].

Classical (without augmentation by prostheses) primary reconstructive surgery aimed to restore anatomy and function (if possible) using unsuitable native connective tissue, and this was clinically manifested by a high incidence of recurrence.

Nowadays the rules in urogynecological surgery are very similar to those of hernia surgery, which simply means that after a primary failure, the use of artificial prostheses is almost obligatory. Currently, in hernia surgery, some physicians even call for primary use of mesh augmentation in order to decrease the percentage of recurrence [8]. It is probable that in the near future the same trend will be observed in urogynecological surgery, but at present there is a lack of standardized recommendations in the case of POP treatment.

Moreover, during POP surgery, the goal is not only anatomical restoration but also (and this is even more important from patients' point of view) functional restoration of urine and fecal continence, with preservation of vaginal coital capacity as well. Currently, the monofilament polypropylene is the most commonly used type of prosthesis due to its biocompatibility and biomechanical characteristics [8].

It is a commonly known fact that prophylaxis is the best strategy in the treatment of any disease. This is exactly the same when considering vaginal mesh surgery. Some prophylactic measures should always be undertaken in order to minimize the risk of complications.

T. Rechberger
2nd Department of Gynecology, Medical University of Lublin, Poland

G.A. Santoro, A.P. Wieczorek, C.I. Bartram (eds.) *Pelvic Floor Disorders*
© Springer-Verlag Italia 2010

Proper Patient Selection

Selection of suitable patients is definitely the best way to avoid unnecessary complications. Moreover, when making a decision concerning the type of operation to be performed, it is important to address (if possible) all the patient's expectations concerning the possible final postoperative outcome. As mentioned earlier, modern urogynecological surgery is mainly reconstructive and, therefore, the goal is to restore not only anatomy but also function, with preservation of coital capacity as well. However, at this point in time, it is my belief that vaginal meshes should not be used in all patients who present with prolapse. In geripausal women with bad general health conditions, some older techniques such as colpocleisis are still valuable. Thus, meshes should be used selectively in patients who will benefit from their use and where the benefits outweigh the potential risks.

Therefore, proper patient selection and preoperative evaluation are imperative in order to reduce complications such as postoperative infections and mesh erosions. All patients with severe urogenital atrophy should be treated preoperatively with vaginal estrogen preparations, in order to restore the vaginal epithelium and proper vaginal flora. A vaginal pH (which is easily measurable) below 5 is a prerequisite for proper wound healing and graft incorporation. Who is the best candidate to benefit most from mesh implantation in order to decrease the probability of recurrence? All patients with recurrent prolapse and postmenopausal women with advanced prolapse (stage III or IV), as well as all women with poor tissue quality.

What to Do with Unexpected Postoperative Complications

Complications of Midurethral Sling Surgery

Typical complications after midurethral sling surgery (tension-free vaginal tape (TVT) and TVT-like) encountered after retropubic or transobturator tape placement are presented in Table IX.1 [9–22].

Table IX.1 Complication rates after midurethral sling placement

Type of complication	Retropubic tape placement	Transobturator tape placement
Bladder perforation	4.5%, Fischer et al, 2005 [9]; 10%, David-Montefiore et al, 2006 [10]	0.5%, Fischer et al, 2005 [9]; 0%, Spinosa and Dubuis, 2005 [11]
Excessive hemorrhage	1.9%, Kuuva et al, 2002 [12]	0.8%, Spinosa and Dubuis, 2005 [11]
Retropubic hematoma	1.9%, Karram et al, 2003 [13]	Case reports (pelvic hematoma)
Urinary tract infection	8%, Fischer et al, 2005 [9]	8.3%, Fischer et al, 2005 [9]
Nerve injury	Single cases	Not encountered, hypothetically possible
Vascular injury	Single cases	Single cases
Tape erosion	1.2%, Hammad et al, 2004 [14]; 4.2%, Rechberger et al, 2006 [16]	5.4%, Deval et al, 2006 [15] ; 13.8%, Domingo et al, 2005 [17] ; 3.2%, Rechberger et al, 2006 [15]
Problems with micturition (with temporal catheterization)	2.3 %, Kuuva et al, 2002 [12]; 10.7%, Deval et al, 2006 [15]	2.0%, Davila et al, 2005 [18]; 6.6%, Hodroff et al, 2005 [19]
De novo urgency	8.3%, Levin et al, 2004 [20]; 21%, Deval et al, 2006 [15]	2.5%, Spinosa and Dubuis, 2005 [11]; 15.6%, Delorme et al, 2004 [21]
Bowel injury	Single cases	Not encountered
Treatment failure	17%, de Tayrac et al, 2004 [22]; 7%, David-Montefiore et al, 2006 [10]	10%, de Tayrac et al, 2004 [22]; 10.1 %, Deval et al, 2006 [16] ; 6%, David-Montefiore et al, 2006 [10]

Certainly the majority of the above-mentioned complications (bladder injury, urethral injury, retropubic hematoma, urinary tract infections, and bowel injuries) are typical surgical complications which also occur regardless of tape use. However, problems with micturition (post-void residue (PVR) > 100 mL or even inability to void) are usually the result of too high tension under the urethra, and should be corrected in the early postoperative period (up to 3 days). Urethral dilatation is performed. A Hegar dilator covered with 1% lidocaine gel is introduced into the urethra, and pressure is exerted over the tape. This results in tape loosening and usually restores a patient's ability to void. This is effective in the first three days after surgery; therefore, PVR should always be checked before a patient is discharged from hospital. If PVR > 100 mL is found during the first postoperative check-up 4–6 weeks after the surgery, and this is not responding to pharmacotherapy (Ubretid, distigmine bromide), it is necessary to cut the tape in order to loosen it. This is done under local anesthesia, and the risk of incontinence recurrence is about 20%. Of course, from a patient's point of view, the worst postoperative complication is treatment failure. For this reason, the treatment of recurrent or persistent stress urinary incontinence (SUI) after primary sling surgery is a new clinical dilemma. It has been shown in several papers that both the techniques of tape placement that are currently most popular, retropubic and transobturator, are equally effective in SUI caused by urethral hypermobility (UH); however in the case of SUI caused by intrinsic sphincter deficiency (ISD), retropubic tape placement is more effective [23–30]. Consequently, when failure occurs, the patient should again be evaluated clinically and urodynamically. Moreover, ultrasonography should be performed in order to re-evaluate the tape position (see Chapter 17). Based on all these findings, a surgeon should make a decision concerning the tape used for reoperation, although the general rule is that if the underlying cause of incontinence is urethral hypermobility, and the failure was caused by tape slippage or loose tape, the same type of sling may be used. If the underlying cause was ISD, and primary surgery used a transobturator tape (TOT), a retropubic sling should be considered for the second operation.

Mesh Extrusions and Exposure

Bacterial contamination during surgery may result later in mesh erosion or even extrusion, and this is strongly dependent on mesh porosity and its properties of adhesion to microorganisms. The reported rate of mesh erosion in urogynecology ranges from 1% for polypropylene to 6–12% for Goretex [31]. This is, of course, not satisfactory, and work to develop better synthetic and/or xenogenic prostheses is in progress.

As was mentioned earlier, a proper patient selection and preoperative local estrogen treatment markedly decreases the probability of late mesh extrusion. After the tape placement, there is always a risk of graft rejection but this is extremely rare and is usually caused by infection. In this type of surgery, tape rejection usually occurs 14–21 days postoperatively. As was shown by Persson et al, the main risk factor leading to tape or mesh erosion is infection, and therefore proper preparation of the operation site, accompanied by prophylactic antibiotic therapy play a crucial role in prevention [32]. Monif et al have shown that local vaginal wash with povidone decreases the number of vaginal bacteria by 106, but the number of vaginal microorganisms reverts to its initial value after 30 to 120 minutes, which clearly demonstrates the influence of time of surgery on the risk of infection [33]. Surgical techniques for mesh placement accompanied by rigorous antiseptic rules and the characteristics of the mesh itself (only type I macroporous should be used) decrease the possibility of graft contamination and, at the same time, the probability of its late exposure. However, even in the most experienced urogynecological centers such complications still occur, and one must be ready to handle them when they do. When the proper mesh is used (a type I, soft, macroporous, monofilament polypropylene), the number of exposures is typically small and they are easily handled. As was mentioned earlier, in most cases, surgical skill and antiseptic prophylaxis avoid such a complication. The vaginal incision should be deep enough to also include underlying fascia. Moreover, it should be kept to the smallest possible size and should not be taken all the way up to the cuff on either the anterior or posterior wall. Dissection of the remaining vaginal wall can be "tunneled" under the vaginal epithelium and fascia with the use of scissors and the surgeon's finger. This concept is very simple: the smaller the size of the incision, the less risk there is of a healing defect or mesh exposure through the incision. Concomitant hysterectomy (if necessary due to uterine or cervical pathology) is definitely a risk factor for subsequent mesh erosion, and therefore special measures should be undertaken in order to decrease such a possibility. The vaginal cuff should be closed separately and the incisions should not be a "T" shape at the cuff [34]. A margin of 2–3 cm of vaginal wall should be left between the incisions. As already mentioned, a thicker dissection plane (including vaginal epithelium and fascia) should always be used, as this will minimize the risk of mesh extrusion through a thin vaginal epithelium. No vaginal skin should be excised after the repair and prior to the closure, because this will increase the risk of mesh extrusion as the patient heals. In hypoestrogenic women, the vaginal skin should be estrogenized both pre- and postoperatively with local estrogen administration. Surgical tips to minimize the probability of tape or mesh exposure are as follows:

- use hydrodissection and maintain a thick dissection plane (incision of the vaginal wall should include both vaginal epithelium and underlying fascia)
- keep incisions as small as possible (use a "tunneling" technique whenever possible)
- excise minimal or no vaginal skin in order to decrease tension on the tissue
- when concomitant hysterectomy is indicated (only due to cervical or uterine pathology), no "T" incisions should be performed
- use only type I soft macroporous mesh
- pre- and postoperative local estrogen administration facilitates wound healing and proper graft incorporation.

How to Manage Postoperative Tape or Mesh Extrusions

If mesh extrusions or exposures occur, they are typically handled very easily. In the case of uninfected type I macroporous mesh, there is no need for the entire graft to be removed. It is enough to use vaginal antibiotic for 3–7 days (such as clindamycin or metronidazole), followed by daily local vaginal estrogen for 2–4 weeks. If the graft is not covered by vaginal epithelium, the exposed mesh will need to be excised, and this can be carried out under a local anesthetic injection. In some cases, the exposed mesh should be excised, and the edges of the vaginal epithelium freshened, and then closed primarily with interrupted absorbable sutures. Since type III tapes and meshes were in clinical use in the past, there are still women who

present with late vaginal or vulvar erosions caused by infection of implanted material. In such circumstances, complete removal of the mesh or tape followed by antibiotic treatment is obligatory.

How to Prevent and Manage Dyspareunia and/or Vaginal Pain after Graft Surgery

Dyspareunia or vaginal pain after the use of synthetic prostheses occurs at a rate of 15–20%, and therefore every patient should be informed about such a possibility before the operation. This is not very surprising, since the risk of such complications is also fairly high with many of the so-called "traditional repairs" with a patient's native tissue. It has been reported that the rate of dyspareunia when using fascial or levator plications for traditional posterior repair varies from 15% to 25%, and this percentage has risen to 38% when additional Burch colposuspension is performed simultaneously [35, 36]. In fact, graft use without any tension on the levators or the ligamentous attachments, and without tissue plication in the midline, is likely to result in less risk of pain with intercourse. Therefore, when performing reconstructive operation with the use of so-called "vaginal mesh kits", no tension should be placed on the mesh arms and this should be rigorously checked before completion of the procedure. A proper dissection plate creates a good cover over the mesh, which cannot be palpated by the patient or the partner, and the mesh should lie flat with no tension and not be bunched up at all. Good estrogenization of the vagina, both pre- and postoperatively, is a prerequisite for proper wound healing. It is clear that every patient experiences postoperative vaginal or buttock/leg pain to some extent, but this should subside quickly following surgery. However, when the technique used to restore the posterior vaginal wall utilizes placement of mesh arms through the sacrospinous ligament, and the patient shows signs of a pudendal neuropathy (vaginal pain, buttock pain shooting down the back of the leg) and this does not resolve within 7 to 10 days, the mesh arms should be removed from the ligaments. This is necessary in order to avoid creation of a chronic nerve injury and, subsequently, protracted chronic pelvic pain. A very similar clinical situation concerns severe groin pain following passage of a transobturator needle. If the pain is mild to moderate, anti-inflammatory medications as well as trigger point steroid injections vaginally can be very helpful. Additionally, pelvic floor physical therapy, biofeedback, and electrical stimulation are typically very successful in pain reduction and may help to avoid operative intervention. However, if there is no improvement, and if a "tight" band of mesh can be palpated in the vagina (where the arms are penetrating the pelvic side walls or the ligaments), these will need to be released. Usually it is enough to cut the mesh arms close to the pelvic sidewall, but if the pain is in the midline of the vagina and the mesh can be palpated through the vagina, the mesh will need to be removed in this region. Therefore whole-mesh removal is only necessary in the situation of generalized infection of the entire mesh (which is an extremely rare clinical situation). Typically, only arms under tension or folded or bunched up parts of the mesh should be excised in order to reduce a patient's pain.

How to See What Went Wrong and Why

In the majority of cases, qualification for the modern urogynecological procedures is still based on patient history, clinical examinations, and urodynamics. To avoid and/or reduce the risk factors responsible for surgical failure after primary repair in urinary incontinence and POP patients, wider use of imaging modalities should be considered. Proper patient selection relies on assessment and consideration of both clinical and imaging findings.

The most available technique for clinicians is transperineal ultrasonography (TPUS) [37]. One of the advantages of this method is its accessibility. The wide range of different types of transducers available in gynecology/coloproctology units encourages their use. The ease of use could be very helpful in enriching our knowledge about the clinical status of patients. In the majority of cases, a simple two-dimensional (2D)-TPUS can provide important information about the position of the urethra and its behavior during functional tests such as Valsalva and squeeze maneuvers. These functional tests could yield information about subclinical pathology, such as small cystocele, recto/enterocele. In some cases, where posterior and anterior defects coexist, ultrasonography could suggest performing a multicompartmental repair during one procedure instead of a single-compartment operation with reoperation after a second defect appears following repair of only one compartment. Additionally, TPUS allows

visualization of urethral diverticula, calcifications in the midurethra, and hypertrophy of the bladder neck, which may be clinically insignificant but might influence future treatment. In such cases, ultrasonography is a method of extension of clinical examination that should be broadly used in patients with pelvic floor problems.

Preoperative TPUS can always be compared with postoperative status. Restoration of urethral position and POP after mesh insertion can be easily checked by 2D TPUS or its modification, three- or four-dimensional (3D/4D)-TPUS [38]. These ultrasound options are very helpful in localization of any plastic elements inserted in the pelvic floor area. To reduce the rate of complications caused by abnormal (too caudal or too cephal) positioning of the tape or mesh, TPUS can even be done in the operating room. The functional character of TPUS may show not only the position but also the symmetry of both ends of the tapes/meshes and their effectiveness. Too-tight placement of TVT/TOT or mesh is easily visible by TPUS during a first postoperative assessment, and in the case of urethral obstruction it could be immediately released. Too-loose insertion of the tape can also be seen by TPUS. The same ultrasound transducer may be used in abdominal scanning to assess post-voiding residual bladder volume. 3D-TPUS with multiplanar and volume reconstruction of plastic elements also allows visualization of their elongations, which can be a source of a complication such as tape extrusion. 3D-TPUS could be a source of axial information about organs creating a urogenital hiatus. Symmetry of the urethra and anal canal could give important information about their support. Render mode options in 3D-TPUS could also give information about levator ani defects and their distribution, helping to improve understanding of pelvic floor disorders.

3D endovaginal ultrasonography (EVUS) with axial imaging of the pelvic floor, working with high frequency over 10 MHz, could significantly enrich our knowledge about the support and morphology of the urethra: the rhabdosphincter, smooth muscle layers, and their connections [39]. Hypotrophy of the rhabdosphincter, fibrotic tissue, and the presence of diffused calcifications especially in the midurethra could predict lack of success of a surgical trial of restoration of urethral position [40]. Color/power Doppler modes allow analysis of urethral vascularity [41]. These valuable imaging assessments carry a huge amount of information that could be helpful in reducing the rate of complications or treatment failure, as a result of inadequate assessment of suitability for surgery. In the case of complications of surgical treatment such as hemorrhage, EVUS gives an anatomical approach allowing visualization of even a small fluid collection with its distribution. 3D cubes with pelvic floor structures after surgical complications and the appearance of fistulae, enables their progress and distribution to be followed. Color/power Doppler modes could be helpful in localizing hypervascularity of pelvic floor tissue in the case of postsurgical infections, which can become a source of perineal pain, even without significant clinical correlation. The above-mentioned ultrasonography options are very easy to access in all the pelvic floor units, which makes them the first-choice imaging techniques, particularly since, in many cases, the imaging may be performed by the same person who selected and operated the patient. In case of existing problems, patient complaints, lack of abnormal ultrasound findings, and unclear status, magnetic resonance (MR) could also be considered. Proper MR assessment of patients with complications after pelvic floor repair needs a very close cooperation between the surgeon and radiologist. The main limitation of this method is still the limited accessibility and, in many cases, lack of functional assessment.

It is probable that in the near future, cooperation between visualizing modalities and qualification and follow-up treatment of patients with pelvic floor problems will become more frequent and fruitful, helping to reduce the rate of complications and increase the cases of effective treatment.

Conclusions

Complications are fundamental to every surgeon's life and this is also true for pelvic reconstructive surgery. Traditional repairs have an unacceptably high rate of failure and, as for any other kind of surgery, are also not free of common complications such as bleeding, infections, or pelvic organ (bladder and rectum) injuries. During the last ten years, the field of urogynecology has been revolutionized by graft augmentation of native patient's tissue in order to achieve a higher cure rate and ultimately achieve better long-term anatomic results for women following prolapse surgery. There is no doubt that synthetic grafts used vaginally have been proved to have higher cure rates than traditional vaginal repairs. However, these new methods of reconstructive surgery are not free of the complications

seen after traditional repair methods, such as risk of failure or recurrence of the original defect, sexual dysfunction, pain, and/or visceral dysfunction and, additionally, infection or rejection of any graft or sutures utilized. Therefore, the specific role of synthetic graft in vaginal reconstructive surgery remains to be defined [42]. The introduction into clinical practice of so-called "surgical kits" for graft placement was an attempt to standardize the techniques and make the vaginal approach less invasive and safer for the patients. However, it is obvious that the clinical studies that create a background for introduction of a global "mesh kit" were conducted by expert surgeons with extensive experience of graft use and knowledge of female pelvic anatomy. Nevertheless, studies need to be continued to evaluate cure rates, complications, and long-term benefits prior to making universal recommendations on "kit surgery" in general practice performed by every surgeon [43]. At this point in time, we can conclude that when used by an experienced and advanced pelvic surgeon, in the proper clinical situation, with an appropriate patient selection, the benefits of graft use do seem to outweigh the risks. Of course, complications do still occur, even in the most experienced surgeon's hands, but these seem to be minimal and not life threatening. However, there is no doubt that we have to continue research on better graft composition, and we must continue to develop techniques to minimize the complications of blind needle passage for mesh placement. Moreover, based on well-designed multicenter clinical studies, recommendations should be made, not only for correct patient selection, but also for correct surgeon selection, since there is no doubt that only properly trained urogynecologists can successfully complete these kinds of repairs with minimal complications and satisfactory anatomical and functional outcome.

Synthetic prostheses are commonly used nowadays in pelvic reconstructive surgery. The occurrence of erosions as well as the danger of excessive fibrosis after polypropylene graft placement is the reason for the current search for better implant material. Preventive measures are the best way to decrease the rate of complications, as well as the risk of failure after any kind of surgery, but this is especially true for synthetic graft usage. Proper patient selection, local estrogen treatment before operation in patients with severe urogenital atrophy, and proper surgical technique accompanied by strict following of antiseptic rules and antibiotic prophylaxis, with more frequent use of imaging modalities, are the keys to success.

References

1. Paraiso MFR, Ballard LA, Walters MD et al. Pelvic support defects and visceral and sexual function in women with sacrospinous ligament pelvic reconstruction. Am J Obstet Gynecol 1996;175:1423–1431.

2. Olsen AL, Smith VG, Bergstrom JO et al. Epidemiology of surgically managed pelvic organ prolapse and incontinence. Obstet Gynecol 1997;89:501–506.

3. Macer GA. Transabdominal repair of cystocele, a 20 years experience, compared with the traditional vaginal approach. Am J Obstet Gynecol 1978;131:203–207.

4. Kholi N, Sze EHM, Roat TW, Karram M. Incidence of recurrent cystocele after anterior colporrhaphy with and without concomitant transvaginal needle suspension. Am J Obstet Gynecol 1996;175:1476–1482.

5. Luber KM, Boero S, Choe JY. The demographics of pelvic floor disorders: current observations and future projections. Am J Obstet Gynecol 2001;184:1496–501.

6. Srikrishna S, Robinson D, Cardozo L, Thiagamoorthy G. The vagina dialogues: Womens expectations of prolapse treatment. Int Urogynecol J 2009;20(suppl 2):S174.

7. Vakili B, Zheng YT, Loesch H et al. Levator contraction strength and genital hiatus as risk factors for recurrent pelvic organ prolapse. Am J Obstet Gynecol 2005;192:1592–1598.

8. Luijendij R. A comparison of suture repair with mesh repair for incisional hernias. N Engl J Med 2000;243:292–298.

9. Fischer A, Fink T, Zachmann S, Eickenbuch U. Comparison of retropubic and outside-in transobturator sling systems for the cure of female genuine stress urinary incontinence. Eur Urol 2005;48:799–804.

10. David-Montefiore E, Frobert JL, Grisard-Anaf M et al. Perioperative complications and pain after suburethral sling procedure for urinary stress incontinence: a French prospective randomized multicenter study comparing the retropubic and transobturator routes. Eur Urol 2006;49:133–138.

11. Spinosa JP, Dubuis PY. Suburethral sling inserted by the transobturator route in the treatment of female stress urinary incontinence: preliminary results in 117 cases. Eur J Obstet Gynecol Reprod Biol 2005;123:212–217.

12. Kuuva N, Nilsson CG. A nationwide analysis of complications associated with the tension-free vaginal tape (TVT) procedure. Acta Obstet Gynecol Scand 2002;81:72–77.

13. Karram MM, Segal JL, Vassalo BJ, Kleeman SD. Complications and untoward effects of the tension-free vaginal tape procedure. Obstet Gynecol 2003;101:929–932.

14. Hammad FT, Kennedy-Smith A, Robinson RG. Erosions and urinary retention following polypropylene synthetic sling: Australasian survey. Eur Urol 2005;47:641–7.

15. Deval B, Ferchaux J, Berry R et al. Objective and subjective cure rates after transobturator tape (OBTAPE) treatment of female urinary incontinence. Eur Urol 2006;49:373–377.

16. Rechberger T, Adamiak A, Miotla P et al. Risk of tape rejection in urogynecological surgeries. Int Urogynecol J Pelvic Floor Dysfunct 2006;17(suppl. 2):302.

17. Domingo S, Alama P, Ruiz N et al. Diagnosis, management and prognosis of vaginal erosion after transobturator suburethral tape procedure using a nonwoven thermally bonded polypropylene mesh. J Urol 2005;173:1627–1630.

18. Davila GW, Johnson JD, Serels S. Multicenter experience with the Monarc transobturator sling system to treat stress urinary incontinence. Int Urogynecol J Pelvic Floor Dysfunct 2006;17:460–465.

19. Hodroff MA, Sutherland SE, Kesha JB, Siegel SW. Treatment of stress incontinence with the SPARC sling: intraoperative and early complications of 445 patients. Urology 2005;66:760–762.

20. Levin I, Groutz A, Gold R et al. Surgical complications and medium-term outcome results of tension-free vaginal tape: a prospective study of 313 consecutive patients. Neurourol Urodyn 2004;23:7–9.

21. Delorme E, Droupy S, de Tayrac R, Delmas V. Transobturator tape (Uratape): a new minimally-invasive procedure to treat female urinary incontinence Eur Urol 2004;45:203–207.

22. de Tayrac R, Deffieux X, Droupy S et al. A prospective randomized trial comparing tension-free vaginal tape and transobturator suburethral tape for surgical treatment of stress urinary incontinence. Am J Obstet Gynecol 2004;191:1868–1874.

23. Neuman M. TVT and TVT-O obturator: comparison of two operative procedures. Eur J Obstet Gynecol Reprod Biol 2007;131:89–92.

24. Meschia M, Pifarotti P, Bernasconi F et al. Tension-free vaginal tape (TVT) and intravaginal slingplasty (IVS) for stress urinary incontinence: a multicenter randomized trial. Am J Obstet Gynecol 2006;195:1338–1342.

25. Rechberger T, Jankiewicz K, Adamiak A et al. Do preoperative cytokine levels offer a prognostic factor for polypropylene mesh erosion after suburethral sling surgery for stress urinary incontinence? J Pelvic Floor Dysfunct 2009;20:69–74.

26. O'Connor RC, Nanigian DK, Lyon MB et al. Early outcomes of mid-urethral slings for female stress urinary incontinence stratified by Valsalva leak point pressure. Neurourol Urodyn 2006;25:685–688.

27. Costantini E, Lazzeri M, Giannantoni A et al. Preoperative Valsava leak point pressure may not predict outcome of mid-urethral slings. Analysis from a randomized controlled trial of retropubic versus transobturator mid-urethral slings. Int Braz J Urol 2008;34:73–81.

28. Charalambous S, Touloupidis S, Fatles G et al. Transvaginal vs transobturator approach for synthetic sling placement in patients with stress urinary incontinence. Int Urogynecol J Pelvic Floor Dysfunct 2008;19:357–360.

29. Daraï E, Frobert JL, Grisard-Anaf M et al. Functional results after the suburethral sling procedure for urinary stress incontinence: a prospective randomized multicentre study comparing the retropubic and transobturator routes. Eur Urol 2007;51:795–801.

30. Rechberger T, Futyma K, Jankiewicz K et al. The comparison of the clinical effectiveness of retropubic (IVS-02) and transobturator (IVS- 04) midurethral slings - randomized trial. Eur Urol 2009;56:24–30.

31. Birch C, Fynes MM. The role of synthetic and biological prostheses in reconstructive pelvic floor surgery. Curr Opin Obstet Gynecol 2002;14:527–535.

32. Persson J, Iosif C, Wolner-Hanssen P. Risk factors for rejection of synthetic suburethral slings for stress urinary incontinence: a case-control study. Obstet Gynecol 2002;99:629–634.

33. Monif GRG, Thompson JL, Stephens HD, Baer H. Quantitative and qualitative effects of Povidone-iodine liquid and

gel on the aerobic and anaerobic flora of the female genital tract. Am J Obstet Gynecol 1980;137:432–438.

34. Collinet P, Belot F, Debodinance P et al. Transvaginal mesh technique for pelvic organ prolapse repair: mesh exposure management and risk factors. Int Urogynecol J Pelvic Floor Dysfunct 2006;17:315–320.

35. Kahn MA, Stanton SL. Posterior colporrhaphy: its effects on bowel and sexual function. Br J Obstet Gynecol 1997;104:82–86.

36. Weber AM, Walters MD, Piedmonte MR. Sexual function and vaginal anatomy in women before and after surgery for pelvic organ prolapse and urinary incontinence. Am J Obstet Gynecol 2000;182:1610–1615.

37. Dietz HP. Ultrasound imaging of the pelvic floor. Part I: two-dimensional aspects. Ultrasound Obstet Gynecol 2004;23:80–92.

38. Dietz HP, Barry C, Lim YN, Rane A. Two-dimensional and three-dimensional ultrasound imaging of suburethral slings. Ultrasound Obstet Gynecol 2005;26:175–179.

39. Santoro GA, Wieczorek AP, Stankiewicz A et al. High-resolution three-dimensional endovaginal ultrasonography in the assessment of pelvic floor anatomy: a preliminary study. Int Urogynecol J Pelvic Floor Dysfunct 2009; 20:1213–1222.

40. Digesu GA, Robinson D, Cardozo L, Khullar V. Three-dimensional ultrasound of the urethral sphincter predicts continence surgery outcome. Neurourol Urodyn 2009; 28:90–94.

41. Wieczorek AP, Woźniak MM, Stankiewicz A et al. The assessment of normal female urethral vascularity with Color Doppler endovaginal ultrasonography: preliminary report. Pelviperineology 2009;28:59–61.

42. Dwyer PL. Evolution of biological and synthetic grafts in reconstructive pelvic surgery. Int Urogynecol J Pelvic Floor Dysfunct 2006;17(suppl 1):S10–15.

43. Davila GW. Introduction to the 2005 IUGA Grafts Roundtable. Int Urogynecol J Pelvic Floor Dysfunct 2006;17(suppl 1):S4–5.

Imaging and Management of Complications of Urogynecologic Surgery

60

S. Abbas Shobeiri

Abstract We engage in "repair" of the pelvic floor by surgical means. To accomplish this, we utilize different biomaterials and meshes to reconstitute pelvic floor anatomy. The goal of the current chapter is to introduce the reader to modalities used in imaging surgical complications. Some treatment modalities are also discussed.

Keywords Fistula • Mesh • Prolapse • Ultrasound • Vaginal stenosis

60.1 Introduction

When one looks at the older urogynecology textbooks, the complications of surgical procedures were mostly limited to postoperative medical complications such as pulmonary embolus, myocardial infarctions, and deep venous thrombosis. With the introduction of bio-materials and mesh kits into vaginal reconstructive surgery over the past decade, unprecedented and un-expected complications have occurred that require in-novative solutions, or, more aptly put, a visit to our old surgical masters.

Increase in the use of biomaterials and mesh kits occurred rapidly. In October 2008, the United States Food and Drug Administration (FDA) issued an alert to patients and practitioners informing them of po-tential complications associated with transvaginal use of mesh in surgery for incontinence and prolapse. Mesh complications have been divided into extrusions "when mesh migrates into the vagina", and erosions "when mesh moves into visceral organs" (e.g. the bladder, urethra, and rectum).

This chapter introduces the reader to imaging urogy-necological complications and surgical remedies that may exist.

60.2 Intra-operative Complications Involving Anti-incontinence Procedures

60.2.1 Overview

Over the past decade substantial advances have been made in the treatment of incontinence. Retropubic procedures have been mostly replaced by mesh slings. The tension-free vaginal tape (TVT) sling procedure (Gynecare, Ethicon Inc., Somerville, NJ) has been popular in the United States since late 1998. This pro-cedure was developed based on "Integral Theory" to represent an easily performed, ambulatory, minimally invasive surgical procedure for the treatment of female genuine stress urinary incontinence [1, 2]. Sling pro-cedures with other names have been mass marketed by the device manufacturers to generalist urologists and gynecologists.

S. Abbas Shobeiri
Section of Female Pelvic Medicine and Reconstructive Surgery,
Department of Obstetrics and Gynecology,
The University of Oklahoma Health Sciences Center,
Oklahoma City, OK, USA

G.A. Santoro, A.P. Wieczorek, C.I. Bartram (eds.) *Pelvic Floor Disorders*
© Springer-Verlag Italia 2010

60.2.2 Slings

The slings currently available are mostly applied retropubically or via a trans-obturator approach. Bladder injury is a constant worry with these slings [3] (Fig. 60.1). One of the common complications of these slings is urinary retention or persistent urinary incontinence [3].

Patients with urinary retention or dysfunctional voiding will do well if their slings are released within two weeks after surgery [4]. Persistent stress urinary incontinence may be managed with bulking agents such as Macroplastique®, but their success rate varies between 8% and 37% [5, 6].

In a study involving retropubic mesh slings, we followed the anatomical path of TVT slings in fresh-frozen pelvises [7]. As recognized in our fresh cadaveric dissections, it is hard to avoid the paraurethral vessels, and therefore these vessels are at a high risk of injury. Disruption of the paraurethral vascular plexus normally responds to intraoperative manual compression or vaginal packing to achieve transvaginal tamponade.

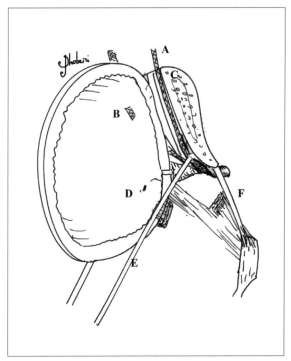

Fig. 60.1 Sagittal anatomy detailing the tension-free vaginal tape position (*A*); the site of bladder injury with TVT in place (*B*); the pubic symphysis (*C*); the bladder cavity (*D*); the arcus tendineus fasciae pelvis (*E*) and the urethral opening (*F*)

Bleeding can also occur in the retropubic space during blind passage of the trocar. The pubic vein, as identified in Fig. 60.2, can potentially be injured resulting in hematoma formation. Most postoperative hematomas present within the first 12 hours as suprapubic discomfort.

Trans-obturator tapes have their own set of unique intraoperative complications, which include bladder and urethral injury. The bladder injuries can be managed conservatively by removal and replacement of the trocars [3].

Another issue to consider is the kind of mesh used in slings. We reported a case of suburethral sinus formation after insertion of a silicon-coated mesh sling (American Medical Systems, Minnetonka, MN) in 2003 [8]. The sling reported in this case has a polyester backbone coated with medical grade silicon. The same material is utilized in a mesh marketed by the same manufacturer for performing sacrocolpopexy. The manufacturer reported that the design made the sling stronger and easier to slide during the insertion process.

The erosion of the sling material can be due to rejection of the material by the host, inappropriate closure or insertion technique, and infection. The cultures obtained were negative in our case [9]. The sling in our case report had no ingrowths of tissue in it and simply fell out after opening of the midline incision. Lack of tissue incorporation could be an etiological factor in sinus formation (Fig. 60.3). Another sling that had significant problems with infection and extrusion was the OBtape® (Mentor Inc., California), which has been withdrawn from the market. The mesh was speculated to be tight knit, allowing the bacteria to infect it easily. An extensive colonization of the surgical mesh with autologous fibroblasts may reduce complications [10].

Imaging techniques may be useful prior to attempting to repair an urethrovaginal fistula to ascertain the location of a fistula in relation to a sling (Fig. 60.4). Frequently, in addition to sling removal (Fig. 60.5), the urethral fistula repair is complicated by the lack of healthy tissue to be reapproximated over the fistula site. We utilize a Martius flap [11, 12] to prevent recurrent urethrovaginal fistula formation.

There are many established materials for performing the sling procedures. New materials should not be used in a clinical setting unless proven safe and effective after undergoing clinical trials.

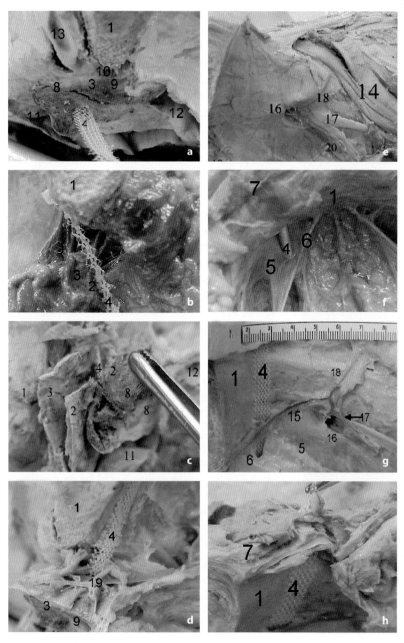

Fig. 60.2 TVT anatomy. **a** Right hemipelvis: sagittal view of the sling entering the suburethral tissue. **b** Right hemipelvis: sagittal view of sling coursing through the extrinsic continence mechanism (numbers *2* and *3*) in a fresh-frozen pelvis. The urethra has been removed and the sling can be seen piercing through the extrinsic sphincter muscles. **c** Right hemipelvis: plantar view of the extrinsic continence mechanism in a formalin-immersed pelvis. The urethra is deflected by forceps to show the underlying extrinsic sphincter muscles. Note the sling coursing through the urethrovaginal sphincter and the compressor urethrae muscle. **d** Right hemipelvis: sagittal view of the paraurethral vascular plexus in a fresh-frozen pelvis lightly sprayed with formalin. A yellow ribbon has been inserted between the extrinsic sphincter muscles and the vascular plexus to demonstrate the paraurethral vascular plexus better. **e** Right hemipelvis: sagittal view of the lateral blood vessels and nerves. **f** Retropubic view of an intact fresh-frozen pelvis as the trocar enters the retropubic space. **g** Right hemipelvis: sagittal view of the sling as it enters and exits the retropubic space. **h** Right hemipelvis: sagittal view of the sling traversing the anterior abdominal wall. *1*, pubic symphysis; *2*, urethrovaginal sphincter; *3*, compressor urethrae; *4*, TVT; *5*, arcus tendineus levator ani; *6*, arcus tendineus fasciae pelvis; *7*, anterior abdominal wall; *8*, urethra; *9*, sphincter urethrae; *10*, puborectalis; *11*, vagina; *12*, bladder; *13*, clitoris; *14*, iliac vessels; *15*, pubic vein; *16*, obturator canal; *17*, obturator nerve; *18*, accessory obturator vein; *19*, paraurethral vascular plexus; *20*, obturator vessels; *21*, inferior epigastric vessels

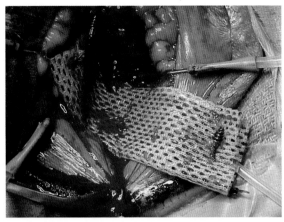

Fig. 60.3 Silicone sling with the bone anchors attached as it is being removed through the vaginal extrusion site

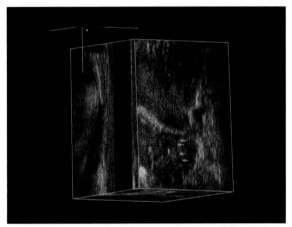

Fig. 60.4 Ultrasound axial view of the tape. The *yellow arrows* demonstrate the fistula tract. The image was obtained with an 8842 BK transducer

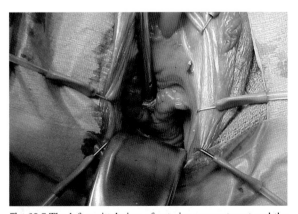

Fig. 60.5 The left sagittal view of anterior compartment and the urethra. This is a rendered view of a sling in relation to a urethrovaginal fistula. The *yellow arrow* points to the fistula tract. The *double arrow* is pointing at the sling. *A*, anterior; *P*, posterior; *PB*, pubic bone; *F*, Foley bulb; *U*, external urethral meatus. The image was obtained with an 8842 B-K transducer

60.2.3 Retropubic Procedures

Complications of retropubic surgery for incontinence include injury to the ureters or the bladder, dysfunctional voiding, and pain.

One major subset of complications specific to retropubic procedures involves ureteral injury. Gynecologic surgery is responsible for up to 75% of cases of iatrogenic injury to the ureter [13]. Risk factors for intraoperative injury to the urinary tract include malignancy, endometriosis, prior surgery, and surgery for prolapse [14, 15]. Patients with undiagnosed injuries can have a highly variable course, causing diagnostic delay, which results in additional hospitalization, prolonged catheterization, and multiple additional procedures [16]. As a result, urinary tract injury during gynecologic surgery may result in medicolegal action [17]. In a study consisting of a large prospective series to assess the incidence of urinary tract injury, utilizing universal cystoscopy, we found the total urinary tract injury rate to be 4.8% [18]. Injuries occurred in 7.6% of total vaginal hysterectomies, 4.0% of total abdominal hysterectomies, and 2.0% of laparoscopic hysterectomies (P = 0.156) [18]. Concurrent prolapse surgery was associated with an increased risk of urinary tract injury (14.6% vs. 4.0%; P = 0.01). Not all urinary tract injuries are detected intraoperatively, as demonstrated by our 30% detection rate prior to cystoscopy. The presence of peristalsis is a poor marker for ureteral integrity. In addition, undetected injuries are not all symptomatic, resulting in silent injuries that can have significant consequences [15, 18]. Although we discuss imaging and management of such complications in this chapter, it is certainly preferable to detect and repair these injuries intraoperatively.

Procedures such as Burch [19] and Marshall-Marchetti-Krantz (MMK) urethropexy carry with them the inherent risk of ureteral, bladder, and urethral injuries. The bladder injuries identified at the time of surgery need to be managed by primary closure [20]. If such injuries go unrecognized at the time of surgery, they may result in urinomas or fistulae (Fig. 60.6). The bladder fistulae can be differentiated from ureteral fistulae by the use of retrograde filling of the bladder with a blue dye such as indigo carmine [21]. The upper genitourinary tract should be imaged with the use of an intravenous pyelogram, ultrasound, or a computed tomography (CT) scan (Fig. 60.7). The bowel and ureteral injuries, if unrecognized, can

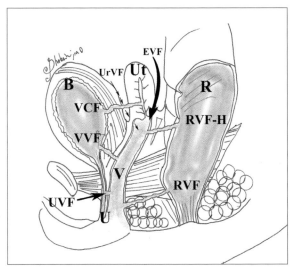

Fig. 60.6 Drawing of various vaginal fistulae. *EVF*, enterovaginal fistula; *R*, rectum; *RVF*, rectovaginal fistula; *RVF-H*, high rectovaginal fistula; *U*, urethra; *Ut*, uterus; *UrVF*, ureterovaginal fistula; *UVF*, urethrovaginal fistula; *V*, vagina; *VCF*, vesicocervical fistula; *VVF*, vesicovaginal fistula

be catastrophic, culminating in a genitourinary fistula, rectovaginal fistula, or overt sepsis and death.

The distal ureter can be injured at the time of retropubic procedures. These injuries can go unnoticed and result in hydronephrosis and gradual renal death. One such patient presented to us for pelvic organ prolapse evaluation. She had had an MMK procedure 20 years earlier. Ultrasound imaging revealed hydronephrosis and a non-functioning right kidney (Figs. 60.8–60.10). Unfortunately for this patient, detection of the ureteral injury came too late, long after she had lost the function of her right kidney. We were meticulous in our intraoperative dissections to protect the contralateral ureter with the use of an intraoperative catheter. These patients may create a medicolegal dilemma, because if the old injury is not detected preoperatively, or

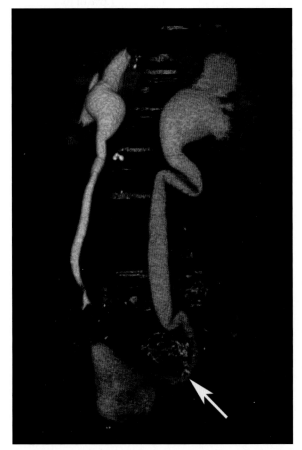

Fig. 60.7 The *arrow* in this CT reconstruction shows the level of distal obstruction, and a dilated left ureter

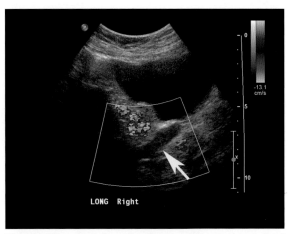

Fig. 60.8 Ultrasound view of a dilated right ureter due to distal obstruction. The *arrow* points at the dilated ureter

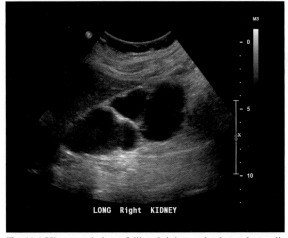

Fig. 60.9 Ultrasound view of dilated right renal calyces due to distal obstruction

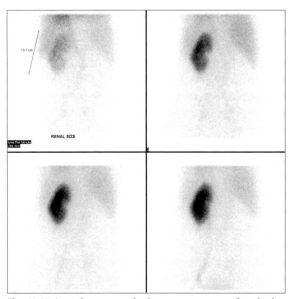

Fig. 60.10 A nuclear tag study demonstrates a non-functioning right kidney

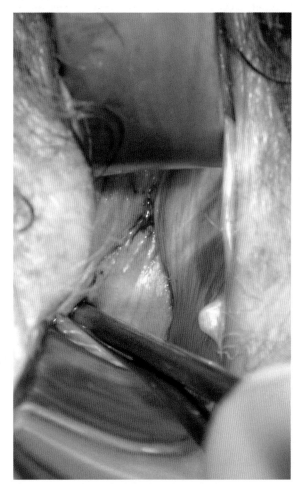

Fig. 60.11 A vesicovaginal fistula at the vaginal apex

intraoperatively, the unsuspecting pelvic surgeon may be the one to take the blame for an old injury.

There are fistulae that result from placement of sutures that go through both the bladder and the vagina at the time of concomitant hysterectomy, or retropubic procedures [18] (Fig. 60.11). The less common ureteral injuries result from clamping or suture placement which has obstructed the ureter at the level of the external and internal iliac bifurcation at the time of salpingo-oophorectomy or sacrocolpopexy. Such injuries may require a Boari flap, which was first described in 1894. Tubulerization of the bladder can bridge a 10–15 cm defect of the ureter with ease. The base of the flap should be 4 cm wide, and the tip 3 cm wide. The flap is fixed to the psoas major muscle and ureteroneocystostomy is completed [22]. Placement of a ureteral stent for six weeks and a retrograde cystography are advocated (Fig. 60.12).

Complex fistulae can also be evaluated by the use of retrograde techniques. We have described a technique for diagnosis of hard-to-find vesicocervical and vesicovaginal fistulae [23] (Fig. 60.13).

The two biggest risks of any anti-incontinence procedure are the facts that the procedure may not work, or may result in obstructed voiding. Obstructed voiding should be dealt with by the use of a protocol to adjust the sling or cut the sling within two weeks [24]. For patients remote from their original surgery date who

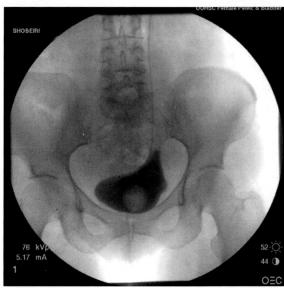

Fig. 60.12 Fluoroscopic view of a retrograde cystogram demonstrating a left ureteral stent six weeks after a psoas hitch and Boari flap

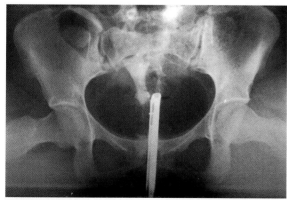

Fig. 60.13 Cystoscopic fistulogram. The contrast dye that was injected into the vesical end of the fistulous tract has filled the uterine cavity giving it the appearance of a hysterogram

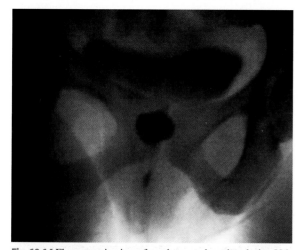

Fig. 60.14 Fluoroscopic view of an obstructed urethra during Valsalva maneuver. Note that because of the obstruction the picture simulates a urethral diverticulum

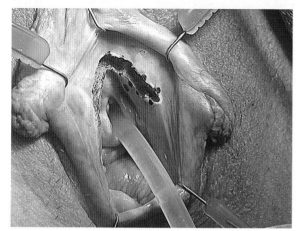

Fig. 60.15 Intraoperative view of a suprameatal urethrolysis. A reverse U incision is made between the urethra and the pubic bone

present with voiding dysfunction as a result of urethral obstruction (Fig. 60.14), a urethrolysis can be performed retropubically or transvaginally. Retropubic urethrolysis may face dense adhesions, resulting in severe blood loss and bladder injury. We advocate a suprameatal urethrolysis approach [25] (Fig. 60.15). After a reverse U incision is made over the urethral meatus, dissection is continued over the urethra, lysing the adhesions to the retropubic area cephalad to the suprapubic area, and laterally to the obturator foramens. In our hands this technique has resulted in 90% resolution of the voiding dysfunction and no occult urinary incontinence. It is important to place an anti-adhesive barrier in the retropubic area, and use a vaginal packing to prevent hematoma formation.

A less common risk of retropubic procedures is pain, oseitis pubis, and osteomyelitis [25–27]. The classic presentation of osteitis pubis is suprapubic discomfort, wide-based gait due to the pain with ambulation, and, frequently, systemic symptoms, such as low-grade fever, malaise, and general debility. Signs of osteitis pubis include irregular margins with a widened symphysis pubis on plain radiographs and, frequently, frank bony destruction associated with involucrum of the pubic bone. Osteomyelitis may be indistinguishable from osteitis pubis in its early stages. Pubic bone pain conditions are mostly associated with MMK procedures or bone anchor sling procedures (Fig. 60.16).

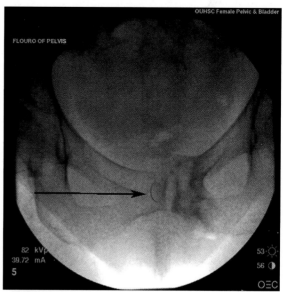

Fig. 60.16 Fluoroscopic view of a needle (*arrow*) found in the retropubic space in a patient subsequent to a MMK procedure

60.3 Complications of Pelvic Organ Prolapse Surgery

60.3.1 Overview

One of the problems associated with pelvic organ prolapse surgery is recurrence of prolapse (Fig. 60.17). As such, the surgeon has to spend significant amount of time with the patient managing expectations, and educating the patient about the pathophysiology of pelvic organ prolapse.

The surgeon who tries to deal with complications of urogynecological procedures has to keep in mind that the correction of complication has to result in a functional vagina if the patient desires vaginal intercourse. In order to create a functional vagina and decrease risk of vaginal narrowing, surgeons have looked for bioidentical material to be used for repair. The only true bioidentical material is the patient's own tissue. The use of other material such as pig tissue, cadaveric tissue, and mesh has resulted in unexpected complications. Managing exposed implanted graft material should result in resolution of pain and vaginal discharge, while restoring normal anatomy.

60.3.2 Apical Segment Complications

Apical vaginal failure is amendable to sacrocolpopexy, suture closure of the enterocele, sacrospinous ligament suspension, and uterosacral plication. The complications of these procedures include pudendal neuropathy, apical prolapse after vaginally implanted graft material, extrusion of abdominally implanted polypropylene mesh, extrusion of vaginally implanted graft material, and vaginal stenosis.

Should pudendal neuropathy occur as a result of trocar injury or suture entrapment, the patient may present with pain and spasm of the pelvic floor, presenting as voiding and defecatory dysfunction. The patient's pain is exacerbated with sitting down and pressure on the perineal area. In such cases, the offending mesh or suture has to be removed as soon as possible before the pain becomes chronic [28, 29].

Another complication of pelvic organ prolapse surgery is recurrence of the prolapse. Patients may experience symptoms of prolapse and herniation before they become evident during pelvic examination. In such cases, dynamic magnetic resonance imaging (MRI) or dinamic 3D ultrasound imaging may be useful (Fig. 60.18). The in-

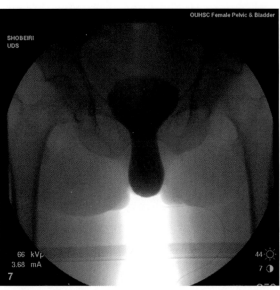

Fig. 60.17 Fluoroscopic view of a stage IV cystocele subsequent to a sacrocolpopexy. In this patient the apical support provided by the sacrocolpopexy was intact

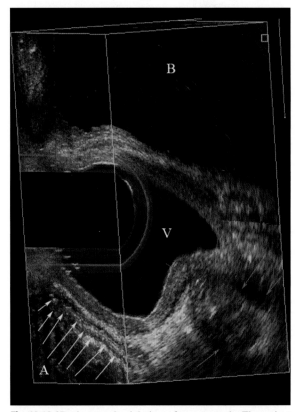

Fig. 60.18 3D ultrasound axial view of an enterocele. The patient had had posterior and apical reconstruction with Pelvicol®. The enterocele is noted herniating through the right side of the vaginal apex. The *yellow arrows* show posteriorly implanted material and *red arrows* mark the enterocele. *A*, anus; *B*, bladder; *V*, vagina

formation obtained from the ultrasound image in Figure 60.18 was useful as we knew the biomaterial implanted was not absorbed by the body and that there was an enterocele to the right of the previous prolapse surgery. During our laparoscopic sacrocolpopexy we took meticulous care to cover the right side of vaginal apex.

Mesh extrusion after past surgical procedures such as abdominal or laparoscopic sacrocolpopexy, especially with silicone and Gore-Tex grafts, is well described [30–32].

Abdominal mesh extrusions are easily fixed with vaginal resection of the exposed mesh. Extrusion of vaginally implanted mesh, on the other hand, may not respond to estrogen cream application and require removal of the exposed mesh. If enough mesh is exposed apically, complete collapse and closure of the upper half of the vagina may result, making intercourse impossible (Fig. 60.19). We have performed surgery in a large cohort of such patients with upper vaginal stenosis where a variety of full-thickness skin grafts from the abdomen were used to recreate the upper vagina (Figs. 60.20, 60.21).

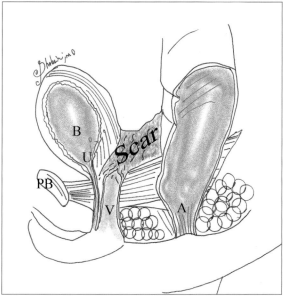

Fig. 60.19 Drawing depicting stenosis of the upper half of the vagina. *A*, anus; *B*, bladder; *PB*, pubic bone; *U*, uterus; *V*, vagina

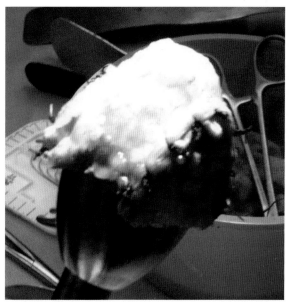

Fig. 60.21 The skin cap measuring 5 cm in length is fashioned with epithelium facing inward

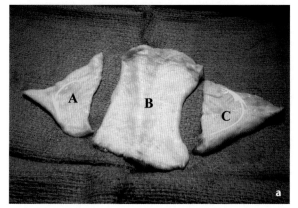

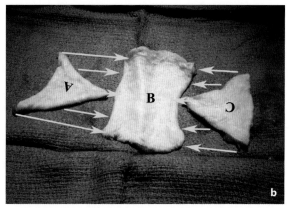

Fig. 60.20 a The harvested skin is cleaned of adipose tissue and cut into three pieces. The end triangles *A* and *C* are rotated in the direction of the *arrows*. **b** The triangular edges of the harvested skin are rotated in preparation to be tailored in to a cap. The skin is sutured along the direction of the arrows, with the epithelium facing towards the vagina, and the suture knots facing towards the pelvic cavity

60.3.3 Lateral Vaginal Complications

Traditionally, posterior compartment defects were addressed with a posterior repair, and those of the anterior compartment with an anterior repair, which occasionally resulted in excessive tightening of the mid-vagina (Fig. 60.22) and consequent dyspareunia. Sometimes, a mid-vaginal stenosis can be addressed with a relaxing incision of the scar tissue vertically, which can be left to close with secondary intention, or closed horizontally after undermining the surrounding vaginal epithelium. However, transfer of adjacent tissue may sometimes be needed to widen the vagina. If this is not possible, full-thickness skin grafts from the buttocks or groin can be used and placed in an elliptical fashion over the exposed area of each relaxing incision (Fig. 60.23). To avoid mid-vaginal stenosis, urogynecologists have been searching for other tissue to patch the defects. The best tissue to use is the patient's own tissue. More and more urogynecologists are being trained in these advanced techniques. Consequently, to reduce the high failure rates of pelvic floor repairs, and to avoid mid-vaginal stenosis formation after a traditional anterior and posterior repair, focus has turned to the use of mesh, porcine tissue, or cadaveric tissue, which carry their own unique risks and complications. The ideal material needs to be strong, easy to handle, and biocompatible, while supporting growth of new tissue with minimal inflamma-

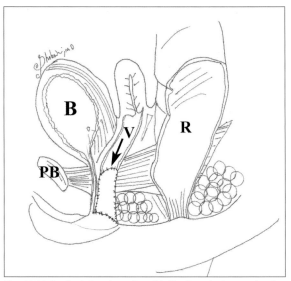

Fig. 60.23 Sagittal drawing of a mid-distal vaginal stenosis after lateral release and application of the graft. The *arrow* points to the graft. Generally, bilateral graft application is needed. *B*, bladder; *PB*, pubic bone; *R*, rectum; *V*, vagina

tory response. Porcine intestinal submucosa tissue (SIS®) is one of the available biomaterials that undergoes complete remodeling within 30 days [33, 34].

60.3.4 Anterior Compartment Complications

Weakness of the pubocervical fibromuscularis (PCFM), and lateral detachment of the PCFM from the arcus tendeneus or the cervical ring predisposes the anterior compartment to failure. The first step in repair of this compartment should be focused repair of damaged tissue by suture reapproximation. In cases where there is a lack of native tissue, reapproximation can result in mid-vaginal stenosis. More recently, surgeons have used a variety of mesh kits and biomaterial to patch the anterior compartment. The space between the bladder and the anterior vaginal epithelium is confined, increasing the risk of implant material showing through the bladder (Fig. 60.24) or the vagina (Fig. 60.25), or creation of a vesicovaginal fistula [35]. In the short term, when these complications occur, they result in tremendous suffering on the patient's part. Either of these problems requires removal of mesh. Despite the surgeon's best attempt, a patient may go to the operating room multiple times to achieve complete removal of the mesh that extrudes or erodes repeatedly.

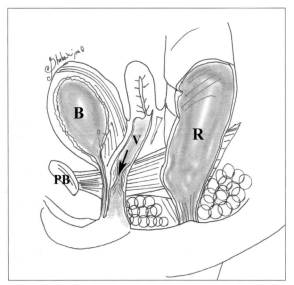

Fig. 60.22 Sagittal drawing of a mid-vaginal stenosis. The *arrow* points to the area of stenosis. *B*, bladder, *PB*, pubic bone; *R*, rectum; *V*, vagina

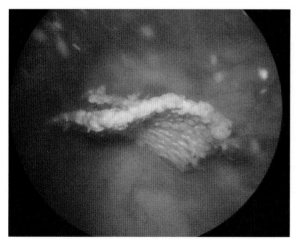

Fig. 60.24 Cystoscopic view of a silicone mesh eroded into the bladder subsequent to a robotic sacrocolpopexy

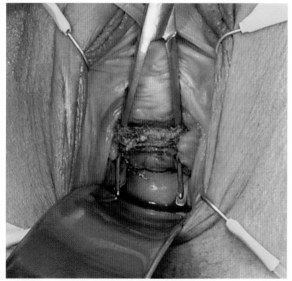

Fig. 60.25 An anterior Prolift® with extrusion into the vagina. The entire anterior compartment is devoid of vaginal epithelium and the chronically exposed mesh is calcified

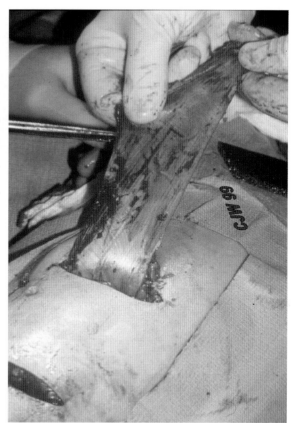

Fig. 60.26 A 20–22 cm by 4–6 cm fascia lata can be harvested

Bladder erosions require removal by laparotomy and cystotomy, or, if a minimally invasive route is chosen, we advocate a combined cystoscopic/laparoscopic approach where the endoshear enters via a 5 mm laparoscopic port that enters directly into the bladder, and the camera is attached to the operative cystoscope with a grasper.

The dilemma with removal of anteriorly implanted material is that the patient may have a recurrent anterior and/or apical prolapse subsequent to removal. It is good to return to basics and use the patient's own fascia lata for an anterior hammock procedure [36].

In this procedure, a large piece of fascia lata is harvested and fashioned into a trapezoid which subsequently is sutured laterally to the arcus tendineus, apically to the sacrospinous ligament [37] and the vaginal cuff, and distally to PCFM at the level of the urethrovesical junction (Fig. 60.26). This is the technique we use for repair of recurrent anterior prolapse. With use of the patient's own fascia lata, there is no risk of extrusion or erosion. In selected patients with deficient vaginal epithelium, if some of the fascia lata is left exposed it will be covered with vaginal epithelium over time, provided regular vaginal dilation is maintained.

60.3.5 Posterior Compartment Complications

The posterior vagina is supported by connections between the vagina, bony pelvis, and levator ani muscles. The lower one-third of the vagina is fused with the perineal body. During vaginal repair, the anatomical

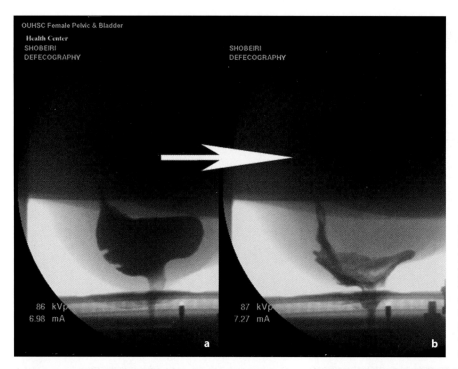

Fig. 60.27 Defecography images of a rectocele. In this patient with prior posterior repair with a mesh kit, the apical portion is not attached, resulting in a high enterocele (**a**). The caudal portion is not attached, causing incomplete evacuation of the stool (**b**)

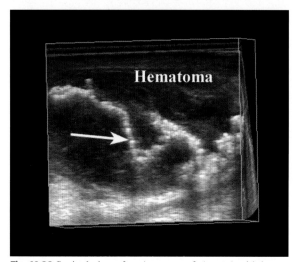

Fig. 60.28 Sagittal view of an Apogee graft (*arrow*) with hematoma

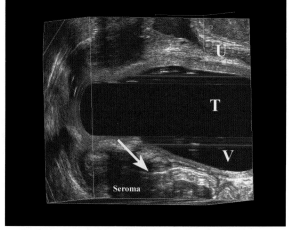

Fig. 60.29 Sagittal view of an SIS® graft (*arrow*) with seroma formation three weeks after surgery. *T*, ultrasound transducer in the vagina; *U*, uterus; *V*, vagina

relationships should be maintained. The use of mesh or biomaterial does not ensure successful repair (Fig. 60.27).

During placement of material in this compartment, brisk bleeding can be encountered. Additionally, the passage of trocars through the sacrospinous ligament, or placement of sutures in this compartment can result in bleeding from the inferior gluteal and pudendal vessels [38] (Fig. 60.28).

Because the posterior compartment is narrower, SIS® tissue has adequate tensile strength to be used to bridge the gap between the posterior arcus laterally, the sacrospinous or uterosacral ligaments as anchoring points, and the vaginal cuff or the cervical ring apically. SIS® is associated with seroma formation, even after vaginal packing is used for 24–48 h [39] (Fig. 60.29).

Whether a direct repair is done or implanted material is used, there is always a risk of rectovaginal fistula de-

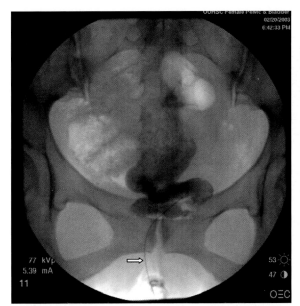

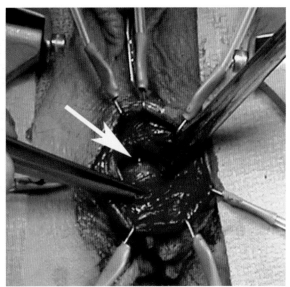

Fig. 60.30 Course of the fistula tract that the glide wire passes through. The *arrow* indicates the point of entry of the wire

Fig. 60.32 Intraoperative rectovaginal fistula glide wire is used to track the fistula and remove it in its entirety. The *arrow* points to the wire

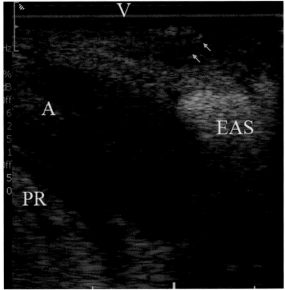

Fig. 60.31 3D ultrasound sagittal view of a rectovaginal fistula. The *arrows* demonstrate the fistula tract. *A*, anus; *EAS*, external anal sphincter; *PR*, puborectalis muscle; *V*, vagina

velopment [40]. Such fistulae develop if a suture is placed through the ano-rectum, if the ano-rectum is injured, or if mesh erodes into the ano-rectum or vagina. Patients present with passage of air, mucus, or frank feces per vagina.

Complex fistulae can also be evaluated by the use of CT scan, ultrasonography, or intraoperative retrograde techniques. We have described a technique for diagnosis of hard-to-find rectovaginal fistulae [41] (Fig. 60.30). Endovaginal ultrasonography with injection of hydrogen peroxide into fistula tracts can be used in the same manner, to visualize the rectovaginal fistula tract (Fig. 60.31).

If these fistulae are associated with mesh use, the repair attempt is more difficult. We generally use a glide wire to ascertain the course of these complex fistulae.

Depending on its location the fistula repair can be performed transperineally (Fig. 60.32), transvaginally, or transanally.

60.3.6 Introital Vaginal Complications

Perineorrhaphy is a traditional part of pelvic floor repair. A traditional perineorrhaphy repair involves making a diamond-shaped incision over the perineal skin and reapproximating the underlying tissue with sutures. This may result in stenosis of vaginal introitus [42] (Fig. 60.33). Addition of mesh to the posterior repair that extends to the perineal body, or the mesh that extends to under the urethra, and is subsequently exposed, complicates the attempts to repair introital vaginal stenosis (Fig. 60.34). Posterior compartment

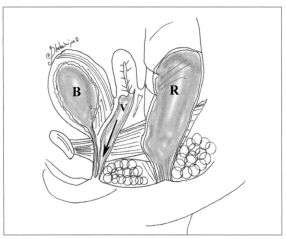

Fig. 60.33 Right sagittal drawing of an introital vaginal stenosis. The *arrow* points to the area of stenosis. *B*, bladder; *R*, rectum; *V*, vagina

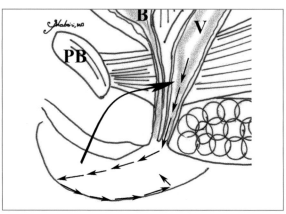

Fig. 60.36 Sagittal drawing of right introital stenosis. The *arrows* point to the line of z-plasty incision in preparation for the rotational vulvovaginal skin flap which results in widening of the vaginal introitus as seen in Fig. 60.37. *B*, bladder; *PB*, pubic bone; *V*, vagina

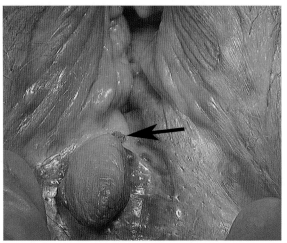

Fig. 60.34 Introital scarring and posterior mesh exposure (*arrow*), also note that the right labia minora is detached anteriorly

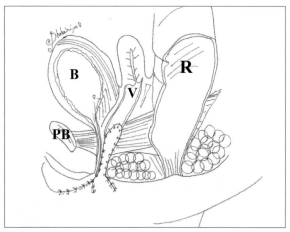

Fig. 60.37 Sagittal drawing of a right side view of a completed vulvovaginal skin flap for an introital vaginal stenosis. *B*, bladder; *PB*, pubic bone; *R*, rectum; *V*, vagina

scarring and narrowing can be surgically addressed with a vulvovaginal skin flap (Figs. 60.35–60.37). An anterior vaginal stenosis can be addressed with a reverse vulvovaginal skin flap. There are cases where there is extreme stenosis of the distal two-thirds of the vagina, and these may be addressed with transposition of bowel (Figs. 60.38, 60.39). These repairs are plagued with excess mucus production, stenosis of transposed bowel, and the need for surveillance to avoid the development of colon cancer in the neovagina.

Repair of a stenosed introitus requires reapproximation of the superficial transverse perinei, bulbospongiosus, puboperinealis, puboanalis, and rectovaginal septum for the best functional results.

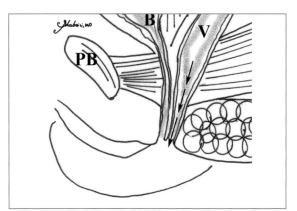

Fig. 60.35 Sagittal drawing of right introital stenosis. The *arrows* point to the line of relaxing incision in the lateral vagina in preparation for a skin graft. *B*, bladder; *PB*, pubic bone; *V*, vagina

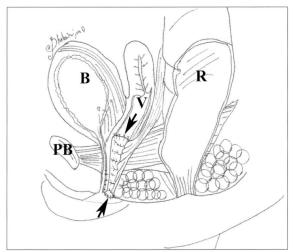

Fig. 60.38 Sigmoid colon transposition for introital vaginal stenosis. *Arrows* point to the sigmoid colon in place with its own blood supply. *B*, bladder; *PB*, pubic bone; *R*, rectum; *V*, vagina

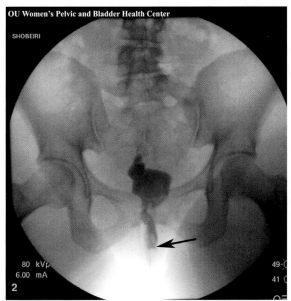

Fig. 60.39 Fluoroscopic image of a transposed sigmoid colon for vaginal agenesis. The *arrow* points to the area of introital stenosis

60.4 Summary

Knowledge of pelvic floor anatomy and function is essential for effective imaging and repair of complications of pelvic floor surgery. With advances in technology, MRI and 3D ultrasound techniques have increased our ability to detect pelvic floor complications and helped us to pose reasonably sound solutions to anatomically difficult problems.

References

1. Petros PE, Ulmsten U. An integral theory and its method for diagnosis and management of female urinary incontinence. Scand J Urol Nephrol 1993;153(suppl):1–89.
2. Ulmsten U, Petros P. Intravaginal slingplasty (IVS): An ambulatory surgical procedure for treatment of female urinary incontinence. Scand J Urol Nephrol 1995;29:75–82.
3. Shobeiri SA, Garely AD, Chesson RR et al. Recognition of occult bladder injury during the tension-free vaginal tape procedure. Obstet Gynecol 2002;99:1067–1072.
4. Shobeiri SA, Nihira MA. Attachment of a sling rescue suture to midurethral tape for management of potential postoperative voiding dysfunction. Neurourol Urodyn 2009;28: 990–994.
5. Maher CF, O'Reilly BA, Dwyer PL et al. Pubovaginal sling versus transurethral macroplastique for stress urinary incontinence and intrinsic sphincter deficiency: a prospective randomised controlled trial. BJOG 2005;112:797–801.
6. Skala CE, Petry IB, Gebhard S et al. Isolation of fibroblasts for coating of meshes for reconstructive surgery: differences between mesh types. Regen Med 2004;4:197–204.
7. Shobeiri SA, Gasser RF, Chesson RR, Echols KT. The anatomy of midurethral slings and dynamics of neurovascular injury. Int Urogyn J 2003;14:185–190.
8. Shobeiri SA, Echols KT, Franco N. Sinus formation after insertion of a silicone-coated suburethral sling. Int Urogynecol J Pelvic Floor Dysfunct 2003;14:356–7.
9. Bent AE, Ostegard DR, Zwick-Zaffuto MT. Tissue reaction to expanded polytetrafluoroethylene suburethral sling for urinary incontinence: clinical and histologic study. Am J Obstet Gynecol 1993;169:1198–1204.
10. Yamada B, Govier F, Stefanovic K, Kobashi K. High rate of vaginal erosions associated with the Mentor ObTape™. J Urol 2006;176:651–654.
11. Martius, H. Die operative Wiederherstellung der vollkommen fehlenden Harnrohare und des Schliessmuskels derselben. Zentralb Gynakol 1928;52:480.
12. Petrou SP, Jones J, Parra RO. Martius flap harvest site: patient self-perception. J Urol 2002;167:2098–2099.
13. Dowling RA, Corriere JN, Sandler CM. Iatrogenic ureteral injury. J Urol 1986;135:912–915.
14. Daly JW, Higgins KA. Injury to the ureter during gynecologic surgical procedures. Surg Gynecol Obstet 1988;167:19–22.
15. Harris RL, Cundiff GW, Theofrastous JP et al. The value of intraoperative cystoscopy in urogynecologic and reconstructive pelvic surgery. Am J Obstet Gynecol 1997;177:1367–1369.
16. Selzman AA, Spirnak JP. Iatrogenic ureteral injuries: a 20 year experience in treating 165 injuries. J Urol 1996;155:878–881.
17. Brudenell M. Medico-legal aspects of ureteric damage during abdominal hysterectomy. Br J Obstet Gynecol, 1996; 103:1180–1183.
18. Vakili B, Chesson RR, Kyle BL et al. The incidence of urinary tract injury during hysterectomy: a prospective analysis based on universal cystoscopy. Am J Obstet Gynecol 2005;192:1599–1604.
19. Burch JC. Urethrovaginal fixation to Cooper's ligament for correction of stress incontinence by simple vesicourethral suspension. Am J Obstet Gynecol 1961;81:281.
20. Morton HC, Hilton P. Urethral injury associated with minimally invasive mid-urethral sling procedures for the treatment

of stress urinary incontinence: a case series and systematic literature search. BJOG 2009;116:1120–1126.

21. Lee RA, Symmonds RE, Williams TJ. Current status of genitourinary fistula. Obstet Gynecol 1988;72:313–319.

22. Konigsberg H, Blunt K, Muecke E. Use of Boari flap in lower ureteral injuries. Urology 1975;5:751–755.

23. Shobeiri SA, Chesson RR, Echols KT. Cystoscopic fistulography: a new technique for the diagnosis of vesicocervical fistula. Obstet Gynecol 2001;98:1124–1126.

24. Petrou S, Brown J, Blaivas J. Suprameatal transvaginal urethrolysis. J Urol 2002;161:1268–1271.

25. Sexton DJ, Heskestad L, Lambeth WR et al. Postoperative pubic osteomyelitis misdiagnosed as osteitis pubis: report of four cases and review. Clin Infect Dis 1993;17:695–700.

26. Graham CW, Dmochowski RR, Faerber GJ et al. Pubic osteomyelitis following bladder neck surgery using bone anchors: a report of 9 cases. J Urol 2002;168:2055–2057.

27. Roth TM. Management of persistent groin pain after transobturator slings. Int Urogyn J 2007;18:1371–1373.

28. Bohrer JC, Chen CC, Walters MD. Pudendal neuropathy involving the perforating cutaneous nerve after cystocele repair with graft. Obstet Gynecol 2008;112:496–498.

29. Alevizon SJ, Finan MA. Sacrospinous colpopexy: management of postoperative pudendal nerve entrapment. Obstet Gynecol 1996;88:713–715.

30. Begley JS, Kupferman SP, Kuznetsov DD et al. Incidence and management of abdominal sacrocolpopexy mesh erosions. Am J Obstet Gynecol 2005;192:1956–1962.

31. Nygaard IE, McCreery R, Brubaker L et al. Abdominal sacrocolpopexy: a comprehensive review. Obstet Gynecol 2004;104:805–823.

32. Stepanian AA, Miklos JR, Moore RD, Mattox TF. Risk of mesh extrusion and other mesh-related complications after laparoscopic sacral colpopexy with or without concurrent laparoscopic-assisted vaginal hysterectomy: experience of 402 patients. J Minim Invasive Gynecol 2008;15:188–196.

33. Claerhout F, Verbist G, Verbeken E. Fate of collagen-based implants used in pelvic floor surgery: a 2-year follow-up study in a rabbit model. Am J Obstet Gynecol 2008;198:94.e1–94.e6.

34. Zheng F, Lin Y, Verbeken E et al. Inflammatory response after fascial reconstruction of abdominal wall defects with porcine dermal collagen and polypropylene in rats. Am J Obstet Gynecol 2004;191:1961–1970.

35. Yamada BS, Govier FE, Stefanovic KB, Kobashi KC. Vesicovaginal fistula and mesh erosion after Perigee (transobturator polypropylene mesh anterior repair). Urology 2006;68:1121.e5–7.

36. Chesson RR, Schlossberg SM, Elkins TE et al. The use of fascia lata graft for correction of severe or recurrent anterior vaginal wall defects. J Pelvic Med Surg 1999;5:96–103.

37. Shobeiri SA, Elkins TE, Thomas KA. Comparison of sacrospinous ligament, sacrotuberous ligament, and 0 polypropylene suture tensile strength. J Pelvic Surg 2000;6:261–267.

38. Barksdale PA, Elkins TE, Sanders CK. An anatomic approach to pelvic hemorrhage during sacrospinous ligament fixation of the vaginal vault. Obstet Gynecol 1998;91:715–718.

39. Deprest J, Zheng F, Konstantinovic M et al. The biology behind fascial defects and the use of implants in pelvic organ prolapse repair. Int Urogynecol J 2006;17(suppl 1):S16–25.

40. Hilger WS, Cornella JL. Rectovaginal fistula after posterior intravaginal slingplasty and polypropylene mesh augmented rectocele repair. Int Urogynecol J Pelvic Floor Dysfunct 2006;17:89–92.

41. Shobeiri SA, Quiroz LH, Nihira MA. Rectovaginal fistulography: a technique for identification of recurrent elusive fistulas. Int Urogynecol J Pelvic Floor Dysfunct 2009; 20(5)571–2.

42. Vassallo BJ, Karram MM. Management of iatrogenic vaginal constriction. Obstet Gynecol 2003;102:512–520.

Invited Commentary

G. Willy Davila

We have witnessed marked advances in pelvic reconstructive surgery over the past decade. These advances have been most notable in the areas of imaging, with the introduction of 3D ultrasound and dynamic magnetic resonance imaging (MRI), as well as in the use of novel materials and kits for pelvic reconstructive surgery. Imaging techniques have been primarily focused on diagnostic approaches, and materials and kits obviously for therapeutic surgical approaches. Blending of these two novel tools can in fact be very helpful for the pelvic surgeon – both in fine tuning implantation techniques as well as in evaluation of post-operative results and complications.

In this chapter on Imaging and Management of Complications of Urogynecologic Surgery, Dr Shobeiri shares a wealth of experience in the use of pelvic 2D and 3D ultrasound for the evaluation and management of pelvic surgical complications. He focuses on using imaging techniques to identify the nature of the complications and to develop an appropriate treatment plan. This, in fact, expands the horizons of imaging techniques in pelvic floor medicine. Although this application of imaging is still in its infancy, the numerous cases that are illustrated in this chapter should help expand the surgeon's horizons in applications of new imaging modalities. The vast number of illustrations in this chapter makes it a valuable resource for any surgeon planning on adding imaging techniques for the post-operative management of his/her patients.

Like any new and innovative surgical technique, the use of mesh and grafts for pelvic reconstruction has certainly has been fraught with controversy. Unexpected complications have been identified – particularly due to abnormalities in tissue healing – although the wealth of published data would suggest that anatomic and functional outcomes are improved with the use of mesh in pelvic reconstruction, relative to traditional techniques.

With the identification of type 1 polypropylene mesh as the only mesh that is applicable for surgical use in the pelvis, many of the previously identified complications related to infection, inflammatory reaction, and lack of incorporation other types of mesh have not required further attention.

Type 1 mesh is very well incorporated, and erosions are likely due primarily to technical factors such as hematoma formation, suture line breakdown, and urogenital atrophy.

Simplification of the management of mesh erosion/exposure without jeopardizing satisfactory long-term outcomes is thus highly desirable. It is rare to need to remove the entire graft in a patient with a mesh erosion [1].

Identification of mesh contraction as a cause of pelvic pain and dyspareunia has been limited to a clinical evaluation [2].

The role of imaging in identifying mesh contraction is expanding, with the hope of identifying those patients who require removal of a segment of the graft versus removal of the entire graft for resolution of pain symptoms. Since mesh contraction may be due to over-tensioning of the mesh during implantation, it is likely that imaging techniques could be valuable in guiding surgeons to achieve appropriate tensioning of mesh – avoiding over-tensioning – to avoid significant

G.W. Davila
Department of Gynecology,
Urogynecology and Reconstructive Pelvic Surgery, Cleveland Clinic Florida, Weston, FL, USA

contraction during the incorporation phase of the implanted mesh.

It is certain that imaging techniques will have greater applications in the evaluation of pelvic anatomy and identification of mesh complications related to pelvic surgery, and eventually in the prevention of complications relative to mesh use.

References

1. Hamilton Boyles S, McCrery R. Dyspareunia and mesh erosion after vaginal mesh placement with a kit procedure. Obstet Gynecol 2008;111:969–975.
2. Finer B, Maher C. Vaginal mesh contraction: definition, clinical presentation and management. Obstet Gynecol 2010; 115:325–331.

Investigation and Management of Complications after Coloproctological Surgery

61

Tim W. Eglington and Frank A. Frizelle

Abstract Coloproctological surgery is associated with a range of possible complications. This chapter reviews the incidence and management of complications specific to colorectal surgery and offers methods to assist in preventing their occurrence.

Keywords Colorectal Surgery • Intraoperative complications • Postoperative complications

61.1 Introduction

Patients undergoing major resectional colon and rectal surgery face a number of possible complications and the risk of perioperative mortality. In addition to the usual problems associated with any major surgery, colorectal resection can result in a number of specific infections, organ injuries, and stomal, thromboembolic and functional problems.

In addition to resectional surgery, this chapter will also discuss complications after surgery for colorectal functional disorders such as fecal incontinence and obstructive defecation, in particular the approach to failure of surgery with the persistence of symptoms.

61.2 Infection-related Complications

Specific infection-related complications include wound infection, intra-abdominal abscess, and anastomotic leak.

61.2.1 Anastomotic Leak

Of these complications, anastomotic leak is the most significant and feared, with the potential for considerable morbidity and mortality. A recent systematic review of the postoperative complication rates of rectal cancer surgery in the literature looked at 53 prospective cohort studies and 45 randomized controlled studies with 36,315 patients, of whom 24,845 patients had an anastomosis. The review found that the anastomotic leak rate, reported in 84 studies, was 11% (95% confidence interval, CI: 10–12); the pelvic sepsis rate, in 29 studies, was 12%; and the postoperative death rate, in 75 studies, was 2% [1]. In a univariable analysis, average age, median tumor height, and method of detection (clinical versus radiologic) were associated with different anastomotic leak rates. The year of publication, use of preoperative radiation, use of laparoscopy, and use of protecting stoma were not significant variables.

With respect to perioperative mortality, the year of publication, geographical study origin, average age, and use of laparoscopy were significant factors; however, median tumor height and preoperative radiation use were not. With multivariable analysis, only average age for anastomotic leak and year of publication for

F.A. Frizelle
Division of Colorectal Surgery, Department of Academic Surgery, University of Otago, Christchurch, New Zealand

G.A. Santoro, A.P. Wieczorek, C.I. Bartram (eds.) *Pelvic Floor Disorders*
© Springer-Verlag Italia 2010

Table 61.1 Complication rates of rectal cancer surgery (reproduced from [1], with permission)

Complication	Rate	95% CI	Number of studies
Wound infection	0.07	0.05–0.08	50
Anastomotic leak	0.11	0.10–0.12	84
Pelvic sepsis	0.12	0.09–0.16	29
Postoperative death	0.02	0.02–0.03	75

postoperative death remained significant [1] (Table 61.1). In 1991 the United Kingdom Surgical Infection Study Group defined anastomotic leak as the "leak of luminal contents from a surgical join between two hollow viscera" [2]. Many experts divide anastomotic leak into two categories based on presentation: subclinical and clinical anastomotic leak. Subclinical anastomotic leaks are leaks detected radiographically in patients with no abdominal signs or symptoms. These types of leaks are most commonly recognized

in diverted patients prior to takedown of a protective, diverting colostomy or ileostomy. Clinical anastomotic leakages are accompanied by signs of peritonitis or abscess, septicemia, and fecal or purulent discharge from the wound, drain, or anus. The incidence of anastomotic leak following colorectal surgery varies with the clinical scenario and the location of the anastomosis. The reported incidence of colorectal or colo-anal anastomotic leak ranges from 1% to 19%, colo-colic leak from 0% to 2%, ileo-colic leak from 0.02% to 4%, and ileo-ileal leak is around 1%.

The management of anastomotic leak also varies with the clinical scenario, and may range from a conservative approach with antibiotics to laparotomy, drainage, and takedown of the anastomosis with stoma formation. In 2008 the International Anastomotic Leak Study Group produced algorithms for the management of anastomotic leak according to the clinical scenario [3] (Figs. 61.1–61.3).

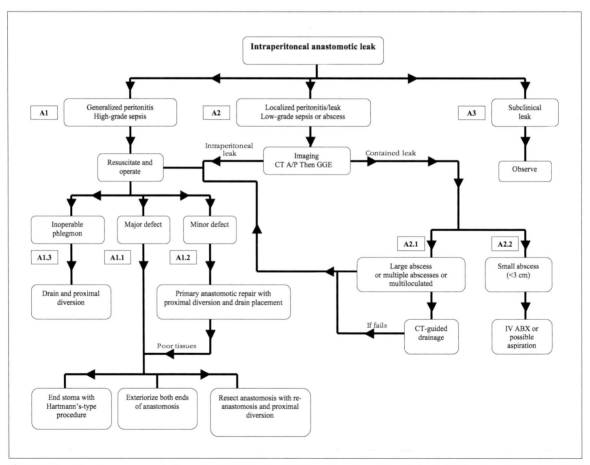

Fig. 61.1 Algorithm for management of non-diverted patients with intraperitoneal anastomotic leak. *GGE*, gastrografin enema. *ABX*, antibiotics. Reproduced from [3], with permission

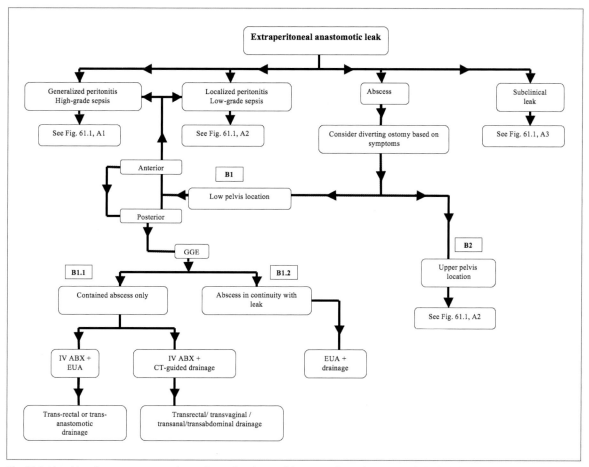

Fig. 61.2 Algorithm for management of non-diverted patients with extraperitoneal anastomotic leak. GGE, gastrografin enema. Reproduced from [3], with permission

61.2.2 Abscesses

61.2.2.1 Small Perianastomotic Abscess (< 3 cm)

If a small abscess (< 3 cm in size) is observed on computed tomography (CT) imaging, broad-spectrum intravenous antibiotics are recommended. Aspiration of the abscess can be performed if possible, as these collections are often too small for insertion of a drain. Many of these small abscesses will respond to broad-spectrum intravenous antibiotics alone, such as a second- or third-generation cephalosporin. Patients with a small abscess following colorectal anastomotic leak may also require bowel rest, with consideration for total parenteral nutrition. In the majority of cases though, enteral feeding and broad-spectrum intravenous antibiotic therapy against Gram-negative and anaerobic organisms are sufficient.

61.2.2.2 Larger Perianastomotic Abscess (> 3 cm)

Abscesses larger than 3 cm may be candidates for CT-guided drainage of the abscess cavity via a transabdominal, transvaginal, transanal, or transrectal pathway.

Low pelvic abscesses may require trans-sciatic or transgluteal approaches; however, these can be associated with sciatic neuritis or local dissemination of the abscess into the gluteal region. If CT-guided drainage fails or is not feasible, examination under anesthesia (EUA) may also permit transrectal or trans-anastomotic drainage. If it is unclear whether or not the abscess is in continuity with the anastomotic leak, the authors recommend that it is assumed that the abscess is in continuity and proceed with management within this context.

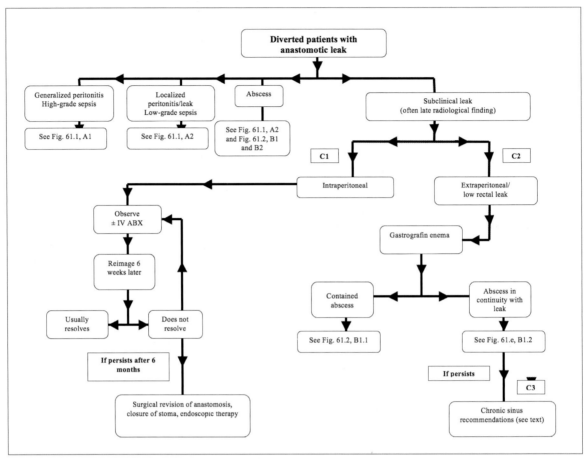

Fig.61.3 Algorithm for management of diverted patients with anastomotic leak. Reproduced from [3], with permission

61.2.2.3 Abscess in Continuity with Leak

If the abscess is in continuity with the anastomotic leak, and the anastomosis is low enough to be accessed transanally, then an EUA allows effective transanal drainage of the abscess with minimal risk of fistula development.

There are several options for transanal drainage. Firstly, it is possible to make a wide opening in the anastomosis with a finger or surgical instrument to allow drainage. An alternative approach is to make a small opening and insert a mushroom-tipped or other type of catheter, which can be sutured in place and made to exit through the anal canal. The drain can then be left in place for several weeks, with or without irrigation through the catheter. Prior to drain removal, repeat EUA or imaging should be considered to ensure resolution of the collection and absence of anastomotic stricture.

61.2.3 Low Rectal Anastomotic Sinus

A low rectal anastomotic sinus may be detected in an asymptomatic patient on luminal imaging prior to de-functioning stoma closure, or it may be identified in a symptomatic patient. The management depends on the size of the sinus and the overall clinical status of the patient. If the patient is asymptomatic and the sinus cavity is small, the patient can be observed, as such sinuses frequently resolve without intervention. If a small (< 1 cm in size) sinus cavity persists after 3 months from the initial surgery, there is usually no contraindication to reverse the stoma.

If the patient is symptomatic or the sinus cavity is large, a mushroom-tipped catheter may be inserted through the defect, with regular EUA every 3–4 weeks to allow the catheter to be gradually downsized. An alternative is to irrigate the abscess cavity with saline using a catheter placed through the defect.

It is important to note that the cavity behind the distal rectum has the potential to be large with rigid boundaries (pelvic sidewalls and sacrum). Therefore, the abscess cavity will often fail to shrink, even though it may be adequately drained. One option to deal with this difficult problem is to divide and marsupialize the posterior wall of the neo-rectum or ileal pouch using scissors or electrocautery. Great care must be taken to avoid injury to other structures that may form the wall of the cavity, such as the small intestine. This technique allows the cavity to granulate in, and the stoma is then closed some weeks later. Recently, the use of an endosponge suction dressing placed in the cavity via a transanal approach and changed at regular intervals has been reported to lead to more rapid collapse of the cavity [4]. Finally, if these less-invasive options fail, a redo anal anastomosis with diverting stoma may need to be considered.

61.2.4 Anastomotic Stricture

61.2.4.1 Colonic

Anastomotic strictures proximal to sigmoid colon are usually associated with Crohn's disease. If present,

such strictures rarely produce significant symptoms, because of the fluid consistency of the stool. When not associated with Crohn's disease they often occur in the setting of a previous anastomotic leak or an ischemic anastomosis. Short strictures may respond to colonoscopic dilation and, if malignancy has been excluded, a prolonged period of conservative management is reasonable as the stricture may soften and dilate. However, if this conservative approach fails, symptomatic patients will require surgical revision.

61.2.4.2 Rectal

Up to 50% of rectal anastomoses may be associated with a minor degree of stricturing; however, this rarely causes a problem. The key to management of a clinically significant stricture is to determine if the stricture is long or short. A pelvic magnetic resonance imaging scan (MRI) may well clarify this. In the case of late strictures and malignant disease, the other issue of concern is that of recurrent disease.

A clinically significant long stricture is usually associated with proximal limb ischemia, leading to anastomotic leak, pelvic sepsis, and subsequent stricture. This is worse if the patient had preoperative radiotherapy. Long strictures usually do not respond to di-

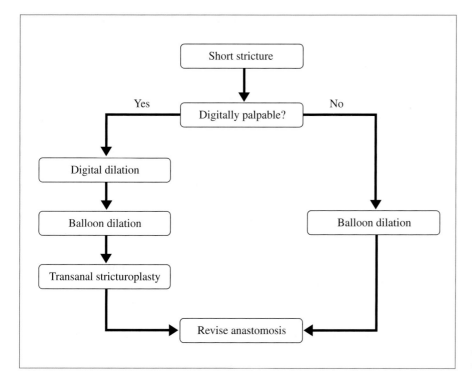

Fig. 61.4 Management of anastomotic stricture; short stricture

lation, and are usually associated with considerable surrounding fibrosis and scar tissue. Revision of these is difficult and often associated with considerable collateral damage, i.e. impotence, bleeding, ureteric injury, and poor function. Often the best solution is to leave the anastomosis defunctioned or to convert to abdominal perineal resection. Revision can be undertaken but is often technically challenging and requires considerable expertise in revisional pelvic surgery. In low hand-sewn anastomoses, a stricture may develop in up to 90% of cases, but when defecation is re-established the stool dilates the anastomosis adequately.

The management of short anastomotic stricture is summarized in Fig. 61.4.

61.2.5 Fistula

See Section VIII.

61.2.6 Wound Infection

The use of preoperative prophylactic antibiotics to reduce postoperative wound infection is well established. A recent systematic review of the postoperative complication rates of rectal surgery analyzed 53 prospective cohort studies and 45 randomized controlled studies with 36,315 patients; the wound infection rate, in 50 studies, was 7%, with two-thirds of infections occurring after discharge [1]. While inpatient wound-infection rates fit known risk factors, postdischarge wound-infection rates do not. A full discussion about the role of antibiotics and wound infection is beyond the scope of this chapter.

61.3 Intraoperative Organ Injury

61.3.1 Ureteric Injury

Iatrogenic ureteral injury occurs in 0.3–1% of primary colorectal pelvic surgery, and may be up to ten times higher in recurrent pelvic surgery. Intraoperative recognition of ureteric injury is an important factor in patient outcome. The morbidity and mortality are significantly higher when the diagnosis is delayed. Only 25–50% of injuries are recognized at the time of surgery. The use of preoperatively placed urethral catheters in selected cases, although not proven to prevent injury, can certainly aid in the recognition of the operative injury. In assessing intraoperative urethral injury, knowledge of the functional status of both the injured renal unit and the contralateral side is most helpful, especially in cases of extensive injury, where nephrectomy may be contemplated.

Repair of urethral injury depends on the area of the ureter injured and the extent of the injury. Injuries above the pelvic brim are generally repaired with uretero-ureterostomy, anastomosing the spatulated ends with fine absorbable interrupted sutures over a double J stent. Injuries within 5 cm of the ureterovesical junction are best managed by ureteroneocystotomy. A psoas hitch or Boari flap may be needed to provide adequate length. Transuretero-ureterostomy may be used as a method of reconstruction in cases of extensive ureteral resection in the region of the pelvic brim. The major concern with this solution is the involvement of the normal contralateral ureter.

When ureteral ligation is suspected, the entire course of the ureter may need to be dissected in the operative field. In this situation, a cystotomy and intraoperative insertion of ureteric catheters may be needed to define the site of ligation.

All repairs should be drained, and double J stents inserted for six weeks. In difficult repairs such as in irradiated fields, the repair should be supported with well-vascularized tissue, such as an omental pedicle.

61.3.2 Splenic Injury

Incidental injury occurs in cases in which splenic flexure mobilization is required. Previous abdominal operations, neoplastic or inflammatory involvement of the spleen, and advanced age all predispose to iatrogenic splenic injury. The majority of splenic injuries result from traction with avulsion of the capsule of the inferior pole. These injuries can usually be managed adequately by packing alone. The application of hemostatic agents such as microcrystalline collagen or topical thrombin in minor capsular tears may prove effective when packing alone fails. The much less frequent injury to the splenic hilum requires full mobilization of the spleen to precisely identify the location and extent of injury. Splenectomy may be required to control bleeding in some cases (15–20%). The concern about such radical measures includes the occurence of post-splenectomy sepsis. In addition, there is some evidence of reduced long-term survival in patients requiring splenectomy after adjustment for cancer stage [5].

61.4 Stomal Complications

61.4.1 Stoma Retraction

Stoma retraction is due either to a poorly placed stoma or to tension. Ischemia due to compromised blood supply, due to either excessive trimming of the mesentery or tension at the fascial level, may lead to necrosis with subsequent retraction at the site of demarcation. The incidence of stoma retraction is 1–6% in most series. This complication is usually avoidable with careful surgical technique and preoperative planning. The bowel should be adequately mobilized, and the vascularity preserved. The opening in the abdominal wall should be wide enough to accommodate the intended bowel. It is best to have a few centimeters of bowel protruding from the opening, which can be trimmed after abdominal wound closure. Suturing of the seromuscular layer to the fascia or elsewhere does not prevent retraction.

Early retraction may be noted in the immediate postoperative period. Usually the retraction is due to ischemia of the terminal portion of the bowel. When necrosis extends proximal to the fascia, surgical revision is usually necessary. Late retraction presents as a dimpled or recessed stoma, usually in an obese patient. It is often associated with stenosis, and the examiner is unable to insert their finger. When the stoma is buried between heavy skin folds and is almost invisible causing leakage around the appliance, revision is necessary.

61.4.2 Peristomal Skin Complications

Peristomal skin complications are common. Contact dermatitis is due to inflammation of the skin as a result of contact with an external agent such as stool, urine, pastes, solvents, soaps, or deodorants. The solution is to identify and avoid the agent. Chemical irritant contact dermatitis is the most common peristomal skin complication, and is usually due to a poor-fitting appliance.

61.5 Thromboembolic Complications

Pelvic surgery increases the risk of thromboembolic complications (deep venous thrombosis, DVT, and pulmonary embolism, PE). This risk is further increased in patients with malignancy or inflammatory bowel disease. A Cochrane review has established that the best prophylaxis in general surgery is heparin and graded compression stockings [6].

61.6 Sexual Dysfunction

Surgery to remove the rectum may cause a loss of sexual function due to autonomic nerve damage. Advancing age and surgery for malignant disease are associated with an increased risk of postoperative problems.

The sympathetic and parasympathetic nervous systems are required for sexual function. In males, sacral parasympathetic fibers carry the neural outflow that mediates dilatation of the vascular inflow to the corpora cavernosa that results in penile erection. The neuronally mediated vasodilatation responsible for erection is dependent on nitric oxide (NO)-induced relaxation of the cavernosal sinusoids. Sympathetic fibers are responsible for emission of semen from the seminal vesicles into the prostatic urethra. In addition, sympathetic fibers innervate the vasa, prostate, urethra, and internal urethral sphincter, a small collection of smooth muscle fibers located at the bladder neck that prevent retrograde ejaculation. Simultaneous sympathetic activation of the muscular components of these structures, together with rhythmic stimulation of the bulbospongiosus and ischiocavernosus muscles that surround the bulbar urethra and the corpora in the superficial perineal pouch, results in ejaculation. The sacral spinal cord is responsible for coordination of the sexual response. Afferent fibers travel to the cord in the pudendal nerve from the dorsal nerve of the penis (clitoris); descending input arrives from higher centers, and efferent fibers travel in the sympathetic, parasympathetic and pudendal nerves [7].

In women, parasympathetic activation mediates the release of vasoactive intestinal polypeptide from nerve endings in the vagina, which results in a marked increase in vaginal transudation of fluid, which, together with Bartholin gland secretion, permits successful vaginal lubrication. In addition, parasympathetic stimulation causes vascular engorgement of the clitoris and labia, analogous to the situation in men. Autonomic damage results in vaginal dryness and dyspareunia [7].

Isolated sympathetic denervation is identified in men by failure to ejaculate despite being able to achieve a satisfactory erection. Such isolated sympathetic damage may occur anywhere from the pre-aortic plexus to the confluence of sympathetic and parasympathetic fibres at the inferior hypogastric plexus, but is less likely to occur distal to that point. In support of this argument, the incidence of isolated ejaculatory failure appears independent of the type of operation performed for rectal cancer – either abdominal perineal excision or low or high anterior resection – suggesting that it is that part of the operation common to all three in which damage occurs [7].

61.6.1 Sympathetic Damage

The sympathetic fibers may be inadvertently damaged at a number of points [7], as the followings.

1. On the aorta during ligation of the inferior mesenteric artery (IMA): the pre-aortic plexus may be damaged during ligation of the IMA at its origin on the anterior surface of the aorta. The IMA plexus forms a fine network of fibers on the vessel as it arises from the anterior aspect of the aorta. The superior hypogastric plexus and the origin of the hypogastric nerves are directly posterior in relation to the IMA and the superior rectal artery as it travels caudally. These sympathetic fibers are easily incorporated in the IMA pedicle if blunt or finger dissection is used to sweep the IMA off the front of the aorta. Damage at this site can be avoided by the use of sharp dissection under direct vision with either diathermy or scissors.

2. At the pelvic brim: sympathetic fibers are also at risk at the pelvic brim as they pass medial to the ureter and tangentially to the lateral edge of the mesorectum where the fascia covering the latter is less well developed. Inadvertent division here is avoided by sharp dissection with adequate traction and counter traction, while keeping the nerves in view.

61.6.2 Parasympathetic Damage

Parasympathetic or combined damage results in impotence in men and vaginal dryness and consequent dyspareunia in women. Controversy exists as to the precise site of parasympathetic damage but essentially there are four possible locations.

1. Damage during perineal dissection: the parasympathetic fibers may be avulsed close to their origin if the perineal operator strips the presacral fascia off the sacrum in abdomino-perineal excision; however, this is unlikely to be a common mechanism of injury in contemporary practice.

2. Damage during lateral pelvic wall dissection: the extensive lateral pelvic sidewall lymphadenectomy practiced by Japanese groups results in a very high rate of impotence and bladder dysfunction due to damage to the inferior hypogastric plexus as its fibers lie superficial to the pelvic vessels and associated nodes; when conventional rectal dissection is practiced by the same authors, rates of impotence are significantly lower and bladder dysfunction is uncommon; the routine use of large clamps to ligate the lateral ligaments is unnecessary and is likely to increase the risk of damaging the plexus, and should be avoided.

3. Damage during anterior rectal dissection: an important site of damage appears to be the delicate cavernosal fibers that pass anterolateral to the rectum on their way to pierce the urogenital diaphragm before entering the corpora. The autonomic fibers at this level are not visible to the naked eye due to their small size. Particular attention must be paid to the 2 and 10 o'clock positions, as this is where the cavernosal fibers are at greatest risk. Division of Denonvilliers' fascia proximal to the base of the prostate avoids damage to the cavernosal fibers.

4. Perimuscular and intersphincteric dissection: while conservative peritoneal incisions laterally and anteriorly around the pelvis keep dissection away from the autonomic nerves, most groups have abandoned the time-consuming and more vascular perimuscular dissection through the mesorectum on the posterior aspect of the rectum. Provided the hypogastric nerves are identified at the start of rectal dissection as previously described, and conservative peritoneal incisions are made, the dissection of the rectum is easier, quicker and less bloody if the mesorectum is removed with the specimen, even in benign disease. Such an approach does not appear to increase the risk of impotence following

restorative proctocolectomy. Close dissection on the muscle of the rectum is, however, essential anteriorly and anterolaterally from the peritoneal reflection down to the pelvic floor, thus avoiding the cavernosal fibers by staying behind Denonvilliers' fascia. Removing the mesorectum has the added advantage of providing room for an ileo-anal pouch to sit comfortably in the pelvis.

61.6.3 Treatment of Postoperative Sexual Dysfunction

In those men who are unable to achieve an erection after rectal excision, parasympathetic denervation is the likely cause. However, in a significant proportion of men, spontaneous recovery has been recorded up to 2 years after surgery. A period of observation and encouragement may therefore be appropriate initially. If the physical nature of the problem is in doubt, an absence of or a reduction in nocturnal tumescence, as measured by the 'Rigiscan' device (Dacomed Corporation, Minneapolis, MN, USA), will confirm its organic nature.

In patients with established neurogenic impotence, physical treatments, with either implanted silicone rods or inflatable penile implants, have largely given way to pharmacological approaches, although vacuum assist devices are effective and popular with some patients. The current mainstay of treatment is oral sildenafil (Viagra; Pfizer, New York, NY, USA), which is effective in up to 80% of patients who are impotent after surgery for rectal resection.

Intracavernosal injection of prostaglandin E1 (Caverject; Pharmacia and Upjohn, Crawley, UK), which can be combined with papaverine and phentolamine, will produce an erection sufficient for vaginal penetration in up to 70% of men. Unwanted effects, however, include pain at the injection site, corporal fibrosis, and priapism, and it is limited to second-line therapy.

A number of simple measures can ameliorate sexual problems after rectal excision in women. Personal lubricants are of value in vaginal dryness due to parasympathetic denervation. A change in position during intercourse can help reduce pain and discomfort when this is a problem. A reduction in oral intake and emptying the pouch before intercourse can prevent pouch leakage during intercourse [7].

61.7 Fecal Incontinence

Fecal incontinence after sphincter-saving surgery for rectal cancer is relatively common and troublesome, but its occurrence can be decreased with careful patient selection, appropriate use of adjuvant therapy, and operative approaches. The same systematic review cited earlier, of 53 prospective cohort studies and 45 randomized controlled studies with 36,315 patients after rectal cancer surgery [1], found incontinence rates reported in 12 of these studies ranging from 1% to 63%. However, as the fecal incontinence rates were reported in so few studies and so heterogeneously, the authors concluded that numerical summarization was inappropriate.

Patients with pre-existing incontinence and poor sphincter function preoperatively, particularly elderly, multigravid females, are likely to have worse function postoperatively if a restorative procedure is performed; hence, adequate preoperative assessment is important. The timing of preoperative incontinence is important to assess, as in some circumstances the tumor itself, rather than any underlying sphincteric or neural mechanism, may produce symptoms of urgency and incontinence, and these symptoms will resolve with resection. Postoperative radiotherapy is associated with worse functional outcome and, where possible, adjuvant radiotherapy should be administered preoperatively such that the radiotherapy-affected tissue is removed at subsequent surgery.

The technique of anastomosis has an important impact on function. In the early postoperative period, a colonic J pouch has been shown to decrease stool frequency, urgency, and nocturnal bowel movements, although by two years postoperatively there is little difference in these outcomes whether a pouch or straight anastomosis has been employed. A small percentage of patients will have debilitating incontinence and require stoma formation.

61.8 Complications after Surgery for Functional Disorders

61.8.1 Fecal Incontinence

The mainstay of surgical therapy for fecal incontinence associated with sphincter injury is sphincter repair. This technique is associated with the usual immediate complications of infection and hemorrhage. However, more significantly, sphincter repair is associated with a failure rate of up to 30% in the early stages, and recent evidence suggests that in the long term, less than half of patients will have sustained benefit [8]. Co-existing pudendal neuropathy has not consistently been shown to be a predictor of worse outcome; hence, in the presence of a sphincter defect, most will proceed with sphincter repair irrespective of the results of pudendal nerve terminal motor latency tests. In the past, surgical intervention after failed sphincter repair has been approached with either a repeat repair in the presence of a documented persisting sphincter defect or, failing that, colostomy.

There are now a number of novel therapies available and of these, sacral nerve stimulation (SNS) now provides an alternative in this group of patients. SNS applies a low-amplitude electrical current to a sacral nerve via an implantable stimulator. Multiple case series and two randomized studies have demonstrated improvement in continence in up to 80% of patients [9, 10]. Early studies required an intact sphincter mechanism for inclusion; however, more recent work has shown efficacy in patients with sphincter defects and after failed sphincteroplasty [11]. Hence SNS shows promise in this group of patients, although data on long-term outcomes are still required.

61.8.2 Rectal Prolapse

There is a huge variety of approaches to surgery for full-thickness rectal prolapse and these are broadly categorized into perineal and abdominal operations. Perineal approaches include Delormes' and Altemeirs', whereas suture rectopexy, resection rectopexy, and ventral mesh rectopexy are examples of commonly used abdominal approaches.

Traditionally, perineal approaches such as Delormes' or Altemeirs' are utilized in the elderly with comorbidity as they can be performed under regional anesthesia and do not carry the major complications seen after abdominal procedures. Bleeding, infection, obstructed defecation, and incontinence can all occur after these approaches. In addition, due to the low colo-anal anastomosis, Altemeirs' procedure also carries the risk of leak and pelvic sepsis, which requires management along the lines described above. The achilles heal of the Delormes' procedure is recurrence, which occurs in 30% or more.

Abdominal procedures are associated with a lower recurrence rate but carry additional risks. In addition to the risks associated with laparotomy, these include autonomic nerve damage leading to sexual and urinary dysfunction and, most significantly, worsening or de novo constipation. Resection rectopexy has been advocated in patients with constipation; however, it carries the risk of anastomotic dehiscence which many surgeons find unacceptable in the setting of benign disease. A number of groups have recently shown that laparoscopic ventral mesh rectopexy is associated with a low rate of constipation and avoids the need for anastomosis [12]. The laparoscopic approach also avoids the requirement for major laparotomy and is generally well tolerated even in elderly patients.

When dealing with recurrence after prolapse surgery, the approach will depend on the previous surgery and the clinical setting. Recurrent prolapse after Delormes' procedure can be approached with a redo Delormes' procedure; however, the submucosal plane is often difficult to establish and further recurrence is common. Where possible, an abdominal procedure avoids this problem due to the virgin state of the extra-rectal pelvic tissue planes. Conversely, after a failed abdominal approach, a Delormes' procedure may be a simpler and safer option than complex redo pelvic surgery.

61.8.3 Obstructed Defecation

As with surgery for overt rectal prolapse, there are a number of different management options for patients with obstructive defecation (OD) syndrome. The mainstay of therapy for OD includes dietary modification, laxatives, and biofeedback. If this conservative management fails and there are anatomical abnormalities detected in association with the OD, surgery may be considered.

Options include rectocele repair via transvaginal, transanal, or transperineal approaches. Morbidity with conventional rectocele repair is low however; recurrence and persistent OD symptoms are a significant problem. For this reason, stapled transanal resection of the rectum (STARR) has become increasingly popular. This operation addresses rectal intussusception in addition to rectocele. The European STARR registry recently published complications after STARR in a series of 1456 patients [13]. Unexpected pain was most common (8%), followed by urinary retention (7%), bleeding (4.5%), staple line complications (3.2%), and sepsis (1.4%) A number of serious complications of the procedure have been reported, including rectal necrosis and rectovaginal fistula. The same registry data suggested efficacy of 85–93%. If symptoms persist following unsuccessful STARR, conservative management with biofeedback should be revisited. Further surgery is dependent on persisting anatomical abnormalities. Some authors report successful repeat STARR procedures, for persisting rectocele; however, significant persisting rectal intussusception or additional problems such as enterocele may be better dealt with by an alternative approach such as ventral rectopexy. The key to avoiding complications with OD surgery is careful patient selection, and all patients being considered for surgery should be carefully investigated to rule out a proximal cancer, slow-transit constipation, irritable bowel syndrome, and anismus.

Acknowledgement

Section 61.6 was reproduced (modified) from [7], with permission.

References

1. Paun BC, Cassie S, MacLean AR et al. Postoperative complications following surgery for rectal cancer. Ann Surg 2010;251:807–818.
2. Peel AL, Taylor EW. Proposed definitions for the audit of postoperative infection: a discussion paper. Surgical Infection Study Group. Ann R Coll Surg Engl 1991; 73:385–358.
3. Phitayakorn R, Delaney CP, Reynolds HL et al. International Anastomotic Leak Study Group standardized algorithms for management of anastomotic leaks and related abdominal and pelvic abscesses after colorectal surgery. World J Surg 2008;32:1147–1156.
4. Bemelman W. Vacuum assisted closure in coloproctology. Tech Coloproctol 2009;13:261–263.
5. Wakeman CJ, Dobbs BR, Frizelle FA et al. The impact of splenectomy on outcome after resection for colorectal cancer: a multicenter, nested, paired cohort study. Dis Colon Rectum 2008;51:213–217.
6. Wille-Jørgensen P, Rasmussen MS, Andersen BR, Borly L. Heparins and mechanical methods for thromboprophylaxis in colorectal surgery. Cochrane Database Syst Rev 2003;(4):CD001217.
7. Keating JP. Sexual function after rectal excision. ANZ J Surg 2004;74:248–259.
8. Malouf A, Norton C, Engel AF et al. Long term results of anterior overlapping sphincter repair for obstetric trauma. Lancet 2000;355:260–265.
9. Jarrett M, Mowatt G, Glazener C et al. Systematic review sacral nerve stimulation for faecal incontinence and constipation. Br J Surg 2004;91:1559–1569.
10. Mowatt G, Glazener C, Jarrett M. Sacral nerve stimulation for faecal incontinence and constipation in adults. Cochrane Database Syst Rev 2007;(3):CD004464.
11. Brouwer R, Duthie G. Sacral nerve neuromodulation is effective treatment for fecal incontinence in the presence of a sphincter defect, pudendal neuropathy, or previous sphincter repair. Dis Colon Rectum 2010;53:273–288.
12. Collinson R, Wijffels N, Cunningham C, Lindsey I. Laparoscopic ventral rectopexy for internal rectal prolapse: short term results. Colorectal Dis 2010;12:97–104.
13. Jayne D, Schwander O, Stuto A. STARR for obstructed defaecation syndrome (ODS): 12 month follow-up. Dis Colon Rectum 2008;51(Suppl):16.

In addition to those illustrated by the authors of this chapter, the complications following colorectal and proctocological surgery are various and related to the indication, to the choice of treatment, and to the general clinical condition.

Under a series of subheadings, the authors have correctly addressed all the complications related to:

- anastomotic complications
- stomal problems
- injury to other organs
- thromboembolic problems
- functional complications.

Their discussion is supported by a large number of valid recent and important publications, in particular regarding the incidence and management of these complications; however, there is not a great deal in the text regarding investigation of the timing for a correct and opportune diagnosis.

Anastomotic Complications

The authors emphasize the difference between clinical and subclinical conditions and, in this case, it is appropriate to acknowledge the role of imaging (from ultrasound to computerized tomography, CT), without neglecting traditional radiology). My experience is totally in accord with that described in the text as well as with international reports, and reinforces the evidence for conservative management of patients with

F. La Torre
Department of Surgical Sciences, University "La Sapienza", Roma, Italy

subclinical status. A non-invasive treatment in all the clinical conditions with poorly defined symptoms is always considered, while invasive treatment is mandatory in all remaining conditions, beginning with ultrasonography or CT-guided treatment with explorative laparotomy, and progressing to diverting stoma in the case of large peri-anastomotic abscesses. In all cases of anastomotic strictures, our first choice must be endoscopic dilatation – of course for those that are no longer than 5–7 cm, and without local malignancy. On the other hand, we can use an endoscopic prosthesis and re-operative treatment with resection and re-anastomosis in colonic and proximal rectal strictures, or a Hartmann's procedure or abdominal-perineal procedure in lower rectal anastomotic stenosis, particularly in post-radiation patients.

Stomal Problems

Creation of a perfect stoma is fundamental for the future of individual patients, and this is also true of a protection stoma. This is because all the complications related to stomas are very disabling, in addition to the disabling nature of the stoma itself; therefore, it is essential that all techniques that help to avoid any problems are used in our surgical practice. Beginning with a correct and long vascular preparation, with a stump that is more than adequate, we also need to perform a regular closure and fixation of the intestine to the abdominal wall. According to these procedures, we can avoid the majority of ischemia-necrosis responsible for retraction and early re-operation, as well as hernia and prolapse. All types of skin complications are related and secondary to a badly constructed stoma, and result in difficult and disabling stoma care.

Splenic and Ureteric Injuries

When performing major colorectal surgery, abdominal complications are observed and frequently described in the international literature. In the case of splenic injury, the surgical procedure has changed in recent years, in favor of a conservative approach rather than splenectomy. With packing and the appropriate use of haemostatic agents, the incidence of splenectomy has dropped to 15–20%. Ureteric injuries are more frequent in the case of a re-operation: early identification of this kind of lesion is very important, because it allows direct ureteric repair and the use of a double J stent which are associated with few problems; all the major morbidity and the mortality results from a late identification.

Thromboembolic Complications

The use of heparin and graded compression stockings, as prophylaxis of deep venous thrombosis and pulmonary embolism, are mandatory in pelvic surgery, particularly in cases of malignancy and inflammatory bowel disease, and have significantly reduced the incidence of mortality.

Functional Complications

A long discussion has been reserved for functional complications. In a high proportion of cases treated for malignant or functional disease, additional functional complications are also observed. These kinds of complications are more justified when they occur after major surgery for cancer, but not in the case of functional surgery. Sexual problems are observed with lesions of the sympathetic and parasympathetic nervous system, and in males result in a defect of erection, while in females they lead to dyspareunia and vaginal dryness. This is observed more frequently during rectal isolation from the sacral wall or with a perineal approach, or because of lymphoadenectomy which occurs with rectal cancer and, more frequently, during re-operations.

Other problems following nervous lesions are observed in the case of "neurological bladder". More than 30% of sexual problems show spontaneous remission within 2 years after surgery. In males, the treatment of sexual complication is based on the use of sildenafil and penile prosthesis implant, while in females it is based on the use of lubricants.

Fecal incontinence is often the price of sphincter-saving procedures for distal rectal cancer. An appropriate pre-operative functional evaluation, as well as the use of postoperative radiation, can help in avoiding the occurrence of fecal incontinence; poor sphincter function is a bad prognostic indicator for restorative surgery. Different evaluations are needed for combined approaches, pull-throughs, and colonic and ileal pouches. On the other hand, fecal incontinence may occur following functional surgery as well as after direct sphincter repair. The importance of perineal rehabilitation (electrostimulation and biofeedback) and the use of sacral nerve stimulation must be emphasized. Full-thickness rectal prolapse may be treated by an abdominal or a transanal surgical approach. Abdominal approaches are described with and without resection and with and without meshes. The incidence of recurrence is high but less than in the perineal approach, which is reserved mostly for elderly individuals with comorbidity.

Obstructed defecation requires important discussion regarding the possibility of an invasive treatment. In my opinion, a large number of procedures are performed without an appropriate preoperative evaluation and, mostly, without a correct and prolonged medical treatment. All surgical procedures performed for an indication of obstructed defecation may have several complications related to the physiology of defecation as well as to anal and pelvic pain and to bleeding, so that, in our opinion, more consideration must be given to this kind of indication, as in all fields of functional surgical treatment.

Invited Commentary

Iwona Sudoł-Szopińska and Małgorzata Kołodziejczak

The authors of this chapter should be congratulated on a well-presented summary of complications after colorectal surgery. Their thorough overview ranges from presenting the statistics of these complications to the algorithms for their management. Without a doubt this work would have greater didactic value if it mentioned the examinations to be performed in diagnosing the presented complications. Also lacking were complications of surgery or procedures on the anal canal, such as incontinence of gas and stool, the recurrence of a fistula-in-ano or an abscess, and strictures and deformations of the anal canal.

Incontinence

Anal sphincters may be damaged in the course of a careless hemorrhoidectomy, through cutting of the internal anal sphincter during a fissurectomy, as well as while operating on an anal fistula, particularly the high kind.

An underestimated cause of postoperative incontinence is a too extended resection of the anal canal's mucous membrane, along with the transition zone that contains receptors differentiating loose stool from liquid and gases; the absence of these receptors results in sensory fecal incontinence. This could occur after an extensive hemorrhoidectomy or an unskillfully-performed operation with the Longo technique. Bilateral damage to the inferior rectal nerves, which could occur during operations of horseshoe fistulae or abscesses, is a rare cause of incontinence. The authors did not encounter this complication in their own surgical practice.

In the diagnosis of incontinence, endoanal ultrasonography (EAUS) is the method of choice for classifying patients with signs and symptoms of incontinence into those with normal anal sphincters or damaged ones. In the case of the latter subgroup, this imaging modality is used to evaluate the extent of the injury, which is necessary in qualifying a patient for surgery and for its planning. After a successful operation of a fistula, scarring of the external anal sphincter and the puborectalis muscle are commonly observed, as is a defect in the continuity of the internal anal sphincter, associated with its partial resection in the course of removing the fistula. A similar focal discontinuity of the internal anal sphincter is frequently seen after an internal sphincterotomy, performed for the treatment of an anal fissure. The consequence of this complication is incontinence and soiling [1]. Of course on the basis of the EAUS image alone it is not possible to conclude whether the visualized physical damage of the internal sphincter is responsible for the reported incontinence symptoms. Integrating the result of a preoperative proctological examination with the EAUS picture, as well as sphincter function from anorectal manometry, allows differentiation of a morphological injury from a neurogenic one.

Recurrence of the Disease

The most common reason for the early recurrence of an abscess (i.e. within 2 weeks from the procedure) is an incision that is too small and inadequate drainage. According to Onaka et al, this occurs in 7.6% of patients [2]. Usually this is due to evacuating only the

I. Sudoł-Szopińska
Department of Diagnostic Imaging, Medical University of Warsaw, Poland

G.A. Santoro, A.P. Wieczorek, C.I. Bartram (eds.) *Pelvic Floor Disorders*
© Springer-Verlag Italia 2010

lower chamber of an hourglass-shaped abscess.

The most frequent cause of fistula recurrence is errors in operative technique, such as not identifying the internal opening, leaving part of the main track and its branches, too tight suturing of the wound, inadequate drainage, or formation of a new inflammatory channel.

The majority of recurrences occur within 1 year of the operation, and according to various authors this pertains to 0–26% of cases [3–5]. In our opinion, the way the patient is managed postoperatively is extremely important. In most cases, wounds should be left to heal per secundam, which prevents the formation of a new fistulous track.

The recurrence of hemorrhoid disease is rare and results from the procedure being insufficiently radical. It is more often associated with alternative treatment methods, which are used in the second and third stages of the disease. For example, after the DGHL method (Doppler-guided hemorrhoidal artery ligation), hemorrhoidal recurrence is approximately 12% [6].

EAUS is the imaging modality of first choice for diagnosing complications after operations of anal fistulae and abscesses. In our center it is routine to perform a 3D EAUS examination 3 months after an anal fistula operation, as well as after incising a complicated anal abscess; this imaging is done earlier in the case of signs and symptoms suggesting a recurrence or inadequate drainage of an abscess. An important goal of control visits by patients with an abscess is early recognition of anal fistula formation, often not yet fully complete. In the case of recurrent fistulae, the endosonographic picture is usually unambiguous. Our latest studies, like those of other authors [7], do not show any significant advantage of EAUS in diagnosing primary and recurrent fistulae; the fistulae appear hypoechoic more frequently than a postoperative scar, although at times they can be anechoic, as described by Law et al [8]. Several authors have experienced difficulties in recognizing this complication [9–11]. Yet after applying a 3% hydrogen peroxide solution through the external opening of the fistula (hydrogen peroxide-enhanced ultrasound, HPUS), an improvement in the accuracy of EAUS is achieved [9, 12–14]. Nonetheless, this improvement is not great enough to deem HPUS as the method of choice for preoperative diagnosis of a recurrent fistula. The efficacy of HPUS with contrast depends on the patency of the fistula and its branches on the day of examina-

tion, as well as their level with respect to the anal sphincters. Additionally, quite often recurrent fistulae may not have an external opening.

The fistula can be differentiated from a scar through magnetic resonance imaging (MRI). The scar gives off a low signal in T1 and T2 images, as well as in STIR sequences. In contrast, given the presence of inflammatory changes, the fistulae or abscesses in most cases present an increased signal on T2-weighed images, and show increased enhancement of their walls after intravenous contrast administration [15–17].

Another useful modern imaging modality is 3D EAUS, along with various post-processing techniques of 3D data. Although their diagnostic value is yet to be determined, initial studies show the volume render mode (VRM) post-processing technique to be more sensitive than the standard examination in B-mode grayscale for locating the fistula's internal opening [18]. Our own studies support the use of the VRM technique in diagnosing residual abscesses, retro-anal inflammatory changes, differentiating scars from recurrent fistulae, and in the diagnosis of anal sphincter injury.

In our opinion, a necessary supplement to the endosonographic evaluation of the anal canal is transperineal ultrasonography (TPUS). This imaging is not commonly used in most centers, whereas we perform it for the diagnosis of superficial fistulae and anal abscesses, including recurrent ones. TPUS allows localization of subcutaneous extensions to the perineum, base of the scrotum, etc, not seen in EAUS. On the other hand, EAUS is a necessary supplement to TPUS to exclude the fistula coexisting with advanced changes in the course of hidradenitis suppurativa, or in differentiating this entity or a pilonodal cyst from an anal fistula, when the skin changes are not characteristic.

Stenosis of the Anal Canal

This complication could occur after any operation on the anal canal. Most often it is seen after hemorrhoidectomy, fissurectomy, or after low anterior resection of the rectum [19, 20]. It may also be the result of a postoperative infection or the organism's natural tendency for stenosing scar formation. It could be due to errors in the surgical technique, such as not preserving some healthy anoderm bridges in the anal canal, or too tight suturing of the wound. Frequent postoperative control visits allow for earlier diagnosis of stenoses as they form and thus make possible their conservative management, i.e. with an appropriate diet. High-degree stenoses require operative treatment via sphincterotomy or plastic surgery of the anal canal. These operations are performed from the perineal approach or from an abdominal one (where the formation of a temporary colonostomy may be required), depending on the level of the stenosis [19].

The diagnosis of high-grade stenosis necessitates examination under anesthesia. In our center, aside from proctography with a thin catheter, we use 3D EAUS with a 3D endorectal probe (3.3–10 MHz) placed on the skin around the anus. With the help of post-processing techniques, this examination provides a precise preoperative assessment of the stenosis anatomy, including its length and level, as well as any coexisting morphological changes in the anal sphincters.

Deformation of the Anal Canal

This complication occurs most frequently after removal of a fistula with the Hippocrates technique, or after an open internal sphincterotomy. It has both cosmetic and functional consequences. A significant deformity, such as a keyhole deformation, makes cleaning of the area difficult, and patients report fecal soiling and pruritus or burning of the perianal skin. Its treatment is surgical.

In conclusion, as stated by the authors of this chapter, patients undergoing coloproctologic surgery face a number of possible complications – those typical for any surgery plus those specific to the treatment of coloproctologic diseases, including permanent disorders of ano-rectal function. These must be borne in mind by the surgeon operating such patients. In many cases, imaging techniques assist in minimizing the number of complications by allowing for appropriate planning of the treatment.

References

1. Ratto C. Invited commentary. Surgical and endosonographic anatomy of the rectum. In: Santoro GA, Di Falco G (eds) Atlas of endoanal and endorectal ultrasonography. Springer-Verlag Italy, Milan, 2004, pp 42–48.

2. Onaca N, Hirhberg A, Adar R. Early reoperation for perirectal abscess: a preventable complication. Dis Colon Rectum 2001;44:1469–1473.

3. Ramanujam PS, Prasad M, Abcarian H, Tan AB. Perianal abscesses and fistulas. A study of 1023 patients. Dis Colon Rectum 1984;27:593–597.

4. Lunnis DJ, Kamm MA, Phillips RKS. Factors affecting continence after surgery for anal fistula. Br J Surg 1984; 81: 1382–1385.

5. Garcia-Aguilar J, Belmonte C, Wong WD et al. Anal fistula surgery: factors associated with recurrence and incontinence. Dis Colon Rectum 1996;39:723–729.

6. dal Monte PP. Transanal hemorrhoidal dematerialisation: non-excisional surgery for the treatment of haemorrhoidal disease. Tech Coloproctol 2007;11:37–46.

7. Fernández-Frías AM, Pérez-Vicente F, Arroyo A et al. Is anal endosonography useful in the study of recurrent complex fistula-in-ano? Rev Esp Enferm Dig 2006;98(8):573–581.

8. Law PJ, Talbot RW, Bartram CI, Northover JMA. Anal endosonography in the evaluation of perianal sepsis and fistula in ano. Br J Surg 1989;76:752–755.

9. Santoro GA, Ratto C. Accuracy and reliablity of endoanal ultrasonography in the evaluation of perianal abscesses and fistula-in-ano. In: Santoro GA, Di Falco G (eds) Benign anorectal diseases. Diagnosis with endoanal and endorectal ultrasound and new treatment options. Springer-Verlag Italy, Milan, 2006, pp 141–183.

10. Choen S, Nicholls RJ. Anal fistula. Br J Surg 1992; 79:197–205.

11. Cheong DMO, Nogueras JJ, Wexner SD, Jagelman DG. Anal endosonography for recurrent anal fistulas: image enhancement with hydrogen peroxide. Dis Colon Rectum 1993; 36:1158–1160.

12. Halligan S, Stoker J. Imaging of fistula in ano. Radiology 2006;239:18–33.

13. Kruskal JB, Kane RA, Morrin MM. Peroxide-enhanced anal endosonography: technique, image interpretation, and clinical applications. Radiographic 2001;21:51–73.

14. Ratto C, Gentile E, Merico M et al. How can the assessment of fistula in ano be improved? Dis Colon Rectum 2000; 43:1375–1382.

15. Ziech M, Felt-Bersma R, Stoker J. Imaging of perianal fistulas. Clin Gastroenterol Hepatol 2009;7(10):1037–1045.

16. Sabir N, Sungurtekin U, Erdem E, Nessar M. Magnetic resonance imaging with rectal Gd-DTPA: new tool for the diagnosis of perianal fistula. Int J Colorectal Dis 2000;15(5–6):317–322.

17. Stoker J, Rociu E, Wiersma TG, Laméris JS. Imaging of anorectal disease. Br J Surg 2000;87(1):10–27.

18. Santoro GA, Fortling B. The advantages of volume rendering in three-dimensional endosonography of the anorectum. Dis Colon Rectum 2006;50:359–368.

19. Liberman H, Thorson AG. Anal stenosis. Am J Surg 2000;179:325–329.

20. Oh C, Divino CM, Steinhagen RM. Anal fissure. 20-year experience. Dis Colon Rectum 1995;38:378–382.

Subject Index